Practical Psychopharmacology

Practical Psychopharmacology

Translating Findings from Evidence-Based Trials into Real-World Clinical Practice

Joseph F. Goldberg, M.D., M.S.
Clinical Professor of Psychiatry, Icahn School of Medicine at Mount Sinai, New York

Stephen M. Stahl, M.D., Ph.D., D.Sc.(Hon)
Professor of Psychiatry and Neuroscience, University of California Riverside and University of California San Diego

Foreword by Alan F. Schatzberg, M.D.

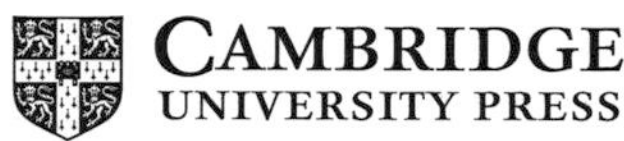

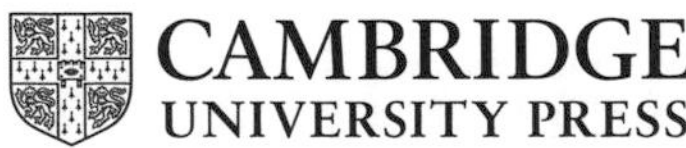

Shaftesbury Road, Cambridge CB2 8EA, United Kingdom

One Liberty Plaza, 20th Floor, New York, NY 10006, USA

477 Williamstown Road, Port Melbourne, VIC 3207, Australia

314–321, 3rd Floor, Plot 3, Splendor Forum, Jasola District Centre, New Delhi – 110025, India

103 Penang Road, #05–06/07, Visioncrest Commercial, Singapore 238467

Cambridge University Press is part of Cambridge University Press & Assessment, a department of the University of Cambridge.

We share the University's mission to contribute to society through the pursuit of education, learning and research at the highest international levels of excellence.

www.cambridge.org
Information on this title: www.cambridge.org/9781108450744
DOI: 10.1017/9781108553216

First published 2021 (version 2, April 2023)

Printed in Great Britain by Ashford Colour Press Ltd., April 2023

A catalogue record for this publication is available from the British Library

ISBN 978-1-108-45074-4 Paperback

To my wife, best friend, trusted source, and most-beloved critic Carrie; and to Joshua, Brian, Hannah, and Jonah, for their limitless support, patience, and encouragement throughout the conception, gestation, and delivery of this work.

- J.F.G.

In memory of Dr. Daniel X. Freedman, mentor, colleague, and scientific father;

to Shakila Marie

- S.M.S.

Contents

Foreword

Over the past four decades, psychopharmacology has become a major tool in the treatment armamentarium for patients with psychiatric disorders. The early days revolved around the first-generation antipsychotics and antidepressants. Since then we have seen the introduction of a number of drugs with different mechanisms of action such that today we have many more tools in our toolbox. Still, we have many patients with so-called refractory disorders necessitating the need for even more agents with unique mechanisms of action. Such efforts offer considerable hope for both clinicians and patients alike. But as we develop new agents we need to be able to evaluate the data that have been used to support their approval. This is even more important today when we are seeing drugs approved with less than the previous standard of two positive Phase III trials. Academics and clinicians both need to have a knowledge base to assess these new data to guide their decision-making. Where are we going to get it? Now we have a textbook – *Practical Psychopharmacology* – that can help guide readers through this area and potentially other domains that affect research and treatment. The Goldberg and Stahl book is a tremendous resource for enhancing evidence-based psychopharmacologic care.

The text elegantly bridges key aspects of preclinical and clinical pharmacology, biostatistics, pharmacogenetics, and clinical practice, and this bridge will enable the reader to understand the key issues in research and drug assessment that determine whether an agent or a laboratory test is accepted into clinical practice and ultimately used in daily practice. The book consists of two major sections (General Principles and Targets of Pharmacotherapy). The first section – General Principles – contains 12 chapters that include amongst others: Targets of Treatment: Categories versus Dimensions of Psychopathology; Placebo and Nocebo Effects; Tailoring the Fit: Moderators and Mediators of Treatment Outcome; Pharmacogenetics: When Relevant, When Not, etc. The second section on Targets of Pharmacotherapy contains 10 chapters and is more traditional in coverage, including, amongst others: Disordered Mood and Affect; Psychosis; Cognition, etc.

The General Principles section is what sets this book apart. It builds the bridge from research to better practice. It elucidates issues in each of these key areas and explains them in an intelligible manner for the reader to digest. It makes it easy to understand why these areas are important for the clinician. That is no easy task and I found myself getting a super refresher course in key research areas related to psychopharmacology and learning a lot about some domains that I probably should have known more about.

Let me give some examples of key areas covered in the book. Goldberg and Stahl go beyond using simple p-values to judge efficacy and give us a precis on effect sizes. Effect sizes are measures of clinical relevance of a drug–placebo difference that are independent of the p-value and the size of the study. This book explains in an intelligible way what an effect size is, how it is determined, and the relevance to clinical effect. It then gives examples of effect sizes of known agents – e.g., memantine for depression, esketamine, etc. The reader will be somewhat surprised that agents we prescribe all the time (e.g., some antidepressants) actually exert small effects. Taken to an extreme in assessing some drugs in specific types of patients (e.g., some antidepressants in milder depressives), investigators have argued the agents are not effective. The authors review this literature in sufficient detail and in a clear manner such that the reader can then judge the clinical significance of specific clinical trials. And that is the point of this book. It gives the practitioner the information from the research literature to better select an individual treatment for a particular patient, making personalized medicine ultimately achievable.

Another example of helping to bridge from studies to practice is the chapter on mediators and moderators. This work was pioneered by my colleague at Stanford – Helena Kraemer – who developed a method of analysis that goes beyond the drug versus placebo comparison to attempt to ferret out the moderators of response to a particular agent, such as age, gender, or some other clinical or biologic feature. That helps the clinician to determine who best to treat with a particular agent. Mediators are those variables that change with a particular treatment and indicate the key parameters that are affected in the course of response, either positive or negative. For example, a change in plasma catecholamines could mediate the response to clozapine or a change in weight on an atypical might mediate developing insulin resistance or diabetes. Again, the authors do a fine job in teaching us how to apply these types of analyses.

A third example is the development of pharmacogenetics to predict efficacy or side effects. In some ways, specific genetic variants are moderators of response. These tests have become increasingly used by clinicians, although there are a number of researchers who question their clinical utility. The authors do an excellent job explaining what a gene is, what an allele is, what SNPs are, how studies are performed, and how we should interpret results to date. The chapter is clear and reviews a number of important and potentially useful markers of both response and side effects. And there are many other examples in the remaining nine chapters in this section.

Crossing over to specific types of agents and disorders, Goldberg and Stahl place the data on specific agents in the context that they have brilliantly laid out for us in Part I on General Principles. We now see what the issues are with the available agents and those being developed that will inform practice today and for the future. This is a book that is worth owning by any practitioner or student of clinical psychopharmacology. Kudos to Goldberg and Stahl for enhancing the literature in this important area.

Alan F. Schatzberg, MD

Kenneth T. Norris, Jr. Professor of Psychiatry and Behavioral Sciences

Stanford University School of Medicine

Stanford, CA

Preface

The impetus for this book comes from our perception of a distinct unmet need in the world of clinical psychopharmacology, that of a marriage between clinical neuroscience and evidence-based trials, brokered by the matchmaker of pragmatism. There is, on the one hand, an ever-growing literature of randomized controlled trials, crossover trials, open case series, proof-of-concept studies, and case reports that lend varying degrees of support for innovative therapeutic strategies; on the other hand, there exists a clinical reality in which patients frequently start and stop drugs not always for compelling reasons, where everyday practitioners manage patients on extensive polypharmacy regimens that may at times look like random assemblages, pharmacodynamic rationales are not always purposeful, mechanisms of action can be unwittingly redundant or contradictory, and ineffective treatments may senselessly get retained (sometimes perhaps even hoarded) rather than deprescribed.

Simultaneously, there is often a mismatch between the crisp diagnostic entities enrolled in industry-based large-scale randomized trials and the often more ill-defined patient presentations that many clinicians encounter in more real-life, nonspecialized treatment settings. While clinical trialists agonize over whether each and every prospective research subject fully meets DSM-5 or ICD-10 diagnostic symptom and duration criteria based on a detailed structured clinical interview – often having to account for the presence of many co-occurring disorders – real-world practitioners generally lack the time, resources, and often the training to apply rigorous diagnostic criteria to rule in or rule out well-defined categorical disorders.

To make matters murkier, the National Institute of Mental Health (NIMH) opted in 2013 to discard DSM-5 diagnostic categories and their inclusion or exclusion criteria altogether, instead favoring a more dimensional than categorical framework meant to reflect suspected underlying neurobiological processes. Making "accurate" diagnoses has never been harder, as the field evolves in its thinking about what constitutes a true clinical entity and its consequent targets of therapy. In a kind of weird parallel process, the traditional nomenclature for classifying psychotropic drugs has come under greater criticism based on outcomes from both controlled and observational treatment studies (such as STAR*D and CATIE), and evolving hypotheses about disease processes and drug mechanisms that render simplistic theories about neurotransmitter "imbalances" archaic and obsolete. Drugs once called antidepressants seem not to treat depression in reliable and robust ways, drugs called antipsychotics treat more than psychosis, certain blood pressure drugs have found new life treating symptoms of anxiety and posttraumatic stress disorder, and (at least some) anticonvulsants possess varied psychotropic properties unrelated to their antiseizure efficacy. New psychotropic properties are being recognized in old drugs (such as prazosin, ketamine, isradipine, scopolamine, anti-inflammatories, and immunomodulators), while novel therapeutics have prompted growing interest in new potential mechanisms of action (such as opioid receptor modulation for depression (e.g., buprenorphine), $5HT_{2A}$ blockade for psychosis (e.g., pimavanserin), GABA modulation and second-generation neurosteroids for postpartum depression (e.g., brexanolone), and VMAT2 inhibition for movement disorders (e.g., valbenazine, deutetrabenazine), among other innovative treatment strategies.

Busy practitioners often find it hard to stay current with the literature. They may be less familiar with the data to support or refute particular drug choices in particular settings, and they may choose medications for their intended or hoped-for effects on specific symptoms (such as inattention, or impulsive aggression, or anxiety, or insomnia) rather than on coherent constellations of signs and symptoms that form a recognizably distinct entity. When clinical presentations are diagnostically ambiguous, there is often the urge to shoe-horn or force-fit an overarching (and reimbursable) diagnostic label upon patients whose problems may simply not be well captured by existing nomenclature. Meanwhile, clinical neuroscientists concern themselves with putative mechanisms of drug action, brain circuitry relevant to clinical phenotypes, and possible pharmacogenetic considerations that might one day meaningfully help to refine precision medicine on a case-by-case basis.

This book seeks to bridge the many gaps that now exist between the activities of everyday clinical practice and findings from evidence-based trials, between the language of neuropharmacology and the language of symptom-targeted interventions, between systematic approaches to iterative, synergistic pharmacotherapies and the accrual of irrational, overextensive polypharmacies. Throughout the pages ahead, our aim is to articulate a scientifically informed approach to clinical psychopharmacology, distilling generalizable information from clinical trials in ways that might help the extrapolation process from the clinical trials database to everyday practice. In a way, this conceptual merger invites the practitioner to assume the role of clinical trialist, viewing every patient as a subject for whom target symptoms are objectified, outcomes are tracked, and rationales form the basis for decision-making about drug therapies.

We also hope to reorient the clinician's attention *away* from the scienceless concept of whether or not a drug is FDA-approved for a particular condition as an organizing principle for pharmacological decision-making. While the drug regulatory approval process provides a public service for quality assurance of drug manufacturing and safety, it is fundamentally an enterprise driven more by commercial interests than neuroscience. At best, it applies neuroscientific concepts for the purposes of substantiating a pharmacodynamic or pharmacokinetic claim for the relevance of a given compound for a particular use. Regulatory approval means that pharmaceutical manufacturers have legal permission to advertise a proprietary compound; it is not built around advancing knowledge for the sake of knowledge about how the brain works. Plenty of generic, nonproprietary compounds have plausible rationales for deployment in particular clinical situations but such an "off-label" status means nothing about whether or not a scientific database exists. Lithium carbonate and thyroid hormone are both examples of highly evidence-based adjunctive strategies for treatment-resistant depression, but neither has or likely ever will receive regulatory agency approval for that purpose unless some commercial interest invents a new proprietary formulation or mode of delivery that could justify return on the sizable investment needed for product development. Industry focuses on patented agents for which a lucrative market share is anticipated; clinicians, hopefully, study whether or not a molecule exerts an important pharmacodynamic or pharmacokinetic effect on a definable collection of signs and symptoms.

There is a popular notion in some circles that pharmacotherapy decision-making is largely a trial-and-error process, with little if any guidance from scientifically meaningful parameters to inform treatment choices. Cynics often point to the relative absence of laboratory measures to benchmark treatment success; there is no equivalent of a viral load, white cell count, tumor burden, or ejection fraction to track the impact of a given treatment on the trajectory of a disease process. Yet, clinical yardsticks for measuring success are no different than in other specialties for conditions that lack biomarkers for gauging longitudinal change, as when neurologists judge improvement from chronic headaches (or alleviation of pain in general), or sleep medicine specialists judge efficacy when treating narcolepsy, or otolaryngologists try to ameliorate tinnitus. Even ophthalmologists rely on patient self-report of perceived visual acuity when refracting for corrective lenses. Mental health is no less tangible than other brain functions.

If one insists on iterative psychopharmacology as being a trial-and-error enterprise, we would counter that the notion of "educated guesswork" comes closer to the true nature of informed (rather than random) decision-making. Like the board game Battleship®, in which successive moves against an opponent are made based on knowledge gained from the outcome of previous maneuvers, decisions about "which drug to try next" after an inadequate response to a particular intervention should involve Bayesian analysis – i.e., reflecting the wisdom gained from past efforts and likely reasons for bad outcomes (e.g., drug intolerances, nonadherence, poor symptom targeting, or too narrow a breadth of spectrum, etc.). And, like a good chess player, one is always thinking about the implications of the current move vis-à-vis the next one.

The book is divided into two main sections. The first addresses broad fundamental concepts that inform decision-making in psychopharmacology, including:

- defining evidence-based principles
- how to read and interpret the clinical trials literature, including how to understand study designs, effect sizes, placebo effects, and ways to extrapolate clinical trial findings to routine practice
- understanding dimensions versus categories of psychopathology as the "true" targets of pharmacotherapy, as described in the NIMH Research Domain Criteria (RDoC)
- understanding pharmacodynamic effects as described in the evolving neuroscience-based nomenclature (NbN)
- accounting for drug interactions and cross-tapering strategies
- recognizing when laboratory or other end-organ monitoring is and is not clinically relevant
- recognizing patient-specific moderators and mediators of treatment outcome that can help tailor individualized regimens

- crafting logical and strategic combination drug regimens
- knowing the strengths and limitations of pharmacogenetic testing

When it comes to pharmacotherapy, our sense is that there is all too often a tendency in busy clinical practices to shoot first and ask questions later – that is, an impetus to formulate rapid diagnostic impressions and then let loose with whatever medication strategies seem most expedient to subdue the most offensive symptoms. We favor a more paced and calculated approach when battling psychopathology, one in which the huntsman more stealthily sizes up his quarry, gains familiarity with its habits, behaviors, and relevant characteristics, assures the identified target has indeed been correctly identified, chooses the appropriate weaponry for the task at hand, carefully aligns the crosshairs within his sights before pulling any triggers, and then inflicts as surgically precise an assault with minimal collateral damage as possible. Sir Francis Bacon's adage, "cure the disease and kill the patient" has no place in our concept of sophisticated psychopharmacology. Although our knowledge of disease mechanisms and treatment effects in many ways remains primitive, the maxim *primum non nocere* remains paramount.

It is impossible for any one psychiatrist, no matter how devoted and astute, to grasp the ever-expanding body of relevant research findings. With hundreds if not thousands of clinically relevant peer-reviewed papers appearing in the literature every year, coupled with the challenge of judging quality, relevance, credibility, and distinguishing the compelling from the spurious, the volume of information is crushing. From our perspective, it is more useful to know where to find information and how to apply new knowledge as it emerges, rather than imagining that the corpus of relevant information can be found in a single repository. This book by no means aims to capture every possible morsel of current knowledge (the half-life of which being an iffy proposition in itself), but rather strives to foster for the reader a sense of how to stay up to date and to put basic principles of evidence-based medicine into daily practice. The phrase "I don't know, but I can look it up" is a favorite and empowering statement to tell patients, trainees, and especially ourselves; more than conveying humility, it imparts a disdain for guesswork. Knowing where and how to find and apply accurate information is one of the many no-longer-kept secrets of psychopharmacology that we have tried to share in the pages ahead.

Part II of this book provides specific detail and information on the evidence base and rationales for specific interventions. We seek to focus on the targets of treatment as described in Part I based on their clinical and neuroscientific bases, drawing on dimensions of psychopathology as phenomena that cut across diagnoses (e.g., problems with attention, impulse control, mood, motivation, perception, anxiety, and self-harm). Throughout, our goal is to draw upon the evidence-based clinical trials literature and translate findings into pragmatic takeaways for the busy everyday practitioner. Often this has proven to be harder than we wish it were, especially when the characteristics of our patients only faintly resemble those of research study subjects. Much the way geneticists trying to reconstruct the genome of an extinct species must sometimes "fill in" missing stretches of DNA with data from a next-nearest species, we have tried to use logic and extrapolation to extend our reach in the clinical realm, applying knowledge about the known to the unknown in order to make judicious decisions in managing complex psychiatric presentations.

How best to present all the information in this text in a reader-friendly and clinically pragmatic way? There is no way around detail when discussing the evidence base for a given psychiatric ailment. Our strategy has been to make the process for the reader as engaging and painless as possible through lively text, illustrative cases, figures, plentiful cartoons, lots of "tip" boxes, and interesting facts along the way. Detailed tables that summarize large swaths of information purposely appear at the end of each chapter rather than dispersed within – allowing those who want a deeper dive to do so without breaking the sense of narrative flow for those who may instead prefer more of a gestalt. We are both as deeply committed to how clinicians learn as to *what* they learn. The ability to stay engaged with complex material is no easy task. We hope that our approach successfully stimulates the paralimbic "oh wow!" and "clinical reasoning" circuitry within all learners.

We have both had the good fortune to know and work with many colleagues, mentors, mentees, and patients, who in varied ways provided us with the curiosity, inspiration, and stimulation, to undertake this project. We are especially grateful to many colleagues who have kindly read segments of this book as a work in progress and offered helpful and useful feedback. Lastly, we cannot begin to express proper appreciation to our families, who have so kindly and selflessly been supportive of our professional strivings and inherent drive to educate, advance knowledge, and deliver to our patients the best care possible.

Abbreviations

5HT	serotonin
5HTP	5-hydroxytryptophan
α_7 nAChR	α_7-nicotinic acetylcholine receptor
AA	Alcoholics Anonymous
AAAD	aromatic amino acid decarboxylase
ACC	anterior cingulate cortex
ACE	angiotensin-converting enzyme
ACh	acetylcholine
AChI	acetylcholinesterase inhibitor
ADD	attention deficit disorder
ADHD	attention deficit hyperactivity disorder
AIDS	acquired immune deficiency syndrome
AIMS	Abnormal Involuntary Movement Scale
ALT	alanine transaminase
AMPA	α-amino-3-hydroxy-5-methyl-4-isoxazolepropionic acid
ANA	antinuclear antibody
ANC	absolute neutrophil count
ANOVA	analysis of variance
ASCVD	atherosclerotic cardiovascular disease
ASD	autism spectrum diorders
ASHP	American Society of Hospital Pharmacists
asp	aspartate
AST	aspartate aminotransferase
ATP	adenosine triphosphate
AUC	area under the curve
BAC	blood alcohol content
BBB	blood–brain barrier
BDD	body dysmorphic disorder
BDNF	brain-derived neurotrophic factor
BEN	benign ethinic neutropenia
BID	twice a day
BMI	body mass index
BMJ	British Medical Journal
bp	base pair
BP	bipolar disorder
BPD	borderline personality disorder
BPDSI	Borderline Personality Disorder Severity Index
BPRS	Brief Psychiatric Rating Scale
BSPS	Brief Social Phobia Scale
CANMAT	Canadian Network for Mood and Anxiety Treatments
CAPS	Clinician-Administered PTSD Scale
CaSR	calcium sensing receptor
CATIE	Clinical Antipsychotics Treatment Intervention Effectiveness
CATIE-AD	Clinical Antipsychotics Treatment Intervention Effectiveness-Alzheimer's Disease
CBC	complete blood count
CBD	cannabidiol
CBI	combined behavioral intervention
CBT	cognitive behavioral therapy
CCK	cholecystokinin
CCPGQ	Criteria for Control of Pathological Gambling Questionnaire
CDP	cytidine-5′-diphosphate
CDT	carbohydrate-deficient transferrin
CGI	Clinical Global Impressions
CGT	complicated grief treatment
CHF	congestive heart failure
CI	confidence interval
CIWA-Ar	Clinical Institute Withdrawal Assessment for Alcohol Revised
CK	creatine kinase
CKD	chronic kidney disease
C-L	consultation-liaison
Cl_{int}	intrinsic clearance
CM	contingency management
CNS	central nervous system
COMT	catechol-*O*-methyltransferase
CONSORT	Consolidated Standards of Reporting Trials

COPD	chronic obstructive pulmonary disease
CoQ	coenzyme Q
COWS	Clinical Opiate Withdrawal Scale
CPIC	Clinical Pharmacogenetics Implementation Consortium
c-PTSD	complex post-traumatic stress disorder
CRD	Centre for Reviews and Dissemination
CRF	corticotropin-releasing factor
CrI	credible interval
CRP	C-reactive protein
CSF	cerebrospinal fluid
CSI	crime scene investigation
CSTC	cortico–striatal–thalamo–cortical
CV	coefficient of variation
cys	cysteine
DA	dopamine
DAAO	*D*-amino acid oxidase
DARE	Database of Abstracts of Reviews of Effects
DAT	dopamine transporter
DBP	diastolic blood pressure
DBT	dialectical behavior therapy
DDI	drug–drug interaction
DHA	docosahexanoic acid
DHEA	dehydroepiandrosterone
DID	dissociative identity disorder
DLPFC	dorsolateral prefrontal cortex
DMPFC	dorsomedial prefrontal cortex
DNA	deoxyribonucleic acid
DOPAC	3,4-dihydroxyphenylacetic acid
DORA	dual orexin receptor antagonist
DRESS	drug reaction with eosinophilia and systemic symptoms
DSHEA	Dietary Supplement Health and Education Act
DSM	Diagnostic and Statistical Manual of Mental Disorders
DSM-IVTR	Diagnostic and Statistical Manual of Mental Disorders, 4th edition, text revision
DST	dexamethasone suppression test
DSST	Digit Symbol Substitution Task
DTs	delerium tremens
DTI	diffusion tensor imaging
DUI	duration of untreated illness
EBM	evidence-based medicine
EC	excitement components
ECNP	European College of Neuropsychopharmacology
ECG	electrocardiogram
ECT	electroconvulsive therapy
EE	expressed emotion
EEG	electroencephalography
eGFR	estimated glomerular filtration rate
EM	extensive metabolizer
EMDR	eye movement desensitization and reprocessing
EPA	eicosopentanoic acid
EPS	extrapyramidal side effects
ER	estrogen receptor
ERP	event-related potential
ES	effect size
ESR	erythrocyte sedimentation rate
ESRD	end-stage renal disease
FA	fractional anisotropy
FDA	US Food and Drug Administration
FDR	false discovery rate
fe	fraction excreted unchanged
FEWP	Free and Easy Wanderer Plus
FGA	first-generation antipsychotic
fMRI	functional magnetic resonance imaging
FOSHU	foods for special health use
FTD	formal thought disorder
FTDR	fixed-tapering-dose regimen
FtM	female to male
FWER	family-wise error rate
GABA	gamma aminobutyric acid
GAD	generalized anxiety disorder
G-CSF	granulocyte colony stimulating factor
GEE	generalized estimating equations

GENDEP	Genome-Based Therapeutic Drugs for Depression Project
GFR	glomerular filtration rate
GGT	gamma-glutamyl transpeptidase
GI	gastrointestinal
GLP-1	glucagon-like peptide 1
glu	glutamate
gly	glycine
GSAS	Gambling Symptom Assessment Scale
GSH	glutathione
GUIDED	Genomics Used To Improve Depression Decisions
GWAS	genome-wide association studies
HAM-A	Hamilton Ratings Scale for Anxiety
HAM-D	Hamilton Ratings Scale for Depression
HAM-$_{D17}$	17-item Hamilton Rating Scale for Depression
HAART	highly active antiretroviral therapy
hGH	human growth hormone
HIV	human immunodeficiency virus
HLA	human leukocyte antigen
HR	hazard ratio
hs-CRP	high-sensitivity C-reactive protein
HVA	homovanillic acid
HWE	Hardy–Weinberg equilibrium
IBS	irritable bowel syndrome
ICD	International Classification of Diseases
ICGDA	International Consensus Group on Depression and Anxiety
ICU	intensive care unit
IED	intermittent explosive disorder
IES	Impact of Events Scale
IL	interleukin
IM	intramuscular
IN	intranasal
IR	immediate release
ISBD-IGSLi	Bipolar Disorders-International Group for the Study of Lithium Treated Patients
iSPOT-D	International Study to Predict Optimised Treatment in Depression
ITT	intent-to-treat
IU	international unit
LAI	long-acting injectable
LD	linkage disequilibrium
LDT	laterodorsal tegmental nuclei
LEE	Level of Expressed Emotion
LHH	likelihood to be helped or harmed
LOCF	last observation carried forward
LSAS	Liebowitz Social Anxiety Scale
LSD	D-lysergic acid diethylamide
MADRS	Montgomery–Åsberg Depression Rating Scale
MAO	monoamine oxidase
MAO-A	monoamine oxidase A
MAO-B	monoamine oxidase B
MAOI	monoamine oxidase inhibitor
MAR	missing at random
MBC	measurement-based care
MCAR	missing completely at random
MCT-1	monocarbylase transport type 1
MCV	mean corpuscular volume
MDD	major depressive disorder
MDD-MF	major depressive disorder with mixed features
MDE	major depressive episode
MDMA	3,4-methylenedioxy-methamphetamine
met	methionine
MFQ	Marks Fear Questionnaire
MGH	Massachusetts General Hospital
mGluR	metabotropic glutamate receptors
MHC	major histocompatibility complex
MI	myocardial infarction
MMRM	mixed models for repeated measures
MMSE	Mini-Mental Status Exam
MOA	mechanism of action
MoCA	Montreal Cognitive Assessment
M/P ratio	maternal milk to plasma ratio
MRI	magnetic resonance imaging
MtF	male to female
MTHFR	methylene tetrahydrofolate reductase
MUPS	medically unexplained symptoms

NAc	nucleus accumbens
NAC	*N*-acetyl-cysteine
NADH	nicotinamide adenine dinucleotide
NaSSA	noradrenergic and specific serotonergic antidepressant
NbN	neuroscience-based nomenclature
NCA	necessary clinical adjustment
NCE	new chemical entity
NDI	nephrogenic diabetes insipidus
NE	norepinephrine
NERI	norepinephrine reuptake inhibitor
NET	norepinephrine transporter
NIAAA	National Institute on Alcohol Abuse and Alcoholism
NIMH	National Institute of Mental Health
NMDA	*N*-methyl-D-aspartate
NMS	neuroleptic malignant syndrome
NNH	number needed to harm
NNT	number needed to treat
NO	nitric oxide
NPD	narcissistic personality disorder
NPV	negative predictive value
NSAID	nonsteroidal anti-inflammatory drug
NSDUH	National Survey on Drug Use and Health
NSSI	nonsuicidal self-injury
OCD	obsessive-compulsive disorder
ODD	oppositional-defiant disorder
OFC	orbitofrontal cortex OR olanzapine/fluoxetine combination
OGT	oxygenated glycerol triester
OR	odds ratio
ORA	orexin A
ORB	orexin B
OROS	osmotic-release oral delivery system
pANCA	perinuclear antineutrophil cytoplasmic antibodies
PANSS	Positive and Negative Syndrome Scale
PAPS	3′-phosphoadenosine-5′-phosphosulfate
PAS	Panic and Agoraphobia Scale
PBA	pseudobulbar affect
PCL-C	PTSD Checklist-Civilian Version
PCL-M	PTSD Checklist-Military Version
PCOS	polycystic ovarian syndrome
PCP	phencyclidine
PDE	phosphodiesterase
PDRS	Panic Disorder Rating Scale
PET	positron emission tomography
PFC	prefrontal cortex
PG-CGI	pathological gambling Clinical Global Impressions scale
PG-YBOCS	pathological gambling modification of the Yale–Brown Obsessive-Compulsive Scale
PIM	potentially inappropriate medication
PK	pharmacokinetic
PKC	protein kinase C
PGx	pharmacogenetics
PM	poor metabolizer
PMDD	premenstrual disphoric disorder
PO	by mouth
PPD	postpartum depression
PPHN	persistent pulmonary hypertension in the newborn
PPT	pedunculopontine nuclei
PPV	positive predictive value
PRISMA	Preferred Reporting Items for Systematic Reviews and Meta-analyses
PRN	as needed
pro	proline
PROSPERO	International Prospective Register of Systematic Reviews
p-SAPK	phosphorylated stress-activated protein kinase
PSM	propensity score matching
PTH	parathyroid hormone
PTSD	post-traumatic stress disorder
qDay	once daily
qEEG	quantitative electroencephalography
qHS	every night at bedtime
QID	four times a day
QTc	corrected QT interval

RBC	red blood cell
RCT	randomized controlled trial
RDC	Research Diagnostic Criteria
RDoC	NIMH Research Domain Criteria
REMS	Risk Evaluation and Mitigation Strategy
RID	relative infant dose
RIMA	reversible inhibitor of MAO-A
RNA	ribonucleic acid
ROC	receiver operating characteristic
RR	relative risk
rTMS	repetitive transcranial magnetic stimulation
SAD	social anxiety disorder
SAH	S-adenosylhomocysteine
SAMe	S-adenosylmethionine
SAMSHA	Substance Abuse and Mental Health Services Administration
SANS	Schedule for the Assessment of Negative Symptoms
SAPK	stress-activated protein kinase
SARI	serotonin antagonist and reuptake inhibitor
SBP	systolic blood pressure
SCIP	Screen for Cognitive Impairment for Psychiatry
ser	serine
SERM	selective estrogen receptor modulator
SERT	serotonin reuptake transporter
SES	socioeconomic status
SGA	second-generation antipsychotic
SHI	Self-Harm Inventory
SIB	self-injurous behavior
SIADH	syndrome of inappropriate antidiuretic hormone secretion
SMD	standard mean difference
SMVT	sodium-dependent multivitamin transporter
SNP	single nucleotide polymorphism
SNRI	serotonin-norepinephrine reuptake inhibitor
SPAI	Social Phobia and Anxiety Inventory
SPECT	single photon emission computed tomography
SPIN	Social Phobia Inventory
SSRI	selective serotonin reuptake inhibitor
STAI	State–Trait Anxiety Inventory
STAXI	State–Trait Anger Expression Inventory
sTNF-R2	soluble tumor necrosis factor receptor 2
STR	symptom-triggered regimen
SUCRA	surface under the cumulative ranking curve
SUD	substance use disorder
SZ	schizophrenia
T_3	triiodothyronine
T_4	thyroxine
TAAR1	trace amine-associated receptor 1
TAU	treatment as usual
TBI	traumatic brain injury
TCA	tricyclic antidepressant
TCI	Temperament and Character Inventory
TD	tardive dyskinesia
TDM	therapeutic drug monitoring
TEAS	treatment-emergent affective switch
TEN	toxic epidermal necrolysis
THC	tetrahydrocannabinol
THF	tetrahydrofolic acid
TID	three times a day
TiME	Time until the need for Intervention for an emerging Mood Episode
TNF	tumor necrosis factor
ToM	theory of mind
TPO	thyroid peroxidase
TPQ	Tridimensional Personality Questionnaire
TRD	treatment-resistant depression
TSH	thyroid-stimulating hormone
UDP	uridine diphosphate
UGT	UDP-glucuronosyl transferase
URM	ultra-rapid metabolizer

VA	US Department of Veterans Affairs
Vd	volume of distribution
VLPFC	ventrolateral prefrontal cortex
VLPO	ventrolateral preoptic nucleus
VMAT2	vesicular monoamine transporter 2
VMPFC	ventromedial prefrontal cortex
VNTR	variable number of tandem repeat
VNS	vagal nerve stimulation
VPC	ventricular premature complexes
VTA	ventral tegmental area
WBC	white blood cell
WCA	World Council of Anxiety
XR	extended release
YBOCS	Yale–Brown Obsessive Compulsive Scale
YMRS	Young Mania Rating Scale
ZAN-BPD	Zanarini Rating Scale for Borderline Personality Disorder

PART I General Principles

1 Core Concepts of Good Psychopharmacology

LEARNING OBJECTIVES

- ☐ Recognize cause-and-effect relationships in psychopharmacology
- ☐ Adopt an investigative "forensic" mindset to assess psychopathology and match symptom constellations to the best-fitting treatment
- ☐ Recognize levels of empirical evidence that support any given pharmacotherapy intervention before making conclusions about generalizability or likelihood of a meaningful effect
- ☐ Know appropriate benchmarks and timepoints for judging if and when to alter medication dosages or otherwise adjust a treatment regimen
- ☐ Focus on putative drug mechanisms, underlying dysfunction of neural networks, and findings from empirical trials, rather than simply on whether or not a drug carries "on"- or "off"-label regulatory agency approval
- ☐ Always strive to define as clearly as possible the intended symptom targets of any treatment

It is a capital mistake to theorize before you have all the evidence.
It biases the judgment.

- Sir Arthur Conan Doyle

A CAUSE AND EFFECT

When someone takes a medication for depression, anxiety, or any other psychiatric problem, how do they or the prescriber know for certain if they are actually better or worse? And in either instance, whether to credit (or blame) the drug? If depression gets better 4–6 weeks after taking an antidepressant, how confidently should we attribute improvement to the drug rather than to serendipity? What if the patient gets better only after 14–16 weeks – is that too far in time to distinguish a plausible drug effect from spontaneous remission? Or, when can we assume the outcome was still a likely drug effect, given that an adequate trial may take longer in some people than others? If they felt better in just a few days, is that evidence of a placebo effect? Or, if they became suicidal or agitated, how do we know if that reflects an adverse drug effect or simply a worsening due to the natural course of illness?

Cause-and-effect relationships are often presumed throughout medicine, even though drugs can have unpredictable effects and despite the fact that numerous biological, psychological, and environmental factors contribute to outcomes. Causality is all the more difficult to infer when a patient receives more than one treatment (as occurs not infrequently in real-world practice), or other psychoactive factors complicate the picture (such as alcohol or drug abuse, or sleep deprivation, or life catastrophes). How do we account for subjective versus objective signs of improvement, while considering the effects of time alone, placebo and nocebo effects, the therapeutic alliance, variable pharmacodynamic drug effects, pharmacokinetic interactions, comorbidities, dosing effects, and – not of least importance – whether the prescribed treatment is even appropriate to the presenting ailment?

Psychiatric drug effects are remarkably varied and unreliable. Contrast the poorly predictable outcome of giving someone a selective serotonin reuptake inhibitor (SSRI) for depression versus the relative certainty of administering general anesthesia for surgery. No anesthesiologist ever tells their patient they have about a 6 in 10 chance that the medication they are about to receive will make them go to sleep. Admittedly, the sleep-inducing effects of halothane produce a safer and more reliable result than having the patient inhale an ether-soaked rag (and halothane is no picnic if the patient has an unrecognized susceptibility to malignant hyperthermia). But can psychotropic drugs ever deliver the same kind of causal precision and reliability for producing an intended effect as occurs with anesthesia induction?

Causal inferences are vulnerable to the so-called *post hoc ergo propter hoc* or logical fallacy phenomenon, in which one concludes that whatever happens after a temporal sequence of events (e.g., taking a medication and then feeling better or worse) necessarily reflects cause and effect. The hazards of spurious associations and outright superstitions abound in psychopharmacology, where both doctor and patient perceptions about cognitive and emotional processing are colored by pre-existing beliefs and expectations. More scientifically, causal relationships in medicine are sometimes judged according to criteria such as those described by Hill (1965), as summarized in Box 1.1.

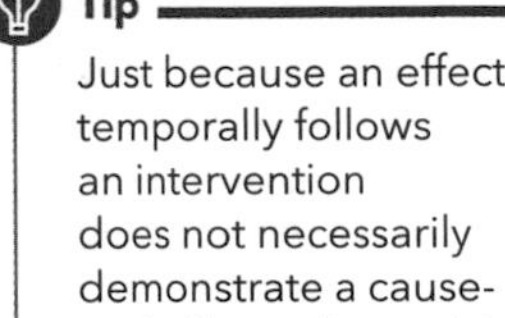

Tip

Just because an effect temporally follows an intervention does not necessarily demonstrate a cause-and-effect relationship.

Additionally, one must consider the presence of confounding factors or potential biases (e.g., different susceptibilities or degrees of responsivity/nonresponsivity across individuals – as when antibiotics may be less effective in someone who is immunosuppressed, or poorly adherent, or has a superinfection), and the impact of other simultaneous interventions that could interact and alter efficacy or tolerability.

Observed Outcomes

Prescribers and patients do not necessarily look for the same tangible results when judging pharmacotherapy effects. For example, surveys show that depressed patients' main therapeutic goals are to feel that life is meaningful and enjoyable, and to feel satisfied with themselves. Doctors, by contrast, set out to eliminate negative feelings such as depression, despair, or hopelessness, and help patients regain interest or pleasure from doing things. These differences may seem nuanced, and could just be a matter of semantics, but they set the stage for how success gets measured, and what kinds of expectations all parties bring when a psychopharmacotherapy is undertaken.

Knowingly or otherwise, clinicians who prescribe psychotropic medications must consider a multitude of factors, both biological and nonbiological, for judging drug effects; and, before that, deciding what, when, how, and for whom to prescribe any agent. Good psychopharmacology reflects such an awareness, and at its best, carries as prerequisite a systematic diagnostic assessment, appreciation for relevant dimensions of psychopathology, and the "fit" between symptom profiles and pharmacodynamic properties, as well as economy of scale (as when one drug accomplishes more than one goal), avoidance of redundant or unnecessary or ineffective agents, and ultimately, customer satisfaction.

Consider the fit between prescribed medications and clinical phenomenology in Clinical Vignette 1.1.

James's case illustrates the kind of litany of problems that often afflict real-world patients. First, one must filter a plethora of psychiatric phenomena ranging from trouble with mood and anxiety to illicit substances to

Box 1.1

Bradford Hill Criteria for Judging Cause and Effect

Criteria	Relevance
Strength of apparent association	Bigger associations = bigger effects
Consistency (reproducibility)	Consistent findings across settings = more likely a true association
Specificity	Specific population with specific disease, unlikely other explanations
Temporality	Exposure precedes outcome
Dose effect	Greater exposure imparts greater risk (but, there could also be a necessary threshold level of exposure)
Plausibility	Is there a plausible pharmacological mechanism?
Coherence	An explanation for likely association makes sense given existing knowledge
Experiment	Experimental interventions can alter the conditions
Alternate explanations	Do other likely explanations exist for the observed association?

CLINICAL VIGNETTE 1.1

James was a 24-year-old information technologist who carried diagnoses of bipolar disorder, attention deficit disorder (ADD), stimulant (cocaine) use disorder, cannabis use disorder, nonverbal learning disability, generalized anxiety disorder, and a mixed personality disorder involving narcissistic and histrionic traits. His extensive medication history has included a multitude of drugs from virtually all major classes and combinations over the years, including anticonvulsants, antidepressants, antipsychotics, benzodiazepines, and psychostimulants. During his most recent consultation, the psychiatrist whom he saw reviewed his lengthy medication history, sought to identify which medications he had never taken, and picked lithium largely because it was one of the few medications James had never tried. He now presents for follow-up noting that "the lithium isn't working."

cognitive complaints, all colored by suspected personality characteristics; then, a vast historical pharmacopoeia requires a better understanding – what medications, at what doses, for how long, with what intended symptom targets, and with what observed effects? And, how accurate is the subjective recall of those parameters? Patients with multiple diagnoses pose especially difficult challenges, not simply because of the need to parse transdiagnostic overlapping symptoms (such as inattention due to bipolar disorder versus ADHD, or apathy due to depression versus cannabis abuse), but also because clinical improvement may demand a hierarchical approach to treatment (e.g., detoxification and abstinence as prerequisites for identifying and targeting primary mood symptoms). Lastly, complex cases sometimes invite the strategy employed here of sifting through a lifetime medication history in order simply to find a drug previously untried that is remotely pertinent to any of the key complaints and/or presumptive diagnoses – followed by the dismay of yet another failure.

A logical and systematic approach to appropriate pharmacotherapy in this case, as in any, begins with a careful and sometimes painstaking reassessment of the presenting phenomena and their context, including the chronology of symptoms, their longitudinal course over time, a careful interview to establish the presence or absence of distinct symptom constellations, episodes versus "usual" states, and the criteria by which categorical diagnoses are formulated. Knowledgeable collateral historians are often helpful sources of corroborative information, although their input too may require filtration and their face value cannot necessarily be taken for granted (as when judging the biases of an estranged, resentful, or otherwise dissatisfied partner or other family member). In James's case, declaring lithium a "failure" assumes that his ailment – the object of treatment – conforms to a symptom picture for which lithium renders a known benefit (such as lithium-responsive bipolar disorder, or at least, impulsive aggression, or suicidal behavior) – lest its selection reflect merely an otherwise random choice based on the hearsay of previous diagnoses that may or may not be correct.

B CLINICAL ASSESSMENT: CSI PSYCHIATRY

Good diagnosticians weave together signs and symptoms into a coherent narrative that fits a recognizable pattern. When we play psychiatric detective, diagnostic clues are like persons of interest in a crime scene investigation (CSI), leading us to develop working hypotheses about the most likely culprit(s). No clinician worth his or her salt can deny the thrill of discovery when medical sleuthing leads to the realization of a disease-defining symptom constellation. But when no clear-cut pattern is evident, sharp psychiatric detectives realize that absence and formulate an impression based on possible *form fruste* presentations, or dimensions of psychopathology that most closely approximate a categorically defined symptom profile. In either instance, appropriate treatments should conform to rigorous clinical appraisals the way a jury might consider whether or not there exists a preponderance of evidence, or even more rigorously, certainty beyond a reasonable doubt.

Definition

Form fruste conditions refer to clinical presentations in which only some of the defining elements of a disease state are evident. (More on this in Chapter 2.)

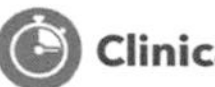

Clinical Tells

Clinical powers of observation are as vital to psychopharmacology as to any other area of medicine. One would be remiss not to notice exophthalmos and a bulging lower neck in someone complaining of depressed mood and fatigue, or impoverished or concrete thinking (schizophrenia? traumatic brain injury? low intellectual functioning? cultural unfamiliarity?), or lack of eye contact, stereotypies, verbosity, mood-incongruent affect, perseveration or difficulty shifting sets, and mismatches between objective functioning and subjective complaints. Such observable clues are the stock-in-trade of CSI psychiatry, juxtaposed alongside a patient's subjective self-report. Only after one formulates a clear impression of the true nature of the problem can one speak of choosing from among the most appropriate treatments, and then gauging the likelihood that the "right" intervention will yield the desired result.

Tip

Discordant match-ups between objective signs and subjective symptoms signal diagnostic complexity.

C DECIDING WHEN PHARMACOTHERAPY IS INDICATED

The sheer making of a psychiatric diagnosis does not necessarily or automatically equate to an indication for pharmacotherapy. Judgments in this area typically hinge not only on severity of symptoms, but also the degree to which symptoms cause distress or disrupt functioning, or the presence of certain cardinal symptoms (such as frank psychosis or severe agitation). An implicit assumption is that effective pharmacotherapy exerts a larger effect than that of a placebo. Just as it makes no sense to initiate or continue a medication that yields no discernible benefits, so too should a proposed pharmacotherapy target symptoms unambiguously, and with reasonable expectations for diminishing their intensity if not eradicating them altogether. And the only way to choose purposeful treatments that most reliably fit the bill, short of blind luck, is to base treatment decisions on known outcomes from well-conceived and executed clinical trials in well-characterized patient groups – that is, drawing upon an empirical evidence base.

D EVIDENCE-BASED PSYCHOPHARMACOLOGY

Evidence-based medicine (EBM) simply means having a foundation for choosing among reasonable treatment options, supported by some degree of empirical proof. Large, randomized placebo-controlled trials are generally considered to be the gold standard for judging rigor behind an evidence base, because they provide sufficient statistical power to differentiate a real effect (or lack of an effect) from a random fluke, and to capture differences that are both statistically and clinically meaningful, even if the magnitude of those differences is subtle. However, as noted in an early editorial describing EBM by Sackett and colleagues (1996, p. 72), "Evidence based medicine is not restricted to randomised trials and meta-analyses. It involves tracking down the best external evidence with which to answer our clinical questions." In other words, even if just a single patient has an extremely favorable and enduring improvement with a medication, without any corroborative proof from other sources or outside studies, that observation alone constitutes evidence of efficacy – *for that one patient*. The problem comes if one tries to generalize about that singular result to other patients with a broader basis.

The Shortfall of Purely Observational Studies

A famous review in the British Medical Journal (BMJ) once noted that no randomized controlled trials (RCTs) have been conducted to prove that parachutes prevent death or major trauma during free fall from an airplane. The authors opined that "everyone might benefit" if ardent critics of purely observational studies devised and participated in such a double-blind, randomized crossover trial (Smith and Pell, 2003).

Traditionally, levels of evidence are described hierarchically, as shown in Figure 1.1.

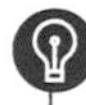

Tip

Meta-analyses and large RCTs represent the most rigorous levels of evidence.

With this framework, one must distinguish the degree of rigor and generalizability (or relative lack thereof) of studies that have been undertaken – and the extent to which an existing database is more provisional or definitive. For example, small open case series or even small RCTs may be undertaken more as *proof-of-concept* studies intended to demonstrate feasibility or anticipate likely within-group effect sizes (as explained in Chapter 3), from which future, more definitive studies can be planned and executed. A small-scale provisional study of a novel compound that shows a significant improvement from baseline in a particular measure of psychopathology may be intended more to help frame the logistics of a larger RCT, rather than to inspire immediate uptake in routine clinical practice. Similarly, small studies that are not intentionally designed to test a hypothesis are sometimes

Figure 1.1 Levels of evidence in clinical trials.

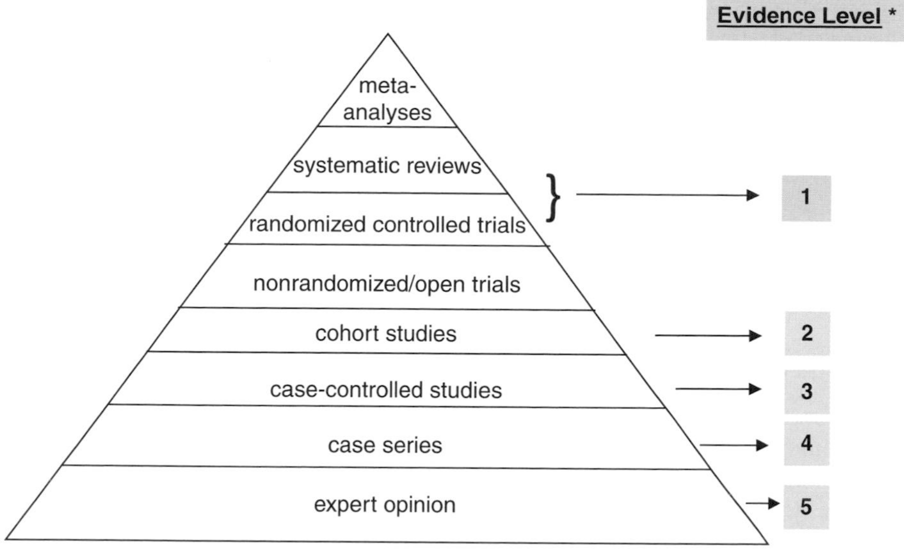

referred to as *hypothesis-generating* – think of a manufacturer beta-testing several prototypes before devoting greater resources to final product development, or a film's producer showing previews that feature alternate endings to gauge audience response before deciding on the final cut.

Tip

Case reports and open trials serve more as hypothesis-generating than hypothesis-testing components of a treatment database. This means that they suggest ideas about viable therapies, rather than demonstrate that they are valid or reliable.

Relatedly, investigators in large RCTs sometimes undertake planned interim analyses to gauge the progress of an ongoing study – rather like peeking at a cake in the oven half way through the baking process, or sampling a stew before it is fully cooked simply to check whether the ingredients are coming together as intended. It would be quite the culinary gaffe to serve a half-baked meal to one's guests, just because an early sampling seemed promising.

E THE COURSE OF TREATMENT

Once a medication that befits a clinical symptom profile has been chosen and begun, how does one decide what comes next? On what timescale is progress reasonably tracked, and how is it quantified? Short of intuition, what parameters help guide decisions about whether dosage adjustments should be made, and when? At what point might additional pharmacotherapies be appropriate? And, when can meaningful conclusions be drawn about the likelihood of seeing further drug effects – that is, when to decide if a drug trial is ineffective or partially effective, and whether to discontinue it, replace it, or retain and augment it?

Circumstances that influence the above considerations vary from ailment to ailment, as well as from drug to drug. Some agents have identified target doses or dosing ranges, and may require titration schedules that are often limited by safety or tolerability issues. Other medications can essentially be "loaded" or dosed rapidly from the outset without jeopardizing tolerability, and possibly leading to a faster onset of efficacy.

As a rule of thumb, adequate medication trials usually take longer and may often involve higher doses in chronic, highly recurrent, or otherwise complex conditions, as compared to relatively "simpler" presentations with less entrenched and enduring stigmata of an underlying disorder. Symptoms that are ego-alien may be easier to dislodge than those which become more engrained or are fundamentally consistent with a patient's basic view of himself and the world. Here, concepts involving personality traits, core beliefs, and self-image, as described further in Chapter 2, can color how any given patient uniquely presents with a "generic" disorder of mood, anxiety, behavior, or cognition; such overtones bear on course and prognosis, as well as distinctions between the *more*-likely viable targets of pharmacotherapy (such as vegetative signs, or poor impulse control, or panic attacks) from those that are *less*-likely viable (such as poor distress tolerance or coping skills, general mistrust of others, long-standing feelings of injustice or envy, or emotional dysregulation linked to interpersonal sensitivities).

F THE TWO-WEEK/20% RULE

While different mental health disorders vary greatly in their features and treatment response, and the trajectory of pharmacotherapy outcomes can vary by patient-specific factors (such as severity, chronicity, pharmacokinetics (e.g., ultrarapid metabolizer phenotypes) and degree of previous treatment resistance), it is nevertheless reasonable to consider the two-week mark as perhaps the first decision-making milestone in the time course for judging a drug's effect on a major psychiatric condition. Responses within one week or sooner generally raise suspicions about transient placebo effects, albeit with some exceptions (notably, rapid antidepressant response to intravenous ketamine); steady-state pharmacokinetics often are not achieved until 5–14 days with many psychotropic medications across classes, making sooner attributions less reliable.

Tip

A measurable improvement of at least 20% from baseline after two weeks of treatment may predict eventual robust response after an adequate trial has elapsed.

Several lines of evidence suggest that by two weeks, at least *minimal improvement* – visible like the sprouting of a seedling, and quantifiable by at least a 20% improvement in symptom severity from baseline – predicts subsequent stable response or remission, at least in the cases of major depression (Papakostas et al., 2006; Szegedi et al., 2009), bipolar depression (Kemp et al., 2011), schizophrenia (Leucht et al., 2007; Samara et al., 2015), panic disorder (Pollack et al., 2002), and generalized anxiety disorder (Rynn et al., 2006). There are conflicting findings about whether signs of improvement in just the *first* week more likely reflect placebo than pharmacodynamic effects, particularly in light of concerns that early placebo effects can be transient. (Hence the basis for single-blind one-week placebo lead-in periods in clinical trials striving to minimize placebo responsivity.) Further complicating debates over possible placebo transience in early responders is the notion of an additive effect between initial placebo-responsiveness and subsequent pharmacodynamic efficacy; in other words, placebo- and drug-response may not be mutually exclusive phenomena during treatment with an active psychotropic agent, and it is possible at least in some instances that even if a brisk initial improvement did reflect a placebo mechanism, that phenomenon does not prohibit subsequent and more enduring pharmacodynamic efficacy from the actual drug. Said differently, across multiple disorders there is a high *negative predictive value* for lack of minimal response in the first two weeks; absence of detectable signs of improvement in that time therefore makes it advisable to alter an existing treatment regimen in some way (via dosing changes, augmentations, or substitutions).

Tweaking

There has been remarkably little study to examine when and how clinicians decide to alter an existing drug regimen. In formal clinical trials, decision points are sometimes algorithmic: if a milestone for improvement is not met by a certain timepoint, adjustments may be protocol-driven (usually dosage increases; sometimes measurement of serum drug levels or reassessment of confounders such as poor adherence or illicit substance use). In real-world practice, rules are looser, seldom evidence-based, and often nonexistent for deciding if and when to alter a drug dose or stop or start a medication. Occasionally, titration schedules are dictated by a drug manufacturer, if not by scientific rationale, for a particular treatment. For example:

- lamotrigine upward dosing in bipolar disorder (see Chapter 13);
- oral loading of divalproex (20–30 mg/kg) in acute mania may yield a faster onset of symptom resolution than more gradual dose escalations, balanced against tolerability (chiefly, gastrointestinal (GI) upset);
- there is little rationale, barring toxicity, for changing lithium doses based on serum lithium levels before the elapse of five days since the last dosage change (i.e., five half-lives to reach steady-state);
- carbamazepine may require up-dosing within several weeks of its initiation due to autoinduction of its metabolism;

- rapid dosing of antipsychotic drugs, particular those with strong D_2 binding affinity, increases the risk for dystonic and other serious adverse motor reactions;
- expected "target" doses may vary from person to person for a wide variety of reasons, limiting the extent to which inexorable dose escalations may be necessary or wise.

Tip

Beware, excessive tweaking of a drug regimen may itself be an outcome measure that serves as a clue about poor prognosis.

Not surprisingly, in a large clinical trial involving expert care for bipolar disorder, eventual treatment responders had fewer *necessary clinical adjustments* ("NCAs") made to their treatment regimens than did eventual nonresponders; every NCA statistically decreased eventual response status by 30% (Reilly-Harrington et al., 2016). Relatedly, every one-unit increase (i.e., worsening) in a patient's Clinical Global Impressions (CGI) overall severity score was associated with a 13% increase in the likelihood of incurring an NCA (Reilly-Harrington et al., 2013). Of course, correlations between multiple NCAs and poorer outcome may simply be a proxy marker for illness complexity, drug tolerability, or poor prognosis in general, while more straightforward clinical presentations may simply require adjustments to a drug regimen less often.

 Newtonian Psychopharmacology

To paraphrase Newton's first law of motion, the trajectory of response to a psychotropic drug will likely remain in constant motion unless acted upon by an outside force. (Outside forces might include nonadherence, substance misuse, medical comorbidities, or worsening of the natural course of illness.) Generally speaking, improvement from an episode of depression, mania, or psychosis follows a time course for recovery that, while not entirely predictable, follows a fairly constant path. Once an appropriate dose has been achieved and signs of improvement are evident, there is often no rationale to tweak a dose so long as signs of improvement do not plateau and tolerability issues are minimal. Overwatering a plant does not make it grow faster. Supratherapeutic drug dosing before an adequate trial has elapsed also generally has little rationale and may be either unnecessary or counterproductive (as in the case of rapid neuroleptization with first-generation antipsychotics (FGAs) producing acute dystonia), with just a few exceptions:

- oral loading of divalproex (20–30 mg/kg in divided doses) may hasten antimanic response (see Chapter 13);
- a rapid initial dose escalation with olanzapine may yield more rapid and effective treatment for acute agitation as compared to a more usual gradual dosing schedule, with comparable tolerability;
- someone with a known ultra-rapid metabolizer genotype for a pertinent catabolic enzyme (see Chapter 8) may expectably require higher than usual doses (though usually without precise compensatory adjustment).

Tip

Have a clear rationale in mind when making any changes to a treatment regimen.

When should dosing adjustments *logically* be made, short of predetermined dose-titration schedules? There may not always be a "should" to answer this question, given high interindividual variability in drug response. One guiding principle involves responding to trends rather than transient vicissitudes in symptom status, not unlike following the stock market. Certainly, when unambiguous and sustained dips or plateaus are reached and adverse effects are minimal and tolerable, it is reasonable to consider dose changes. At the same time, one must be aware that some agents likely have therapeutic windows, above or below which efficacy may wane. Tricyclics for which serum therapeutic levels distribute along a bell curve distribution represent one such example, as is also the case for bupropion. Lower rather than higher doses of some medications (such as some second-generation antipsychotics (SGAs)) may yield better outcomes in certain subpopulations (e.g., anxious depressed patients), as discussed in Chapter 13).

Dosing: Usual, Homeopathic, Supratherapeutic

There has been surprisingly little formal literature examining the many assumptions clinicians make about dose–response relationships with respect to pharmacodynamic benefits as well as adverse effects. Some of the pertinent questions in this realm for which empirical data are either indirect or limited include:

- If a patient appears to improve on a medication at a lower-than-usual dose, is it unwise to maintain the low dose rather than strive toward usual dosing regardless of apparent improvement in baseline symptoms?

- When using two (or more) pharmacological cotherapies, is optimized dosing more useful or unnecessary for adjunctive as well as primary agents?
- For medications with established therapeutic serum levels (see Chapter 7), should dosing routinely continue toward the therapeutic range if the patient markedly improves at a subtherapeutic dosage?

Supratherapeutic dosing (defined as exceeding a manufacturer's maximum dose as approved by a regulatory agency such as the US Food and Drug Administration (FDA)) is limited pragmatically by drugs with narrow therapeutic indices (such as lithium or tricyclic antidepressants), dose-related adverse effects, or issues such as physiological tolerance or dependence. While *optimized* dosing (defined as achieving a maximally tolerated drug dose within the parameters of a drug manufacturer's label) is common practice in the setting of incomplete responses or loss of efficacy, despite continued pharmacotherapy, evidence to support greater efficacy from *supratherapeutic* dosing in those settings is largely anecdotal, as described more fully in Part II of this book.

G JUDGING TREATMENT EFFECTS: IS THE PATIENT *REALLY* BETTER?

Symptom checklists and rating scales are useful for judging the presence and severity of a disease state at a given time, but they are not as dynamically informative as gauging the impact of symptoms on how a patient navigates everyday stresses. Life itself is a psychiatric stress test, akin to the treadmill used to assess myocardial function. Or, taking an automotive analogy, no matter how appealing and pristine a vehicle looks in the showroom, one cannot *really* know how well it performs until one takes it on the road and puts it through its paces. In the world of mental health, stressful life events are like the everyday potholes and maneuverings that cars endure when being road-tested. If a psychotropic drug is successful in reducing psychiatric symptoms, we learn far more about the breadth and durability of its effect by asking how it helps improve the patient's everyday functioning and capacity for resilience when under pressure – that is, the ability to maintain a sense of equilibrium and relative freedom from psychiatric symptoms in the face of adversity.

Tip

Meaningful improvement is judged not simply by a reduction in symptoms but, as importantly, by the ability to manage life stresses without incurring a resurgence or worsening of psychopathology.

The ability to maintain a sense of mental equilibrium when under stress is in some ways analogous to the function of a gyroscope keeping an airplane level during flight, regardless of weather conditions that might otherwise jeopardize its aeronautical integrity. For an expanded depiction of this concept, see Box 1.2.

Box 1.2

Psychiatric Gyroscopes

The concept of resilience in mental health is rather analogous to the role of a gyroscope in maintaining a level, unswerving flight path for aircraft regardless of encountered turbulence. Whatever psychiatric shearing forces the winds of fate may inflict, we rely on an intact internal guidance system to maintain composure and a sense of forward movement without veering too far off path. Effective psychiatric treatments ought not to simply reduce current symptoms or prevent relapses, but even more critically, help ensure an intact capacity to compensate mentally for normal daily life stresses.

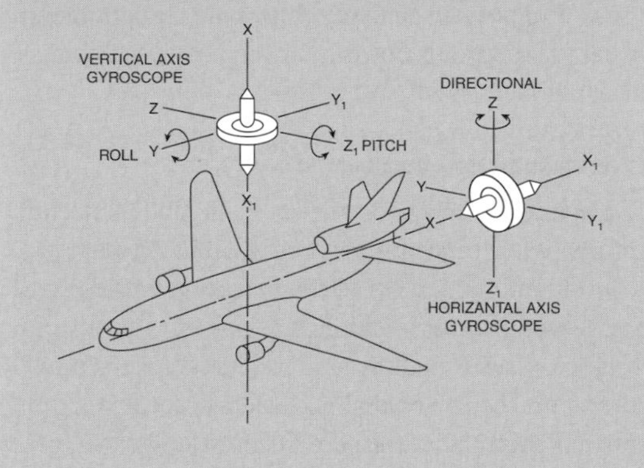

Of course, another way to determine empirically if the patient "really is better" after an adequate trial has elapsed is to stop the treatment in question to find out if clinical symptoms then recur or worsen. The obvious downside to this approach is its risk for clinical deterioration, with no guarantees against further declines if the stopped therapy is restarted. Sometimes this approach can be helpful for giving patients (or practitioners) a more unequivocal appraisal of the effects of a drug whose efficacy and purpose may have thus far been ambiguous.

H IF IT WORKED BEFORE, WILL IT WORK AGAIN?

There is more conjecture than evidence about assumptions that if a psychotropic drug was efficacious at some point in the past, it should expectably evoke the same clinical response on rechallenge after discontinuation. The trouble with questions such as this involves presuming that the clinical profile of a psychiatric problem that occurred in the remote past will re-present with the same characteristics many years later, or, ignoring the impact of new comorbidities, medical problems, concomitant drugs, or changes in hepatic or renal function over time. Nevertheless, there exists at least some data showing that in the case of chronic depression, retreatment with a tricyclic antidepressant after initial response again yielded robust benefit in slightly over 90% of patients (Friedman et al., 1995). In bipolar disorder, some authors have reported cases of lithium discontinuation-induced refractoriness, particularly when cessation is abrupt (over less than two weeks), while others have challenged such observations as being purely anecdotal. A 2013 meta-analysis of five studies involving 212 patients found no statistically significant reduction in lithium's prophylactic efficacy upon reinstitution after discontinuation (de Vries et al., 2013).

Our perception of such reports, particularly in the absence of adequately powered trials designed and devoted to assess true loss of efficacy or tachyphylaxis, is that because many real-world factors confound treatment stops and starts, it is difficult to form reliable generalizations about lesser efficacy upon psychotropic rechallenges. To the extent that clinical circumstances bear sufficient resemblance from one presentation to another in the same patient, a known history of favorable previous response to a given medication likely bodes well for its future success upon reinitiation.

I DO MECHANISMS OF ACTION MATTER?

All psychotropic drugs, from lithium to SSRIs to antipsychotics to psychostimulants to sedative-hypnotics, carry language in their manufacturers' product labels (usually found in Section 12.1) to the effect that the exact mode of therapeutic action for treating [the clinical condition of interest] is not known (or "unclear" or "not fully understood," depending on wording for a given agent). Is this simply a medicolegal disclaimer? Not entirely. While animal or other preclinical studies provide some knowledge about brain structures and neurotransmitter systems affected by a given drug, a considerable inferential leap is often needed to extrapolate those findings to observed human pharmacodynamic effects. Broad pharmacodynamic conclusions based solely on a mechanism of action also run the risk of implying class effects where none may exist. For example, not all GABAergic anticonvulsant drugs have mood-stabilizing, or anxiolytic, or antinocioceptive properties – some do, some do not, and seldom is one drug "within class" interchangeable for another.

Neurotransmitter pathways also may exert different effects in different brain regions (for example, dopamine agonism may promote attentional processing in the prefrontal cortex but have psychotomimetic effects in mesolimbic pathways). Finally, modern thinking about neural circuits points more to broad architectural pathways of circuits that interact with one another across brain regions, rather than "single" regions as a solitary focus of brain function or pharmacodynamic activity.

Some psychotropically active compounds have extremely diverse mechanisms of action (MOAs). In such instances, especially when the putative MOA to explain a particular psychotropic effect could be one of many, it becomes impractical if not senseless to try to formulate a classifiable descriptor based on receptor or enzymatic or neurotransmitter profiles. Consider, for example, the case of ketamine, a multipurpose drug for which its antagonism at the *N*-methyl-D-aspartate (NMDA) receptor is thought to mediate its dissociative anesthetic effects but not necessarily its antidepressant properties. (As described further in Chapter 13, a number of NMDA receptor antagonists other than ketamine have been shown to be no better than placebo for treatment of depression.) It would be mechanistically accurate, but awfully cumbersome and none too pithy to speak of ketamine as an exemplary drug that antagonizes NMDA, μ opioid, α_7 nicotinic, and M_1, M_2 and M_3 muscarinic receptors while agonizing D_2 and σ_1 or σ_2 receptors as well as inhibiting serotonin reuptake inhibitor (SERT), norepinephrine transporter (NET), dopamine transporter (DAT), and acetylcholinesterase.

For that matter, to the extent that every atypical antipsychotic also has a unique molecular signature with respect to its binding affinity and differential ratios of one neurotransmitter system to another (e.g., $5HT_{2A}:D_2$), broad mechanistic classifications may not tell enough of the story to account for relevant psychotropic effects, or even "best in class" designations (e.g., clozapine versus all other atypical antipsychotics). Within a classable MOA, drugs also may vary in their central nervous system (CNS) penetration (e.g., β-blockers crossing the blood–brain barrier), potency (e.g., tramadol and ziprasidone are both serotonin-norepinephrine reuptake inhibitors (SNRIs), albeit weakly so), receptor subtype selectivity/nonselectivity (e.g., α-agonists, monoamine oxidase inhibitors (MAOIs)), or dose-related recruitment of one system over another (e.g., venlafaxine functions predominantly as an SSRI rather than an SNRI at low doses; ziprasidone at low doses (e.g., <120–160 mg/day) functions more as a $5HT_{2C}$ antagonist than a D_2 antagonist (Mattei et al., 2011)).

J NO MORE "CHEMICAL IMBALANCE" OVERSIMPLIFICATIONS

In the 1960s, the so-called catecholamine hypothesis of mood disorders held that relative overabundances or deficiencies of monoamines were responsible for externalizing states (such as mania or psychosis) or internalizing states (such as depression or negative/deficit symptoms), respectively. Such simplified concepts failed to take into account different effects of particular neurotransmission in one brain region versus another (e.g., low hypodopaminergic tone is associated with inattention and low motivation in prefrontal circuitry but parkinsonism in the striatum), or interactions between pathways that might operate through different transmitter systems (e.g., the role of gamma aminobutyric acid (GABA) interneurons that serve to "turn on" or "turn off" other circuits).

Another point of uncertainty involves generalizations about expectable pharmacodynamic effects based on a drug's MOA. Here things can become tricky. For instance, likely all D_2 antagonists have antipsychotic properties, but not all antipsychotic drugs treat depression, and some may even cause or exacerbate depression. Similarly, anticonvulsants vary considerably in their psychotropic effects. In the 1990s, many anticonvulsant drugs were presumed to exert mood-stabilizing effects based on the presence of GABAergic activity (putatively antimanic) or antiglutamatergic activity (putatively antidepressant). This theory neatly fits the biochemical relationship of glutamate and GABA in presynaptic neurons and their respective effects on neuronal excitation or inhibition, but then fails to account for numerous subsequent negative or failed trials of newer anticonvulsants (such as gabapentin, topiramate, tiagabine, and others) in studies to treat mood symptoms in bipolar disorder. The model does help to account for the relative lack of antimanic efficacy of lamotrigine (as an antiglutamatergic but non-GABAergic compound) and the only modest antidepressant impact of divalproex (as a GABAergic agent). However, as a broad concept, it failed to account for the relative absence of mood-stabilizing effects seen in a host of other GABAergic or antiglutamatergic compounds that followed.

Examples of the diversity of relationships between psychotropic agents, their known pharmacodynamic effects, and evidence regarding their putative MOAs are presented in Table 1.8 at the end of this chapter.

K ON-LABEL AND OFF-LABEL DRUG USES

Approval by drug regulatory agencies such as the FDA is not necessarily synonymous with evidence-based medicine or the scientific rationale behind using a particular drug for a unique patient. Drug manufacturers pursue regulatory agency approval for proprietary formulations or molecular compounds for which generic versions are unavailable and sufficient patent life remains active for the drug of interest, usually when there is a large enough market share to justify the enormous expenditure of time and financial resources necessary to obtain regulatory approval.

The pursuit of regulatory agency approval for a new chemical entity (NCE) is a lengthy process divided into phases, as described in Table 1.9 at the end of this chapter. It is important for both clinicians and patients to recognize that distinctions between "on-label" and "off-label" uses according to regulatory agencies such as the FDA mainly reflect the outcome of efforts by drug manufacturers with vested interests in marketing proprietary products. Generic compounds or drugs whose patent lives have expired may indeed have demonstrable efficacy and safety from Level 2- or even Level 1-evidence studies (see Figure 1.1), but without the substantial resources necessary to pursue a regulatory agency-approved indication, many evidence-based treatments remain off label. Given that 95% of drugs tested in Phase 0 and Phase I trials fail to demonstrate adequate safety and efficacy to justify their further development, and that the cost to bring a new drug to market may be as high as $5 billion, one must appreciate the economic versus scientific basis for "on-label" drug designation and marketing as wholly separate from the rigor with which evidence may exist for "off-label" pharmacodynamic efficacy. Examples of such evidence-based but "off-label" drug uses abound within clinical psychopharmacology and include the following:

- **Gabapentin for anxiolysis:** A positive 14-week RCT in social anxiety disorder found a 38% response rate; data are less robust in generalized anxiety disorder (GAD) (Mula et al., 2007);
- **Lamotrigine for acute bipolar depression:** Five randomized placebo-controlled trials collectively demonstrated significant greater likelihood of response with lamotrigine than placebo, specifically in patients with high baseline severity (Geddes et al., 2009);
- **Lurasidone for major depressive disorder with mixed features (MDD-MF):** No psychotropic drug carries FDA approval for this newly described DSM-5 (Diagnostic and Statistical Manual of Mental Disorders) diagnostic entity; however, one six-week RCT showed significant reduction in both manic and depressive symptoms with large effect size, low discontinuation due to intolerance (Suppes et al., 2016);
- **Modafinil for attention deficit hyperactivity disorder (ADHD):** Five multisite RCTs showed significantly greater reduction in ADHD severity scores than placebo with medium-to-large effect size, fivefold decreased appetite, sixfold decreased insomnia, no cardiovascular adverse effects, dropouts due to adverse effects comparable to placebo (meta-analysis by Wang et al., 2017a);
- **Pregabalin for GAD:** Eight placebo-controlled trials demonstrated significant efficacy but with only a small-to-medium effect size, comparable response rates to benzodiazepines, no differences from placebo in dropout due to adverse events (Generoso et al., 2017);
- **Quetiapine for GAD:** Three placebo-controlled trials showed better response and remission rates than placebo for quetiapine XR 50 or 150 mg/day, comparable efficacy and discontinuation due to adverse effects as SSRIs (meta-analysis by Maneeton et al., 2016);
- **Quetiapine for MDD:** Three RCTs showed better response and remission rates than placebo for quetiapine XR 50 or 150 mg/day, comparable efficacy and discontinuation due to adverse effects as SSRIs (meta-analysis by Maneeton et al., 2016);
- **Topiramate for alcohol use disorder:** Seven placebo-controlled trials showed significant improvements with medium effect sizes in heavy drinking days and abstinence, smaller effect/nonsignificant for craving (meta-analysis by Blodgett et al., 2014).

L WHAT'S IN A NAME?

The nomenclature by which we classify psychotropic (and many nonpsychotropic) drugs is often antiquated and increasingly uninformative with respect to the actual specific pharmacodynamic effects of a specific drug. Not all anticonvulsants treat all forms of epilepsy, not all antineoplastic drugs treat all neoplasms, and not all antidepressants treat all forms of depression. Paradigm shifts are far from new in psychiatry, and drug classification by an original indication quickly can become uninformative – MAOIs are no longer called antituberculosis drugs, chlorpromazine is no longer the preanesthetic sedative that it was in the 1950s, and many anticonvulsants are nowadays prescribed for bipolar disorder or migraine or neuropathic pain irrespective of their anticonvulsant origins. Meanwhile, some "non-antidepressants" are evidence-based for some forms of depression, to the consternation of many clinicians wedded to an old and increasingly archaic nomenclature. Consider Clinical Vignette 1.2.

CLINICAL VIGNETTE 1.2

Arthur was a 34-year-old man with bipolar I disorder being treated with lamotrigine 400 mg/day, lurasidone 40 mg/day, armodafinil 250 mg/day, and *N*-acetylcysteine 1800 mg/day. He nevertheless complained of persistent depression and his psychotherapist called his psychiatrist to ask why he was not taking an antidepressant. The psychiatrist, who was thoroughly familiar with the content of Chapter 13 of this book, needed to explain that no "traditional" antidepressant has ever demonstrated efficacy greater than that of a mood stabilizer alone, but that each of the four compounds Arthur was taking had at least one (if not more) randomized, double-blind, placebo-controlled trials to support efficacy for bipolar depression, with at least moderate effect sizes, and nonredundancy (and possible pharmacodynamic synergy) in their respective putative mechanisms of action. The therapist, nevertheless, felt the psychiatrist was still remiss in not prescribing "an antidepressant."

Table 1.10 provides examples of medications whose evidence-based psychotropic drug effects have little or no correspondence with broader "classifications" by which they are often popularly recognized. Drugs that possess multiple evidence-based pharmacodynamic effects hold special importance in the hearts and minds of psychopharmacologists. Like Swiss army knives that do far more than simply perform expected knife duties, or smart phone devices whose functional utility may have little or no relevance to telephone capabilities, our nomenclature is expanding to capture the varied actual psychotropic properties vis-à-vis putative mechanisms of action. Not all antituberculosis drugs treat depression (iproniazid), nor do all antihypertensives treat tremor (propranolol).

M NEUROSCIENCE-BASED NOMENCLATURE (NBN)

In 2010, the European College of Neuropsychopharmacology (ECNP) established a task force to reassess and revise the terminology with which psychotropic drugs are classified. The resulting neuroscience-based nomenclature (NbN) attempts to classify medications based on a drug's pharmacology and putative mode of action, alongside its clinical indication (see www.nbn2.com). Representative examples of this classification system are provided in Table 1.11. (Note that many drugs have multiple mechanisms of action and are thus classifiable under more than one heading.)

In some instances, uncertainty or ambiguity about a drug's mode of action leads to classifications that may not be so directly useful (e.g., the NbN identifies lithium's mode of action as "enzyme interactions"), or a putative mechanism may involve so many receptors as to defy a *general* classification (e.g., vortioxetine). Others may have such elaborate putative mechanisms of action so as to make a broad categorization based on mode of action unduly cumbersome, if not simply overspeculative. Examples here might include topiramate (whose mode of action is described as "facilitation of GABA transmission, receptor antagonist on AMPA or kainic acid"). Ketamine's MOA may vary across its diverse pharmacodynamic properties – its anesthetic effects may stem from its NMDA receptor antagonism, while its analgesic effects may relate to both its anti-NMDA receptor properties plus its μ opioid receptor blockade; its apparent antidepressant effects are presently hypothesized to come from its activation at α-amino-3-hydroxy-5-methyl-4-isoxazole propionic acid (AMPA) receptors or σ_1 and σ_2 receptors more likely than from its NMDA receptor-blocking effects – making it hard to neatly "class" the drug based on numerous mechanisms of action that may pertain to different pharmacodynamic effects (e.g., analgesic versus antidepressant properties).

N DEFINING THE GOALS OF TREATMENT

All too often, patients and clinicians embark on a treatment regimen with little or no explicit discussion about realistic goals and expectations. Seldom does psychopharmacology magically transform all mental health blemishes, particularly when problems are longstanding and complex, making it important to identify specific targets of treatment, acknowledge limitations, agree on practical goals and priorities, and clarify what is and is not likely to be pharmacologically remediable. Staunch refusal to accept or tolerate annoying but medically nonhazardous adverse drug effects often means foregoing aggressive medication regimens. Histories of extreme treatment resistance (involving nonresponses to numerous adequate and appropriate medication trials) portend a low (though not necessarily nil) probability of substantial improvement, as opposed to making less substantial, more modest possible inroads for certain symptoms in managing a chronic condition. Longstanding or deeply engrained negative attitudes or beliefs, unhealthy lifestyle choices, poor adaptation or coping skills, marked distress intolerance, or dissatisfaction with life circumstances all may require interventions other than pharmacotherapy.

In palliative care medicine, the concept of "defining the goals of care" provides a useful example of establishing unambiguous expectations and clear priorities about targeted treatment outcomes. It is a reality that even with excellent pharmacotherapy, response and remission rates for many serious psychiatric conditions are far less than 100%, while relapses and recurrences are sometimes inevitable and unavoidable despite proper care. Particularly in chronic conditions that have not responded to multiple appropriate biological therapies, adopting a "disease management" rather than a "disease modification" approach often becomes an unspoken necessity.

Defining the goals of care in an explicit manner from the outset can help to temper unrealistic expectations and effectively "set the bar" low enough that *any* improvements will be more likely hailed than discounted. Examples of key targets that could serve as goals of treatment unto themselves might include:

- restoring disrupted sleep or appetite
- averting emergency department visits, hospitalizations, or suicide attempts

- maintaining work role functioning and minimizing absenteeism/presenteeism
- maintaining an independent living status
- minimizing the cumulative burden of adverse drug effects by pruning ineffective medications

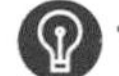

Tip

Know exactly what symptoms are the intended targets of any purposeful intervention.

- strengthening coping skills and striving to improve quality of life despite the incomplete resolution of psychiatric symptoms

In the pages ahead, we urge the reader to keep in mind the particular goals of treatment specific to each patient they encounter, rather than simply the notion of trying to ameliorate a diagnosis as if the process were generic and divorced from the patient-specific characteristics that drive treatment outcome as discussed throughout subsequent chapters.

TAKE-HOME POINTS

- Critically examine the evidence behind suspected cause-and-effect relationships when prescribing medications and judging presumptive efficacy, lack of efficacy, or adverse effects, versus the natural course of illness. Impose Hill criteria for causality.
- Recognize the degree of rigor and evidence base to support the utility of treatment interventions. Randomization is the "great equalizer" that accounts for confounding factors that can differentially influence outcome within clinical subgroups.
- While adequate pharmacotherapy trials often require many weeks to assess, just-noticeable differences often should be apparent by two weeks; their absence at this benchmark may signal the need to alter medication doses or otherwise modify a treatment plan in order to optimize eventual response or remission. By the same token, have a specific rationale in mind to justify decisions behind changes to a treatment regimen.
- When judging treatment efficacy, consider not only symptomatic improvements but also signs that a patient has an improved capacity to withstand normal daily stresses.
- Favor complementary over redundant drug mechanisms of action when combining pharmacotherapies or choosing plausible rationales behind medication decisions.
- Have clear and specific therapeutic goals in mind when making any changes to a treatment regimen.

Table 1.1 Brain distribution of neurotransmitter targets and their pharmacodynamic effects: cholinergic system

Neurotransmitter targets	Regional locations	Putative pharmacodynamic effects
ACh (subtypes: muscarinic: M_1–M_5; nicotinic)	Basal forebrain (i.e., the septal nuclei and the nucleus basalis of Meynert) projections to PFC, hippocampus, and amygdala; the laterodorsal tegmental and pediculopontine nuclei, projecting to thalamus, pons, medulla, cerebellum, and cranial nerve nuclei; and cholinergic projections from the caudate nucleus	M_1 *agonists* (e.g., xanomeline) may enhance attention, verbal reasoning, and memory while *antagonists* (e.g., benztropine, diphenhydramine, oxybutynin, tricyclics) may cause cognitive dulling. M_3 *agonists* stimulate salivary and other glandular secretions; *antagonists* (e.g., oxybutynin) may cause urinary retention. Some nicotinic *agonists* may aid cognition (e.g., galantamine), particularly those binding at the α_7 subunit, at least theoretically, or smoking cessation (e.g., varenicline); *antagonists* may also help smoking cessation (e.g., bupropion) or act as nondepolarizing neuromuscular blockers (e.g., atracurium, pancuronium).

Abbreviations: Ach = acetylcholine; PFC = prefrontal cortex

Table 1.2 Brain distribution of neurotransmitter targets and their pharmacodynamic effects: dopaminergic system

Neurotransmitter targets	Regional locations	Putative pharmacodynamic effects
D_1	Dorsal striatum (caudate, putamen), ventral striatum (NAc, olfactory tubercle), PFC and temporal cortex	*Agonism* in PFC may enhance working memory and social cognition, and in striatum may produce antiparkinsonian effects (e.g., pergolide, rotigotine); *antagonism* may produce antipsychotic effects (most FGAs and SGAs) and sometimes antidepressant effects.
D_2	*Postsynaptic* receptors found in nigrostriatal (substantia nigra pars compacta → caudate and putamen), mesocortical (ventral tegmentum → PFC), mesolimbic (ventral tegmentum → ventral striatum (NAc, olfactory tubercle)), tuberinfundibular (arcuate nucleus of the hypothalamus → pituitary) tracts. Postsynaptic D_2 receptors are also found as heteroreceptors on nondopaminergic neurons. *Presynaptic* D_2 autoreceptors are most densely concentrated in ventral tegmentum and substantia nigra pars compacta	*Agonism* at postsynaptic receptors may enhance attention (PFC) and reward (mesolimbic), diminish parkinsonian movements (nigrostriatal), and counteract hyperprolactinemia (tuberoinfundibular); *postsynaptic antagonism* produces antipsychotic and Parkinsonism effects, hyperprolactinemia; *presynaptic agonism* downregulates DA release, producing similar effects to those seen with postsynaptic antagonism
D_3 (D_2-like)	*Presynaptic*. High concentrations in ventral striatum (NAc, olfactory tubercle), thalamus, hippocampus, motor regions (e.g., putamen)	*Agonists* (e.g., bromocriptine, pramipexole, rotigotine) may enhance motivation or aggravate psychosis; *partial agonism* (e.g., aripiprazole, brexpiprazole, cariprazine) may contribute to antidepressant effects; *selective antagonism* could exert anticraving and antipsychotic efficacy (though lesser affinity than for D_2 receptors; e.g., nemonapride[a]) while potentially sparing adverse cognitive and motor effects associated with D_2 blockade
D_4 (D_2-like)	Frontal cortex, medulla, hypothalamus, striatum, NAc	May play a role in novelty-seeking, working memory, fear-based memory; clozapine potently antagonizes D_4 receptors
D_5 (D_1-like)	Found in PFC, amygdala, hippocampus, thalamus, striatum, cerebellum, basal forebrain	No selective agents available; may be associated with fear-based memory, smoking initiation

[a] Not available in the USA

Abbreviations: DA = dopamine; FGA = first-generation antipsychotic; NAc = nucleus accumbens; PFC = prefrontal cortex; SGA = second-generation antipsychotic

Note: DA concentrations are said to follow a U-shaped curve (∩) in relation to working memory; too high or too low basal DA levels seem to impair cognitive function; optimal functioning occurs in a middle-ground "Goldilocks" zone

Table 1.3 Brain distribution of neurotransmitter targets and their pharmacodynamic effects: serotonergic system

Neurotransmitter targets	Regional locations	Putative pharmacodynamic effects
$5HT_{1A}$	Presynaptic somatodendritic autoreceptors in raphe nucleus; postsynaptic receptors in limbic system, hypothalamus, cortex, dorsal horn	*Presynaptic agonism* downregulates (while *antagonism* upregulates) serotonergic release; *postsynaptic agonism* associated with antidepressant and anxiolytic effects
$5HT_{1B}$	PFC, basal ganglia, striatum, hippocampus	*Antagonism* associated with antidepressant effects
$5HT_{2A}$	PFC, parietal and somatosensory cortex, olfactory tubercle, hippocampus	*Antagonism* increases prefrontal DA release, may enhance attention and working memory; *agonism* associated with psychedelic effects of serotonergic hallucinogens (e.g., LSD), enhanced associative learning, release of oxytocin, prolactin
$5HT_3$	Cortex, hippocampus, NAc, ventral tegmentum, substantia nigra, brainstem (area postrema and nucleus tractus solitarius)	*Agonists* enhance release of DA, GABA, CCK; affects vomiting reflex, cognition, anxiety while *antagonists* (e.g., ondansetron, granisetron, zacopride, phenothiazines) produce antiemetic, anticraving, and possible antipsychotic effects
$5HT_7$	Thalamus, hypothalamus, amygdala, hippocampus, dorsal raphe, caudate, putamen, substantia nigra	*Agonism* enhances GABA-mediated inhibition of 5HT in raphe nucleus (effectively decreasing 5HT release), enhances GABAergic inhibition and increases glutamatergic stimulation in hippocampus, may influence mood, learning and memory, sleep–wake cycle, thermoregulation, nocioception

Abbreviations: CCK = cholecystokinin; DA = dopamine; GABA = gamma-aminobutyric acid; 5HT = serotonin; LSD = D-lysergic acid diethylamide; NAc = nucleus accumbens; PFC = prefrontal cortex

Table 1.4 Brain distribution of neurotransmitter targets and their pharmacodynamic effects: noradrenergic system

Neurotransmitter targets	Regional locations	Putative pharmacodynamic effects
NE	Pons (locus coeruleus)	α_1 *agonists* (e.g., phenylephrine) vasoconstrict; *antagonists* can cause orthostatic hypotension, may reduce nightmares associated with PTSD (e.g., prazosin); α_2 *agonists* (e.g., clonidine) cause sedation and blunt autonomic hyperarousal (e.g., during opiate withdrawal); α_2 *antagonists* (e.g., yohimbine) may counteract erectile dysfunction but increase blood pressure and cause anxiety; β_1 *agonists* (e.g., dobutamine) increase heart rate and cardiac contractility (e.g., to treat congestive heart failure); *antagonists*[a] are cardioselective to treat hypertension and tachycardia; β_2 *agonists* (e.g., albuterol) bronchodilate, delay premature labor (e.g., terbutaline); *antagonists* lack known clinical use

[a] Nonselective β1 and β2 antagonist examples include propranolol, pindolol, nadolol, labetolol, carvedilol

Abbreviations: NE = norepinephrine; PTSD = post-traumatic stress disorder

Table 1.5 Brain distribution of neurotransmitter targets and their pharmacodynamic effects: GABA/glutamate system

Neurotransmitter targets	Regional locations	Putative pharmacodynamic effects
GABA	The major inhibitory neurotransmitter, distributed widely throughout cortical and subcortical (e.g., basal ganglia) brain regions	GABA *agonism* can produce sedative, anxiolytic, and anticonvulsant effects. GABA interneurons often function as "feed forward" or "feed backward" circuit-breakers (meaning, they function like on/off switches) by inhibiting other circuits within a neural network
Glu	Cortico-brainstem, corticostriatal (PFC → striatum and NAc), thalamo-cortical, cortico-thalamic, corticocortical (intra-cortical pyramidal neurons) pathways	Regional binding may influence attention, learning and memory, psychosis, pain perception, parkinsonism

Abbreviations: NAc = nucleus accumbens; PFC = prefrontal cortex

Table 1.6 Brain distribution of neurotransmitter targets and their pharmacodynamic effects: histamine system

Neurotransmitter targets	Regional locations	Putative pharmacodynamic effects
H_1	Highest densities in frontal, temporal and occipital cortices, cingulate gyrus, striatum, thalamus	*Antagonism* associated with sedation, cognitive dulling, weight gain, relief from allergic reactions
H_2	Distributed throughout cortex, caudate, putamen, hippocampus	*Antagonism* may impair memory and cognition
H_3	Prominent in basal ganglia, globus pallidus, hippocampus, cortex	Presynaptic inhibitory heteroreceptor. *Antagonism* may broadly affect cognition via enhancing release of histamine, ACh, NE, DA, among other neurotransmitter systems. Pitolisant, a novel H_3 receptor antagonist/ inverse agonist received FDA approval as a nonscheduled pharmacotherapy for narcolepsy in 2019

Abbreviations: ACh = acetylcholine; DA = dopamine; NE = norepinephrine

Table 1.7 Brain distribution of neurotransmitter targets and their pharmacodynamic effects: melatonin and orexin systems

Neurotransmitter targets	Regional locations	Putative pharmacodynamic effects
Melatonin	Pineal gland	*Agonists* (e.g., ramelteon) may promote sleep by synchronizing circadian rhythms
Orexin	Perifornical area and lateral hypothalamus	*Antagonists* of orexin A (ORA) and orexin B (ORB) receptors (e.g., suvorexant) may promote sleep by downregulating activity of the ascending arousal pathway and upregulating sleep-promoting brain nuclei (notably, the ventrolateral preoptic nucleus (VLPO) of the anterior hypothalamus)

Table 1.8 Diverse relationships between psychotropic drug effects and presumed mechanisms of action

Agent	Clinical disorders of interest	Proposed mechanism(s) of action	Conflicting evidence
Amphetamine	ADD/ADHD, depression	↑ extracellular DA via: (a) decreasing presynaptic DA uptake by competitively inhibiting uptake at the DA transporter, (b) facilitating DA vesicle release into the cytoplasm through VMAT2 binding, and (c) increasing intrasynaptic DA and NE by reversing the direction of transport through DA and NE transport proteins into the synaptic cleft	None
Anticonvulsants	Bipolar disorder, epilepsy, anxiety disorders	GABAergic and antiglutamatergic effects	Most anticonvulsants apart from divalproex, carbamazepine and lamotrigine show no benefit for mood disorders
Ketamine	Depression; depression with suicidal ideation	NMDA receptor antagonism; sigma receptor blockade; μ opioid receptor blockade	Other antiglutamatergic drugs (such as riluzole, memantine and lanicemine) have not demonstrated antidepressant efficacy
Lithium	Bipolar disorder, impulsivity, suicide	Numerous proposed mechanisms involving intracellular second messenger and signal transduction pathways, as well as neurotrophic and anti-apoptotic effects	Not all proposed mechanisms broadly affect mood (e.g., some but not all PKC inhibitors (see Chapter 13))
SNRIs	Depression, anxiety, pain	Increased presynaptic 5HT and NE availability via reuptake inhibition	None
SSRIs	Depression, anxiety	Increased presynaptic 5HT availability via reuptake inhibition	None
DORAs	Insomnia	Suvorexant, lemborexant are dual orexin receptor antagonists	None

Abbreviations: 5HT = serotonin; ADD = attention deficit disorder; ADHD = attention deficit hyperactivity disorder; DA = dopamine; DORA = dual orexin receptor antagonist; GABA = gamma aminobutyric acid; NE = norepinephrine; NMDA = *N*-methyl-D-aspartate; PKC = protein kinase C; SNRI = serotonin-norepinephrine reuptake inhibitor; SSRI = selective serotonin reuptake inhibitor; VMAT2 = vesicular monoamine transporter 2

Table 1.9 Phases of drug development

Preclinical	Phase 0	Phase I	Phase II	Phase III	Phase IV
Animal or in vitro studies conducted to identify pharmacokinetic properties (dosing, metabolism) and determine if a proposed drug is safe for human exposure	Microdosing in a small number of healthy human subjects to obtain further information about pharmacokinetics (e.g., bio-availability, half-life) and drug safety	Somewhat larger trials in healthy human subjects to clarify dosing and safety	Larger trials on a patient population to gauge likely efficacy and adverse effects	Large-scale trials in patient populations to provide a more definitive assessment of drug efficacy and safety	The collection of post-marketing surveillance (also called pharmaco-vigilance) data to gauge long-term effects during routine treatment
			Phase IIa: Pilot trials in selected populations; **Phase IIb**: Rigorous, well-controlled, "pivotal" trials	**Phase IIIa**: Additional safety and efficacy data after initial efficacy has been demonstrated, prior to regulatory submission; **Phase IIIb**: conducted after regulatory submission but prior to approval and launch	

Table 1.10 Distinctions between common drug "classifications" and their evidence-based uses

Classification	Examples	Evidence-based uses unrelated to classification
Anticonvulsants	Carbamazepine	Bipolar disorder; trigeminal neuralgia
	Gabapentin	Neuropathic pain; anxiety; insomnia
	Lamotrigine	Bipolar disorder
	Topiramate	Migraine; weight loss; alcoholism
Antidepressants	Bupropion	Smoking cessation; weight loss
	Duloxetine	Stress incontinence; chronic low back pain
	Nortriptyline	Migraine, neuropathic pain
Antihistamines	Diphenhydramine	Insomnia
	Hydroxyzine	Anxiety
	Trimethobenzamide	Nausea
Antihypertensives	Propranolol	Tremor; performance anxiety; migraine
	Clonidine	ADHD; opiate withdrawal; tics
	Guanfacine	ADHD; tics
Antipsychotics	Aripiprazole	Major depression; bipolar mania
	Brexpiprazole	Major depression; bipolar mania
	Cariprazine	Bipolar mania; bipolar depression
	Lurasidone	Bipolar depression
	Quetiapine	Depression; bipolar mania/depression; anxiety

Table 1.11 Examples of neuroscience-based nomenclature[a]

Putative mechanism	Examples
ACh inhibitor	Donepezil
DA reuptake inhibitor	Modafinil
DA/NE reuptake inhibitor/ releaser	Amphetamine, lisdexamfetamine, methylphenidate
Enzyme inducer	Lithium carbonate (inositol monophosphatase, protein kinase C, glycogen synthase kinase-3)
Enzyme inhibitor	Selegiline (MAO-A, MAO-B)
Irreversible enzyme inhibitor	Isocarboxazid, phenelzine (MAO-A, MAO-B)
Partial agonist	Buprenorphine (μ); buspirone, cariprazine, vilazodone ($5HT_{1A}$); varenicline ($\alpha_4\beta_2$ and $\alpha_6\beta_2$)
Positive allosteric modulator	Acamprosate, alprazolam, clonazepam ($GABA_A$)
Receptor agonist	Clonidine, guanfacine (α_1); melatonin, ramelteon (M_1, M_2); prazosin (α_1); varenicline (α_7 nicotinic)
Receptor antagonist	Buprenorphine (κ, δ); olanzapine, ziprasidone (D_2, $5HT_{2A}$); clozapine, paliperidone, risperidone (D_2, $5HT_{2A}$, α_1); flumazenil ($GABA_A$); diphenhydramine, hydroxyzine (H_1); ketamine, memantine (NMDA); prazosin, quetiapine, risperidone, trazodone (α_1); mirtazapine[†] ($NE\alpha_2$, $5HT_{2A}$, $5HT_3$); nefazodone, pimavanserin, trazodone ($5HT_{2A}$); vortioxetine ($5HT_{1D}$, $5HT_3$, $5HT_7$)
Receptor partial agonist/ receptor antagonist	Aripirazole, brexpiprazole, cariprazine (D_2, $5HT_{1A}/5HT_{2A}$)
Reuptake inhibitor	Atomoxetine, desipramine, maprotiline, nortriptyline, reboxetine (NET); bupropion (NET, DAT); fluoxetine, sertraline, vilazodone, vortioxetine (SERT); clomipramine, duloxetine, imipramine, levomilnacipran, venlafaxine, desvenlafaxine (SERT, NET); suvorexant (OR1, OR2)
Voltage-gated Ca^{++} channel blocker	Carbamazepine, gabapentin, oxcarbazepine, pregabalin
Voltage-gated Na^+ channel blocker	Acamprosate, divalproex

[a] As modified from www.nbn.com

[†] Mirtazapine is sometimes referred to as a noradrenergic and specific serotonergic antidepressant (NaSSA)

Abbreviations: 5HT = serotonin; DA = dopamine; DAT = dopamine transporter; GABA = gamma aminobutyric acid; MAO = monoamine oxidase; NE = norepinephrine; NET = norepinephrine transporter; NMDA = *N*-methyl-D-aspartate; OR = orexin; SERT = serotonin reuptake transporter

2 Targets of Treatment: Categories versus Dimensions of Psychopathology

LEARNING OBJECTIVES

- ☐ Identify *dimensions* as well as *categories* of psychopathology related to mood, thinking, perception, and behavior that may cut across diagnoses and correspond more directly to disordered underlying neural circuitry; at the same time, whenever possible, look for recognizable constellations of symptoms that track together as coherent clinical entities
- ☐ Recognize *form fruste* (or, partial) presentations of major clinical syndromes; course over time may help to validate diagnostic constructs and their longitudinal stability
- ☐ Use knowledge of common comorbidities to corroborate likely diagnostic impressions
- ☐ Appreciate that transdiagnostic features such as autonomic hyperarousal, distress intolerance, executive dysfunction, and emotional lability may in themselves pose relevant targets for pharmacotherapy

> We are much too much inclined in these days to divide people into permanent categories, forgetting that a category only exists for its special purpose and must be forgotten as soon as that purpose is served.
>
> *– Dorothy L. Sayers*

Diagnostic systems such as the DSM have long struggled over whether to organize psychiatric disorders as black-and-white *categories* defined by operational criteria (where "casehood" is unambiguously either present or absent) versus *dimensions* of psychopathology (where certain clinical elements are present but insufficient in number or duration to meet minimum criteria that define a particular clinical condition). Clinicians, meanwhile, often tend to identify and treat prominent symptoms, with varying degrees of awareness and concern about their broader context for defining the presence or absence of a distinct syndrome. In this chapter we will examine when pharmacological treatment targets can or should be thought of as unambiguous disease categories as opposed to dimensions of psychopathology that may not always be so clear-cut.

Diagnoses are clusters of signs and symptoms that should form a coherent constellation based on their inter-relationships. Often, no single symptom in itself defines one diagnosis over another, although some cardinal features may point more compellingly toward a particular diagnosis (e.g., suicidality is more diagnostically suggestive of depression than is, say, insomnia). Diagnostic validity becomes especially challenging when no pathognomonic features exist and fundamental symptoms overlap across multiple disorders. Parsimony always favors finding an overarching diagnosis rather than tackling individual symptoms piecemeal, at least when a unifying pathophysiological process can be identified – but it becomes especially difficult to pronounce diagnostic categories as valid when the etiology of most forms of mental illness remains unknown.

Symptom constellations sometimes fall together neatly and nonarbitrarily, as, for example, in eponymous conditions defined by unique symptom conglomerations (e.g., the triad of ptosis + miosis + anhydrosis = Horner's syndrome; or, ophthalmoplegia + ataxia + confusion = Wernicke's encephalopathy). Other examples of categorical entities defined by recognizable symptom collections include normal pressure hydrocephalus (the triad of gait abnormalities + urinary incontinence + mental status changes), nephrotic syndrome (defined by proteinuria + hypoalbuminemia + hyperlipidemia + peripheral edema), or multiple sclerosis (characterized by the convergence of weakness, vision changes, paresthesias, and cognitive deficits).

Medical diagnosticians rely on corroborative anatomical or physiological signs and symptoms to affirm a suspected unifying explanation – as when lower extremity edema occurs with rather than without hepatomegaly and pulmonary rales (suggesting congestive heart failure), or when it occurs with rather than without femoral lymphadenopathy (suggesting lymphedema from a possible malignancy). In much the same way, the basis for a categorical diagnosis in psychiatry can often be deduced by amassing clues and corroborative data that ultimately point to an identifiable suspect.

Psychiatric detective work demands clinical curiosity about which signs and symptoms belong together and which ones seem out of place or fail to add up to a coherent whole. Symptom profiles should follow a logical, nonrandom pattern, and should be commensurate with outward functioning or disability. Sometimes, categorical diagnoses emerge with utter clarity when puzzle pieces fit neatly together to tell a coherent story and support a working hypothesis. For examples, see Clinical Vignettes 2.1–2.3.

CLINICAL VIGNETTE 2.1

In a young adult man with auditory hallucinations, the presence of concrete thinking and poor interpersonal relatedness helps to corroborate hypotheses about schizophrenia, while a more affectively related, fairly abstract thinking version of the same patient would less likely arouse such inklings. Rapid resolution of psychotic symptoms might alternatively prompt speculation about psychoactive substance misuse. Concomitant hemiparesis with an aura and blurry vision might instead suggest hemiplegic migraines.

CLINICAL VIGNETTE 2.2

Preoccupations with jumping out of a high-story window of a tall building fit conceptually with depression when accompanied by anhedonia, hopelessness, and vegetative signs, or with obsessive-compulsive disorder when the thoughts are unmistakably intrusive, ego-dystonic, frightening, and contrary to an emotional state of sadness and despair, or with schizophrenia if the intent is to act on or escape from command hallucinations, or with an anxious-insecure attachment style and poor distress tolerance, in the absence of an affective syndrome, following a romantic rejection.

CLINICAL VIGNETTE 2.3

A young adult with complaints of incessant anxiety unrelieved by SSRIs might draw skepticism about the legitimacy of her symptoms when there is also a history of sedative-hypnotic abuse, particularly if the patient claims ardently that only benzodiazepines are helpful, or expresses an intense lack of interest in rigorously exploring pharmacotherapies that are not controlled substances or in considering nonpharmacological treatment options.

A SYMPTOM OVERLAP: WHEN CATEGORIES BREAK DOWN

DSM psychiatric diagnoses are grounded in phenomenology and make no pretense about knowing the real cause of any mental illness. For all the biological correlates espoused about disease states and their viable remedies – from neurotransmitter systems to aberrant brain circuitry to genetics or endocrinological or inflammatory processes – modern nosology remains atheoretical with respect to the etiology of psychiatric disorders. Biological or laboratory markers sometimes help to affirm suspected diagnoses elsewhere in medicine, although the absence of biomarkers to help validate distinct diagnostic entities is not unique to psychiatry – there are no laboratory or other biological measures to help differentiate migraine from cluster or tension headaches, or Meniere's disease from vestibular labyrinthitis, or Raynaud's phenomenon from complex regional pain syndrome. The hunt for biomarkers of mental illness has long been elusive, and tends to ignore the psychological dimensions and context of symptom presentations. Some clinicians and investigators think that until valid biomarkers are identified, the quest for personalized medicine and predictable pharmacodynamics will remain plagued by insurmountable guesswork. We maintain that clinical psychopharmacology need not and should not involve guesswork, and can be pursued using a systematic approach informed by a sufficiently thorough initial clinical assessment.

It is harder to think of diagnostic categories as clearly separable if and when their defining criteria share many overlapping elements such as "psychosis" or "anxiety" or "inattention" or "low motivation" or "mood instability." Symptom collections that present in unrecognizable or haphazard patterns often defy diagnostic categorization during structured clinical interviews. For practical purposes, such mosaicism often leads clinicians to think about treatment targets as psychopathology dimensions along spectra, rather than trying to spot whether or not a particular category is unambiguously present. And, unlike antibiotics or antineoplastics or antianginal drugs, ameliorative psychotropic drugs do not necessarily correct underlying pathophysiologic processes as much as compensate for them, in much the same way that guaifenesin eases symptoms of a cough but does not fundamentally treat its etiology.

Table 2.1 presents representative examples of overlapping symptoms domains – ranging from sleep/wake cycling disruptions to affective, cognitive, and behavioral phenomena – across varied psychiatric diagnostic categories.

Psychiatric diagnostic criteria can be fickle and may not always fit together so neatly. They are usually developed by consensus agreement among expert work groups, rather than "discovered" as the natural assemblage of a disease state in the wild. Diagnoses are sometimes voted by committees into or out of existence (e.g., disruptive mood dysregulation disorder and Asperger's syndrome, respectively). In fairness, though, the defining criteria for some nonpsychiatric medical conditions also can evolve as key elements are thought to assume greater or lesser nosological importance. Examples here would include the American Diabetes Association criteria for Type II diabetes, or the Androgen Excess PCOS Society Criteria for polycystic ovarian syndrome, or the American–European Consensus Sjögren's Classification Criteria. In both psychiatric and nonpsychiatric medical conditions, consensus-based criteria for a categorical diagnosis often undergo periodic revision as knowledge advances about the relative importance of certain cardinal features. (For example, in 2010 the standardized criteria for Marfan syndrome placed new emphasis on the presence of certain cardiovascular and ophthalmological signs; in schizophrenia, bizarre delusions were at one time considered to hold particular nosologic importance.) Diagnostic criteria are also sometimes revised to reflect changing thresholds for determining when intervention is appropriate (as in the case of revised guidelines for the detection, prevention and management of hypertension by the American College of Cardiologists/American Heart Association).

Tip

Psychiatric diagnoses are defined by symptom clusters according to consensus opinion, making their "accuracy" more relative than absolute.

Also similar to nonpsychiatric medical conditions, cross-sectional symptoms comprise only one leg of diagnostic validity, alongside such corroborative features as:

- *age at onset* (e.g., first episodes of psychosis or bipolar mania are rare after middle age),
- *longitudinal course* (schizophrenia tends more often to involve persistent symptoms and chronic disability; childhood ADHD remits about one-half to two-thirds of the time into adulthood (Kessler et al., 2005a)), and
- *family history* (which again may reflect symptom clusters (such as suicidal behavior, impulsivity, or social aversion) more accurately than syndromes being categorically present or absent).

Psychiatric diagnostic categories tend to be reliable (meaning observers can reasonably agree on their presence or absence) more than valid (meaning they accurately discriminate one genuine underlying process from another). Even when there exists a *sine qua non* individual symptom that defines a condition, constellations with other symptoms often remain important. When does inattention denote ADHD, or when is it merely the symptom of a broader construct? Like the showy lead singer of a band, or the soloist in a choral ensemble, one highly prominent symptom could easily unduly overshadow other aspects of a constellation. Here one runs the risk of overgeneralizing the importance of a particular clinical feature, then jumping the gun pharmacologically, and neglecting altogether the concept of differential diagnosis. Examples include presumptions such as:

- self-injury or self-mutilation behavior equates to borderline personality disorder
- mood swings equate to bipolar disorder
- inattention or poor concentration means ADHD
- bizarre delusions or first-rank symptoms equate to schizophrenia
- a history of trauma automatically equates to post-traumatic stress disorder (PTSD)

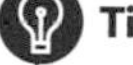

Tip

A single symptom, however prominent, does not in itself equate to a psychiatric diagnosis.

B DO DIAGNOSES REALLY MATTER?

Categorical diagnoses matter most when a particular disease entity exists that is defined not just by its obvious symptoms but by additional features that make it a coherent and valid construct. These include:

- an expectable prognosis and course over time
- a predictable epidemiology with recognizable at-risk groups
- a unique underlying pathophysiology
- a specific treatment (especially if withholding the "right" treatment worsens prognosis and course)

In the case of psychiatric diagnoses, reliability is often easier to establish than validity, because it pertains only to the reproducibility and consistency of a conclusion (the diagnosis) irrespective of its accuracy. Some diagnostic constructs are more reliably recognizable than others. Table 2.2 provides examples of diagnostic reliability from the DSM-5 field trials (comparing diagnostic impressions between interview raters across 11 academic centers). Diagnoses nearer the end of the table in more darkly shaded cells represent conditions with the poorest inter-rater reliability from among those conditions studied – notably, mixed anxiety-depression as a distinct entity, generalized anxiety disorder, and even major depressive disorder.

Tip

Reliability refers to the *consistency* with which an observation is made from one assessment point to another without great variation.

Validity refers to whether an observation accurately reflects a well-founded conclusion that is objectively true.

Are anxiety and depression not valid diagnostic entities?

It's not about their validity, but their reliability – those conditions can be hard to differentiate clearly from other similar-looking disorders.

Symptom-based (rather than diagnosis-based) treatment approaches can be fairly benign endeavors when an appropriate treatment is unrelated to a unique causal disease process – for instance, diuretics often produce equivalent results for treating peripheral edema regardless of its cause, and acetaminophen treats a variety of minor aches and pains with little danger of worsening an underlying or occult pathophysiology. Superficial similarities across some psychiatric conditions matter less when symptomatic relief can be achieved in a generic, relatively safe manner (e.g., benzodiazepines can treat insomnia or anxiety caused by a wide variety of problems; antipsychotics can help to manage agitation that may have one of many etiologies; stimulants can promote alertness in virtually anybody). However, symptom-based treatment approaches are a riskier proposition when underlying pathophysiologies differ across conditions that share only superficial resemblances and the treatment is tied to a unique underlying process. Increased abdominal girth caused by obesity versus pregnancy versus ascites obviously requires very different treatment approaches. Shortness of breath is managed differently when it is caused by a mechanical obstruction or cardiogenic or bronchospastic or infectious or anaphylactic origins. Similarly, there are vastly different treatments for chest pain caused by angina, peptic ulcer disease, gastroesophageal reflux, or a pulmonary embolism. Anxiety caused by a pheochromocytoma requires treatment of the underlying adrenal medullary tumor, and depression caused by hypothyroidism will not budge much with antidepressants instead of exogenous thyroid hormone.

In the absence of a clear-cut, unambiguous psychiatric diagnosis, it is no less important to have a working hypothesis about the likely basis for a symptom profile before embarking on a treatment, even if one is taking an empirical rather than a definitive approach.

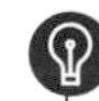

Tip

Have at least a working hypothesis about the likely cause of a symptom presentation, and a basis for that hypothesis over others.

C "...THE DISORDER IS NOT BETTER ACCOUNTED FOR BY ANOTHER CONDITION..."

When making a categorical diagnosis, all editions of the DSM note that "the disturbance is not better accounted for by another mental disorder..." This means that clinicians should be aware that certain signs and symptoms are epiphenomena related to a core diagnosis, rather than invoke additional separate disorders to explain the totality of symptoms present. (Chances are, someone with muscle aches and weakness as part of the flu has not coincidentally additionally developed fibromyalgia or chronic fatigue syndrome.) Consider these examples in psychiatry:

- In schizophrenia, avoidance of social interactions and poor interpersonal functioning are more likely manifestations of paranoia and/or negative symptoms than truly comorbid social phobia

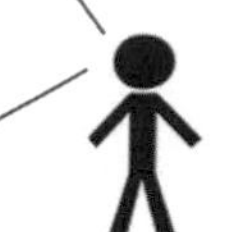
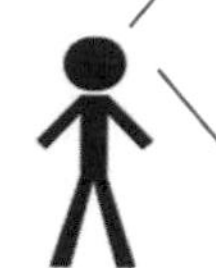

Y'know, I don't treat schizophrenia or major depression.
Oh? Why's that?
I treat symptoms. Delusions, hallucinations, sadness, guilt…
Ok, but, you want to have some idea about what's going on in terms of underlying cause. Hallucinations in psychosis are different from hallucinations in delirium or intoxication or epilepsy. Social avoidance is different in somebody who's paranoid versus phobic. Inattention is different in ADHD versus in a stroke or dementia patient…

- Depressed patients may have poor concentration and sustained attention as signs of their depression, without the need to speculate about concurrent ADD as another separate problem
- Loss of appetite commonly occurs during depressive episodes without the need to invoke a comorbid diagnosis of anorexia nervosa
- Paranoia in the context of hypervigilance associated with PTSD may not reach delusional proportions; labeling such features as "comorbid" unspecified psychosis generally makes little sense

D *FORM FRUSTE* PRESENTATIONS AND "SPECTRUM" DIAGNOSES

Given that bona fide psychiatric problems can and do present with fewer than the requisite number or duration of symptoms specified by DSM or similar nosologic systems, it can be difficult to formulate the best (or even appropriate) pharmacotherapy for a condition that cannot be operationally defined. It is obviously preferable not to misattribute a symptom to one condition when it is better accounted for by another (such as a substance-induced mood disorder versus major depression, or disturbing thoughts driven by obsessive versus delusional thinking); additionally, most large-scale RCTs reflect outcomes of an intervention when used for a specific, well-defined patient group, leading to unpredictability and loss of evidence base when extrapolating to more nebulous, diminutive or ill-defined clinical groups. The DSM-IV diagnosis of "not otherwise specified" (NOS) was meant to capture such instances, at least as a mental placeholder subject to future revision, for patients who manifest some but not all features of a diagnosable entity (i.e., *form fruste* presentations). DSM-5 and ICD-10 replaced this terminology, but not its nosological intent, with the designation of "unspecified" mood, anxiety, psychotic, or other comparable major disorders.

Tip

Ambiguous diagnoses often can be clarified based on course over time.

There is not much of a formal evidence base for treating ambiguous or *form fruste* presentations of any form of mental illness. (Partly, that may be an artifact of the impracticality of identifying and enrolling prospective subjects whose exact ailment is hard to specify.) But, given that many busy practitioners likely assign diagnoses with less formal rigor than occurs in research trials, this gap is perhaps one of the greatest shortcomings in applying evidence-based empirical literature.

Tip

Treating *form fruste* presentations requires substantial extrapolation from studies of more well-defined conditions, possibly yielding different outcomes.

Some authors point out that committing a patient to a long-term or possibly indefinite course of treatment (such as lithium for bipolar disorder, or long-acting antipsychotics in schizophrenia) discourages clinicians from re-evaluating or reconsidering an initial working diagnosis, or may impart assumptions about long-term course and outcome that may not necessarily be valid. Adverse effects also may not translate neatly from one illness subtype to another. (For example, antidepressant-associated mania appears to be more likely to occur in bipolar I than bipolar II or bipolar disorder unspecified (formerly designated as bipolar disorder not otherwise specified (NOS) patients.) Given the inevitable balance of risks and benefits of all medications, clarity of diagnosis is especially important when considering the indefinite use of drugs whose long-term use may incur more serious adverse effects (e.g., renal or hepatic dysfunction, tardive dyskinesia, metabolic syndrome, leukopenia).

Nonresponse to multiple appropriate psychotropic drug trials for a particular disorder typically leads to pronouncements of a pharmacologically unresponsive or treatment-resistant form of the presumed condition, or else fundamental reconsideration of the original diagnosis. The overzealous pursuit of a specific pharmacotherapy approach can equally lead one to ignore the possibility of a wrong diagnosis from the outset (especially if presenting symptoms conform poorly to an established condition, and the original diagnosis may have been a force-fit), or a failure to recognize important collateral features that require independent attention. Examples of the latter might include:

- depression that fails to remit in the setting of active alcohol or illicit substance use, unrecognized hypothyroidism, or significant anxiety
- presumptions that substance misuse represents "self-medication" of another psychiatric disorder, rather than an addiction needing its own independent treatment
- paranoia and mistrust that are misidentified as "anxiety" and treated solely with SSRIs, beta-blockers and benzodiazepines rather than antipsychotics
- negative/deficit symptoms (characterized by affective flattening and an absence of expectable cognitive or emotional processes) misconstrued as depression (where one expects the "feelingful," demonstrable presence of negative thoughts and emotions)
- internal preoccupations and poor awareness of social cues due to a developmental disability that becomes misidentified as schizophrenia
- anxiety and avoidance of social interactions labeled as social phobia which may actually be driven by psychosis
- akathisia misidentified as anxiety or hypomania
- compulsive gambling mislabeled as mania
- pseudoseizures (psychogenic nonepileptiform seizures) misidentified as epilepsy

E NON-CATEGORICAL CONCEPTS ABOUT PSYCHOPATHOLOGY

There are many frameworks for conceptualizing dimensions of psychopathology, as described below. At an initial level, one can differentiate psychiatric conditions that overtly manifest themselves as *externalizing* versus *internalizing*. Characteristics along this dichotomy are summarized in Table 2.3 at the end of this chapter.

Homotypic Comorbidity

Externalizing disorders tend to co-occur with other externalizing disorders, while internalizing disorders tend to co-occur with other internalizing disorders (the comorbidities are said to be "homotypic"); externalizing + internalizing comorbidities ("heterotypic") are uncommon.

F LONGITUDINAL STABILITY OF PSYCHIATRIC DIAGNOSIS

The validity of a psychiatric condition is partly affirmed or corroborated by its consistency over time as a stable construct. To the extent that many if not most psychiatric problems are associated with recurrence, successive episodes provide the opportunity to appraise similarities and differences across acute presentations. Accurately tracking the stability of a psychiatric diagnosis over time can be difficult, in part owing to imprecise retrospective recall, variable follow-up durations, the impact of treatment and adherence, and the natural evolution of a disorder and its comorbidities (e.g., some proportion of unipolar depressed patients may not have a first lifetime mania or hypomania until many years after an index depression; schizophreniform patients may or may not develop schizophrenia).

G WHAT'S KNOWN FROM FOLLOW-UP STUDIES OF FIRST-EPISODE PRESENTATIONS?

A meta-analysis of 42 studies of first-episode psychosis (Fusar-Poli et al., 2016) examined the longitudinal stability of initial psychiatric diagnoses among 14 484 cases reassessed over a mean of 4.5 years. Point estimate concordance rates between index and subsequent episodes, in descending order, are summarized in Table 2.4. Note the wide range from schizophrenia and affective disorders (diagnostic correlations >0.80) to schizophreniform disorder and unspecified forms of psychosis (correlations <0.40) for which longitudinal course may be especially critical to diagnostic validation.

First-episode psychoses also rarely transformed to primary affective disorder diagnoses, and vice versa. In the case of substance-induced psychosis, findings elsewhere (Starzer et al., 2018) have shown that about one-third of such patients converted diagnostically either to bipolar disorder or schizophrenia, typically within three to five years after an index presentation. Famously, tendencies were observed prior to the DSM-III era for American psychiatrists to identify schizophrenia when rating interviews with psychosis patients while British psychiatrists more often characterized the same patients as having bipolar disorder (Kendell et al., 1971), suggesting geographic or cultural biases in diagnostic perception.

H SUPERFICIAL SIMILARITIES, DIFFERENT UNDERLYING PROCESSES

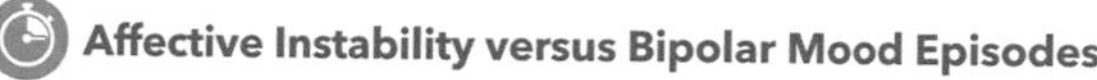

Affective Instability versus Bipolar Mood Episodes

Moment-to-moment shifts in mood, particularly involving sudden disproportionate anger (and seldom euphoria) arising in response to heightened interpersonal sensitivities, tend to be hallmark features of borderline personality disorder more than an affective illness such as bipolar disorder. The term "mood stabilizer" is itself something of a misnomer in that there has been almost no formal research with agents such as lithium or divalproex specifically to examine their impact on affective lability per se (that is, sudden shifts in mood or moment-to-moment variations in emotions that may occur in response to environmental stresses, frustrations, or interpersonal conflicts). In fact, mood stabilizers may more successfully target motor signs of mania (such as increased energy and rapid speech or thinking) than tendencies toward disrupted mood states – much the way antidepressants may more dramatically help vegetative or psychomotor symptoms of depression with often less clear impact on negative self-worth or sad mood.

Tip

"Mood stabilizers" target psychomotor signs of mania more than vicissitudes of mood.

Tip

Mood "swings" in borderline personality disorder involve sudden, interpersonally triggered anger or rage more often than euphoria.

Negative Symptoms versus Depression

In distinguishing depression from schizophrenic negative symptoms, one might consider that while "depression" or dissatisfaction may be complaints voiced in either situation, depression is the "feelingful" presence of strongly unpleasant emotions focused on themes of despair, sadness, melancholy, low self-worth, and often loss; negative symptoms, by contrast, involve the relative absence of emotion per se, with a flat (rather than sad) or dull (rather than emotive) conveyance of an inner state. Depressive themes contain sad content, while negative symptoms may lack themes of any kind altogether or reflect emptiness more than despair or global impoverishment more than dismay or despondency. Antidepressants tend to exert relatively modest effects for negative symptoms as opposed to frank depression (Helfer et al., 2016).

Tip

Depression involves the *presence and expression* of sad feelings whereas negative symptoms involve the *absence* and *nonexpression* of emotions.

Cognitive Disorganization: Psychosis, Delirium or Dementia?

Form of thinking (irrespective of content) can be disorganized across an array of psychiatric conditions. Once considered more a hallmark of schizophrenia (classically defined as the "splitting of fibers of thought"), formal thought disorder (FTD) can encompass loosening of associations, circumstantiality, tangentiality, derailment, perseveration, illogicality, thought blocking, and impoverished content of thought. Thinking is traditionally inferred from language, at times making it difficult or even circular when distinguishing an FTD from a speech disorder. As an indicator of global cognitive dysfunction (i.e., difficulty formulating, conceptualizing, organizing, and expressing logical ideas), the presence of an FTD quickly draws clinical attention as a prominent domain and potential focus of treatment. Its presence may also help to rule out other significant psychiatric disorders where FTD is generally absent (such as personality disorders and most anxiety disorders, barring highly agitated or regressed states).

In addition to primary psychotic disorders such as schizophrenia/schizophreniform or schizoaffective disorder, FTDs may also be evident in patients with other neuropsychiatric conditions, such as:

- delirium or psychosis secondary to general medical conditions (e.g., lupus cerebritis, limbic encephalopathy, CNS Lyme)

- acute intoxication/withdrawal states
- frontotemporal and other dementias
- epilepsy
- stroke
- psychotic depression
- psychotic mania
- dissociative states
- autism spectrum disorders (e.g., illogical thinking and loose associations related to cognitive dysfunction) (Solomon et al., 2008)

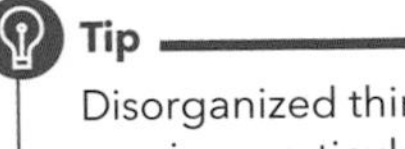

Tip

Disorganized thinking requires particular scrutiny to determine a likely underlying cause.

Transient or varying manifestations of FTD tend to reflect more state- than trait-dependent phenomena (e.g., intoxications rather than dementias) that eventually remit either spontaneously or via treatment of an underlying medical etiology. Psychopharmacological interventions aimed purely at symptomatic treatment for FTD therefore requires careful assessment of possible underlying correctable medical etiologies.

COMORBIDITIES: MANY DIFFERENT CO-OCCURRING DISORDERS, OR PLEIOMORPHIC HETEROGENEITY?

Having one psychiatric diagnosis greatly increases the likelihood of having additional diagnosable conditions.

Tip

Comorbidity is not random; certain psychiatric conditions are more likely than others to arise as co-occurring disorders.

Diagnostic subgroups also may differ in their comorbidities – for example, alcohol or other substance use disorders are considerably (~20%) more likely among bipolar I than bipolar II disorder patients (Merikangas et al., 2007). Examples of lifetime prevalence rates of specific comorbid conditions associated with several psychiatric disorders, based on findings from the National Comorbidity Survey Replication Study, are shown in Figures 2.1–2.4.

Box 2.1

Psychiatric Comorbidity is Common

In the National Comorbidity Survey Replication, about half of adults with one psychiatric disorder will have at least one other (Kessler et al., 2005c). In fact, according to epidemiological studies, *three or more* additional psychiatric diagnoses were evident in:

- 70% of bipolar disorder patients (Merikangas et al., 2007)
- 47% of adults with nonaffective psychotic disorders (Kessler et al., 2005b)
- 34% of adults with anorexia nervosa (Hudson et al., 2007)
- 64% of adults with bulimia nervosa (Hudson et al., 2007)
- 49% of adults with binge eating disorder (Hudson et al., 2007)

Figure 2.1 Comorbid conditions in adults with ADHD. Data based on Kessler et al., 2006.

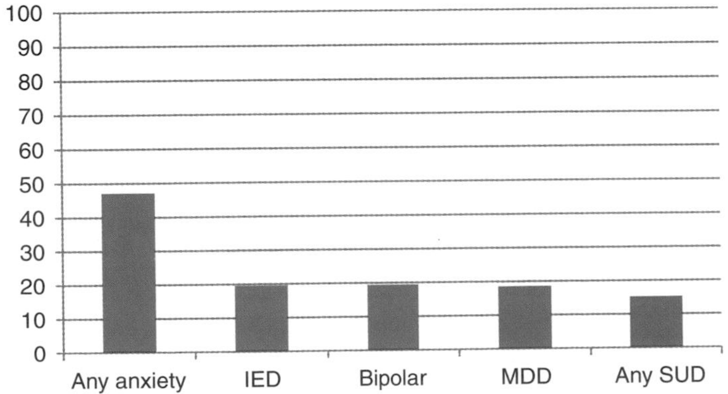

Abbreviations:
IED = intermittent explosive disorder;
MDD = major depressive disorder;
SUD = substance use disorder

Figure 2.2 Comorbid conditions in adults with binge eating disorder. Data based on Hudson et al., 2007.

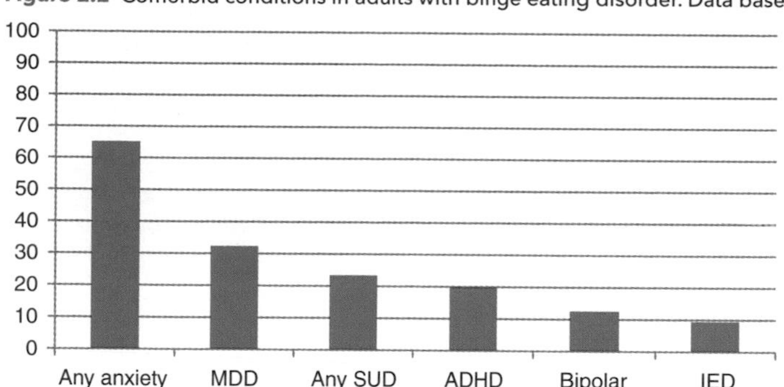

Abbreviations:
ADHD = attention deficit hyperactivity disorder
IED = intermittent explosive disorder;
MDD = major depressive disorder;
SUD = substance use disorder

Figure 2.3 Comorbid conditions in adults with nonaffective psychotic disorders. Data based on Kessler et al., 2005b.

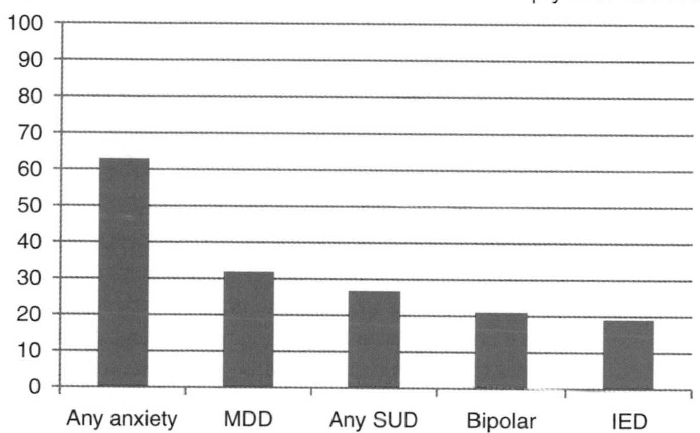

Abbreviations:
IED = intermittent explosive disorder;
MDD = major depressive disorder;
SUD = substance use disorder

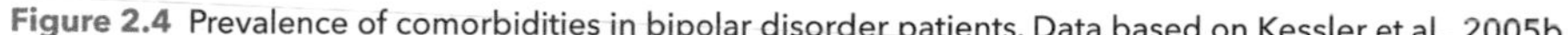

Figure 2.4 Prevalence of comorbidities in bipolar disorder patients. Data based on Kessler et al., 2005b.

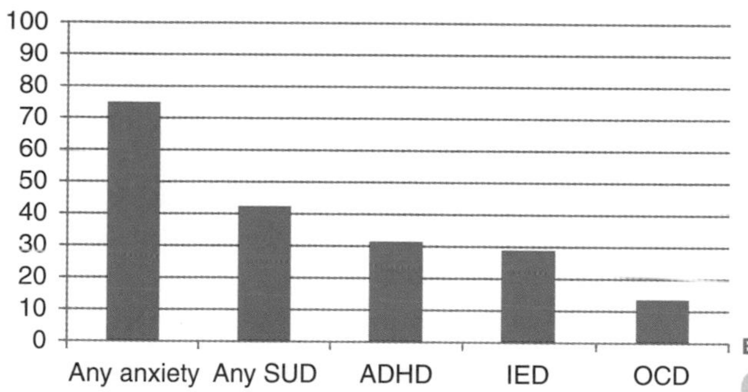

Abbreviations:
SUD = substance use disorder;
ADHD = attention deficit hyperactivity disorder;
IED = intermittent explosive disorder;
OCD = obsessive-compulsive disorder

Box 2.2

Facts About Comorbidity

- Bipolar probands have an increased risk for panic disorder among first-degree relatives (MacKinnon et al., 2002)
- A family history of an alcohol use disorder is more common in bipolar probands (OR = 14.5) than unipolar depression probands (OR = 1.7) (Preisig et al., 2001)
- Probands with ADHD are more likely to have first-degree family members with substance use disorders
- Parental alcoholism may increase the risk for ADHD in offspring by two- to threefold (Sundquist et al., 2014)

E THE GENETICS OF COMORBIDITY

The idea that two frequently co-occurring disorders spring from a common underlying process is bolstered by family and genetic data.

From a molecular-genetic standpoint, the Cross-Disorder Group of the Psychiatric Genomics Consortium

Figure 2.5 SNP-based coheritabilities ($r_{g\ SNP}$) between disorders.*

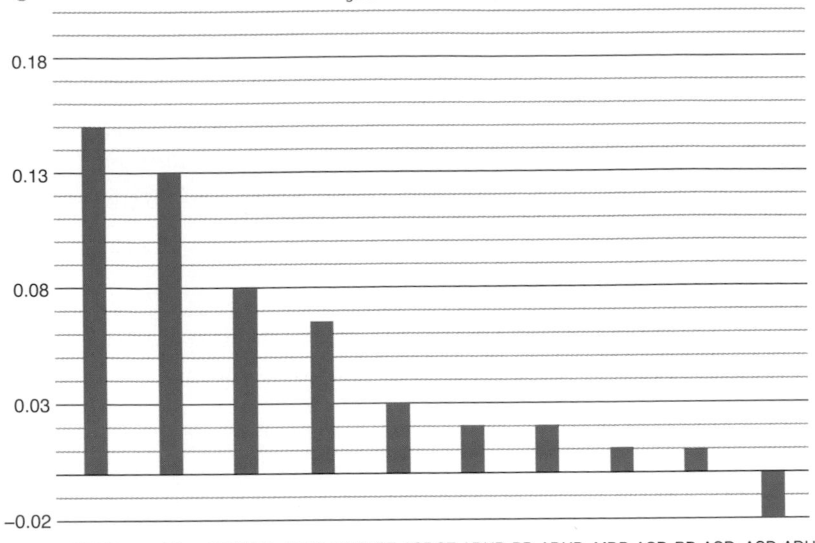

Abbreviations:
SZ = schizophrenia;
BD = bipolar disorder;
MDD = major depressive disorder;
ADHD = attention deficit hyperactivity disorder;
ASD = autism spectrum disorders

* based on findings from Cross-Disorder Group of the Psychiatric Genomics Consortium, 2013

(2013) estimated genetic variation within and between psychiatric diagnostic groups and found high or moderate significant associations between identified single nucleotide polymorphisms (SNPs) in *schizophrenia and bipolar disorder, schizophrenia and major depressive disorder, bipolar disorder and major depressive disorder*, or *ADHD and major depressive disorder* (see Figure 2.5). Other pairings of disorders had low, nonsignificant correlations.

Geneticists speak of pleiomorphic heterogeneity when referring to a common underlying genetic entity that can give rise to several or more phenotypes. Further clues about whether comorbidities could actually be pleomorphic manifestations of just one condition come from studies of familial psychiatric conditions. For example, ADHD patients have high rates not only of familial ADHD but also of familial substance use disorders (ORs ~2.2; Skoglund et al., 2015; Biederman et al., 2008a), schizophrenia (OR = 1.7–2.2; Larsson et al., 2013) or mood disorders (bipolar disorder: OR = 1.8–2.5; Larsson et al., 2013), but fairly low rates of familial anxiety disorders (Biederman et al., 1991a, 1991b).

J SYMPTOM SUBCOMPONENTS WITHIN A CATEGORICAL DISORDER

Common threads of psychopathology also can be found to run *within* an overarching diagnosis. Consider, in the case of depression, the role of its affective, cognitive, behavioral, and somatic components. Does pharmacotherapy equally target all such domains? If, for instance, sleep and appetite improve with a given treatment but concentration and motivation lag, when should that prompt simply a dosage increase for an incomplete response as opposed to augmentation with another medication that might more successfully target specific residual symptoms (such as – if MOAs at least *hint* at underlying processes – an antihistaminergic drug for insomnia, a GABAergic agent for anxiety, lithium or divalproex for poor impulse control, or a stimulant or other pro-dopaminergic drug for arousal and attention)? While there is no one-size-fits-all answer, such questions should at least enter into the thought process behind modifications to a pharmacotherapy regimen.

The use of psychometric rating scales to track changes in overall symptom severity and individual subcomponents (so-called "measurement-based care") offers an empirical approach for discerning changes over time in relevant subelements of an overall disorder. Statistical approaches such as factor analysis, principal components analysis, regression models, or latent class analyses can sometimes "boil down" a complex collection of symptom domains and have been used to find common comorbidity patterns across multiple separate disorders, yielding further clues about common psychopathological processes – such as the cognitive versus physical aspects of depression, the psychic versus somatic aspects of anxiety, or positive versus negative versus cognitive symptoms of schizophrenia.

K SUBSTANCE MISUSE AS A DIAGNOSTIC WILDCARD

Substance use disorders that co-occur with other psychiatric disorders pose unique challenges for diagnostic classification and treatment. On a practical level, it is often difficult if not impossible to tell when substance misuse (or a behavioral addiction) is the direct product or manifestation of a more overarching psychiatric condition (such as stimulant misuse arising after the onset of a new manic episode) or as the mimic of a suspected dual diagnosis (such as cocaine intoxication that results ostensibly in compulsive gambling and psychomotor signs resembling mania, followed by a depressive crash when the drug wears off) or as a truly separate phenomenon. Establishing chronology sometimes helps but is not always feasible. Family history may help to corroborate the "independence" of one set of symptoms relative to another, but again this may not always be revealing.

In the National Comorbidity Survey Replication study of US households, substance use disorders arose *after* the onset of anxiety disorders or externalizing disorders more than half the time, although in the case of mood disorders more variability was observed in the chronology of substance misuse, with alcohol or illicit substances more often arising before the onset of unipolar or bipolar disorder (see Figure 2.6).

L NEUROSCIENCE-BASED PSYCHIATRIC DIAGNOSES: ARE WE THERE YET?

Contemporary thinking about psychopathology in general increasingly leans toward considering symptom domains along continua, finding common phenomenological threads that cut across different recognized disorders. Such threads are diagnostically nonpathognomonic (like fever) but may help tease apart underlying neurobiological mechanisms (such as infectious versus autoimmune etiologies). Recognizing prominent threads may, in fact, more closely approximate the way many clinicians actually make treatment decisions, consciously or otherwise, when they envision the kinds of results they expect their interventions to produce.

Dimensions of psychopathology are thought to conform or "map" to neural circuitry more accurately than the categorical entities we define by consensus as diagnoses. Efforts such as the NIMH Research Domain Criteria (RDoC) represent one attempt to describe dimensions of human behavior and mentation that cut across possible diagnostic constructs and may better approximate the neurobiological substrates of psychopathology – and potential targets of psychopharmacology. The original matrix described under the RDoC system includes five components, as described in Table 2.5 at the end of this chapter.

Temperamental characteristics can color, or even mimic, the presentation of mood, psychotic, anxiety or

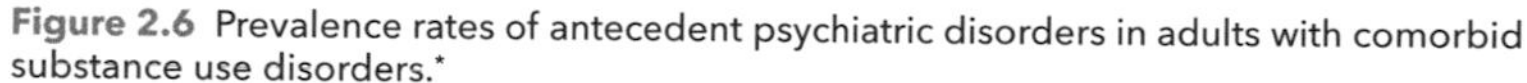

Figure 2.6 Prevalence rates of antecedent psychiatric disorders in adults with comorbid substance use disorders.*

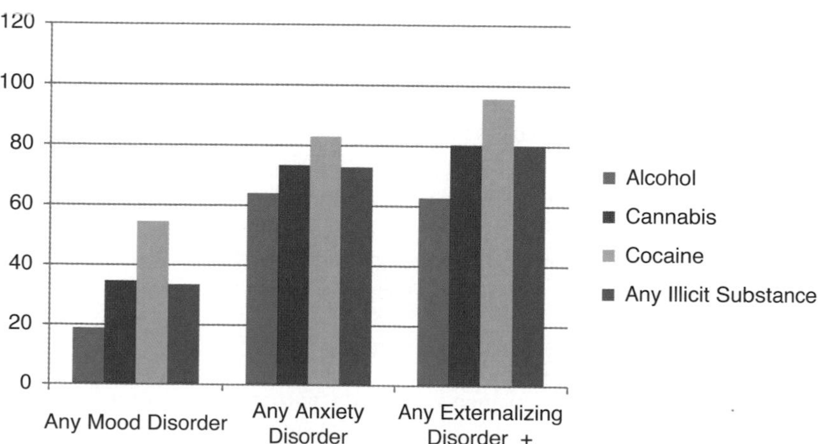

* National Comorbidity Survey Replication (Glantz et al., 2009)

\+ Externalizing disorders include intermittent explosive disorder, conduct disorder, oppositional-defiant disorder, and attention deficit hyperactivity disorder other psychiatric disorders. The "five-factor model" of personality, as articulated by Cloninger et al. (1991), provides one framework for considering the impact of temperamental traits on psychiatric diagnosis and psychopharmacology. It focuses on components involving "openness to experience," "conscientiousness," "extraversion," "agreeableness," and "neuroticism," as elaborated in more detail in Table 2.6 included at the end of this chapter.

Tip

Remember the five-factor model of personality by the mnemonic *OCEAN* (openness, conscientiousness, extraversion, agreeableness, and neuroticism).

Additional dimensions of personality and temperament were later captured in the Tridimensional Personality Questionnaire (TPQ; Cloninger et al., 1991) and the Temperament and Character Inventory (TCI; Cloninger, 1994). This framework captures elements such as "harm avoidance," "novelty-seeking," "reward dependence," and "persistence," (as described further in Table 2.7 at the end of this chapter), which can lend further clarity in understanding how psychopathology presents within an individual, and may help to identify appropriate substrates for pharmacology. By way of example, in some clinical trials, secondary analyses have found that extensive polypharmacy in bipolar disorder patients may be associated with comparatively low levels of openness, extraversion, and conscientiousness (Sachs et al., 2014).

The evidence base for or against the use of psychopharmacology to modify temperamental and/or personality characteristics such as those described above is discussed at length in Chapter 20.

Finally, in the following sections we invite consideration of a number of additional dimensions of psychopathology that cut across traditional diagnostic boundaries and are often taken as the basis for devising and implementing psychopharmacological interventions.

M AFFECTIVE INSTABILITY OR LABILITY

As noted in earlier sections, mood dysregulation, affective instability, or high moment-to-moment variability of mood or affect are not synonymous with any one disorder.

N ATTENTIONAL PROCESSING

Inattention is among the most ubiquitous symptoms cutting across psychiatric disorders. It may derive from numerous underlying processes – from the distractibility of ADHD to the preoccupation of intrusive thoughts in OCD or anxiety disorders to the "deer in the headlights" phenomenon of autonomic hyperarousal to intoxication with alcohol or other CNS depressants. As such, it would be erroneous to declare all of inattention as "ADD spectrum" or to think reflexively that a psychostimulant trial is automatically warranted to address "an ADD component" whenever subjective or objective manifestations of inattention are noted. Chapter 21 systematically discusses pharmacotherapy targets of impaired attention and cognitive functioning.

Box 2.3

Structural Components of Personality: the DSM-5 Perspective

The Personality and Personality Disorders Work Group for DSM-5 developed an "alternative model" for personality "dispositions" encompassing five domains meant to be amalgams of previous dimensional and categorical constructs. These included:

- *Negative Affectivity*: reflecting frequent high levels of intense negative emotions (e.g., depression, anxiety, anger) potentially linked with self-harming behaviors
- *Detachment*: involves the avoidance of social interactions and emotional connections and restricted displays of affect
- *Antagonism*: reflecting hostility or opposition; may include an exaggerated sense of self-importance and expectations of special treatment, with relative lack of empathy toward the needs and feelings of others
- *Disinhibition*: reflecting loss of impulse control and a lack of restraint in decision-making and other behaviors; focus may be on immediate gratification and disregard for consequences
- *Psychoticism*: reflecting peculiar, odd, eccentric elements in the form or content of thinking that are not congruent with cultural norms

O EXECUTIVE DYSFUNCTION

As the seat of planning, organization, and logical reasoning, brain regions associated with executive function exert fundamental control over higher cortical functions. "Cold cognition" refers to information processing minimally influenced by emotion, driven mainly by prefrontal circuitry (in contrast to "hot cognition" involving immediate emotional experiences, driven subcortically by limbic structures). Deficits may be evident in a wide range of conditions, including primary cognitive disorders (e.g., ADHD), impulse control disorders, mood disorders, learning disorders, trauma-related phenomena, OCD, and anxiety disorders (e.g., the inability to ignore extraneous or unwanted information, consequently leading to increased distress and thereby reciprocally impacting mood, behavior, and impulse control). Pharmacologies that specifically target executive dysfunction (as opposed to attentional processing) have not as yet been well described.

P IMPULSIVITY

Impulse control is one specific component of executive function, although its potential links with mood, aggression, and other domains warrant its separate elaboration. Poor impulse control occurs along a gradient of intensity. At one end it may include the failure to recognize and suppress an overly candid or socially inappropriate remark, or to make a hasty low-stakes decision that carries the potential for minimal negative ramifications, if any (such as not bothering to check a train schedule, instead relying on chance timing), progressing to larger-scale gaffes or more egregious transgressions of judgment.

Impulsive behavior generally reflects failure of "top down" "cold cognitive" regulation by prefrontal executive control circuitry over "bottom up" "hot cognitive" limbic activity as described in more detail in Chapters 13 and 14. Impulsivity can occur in the context of heated emotion (e.g., the fight of a fight/flight/freeze situation) or can also sometimes occur less emotively – as when failing to recognize risks that may not be so obvious (e.g., clicking on a malware website whose suspiciousness may only be apparent in hindsight), miscalculating the magnitude and degree of risk or its consequences, or it may entail outright ignoring a known hazard (sometimes for compelling reasons – such as driving far above the speed limit because of a medical emergency, and sometimes out of sheer recklessness, sensation-seeking or social defiance, or sometimes for no understandable or explicable reason at all (as in the case of cognitive disorganization)).

Q SOCIAL COGNITION AND THEORY OF MIND

Social cognition, and its closely linked construct theory of mind (ToM), together capture the awareness of social cues, nonverbal communication, and the ability to attribute mental states to others (e.g., comprehending what one person thinks of another). The ToM neural network is thought to encompass the left and right temporo-parietal junction, medial parietal cortex (including the precuneus and posterior cingulate gyrus), and the rostral anterior cingulate and medial PFC. Deficits (as might occur in autism, schizophrenia, traumatic brain injury) may in turn exacerbate problems with social behavior, mood, empathy, inferential thinking, and associated behaviors.

R PSYCHOSIS

The capacity to discern reality from nonreality is perhaps one of the best examples of a dimensional construct. Factor analytic studies of psychosis as a dimensional construct have identified several key domains, including positive symptoms (delusions, hallucinations, reality distortions), negative symptoms (affective flattening, alogia, impoverished thinking), disorganization (incoherence, tangential or illogical thinking, circumstantiality, bizarre behavior), and affective symptoms (anxiety, depression, hostility, impulsivity, uncooperativeness) (reviewed by Potuzak et al., 2012). On the surface it would seem entirely obvious to know whether a perceptual or ideational experience is or is not real, but anyone who has awoken from a lucid dream, stared at an optical illusion, been bamboozled by a magic trick, or tried to feel a limb that has fallen asleep knows that our capacity for judging reality is at the mercy of our senses. Senses play tricks, and the only way we can really judge their accuracy is to impose doubt. In full-on psychosis, perceptions are fixed convictions and there *is* no doubt, nor much capacity even to consider the *possibility* that things could be anything other than the way they appear to be. Cognitive rigidity becomes a cornerstone of psychotic experiences, as the lines between plausible and implausible blur without one's own realization. Vague inklings and suspicions give way to entrenched misperceptions that, by definition, defy challenges from logical reasoning or the consideration of alternative explanations.

Psychosis is sometimes viewed as a phenomenon based more in abject fear than worry, the former reflecting limbic hyperarousal while the latter involves a more tempered and contained kind of anxiety or apprehension. Reality testing is usually more intact in worry than psychosis, with a capacity to anticipate ramifications of an idea or perception with less fixed conviction (e.g., "what if this is a tumor?" versus "I know this is a tumor and the doctors are lying to me").

Loss of insight is often taken as a key component of psychosis; when reality testing is impaired, it almost follows automatically that one is unaware of their distorted perception. Indeed, if someone had sufficiently intact insight to recognize a false belief or perception as false, that capacity alone would essentially "downgrade" the experience from a delusion or hallucination to a worry. *Bizarre* thought content was at one time taken to be highly suggestive of a process related to schizophrenia, but debate about poor diagnostic specificity of this feature led to its lesser emphasis in modern nosology systems regarding psychotic disorders.

In a dimensional or continuum model, one might consider features such as those described in Box 2.4.

Box 2.4

Considerations for a Dimensional Model of Psychosis

- it may be hard for the person to recognize that the experience is abnormal, or may seem strange to others
- the degree to which an aberrant idea or perception is fixed (thinking is rigid); there is little curiosity about the basis for the experience, or capacity to subject the content to scrutiny or doubt
- it is hard for the person to generate, or at least entertain, alternative explanations for the basis of the idea or perception
- the phenomenon causes distress

From the above, one could judge a clearly psychotic phenomenon to be of mild, moderate, or severe intensity; separately, one could gauge the degree to which someone is able to fathom that an idea or perception is even *possibly* inaccurate, and share in the clinician's desire to vet the basis for the phenomenon.

S PSYCHOSIS VERSUS OBSESSIONS

Some would contend that obsessions differ from delusions based on a less intense degree of belief-conviction ("I can't help but feel as if something is not right…") and an intact capacity to recognize the peculiarity or implausibility of an obsessive thought (e.g., "I know this makes no sense, but…"). The degree of distress associated with either a psychotic or an obsessional symptom can vary in intensity; some presentations of psychosis may involve a relatively blasé sense of fateful resignation, while obsessional thoughts usually are by definition unwanted, intrusive, and disturbing to the person who is experiencing them. Suggesting a continuum, the term "schizo-obsessive" has garnered interest among clinicians and investigators, but eluded inclusion in any edition of the DSM.

T AUTONOMIC HYPERAROUSAL

Spanning constructs from PTSD to phobias to paranoid or persecutory psychosis, autonomic hyperarousal represents an individual's general state of acutely heightened awareness of the environment and its potential threats.

U DISTRESS INTOLERANCE

Perhaps one of the most ubiquitous problems that leads people to seek mental health treatment, yet one that is seldom identified as a problem to be addressed in its own right, is the capacity to tolerate emotional distress. Everyone has their own threshold for tolerating physical or emotional pain, or the discomfort of ambiguity and uncertainty. That inter-individual variability makes it hard to judge whether and when the magnitude of a distress response is excessive versus "reasonable" and commensurate with a given stress, and potentially even meaningless if there is little knowledge of the sufferer's past experience. Standards may differ across, say, survivors of bullying or chronic emotional deprivation versus repeated childhood physical or sexual assault versus trained military combatants versus phobics who have undergone exposure therapy with response prevention. The psychological and behavioral tools with which one strives to cope with adversity tend to be the cornerstones of managing distress intolerance, usually more so than pharmacological interventions.

Linked conceptually with the notion of resilience – the ability to withstand adversity without its provoking psychopathology – distress intolerance manifests itself through a variety of overt behaviors and subjective complaints. Those behaviors and complaints typically coalesce around intense discomfort, helplessness, and at times outright demands that the environment acknowledge and "do something" to alleviate not simply a perceived cause of suffering but, more specifically, the sufferer's emotional inability to tolerate and manage negative emotional reactions to the experiences they endure. For some people, everyday life may seem unduly filled with injustices and discomforts inflicted upon them by agents outside of their own control. (We might call this an external locus of control.) Others, who may feel less subjugated by the forces of nature, likely experience a greater sense of personal agency over the events and emotional reactions that come their way. (That is, they possess a more internal locus of control.) Counterbalances to emotional distress involve elements that bear on developmental–psychological constructs (e.g., the capacity to self-soothe, the ability to use developmentally mature defense mechanisms), temperament (e.g., predilections to openness versus risk aversion/harm avoidance), cognitive processes (e.g., the ability to anticipate future solutions and resolutions to current problems, executive tasks related to problem-solving, the ability to compartmentalize, the capacity to perceive and appreciate alternative points of view), and pure neurobiological processes (e.g., high emotional distress likely reflects limbic hyperactivity, whereas more stoical reactions to intense stimuli may correlate with underactive limbic functioning).

V DISTRESS INTOLERANCE AFTER TRAUMATIC EXPERIENCES

Distress intolerance that follows repeated trauma can be especially difficult to "fit" into a diagnostic model, apart from that of PTSD, because repeated exposures to noxious stimuli essentially represent operant conditioning paradigms. Viewed within the model of learning theory, expectations of a pleasurable experience (e.g., sexual arousal, or salivation when smelling freshly baked bread) or of aversive stimuli (e.g., helplessness and anger when shamed, anticipatory nausea before repeated cancer chemotherapy) elicit a fairly predictable and normal set of emotional and physiological reactions. When someone manifests emotional dysregulation (e.g., anger outbursts, impulsive aggression, self-injury, marked distress) or even suspiciousness and distrust of one's own instincts elicited from noxious learning paradigms and repeated aversive conditioning (think of the phenomenon of gaslighting), a diagnostically contextual gray zone often occurs between normality and pathology – just as the products of classical conditioning are not frank disease states (Pavlov's dog did not develop a hypersalivation disorder). The substrate of treatment may then become ambiguous – is pharmacotherapy indicated mainly for symptom relief of intense emotional distress responses, or is there a core illness state for which pharmacotherapy is meant to deliver more than symptom relief? The optimal remedy for operant conditioning is extinction learning, or exposure therapy with response prevention, essentially to "unlearn" a normal but maladaptive emotional–physiological response to aversive stimulus exposure.

If and when the psychopharmacologist is called upon to provide remedies for contextually bound distress intolerance, one must be cautious about the temptation to force-fit that phenomenon into a necessarily broader diagnostic category if none exists. One might rightfully screen for a prior history of any definable psychiatric ailment, and recognize the potential for such a diathesis to become exacerbated by an environmental catalyst. But life's misfortunes in and of themselves do not expectably cause major depression, nor do bipolar mixed states suddenly emerge de novo simply because a financial or emotional caretaker has abandoned their beneficiary. If no discernible symptom constellation happens to coincide with emotional distress, then raw distress intolerance usually demands its own psychosocial intervention aimed to shore up coping skills and strengthen behavioral management strategies. Pharmacotherapy as a *supplemental* intervention may *sometimes* be relevant, usually on a short-term basis, in the absence of a salient psychiatric disorder, aimed at symptomatic relief for associated features such as insomnia or marked anxiety.

W SUICIDALITY

Suicidal thoughts and behaviors likely represent a final common pathway for multiple aspects of psychopathology. In many ways, suicidality presents a broad and complex interface that links depression with demoralization and hopelessness, desperation, overt and passive aggression, diminished cognitive capacity for problem solving and "seeing beyond" present circumstances, loss of impulse control, loss of the survival instinct, fear circuitry, obsessionality (as in the case of chronic suicidal ideation), distress intolerance, and sometimes an oblique form of interpersonal communication. Suicidal thinking typically precedes suicidal behavior, but their underpinnings may arise from different processes. From a neurobiological perspective, suicidal acts are thought to involve prefrontal hypoactivity and possible decreased serotonergic binding and functioning in prefrontal cortical circuitry; premeditation and loss of impulse control can both contribute to suicidality, alongside executive dysfunction (diminished problem-solving ability, cognitive inflexibility, difficulty weighing pros and cons) and limbic hyperactivity.

Even though suicidality is often linked conceptually with depression, it is important for clinicians not to presume that suicidal features are necessarily *just* a manifestation of depression without investigating other dimensions of psychopathology that could contribute to suicidality independent of depression. For example, while panic disorder notoriously can increase the risk for suicide attempts in depressed patients, multivariate regression models reveal that even while controlling for confounding depressive symptoms, suicidal thoughts or behaviors may be linked independently to other elements of panic itself, such as palpitations and fear of losing control (Lim et al., 2015).

Suicidality also merits consideration in the context of anger, drama, and difficulty self-regulating strong emotional reactions to frustrations, interpersonal conflicts, or reversals of fortune. While many clinicians are quick to associate suicidal statements with the presence of depression, pharmacotherapy (or any other specific treatment) cannot reasonably occur without first establishing any suspected features of an overarching psychiatric diagnosis. Suicide threats made during acute intoxication states are often unfounded, and likely not even remembered after an offending substance has cleared. In the case of an "antagonistic" but persistent, reward-dependent, highly conscientious professional who declares that he would literally rather kill himself than endure the mortification of a job demotion, or make good on a large debt that feels unjust, there may not necessarily be an indication for pharmacotherapy targeting depression or any other major psychiatric condition despite the issuing of an inflammatory suicidal statement, depending on the larger context of symptoms and environmental circumstances in which "suicidal ideation" arose.

TAKE-HOME POINTS

- "Transdiagnostic" treatment approaches encourage thinking about dimensions rather than categories of psychopathology, and ways in which symptom domains may occur in definable constellations across a range of psychiatric disorders. Try to link target symptoms to other symptoms within a constellation (e.g., insomnia with depression versus insomnia with nightmares, or inattention in the context of mania versus dementia versus alcohol intoxication) to help understand underlying processes and inform logical pharmacotherapy strategies.
- Search for recognizable symptom constellations that may form a coherent diagnostic entity. Most evidence-based clinical trials are based on well-defined clinical syndromes but "real-world" patients may require extrapolation from patient groups whose course and outcomes may differ in ways that are not always predictable.
- Recognize common comorbid psychiatric conditions and the ways in which they may color a clinical presentation and treatment response.

Table 2.1 Examples of symptoms and symptom domains found across psychiatric disorders

Symptom/ dimension	MDD	Panic disorder	Bipolar disorder	SZ	ADHD	PTSD	SUDs	BPD	NPD	TBI	Dementia
Euphoria			✓				✓				
Depression	✓		✓			✓	✓	✓		✓	
Affective instability/ lability	±	±	✓		✓	✓	✓	✓		✓	✓
Irritability/ aggression/ rage attacks	✓		✓			✓	✓	✓	✓	✓	✓
Poor impulse control											
Inattention	✓		✓	✓	✓					✓	✓
Executive dysfunction	✓		✓	✓	✓					✓	✓
Paranoia			✓	✓		✓			✓		✓
Psychosis/ perceptual distortions	±		✓	✓		✓	✓	✓			
Disorganized form of thinking			✓	✓						✓	✓
Grandiosity			✓						✓		
Autonomic hyperarousal		✓				✓					
Sleep disruption	✓		✓			✓					✓
Risky/ hedonistic behaviors			✓				✓	✓			
Nonsuicidal self-injurious behaviors								✓			
Suicidal thoughts or behaviors	✓	✓	✓	✓			✓	✓			

Abbreviations: MDD = major depressive disorder; ADHD = attention deficit hyperactivity disorder; NPD = narcissistic personality disorder; PTSD = post-traumatic stress disorder; BPD = borderline personality disorder; SUDs = substance use disorders; SZ = schizophrenia; TBI = traumatic brain injury

Table 2.2 Test-retest reliability of target diagnoses in DSM-5 adult field trials[a]

Target diagnosis	Intraclass kappa	Interpretation
Major neurocognitive disorder	0.78	Very good
Post-traumatic stress disorder	0.67	Very good
Complex somatic symptom disorder	0.61	Very good
Binge eating disorder	0.56	Good
Bipolar I disorder	0.56	Good
Borderline personality disorder	0.54	Good
Schizoaffective disorder	0.50	Good
Mild neurocognitive disorder	0.48	Good
Schizophrenia	0.46	Good
Alcohol use disorder	0.40	Good
Mild traumatic brain injury	0.36	Questionable
Major depressive disorder	0.28	Questionable
Antisocial personality disorder	0.21	Questionable
Generalized anxiety disorder	0.20	Questionable
Mixed anxiety-depressive disorder	-0.004	Unacceptable

[a] Based on findings reported by Regier et al., 2013

Table 2.3 Distinctions between externalizing and internalizing forms of psychopathology

	Externalizing features	Internalizing features
Traditional diagnostic categories	ODD, conduct disorder, ADHD, antisocial personality disorder, borderline personality disorder, substance use disorders, kleptomania, intermittent explosive disorder	Major depression, OCD, anxiety disorders, autism spectrum disorders, schizoid personality disorder, avoidant personality disorder
Clinical components	Aggression, impulsivity, defiance, interpersonal exploitativeness	Negative affect, anxiety, depressed mood, low self-esteem, anhedonia, rumination, low trait impulsivity, inhibition, obsessionality, loneliness, withdrawal/isolation
Stability over time	Tend to persist over time in ~40% of young children (Verhulst and Van der Ende, 1995)	Tend to persist over time in ~40% of young children (Briggs-Gowan et al., 2006)
Potential implications for pharmacotherapy	May favor antipsychotics, sedative-hypnotics, antimanic agents, or stimulants when deemed helpful, non-activating, and not abused	May favor antidepressants, nonsedating anxiolytics, stimulants, or other pro-dopaminergic agents
Prognosis	Poorer	Better

Abbreviations: ADHD = attention deficit hyperactivity disorder; OCD = obsessive-compulsive disorder; ODD = oppositional-defiant disorder

Table 2.4 First-episode psychosis diagnostic correlations with subsequent episodes

Baseline diagnosis	Diagnostic concordance at follow-up	95% CI
Schizophrenia	0.90	0.85-0.95
Affective spectrum psychoses	0.84	0.79-0.89
Schizoaffective disorder	0.72	0.61-0.83
Substance-induced psychotic disorder	0.66	0.51-0.81
Delusional disorder	0.59	0.47-0.71
Acute/transient psychotic disorder or brief psychotic disorder	0.56	0.52-0.60
Psychosis not otherwise specified	0.36	0.27-0.45
Schizophreniform disorder	0.29	0.22-0.38

Table 2.5 Research domain criteria (RDoC)

Domain	Phenomenology	Diagnostic examples	Neurotransmitters	Neural circuitry
Negative valence systems	Fear/threat, anxiety, loss, frustration nonreward (i.e., the inability to obtain positive rewards after repeated efforts)	Depression	Dopamine, GABA, glutamate, serotonin, steroids, vasopressin	Amygdala, hypothalamus, locus coeruleus, OFC, periaqueductal grey, parasympathetic system, septum striatum
Positive valence systems	Positive motivational situations (e.g., reward-seeking, willingness to work, expectancy of reward for effort)	Mania, pathological gambling	Dopamine, serotonin	Anterior medial orbitofrontal cortex, cortico-limbic circuit, ventral limbic striatum, ventral tegmental area/substantia nigra
Cognitive systems	Attention, perception, sensation, memory, language, goal selection	ADHD, autism, narcissism	GABA, glutamate, acetylcholine, dopamine, histamine, serotonin	Basal forebrain limbic systems, ventral and dorsal attention networks, pulvinar, thalamic reticular nucleus
Social processes	Affiliation and attachment, self-knowledge, perception and understanding of others	Autism, bereavement	Dopamine, κ and μ opioid receptors, oxytocin, vasopressin	Amygdala and vasopressin fiber system of the amygdala, bed nucleus of the stria terminalis, fusiform face area, nucleus accumbens, orbitofrontal cortex, ventromedial prefrontal cortex, paraventicular nucleus of the hypothalamus
Arousal and regulatory systems	Circadian rhythms, sleep-wakefulness	Narcolepsy, anorexia, binge eating disorder	Acetylcholine, CRF, cytokines, dopamine, GABA, ghrelin, glutamate, histamine, leptin, orexin, neuropeptide Y, norepinephrine, opioids, oxytocin, serotonin, vasopressin	Basal forebrain nuclei to cortical circuits, brainstem monoaminergic and cholinergic projections to basal forebrain, central amygdala to monoaminergic and basal forebrain cholinergic nuclei, cholinergic and monoaminergic nuclei projections to thalamus and cortex, circadian and sleep-related circuits, fronto-insular and dorsal anterior cingulate, hypothalamic to thalamic and cortical circuits, central nucleus of the amygdala, dorsal raphe nucleus, lateral/perifornical/dorsomedial hypothalamus, LDT, locus coeruleus, PPT, tuberomammillary nucleus, ventral tegmental area

Abbreviations: ADHD = attention deficit hyperactivity disorder; CRF = corticotropin-releasing factor; GABA = gamma aminobutyric acid; LDT = laterodorsal tegmental nuclei; OFC = orbitofrontal cortex; PPT = pedunculopontine nuclei

Table 2.6 Five-Factor Model of Personality

Characteristic	Description	Presumed neurobiological underpinnings	Manifestations within psychiatric diagnostic constructs
Openness to experience	Reflects curiosity, interest in novelty and possible risk-taking	Associated with *appropriate* dopaminergic tone (meaning, neither too much nor too little)[a] in DLPFC (i.e., regulation of cognitive flexibility, ideational fluency and working memory) and ACC (conflict monitoring)	Mania, schizophrenia (Lo et al., 2017); cognitive inflexibility with regard to "set-shifting," coupled with perfectionism, may predispose to anorexia nervosa
Conscientiousness	Reflects dependability and an organized, planned pursuit of goals	Associated with DLPFC function/ executive planning and impulse restraint; middle frontal gyrus, fusiform gyrus (DeYoung et al., 2010)	May help minimize risk for developing depression or anxiety disorders
Extraversion	Reflecting a socially outgoing, high-energy, attention-seeking mode of interacting	Associated with medial OFC function/reward processing; lateral paralimbic regions	Mania, ADHD, negatively associated with depression, anxiety disorders and social phobia (Kotov et al., 2010), as well as antidepressant adherence (Cohen et al., 2004)
Agreeableness	Reflects a cooperative, nonconfrontational, trusting (or overtrusting) stance toward others	Superior temporal sulcus, posterior cingulate, fusiform gyrus (DeYoung et al., 2010)	
Neuroticism	Reflects emotional instability and a proneness toward unpleasant emotional states	DMPFC function, medial frontal gyrus, mid-cingulate gyrus, middle temporal gyrus, precentral gyrus, cerebellum (DeYoung et al., 2010)	Associated with depression, generalized anxiety disorder

[a] For any given cognitive task, optimal dopaminergic tone appears to follow an inverted U-shaped curve, such that either deficiencies or excesses may disrupt normal function (Cools and Robbins, 2004)

Abbreviations: ACC = anterior cingulate cortex; DLPFC = dorsolateral prefrontal cortex; DMPFC = dorsomedial prefrontal cortex; OFC = orbitofrontal cortex

Table 2.7 Temperaments described in the Tridimensional Personality Questionnaire

Characteristic	Description	Presumed neurobiological underpinnings	Manifestations within psychiatric diagnostic constructs
Harm avoidance	Worry, fear of uncertainty, shyness, and fatigue	Hypodopaminergic and high serotonergic tone; ↑ GABAergic and ↓ glutamatergic transmission in anterior cingulate cortex (Kim et al., 2009); possible ↓ OFC, occipital volume (Gardini et al., 2009)	*Harm avoidance + low self-directedness* may predispose to **depression**; *Harm avoidance + low novelty-seeking* may predispose to **obsessive-compulsive features**; *Harm avoidance and reward dependence* may predispose to **social anxiety**; *Harm avoidance + persistence* may predispose to **anorexia nervosa**
Novelty-seeking	Excitement in response to unusual or possible high-reward stimuli ("exploratory excitability" and "extravagance" in approach to reward cues), linked with impulsive decision-making, quick loss of temper, and avoidance of frustration ("disorderliness")	Increased noradrenergic and hypodopaminergic tone; ↑ volume in frontal and posterior cingulate regions (Gardini et al., 2009)	Addictions; borderline personality disorder; minimal association with psychotic disorders (Peritogiannis, 2015)
Reward dependence	High sensitivity to social rewards and attachments	Low noradrenergic tone; ↓ volume in PFC and caudate (Gardini et al., 2009)	Dependent and histrionic personality disorders, addictions; *low* reward dependence linked with autism spectrum disorders, paranoid/schizoid/schizotypal and antisocial personality disorders, social detachment
Persistence	Eagerness, work hardened, ambitious, perfectionistic; associated with conscientiousness	↑ volume in precuneus, paracentral lobule, hippocampal gyrus (Gardini et al., 2009)	Anxiety disorders; OCD; may protect against mood disorders (Cloninger et al., 2012)

Abbreviations: OCD = obsessive-compulsive disorder; OFC = orbitofrontal cortex; PFC = prefrontal cortex

3 Interpreting and Using the Literature: Integrating Evidence-Based Trials with Real-World Practice

LEARNING OBJECTIVES

- ☐ When reading a clinical trial, be able to describe the characteristics of the group being studied, and recognize ways in which they may be comparable or dissimilar to other types of patients (such as those whom you treat) before generalizing findings to a wider potential treatment group
- ☐ Recognize whether a study was purposefully designed from the outset to evaluate the outcome measures being reported, or whether reported findings are secondary and thus only provisional and hypothesis-generating, rather than hypothesis-testing
- ☐ Understand the importance of sample sizes and adequacy of statistical power, prospective versus retrospective designs, post hoc analyses, correction of statistical significance levels for multiple comparisons, noninferiority trials, how to interpret confidence intervals, sample enrichment, attrition, failed versus negative trials, and the difference between p-values (statistical significance) and effect sizes (clinically meaningful differences)
- ☐ Appreciate why the concept of randomization is often referred to as the "great equalizer" in clinical trials methodology (and why nonrandomized trials yield far less compelling data than randomized trials)

All things are subject to interpretation. Whichever interpretation prevails at a given time is a function of power and not truth.

- Friedrich Nietzsche

Many of the groups… are far too small to allow of any definite opinion being formed at all, having regard to the size of the probable error involved.

- Karl Pearson

When investigators report the findings from a clinical trial, the results require interpretation. Peer review is the process through which the structure and execution of a clinical study is judged to be coherent, linear, and logical. The procedure is not unlike conducting a mental status exam: the evaluator is trying to discern if the content is credible at face value, if any underlying factors that could be biasing the results are accounted for, if the observed phenomena are being interpreted accurately, and if the conclusions drawn are valid. With varying degrees of provisionality or certainty, clinical trials give information about the narrow impact of (usually) one intervention versus a comparator (a placebo; an active comparator; or treatment as usual (TAU)) for a circumscribed period of time, with efforts made to hold other relevant variables constant (so, no *other* treatments are begun or altered, adherence must be near-perfect, substance use is grounds for ejection, and major life disruptions could botch the findings).

Clinicians trying to interpret the literature[1] rely on the rigor of peer review and editorial filtering when judging if a finding is "ready for prime time" implementation, or more just an interesting idea or observation that needs further beta-testing and elaboration before it should be taken up into everyday practice. They must also judge how results obtained from a carefully controlled environment using hand-picked cases will translate into less meticulously structured treatment settings.

1 We differentiate the published peer-reviewed literature from the so-called "gray literature," comprising scholarly works that have not been formally published in peer-reviewed journals, such as dissertations, conference proceedings, technical reports, and government reports (described further at www.opengrey.edu).

There is no shortage in the marketplace of simplified digests, newsletters and distillations of current literature that promise to boil down detailed research efforts into a single authoritative soundbite – helpful for gaining quick headline summaries, but also running the risk of equating a "Cliff Notes" version of a novel to actually reading and understanding the novel itself.[2] For the sake of gaining up-to-date knowledge and true expertise, there is really no shortcut to searching, understanding, and applying the primary literature. Therefore, our aim in this chapter is to equip clinician-readers with the tools they need to assess for themselves the claims made by a clinical trial using the same kind of critical, forensic mindset they would apply to the self-reported history of a potentially complex patient during a clinical encounter.

A SHOW YOURSELF THE EVIDENCE

As noted in Chapter 1, varying levels of rigor define the strength of evidence with which an intervention is supported, refuted, or unknown. Large, adequately powered, prospective, randomized, placebo-controlled trials that have been sufficiently replicated provide the most confident information about likely outcomes when a particular treatment is undertaken for a specific ailment. Smaller, underpowered, open-label, nonrandomized trials, case series, or anecdotal observations provide proof-of-concept data that can generate tentative hypotheses that must then be tested more extensively in a-priori-designed large-scale trials. The latter can then yield more definitive conclusions about the appropriateness and expectable effects of an intervention, strengthening the basis for its uptake into clinical practice.

Sourcing the empirical literature directly is the most scientific way a clinician can determine for himself or herself whether a candidate treatment for a particular ailment is evidence-based, and how well an existing evidence base may apply to a specific individual patient (as opposed to just a diagnosis, with no contextual information). Electronic database search engines such as MEDLINE, Ovid, the Cochrane Library, Web of Science, Embase, CINAHL, PsycINFO, PsycLIT, and Science Citation Index Expanded place access to the empirical literature literally at one's fingertips. Do-it-yourself online searches not only allow anyone to find the most up-to-date information, but perhaps even more importantly, enable highly tailored searches and types of studies by specifying relevant search terms (for example, "stroke" + "depression" + "cancer" + "stimulant" + "randomized trial").

To fully appreciate any given evidence base, let us now consider in greater detail the factors that make clinical trial designs and findings interpretable and comprehensible.

B WHO IS BEING STUDIED?

If one has to pick the single most important consideration when reading a clinical trial, it would probably be the description of the study group. Read it carefully, then reread it. Who exactly is being studied? How were diagnoses established, and how were subjects enrolled (sample of convenience? consecutive admissions? treatment-seekers?)? What associated characteristics of the study group are captured in the sample description? Apples-to-apples comparisons are impossible when study groups vary in their severity, chronicity, comorbidity, atypicality, and degree of past treatment resistance. For the clinician-reader, the particular importance of this point involves recognizing how study patients resemble or differ from one's own clinical population. Moreover, the only way one can sensibly draw inferences from study findings to one's own clientele is to apply formal diagnostic criteria to one's own patients in order to validate their comparability to the kind of patients about whom treatment inferences are drawn from a clinical trial. This means, in every instance, imposing DSM-5 symptom and duration criteria to one's own patients, assuring current symptoms are not better accounted for by another (e.g., general medical, substance use, or other psychiatric) condition, and then forming an impression about points of convergence and divergence between a study population and one's own. Otherwise, there may be little to no validity in extrapolating results based on, say, a well-defined group of bipolar I manic inpatients to a more loosely defined group of mood-unstable outpatients that lacks the psychomotor signs of a distinct manic episode, or transposing results in a psychosis population with clear persecutory delusions and hallucinations to a more heterogeneous group with chronic mistrust and paranoid thinking but no frank psychosis.

[2] For those seeking a compromise between original source reports and a third party's critical commentary, we would encourage readers to visit a website sponsored by the National Institute for Health Research and available through the Library of Medicine from the National Institute of Health, called the Database of Abstracts of Reviews of Effects (DARE): Quality-assessed Reviews. Devised and maintained by the Centre for Reviews and Dissemination (CRD) at the University of York, UK, the DARE site provides not only cogent summaries of published reports, but also appraises their quality, highlighting methodological strengths and weaknesses (www.crd.york.ac.uk/CRDWeb/).

C DESIGN CONSIDERATIONS

Variables of interest in a clinical trial are customarily thought of as *independent* (meaning, evident at baseline, and nonvarying – such as treatment arm, or age, or years ill) or *dependent* (meaning, evident at study end, varying in magnitude, and reflecting an outcome state or a parameter thought to be influenced by the effects of one or more independent variables – such as magnitude of change in symptom severity).

> **Tip**
>
> Glean from the Method section of a research report a clear impression of who the study group is, how they were ascertained, and what characteristics make the participants more representative versus unusual.

Successful clinical trials begin with the formulation and appropriate testing of a cogent hypothesis that is matched to well-defined clinical populations. Try to affirm that an explicit research question and hypothesis are articulated; the purpose of a research paper should never be cryptic or mysterious. An equally important up-front issue that often receives too little detail is a clear statement of *who the study group exactly is*. Are subjects well-described? In what ways is the group demographically and clinically similar or heterogeneous? Are subjects consecutively screened, or are they a sample of convenience? How representative are they of real-world patients? Modern clinical trials typically present a flow diagram (called a CONSORT (CONsolidated Standards of Reporting Trials) diagram), which outlines exactly how many prospective subjects were screened and evaluated and what percentage of those who were assessed for their eligibility to enroll in a study actually did – and of those who did not, an accounting for reasons for nonenrollment (such as, withdrawal of informed consent, failure to meet inclusion or exclusion criteria, or other reasons). CONSORT diagrams quickly reveal key aspects about whether a study is large or small, how many potential subjects had to be screened in order to become enrolled (for many psychiatric disorders, screen-to-enrollment ratios can be 10–20:1 or higher), how many left the study before it ended, and reasons why. (See Table 3.3 at the end of this chapter for an illustration of this.)

A typical CONSORT flow diagram is depicted in Figure 3.1.

Figure 3.1 Typical CONSORT flow diagram.

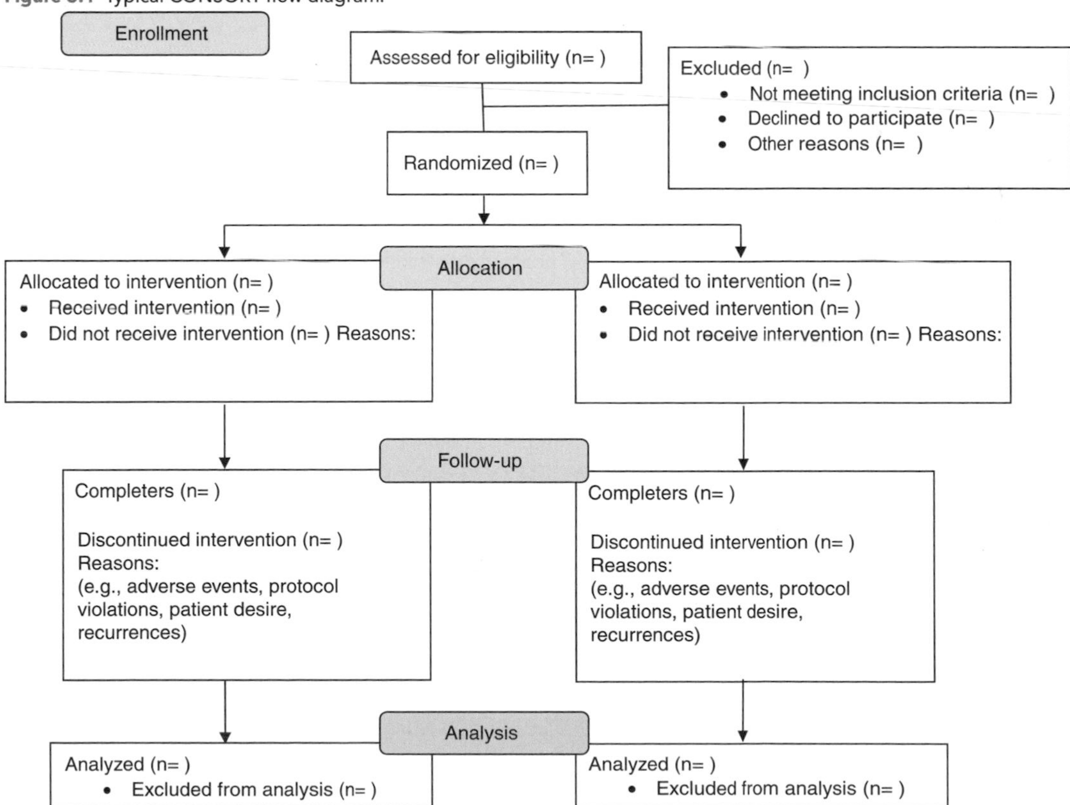

When judging the rigor with which a clinical trial has been performed, a number of key aspects should be considered:

Prospective versus Retrospective Study Designs

Prospective studies involve making planned, direct observations before they occur, with the greatest chance to capture anticipated events and their relevant details. Retrospective studies (e.g., chart reviews) rely on historical recall of past clinical phenomena (e.g., severity of discrete mood episodes, frequency of panic attacks, duration of psychosis, demarcation of full recovery versus partial responses or nonresponses) that may not have been formally identified or recorded in sufficient detail to be unambiguous. So, for example, in a retrospective study, patients might self-report that they have had on average five previous episodes – but we do not know if formal operational criteria were met to define an episode, if the "episodes" were true events or just waxing and waning continuous symptoms from a single unresolved event, if the phenomenon was secondary to psychoactive substances or a medical condition, or if a patient's subjective recall of symptoms and their duration is even remotely accurate. Outcomes (e.g., "recovery") can be hard to quantify or judge with confidence in the absence of firsthand observation, formal rating scales, or systematic symptom assessments.

Observational or Naturalistic Studies

When treatment interventions and their parameters are not chosen by the investigators or according to a specified protocol, but instead just observed under ordinary or naturalistic conditions, a study of treatment outcomes under such circumstances is termed observational or naturalistic. In such situations, inferences about cause-and-effect relationships with treatments may be impossible to infer because treatment "assignment" can itself become an outcome state.

Parametric and Nonparametric Tests

Statistical tests depend on assumptions about the groups being analyzed. One such assumption involves whether the values or scores obtained on a variable of interest (say, hours of sleep) within a study sample (say, a group of insomniacs enrolled in a particular clinical trial) reflect a pattern of score distributions similar enough to that seen in the broader population of interest (say, the universe of all insomniacs). A normal distribution follows a bell-shaped curve (see Figure 3.2), symmetrically around a mean score, with one standard deviation from that mean describing 68% of the data, two standard deviations capturing 95% of the data, and three standard deviations encompassing 99.7% of the data.

Figure 3.2 Normal curve distribution.

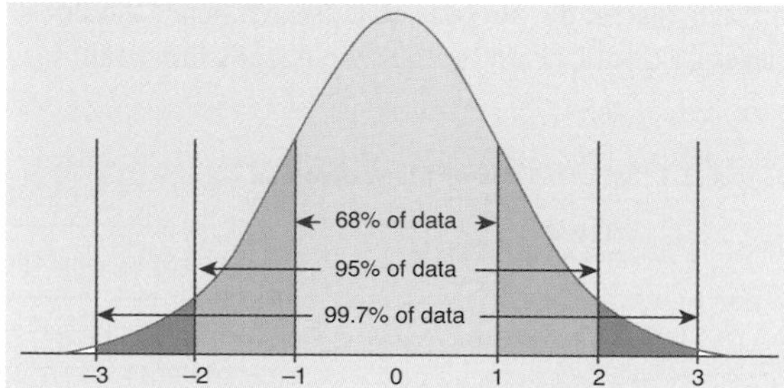

Parametric tests assume that in the population from which a sample is drawn, the variable of interest is normally distributed, and variance is homogeneous.

Box 3.1

Example: Confounding By Indication

Consider a large observational study of suicide attempts among bipolar disorder patients drawn from a large health plan database, comparing patients who had been prescribed lithium or divalproex (Goodwin et al., 2003). Imagine observing nearly a threefold higher rate of suicide attempts among those who took divalproex and not lithium over an eight-year period. Sounds like lithium is the better bet for keeping suicide at bay? Not necessarily. If assignment to lithium was not a randomized decision, it becomes hard to know cause versus effect. It is *possible* that patients who took lithium consequently had three times fewer suicide attempts, but because confounding factors (such as previous suicide attempts) might have influenced prescribers' decisions about what drug to prescribe, it is equally possible that prescribers may have been more reluctant to put patients whom they deemed to be at higher risk for suicide on lithium, and therefore instead favored giving such higher-risk patients a drug with less lethality risk in overdose (divalproex) while selecting lower suicide-risk patients to receive lithium – making "treatment arm" more of a marker for perceived suicide risk at baseline rather than a potential cause versus protectant against later attempts.

They are used when the parameters of the population (such as the population mean value on the variable of interest) are known and a normal distribution can be safely assumed. *Nonparametric* tests are used when one cannot assume that the population data are normally distributed. They are used when the variables of interest are ranked parameters or are known to follow a skewed distribution, when variance is not homogeneous, or when sample sizes are relatively small. Examples of parametric and nonparametric tests are described in Table 3.1 at the end of this chapter.

Tip

An "omnibus test" refers to an overall statistical test of significance that tells whether explained variance is greater than unexplained variance – i.e., observed findings are nonrandom.

If an overall statistic in a comparison of three or more groups is significant, post hoc between-group comparisons are sometimes needed to tell "which" between-group differences are or are not significant. For instance, if an ANOVA (ANalysis of VAriance) comparing means (say, number of hours slept) across three groups (say, diagnoses of insomniacs, narcoleptics, and depressed patients) produces an overall significant value (the F-statistic), that alone does not tell whether each and every group is significantly different from one another, or if only some of the groups may differ significantly from one another. Box 3.2 lists commonly used post hoc tests to discern pair-wise differences between groups when an overall test statistic is significant.

Tip

Post hoc analyses refer to statistical tests undertaken after a study has been completed and the main findings are already known.

Odds Ratios and Confidence Intervals

Odds ratios (ORs) and their accompanying confidence intervals (CIs) refer to the range of values for a parameter of interest (say, likelihood of response) that provides a certain probability (often, 95%) that the true value of interest falls within that range. Say that the odds of antidepressant response to lithium augmentation of an SSRI is roughly threefold higher than taking an SSRI alone; an OR of 3.06 with a 95% CI of 1.4–5.6 means that the actual probability lies between 1.4 and 5.6-fold. The wider the CI (e.g., if the CI = 1.4–68.6), the harder it then becomes to identify the reported OR as a reliable estimate: here, it could be anywhere from 1.4 to 68.6 – nearly a 50-fold difference in magnitude. Hence, findings that involve "tight" CIs are considered to be especially compelling because the actual likelihood for the event of interest occurring is fairly circumscribed within a narrowly defined range.

CIs that do not cross "zero" are deemed statistically significant, while those that include zero within the CI are nonsignificant. These are easily depicted in so-called Forest plots as presented in meta-analyses (see, for example, Chapter 10, Figure 10.1). CIs that overlap (as in the case of two treatment arms) are said not to differ significantly from one another (again, see Figure 10.1).

Randomization

Statistically speaking, randomization is considered the great equalizer among treatment groups within a study. It is the process whereby potentially unrecognized clinically important differences between two or more treatment groups become equally distributed among all groups. Successful randomization means that potentially important sources of systematic bias (that could affect the study outcome) are not over-represented in one group relative to another. Such variables are called *confounding factors*. When unrecognized, they can lead to mistaken conclusions, as illustrated by the example in Box 3.3.

Box 3.2

Common Post Hoc Tests for Significant Pairwise Differences Among Multiple Groups When an Overall Test Statistic is Significant

Overall test	Post hoc comparisons test
ANOVA	Scheffe test
Kruskal-Wallis	Tukey comparisons
Chi-square (involving ≥3 groups, i.e., >1 degree of freedom)	"Calculation of residuals" (the differences between observed and expected values of a cell in a contingency table), or "ransacking," or "partitioning"

Box 3.3

Example

In bipolar disorder, lithium responsivity is influenced by a number of known factors, including the number of past episodes, a history of past-year rapid cycling, normal renal function, and an absence of mixed affective features during an episode. In a hypothetical study of lithium versus placebo for older adult mania, the excessive presence of any of these known relevant factors in one group versus the other could unbalance the study arms and pose a confounding effect on treatment outcome (e.g., lithium will appear to underperform relative to placebo if there are more rapid cyclers assigned to lithium than placebo, or the placebo group has a fewer mean number of lifetime episodes).

When factors such as these are known before the study is undertaken, subjects who have a characteristic of interest can deliberately be randomized equally to each study arm. This is called *stratification*. But, it is impractical to stratify treatment arms by randomization that takes into account each and every potential confounding factor. Therefore, randomized trials typically compare the treatment groups on key demographic or baseline clinical variables (often presented in a first table of a report). Randomization is said to be "successful" if the treatment groups do not differ significantly in any baseline characteristics that are known to influence outcomes. If, after the study was completed, any noteworthy characteristics were found to differ between the treatment groups, all is not lost – one can statistically control after the fact (i.e., post hoc) for possible confounding effects of a relevant variable that differs between the treatment groups (say, age at onset, or baseline severity, or chronicity of illness). If an observed difference in outcomes between study groups is sustained after controlling for potential confounders, the effect is considered to be more robust and not spurious (assuring, for example, that an observed lower relapse rate with lithium than placebo is not merely an artifact of the lithium group having an inherently lower risk for relapse to begin with because they were less chronic, less severe, or less confounded by markers for poor lithium response than seen in the comparator arm).

Tip

In a "successfully" randomized trial, treatment arms do not differ significantly from each other at baseline on variables known ahead of time to affect treatment outcome.

Sometimes, two or more known viable treatment options exist for a condition but there is uncertainty among experts about whether one likely differs from another in overall benefit or harm. Such situations are called "clinical equipoise" – a condition that should be established on ethical grounds before a randomized trial is undertaken. When several competing viable treatment options do exist, "equipoise randomization" means that subjects could be randomized to one of potentially several active treatment arms.

Parallel versus Crossover Designs

When two separate groups, matched on key demographic or baseline clinical features, are randomized to undergo treatment with an active intervention versus a comparator or placebo, inferences can be drawn about the relative effects of one treatment arm versus another. This is known as a parallel design. However, if the same study group is exposed to one arm and then crossed over by randomization to the other arm, this is a "crossover design." Its advantages are economy (half as many subjects are needed as in a two-arm parallel design) and homogeneity of between-group confounding factors (each subject serves as its own control); its main disadvantages have to do with *carryover effects*, meaning that the impact of the treatment arm prior to the crossover may account for some or much of the effect seen afterward (see Figure 3.3). The carryover effect of one treatment arm also may differ from that of another arm (e.g., with respect to adverse effects), potentially causing inadvertent unblinding of a randomized trial (see Chapter 4). Washout periods between the first and second phases (e.g., ideally lasting five half-lives of the longest-acting active treatment) can partially help to diminish carryover effects, although parallel designs usually produce more reliable outcomes, particularly when carryover effects may be substantial.

Tip

Carry-over effects in crossover trials may confuse the treatment effects attributable to one intervention versus another.

Single-group Open Trials

When all subjects receive only one intervention and there is no comparator group or other treatment arm, changes are measured within subjects (rather than

Figure 3.3 Crossover study design.

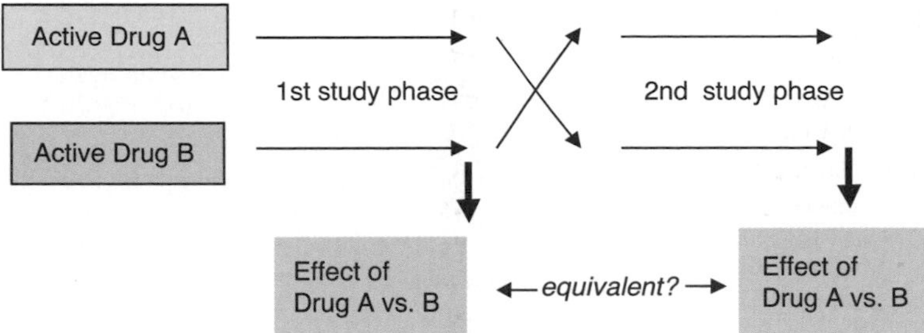

between subjects) from baseline to study end. Inferential statistics can be performed using dependent (rather than independent) measures (such as dependent t-tests for continuous variables (e.g., scores on a symptom severity scale) number of events (e.g., number of panic attacks or suicide attempts)) to tell if there has or has not been a significant change since the treatment was begun. Open trials are somewhat more informative when using a mirror-image design, meaning that the time period of observation with an intervention is compared retrospectively to a comparable period of time preceding the start of the intervention.

The adequacy of rigor in a clinical trial is sometimes rated quantitatively using a measure called the Jadad scale, as described in Box 3.4.

Box 3.4

The Jadad Scale

The methodological quality of a clinical trial is sometimes quantified using the Jadad scale (devised by Colombian physician-investigator Alejandro Jadad-Bechara), scored from 0 (poor) to 5 (rigorous) based on yes/no answers to three questions:

1. Was the study described as randomized? Was it appropriate? (2 points)
2. Was the study described as double-blind? Was the method of blinding described, and appropriate? (2 points)
3. Was there a description of withdrawals and dropouts? (1 point)

A criticism of this rating system has been that it does not fully take into account additional pertinent aspects of clinical trial rigor, such as intent-to-treat (ITT) and management of dropout, diagnostic criteria, treatment adherence, assessment measures, and trial duration, among others.

The clinical meaningfulness of an intervention in a single group "before and after" treatment, with no comparator group, is expressed as a *within-group effect size* – a measurement which can then be used subsequently to estimate how much *power* (i.e., the number of subjects) is needed when calculating the sample size necessary to detect a meaningful treatment effect in a future between-group comparison (e.g., active drug versus placebo). If a within-group effect size is moderate or large, after accounting for anticipated dropout, fewer subjects will expectably be needed to show a meaningful between-group effect. If a within-group effect size is fairly small, then the anticipated impact of the intervention would be considered subtle, and a larger sample size (more power) will be needed to detect a meaningful between group difference when compared to placebo. This now brings us to a proper discussion of statistical power and effect sizes.

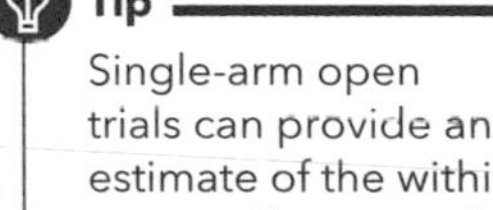

Tip

Single-arm open trials can provide an estimate of the within-group effect size of an intervention.

D STATISTICAL SIGNIFICANCE AND POWER

If a study shows a difference in effects between a drug and a placebo, or a drug and an active comparator, how confident are we that the findings were not a fluke? Or for that matter, if no difference is found, how certain can we be that the absence of a difference is a true absence and not a random occurrence? Here we must consider not only the concept of statistical differences, but also of clinically meaningful differences, as described in Box 3.5.

A finding is said to be *statistically significant* when the probability that an observed difference between a drug and its comparator simply happened by chance is considered quite small. A p-value (probability) tells whether or not an observed difference between two or

Box 3.5

The So-What Factor: When Does Size Matter?

If a between-group effect size is small, a larger sample size will be needed to detect a difference from placebo - but, if an effect is statistically *significant* (not random) *but small in size*, perhaps from an overpowered study, does it matter? For example, the Empire State Building is taller (but not by much) than the Chrysler Building, and both are dwarfed by Tapei 101 in Taipei which in turn is even more dwarfed by the Burj Dubai building in Dubai. All of these structures are vastly taller than was the Home Insurance Building in Chicago (42 m), which in 1885 was the tallest building in the world.

Everything is relative. If one intervention significantly reduces a symptom severity score by only 1 or 2 points more than another intervention, is that consequential? It could be, if the scale represented deaths per unit time, or disability-adjusted life years, or years of life.

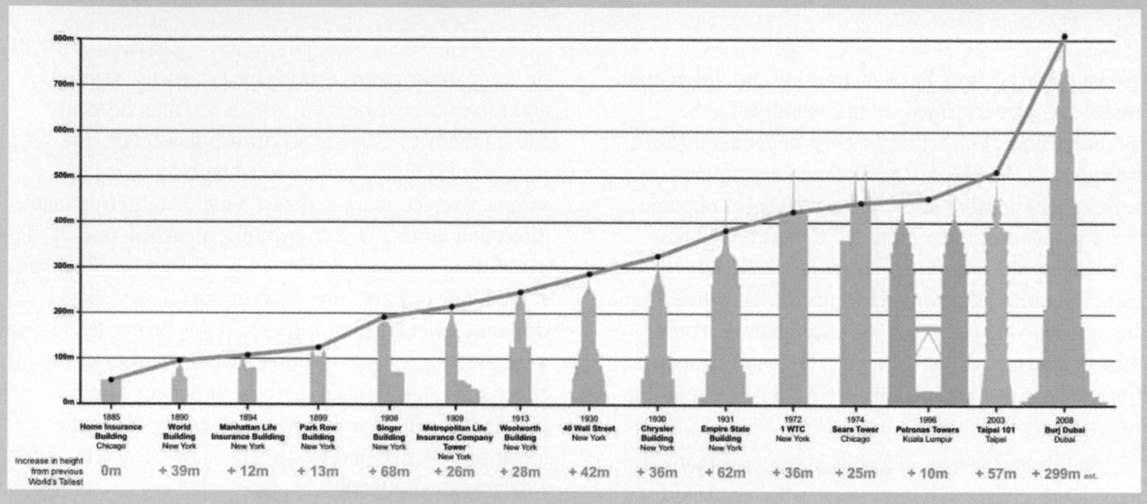

more groups is likely due to random chance; p-values of 0.05 or less mean that 95 times out of 100, one is likely to see the same result.

Suppose that a study showed that a medication significantly improved depression symptom score ratings in major depression as compared to placebo (i.e., low probability the finding is due to chance), but the magnitude of the clinical meaningfulness of the difference was small. A relatively large sample size would be necessary to detect such a difference. By contrast, a smaller sample size is usually needed to reveal a significant difference that imparts a large clinical effect. When a statistically significant finding occurs with a small sample size (meaning, the power to detect a small difference is low because of the N), it runs the risk of a so-called *Type I error ("false positive")* – meaning that a seemingly significant result is actually a fluke, due only to random chance. This issue comes up most often when a small proof-of-concept study identifies a significant relationship between an intervention and an outcome but it is not already known whether the intervention has a large effect (e.g., penicillin for Gram-positive streptococcal pharyngitis), for which few subjects would expectably be needed. *Type II errors ("false negatives")* are the opposite phenomenon, in which there is a failure to identify a true difference between an intervention and a comparator (in other words, a real effect goes undetected).

The rate of Type I errors is referred to as an *alpha level*, and is synonymous with the p-value reported in studies (that is, the probability of wrongly rejecting the null hypothesis). The rate of Type II errors is referred to as *beta*, and the *statistical power* of a test (that is, its ability to detect at least a minimally clinically important difference) is *1 minus beta*. Type I errors are considered to be four times more serious than Type II errors, and hence, when alpha levels are set at 0.05, beta levels are set at 0.20, and power is then established at 0.80.

Things quickly gets more complicated. What if many variables rather than just one are being studied in relation to an outcome of interest? The dilemma of multiple comparisons or simultaneous inference (also known as multiplicity) then arises, where the p-value that reflects statistical significance for one test suddenly loses its stringency. Suppose the univariate associations between treatment response and 10 variables were separately examined and the resulting p-value for each analysis was <0.05. Because multiple comparisons have been made, these would each be considered *nominal* p-values (meaning, assumptions about the probability that the null hypothesis is true (i.e., no true difference exists) may not be valid) – so the false positive rate (Type I error) may be high. The "real" p-value must take into account the multiple comparisons that were made, a dilemma also known as simultaneous inference, or multiplicity. When two or more statistical tests are performed on the same dataset, the adjusted probability of a Type I (false positive) error is sometimes referred to as a joint significance level, or *family-wise error rate* (FWER).

Tip

When multiple statistical tests are performed, uncorrected (nominal) p-values could inflate the chances of a false positive finding.

There are different ways of correcting a p-value for multiple comparisons, using varying degrees of rigor. Many clinicians are probably already familiar with Bonferroni correction, in which an alpha level is simply divided by the total number of statistical tests performed – often whittling down a corrected p-value to a quite miniscule value. These and other methods of correction for multiple comparisons are described in Table 3.2 at the end of this chapter.

Tip

Independent (baseline) variables are studied to determine if they can predict a *dependent* (outcome) variable.

When multiple hierarchically ordered objectives are being evaluated in a clinical trial (e.g., comparing several fixed doses of a medication versus placebo), multiple null hypotheses are again being tested, inflating the chances of a Type I error. To help control the family-wise Type I error rate, a technique known as "tree-structured gatekeeping procedures" has been described. Using a technique called *Hommel-based gatekeeping*, null hypotheses are hierarchically ordered into families that are then tested sequentially for acceptance or rejection of a null hypothesis.

Dilemma

When multiple statistical tests have positively correlated results, Bonferroni correction for multiplicity may be overly conservative. Some authors have therefore suggested simpler correction factors (e.g., based on intraclass correlations) but the subject remains a point of debate (see, e.g., Shi et al., 2012)

 Noninferiority, Superiority, and Assay Sensitivity

Clinicians often express a desire to see head-to-head comparison trials of one drug versus another, but an important limiting factor in such studies has to do with the expected size of the effect for one treatment relative to another. If two distinct interventions each are known to have a substantial impact, it would take a lot of statistical power to detect a meaningful difference (see Box 3.5). Powering an RCT for *superiority* of one known efficacious treatment over another poses practical issues because a much larger sample size will be needed than if the goal were to show that the drugs' effects are roughly similar. More often, and more feasibly, head-to-head comparison studies are therefore powered for *noninferiority*, intended not to show whether one efficacious treatment is better than another, but rather, that *neither is worse than the other*. Such designs also should not be confused with situations in which an active comparator drug is used for purposes of *assay sensitivity*, which means that its role is solely to assure that the impact of a placebo arm is not unduly and unexpectedly high (see section "Placebo-Controlled Trials and Active Comparators"). Decisions about what minimum sample size is needed in order to show superiority or noninferiority or equivalence are made based on the overlap of confidence intervals relative to upper and lower limits (margins) of a drug's effect, as illustrated in Figure 3.4.

 Tell Tails

Statistical tests of significance may intentionally focus on the possibility that a "real" (nonrandom) difference between treatment arms is expected to occur if the active treatment arm either has no effect or an effect in only *one direction* (for example, giving acetaminophen is unlikely to *increase* body temperature in a febrile patient more than would be expected by chance alone). Such a test for change in only one direction would be called a one-tailed test. On the other hand, if it is possible that an active treatment might outperform or underperform relative

Figure 3.4 Overlapping confidence intervals for determining noninferiority.

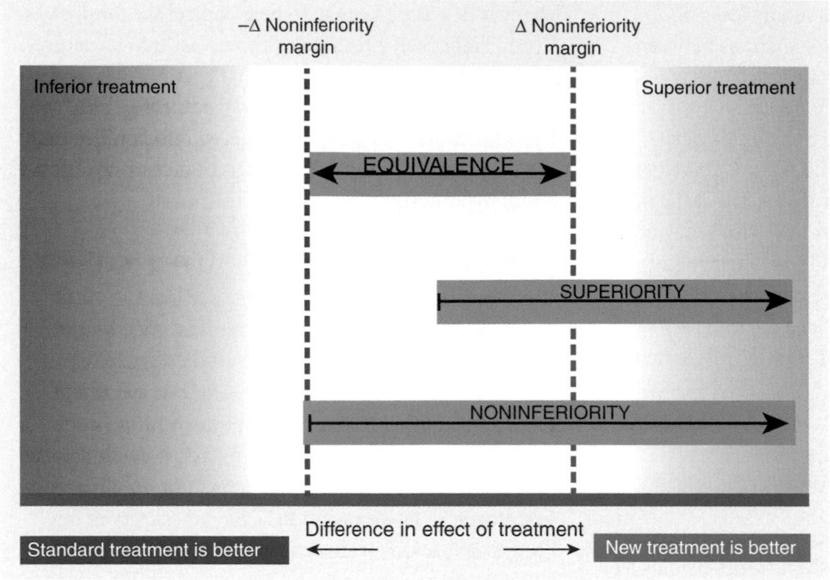

−Δ Noninferiority margin
Δ Noninferiority margin
Inferior treatment
Superior treatment
EQUIVALENCE
SUPERIORITY
NONINFERIORITY
Difference in effect of treatment
Standard treatment is better
New treatment is better

to a placebo or other comparator (which often ends up being a plausible possibility), two-tailed tests are performed for measuring possible bidirectional change in a dependent variable of interest.

Tip
One-tailed p-values assess change in only one direction; two-tailed tests assess possible increases or decreases in a variable of interest.

 Is an Observed Effect Clinically Meaningful?

There are several ways to quantify how large or clinically meaningful the impact of a treatment is, regardless of its statistical significance. Effect sizes are one common statistical means for expressing the magnitude of a clinical effect. *Cohen's d* (sometimes also called the standard mean difference, or SMD) is a measure of effect size that is calculated by dividing the pooled mean by the pooled standard deviation, creating a decimal to small, medium, and large effects. When the study groups differ substantially in size, each group's standard deviation is sometimes weighted by its sample size; this produces a measure of effect size analogous to Cohen's *d* called *Hedges's g*.

Tip
Effect sizes describe how much the impact of a treatment is clinically meaningful.

Effect sizes can be calculated for just a treatment itself (comparing final outcome ratings to baseline ratings), where it is referred to as a within-group effect size. Alternatively, a so-called "between-group" effect size can be calculated to compare the magnitude of difference between a treatment of interest and a comparator group (such as a placebo). A within-group effect size obtained from an open trial of a drug can give an estimate of whether the drug may be worth studying using a larger and more rigorous design. The within-group effect size of the experimental treatment can give an estimate of how large a sample size would be needed to detect a significant and clinically meaningful

Tip
"To assess clinical significance, every p-value (significant or not) should be accompanied by an effect size that indicates clinical significance and a confidence interval that indicates estimation precision" (Kraemer, 2016, p. 674)

Tip
Kraemer (2016) points out that a small effect size corresponds to an NNT of about 9, a medium effect size corresponds to a NNT of about 4, and a large effect size would equate to an NNT of about 2.

difference as compared to a placebo (or other comparator intervention) – that is, the between-group effect size.

Another way of expressing the clinically meaningfulness of an effect is the concept of *number needed to treat (NNT)*, which tells how many additional cases must receive a particular intervention before one additional beneficial outcome is observed. NNT is calculated by subtracting the inverse of the response or remission rate in a comparator group from that of a treatment group. Single-digit NNTs are optimal; an NNT of 1 means that everyone who receives a treatment of interest will benefit. The higher the NNT, the less clinically impactful the drug's actual effect.

Tip

NNT does not account for baseline individual risk.

For example:

	Response	Remission
Drug X	54%	35%
Placebo	21%	25%

NNT for response = 1/(0.54 - 0.21) = 3.03 ~ 3 NNT for remission = 1/(0.35 - 0.25) = 10

Examples of NNTs throughout medicine can be found at www.thennt.com. Interested readers of the literature can also calculate an effect size for themselves, if it is not provided in a publication, based on t-tests, ANOVAs, or most other commonly presented statistics, through one of many available online websites (e.g., www.psychometrica.de/effect_size.html) (Lenhard and Lenhard, 2016).

Tip

An NNT pertains to treatment effects *over a specified study period.* The same treatment may have a different NNT over, say, 3 weeks versus 8 weeks versus 24 weeks.

Tip

Effect sizes (such as Cohen's *d*) are calculated for a continuous variable (e.g., a change in severity scores); NNTs are calculated based on categorical outcomes (e.g., response or remission rates).

Box 3.6 presents a summary of effect sizes as reported across randomized trials for an array of psychotropic compounds across diverse psychiatric conditions. Readers may find the magnitude of effect for some reported compounds surprisingly lower than they might have expected.

E WHY PSYCHOPHARMACOLOGISTS NEED TO KNOW ABOUT BAYESIAN ANALYSIS

Thomas Bayes was an eighteenth-century English statistician whose work on probability theory focused on the idea that the likelihood of an event happening was influenced by knowledge of the conditions that might predispose to it. The more one knows about the factors associated with an event, the more likely the event is to occur – but also, the more likely one might knowingly or unknowingly bias a situation in favor of the expected outcome. Bayesian approaches to drawing inferences about a phenomenon contrast with *frequentist statistics*, which simply describe the chances that an event will occur (such as remission from depression with an SSRI) no matter how many times an experiment is performed (e.g., taking an SSRI) and without being privy to additional information that could influence the outcome (e.g., how many SSRI trials have already occurred?) A frequentist statistical approach to pharmacology makes no distinction between Trial #1 and Trial #6 or Trial #60.

Tip

Bayes' theorem holds that decisions are influenced by updated knowledge about the chances of an event's occurrence, based on information from past experiences.

In the world of Bayesian psychopharmacology, treatment decisions are usually influenced by past experiences (responses, intolerances) that in turn influence expectations, which introduce biases on the part of the treater or the patient – such as the idea of abandoning a treatment if a desired result doesn't happen soon enough, or hesitation to increase a medication dose because an undesired side effect is believed to be dose-related, or to use a different dose in younger versus older patients, or to pursue supratherapeutic doses based on past experience that higher doses are more effective in treatment-resistant cases. Past experiences can update our knowledge about judging probabilities (called *posterior probabilities* in Bayesian language), and are obviously more valuable if they are accurate, based on empirically observed findings, as opposed to *wrong inferences* drawn from past experiences (such as, SSRIs work better if started on a Monday). A range of likely values for a given

Box 3.6

Effect Sizes Expressed As Cohen's *d* or Hedges's *g* [a]

Value of *d*	Description	Clinical Examples
0.20	Small	Lamotrigine for bipolar depression: ***d* = 0.13** (Selle et al., 2014)
		Buspirone for GAD: ***d* = 0.17** (Hidalgo et al., 2007)
		SSRIs added to antipsychotic for schizophrenic negative symptoms: ***g* = 0.18** (Sepehry et al., 2007)
		Memantine for cognitive symptoms in Alzheimer's dementia: ***d* = 0.27** (Matsunaga et al., 2015)
		Antidepressants in major depression: ***d* = 0.31–0.41** (Turner et al., 2008)
		SSRIs for GAD: ***d* = 0.33** (Gomez et al., 2018)
		Pregabalin for GAD: ***g* = 0.37** (Generoso et al., 2017)
		Lithium in mania: ***g* = 0.39** (Yildiz et al., 2011a)
		SSRIs for OCD in children: ***g* = 0.39** (Locher et al., 2017)
		Buprenorphine for opiate withdrawal: ***d* = 0.43** (Gowing et al., 2017)
		Olanzapine-fluoxetine combination in bipolar depression: ***d* = 0.45** (Selle et al., 2014)
		Atypical antipsychotics for agitation in dementia: ***d* = 0.45** (Yury and Fisher, 2007)
		Antidepressants for schizophrenic negative symptoms: ***d* = 0.48** (Singh et al., 2010)
		Methylphenidate for adult ADHD: ***d* = 0.49** (Cortese et al., 2018)

parameter that falls within the distribution of a posterior probability is called a *credible interval* (CrI; analogous to the confidence interval described earlier in frequentist statistics).

The likelihood of an event happening (e.g., treatment response) *uninformed by the experience of past events* (e.g., is response different when dosing is begun slowly rather than by rapid titration?) is

Value of *d*	Description	Clinical Examples
0.50	Medium	Bupropion for adult ADD: ***d* = 0.50** (Verbeeck et al., 2017)
		SSRIs for panic disorder: ***d* = 0.55** (Otto et al., 2001)
		Carbamazepine in mania: ***g* = 0.61** (Yildiz et al., 2011a)
		Antipsychotic augmentation of SSRIs in OCD: ***g* = 0.64** (Dold et al., 2015a)
		Esketamine in MDD (24 hours): ***d* = 0.65** (Canuso et al., 2018)
		Clomipramine in trichotillomania: ***d* = 0.68** (Bloch et al., 2007)
		Modafinil in ADHD: ***d* = 0.71** (Wang et al., 2017a)
		Amphetamine in adult ADHD: ***d* = 0.79** (Cortese et al., 2018)
0.80	Large	Benzodiazepines for insomnia (sleep quality): ***g* = 0.81** (Winkler et al., 2014)
		Clozapine in schizophrenia: ***d* = 0.88** (Leucht et al., 2013a)
		Intravenous ketamine in major depression: ***d* = 1.01** (Lee et al., 2015)
1.10	Very large	Lisdexamfetamine for ADHD: ***d* = 1.21–1.60** (Biederman et al., 2007)
≥1.40	Extremely large	

[a] Based on findings from reported meta-analyses

Uh, so most psychotropics… their effect sizes are, uh, not so big…
Shhhhh!

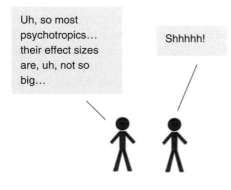

called the *prior probability* or simply the *prior*. When the prior probability of an event happening becomes modified by experience, the prior now becomes the new, revised posterior probability. Accurate posterior probabilities can form the foundation of tailoring a treatment to a given individual based on their unique characteristics (see Chapter 5) – but before such impressions can be taken as empirically valid conclusions (e.g., "divalproex works better than lithium in mixed manic episodes" or "tricyclics work better than SSRIs in melancholic depression") they must be tested as a priori hypotheses.

Bayes' theorem hinges on posterior probabilities to update and inform iterative decision-making. As discussed more fully later in this chapter, it is in that way analogous to the concept of "enriching" a study sample for features that will increase the likelihood of a desired outcome (e.g., what is the chance a particular drug will improve negative symptoms of schizophrenia given more than a certain number of previous treatment nonresponses, a particular duration and severity of illness, and the presence of comorbid cannabis use). **Skillful awareness and use of posterior probabilities is perhaps *the secret* of successful psychopharmacology.**

Attrition and Missing Data

A significant problem when conducting and interpreting clinical trials is the dropout of patients who begin but do not finish a study, or patients who have missing data during assessment points over the course of their participation. As a practical matter, it is difficult to retain patients in a long-term treatment study, especially if it is a randomized trial with a placebo comparator arm.

Dropout from long-term randomized trials is common, often unavoidable, causes loss of statistical power, and often makes it hard to know what to make of the rarified patients who stay till the end. Subjects prematurely discontinue long-term study participation due to factors such as worsening of clinical symptoms, intolerance to treatment, poor treatment adherence, violations of study protocol procedures, withdrawal of consent to continue, moving away, or simply opting to discontinue participation for no declared reason.

An *intent-to-treat (ITT)* sample refers to all patients who were randomized (for whom the intention was to undergo study treatment). The "ITT" sample is thus comprised of all randomized subjects, regardless of how far they proceeded in the study protocol. Some subjects prematurely leave at random intervals for random reasons (e.g., dissatisfaction with their personal results thus far, dislike of adverse drug effects, inconvenience of study visits, feeling better and perceiving no need for ongoing treatment), while others may prematurely exit a study in a way that reflects systematic bias (such as the emergence of serious adverse events, or significant worsening of their underlying condition). The premature loss of study subjects reduces statistical power over the course of the study but even more importantly, if attrition is not random, it introduces a source of systematic bias that can compromise the integrity of the study findings. In other words, if the study results pertain mainly or solely to study completers, they will not be generalizable to patients who left early, and their characteristics (e.g., severity, complexity) might differ from those who remained in the study longer. If there is no systematic bias leading to missing data, they are then assumed to be *missing at random (MAR)* or *missing completely at random (MCAR*; meaning that dropout is *completely unrelated* to factors such as illness severity, worsening symptoms, or adverse effects). MAR is usually more likely to be a valid assumption, whereas MCAR may not be.

Tip

"Completer" analyses, also termed "per protocol" analyses, count only subjects who complete their assigned treatment arm; they may be appropriate for noninferiority analyses but introduce bias against dropouts in superiority trials.

Examples of completion rates and dropout rates for reasons other than reaching primary endpoint (e.g., relapse) in contemporary long-term RCTs for affective disorders are shown in Table 3.3 at the end of this chapter.

One approach to missing data is to count only the patients who actually finish the study (called *observed cases* or "completer analyses"), which has the advantage of providing full information for all subjects, but the substantial disadvantage of omitting information about premature dropouts, and their status at the time they left the study. One way for clinical trials to manage attrition is to use symptom ratings obtained from the last assessment and carry that rating "forward" to the end of the study, imputing later scores by maintaining a subject's last assessment rating regardless of when they left the study, the same as if they had finished it entirely (known as *last observation carried forward*, or LOCF – meaning that a subject's assessment when last seen is imputed or carried forward and counted as if it were their planned final assessment). Through the early 2000s, the US FDA tended to prefer LOCF analyses over observed cases as a more conservative method that captures more information about all subjects. From about 2009 onward, likelihood-based models, or *multiple (rather than single) imputation methods*, have become the preferred modality for analyzing incomplete datasets. Examples are *mixed models for repeated measures (MMRM)* or *generalized estimating equations (GEE)* in which data from all subjects and all data points are used.

To summarize, clinical trials may report findings that account for or otherwise manage missing data in one of several ways:

1. One can examine the *last observation carried forward (LOCF)*. This means that the last data point available for every patient is the one used for purposes of comparative analyses at study endpoint – that is, the final assessment value is *imputed*, or carried forward as if it were the same thing as the planned final visit of the study. *Advantages* are that this method is conservative, and treatment effects, if anything, are underestimated. *Disadvantages* are that there arises a greater risk for a Type I error (can underestimate within-group mean changes), accurate outcomes may not be captured if, say, a disease course is rapidly deteriorating (e.g., acutely suicidal depression), LOCF may also under-report adverse effects that occur later rather than sooner in the course of a clinical trial.
2. *Observed cases*. This means that only subjects who fully complete a study are analyzed (no early dropouts). *Advantages* are mainly that it becomes convenient to manage missing data by ignoring it. *Disadvantages* are that "observed cases" assumes data are MCAR (i.e., no dropouts due to lack of efficacy); tends to overestimate within-group changes.
3. One can perform a *mixed model repeated measures (MMRM)* analysis or a *generalized estimating equations (GEE analysis)*. In these statistical approaches to missing data, multiple imputations are made based on all available data. *Advantages* are that such models account for all available data points. *Disadvantages* are that MAR assumptions must be valid.

F MEASURING OUTCOMES

Univariate and Multivariate Analyses

A first pass through the reported findings of a dataset usually involves univariate statistics, which may be *descriptive* (e.g., continuous measures such as mean age, mean years ill, mean number of prior episodes, or categorical measures such as percent female, percent white, percent employed) or *inferential* (e.g., making comparisons between two or more groups on a given variable of interest – such as assessing for differences among diagnostic groups in mean age at illness onset.) "Univariate" means focusing on just one variable without regard to its relationship to any other variables. Between-group comparisons of demographic or baseline clinical characteristics are usually presented using univariate tests (t-tests for mean differences between two groups, chi-squares for comparing categories, or analyses of variance (ANOVAs) if comparing three or more groups). Let us illustrate this issue with the example in Box 3.7.

Box 3.7

Example

A group of patients with panic disorder is given an SSRI or a placebo for six weeks. The mean change in scores on the Panic Disorder Rating Scale (PDRS) is significantly greater for subjects taking drug than placebo. However, if the SSRI recipients turned out to have a mean older age at onset than the placebo group, then that factor must be taken into account ("covaried" or controlled for) using a multivariate statistical model (such as regression analysis) to determine if the observed significant univariate association between treatment group and PDRS score reduction is sustained after accounting for the possible moderating impact of age at onset. If the difference is no longer significant, the findings become more provisional, and a next step would be to perform a new study in which treatment arms are stratified (equally distributed) at the beginning in their proportion of subjects with early age at onset to clarify more definitively if the SSRI is ineffective, or if it just works better in panic disorder patients with an older age at onset.

Analysis of Variance

While t-tests measure mean differences between two categorical groups for a dependent variable of interest, the mean-group comparison of three or more independent groups is calculated using either analysis of variance (ANOVA; a parametric test statistic that is appropriate when assumptions of a normal population distribution are valid) or a Kruskal–Wallis test (the nonparametric counterpart to ANOVA). A one-way ANOVA conducted on three (or more) independent variables is kind of like running three (or more) separate t-tests on each of three independent variables, but without inflating the Type I error rate that would otherwise occur from making multiple comparisons. In a two-way ANOVA, two independent variables ("factors," each having two or more levels; e.g., "treatment arm" = drug X or placebo; "visit" = each assessment point) are tested for their effect on a dependent (outcome) variable. Tests of significance for each factor are expressed as an F-statistic. A *main effect* examines the impact of each factor by itself on the dependent variable, and an *interaction effect* (e.g., treatment-arm by visit) tells whether one factor has an effect on the other. A *repeated measures ANOVA* would be a technique for measuring mean differences in a dependent variable of interest (say, depression severity score) for three or more groups at multiple time points (say, baseline, end of Phase I, end of Phase II), or when using a crossover design (see Figure 3.3) to compare mean scores for the same group of patients during three or more conditions (say, baseline, end of Trial 1, end of Trial 2).

G REGRESSION MODELS

If randomization is the great equalizing accountant among treatment groups, then regression is the great bookkeeper that assures proper accountability and apportionment of many independent variables potentially impacting treatment outcome. Regression models examine the strength of association or correlations between each independent variable of interest and the dependent/outcome variable, while accounting for the relative contribution of each of the other independent variables in the model. In other words, regression models control for the relative impact of each variable of interest in the context of all the variables being considered. *WOW!!*

One in Ten Rule

As a rule of thumb at least 10 subjects are required for each independent variable entered into a regression model. Also known as the "one in ten" rule (Peduzzi et al., 1996).

In *multiple or linear regression*, the outcome measure is a continuous variable (say, a symptom severity score rating) and the strengths of association between it and each individual independent variable is expressed as a partial correlation coefficient (β) with an accompanying level of significance (p-value).

The power of the model as a whole to explain or account for the variability seen in the dependent variable is called the proportion of explained variance, expressed as a decimal quantity called R^2. Powerful models that can strongly predict an outcome of interest have a high R^2.

If the dependent/outcome variable of interest is dichotomous rather than continuous (say, "response" scored as yes/no), then logistic regression models are used. Here, the strength of association between each independent variable and the designated outcome variable is expressed as an odds ratio with an accompanying 95% confidence interval. Again, the model allows one to measure strengths of association variable by variable, while simultaneously controlling for the relative contribution made by the other independent variables within the model. *WOW again.*

H POST HOC AND MODERATOR ANALYSES

What if the possible contributions made by other variables on an outcome measure are not considered a priori? Suppose Drug X significantly improves anxiety symptoms as compared to placebo in a group of GAD patients, but we then wonder if it worked especially well in certain subgroups – say, women versus men, or nonchronic versus chronically ill patients, or Democrats versus Republicans. One could pose such questions even after the study was undertaken using *post hoc analyses*. On the up side, when an overall hypothesis test shows a significant treatment effect, it can be useful to further identify and refine subpopulations whose response may be especially robust, or to determine if there are clinically important subgroups for whom treatment responsivity warrants special attention. An example is provided in Box 3.8.

Box 3.8

Example

In a statistically significant RCT of quetiapine for bipolar depression, favorable *post hoc* analyses were subsequently published to "demonstrate" that efficacy relative to placebo was observed in the study subgroup with bipolar II depression (Suppes et al., 2008) and in the subgroup with a history of past-year rapid cycling (Vieta et al., 2007). While these post hoc analyses imbue optimism about the possibly special value of quetiapine in the next rapidly cycling bipolar II depressed patient who comes along, it is not quite synonymous with having set out to undertake a prospective RCT of quetiapine in known bipolar II depressed patients, or a group of rapidly cycling bipolar depressed patients. The post hoc findings are therefore more provisional than definitive because of their increased risk for Type I error due to multiplicity in assumptions made around hypothesis testing.

Post hoc analyses are legitimate strategies to discern whether a relationship between an independent and dependent variable is influenced by a third intervening variable – called a *moderator* variable. For example, suppose lithium works better than a placebo to treat acute mania, but only in patients with fewer than three lifetime episodes. One could examine the relationship between treatment (lithium or placebo) and responder status while controlling post hoc for lifetime episode number as a possible moderating variable.

Investigators often "data mine" a dataset after the primary outcome analyses have been completed, planning and undertaking post hoc analyses to search for possible interesting associations that might generate hypotheses for future prospective studies. Excessive data mining is sometimes dubbed data dredging or "fishing expeditions" in which no hypotheses govern the conceptualization and implementation of test efforts. While frowned upon by methodological purists (because of an inflated risk for Type I error), others within the scientific community sometimes fondly point out that without fishing expeditions, how else can one hope to catch any fish?

Suppose one wonders if a outcome state in a clinical trial is simply the artifact of having treated an overarching condition, as opposed to delivering a specific effect on a free-standing target symptom falling within the broader symptom constellation of interest. For that dilemma we must consider the concept of pseudospecificity, discussed in Box 3.9.

Box 3.9

What is Pseudospecificity?

The term "pseudospecificity" was coined by the FDA in 2001 to describe situations in which the effect of a drug on a particular symptom that occurs as part of a broader diagnostic syndrome could be construed as having a distinct effect on that one symptom, irrespective of its presence in other syndromes. Examples would be claims that a drug treats cognitive symptoms of depression (independent of resolving other symptoms in a major depressive episode (MDE)), or treating agitation or hallucinations in schizophrenia (without clarifying if it treats those symptoms when they arise in disorders other than schizophrenia), or even claiming that treatment for a particular condition (such as an antidepressant for major depression) exerts its effect uniquely for a given population (e.g., poststroke depression). Or, amoxacillin could have an antitussive effect by virtue of treating bronchitis or pneumonia, but its antitussive effect is specific (to the infectious disease state) rather than pseudospecific, because it does not treat any and all forms of cough. Pharmaceutical marketers hold an obvious stakeholder interest in differentiating their products from others within the marketplace, and concerns about "pseudospecific" claims require careful analyses in order for prescribers to understand the likelihood that a touted target of treatment for a particular population is genuinely unique to that population, or merely an artifact of treating a broader clinical condition for which the target symptom is not *specific*.

 META-ANALYSES

While meta-analyses are often considered the highest level of evidence (see Chapter 1), they are not infallible and are subject to biases of their own if carried out improperly. Meta-analyses are traditionally conducted in accordance with guidelines (described in the Preferred Reporting Items for Systematic Reviews and Meta-analyses (PRISMA)) and should be registered in the International Prospective Register of Systematic Reviews (PROSPERO; www.crd.york.ac.uk/Prospero/) to avoid duplication of efforts by multiple teams, as well as minimize the risk for contradictory findings by different investigators examining the same topic.

Meta-analyses provide an aggregate or pooled estimate of the effect of an intervention, involving a weighted mean (and standard deviation) of the individual studies included. *Heterogeneity* is a term used to describe how much the observed effect sizes seen in a meta-analysis vary across the different populations included. Statistically, heterogeneity is expressed as *Cochran's Q*, a parameter that is dependent on the number of studies included in the meta-analysis. Another statistic, I^2 (with an accompanying confidence interval), describes how much the variation observed across studies is due to heterogeneity rather than to chance. Meta-analysis models involve either *fixed effects* (appropriate when I^2 is low, meaning that the methodologies, conditions, and subject characteristics from across all included studies were very similar), or, more usually, *random effects* (in which no assumptions are made about variability in methodologies across studies). *Mixed effect models* contain both fixed and random effects; for example, fixed effects might include treatment arm, age group, and baseline severity, while the random effects might include medication dose, adherence, and the use of adjunctive "rescue" pharmacotherapies.

Cautionary issues involving meta-analyses and their interpretation are summarized in Table 3.4 at the end of this chapter.

 Network Meta-analyses

While traditional meta-analyses make pairwise comparisons of an intervention (e.g., one-by-one

Figure 3.5 Illustration of funnel plots.

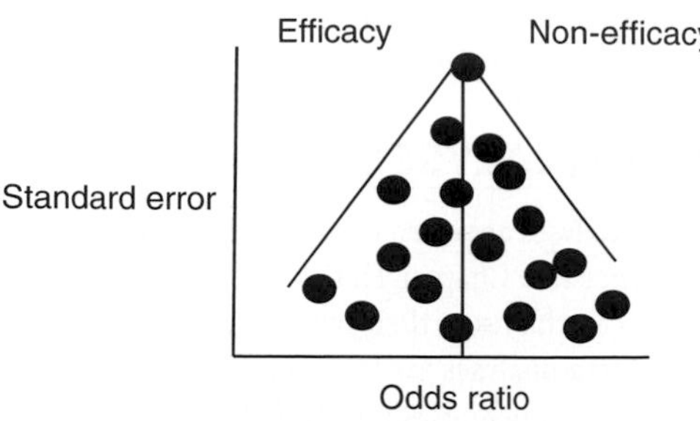

Symmetrical; low likelihood of publication bias

Efficacy
Non-efficacy
Standard error
Odds ratio

Asymmetrical; likely not so unbiased

versus placebo), network meta-analysis involves comparisons among a large group of available RCTs, typically with rankings of how well interventions perform from best to worst. Those rankings are presented as a cumulative ranking curve, with the "surface under the cumulative ranking curve" (termed "*SUCRA*") representing a series of single numbers ranging from 0 to 100%, with the highest percentages being in the top rank. Mean differences between studies are usually presented alongside 95% credible intervals (CrIs).

Reminder

Credible intervals are the Bayesian counterpart to confidence intervals, as reported in frequentist statistics.

However, SUCRA rankings can have a number of important limitations:

- they do not necessarily take into account the quality of the evidence behind individual studies (which may vary based on factors such as sample size, successful blinding of study drug, width of confidence intervals, study durations, and attrition);
- they do not account for potential adverse effects of one intervention relative to another;
- the degree or magnitude of difference between one ranking and another is not captured, making it hard to know if the higher ranking of one treatment versus another reflects a substantial or only a marginal difference.

J FIXED VERSUS FLEXIBLE DOSE STUDIES

In flexible dose studies, the treating clinician is encouraged to dose a study drug to a minimum threshold dose and thereafter use their discretion (or, follow a specified protocol based on whether or not benchmarks for improvement have been reached) to continue an upward dosing titration based on response criteria. It is difficult to infer dose–response relationships from flexible dose studies because of the potential for selection bias based on prior observations (posterior probabilities); specifically, dosages are chosen based on the prescriber's expectations about minimum necessary dosages for efficacy as well as anticipation of possible dose-related adverse effects. A statistical technique known as marginal structural modeling has been described involving weighted pooled repeated measures analysis that account for dose effects based on dosing patterns prior to the time of assessment (Lipkovich et al., 2012).

K INFERENCES FROM CLINICAL TRIALS: PRIMARY AND SECONDARY OUTCOMES

Evidence-based medicine draws from the systematic findings of clinical trials, where a priori-defined outcomes help practitioners know what kind of results to expect. Returning to our automotive road test analogy from Chapter 1, outcomes might include acceleration time from zero to 60 miles per hour, speed of arrival time, smooth handling through hairpin turns and adequate shock absorption on rough terrain, chassis wear-and-tear, performance consistency, road sway and veering, and general customer satisfaction. So too, pharmacotherapies can differ in their speed of onset, need for titration, efficacy across broad clinical subgroups, reliability, adverse effects, specificity for distinct symptom targets, and global improvement. All of these characteristics collectively bear on conclusions about whether a treatment is deemed to be appropriate, desirable, and preferred over other options.

"Primary" outcomes are the main focus of interest in a clinical trial, using a designated measure (such as symptom severity or global improvement). Treatments sometimes perform better than a placebo or an active comparator on measures other than a primary outcome, which often greatly interests a clinician but unfortunately usually does not "count" toward declaring whether a study is a success or failure, as defined a priori before the study has begun. A notable example is the first of the five RCTs of lamotrigine intended for regulatory registration for acute bipolar depression. Separation from placebo was not evident by study end on the Hamilton Ratings Scale for Depression (HAM-D), the measure chosen a priori as the primary outcome, making this a negative study. However, a significant difference was observed using a secondary outcome measure for depression (the Montgomery–Åsberg Depression Rating Scale (MADRS); Montgomery and Åsberg, 1979). This event led the investigators to reconceptualize the first (negative) study as "exploratory" in nature (presuming that the MADRS must have been more sensitive than the HAM-D for revealing lamotrigine's efficacy) and design four subsequent studies to use the MADRS as their primary outcome. Unfortunately, all those studies also showed no differences between lamotrigine and placebo.

Clinical trials sometimes identify primary outcomes as "response" or "remission" or "recovery" (often given by group percentages), in addition to the reporting of raw changes in a rating scale score from baseline or a reporting of effect sizes. Each of these concepts is defined along with its relative advantages and disadvantages in Table 3.5.

"Secondary outcomes" may pertain to one of several constructs. A secondary outcome measure could mean that, in addition to the specific rating scale or operational outcome definition chosen a priori as the main focus of a study, the investigators may also have included additional scales or measures of the phenomenon of interest (e.g., symptoms, or performance on a task such as a cognitive measure) or a related phenomenon (e.g., global improvement, or a global assessment of functioning). (A vexing problem occurs when a chosen primary outcome measure fails to separate from placebo but a secondary outcome measure proves to be significant – does that mean the study is simply negative because our favored horse lost the race, or does it mean our horse was a poor choice to begin with and there is a better candidate able to reveal our horsemanship prowess?[3]) Secondary outcomes also could mean incidental phenomena that are of interest in the context of treating the ailment being studied – for example, quality of life, or work and social functioning, or service utilization.

L EFFICACY VERSUS EFFECTIVENESS

Efficacy is a term used to describe whether or not an intervention is better than a placebo, under well-controlled conditions. *Effectiveness* is a term that describes how well an otherwise-efficacious treatment performs under ordinary clinical circumstances (where one must take into account additional factors such as tolerability, cost, ease of administration, and other possible patient burdens). Effectiveness is often measured as "all-cause discontinuation" or time until study dropout (as was the primary outcome measure in the NIMH CATIE trial; see Chapter 15, "Psychosis").

M TIME-UNTIL-EVENT ANALYSES

Survival analysis is a statistical method for comparing differences between two or more categorical groups (e.g., treatment arms, or diagnoses) in their time until an event, generating a graph known as a Kaplan–Meier curve, with an accompanying log-rank statistic. Two matched groups might be compared in time till recovery, or time until relapse. Subjects who never incur the outcome event of interest are classified as "censored" cases.

Cox proportional hazard models are a specialized case of survival analysis in which the time until the occurrence of an event (e.g., relapse) is predicted by a number of noncategorical (continuously scored) independent variables (termed "covariates," such as age, baseline severity, medication dose, or lifetime number of episodes), simultaneously accounting for the relative impact of each covariate on the dependent variable/ outcome event of interest.

3 For further discussion on what happens when a secondary but not the primary outcome measure is efficacious in a clinical trial, see the section "Why Lamotrigine Isn't Considered An Antidepressant" (Chapter 13). Subjects who never incur the outcome event of interest are classified as "censored" cases.

N PLACEBO-CONTROLLED TRIALS AND ACTIVE COMPARATORS

In the United States, regulatory agency approval generally requires two placebo-controlled trials that yield positive results on the primary outcome measure that was chosen before the study begins. Head-to-head comparisons between psychotropic drugs are less commonly undertaken in the USA. Sometimes, an active comparator drug is included as a third arm in a randomized placebo-controlled trial for purposes of "assay sensitivity" – that is, to assure the study findings are interpretable if the experimental treatment proves to be no different from placebo. In that instance, if another established treatment for the ailment of interest is efficacious when placebo is not, we conclude that the *trial is negative*, but if both the experimental drug and the active comparator are no different from placebo, the *trial is failed*, and not much can be inferred about the utility of either drug because of the high placebo effect.

Tip

A *negative* trial means a treatment was no better than a placebo. A *failed* trial means a high placebo response rate could have obscured the true potential efficacy of the active treatment.

Enriched Designs

Judging initial responsiveness to a particular drug before embarking on its long-term use for relapse prevention is a little like dating before marriage. Imagine entering into a committed relationship without first finding out if there is a good fit. Chances are, a long-term relationship (the maintenance phase) will be more successful if there is first an initial exposure (acute phase, the dating period) before making a longer-term commitment. Settling down for good with someone you barely know may make for an all-too-brief union.

Tip

Enriched design studies are those in which a treatment is continued only in acute responders; they tell more about optimal efficacy than generalizability.

Clinical trials that first judge whether a patient has an initial response to a particular treatment utilize *enriched designs*. If, for example, a drug was known to work better in women than men, or in patients with a particular family history or subtype of an illness, then the deck becomes stacked in favor of the experimental drug if a disproportionate number of such patients is over-represented in the active arm of a treatment study. Consider the example presented in Box 3.10.

Box 3.10

Example

The manufacturer of divalproex designed a study in which prevention of manic or depressive episodes in bipolar disorder was evaluated with divalproex or placebo (with lithium as an active comparator) in all-comers with bipolar disorder who had recently recovered by whatever means from a manic episode. The results showed no differences among the three groups (Bowden et al., 2000). However, when the investigators looked back and selected out only those patients who had initially gotten better with divalproex, they indeed were the ones more likely to stay well over the long run by continuing the drug that helped them originally (McElroy et al., 2008). Had the study sponsor chosen to enrich their relapse prevention protocol by enrolling only acute responders to divalproex, the drug may very likely have successfully defeated the placebo arm, leading to an FDA indication for maintenance treatment of bipolar disorder.

Some researchers criticize the "enriched design" methodology because it provides less generalizable information about how well a medication can prevent new episodes than would be the case if, instead, "all comers" were enrolled from the outset in a relapse-prevention study. The problem with such a criticism, though, is that it may make perfect sense to study relapse prevention specifically in patients for whom an initial response has already been established, rather than in patients for whom there is not necessarily any reason to think the study drug will provide a sustained effect. Enriched designs are good for what they are good for. Knowing the earmarkings of a likely responder profile (not just a diagnosis per se) matched to a particular medication can make for prescient psychopharmacology. Embarking on a long-term treatment regimen without having some idea of how useful and acceptable it is at the outset is over-reliance on serendipity. Consider the example presented in Box 3.11.

Box 3.11

Enrichment: Case in Point

Aripiprazole long-acting injectable (LAI) was studied as compared to placebo in a 52-week RCT for relapse prevention following an acute index manic episode (Calabrese et al., 2017b). Time until the recurrence of a manic or mixed episode was significantly longer with aripiprazole LAI than placebo, but time until a depressive episode was not. One might conclude that aripiprazole LAI is more effective to prevent manias than depressions, but the study design does not really allow for that inference because the enrollment of patients with index manic (not depressed) episodes enriched the study design for a greater proclivity toward manic rather than depressed phase recurrences in the ensuing months. How do we know this is true? By looking at the placebo arm to judge natural course. The rate of mania relapses on placebo was 30%, but depressive recurrences occurred in only 14%, which was not significantly different from active drug. A more fair appraisal of the value of aripiprazole LAI for depression prophylaxis would have required equivalent randomization of index depressed phase study entrants.

0 SENSITIVITY, SPECIFICITY, PPV, NPV

When performing tests to screen for a diagnosis or a diagnosis-related condition, parameters known as "classification functions" are often calculated to give an estimate of the likelihood of the presence or absence of the phenomenon of interest, based on the test result. High sensitivity essentially means that the great majority of individuals who have the condition will be identified – but casting a wide net means also increasing the risk for including people who do not really have the feature of interest (false positives). High specificity means that if the test is positive, it is quite specific in detecting only the item of interest (*false* positives are few if any), but not everyone with the condition will necessarily be captured (false negatives can be high). Positive and negative predictive values (PPV, NPV) further refine these parameters; a test with high PPV means that it is very good at capturing the phenomenon of interest, and only that phenomenon; a high NPV means that if the test is negative, then it is extremely unlikely the condition is present. These items are further described in Box 3.12.

Box 3.12

Classification Functions of Diagnostic Screening Tests

Test	Definition	Clinical Meaning
Sensitivity	True positives/ (true positives + false negatives)	If someone has a disorder, how often will the test be positive?
Specificity	True negatives/ (true negatives + false positives)	If someone does not have a disorder, how often will the test be negative?
Positive predictive value (PPV)	True positives/ (true positives + false positives)	If someone has a positive screening test result, what is the probability that the patient actually has the condition being screened for?
Negative predictive value (NPV)	True negatives/ (true negatives + false negatives)	If someone has a negative screening test result, what is the probability that the patient truly does not have the condition being screened for?

It is important to remember that a screening test for a disorder is just that, a screen, and not synonymous with "casehood" or the unequivocal establishment of a diagnosis (the same way a positive Pap smear is not synonymous with cervical carcinoma – but demands closer scrutiny and surveillance). Beware of research studies that may use diagnostic screens as proxies for conducting formal diagnostic interviews – they may poorly discriminate true cases from near-lookalikes.

P RECEIVER OPERATING CHARACTERISTIC CURVES

What if you wanted to estimate how well a continuous independent variable (say, antidepressant blood levels) could discriminate a yes–no outcome variable (say, antidepressant response status)? You may wonder how to tell if there is a threshold or cut-off score that could optimally identify a "yes" (e.g., responder) versus a "no" (e.g., nonresponder). A common statistical strategy for this is to graph sensitivity (true positives) along the *y*-axis and specificity (true negatives) along the *x*-axis in order to generate a graph known as a *receiver operating characteristic* (ROC) curve. The resulting area under the curve (AUC) reflects how well the independent variable predicts or discriminates responders from nonresponders, with a perfect relationship being equal to 1.0 (100% sensitivity and 100% specificity). An optimal trade-off between sensitivity and specificity would occur around where the highest point of the vertical and horizontal portions of the curve meet, as depicted in Figure 3.6. AUCs >0.75 are generally considered to have clinically meaningful discriminatory value. In Chapter 7, we shall revisit the use of ROC curves as a tool for judging whether and when specific medications have therapeutically meaningful blood levels.

Figure 3.6 A receiver operating curve.

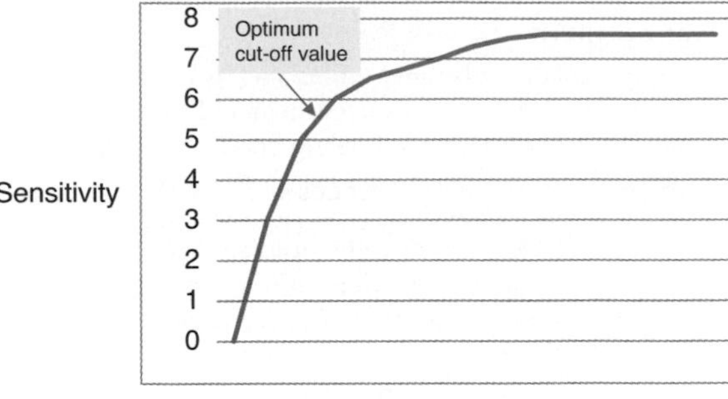

> **Etymology**
>
> "Receiver operating characteristic" curves were so named during World War II when referring to how accurately radar operators (receiver operators) could discriminate true versus false positive signals on radar screens.

TAKE-HOME POINTS

The Quick and Dirty Summary: A Checklist for How to Read a Research Study

- Are the study objectives clearly stated, and is there a stated hypothesis? Does it make clinical sense?
- Who are the subjects and how were they ascertained? Are they treatment-seeking, a sample of convenience, or actively recruited? How well do their clinical characteristics resemble or differ from your own patients?
- Is the study sample generalizable and representative? Treatment-naive or treatment-resistant?
- What are the sample sizes? If a comparative study, was it powered adequately (Method section) or is this a preliminary proof-of-concept study? Are p-values nominal or adjusted for multiple comparisons?
- Are diagnoses well-defined, and were they established by formal systematic interviews?
- Check the CONSORT diagram; how many ITT subjects completed or dropped out prematurely?
- If an RCT, was randomization successful? If not, did the authors account for possible confounding factors in post hoc analyses? How was the comparison/healthy control group chosen?
- In pharmacotherapy trials, was dosing adequate and appropriate? If cotherapies were allowed, were they balanced between treatment groups and were relevant pharmacokinetic interactions considered (e.g., CYP450 inducers or inhibitors)?
- If an intervention trial, were any pre-enrollment cotherapies held constant?
- If a crossover design was used, how were potential carryover effects addressed?
- How was treatment adherence monitored?
- How was premature dropout handled? Were data MAR/MCAR? Are analyses based on observed cases, LOCF, or were mixed models used?
- If parametric statistics were used, are normality assumptions justified?
- If a meta-analysis, were potential sources of bias and study heterogeneity adequately addressed?

Table 3.1 Parametric and nonparametric tests

What's being studied?	Parametric tests	Nonparametric tests
Comparison of mean differences between two independent groups	Independent t-test	Wilcoxon rank-sum test (aka Mann-Whitney U test)
Comparison of mean differences in a continuous variable within the same subjects over time	Dependent t-tests	Wilcoxon signed-rank test
Comparison of mean differences in a continuous variable over time among three or more groups	Analysis of variance (ANOVA); effect size may be expressed as eta squared (η^2)	Kruskal-Wallis test
Comparison of proportions in a 2×2 or similar contingency table (e.g., comparing diagnosis by sex, or current smoking status)	None	Chi-square test, Fisher's exact test (sometimes recommended if a cell size is <5), McNemar's test (measures consistency in responses across two variables), Cochran's Q (used for binary outcomes with ≥3 comparably sized groups)
Degree of association between two variables scored as *continuous* variables (e.g., age, height, weight)	Pearson correlation	Spearman's rank correlation (ρ)
Comparison of ranked *ordinal* variables (ranked correlation) (e.g., ratings of 1st, 2nd, 3rd,…)	None	Kendall's tau (τ) Spearman's rank correlation (ρ)

Table 3.2 Common methods of alpha correction for multiple comparisons

Correction method	Description
Bonferroni	This method involves dividing the initial alpha level by the number of tests performed to obtain a new, Bonferroni-corrected alpha level. For example, if an initial alpha level is 0.05 and eight independent variables are tested for their associations with a dependent variable of interest, the Bonferroni-corrected alpha level would be 0.5/8 = tests performed = 0.00625. Bonferroni is considered an especially conservative method, but comes with a great reduction in statistical power (possibly inflating the chance for a Type II error (rejecting a true finding)).
Holm–Bonferroni	A modification of the Bonferroni method, this is a sequential or rank-ordered procedure to address FWER that retains more statistical power than a Bonferroni correction. First, rank order the observed p-values from lowest to highest for all the tests performed. Then, divide the desired alpha level (say, 0.05) by the number of tests performed minus the rank number (i.e., "1") + 1. Then, compare the lowest-ranked (smallest) p-value from the series to the just-calculated Holm–Bonferroni alpha. If the p-value is smaller, reject that test. Then repeat the calculation successively for each rank number in the denominator (2, 3, 4, etc.), accepting p-values that are smaller and rejecting those that are higher than each calculated alpha.
False discovery rate (FDR)	This statistic tells what proportion of rejected null hypotheses are actually true; i.e., the ratio of falsely rejected hypotheses to all rejected hypotheses. It runs the risk of inflating the chances for a Type I error.

Table 3.3 Premature dropout from published long-term modern randomized clinical trials of affective disorders

Condition	Change from ITT sample size to sample size at study end	Study duration	Percentage completing entire study	Percentage premature dropout for reasons other than reaching primary endpoint
Bipolar relapse	Aripiprazole N = 78→7 vs.	100 weeks	9%	72%
	Placebo N = 83→5		6%	91%
	(Keck et al., 2007)			
	Divalproex N = 187→71 vs.	52 weeks	38%	38%
	Lithium N = 91→22 vs.		24%	45%
	Placebo N = 94→23		25%	37%
	(Bowden et al., 2000)			
	Lamotrigine N = 59→18 vs.	18 months	31%[a]	22%
	Lithium N = 46→10 vs.		22%[a]	39%
	Placebo N = 70→11		16%[a]	14%
	(Bowden et al., 2003)			
	Lamotrigine N = 221→38 vs.	18 months	17%	31%
	Lithium N = 121→20 vs.		28%	37%
	Placebo N = 121→12 (Calabrese et al., 2003)		10%	36%
	Olanzapine N = 225→48 vs.	48 weeks	21%	32%
	Placebo N = 136→9		7%	13%
	(Tohen et al., 2006)			
	Lithium/Divalproex + olanzapine N = 51→16 vs.	18 months	31%	43%
	Lithium/Divalproex + Placebo N = 48→5		10%	54%
	(Tohen et al., 2004)			
Major depression	Fluoxetine N = 70→49 vs.	48 weeks	70%	24%
	Placebo N = 70→29		41%	10%
	(Gilaberte et al., 2001)			
	Sertraline 50 mg/day N = 95→58 vs.	18 months	61%	39%
	Sertraline 100 mg/day N = 94→57 vs.		61%	39%
	Placebo N = 99→50		51%	49%
	(Lépine et al., 2004)			
	Escitalopram N = 74→37 vs.	12 months	51%	32%
	Placebo N = 65→12 (Kornstein et al., 2006)		18%	46%
	Venlafaxine ER N = 160→66 vs.	12 months	41%	41%
	Placebo N = 164→37		23%	60%
	(Kocsis et al., 2007)			
	Vortioxetine N = 204→125 vs.	64 weeks	61%	39%
	Placebo N = 192→104 vs. (Boulenger et al., 2012)		54%	46%

[a] The study was prematurely discontinued before all subjects completed; study endpoint therefore reflects participants' termination at the time the protocol was discontinued.

Table 3.4 Potential pitfalls of meta-analyses

Problem area	What it means	Strategy to resolve
Heterogeneity	Different studies may use different methodologies and measures that may not uniformly capture the same outcome of interest; findings across studies may vary considerably in their direction, and confounding biases are no longer controlled for by randomization.	Check Cochran's Q and I^2 (customarily reported in a meta-analysis) to gauge the extent of heterogeneity. *Meta-regression* is a technique that extends a meta-analysis, providing a method to control for potential confounding variables that could affect the magnitude of the effect of included studies. It examines possible methodological differences across studies ("methodological diversity") or in study populations that have been combined ("clinical diversity").
Restricted scope of included studies	May not include all available studies (e.g., restricted to English language, omission of unpublished data).	Meta-regression may help to detect language bias, citation bias, or other sources of reporting bias.
Substantially uneven distribution of subjects across included studies	If a majority of the data in a meta-analysis comes from a disproportionately low number of studies (e.g., one, or only a few), the results may not be as meaningful and meta-analysis itself may be inappropriate.	Difficult to "resolve." If an inordinate proportion of the data included in a meta-analysis comes from only one or a few of many included studies, the findings may simply be less valid and generalizable.
Small study effects	Smaller studies tend to report larger effects than do larger studies (i.e., smaller studies require larger effects in order to be statistically significant).	Weighted regression methods can detect bias from small studies where treatment effects are low, but not moderate or large (Sterne et al., 2000).
Publication bias	Positive studies and large studies are more likely to be published than negative ones or small ones.	A *funnel plot* is a graphical depiction of effect sizes, or odds ratios, or percent differences (along the *x*-axis) plotted against a measure of precision, such as sample size or the reciprocal of their standard errors (along the *y*-axis). When the resulting plot is symmetrical or "funnel shaped," the likelihood of publication bias is low (see Figure 3.5). However, an asymmetrical funnel plot may not necessarily indicate bias if large observed treatment effects are based on smaller trials (Sterne et al., 2000).

Table 3.5 Outcomes described in clinical trials

Outcome	Definition	Pros	Cons
Response	In mood and anxiety disorders, usually ≥50% reduction from baseline in symptom rating scale. Lower thresholds often used in other conditions (e.g., schizophrenia or PTSD may be 20 or 30% reductions from baseline, respectively)	A common metric for clinically meaningful improvement	May fall short of a desired outcome; substantial improvement could occur but patients may still remain highly symptomatic
Remission	Sufficient resolution or reduction of symptoms such that any remaining features are judged to be within the realm of normal, or not of clinical importance; often operationally defined by convention as a rating scale score falling below a specified maximum for a minimum time duration, e.g., a MADRS depression score ≤10 for two consecutive visits, a CGI severity score ≤2, a BPRS score ≤30, or a YMRS score ≤12	A more rigorous measure of improvement than "response;" implies *sustained* improvement	Harder to achieve, may be unrealistic in more chronic or treatment-resistant conditions
Recovery	An all-encompassing term that captures minimal-to-no clinically meaningful symptoms plus achievement of adequate psychosocial functioning for a minimum specified time period	A more comprehensive "real life" measure of overall improvement than simply gauging symptom severity	A rigorous benchmark that can be difficult to achieve, may portray an effective treatment as less valuable than it might actually be
Mean reduction in symptom score from baseline	Mean change in rating scale scores from baseline/study entry to study end	Common primary outcome measure in FDA registration trials; allows for determination of effect size	Less tangible than "response" or "remission" rates, less informative about absolute level of wellness or degree of improvement
Effect sizes (ES) and number needed to treat (NNT)	Provides a quantifiable description of the magnitude of clinically meaningful change associated with a given treatment either from baseline ("within-group ES") or relative to a placebo or comparator treatment ("between-group ES")	ES is calculable from mean change in symptom severity ratings for treatment arm vs. comparator; NNT can be derived from the inverse of response (or remission) rates	There is no perfect metric to express clinical magnitude of effect

Abbreviations: BPRS = Brief Psychiatric Rating Scale; CGI = Clinical Global Impressions Scale; ES = effect size; MADRS = Montgomery–Åsberg Depression Rating Scale; NNT = number needed to treat; YMRS = Young Mania Rating Scale

4 Placebo and Nocebo Effects

LEARNING OBJECTIVES

- [ ] Understand the clinical importance of the placebo effect, its magnitude and known clinical and neurobiological (e.g., pharmacogenetic) determinants across major psychiatric disorders, and how it differs from "no treatment"
- [ ] Differentiate relatively high- versus low- placebo-responsive forms of psychopathology
- [ ] Recognize the controversy within the literature about rising placebo response rates in clinical trials and how these may influence "failed" rather than "negative" study outcomes
- [ ] Understand the role of baseline severity as a factor influencing drug–placebo response rates across psychiatric disorders
- [ ] Describe the nocebo effect and its known clinical determinants
- [ ] Describe strategies to minimize placebo response rates in psychopharmacology clinical trials

The art of medicine consists in amusing the patient while nature cures the disease.

- Voltaire

If a person is (a) poorly, (b) receives treatment intended to make him better, and (c) gets better, then no power of reasoning known to medical science can convince him that it may not have been the treatment that restored his health.

- Sir Peter Medawar

If the placebo effect is not the bane of every psychopharmacologist's existence, it probably should be. Placebo responses largely negate all rules of pharmacodynamics, undermine theories about drug mechanisms of action, ruin clinical trials by causing failed (rather than negative) findings that mask the true potential for otherwise promising compounds, inflate costs for drug research and development, and generally give a black eye to neuroscience-based explanations for psychopathology. They also lend humility to clinicians' assumptions that psychopharmacology reliably holds the upper hand when dealing with any and all matters of mental illness. In this chapter we will review known clinical features and correlates (if not actual predictors) of placebo responsivity across major psychiatric conditions, and offer guidance about how clinicians can anticipate, recognize and manage placebo effects – rather than ignore, dismiss, or otherwise struggle against them.

"Placebo" literally means "I shall please" and historically has been a descriptor for any treatment intended mainly to provide psychological benefit rather than physiological efficacy. For the purposes of this discussion we use the term to define a pharmacodynamically inert or psychotropically inactive substance. That said, we would challenge the frequent assertion that a placebo is a substance having no intended therapeutic value; on the contrary, it is precisely because placebo effects account for so annoyingly large a proportion of the variability in psychiatric treatment outcomes that clinicians must understand their therapeutic role. This means recognizing characteristics of a placebo versus pharmacodynamically mediated response, anticipating factors that could predispose to placebo effects, and – for clinicians, but not clinical trialists – capitalizing on their potential contribution to overall outcome whenever and wherever opportunity permits. *Strangely enough, investigators strive intentionally to minimize placebo effects in RCTs while clinicians strive unintentionally to maximize them in real-life practice.* Particularly in highly treatment-resistant patients, the clinician's ability to breathe life into an otherwise inert substance – in no small part via the therapeutic alliance – may be the very glue that keeps fragile patients engaged and able to persevere despite the pull toward demoralization and defeat.

Tip

"Regression to the mean" means that repeated measurements of a variable within a studied sample will eventually fall back ("regress") to the mean value of the population from which the sample was derived.

A PLACEBO EFFECTS VERSUS REGRESSION TO THE MEAN

Perhaps the most obvious and important criticism one can levy against the placebo effect is the claim that it does not exist – or, more specifically, that it is no more than an artifact of a phenomenon called *regression to the mean*. This is the statistical observation that when extreme values on a complex measure of interest (e.g., symptom severity) are observed in a study sample, subsequent or repeated measurements are likely to be less extreme and closer to the true average value simply due to chance variation. Regression to the mean is particularly operative when comparing two variables that are poorly correlated. The risk is especially true in the case of small sample sizes, which increases the chance of Type II (false negative) errors. It is more likely to occur if treatment allocation is not by randomization (so, for example, regression to the mean is of greater concern in observational studies such as the comparison of suicide risk in bipolar patients nonrandomly assigned to lithium or divalproex, as described in Chapter 3, Box 3.1). Risk of regression is greater for disease states that are inherently variable in course, where symptoms are more prone to come and go, or wax and wane (such as rapid cycling bipolar disorder, or panic disorder, or relapsing binge drinking) than is the case for more persistent, nonepisodic, and unvarying conditions (such as persistent/chronic depression, obsessive-compulsive disorder, or generalized anxiety disorder).

Tip

A baseball player at the start of the season who gets three hits in his first four at-bats has an impressive 0.750 average. Regression to the mean will nearly always bring that number back down to earth over more at-bat opportunities.

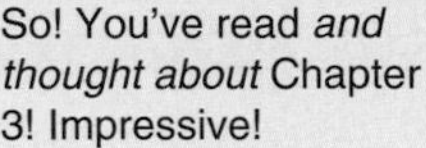
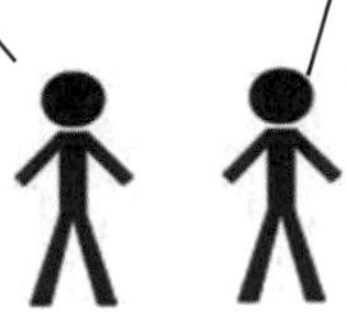

Is that why it's easier to get an inflated-looking big effect with a small sample size? Not enough at-bats yet?
So! You've read *and thought about* Chapter 3! Impressive!
But that'll remain impressive only after you read another 10 chapters and haven't by then regressed to the mean.

It can be hard to know with certainty if a high placebo response rate truly reflects a beneficial effect from the placebo as opposed to random or natural variation in the course of illness. The only way to make such a distinction is to compare placebo to no treatment. Such a meta-analysis was undertaken by a group from the University of Copenhagen, involving 114 RCTs encompassing 40 different general medical or psychiatric conditions (including depression, anxiety, ADHD, schizophrenia, phobias, and insomnia, among others) (Hrøbjartsson and Gøtzsche, 2001). No significant differences were found between placebo and no treatment in any of the psychiatric disorders studied, and the lack of significant differences was not an artifact of higher dropout rates in one group versus another, or whether investigators were unblinded to study conditions.

Tip

The strength of the therapeutic alliance may influence treatment outcomes more strongly during treatment with a placebo than with an active pharmacotherapy.

However – knowing what we know from Chapter 3 – significant heterogeneity was found across trials, and the meta-analysis may not have been adequately powered or sufficiently sensitive to identify small yet meaningful effects from placebo in at least some clinical settings. The meta-analysis also did not account for qualitative aspects of the therapeutic alliance which, as they state, "may be largely independent of any placebo intervention" (p. 1599). Elsewhere, at least in the case of depression, the strength of the therapeutic alliance has been shown to exert a greater mediating effect on outcomes with placebo than with active drug therapy (Zilcha-Mano et al., 2015). Indeed, "placebo effects" for psychiatric disorders, treated within a mental health setting, may very well differ fundamentally from all other clinical situations involving placebo.

In Chapter 1, we examined potential obstacles to drawing accurate causal inferences in the course of pharmacotherapy. Coupling that with the information on Bayesian analysis (i.e., how iterative experiences cause us to revise our estimates of the probability that an event will happen), we can now make things even more complicated when trying to infer cause and effect if we bring in the concept of regression to the mean. If two variables are poorly correlated (say, a treatment and a change in a symptom severity rating), then poor baseline scores can only improve (move closer to the population mean) over time simply due to random variation. Similarly, if an adverse event (especially a rare or unexpected adverse event) temporally follows exposure either to a drug or a placebo, one must consider the possibility that the occurrence is random with no evidence for causality. When successful outcomes occur with unproven compounds (and, especially, when they are extolled in case reports), the same risk surrounding causal inference is unavoidable. However, unlike an RCT, in real-world practice this methodological dilemma is often *irrelevant* to the goals of treatment; unlike the clinical investigator, both the practitioner and the patient for better or for worse generally care less about *why* improvement occurs, so long as it does. This is a fundamental difference in the basic approach of research versus non-research-based treatment delivery.

Particularly in psychiatry, unless the prescriber is an unplugged vending machine, the dispensing of inert substances is *never* devoid of a meaningful placebo effect. Skilled clinicians knowingly or unknowingly capitalize on what psychotherapy researchers sometimes call the "nonspecific" factors that operate in psychotherapy; they actively listen, reassure, validate the legitimacy of concerns, reframe questions, and (intentionally or not) often incorporate psychotherapeutic techniques such as abreaction, clarification, and suggestion – consequently imposing a sense of order and containment over the distress typically associated with most forms of psychopathology. In psychotherapy research, the existence of a positive therapeutic alliance has been found to have an effect size of 0.26 (Horvath and Symonds, 1991). The act of simply asking structured interview questions about a patient's problems has been shown to diminish subjective distress, anxiety and depression in more than half of depressed patients (Scarvalone et al., 1996). So impactful is the sheer act of conducting an assessment interview that some study protocols deliberately restrict time durations for conducting assessments and prohibit empathic statements (e.g., "that must have been very difficult for you…"), lest inadvertent supportive psychotherapeutic exchanges contaminate the assessment à la the "observer effect" (just *assessing* the patient may alter their symptom presentation) plus a smattering of the Hawthorne effect (that is, just *knowing* that they are being assessed may also alter how patients present themselves).

Tip

In physics, the "observer effect" means that the act of measuring a phenomenon, in itself, unavoidably changes it.

Tip

The Hawthorne effect describes a situation in which individuals perform differently when they know they are being observed.

Fun Fact

The term "Hawthorne effect" was coined in 1958 to describe the phenomenon in which employees at the Western Electric factory in Hawthorne, Illinois were found to work harder and perform better when they knew they were being observed.

B CHARACTERISTICS OF PLACEBO RESPONSIVITY

Placebo response rates differ across psychiatric disorders and are influenced by an array of clinical factors, but certain patient-specific characteristics are worth noting that may help clinicians gauge the probability that someone may respond favorably to a pharmacodynamically inert substance – or, of equal importance, the chance that they may experience *adverse effects* when taking a placebo (the so-called *nocebo* effect, discussed further below). There is no consensus in the literature about whether a given patient who responds to a placebo for a particular psychiatric disorder at any one time will remain a "trait" placebo responder across possible future symptom recurrences, or across other psychiatric (or nonpsychiatric) disorders that may arise over time. However, most experts believe that situational factors are important; so much so that patient-specific factors are unlikely to account for enduring placebo effects within an individual over time. (And in part, placebo responsivity involves a learning or behavioral conditioning paradigm: according to Bayesian analysis, past treatment experiences influence outcome expectancies (i.e., revising the posterior probability of response), as new experiences serve to update prior probabilities.)

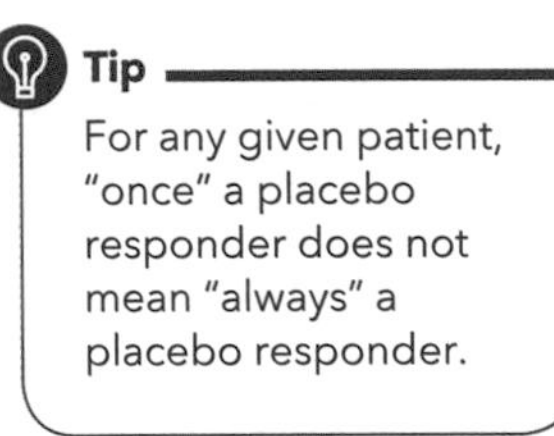

Tip
For any given patient, "once" a placebo responder does not mean "always" a placebo responder.

Formal studies of psychological factors that influence placebo responsivity in psychiatry tend to describe overlapping contributions of personality variables, situational variables, and expectancy factors (not just whether patients think they will or will not get better, or that an intervention is "powerful," but also the impact on patient behavior that comes from the act of observing and monitoring them – i.e., the Hawthorne effect). The interplay of psychological and neurobiological factors thought to underlie placebo responsivity is illustrated in Figure 4.1.

A vivid example of expectancy is illustrated in studies of major depression showing that the magnitude of antidepressant response to *open-label* SSRI is substantially greater than in patients who receive the identical drug without knowing whether it is the active agent or a placebo, particularly in younger patients – suggesting that patient expectancy ("hope induction" or "expectation bias" (Kasper and Dold, 2015)) is a mediator of the placebo effect (Rutherford et al., 2017). On the other hand, patients who have had a

Tip

A given patient's expectations about how symptoms are likely to change over time, and how effectively they can cope with symptoms, are among the strongest patient-specific determinants of placebo responsivity.

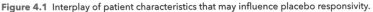

Figure 4.1 Interplay of patient characteristics that may influence placebo responsivity.

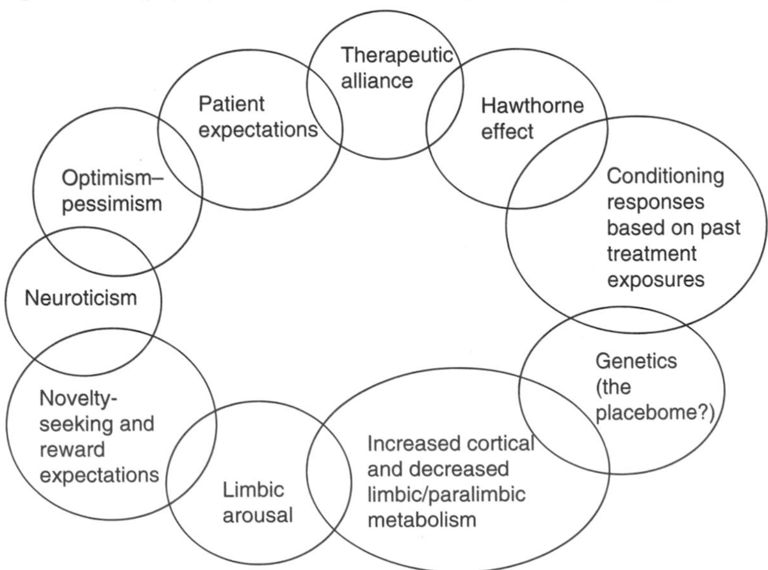

previous favorable response to an active drug may be less prone to a future placebo response, as has been shown in the case of crossover studies (Rickels et al., 1966).

Dosing Frequency

Have you ever dosed a psychotropic drug that has a long elimination half-life (say, olanzapine) more often than once a day, and at some point wondered why you were doing that? Sometimes we divide the dosing of long half-life drugs in the hopes of minimizing adverse effects (e.g., divalproex ER when orally loaded at 20–30 mg/kg for concerns of sedation and nausea, or iloperidone, for concerns about sedation and orthostatic hypotension). In the absence of tolerability concerns, the incentive for clinicians to *favor* otherwise unnecessary multiple daily doses may relate to hopes for optimizing the placebo contribution to outcome. For example, in studies of sham acamprosate in alcoholism, three-times-a-day dosing did not lessen treatment adherence and yielded better outcomes than did behavioral interventions without sham placebo – perhaps as a tangible "reminder of the reason for the pill taking," as noted by the study authors (Weiss et al., 2008). Number and color of pills, as well as dosing frequency, have all been identified in the literature as possible contributors to placebo responsivity.

Psychological and Personality Correlates

There is no well-established or validated "personality type" associated with placebo responsivity. It is intuitively compelling to imagine that traits such as suggestibility, openness to experience, introversion, or the need for social approval would predict placebo responsivity, but no personality characteristics have robustly been shown to determine response versus nonresponse to placebo in the case of analgesia or other clinical situations. Nevertheless, a number of such constructs have received particular attention as possible correlates of placebo and nocebo treatment responses, as summarized in Box 4.1.

Box 4.1

Correlates of Placebo and Nocebo Responses

- *Dispositional optimism* – defined as a generalized positive outcome expectancy, optimists tend to be more placebo-responsive than nonresponsive; similarly, dispositional pessimists are more likely than optimists to experience unpleasant (nocebo) effects from a placebo when apprised of discomfort as a likely consequence (Geers et al., 2005)
- *Low self efficacy* – referring to a person's diminished belief in their ability to execute behaviors that can achieve their desired goals
- Having an *external locus of control* – individuals with an *external* locus of control attribute their experiences and actions largely as *reactions* driven by the influence of the outside world (contrasted with an *internal* locus of control, where one fundamentally believes that his or her own decisions and actions critically shape how their life events unfold). "Externals," as dubbed by social psychologists, may be inclined to rely more on external than internal cues to guide inner experiences. Some authors have further suggested that low self-esteem may moderate the impact of external locus of control on placebo responsivity (Horing et al., 2014)
- *Novelty-seeking* – a personality component involving the predilection for pursuing unusual, complex, and intense experiences
- *Neuroticism* – as defined within the Five-Factor Model of Personality (see Chapter 2, Table 2.6), neuroticism is a trait feature that describes emotional instability, anxiousness, and depression

A related phenomenon that can psychologically influence drug responsivity, in the context of patient expectancies and the therapeutic alliance, is the *paradoxical injunction*. In essence, paradoxical injunctions involve "prescribing" the very symptom(s) the patient seeks to alleviate, structuring the treatment paradigm in such a way that the patient is more likely to defy than accept the clinician's pronouncement or instruction, as illustrated in Box 4.2.

Box 4.2

Clinical Vignette

Mark was a 27-year-old man with chronic (persistent) depression who had had minimal to no response to numerous antidepressant trials that had been thoughtfully and sequentially suggested by his psychiatrist. There was no psychosis, substance misuse, or other comorbidities, and medication adherence was more than adequate. Dispositional pessimism was abundant as were temperamental feelings that no one really cared about him, including his therapist, leading him to declare many times that his fate in life was, no doubt, to suffer interminably without hope for relief. One day he spontaneously mentioned that he had seen an advertisement for a new antidepressant on television and wondered if that might be worth trying. Rather than heaping

Box 4.2 (Cont.)

praise and optimism upon the new drug in hopes to generate expectancy of a success, the prescriber set a very low expectation by remarking that, candidly, he did not think the new drug was "anything special" and would probably not work that well, but Mark could try it if he wanted to. The gauntlet thus thrown down, Mark capitulated in the challenge to prove the prescriber wrong. When he began to report signs of feeling better after just a week, the prescriber scoffed and predicted that the obvious "placebo response" would not last. As Mark's improvement persisted, the prescriber continued to express puzzlement and a defeatism over his prediction that yet another pharmacological failure was inevitable. Put another way, the psychiatrist allowed Mark to regain psychological control over his ill-fated suffering by restoring his internal locus of control.

Neurobiological Correlates

Neurobiological correlates of placebo responsivity likely differ across disorders. In depression, functional neuroanatomical studies suggest that placebo responsivity appears associated with:

- increased metabolism in cortical regions (prefrontal, anterior and posterior cingulate, premotor, parietal, posterior insula), and
- regional decreased metabolism in subgenual cingulate, parahippocampus, thalamus (Mayberg et al., 2002).

Classical studies of analgesia response to placebo implicate the role of endogenous opioids (and their blockade by naloxone), as well as dopaminergic tracts involved in the reward pathway (expectancy of benefit). A handful of studies have examined potential associations between psychotropic placebo responsiveness and known genetic variants in candidate genes involved in catecholamine metabolism. Possible genomic correlates of the placebo response (dubbed by some as the "placebome") include dopaminergic, serotonergic, opioid, and endocannabinoid potential markers (reviewed by Hall et al., 2015). Examples are depicted in Box 4.3.

Tip

Neurotransmitter systems implicated in placebo responsivity include the serotonin, catecholamine, opioid, and endocannabinoid systems.

Box 4.3

Pharmacogenetic Correlates of Placebo Responsivity

- Preliminary studies have linked a known functional polymorphism involved in catecholamine metabolism (the high activity ("G") allelic variant of the *monoamine oxidase A* gene) with a diminished placebo response in depression (Leuchter et al., 2009);
- Homozygosity of the "G" variant in the G-703T polymorphism of the *tryptophan hydroxylase* promoter gene has been linked with greater placebo response in social anxiety than observed in "T" homo- or heterozygotes (Furmark et al., 2008);
- The Val^{158}Met polymorphism of *the catechol-O-methyltransferase (COMT) gene* affects degradation of dopamine; a G→A substitution at codon 158 leads to a Val→Met substitution which, in turn, makes for expression of a lower-activity variant of COMT. Lower COMT activity, in turn, means less dopamine degradation and therefore greater dopamine tone in prefrontal cognitive processing regions. This polymorphic variant has been linked with greater placebo responsivity in irritable bowel syndrome and a number of other disorders (Hall et al., 2012).

Caveat

As discussed further in Chapter 8, the utility of pharmacogenetic testing to help predict psychotropic drug response is limited and currently, like neuroimaging, represents more of a research probe than a practical tool for use in everyday patient care.

C ARE PLACEBO RESPONSE RATES ON THE RISE?

There has been controversy regarding the question of whether differences in response rates between antidepressants and placebo are less robust than has traditionally been thought. One key methodologic point of relevance is that placebo response could be rising over time as more and more industry-based trials strive to increase study enrollment and run the risk of enrolling patients who might meet only minimal entry criteria for depression symptom severity. Conflicting findings have been reported on this issue across meta-analyses. Examples are noted in Box 4.4.

Box 4.4

Examples of Reported Rising Placebo Response Rates Across Clinical Trials

- Rief and colleagues (2009) examined 96 RCTs that enrolled 9566 depressed patients from 1980–2005 and found a strong, significant correlation between publication year and observer-rated placebo-group effect size in RCTs for depression ($r = 0.41$, $p < 0.001$)
- Khan and colleagues (2017) examined 16 antidepressants across 85 FDA trials from 1987–2013 and found that the magnitude of placebo response, but also active drug response, has risen steadily by about 6% since 2000; the net magnitude of antidepressant-placebo differences has remained unchanged over the years
- A still larger meta-analysis of over 250 RCTs from 1978–2015 found that average placebo response rates have actually remained fairly constant over that several decade period (Furukawa et al., 2016)

Why these discrepancies? Furukawa et al. (2018a) found that rises in the year-by-year percentage of symptom reduction from placebo are no longer significant when controlling for the confounding effects of variable study durations, number of study sites, dosing schedules, and when comparing only studies conducted after 1991. In other words, methodological differences in study design over time may have artifactually but proportionally inflated both placebo and active drug response rates in depression.

In the case of antipsychotic RCTs for schizophrenia and schizoaffective disorder, significant increases in placebo response rates also have been observed from 1960 to 2013, despite overall decreases in effective dose medication arms (Rutherford et al., 2014). In a review of placebo versus antipsychotic RCTs from 1970–2010, Agid and colleagues (2013) found that placebo rates increased over the 40-year study period. In their large meta-analysis, extensive heterogeneity was found across studies, a phenomenon that meta-regression analysis identified as resulting from the *number of study sites per trial* and *a decrease in the number of academic sites*. Leucht and colleagues (2013b) point out a vicious cycle in large, multisite industry-sponsored drug trials: because smaller studies tend to report larger effect sizes (see Chapter 3, Box 3.6), multisite trials that strive to recruit larger numbers of subjects (to optimize the chances for statistical significance through adequate power to capture small or medium effects) essentially increase variability (heterogeneity) which, in turn, lowers between-group effect sizes – thereby inflating placebo response rates. Furthermore, acutely ill subjects recruited to participate in clinical trials must still be psychiatrically healthy enough to comprehend lengthy informed consent procedures (even if psychotic), pose no risk for imminent danger or self-harm (even though they may have originally been hospitalized because of such risks), and often have been "pretreated" during a screening period in which they are able to endure washouts of prior pharmacotherapies without gravely decompensating – collectively enriching samples for sufficiently lesser severity so as to enhance placebo responsivity.

D TRIAL DURATION AND PLACEBO RESPONSE

The potential relationship between trial duration and duration and placebo responsivity varies across disorders. In bipolar depression, for example, a meta-analysis and meta-regression of 17 RCTs identified longer trial duration and low baseline severity as the most robust predictors of placebo response. By contrast, in schizophrenia, a meta-regression of 32 RCTs of antipsychotics for primary psychotic disorders (i.e., schizophrenia, schizoaffective disorder, schizophreniform disorder) found an *opposite* effect:

Figure 4.2 Relationship between trial duration and placebo response in schizophrenia, schizoaffective disorder, and schizophreniform disorder.*

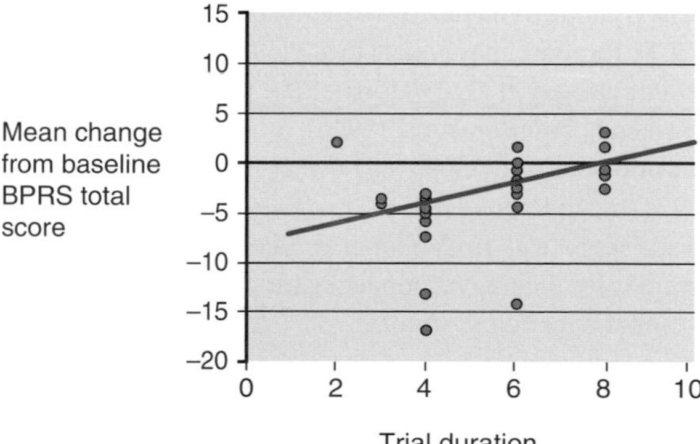

* adapted from Welge and Keck, 2003

The positive slope of the regression line indicates *less* improvement with placebo across successive weeks.

placebo response rates were higher when trials were *shorter* than 6–8 weeks, as depicted by the linear relationship in Figure 4.2 (Welge and Keck, 2003). The average placebo response *decreased* by about one BPRS point per week. In major depressive disorder, a review of 182 RCTs by Papakostas and Fava (2009) found no association with trial duration and magnitude of drug–placebo differences.

In studies of mood disorders, sheer separation of study drug from placebo is usually evident by the third or fourth study week post randomization, casting doubt on the necessity for favoring longer trials just to diminish the magnitude of the placebo effect. Also, as nonresponders tend to drop out prematurely over successive weeks, subjects who remain on placebo (or active drug) until the termination of a trial may in effect be an enriched group more representative of good-prognosis patients. At least some RCTs that had shown clear initial benefits ultimately failed due to loss of prior drug–placebo separation by the final study visit (e.g., as in the case of aripiprazole for acute bipolar depression).

E PREVALENCE ACROSS DISORDERS

Prevalence rates of placebo responsivity vary considerably across clinical trials of most psychiatric disorders. Comparative response rates across disorders also can be hard to judge in part because "response" is often conventionally defined differently across disorders. For example, as noted in Chapter 3, response rates in PTSD are often operationally defined as a rating scale (e.g., the Clinician-Administered PTSD Scale, or CAPS) improvement from baseline of ≥30%, while in OCD, response may equate to a ≥25% improvement (Montgomery et al., 1993) or ≥35% improvement from baseline (Tollefson et al., 1994b), or a Clinical Global Impressions (CGI) score of 1 ("very much improved") or "2" ("much improved"), irrespective of symptom rating scale score (e.g., Hollander et al., 2003a). Variable time frames for judging responder status also bear on making comparisons across studies.

Categorical outcomes such as "response" or "remission" are not always presented for all types of psychiatric disorders – making it hard in such instances to quantify the comparative magnitude of placebo versus active drug effects. For example, in RCTs for addictions, "response" is commonly defined based on time or duration parameters related to abstinence (e.g., zero use in past month, percentage days abstinent in past month). In the treatment of sleep disorders, outcome measures are usually noncategorical, mean group differences (e.g., sleep latency time, total sleep efficiency, number of wakings after sleep onset). In anorexia nervosa, we were unable to locate any published pharmacotherapy RCTs reporting outcomes as "response" or "remission" rates; all presented noncategorical mean differences in caloric intake, or comparative mean time until achieving a target weight.

As a rule of thumb, certain patient-specific characteristics have traditionally been associated with a higher likelihood of placebo responsivity across disorders, particularly low baseline severity. Study design factors linked with placebo responsivity include trials conducted in more recent years, and a greater number of study centers in multisite RCTs (e.g., Yildiz et al., 2015). Unbalanced randomization (that is, proportionally more subjects being assigned to active drug than placebo) has been associated with greater placebo responsivity across most disorders (Mallinckrodt et al., 2010; Weimer et al., 2015).

Table 4.1 at the end of this chapter provides a summary of placebo response or remission rates from RCTs as reported across major psychiatric disorders, alongside known correlates or predictors of placebo response. Note the observed distinctions between conditions associated with relatively low placebo response rates (e.g., bulimia, OCD) and higher placebo response rates (e.g., major depression, PTSD, alcohol use disorders). Note also from the table that social anxiety disorder appears to be the least placebo-responsive anxiety disorder.

High baseline severity appears throughout the literature as a robust moderator of drug–placebo differences, with only a handful of exceptions. Furukawa and colleagues (2018b) conducted an individual participant-level data meta-analysis using antidepressant trials conducted in Japan and found no significant interaction between baseline severity and treatment outcome (suggesting comparable antidepressant benefits in mild, moderate, or severe forms of depression); they argued that relationships based on group-level data pose an "ecological fallacy" that may not accurately reflect true relationships at the individual participant level.

Tip
High baseline symptom severity tends to suppress placebo responsivity.

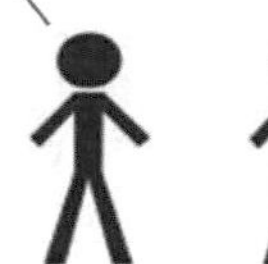

If depression can have such a large placebo effect then why is it so hard to find effective new treatments?
Precisely for that reason – drugs can be inherently quite effective but, if a placebo effect is substantial, even an effective drug may fail to separate from placebo. This brings us to the difference between failed versus negative trials, as previously discussed in Chapter 3. You should really go reread Chapter 3...

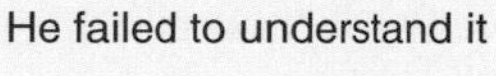

He failed to understand it

How negative

Definition

An *ecological fallacy* means that inferences about individuals cannot necessarily or reliably be drawn from observations about groups to which those members belong.

The observation elsewhere of higher drug–placebo differences in depressed patients with higher baseline severity could be "spun" as if to suggest that a medication works "especially well" in more severely ill cases, when the statistical reality is simply that high baseline severity merely suppresses a placebo response, thereby inflating the between-group effect size between drug and placebo (as opposed to increasing the within-group effect size inherent to the drug itself).

Let us consider a real-life example of a series of failed trials that were shown to be failed rather than negative thanks to careful analyses of the moderating effects of baseline severity (Box 4.5).

F ARE PLACEBO EFFECTS PERSISTENT OR FLEETING?

Despite lore that placebo responses tend to be transient, the limited literature that has empirically examined the longevity of placebo responses (mostly in depression) has been inconclusive. Early work by Quitkin and colleagues (1984), examining week-by-week response patterns, found that when acute antidepressant response occurred sooner than two weeks, effects tended not to endure, whereas responses noted only after two weeks tended to persist – arguing that response in the first two weeks suggested a placebo effect. Subsequently, when studying relapse after apparent initial response to fluoxetine, Stewart and colleagues (1998) observed that depressed patients who responded *only after two weeks* were more likely to sustain benefits for up to 50 weeks ("delayed and persistent," or "true drug response"), whereas those who appeared to "lose" their initial response were more likely to have had an early/nonpersistent ("placebo") response to the active drug.

Box 4.5

Example

In a pooled analysis of five industry-sponsored RCTs of lamotrigine for acute bipolar depression using individual patient-level data, Geddes and colleagues (2009) reported an interaction effect between baseline severity of depressive symptoms and response to lamotrigine versus placebo (meaning lamotrigine was superior to placebo in patients with high, but not moderate, baseline severity). As the authors acknowledge, the higher response rate was not because lamotrigine had an *intrinsically bigger effect* among more severely ill patients (as if to suggest that lamotrigine works especially well in sicker patients), but rather, that placebo response rates were less when baseline severity was high (baseline HAM-D scores ≥24):

	***Moderate* baseline severity**	***High* baseline severity**
Lamotrigine response rate	47.5%	45.4%
Placebo response rate	44.6%	**30.1%**

In contrast, in a review of eight RCTs encompassing 3063 depressed patients collectively randomized to antidepressant pharmacotherapy (about two-thirds) or placebo (about one-third), Khan and colleagues (2008) found that as many as four out of five placebo responders *sustained* their response for up to 12 weeks.

In panic disorder, placebo response has been noted to occur often within the first week and to persist during treatment taper and then at one month follow-up after study termination (Dager et al., 1990).

G ACTIVE VERSUS INACTIVE PLACEBOS

The "blinding" of clinical trials becomes dubious when an active drug commonly has marked or unmistakable adverse effects as compared to an inactive placebo. Features such as sedation, appetite stimulation, cognitive dulling, or nausea can all rather quickly break blinds inadvertently; in turn, clinical trial subjects who early on perceive no adverse effects and no obvious improvement may be more inclined to discontinue their study participation prematurely – that in turn can lead to systematic attrition in the placebo arm and loss of statistical power, as the subjects who opt to continue while on placebo are more likely those who perceive a benefit. For example, in trials of omega-3 fatty acids from fish oil in mood disorders, a simple whiff of study drug will likely end any uncertainty about whether or not the capsules' contents hail from briney origins. Ketamine, used in major depression, commonly causes unmistakable dissociation, while sedation from the antihistaminergic effects of quetiapine is similarly hard not to notice.

It is customary in RCTs to ask subjects to guess whether they think they had been taking placebo or active drug while they were participating in the study. While responses vary across disorders and study drug formulations, more than half of patients often correctly guess that they had been taking placebo, often based on a perceived lack of side effects.

Open-label Placebos

Yet another curiosity involves the outcomes of patients who are on open-label placebos – that is, they are made aware from the outset that they are taking a pharmacodynamically inert substance. In the case of major depression, for example, a randomized pilot study of open-label placebo, as compared to wait-list, observed after four weeks a significant improvement in depression symptom severity scores with a medium effect size ($d = 0.54$) (Kelley et al., 2012). Side-stepping the issue of deception, and capitalizing on the potential power of suggestion, investigators told subjects explicitly that the pills they were going to take had "no medicine in them" but that they might help the body to heal itself, and needed to be taken consistently in order to work. Some authors have advocated that because of their safety and apparent effect sizes, placebos for four to six weeks' duration should be considered among the appropriate first-line treatments for mild to moderate forms of depression (Brown, 1994).

H THE NOCEBO EFFECT

Nocebo effects are *bad consequences* caused by pharmacologically inert substances. In RCTs for major depression, up to nearly two-thirds of patients assigned to placebo report at least one adverse drug effect, and about 1 in 20 discontinues due to a significant side effect while taking placebo (Mitsikostas et al., 2014; Dodd et al., 2015). Few systematic studies have explored its correlates and possible predictors. In bipolar disorder, one meta-analysis of nine RCTs involving olanzapine found that adverse events occurred among 68% of subjects randomized to placebo, most often associated with an absence of treatment naiveté, younger age, having participated in a previous RCT, having a US geographic location, and being classified as obese (Dodd et al., 2019).

> **Tip**
> Nocebo effects refer to adverse (rather than beneficial) experiences attributed to a placebo.

While characteristics of the nocebo effect are vastly understudied, and its determinants remain more speculative than those linked with subjective benefits of placebos, the sheer existence of this phenomenon invites both theoretical and practical speculation about its impact on psychopharmacotherapy outcomes. Borrowing ahead from Chapter 10 ("Managing Major Adverse Drug Effects"), let us consider at least the psychological relationship between beneficial and adverse treatment effects, invoking what we shall call *Newton's Third Law of Psychopharmacology:*

> *For every intended drug effect there is an equal and opposite unintended effect.*

The above concept, more a postulate than a law, is meant to suggest that clinical benefits are often hard to come by without incurring at least some measure of adversity. To our knowledge no empirical studies have yet examined the correlation between nocebo effects and clinical response or nonresponse, but anecdotal observation reveals at least some instances in which RCT participants link the two:

- nocebo responders may construe adverse effects as the *tell* that *proves* they have been assigned to active drug (a phenomenon known as "side effect cueing"). Based on such expectancy (or hope induction), nocebo effects may actually represent welcome affirmation that true pharmacodynamic help must be on the way. Correspondingly, the absence of adverse effects may cause such patients to cast doubt on any previously more optimistic treatment expectations; *or*,
- nocebo effects might sometimes affirm for the patient quite the opposite expectation that help is forthcoming – rather, that they, the patient, are inescapably the object of torture and persecution, nearly always at the mercy of a menacing environment. Such a paranoid stance to the world can easily imbue placebos with as much power to wreak havoc as the sufferer's imagination will allow; *or*,
- somewhat less noxious, but no less potent, is a patient's projection of fear and anxiety onto a placebo as a kind of *tabula rasa*. Individuals with a high internal locus of control, or an ambivalent attachment style, may only grudgingly cede control over their bodily functioning to an external agent (a doctor, a medicine, a study protocol) and nocebo reactions may then serve as psychosomatic expressions of abject distress; *or*,
- the therapeutic alliance can be a mediator of nocebo as much as placebo phenomena, as discussed by Dodd and colleagues (2017); they note that perceived harm from a treatment may be especially likely to occur within the dynamic of a hostile-dependent treatment relationship when patients with an insecure attachment style are forced to rely on the benevolence and competence of the clinician entrusted with their care. Psychologically, such patients might develop adverse effects from placebos as a kind of test of the prescriber: nocebo effects provide a way to gauge whether the clinician possesses sufficient empathy and care-taking skills to notice and validate (and certainly not disavow) the sufferer's suffering, take apologetic ownership of it on their behalf (the prescriber caused it, whether inadvertently or deliberately), and muster some kind of credible reassurance that the victim will survive and go on to thrive despite the perceived hazard; *or*,
- the concept of *somatosensory amplification* refers to the phenomenon of experiencing normal bodily sensations as excessively intense and disturbing, and bears on the expectation of physical symptoms, particularly in the context of perceived threat to the integrity and well-being of one's physical functioning.

While there are no formal systematic studies that explore the psychological and neurobiological mechanisms that underlie nocebo responses, some preliminary CSI-style psychiatric sleuthing may allow us to draw some preliminary inferences.

Table 4.2 at the end of this chapter provides a summary of the most common adverse effects associated with placebo treatment arms across a range of FDA registration trials in psychiatry. From that table, we highlight in Box 4.6 a number of key points, summarizing nocebo effects reported with incident rates ≥10% among placebo recipients drawn from FDA registration trials of active psychotropic agents:

Box 4.6

Nocebo Effects

- *Headache*, *nausea* and *insomnia* comprise the most frequent adverse effects associated with placebo across trials for varied FDA drug indications
- As many as one-third of social anxiety disorder patients report headache while taking placebo, identical to the proportion taking active venlafaxine XR; similarly, in pooled OCD and MDD trials of fluvoxamine, reported incident rates of headache were disproportionately and comparably high for subjects taking either fluvoxamine (22%) or placebo (20%)
- MDD and OCD are among the conditions that appear to incur the most adverse effects from a placebo, while ADHD and bulimia appear to be the least nocebo-prone
- Weight gain was not commonly reported (≥10% incidence) with placebo (i.e., being simply an artifact

of the primary disorder being treated) in any FDA registration trials

- A strikingly high proportion of bipolar-manic or schizophrenia patients taking placebo had a ≥50% increase from baseline in fasting triglyceride levels, while LDL cholesterol levels rose ≥30% from baseline in 14% of placebo recipients, despite a mean weight loss of 0.3 kg (based on pooled data from short-term (six-week) olanzapine registration trials; data not shown in Table 4.2)
- Surprisingly, adverse effects from placebo among GAD patients were relatively infrequent (based on comparative trials with paroxetine, escitalopram, duloxetine, venlafaxine, and buspirone). In fact, "anxiety" or "nervousness" often occurred in <1% – perhaps suggesting a placebo benefit to the underlying condition. Premature trial discontinuations due to adverse events were uniformly <1% among GAD patients or panic disorder patients taking placebo
- In PTSD, sleep disturbances during placebo treatment were not disproportionately high, as one might otherwise expect
- Akathisia was observed in up to almost a quarter of schizophrenia patients taking placebo based on prospective systematic ratings of abnormal movements

In FDA registration trials, manufacturers' reporting of adverse effects of the kind described in Table 4.2 largely reflect subjects' spontaneous reporting rather than systematic prospective surveillance. As such, they are prone to under-reporting – which, for our purposes, means they are, if anything, conservative underestimates. With that in mind, it is noteworthy that *no* spontaneously reported adverse events occurred in ≥10% with placebo during FDA drug registration trials in MDD for escitalopram, fluoxetine, or lisdexamfetamine, or in schizophrenia RCTs, as compared to ziprasidone, brexpiprazole, or lurasidone.

I DRUG DISCONTINUATION EFFECTS

In RCTs, drug washout periods customarily involve cessation of medications that were being taken prior to enrollment in such a way that their discontinuation effects could potentially influence placebo effects after randomization. For example, some authors have argued that in bipolar disorder, abrupt cessation of lithium (over less than two weeks' duration) could hasten time until relapse in subjects subsequently randomized to placebo, as compared to those for whom a more gradual lithium discontinuation had occurred before assignment to placebo, artificially increasing the likelihood of clinical deterioration due to rebound. Similarly, short-half-life serotonergic antidepressants that are abruptly stopped have been associated with discontinuation syndromes involving an array of somatic complaints. Such phenomena could be confused with adverse effects of the next drug started, whether that was an active agent or a placebo, artificially inflating observations of adverse effects otherwise attributed to the study drug.

J MINIMIZING PLACEBO EFFECTS: IMPLICATIONS FOR STUDY DESIGNS

As multisite industry-sponsored clinical trials strive to minimize placebo response rates, no single strategy has been universally adopted, although many elements have been described and are often incorporated. These are summarized in Table 4.3.

In this approach, analyses are performed only on subject cells in the darkened boxes.

This offers the advantage of minimizing placebo effects and controlling for "early" placebo responses which could reflect nonspecific factors related to study participation other than placebo assignment per se. Subjects also may have up to two opportunities to receive active drug.

Figure 4.3 Sequential parallel comparison design.

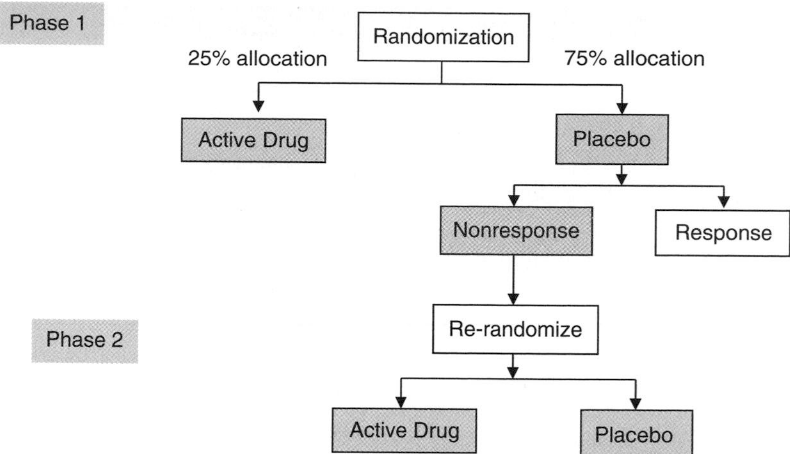

TAKE-HOME POINTS

- Placebo responses in psychiatry are often salient phenomena that can be substantial and vary considerably across disorders.
- They likely reflect a combination of nonspecific factors in the treatment paradigm, including the therapeutic alliance, expectations, conditioned responses to past experiences, and dispositional optimism/pessimism.
- Their effects are not necessarily transient and may endure depending on the clinical situation.

Table 4.1 Reported placebo response rates from clinical trials across disorders

Lower

Disorder	Reported placebo response rates	Reported predictors
Bulimia nervosa	Pooled = 8% (range: 0–11.8%) [1]	- None
OCD	- Range: 8.5% [2] to 26% [3] - Mean weighted ES (g) = 0.49 [4]	- Lower baseline severity [5]
Social anxiety disorder	- Range: 26% [6] to 46.6% [7] - Mean weighted ES (g) = 0.70 [4]	- Lower baseline severity [8] - Duration of disorder *not* predictive [8]
Panic disorder	- Response rate ~34% [9] - Mean weighted ES (g) = 0.94 [4]	- Fewer baseline panic attacks [9] - Less baseline distress, interpersonal sensitivity, paranoia [9] - Baseline severity *not* predictive [8]
GAD	- Response rates: 33.7–54.8% [8] - Mean weighted ES (g) = 1.10 [4]	- Duration of disorder and baseline severity both *not predictive* [8]
Binge eating disorder	- Pooled abstinence = 28.5% [10] - Pooled response = 38% [11]	- Low baseline severity [5,12] - Lower binge frequency at baseline [11] - Longer study participation [11] - Higher body mass index [5]
Bipolar mania	- Pooled response rate = 31% [13]	- Lower baseline severity [13] - Absence of psychosis [14] - Women [13,14] - Older age [13]
Bipolar depression	- Pooled response rate = 39% [15]	- Lower baseline severity (for each point on baseline HAM-D, placebo response decreased by 13.3%) [15] - *Longer* treatment duration [15]
ADHD	- Response range: 17–40% [16] - Placebo ES: g = 0.32 [16]	- Baseline severity (*lower* in some studies, [16] *higher* in others [17]) - Younger age [5] - Shorter duration of illness [5]
Schizophrenia	- 30% by PANSS ≥20%; 14% by PANSS ≥50% [18] - Mean PANSS change from baseline = 6.25 (95% CI = 4.64–7.85) [19]	- Younger age [19] - Baseline severity (*lower* in some studies, [20] *higher* in others [21]) - Shorter duration of illness [20] - *Shorter* study duration [20,22] - Women [23]
MDD	- Pooled response: 35–40%; [24] 22% if chronic [25] - Pooled placebo ES: d = 1.69 (if self-rated: d=0.67), [27] larger in MDD (d = 1.83) than dysthymia (d = 1.11) [26]	- Lower baseline severity [27] - Shorter duration of illness - Early onset (chronic depression) [25]
PTSD	- Response rates: 38% [28] to 43% [29] - Mean weighted ES (g) = 0.97 [4]	- History of sexual trauma [30] - Higher in civilian than combat [31]
Alcohol abuse/ dependence	- Median response rate: 77.5% vs. naltrexone, 39.1% vs. acamprosate [32]	- Placebo response negatively correlated with age or effect size of active drug [32]

Higher

Abbreviations: ADHD = attention deficit hyperactivity disorder; CI = confidence interval; ES = effect size; GAD = generalized anxiety disorder; MDD = major depressive disorder; OCD = obsessive-compulsive disorder; PTSD = post-traumatic stress disorder. Sources: [1] Bacaltchuk et al., 2000; [2] Tollefson et al., 1994a; [3] Montgomery et al., 1993; [4] Sugarman et al., 2017; [5] Weimer et al., 2015; [6] Careri et al., 2015; [7] Stein et al., 2010; [8] Stein et al., 2006; [9] Rosenberg et al., 1991; [10] Reas and Grilo, 2008; [11] Blom et al., 2014; [12] Jacobs-Pilipski et al., 2007; [13] Yildiz et al., 2011b; [14] Welten et al., 2015; [15] Nierenberg et al., 2015; [16] Waxmonsky et al., 2011; [17] Buitelaar et al., 2012; [18] Leucht et al., 2017; [19] Leucht et al., 2018; [20] Agid et al., 2013; [21] Chen et al., 2010; [22] Rutherford et al., 2014; [23] Mallinckrodt et al., 2010; [24] Furukawa et al., 2016; [25] Meister et al., 2017; [26] Rief et al., 2009; [27] Kirsch et al., 2008; [28] Davidson et al., 2001b; [29] Friedman et al., 2007; [30] Connor et al., 2001; [31] Davidson et al., 1997b; [32] Litten et al., 2013

Table 4.2 Most common adverse effects caused by placebo in FDA registration trials across indications for psychotropic agents[a]

	Occurrences in ≥10% of Subjects Taking Placebo										
FDA indication	**Headache**	**Dizziness**	**Nausea**	**Dry mouth**	**Diarrhea**	**Anorexia**	**Insomnia**	**Somnolence**	**Fatigue**	**Sexual dysfunct'n**	**EPS**
Adult ADHD	16–19%										
BP-mania	13-23%	12%	10–13%				11%	12–19%			12%
BP-depression	19%	11-13%	10%	13%				11-15%			
Bulimia			11%				10–13%				
GAD	11-18%	11%	11-17%	11%	12%		10%			25%	
MDD	15-26%		10-12%	12%	10%		11-16%	18%		14-20%	
OCD	20%		10-14%	10%	10-13%	10%	10-22%		10%		
Panic disorder		10%	12-18%	10-11%			10%	11%			
PTSD	14%		11-22%		15%		11%				
Schizophrenia	12-23%		11%				11-21%				15-23%
SAD	16-33%	16%					10-16%	16%			

Abbreviations: BP = bipolar disorder; EPS = extrapyramidal side effects; GAD = generalized anxiety disorder; MDD = major depressive disorder; OCD = obsessive-compulsive disorder; PTSD = post-traumatic stress disorder; SAD = social anxiety disorder

[a] based on data reported in manufacturer's product information insert pages

Table 4.3 Study design strategies to minimize placebo responsivity

Strategy	Description/Rationale	Pros	Cons
Single-blind placebo lead-in period	All subjects initially receive single-blind placebo (typically one to two weeks); nonresponders then randomize to begin active drug versus ongoing placebo	Theoretically enriches study design against subjects more likely to respond to placebo	Has not led to greater drug–placebo differences in MDD trials; may bias clinicians to underestimate early improvement
Use different rating scale to assess baseline severity from symptom change during course of the study	Tracking both baseline severity and improvement with the same scale risks enrolling subjects who "just barely" meet entry or responder criteria	Separate measures for entry eligibility and subsequent improvement minimize capturing equivocal status	Cases of borderline minimum severity for enrollment eligibility may still contribute to inflation of placebo effects
Use of off-site raters of symptom measures at follow-up visits	Independent raters, different from the study interviewer asking assessment questions, perform actual subject ratings based on their observations of the assessment interview	Possibly fosters more neutral or impartial ratings than would be obtained from a rater who has a therapeutic alliance with the subject	A rater who knows the subject well can rate symptoms from a more informed background context
Minimize the number of study sites	More study sites have been associated with higher placebo response rates across disorders	Using fewer carefully chosen investigator sites improves homogeneity	Practical limitations of finding sufficient high-quality sites to keep enrollment feasible and timely
Sequential parallel comparison design (Fava et al., 2003)	In a two-step approach, subjects who are initially randomized to placebo and do not respond are then rerandomized to active drug or placebo (see Figure 4.3).	Excludes patients responding to early effects of placebo, therapeutic alliance, and other nonspecific factors at treatment initiation; efficiently allows "reuse" of some subjects; can reduce needed sample size by 20–50%	Study may take longer; clinicians and investigators may be unfamiliar with methodology; may hamper "apples-to-apples" comparisons with older trials

5 Tailoring the Fit: Moderators and Mediators of Treatment Outcome

LEARNING OBJECTIVES

- ☐ Define and understand the role of moderators and mediators in clinical psychopharmacology trials
- ☐ Discuss the moderating effects on drug treatment outcome with key factors such as baseline clinical severity, demographic factors, age at onset, chronicity, episode number, duration of untreated illness, and history of trauma
- ☐ Recognize the mediating effects on treatment outcome of medication nonadherence, pharmacokinetic interactions, interpersonal factors, and comorbid disorders

I often wonder why the whole world is so prone to generalise. Generalisations are seldom, if ever, true and are usually utterly inaccurate.

- Agatha Christie

It is much more important to know what sort of a patient has a disease than what sort of a disease a patient has.

- Sir William Osler

A ONE SIZE FITS ONE

Previous chapters have described ways in which "real-world" patients usually present with a diversity of psychiatric, medical, psychosocial, and other features that make a "one-size-fits-all" approach to treatment problematic. Large-scale randomized trials typically favor diagnostic uniformity so that all enrolled subjects more or less display the same kinds of symptoms under study. Consequently, the controlled trials literature that informs evidence-based practice largely comes from rarified, homogeneous study groups with rigidly defined diagnostic criteria. As a result, such studies trade off optimal outcomes ("efficacy") for generalizability ("effectiveness") under more ordinary conditions. This is why so-called "effectiveness" studies such as the Clinical Antipsychotics Treatment Intervention Effectiveness trial (CATIE; see Chapter 15) strive to enroll representative patients with comorbidities, imperfect treatment adherence, and issues with drug tolerability, adopting "bottom line" primary outcome measures such as "all-cause dropout." No matter how well a treatment *can work*, the pragmatic concern remains how well it actually *does work* in real-life settings.

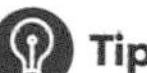

Tip

Treatment *efficacy* refers to how well a treatment can work under optimized conditions; *effectiveness* refers to how well an efficacious treatment actually performs under ordinary clinical conditions.

In routine treatment settings, outcomes can vary greatly when clinicians extrapolate from idealized patient types to more heterogeneous groups, whose actual problems may only faintly resemble those seen in study patients. Obviously, not everyone with the same overarching diagnosis responds to the same treatment, for many reasons. Therefore, we will now consider how to dissect the varied clinical elements that define and make every case unique, and use those characteristics to forecast likely outcomes and inform best pharmacotherapy decisions.

Like fingerprints, most patients have unique identifiable features that distinguish them from other people with the same overall condition. Those unique attributes create a biosignature that discriminates the

Bespoke Psychopharmacology

Like a made-to-measure suit individually tailored to the dimensions of a single wearer, "bespoke" psychopharmacology takes into account each patient's defining characteristics in order to craft the best-fitting regimen *for them*.

individual from the group, and thus may influence (and sometimes even govern) the usefulness of a particular treatment. Knowledge of someone's distinctive clinical features is central to the concept of personalized medicine. It encompasses not only potential biomarkers (e.g., pharmacogenetics, as discussed more fully in Chapter 8) but also a wide range of clinical and demographic characteristics. By creating a case-by-case profile of those patient-specific elements that affect treatment outcome– called moderators and mediators – one can better refine the goodness-of-fit between a specific patient (rather than a general diagnosis) and a candidate therapy.

B MODERATORS AND MEDIATORS OF TREATMENT RESPONSE

Moderators are factors that statistically influence the strength of a relationship between two variables. In clinical trials, moderators are essentially covariates that spell out the characteristics of *who is most likely to benefit from a particular treatment. Mediators* are factors that influence *how to obtain the best treatment outcomes.* Generally speaking, mediators describe events or clinical features that can impact *how the treatment is delivered after it has been started.* They also help to identify possible mechanisms that may explain how a treatment produces a desired effect. (For instance, a drug useful for weight loss could mediate that effect by suppressing appetite (e.g., amphetamine) or curbing the urge to binge-eat (e.g., topiramate) or enhancing insulin sensitivity (e.g., metformin). Or, a stimulant could effectively reduce anxiety if anxiety is mediated by inattention.) As described by Kraemer (2016), moderators and mediators are ways of drawing population inferences with respect to "what might be learned from trial reports that apply to a clinician's own patients"(p. 672). As such, this concept represents a cornerstone for the main thesis of this book – how to translate findings from evidence-based trials into real-world clinical practice.

Tip

A moderator that is *not irrelevant* to treatment outcome is said to be a *predictor*.

Terminology

Moderators are *baseline* (pretreatment) patient characteristics that affect outcome (i.e., who should get the treatment).

Mediators are factors that influence outcomes after a treatment has begun (such as nonadherence, drug–drug interactions or adverse effects).

Moderators can be clinical, demographic, or other patient pretreatment baseline characteristics (such as body weight, family history, or genotype) that can increase or decrease the likelihood of a response to treatment for an otherwise broadly defined ailment. For example, age at illness onset could moderate the effects of an antidepressant on depression symptom improvement, or a poor metabolizer genotype could increase the chances for developing adverse effects of a particular medication in distinct patient subgroups. Interestingly, and surprisingly, in a post hoc hierarchical modeling analysis of STAR*D Level 1 data in MDD, socioeconomic variables (notably, income and education level) were more robust predictors of antidepressant response to citalopram than were symptoms or other clinical factors (Jain et al., 2013). Other known demographic moderators of poor treatment response in MDD include living alone and having less than a high school education (Hirschfeld et al., 1998). Socioeconomic status (SES) can be a spurious covariate of other "good prognosis" moderating or mediating factors, such as access to health care, supportive living arrangements, higher functioning due to employment, and better physical health and nutrition.

Quotable

"Ignored moderators may be one explanation for why so many psychiatric treatments appear to have such low effectiveness." (Kraemer, 2016)

Biomarkers as Treatment Moderators

Psychopharmacology has long aspired to identify laboratory or other biological markers that could predict treatment response, and perhaps help to validate distinct illness subtypes. In the 1970s, such efforts focused heavily on endocrine correlates of depression (such as morning serum cortisol levels, or the dexamethasone suppression test) or urinary or cerebrospinal fluid (CSF) monoamine metabolites; in the 1990s and early 2000s attention turned more to functional and structural neuroimaging, event-related potentials (ERPs, which are measurable EEG (electroencephalography) waveforms in response to auditory or sensory stimuli) and quantitative EEG (qEEG) waveform parameters; more recently, the search for biomarkers has incorporated pharmacogenetics and proteomics (the latter referring to the entirety of proteins synthesized by an individual, and the effort to match optimal treatments with their effects on protein markers).

One example of a systematic undertaking devoted to the search for possible biomarkers of antidepressant drug response is the 17-site International Study to Predict Optimised Treatment in Depression (iSPOT-D). Conducted from 2008–2012, iSPOT-D enrolled 1008 depressed patients with the primary aim to gather prospective data on potential biomarkers such as pharmacogenetics, cognitive styles, emotional resilience, electrophysiology (EEG and ERPs) and neuroimaging to determine their moderating effects on treatment outcomes during standardized open randomized antidepressant trials.

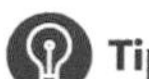

Tip

Hypothesis-generating studies are exploratory investigations meant to gather preliminary observations from which formal hypotheses can then be formulated and tested a priori. Their findings are by definition provisional and intended to prompt future study, rather than provide definitive evidence for uptake into clinical practice.

Elsewhere in medicine, some biomarkers are indisputably well-established (e.g., Gram stain properties of a bacterial culture in choosing an antimicrobial, tumor markers when selecting an antineoplastic). Until the validity of a suspected biomarker is confirmed by replication studies, its potential value is as a tentative "proof-of-concept" finding. As exciting or interesting as a suspected biomarker relationship may be, it is important for clinicians not to embrace prematurely a provisional finding as dogma – recapitulating Sherlock Holmes's admonition at the beginning of Chapter 1 that premature conclusions before one has sufficient data can bias thinking. In the language of EBM, studies that yield provisional findings would be called "hypothesis-generating" rather than "hypothesis-testing." Biomarkers, as yet, remain at best experimental as potential moderators (predictors) of treatment response. As such, we present information about biomarkers more to provide clinicians with a broader context for understanding possible correlates of pharmacodynamics and pharmacokinetics, rather than as a practical tool ready for use at the bedsides – at least, not quite yet.

Examples of representative provisional biomarkers of pharmacotherapy outcomes are described in Table 5.1 at the end of this chapter. In particular, neuroimaging as a possible biomarker of psychotropic drug response often relies on a technique known as diffusion tensor imaging (DTI), which is explained in Box 5.1.

Box 5.1

A Quick Primer on Diffusion Tensor Imaging

Diffusion tensor imaging (DTI) is an fMRI-based neuroimaging technique using the diffusion of water molecules to identify white matter tracts (also called white matter tractography), creating two- and three-dimensional images of cortical and subcortical networks. The term *isotropy* means that a structure has uniform shape in all directions (such as a sphere); in DTI, *anisotropy* refers to the uneven diffusion of water, as might occur due to structural disruption of axonal myelination. *Fractional anisotropy* (FA) is a measure in DTI that describes the degree of intactness of white matter tracts, scored as a ratio from zero (perfectly spherical) to one (perfectly linear). Well-defined fiber tracts generally have FA larger than 0.20. Increases in FA pre- to post-treatment, at least in theory, are thought to reflect improved white matter structural integrity. Whole-brain DTI tractography has been used to model brain structural networks. The term *connectome* has been coined to describe such a comprehensive network map of brain circuitry, and connectomic changes pre- and post-treatment represent a possible biological correlate of pharmacological treatment response.

If a biomarker of an illness is also a moderator of treatment outcome, is that synonymous with its being an intrinsic property that contributes to defining the disease itself, like methicillin-resistant *Staph. aureus*? Not necessarily. An elevated white blood cell count may be one biomarker of an infection, but it could be a sign of many things besides an infection. And the absence of an elevated white blood cell count does not rule out the possibility of an infection, but may be a clue that the patient could be immunocompromised. A disease also could have no measurable biomarkers – such as migraine headaches, or tinnitus – in which case "tailored" therapies depend more on clinical characteristics than on any laboratory guidance.

C RELATIONSHIP CONFOUNDERS AND INTERACTIONS

To further complicate things, one moderator could interact with another in ways that confuse or obscure a "real" relationship – for instance, SSRIs can more effectively reduce drinking behavior in late-onset than early-onset alcoholism, but that relationship, in turn, may be moderated by genotype of the serotonin transporter gene polymorphism (5HTTLPR) (Kranzler et al., 2011). A large multisite study of baseline EEG to predict antidepressant response found that right frontal alpha asymmetry moderated SSRI (but not SNRI) response, but only in women (Arns et al., 2016), whereas a larger N1 amplitude has been shown to moderate venlafaxine response, but only in men (van Dinteren et al., 2015). Greater DLPFC functional activity during a continuous performance task was associated with antidepressant improvement, but only in the absence of childhood maltreatment (Miller et al., 2015).

With respect to clinical moderators, for example, consider the following:

- Rejection sensitivity (within the constellation of "atypical" depressive features) is sometimes considered a possible predictor of a better response to an MAOI than to a tricyclic (e.g., Quitkin et al., 1993), but rejection sensitivity itself also correlates with early age at onset (Benazzi, 2001). Which of these two factors is the more robust predictor of response – or are they additive? Or collinear?
- Suppose that baseline severity of a condition predicts pharmacotherapy response/nonresponse, but a history of childhood trauma and age at illness onset both predict baseline severity. Which of these independent variable(s) then most directly drives treatment outcome, or does collinearity among the predictor variables interfere with demonstrating statistical significance?

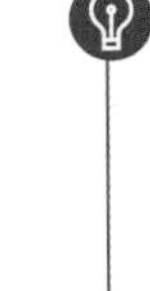

Tip

The statistical term *collinearity* is used to describe situations in which two or more independent/ predictor variables are themselves highly correlated, consequently diminishing their significance to explain the observed variation in a dependent variable.

The kinds of potential moderator variables that we consider in psychiatry are often inter-related and can be organized within broad clusters that overlap at least partially in the cognitive, behavioral, and emotional processes they tap. The mosaic depicted in Figure 5.1 portrays overlaps among various mental constructs that are conceptually related, and therefore potentially collinear as independent variables.

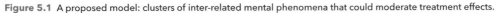

Figure 5.1 A proposed model: clusters of inter-related mental phenomena that could moderate treatment effects.

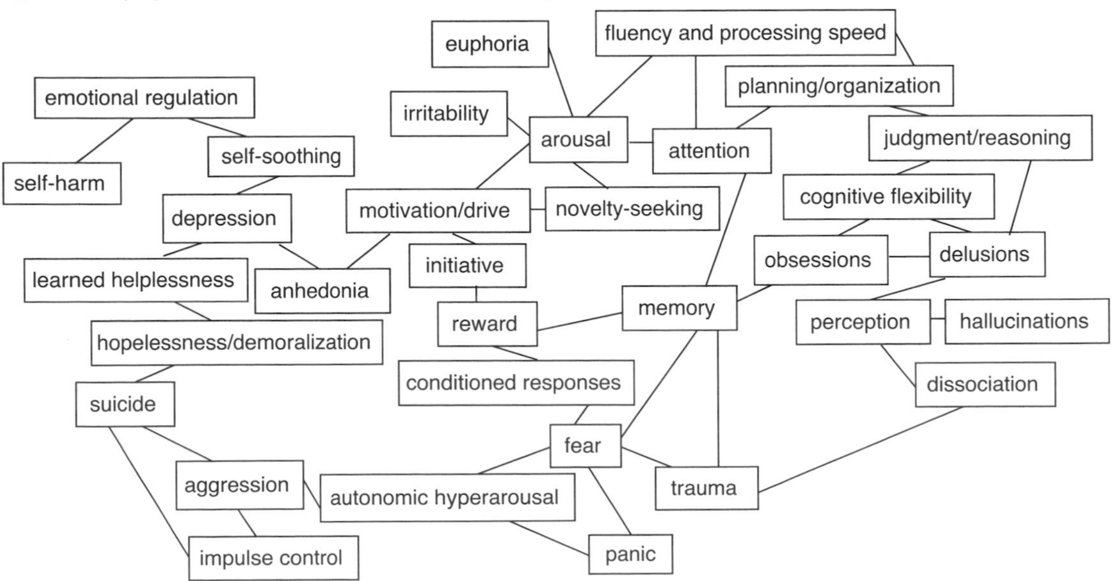

D TRUE OR SPURIOUS RELATIONSHIPS?

When more than one study is done to replicate an initial finding, credibility for a suspected moderating relationship is strengthened. Provisional evidence for a suspected moderating relationship comes not only from preliminary research studies but, no less importantly, from observations made by astute clinicians. Practitioners who suspect that a causal connection may exist between treatment response and a possible moderating factor might usefully ask themselves questions that draw on the Bradford Hill criteria for causation (see Chapter 1), such as an identifiable, plausible cause-and-effect mechanism, or a clear temporal relationship between the suspected moderator and treatment exposure.

In trying to craft an optimal treatment for a single patient based on their clinical characteristics, one could round up more than enough potential treatment moderators to take the bespoke approach to preposterous extremes if the relevance of any given treatment correlate is unclear (as when considering political and religious affiliations, favorite sports teams, and astrological sign; see Box 5.8 for more about the latter). Barring the absurd, let us now systematically consider established moderators of treatment outcome as they may bear individually and collectively for a given patient.

E SPECIFIC EXAMPLES OF TREATMENT MODERATORS

1. Baseline Severity

As noted in Chapter 4, high baseline severity suppresses placebo responsivity, which in turn makes baseline symptom severity a common moderator of drug–placebo differences. A problem related to low baseline severity as a predictor of response involves the "floor effect" posed by not enough variance in the range of scores. It is harder to halve a Hamilton Ratings Scale for Depression score of 8 (defining response) than a score of 28. Higher baseline severity affords the potential for more variance, according to the so-called "law of initial value" (also sometimes called Wilder's law). Thus, it remains at issue whether high baseline severity *diminishes, amplifies,* or *has no effect* on the within-group effect size of *active drugs* for certain psychiatric disorders.

> **Wilder's Law**
>
> Wilder's "law of initial value" states that the larger an initial value on a clinical rating, the greater the potential for observing a larger magnitude of change.

There exists at least some evidence on both sides of this uncertainty. Examples are listed in Box 5.2.

Box 5.2

> **High Baseline Severity Lessens Placebo Effect But *Not* Active Drug Effect**
>
> - Meta-analysis of 35 antidepressant trials (involving fluoxetine, sertraline, paroxetine, nefazodone) for MDD submitted to the FDA (Kirsch et al., 2008)
> - Meta-analysis of five olanzapine trials in bipolar mania (Samara et al., 2017)
> - Patient-level meta-analysis of six antidepressant RCTs for MDD; small between-group effect sizes observed in mild, moderate, or severe depression but larger effect sizes were evident for patients with very severe baseline symptoms (Fournier et al., 2010)
> - Patient-level meta-analysis of five RCTs of lamotrigine for bipolar depression (comparable response rate for high- and low-severity patients on active drug) (Geddes et al., 2009)
> - Patient-level meta-analysis of six RCTs of antipsychotics for schizophrenia demonstrate comparable active drug efficacy regardless of baseline severity (Furukawa et al., 2015)

> **High Baseline Severity Lessens Both Placebo Effect *and* Active Drug Effect**
>
> - Meta-analysis of 19 antidepressant trials in late-life depression; baseline severity moderated improvement with both drug and placebo (Locher et al., 2015)

In fact, following Wilder's law, high baseline severity in RCTs can often be a predictor of *better* response to an active drug, not simply by suppressing placebo responsivity but by allowing for greater variance in the active treatment arm with which to see clinically meaningful change. This aspect of EBM can create an annoying artifact for clinicians, whose concern is less about Wilder's law than about knowing what sort of patient may fare best with what particular drug. High baseline severity fundamentally in no way equates to an inherently better prognosis with a particular drug; rather, it simply means there exists more room for visible improvement to occur as compared to scenarios in which initial symptom severity may be subtler. One must not confuse baseline severity as a potential treatment moderator with a drug having a large or very large effect size. Highly robust, "big gun" interventions such as clozapine in refractory schizophrenia, or olanzapine/fluoxetine combination in treatment-resistant depression (TRD), or even electroconvulsive therapy in severe melancholic depression often become niched as such partly because each may work better and more reliably than most alternative options in more overall severe or treatment-resistant cases.

2. Age

In and of itself, age is a difficult factor about which to draw conclusions regarding treatment effects. Sometimes, extremes of age alter treatment outcomes because of pharmacokinetic rather than pharmacodynamic effects (e.g., impaired hepatic metabolism or renal excretion in the elderly, or immature functioning of Phase I or Phase II hepatic metabolism in youth); sometimes, for reasons not always obvious, certain age groups may demonstrate inherent paradoxical effects with psychotropic medications (such as an increased rather than decreased risk for suicidal thoughts or behaviors in depressed children and adolescents who take an antidepressant). From an EBM perspective, one must also acknowledge that if a drug has not been well-studied in a particular age group, the limitations of extrapolation may make it impossible to know with confidence whether pharmacodynamic effects will or won't be similar to those seen in adults.

Increasing age also poses confounding factors with other issues that influence treatment outcome: for example, older patients have had more time to successfully negotiate their developmental milestones and consequently shore up their equity in terms of occupational, psychosocial, and financial resources. They have usually endured more normal stressful events that could enhance their capacity for resilience. Age also provides a benchmark for gauging whether a particular psychiatric presentation falls within an expectable epidemiologic framework; new-onset psychosis after age 50 is anomalous, as is mania before age 10. Anomalies mean deviation and extrapolation from the more predictable generalizations associated with common clinical presentations.

Age has emerged as a significant moderator of pharmacotherapy response in only a handful of instances. Best-known perhaps is the database leading to the FDA boxed warning regarding the risk for suicidality for all products that have established antidepressant properties: regardless of diagnosis, individuals ≤24 years of age may have an increased risk for developing new suicidal thoughts or behaviors after beginning a medication that treats depression.

3. Early Age at Onset

Arguably, early age at onset may be the most ubiquitous and robust negative predictor of any ailment imaginable. At a biological level, early onset raises question about the idea of genetic anticipation and the possibility of an especially virulent form of illnesses that have at least some heritability. At the same time, early age at onset as a variable is often collinear with a multitude of other poor prognosis variables across many if not most psychiatric conditions, making it difficult for clinicians to know if the presence of early age at onset in and of itself represents a likely negative moderator of treatment response or if, instead, it functions more as a clue about the likely presence of other (collinear) moderating factors that exert a more proximally detrimental effect on outcome (rather like making the observation that people who carry cigarette lighters seem more prone to develop lung cancer).

4. Chronicity

As a rule of thumb, longstanding and entrenched problems tend to be more difficult to leverage. In part, this may reflect disease pathology (e.g., possible neuroprogression with neuronal loss in the case of schizophrenia, dementia, and perhaps some mood disorders) as well as the psychosocial adaptations (or maladaptations) and consequences resulting from persistent disability. Like unwanted houseguests who overstay their welcome, chronic mental illnesses often lead their sufferers (the "hosts") to make lifestyle accommodations and increasingly take for granted the unshakable reality imposed by their symptoms and their consequent circumstances.

On the other hand, longer duration of illness (>10 years) better differentiates antidepressant from placebo response in geriatric depression (Nelson et al., 2013). This could in part have more to do with assuring a lack of placebo in chronic depression rather than the implication that antidepressants in themselves "work better" in chronically ill people. In psychotic depression, duration of the index episode was a strong predictor of relapse after stopping an antipsychotic in favor of continued antidepressant monotherapy (Rothschild et al., 2003).

Other conditions for which chronicity has been recognized as a predictor of poor treatment response include OCD (as shown during open-label fluoxetine trials; Storch et al., 2006).

5. Episode Number

Related to chronicity is the number and cumulative duration of occurrences of a recurring ailment (sometimes also called "illness burden"). The more heart attacks or strokes someone incurs, the harder it usually becomes to fix the underlying problem. In epilepsy, increasing episode number is described in the so-called "kindling" paradigm, in which someone's first few lifetime seizures may be easier to treat than their umpteenth seizure. (Akin to the way a fire eventually results after enough friction and rubbing of sticks has transpired.) The neurological concept of kindling has been borrowed as an analogy to explain the greater treatment challenges frequently seen in multiepisode mood disorders. A linked notion, called behavioral sensitization, also involves the idea that whatever environmental factors may play a role in precipitating the first few occurrences of an illness, such external factors play a lesser and lesser important role as more episodes happen, as the disease process becomes increasingly automatic.

As one common example, consider the frequent observation in the literature that lithium carbonate seems to work better in treating or preventing recurrences in bipolar disorder when it is begun no later than the first few episodes. This represents a specific rationale for favoring lithium in first-episode mania, all else being equal, because the first episode may offer the most robust opportunity for lithium to work. In contrast, divalproex has been shown to be effective for treating mania even after the passage of multiple episodes (Swann et al., 1999). Alternatively, in major depression, the number of past episodes has *not* been shown to moderate drug–placebo differences in comparative studies of SSRIs or SNRIs (Dodd et al., 2013).

6. Duration of Untreated Illness (DUI)

Also conceptually linked to chronicity, there has been ongoing debate in the literature as to whether a prolonged duration of untreated mental illness in itself confers a negative prognosis on treatment outcome. Such a concept is obvious in oncology or infectious diseases, where disease progression inexorably takes its own toll if left unchecked. In psychiatry, more uncertainty exists about whether or not disease progression (sometimes called "neuroprogression") is quite so literally as comparable and inexorable a process as is the case in, say, sepsis. Some researchers believe that mood disorders and psychotic disorders such as schizophrenia unquestionably are not only chronic but also degenerative conditions, where the thinking is that delayed initiation of appropriate treatment doesn't merely cause prolonged suffering and adverse psychosocial consequences, but could in fact make for a poorer outcome because of actual unaverted apoptosis (neuronal death) or loss of neuroplasticity.

Part of the challenge here involves the as-yet undemonstrated role for psychotropic drugs to either arrest or reverse a clear degenerative process – as opposed to serving more as a kind of chemical prosthesis to compensate for impaired function. If someone might develop hypertension in the future, antihypertensive drugs in the present likely confer no physiologically prophylactic benefit. Similarly, wearing eye glasses helps far-sighted people see close-up objects better, but probably does nothing to forestall eventual presbyopia. In the case of psychotropic drugs, this is largely why "neuroprotective" or "neurotrophic" properties are extolled; medications such as lithium that can, in vitro, prevent cell death or increase synaptic sprouting and neuropil density are presumed remedies capable of averting future neural devastation. However, whether or not this truly occurs in actual patients is quite speculative. Indeed, the handful of studies done thus far with atypical antipsychotics in young people "at risk" for psychosis (who may have a strong genetic loading but have not yet manifested a clear psychotic episode) have not been terribly persuasive in showing that early intervention staves off the *risk* for psychosis.

A prolonged rather than brief duration of untreated mood, psychotic, anxiety, or other psychiatric symptoms probably does no one any good, but complications may arise more from psychosocial than neurobiological consequences, as employers and families become less tolerant, and economic and occupational ramifications amplify. DUI also can be confounded by poor premorbid adjustment, inasmuch as the latter carries its own negative prognostic implications and additionally can make patients less inclined to seek or follow through with treatment. Psychologically, a prolonged DUI may also lead patients to find themselves reflexively accepting their "new normal" rather than taking a proactive stance to reverse a deteriorating set of circumstances.

DUI has been identified as an independent moderator of treatment response (while controlling for other baseline predictor variables) in:

- first-episode psychosis (Conus et al., 2017; Marshall et al., 2005) as well as very long-term outcome in schizophrenia (Primavera et al., 2012)
- first-episode MDD (across three pooled studies, relative risk (RR) for response with shorter DUI = 1.70) (Ghio et al., 2014)

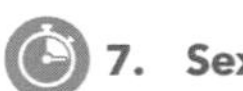

7. Sex

Perhaps surprisingly, there is not an extensive literature to suggest that sex differences in psychotropic drug response are generally robust. Indeed, differential treatment outcomes by sex tend more to be the exception than the rule. For example, adjunctive thyroid hormone in bipolar depression may work better in women than men (Stamm et al., 2014b) – but then again, sex could be a spurious association, if it turned out that women in this particular study had an over-representation of rapid cyclers, or bipolar II patients, or some other unrecognized confounding factor. Sometimes, sex differences artifactually contribute to pharmacodynamic differences, as in the case of women taking estrogen-containing oral contraceptives – or entering the third trimester of a pregnancy – which could induce the Phase I hepatic metabolism of SSRIs and some anticonvulsants, among other agents.

As is the case with many demographic moderators, the demonstrated predictive value of sex differences on psychotropic treatment outcomes is rather limited, and most studies that have included sex among independent variables in devising predictor models of treatment response have revealed nonsignificant findings. Nevertheless, known examples are listed in Box 5.3.

8. Race and Ethnicity

Racial and ethnic differences can exert bona fide effects on how people metabolize a drug or otherwise may be predisposed to unusual reactions – for example, Ethiopian Blacks are much more likely than other groups to be ultra-rapid metabolizers for the cytochrome P450 2D6 genotype, causing them to have little if any effect from drugs metabolized by that liver enzyme. Some Asian groups may be genetically more at risk than other groups for developing Stevens–Johnson syndrome when taking carbamazepine. Extrapyramidal adverse effects from some antipsychotic medications have been shown to be more common among Latin Americans than Whites, and African Americans may be more prone than Whites to develop weight gain or other adverse metabolic effects from atypical antipsychotics such as olanzapine. However, race represents another complex factor with many of its own built-in confounding factors; while it could represent a source for differential pharmacokinetic or even pharmacodynamic effects, racial group differences could also reflect stratification for other important characteristics that affect treatment outcomes, such as access to quality healthcare, nutrition, and general physical health, or socioeconomic factors that in themselves could moderate treatment outcomes.

9. History of Suicide Attempts

Suicidal thoughts or behaviors are sometimes regarded as proxies for illness severity, but in themselves make an independent contribution to treatment responsivity. For example, in first-episode psychosis patients, symptomatic remission was less likely in patients with a history of having made a suicide attempt (independent of, and alongside other studied predictors, such as baseline severity and duration of untreated illness) (Conus et al., 2017).

Box 5.3

Examples Where Sex is a Demographic Moderator

- S-adenosylmethionine (SAMe) for MDD (greater improvement in women > men; Sarris et al., 2015)
- Women may respond more poorly than men to fluoxetine for treatment of GAD (Simon et al., 2006b)
- Women may respond better than men to sertraline for panic disorder (Clayton et al., 2006) and to SSRIs in general for treatment of MDD (Khan et al., 2005)
- Menopausal status may further moderate gender differences in the pharmacotherapy of chronic depression: premenopausal women have been shown to respond better to sertraline than imipramine, while postmenopausal women have shown equivalent response rates to either antidepressant (Kornstein et al., 2000)
- Supraphysiologically dosed levothyroxine in bipolar depression was not different from placebo overall, but was superior to placebo only among women (Stamm et al., 2014b)

10. Baseline Anxiety

High baseline anxiety was notoriously identified as a robust predictor of poor antidepressant response in the STAR*D MDD trials, as well as numerous other individual pharmacotherapy RCTs for depression (reviewed by Bagby et al., 2002, who note that, "There are relatively few studies in which the existence of a comorbid anxiety disorder was not predictive of nonresponse"). See Box 5.4 for a sidebar discussion on the potential association between bupropion and anxiety in the course of treatment for depression.

Box 5.4

> **Is Bupropion Really Anxiogenic?**
>
> Contrary to lore and popular perception, high baseline anxiety or insomnia were found *not* to predict nonresponse to antidepressant outcomes with bupropion (Rush et al., 2005); its effect on anxiety symptoms coexisting with depression appears comparable to that of sertraline (Trivedi et al., 2001). In a review of 10 RCTs in anxious depression, no differences were observed between bupropion and SSRIs in improvement in depression or improvement in anxiety (Papakostas et al., 2008).

11. Childhood Trauma

Childhood trauma has received growing attention in the literature as a negative prognostic factor, and covariate of psychiatric comorbidities and greater treatment complexity, across a variety of conditions. Reasons for this likely range from the neurobiological (e.g., abnormally small amygdala or other limbic structure volumes associated with early life trauma suggest the likelihood of abnormal emotional processing) to the psychosocially developmental (e.g., secure attachments to early caregivers may not form, jeopardizing a sense of basic trust, in turn weakening the capacity for resilience and posing greater vulnerabilities for depression or other internalizing psychological responses to adversity). Across several studies in major depression, antidepressant response to several SSRIs and SNRIs has been demonstrably poorer in patients with histories of childhood physical, emotional, or sexual abuse, particularly occurring before age seven (e.g., Williams et al., 2016). In bipolar depression, as already noted in Chapter 2, an innovative RCT of the monoclonal antibody/antitumor necrosis factor-α drug infliximab showed no significant difference from placebo on an overall basis, but a secondary analysis revealed an interaction effect of treatment × time × history of childhood trauma, suggesting the possibility of a unique advantage for infliximab in the distinct subpopulation of depressed bipolar patients with histories of childhood physical or sexual abuse (McIntyre et al., 2019).

12. Resilience

The capacity to demonstrate resilience, introduced in Chapter 1 as an outcome measure and potential target of pharmacotherapy in and of itself, can also be easily conceptualized as a baseline patient characteristic that could in turn moderate treatment outcomes. For example, Laird and colleagues (2018) examined four subcomponents of resilience (grit, active coping self-efficacy, accommodative coping efficacy, and spirituality) as moderators of antidepressant outcome in older adult depression and found significant predictive value both for response and remission. Specifically, they noted that a 20% increase in baseline resilience led to a nearly twofold increase in the likelihood of remission.

> **Tip**
>
> Resilience refers to the capacity to thrive in the face of adversity, and to experience life stresses without their necessarily leading to or exacerbating psychiatric symptoms.

High baseline resilience also has been identified as a moderator of response to venlafaxine-XR in pooled RCTs for PTSD (Davidson et al., 2012).

13. Past Treatment Response

It is rather interesting that diagnostic nomenclature in psychiatry so seldom, if ever, includes information about previous drug responsivity as part of nosology. By comparison, infectious diseases are often routinely identified or characterized by this criterion (as in the case of methicillin- or vancomycin-resistant staphylococcal infections, or protease inhibitor-resistant acquired immune defiency syndrome (AIDS)). Some psychiatry investigators refer to "lithium-responsive bipolar disorder" or "clozapine-responsive schizophrenia" but imagine the depth of clinical information conveyed if a referring clinician spoke of a "29-year-old third-episode multi-SSRI-resistant, adjunctive-bupropion and -aripiprazole and -lithium-resistant, MAOI-responsive man with nonpsychotic major depression." Pharmacological "staging systems" for depression or schizophrenia tend to notch demerits for successive failed medication trials (with some even rather grimly forecasting a zero probability of remission after a sufficient number of nonresponses to medications and electroconvulsive therapy (ECT); Petersen et al., 2005). Such cataloguing of past treatments, however, often fails to account for confounders such as the presence or absence of adjunctive therapies and their pharmacokinetic/pharmacodynamic influences, the potential necessity for longer treatment trials to judge "adequacy" of a response in more chronically ill populations (e.g., see Koran et al., 2001), or, nowadays, whether pharmacokinetically inappropriate drugs are unfairly counted in the tally (e.g., pro-drugs such as carbamazepine or desvenlafaxine, which cannot be broken down to their active metabolites in patients with slow-metabolizer genotypes for their respective cytochrome P450 enzymes).

14. Familiality

Clinicians often assume that drug response is heritable, although the evidence for this presumption is largely either unfounded, impressionistic, or simply unexplored – with a very few notable exceptions:

- Lithium responsivity appears concordant about two-thirds of the time among first-degree affected relatives within a bipolar pedigree (Grof et al., 2002)
- Antidepressant responsivity to some SSRIs (e.g., fluvoxamine) has empirically shown concordance among affected first-degree relatives within depression pedigrees (Franchini et al., 1998)

15. Patient Treatment Preference

Patient preferences for a particular treatment modality have been examined as possible influences on treatment outcome. Some studies (e.g., Dunlop et al., 2017) have found that in MDD, when patients' treatment preference is concordant with (randomized) assignment to pharmacotherapy versus cognitive behavioral therapy (CBT), study retention is longer (less premature dropout occurs) – suggesting a possible indirect mediating effect of preference on study outcome. However, despite potential higher premature dropout when preferences and treatments are discordant, baseline preference has not been shown to exert a direct moderating effect on treatment outcome for depression.

16. Elevated Inflammatory Markers

There has been growing interest in the relationship between peripheral inflammatory markers (see Table 5.1) not just in mood disorders, but also chronic schizophrenia, anxiety disorders, obsessive-compulsive disorder, and post-traumatic stress disorder, among others. As noted in Table 5.1, baseline elevation of serum inflammatory markers such as hs-CRP has been shown at least in preliminary studies to moderate antidepressant response to specific agents (e.g., nortriptyline over escitalopram). As noted earlier, directional cause-and-effect inferences about inflammation and psychopathology remain poorly understood. While the use of peripheral inflammatory markers to predict or otherwise inform likely treatment outcomes is premature – such studies require extensive replication – early reports inspire the possibility that the presence or absence of baseline inflammation could be a potential innovative way of subtyping certain clinical entities, such as depression and possibly other disorders.

17. Psychosocial Context

Psychosocial factors can catalyze certain illness presentations (e.g., trauma preceding PTSD, cannabis dependence as a "gateway" to the unmasking of a schizophrenia diathesis, sleep deprivation and induction of mania) which, in turn, could have moderating implications for treatment effects (e.g., persisting or chronic stresses such as pending litigations or other forms of secondary gain and adoption of the sick role).

18. Illness Subcharacteristics

Some specific disorders also often have unique characteristics that represent potential moderators of treatment outcome, as illustrated by the examples in Table 5.2 at the end of this chapter.

In RCTs, investigators sometimes try to formally quantify how much a particular individual or group may be predisposed to a certain outcome (such as treatment response) using a statistical method known as *propensity scoring*. Propensity score matching (PSM) is a statistical modeling technique that takes into account the diversity of relevant moderators, confounds, or other individual characteristics between treatment groups that are known to affect the otherwise simple relationship between a patient's diagnosis and their likely treatment outcome. The concepts used in PSM can be applied in general ways for thinking about the relative collective impact of different moderators across various patients who may share the same overarching psychiatric diagnosis.

Consider the following two scenarios:

Case A

Bob, Age 47, White
Dx: Panic disorder, ICD-10 F41.0
Treatment: sertraline 150 mg/day

- symptomatic for >30 years
- two previous suicide attempts
- unresponsive to fluoxetine 20 mg/day for five years
- divorced
- annual income >$150k
- comorbid major depression
- CYP450 2D6 normal genotype
- sporadic alcohol abuse

Case B

Angela, Age 23, Japanese
Dx: Panic disorder, ICD-10 F41.0
Treatment: sertraline 150 mg/day

- symptomatic for one year
- no prior pharmacotherapies
- never suicidal
- steady partner
- unemployed, never finished college
- no psychiatric comorbidities
- CYP450 2D6 poor metabolizer
- sporadic cannabis abuse

If one were placing bets on whether Bob or Angela is more likely to fare well with sertraline, where would your money go? Neither clinical background is glowing in terms of sertraline responsivity, even though the diagnosis itself is unambiguous and straightforward. Subjectively, would you as a clinician prefer to tackle Bob's chronicity, suicide loading, and alcoholism, encouraged instead by his income (a proxy for financial independence and, perhaps, resilience)? Does his longstanding lowish dose of fluoxetine pique your interest and inspire you toward more aggressive treatment? Or, in Angela's case, would the favorable prognosticators of her youth, lack of past treatment failures, and relative absence of chronicity offset your concerns that she will probably not tolerate a usual dose of sertraline, or that her cannabis use may quash her chances for an effective SSRI response? We leave this as an exercise for the reader to render his or her own conclusions.

F MEDIATORS OF TREATMENT RESPONSE

Mediators are factors that influence how well a treatment can work *after it has commenced*. They reflect the kinds of events in real-world settings that could derail or contaminate an otherwise efficacious mode of therapy – or, equally, enhance a treatment's effectiveness by averting obstacles to optimal care. Many such factors are psychosocial more than biological or directly pharmacological (e.g., issues involving finances or access to health care, family support, patients' evolving attitudes about continuing treatment after the acute phase).

Mediators can themselves have predictors, or moderators, and some variables can be moderators (at baseline) as well as mediators (after treatment has begun). An example of the latter is the observation that executive dysfunction can itself *moderate* poor treatment response in MDD (see Table 5.1), while in older adult depression, poor executive function (notably, set-shifting and semantic fluency) has been shown to *mediate* treatment noncompletion, but not nonremission, during open treatment with venlafaxine (Cristancho et al., 2018).

Examples of well-recognized mediators of pharmacotherapy are summarized below.

1. Treatment Adherence

Poor adherence to a treatment regimen is probably the most obvious, if not the most fundamental, mediating factor that can derail an otherwise efficacious treatment once it has been initiated. Many factors, in turn, impact poor treatment adherence, and may vary across diagnoses. Some studies note that the best predictor of future nonadherence to pharmacotherapy is past nonadherence to pharmacotherapy. Collectively, other major recognized contributors to poor adherence include those summarized in Box 5.5.

2. Pharmacokinetic Interactions with Other Drugs

For obvious reasons, coadministration (or subsequent administration) of a drug (or food product) with a second agent that significantly induces or inhibits its metabolism or delays its elimination will alter the pharmacokinetics and potentially the pharmacodynamics of the primary drug of interest. Examples are summarized in Box 5.6.

Box 5.5

Demographic Factors

- Younger age
- Female sex
- Unemployment
- Higher levels of education

Clinical Factors

- Adverse effects (and perceptions of their being unmanageable)
- Cognitive dysfunction
- Depression symptom severity
- Psychosis
- Lack of social supports
- Substance use comorbidity
- Other psychiatric comorbidities
- Poor insight into the need for treatment
- Negative attitudes toward medication
- History of suicide attempts
- Early age at onset
- Short duration of illness

Box 5.6

Examples of Adverse Pharmacokinetic Interations

- Patients stably taking a psychotropic drug that is highly bound (>85%; see Chapter 12, Box 12.12) to plasma proteins (e.g., carbamazepine, divalproex, diazepam, prazosin) who then begin taking another drug that competes for and displaces protein binding (e.g., warfarin, aspirin, naproxen, ibuprofen, indomethacin, furosemide) of the first protein-bound drug, causing increased free drug plasma concentrations and potential pharmacodynamic overactivity or toxicity of the displaced drug[1]
- Patients stably taking a psychotropic drug (e.g., propranolol) that then becomes competitively displaced by another agent (e.g., furosemide), hastening elimination of the first drug causing diminished efficacy
- The introduction of oral contraceptives can interfere with oxidation and clearance of benzodiazepines such as alprazolam, chlordiazepoxide, and diazepam; they may also effectively inhibit the clearance of beta-blockers, tricyclic antidepressants, and corticosteroids
- Addition of a NSAID to lithium can potentially increase serum lithium levels by about 20%, in turn possibly exacerbating adverse effects or risk for toxicity
- Patients who may begin clozapine and then stabilize on it when administered in a nonsmoking environment, and then later begin (or resume) smoking cigarettes, will often "relapse" because of cytochrome P450 1A2 induction of clozapine caused by cigarette smoking. Other nonpsychotropic, not-so-always-obvious culprits for P450 induction or inhibition are summarized in Box 5.7.

Box 5.7

CYP450 Inducers

Broccoli (1A2)
Brussel sprouts (1A2)
Carbamazepine (1A2, 2C9, 2C19, 2D6)
Chamomile tea (1A2)
Charred meat (1A2)
Dexamethasone (2D6)
Modafinil (1A2, 3A4/5)
Omeprazole (1A2)
Phenobarbital (1A2, 2C9, 2D6, 3A4)
Phenytoin (2C9)
Prednisone (3A4)
Primidone (3A4)
Rifampin (2C9, 2C19)
St. John's wort (3A4)
Topiramate (3A4)

CYP450 Inhibitors

Amiodarone (2C9, 3A4)
Cimetidine (2C19)
Ciprofloxacin (1A2)
Clarithromycin, erythromycin (1A2, 3A4)
Corticosteroids (3A4)
Cyclosporine (3A4)
Diltiazem (3A4)
Fluconazole (2C9, 2C19, 3A4)
Grapefruit juice (3A4)
Omeprazole (2C19)
Protease inhibitors (3A4)
Verapamil (3A4)

1 Some authors point out that the clinical implications of displacement of drug protein binding is often overestimated; practically speaking, for situations in which protein binding displacement is of potential concern, one might measure a serum unbound fraction of the drug of interest to obtain a more meaningful estimate of its pharmacokinetic and (possibly pharmacodynamic) bioavailability.

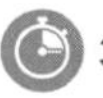 **3. Interpersonal and Psychosocial Life Disruption**

What happens when someone begins a new treatment for depression or anxiety and soon thereafter loses their job, partner, health, or home… or, wins the lottery? It can be hard to account for the confounding effects of unforeseen reversals of fortune or other sudden (or even nonsudden) life events as untoward influences (both for better or worse) on gauging treatment effects for a psychiatric condition. Such factors require qualitative consideration when judging changes in symptoms during the course of a pharmacotherapy regimen.

Related to the impact of interpersonal functioning on outcome is the construct of expressed emotion (EE). Originally described as a relapse factor in schizophrenia and later in major depression and bipolar disorder, EE refers to critical, hostile, or emotionally overinvolved communication styles within families that can undercut otherwise favorable moderators and mediators of successful treatment outcome (such as therapeutic drug doses and levels, or appropriate medication adherence). While research studies formally assess EE via semi-structured interviews, a number of fairly quick self-administered questionnaires have been developed and validated for the purposes of gauging high- versus low-EE patient–relative relationship styles (reviewed by Hooley and Parker, 2006). Astute clinicians can also simply remain attuned to overt data patients may offer about high levels of perceived criticism, arguments, hostility, intrusiveness, and emotional overinvolvement at home, and consider appropriate psychosocial interventions.

> **Getting a Fix on EE**
>
> For a quick-and-dirty appraisal of EE, consider having patients fill out the Level of Expressed Emotion (LEE) Scale, a 10–15 minute, 60-item questionnaire with demonstrated predictive value for relapse across various disorders (Cole and Kazarian, 1988)

 **4. Changes in Cognitive Function**

The cognitive components of depression (attentional processing, executive function and decision-making, reward appraisal, and processing of information with high emotional valence) have received growing interest among mood disorder investigators, representing a distinct component of treatment outcome. In a review of seven randomized pharmacotherapy or other somatic intervention studies for depression, Park and colleagues (2018) observed that *early changes in emotional processing* or "hot" cognition (as measured by a facial emotional recognition task) was a significant predictor of eventual antidepressant response. In examining changes in "cold" cognition as a possible mediator of antidepressant response, early improvements in visuospatial memory emerged as the most robust predictor of eventual treatment response.

>  **Tip**
>
> "Hot" cognition refers to the processing of information with predominantly high emotional content (involving limbic and related subcortical structures). "Cold" cognition describes processing of more emotionally neutral-content material (engaging more prefrontal and related cortical neural networks). More on this in Chapter 14.

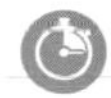 **5. Early Changes in Hedonic Capacity**

Among predictors of antidepressant response, one interesting retrospective study using the melatonin receptor agonist agomelatine found that an *increase in joy* after two weeks of treatment had greater predictive value for eventual antidepressant treatment response or remission than did a reduction in sadness during the same period (Gorwood et al., 2015).

 **6. Pregnancy**

Apart from psychological, psychosocial, and hormonal ramifications, pregnancy also introduces pharmacokinetic changes (e.g., increased volume of distribution, induction of CYP450 enzymes) that consequently affect the metabolism and elimination of pre-existing psychotropic compounds.

7. Psychoactive Substance Misuse

Illicit substances vary in the extent to which they cause CNS elevation or depression, autonomic dysregulation, mood alteration, and potential psychotoxic effects (e.g., alcohol, cannabis, cocaine, hallucinogens) as well as potential hepatotoxic (and metabolic) pharmacokinetic and pharmacodynamic consequences.

G DOES EARLY RESPONSE PREDICT ENDURING RESPONSE?

There are different schools of thought on the relevance of symptom change during the first one to two weeks of psychotropic drug therapy, across various conditions.

In the realm of major depression, as well as bipolar depression and schizophrenia, there is literature suggesting that patients who display at least a 20% improvement from their baseline symptom severity have a greater chance of achieving eventual response if not full remission by the end of an acute trial. In that sense, early signs of improvement could moderate subsequent outcome. Indeed, there is evidence that antidepressant response or remission achieved by week 6 may be one of the strongest predictors (mediators) of 12-month remission status from depression (Ciudad et al., 2012). However, other moderating or mediating factors could in turn affect the robustness of that relationship; for example, the rule may not apply equally in both chronic and nonchronic conditions, or highly comorbid disorders.

Tip

While placebo responses are not necessarily fleeting, a brisk initial drug response that quickly fades may reflect the loss of a placebo effect.

The amount of statistical variance needed to see a 20% change from baseline also differs in high- versus low-severity cases. Someone whose baseline HAM-D score of 20 drops to 14 after two weeks would meet this benchmark, but their symptoms may not outwardly appear all that different; a patient with a HAM-D baseline of 40 whose symptom rating drops to 35 after two weeks may well be on the road to recovery, but falls shy of the statistical benchmark.

Another point of view is that improvements seen in the first one to two weeks of pharmacotherapy may, in some or even many patients, mainly reflect a placebo response that is *unlikely* to endure. For that very reason, some clinical trial designs begin with a one-week single-blind placebo lead-in phase, eliminating from further study those patients who show clear signs of getting better in the first week while on placebo. Some studies of SSRI or other antidepressant loss of response after initial response have suggested that this phenomenon most often may really reflect loss of an initial placebo response, rather than true tachyphylaxis. However, findings have been inconsistent in establishing whether early response in and of itself confers a higher chance for relapse during longer-term maintenance treatment in major depression (McGrath et al., 2006b).

H MORE ABOUT WHEN TO "TWEAK" DOSAGES

In Chapter 1 we touched briefly on the issue of when, how, and why clinicians adjust pharmacotherapy doses. Having now also taken into consideration the impact of placebo effects on both the patient and the prescriber (Chapter 4), let us now expand on the role of dosage tweaking in light of our additional consideration of moderators and mediators of pharmacotherapy outcome.

Tip

Eventual treatment responders usually require fewer dosage adjustments to a medication regimen.

There is no scientific crime in prematurely altering a medication dose or dosing frequency in order to appease patient (or clinician) anguish, provided that one does so knowingly with respect to pharmacodynamic and pharmacokinetic rules of the road. In fact, making pharmacodynamically or pharmacokinetically unnecessary tweaks (e.g., BID (twice a day) or TID (three times a day) dosing of otherwise once-daily extended-release drug preparations, or raising or lowering a dose by a homeopathic amount) might sometimes fall within the service of sustaining a patient's need to perceive activity, and preserving their retention with a given treatment to ensure that enough time elapses to judge that a trial has been of adequate duration.

Some basic factors that should enter this overarching calculus include:

- Has steady state been reached (i.e., have five half-lives elapsed)?
- Is the drug in question known to achieve better results, with acceptable tolerability, via a more rapid dosing titration or even oral loading strategy (e.g., as in the case of divalproex in mania, or olanzapine in acute agitation)?
- Does the symptom severity of a particular patient correspond to better outcomes at higher doses? A start-low-and-go-slow approach makes no sense in fulminant presentations such as agitated psychosis or florid mania.
- Is there reason to suspect that a patient may require higher than usual doses (e.g., based on their past personal history with other medications, or a

suspected ultra-rapid metabolizer phenotype based on clinical and/or pharmacogenetic evidence, or a known pharmacokinetic interaction with a coadministered metabolic pathway inducer)?

- Is there a known target dose, threshold dose, or therapeutic window of a given drug – below which would lessen the chances of improvement, while exceeding a maximum level might yield no greater benefit but might well invite more adverse effects?
- Is the patient taking less than a conventionally recognized threshold or target dose and still symptomatic? Have they been taking an existing dose long enough to judge whether that dose is inadequate to achieve optimal benefit?

I IS IT SCIENTIFICALLY LEGITIMATE TO PARSE TREATMENT-RESPONSIVE SUBGROUPS?

Let us conclude by acknowledging the hazards of identifying treatment-responsive profiles as post hoc characteristics that "point to" subgroups of patients who may be especially good candidates for a particular pharmacotherapy. Imposing post hoc analyses on a study in order to subtype the most highly responsive groups is a hypothesis-generating rather than hypothesis-testing venture. Until a finding is tested as an a priori hypothesis, and replicated, it is risky to form generalizations. This is a scientifically vexing problem because subgroup analyses are in one sense a legitimate way to discover possible patient characteristics that may portend a better or worse treatment outcome, yet on the other hand, it can be difficult to know if characteristics that are found post hoc to correlate with a particular outcome could just be a Type II error (see, for example, Box 5.8).

J ENRICHMENT REVISITED

In Chapter 3 we considered the impact of enriched study designs on treatment outcomes – that is, "preloading" a study with subjects who possess known characteristics that will increase the likelihood of their achieving a desired result. Readers of the literature can form their own appraisals of whether, and how much, a particular clinical trial draws on an enriched study sample versus a more generalizable cohort, based on tallying the identified moderators and mediators of outcome, and gauging whether or not efforts were made to assure their even distribution across treatment arms. On the more literal and concrete side of things, if a clinical trial showed a drug to exert its optimal benefits in first-episode, noncomorbidly ill patients with anorexia, middle insomnia, trait impulsivity, a BMI <30, and an absence of suicidal features, let there be no doubt for whom that drug represents the first-line treatment choice. Use in morbidly obese or suicidal patients would pose an extrapolation, even if the overarching diagnosis (or FDA indication) was the same. The degree to which clinicians find themselves deviating from the archetypal treatment responder plants them on that much less solid ground when it comes to devising a bespoke pharmacotherapy. On the other hand, very broad spectrum drugs that "hit everything" in terms of known moderators and mediators make such an exercise in tailored craftsmanship less necessary or relevant. Until such drugs are invented, though, accomplished craftsmen will likely continue to find ample opportunity to ply their trade.

Box 5.8

The Perils of Spurious Subgroup Analyses

A memorable example of the perils of direct subgroup-specific post hoc analyses and spurious associations can be found in a now-famous large (N = 17 000) one-month study of aspirin for suspected myocardial infarction, in which the authors, perturbed by innumerable requests from the manuscript reviewer to account for more possible covariates, included post hoc subgroup analyses stratifying outcomes by patients' astrological signs: lo and behold, Libras and Geminis who took aspirin fared worse than other astrological groups in surviving an MI (myocardial infarction) (ISIS-2 Collaborative Study Group, 1988).

TAKE-HOME POINTS

- Moderators are baseline patient characteristics that influence treatment outcome. Mediators are factors that affect outcome after a treatment has been initiated. By focusing on moderating and mediating factors that influence treatment outcomes – rather than simply on whether or not a diagnosis is present in a given patient – prescribers can profoundly increase their ability to broker an optimal fit between viable treatment options and the unique clinical profile of a given individual patient.
- The ability to correctly recognize likely moderators and mediators of outcome also permits for a much greater and more critical capacity to interpret and generalize about the validity and applicability of clinical trials in the peer-reviewed literature.

Table 5.1 Provisional biomarker relationships that could moderate psychotropic drug response in depression

Putative biomarker	Examples of findings
Inflammatory markers	
High-sensitivity C-reactive protein (hs-CRP)	- hs-CRP >2.25 mg/L may predict better response to L-methylfolate in MDD (Papakostas et al., 2014) - Low hs-CRP levels associated with better antidepressant response to escitalopram, high levels better response to nortriptyline (Uher et al., 2014)
Interleukin-6 (IL-6) Tumor necrosis factor (TNF)-α Soluble TNF receptor 2 (sTNF-R2)	- High serum levels of IL-6, TNF-α and sTNF-R2 higher in MDD patients with three or more failed antidepressant trials (versus those with one or less failed trial (Haroon et al., 2018) - In MDD, high baseline TNF and sTNF-2 levels associated with antidepressant response to the TNF antagonist infliximab (Raison et al., 2013)
Neurophysiology	
EEG	SSRI responders have greater alpha power (less activity) at occipital sites and over R>L hemispheres (Bruder et al., 2008)
Frontal qEEG	Antidepressant Treatment Response Index at week 1 (a physiological measure) predicts remission by week 7 with 76% positive predictive value (Cook et al., 2013)
Autonomic arousal	SSRI responders or remitters have shown faster decline of CNS arousal at rest (measured by EEG-vigilance); SNRI responders have shown increases in autonomic arousal (Olbrich et al., 2016)
Cognitive performance	Impaired baseline performance on a computerized measure of psychomotor, executive, memory-attention, processing speed, inhibitory and emotional functions predicts poor antidepressant response (Etkin et al., 2015)
Neuroimaging	
PET or fMRI	- Hypermetabolism in pregenual anterior cingulate (Pizzagalli, 2011) associated with SSRI response in depression - In drug-naive MDD, treatment-responsivity associated with a higher *variable coefficient* of the fMRI global signal as compared to patients who went on to manifest treatment-resistant depression (Zhu et al., 2018) - Individual differences in striatal functional connectivity may predict antipsychotic response in first-episode psychosis (Sarpal et al., 2016) - Larger hippocampal tail volumes positively correlated with SSRI or SNRI antidepressant response (Maller et al., 2018) - Left hippocampal, bilateral posterior cingulate, and lower right temporolateral gray matter volumes associated with antidepressant response (Sämann et al., 2013) - Using diffusion tensor tractography (see Box 5.1), "higher global efficiency

Tip

In resting-state fMRI studies, the *global signal* is taken as a measure of "non-neuronal noise." Increased variance in the global signal has been proposed as a biomarker for certain disorders (e.g., schizophrenia).

Putative biomarker	Examples of findings
	in structural connectomes" associated with antipsychotic response in first-episode psychosis (Crossley et al., 2017) - Altered connectivity of the cingulate and stria terminalis, using DTI, predicts SSRI nonresponse in MDD (Korgaonkar et al., 2014; Grieve et al., 2016) - DLPFC activation during response inhibition tasks may predict SSRI remission from depression (Gyurak et al., 2016)
Pharmacogenetics	
SNP associations with treatment response	See examples in Table 8.4 and 8.5 (Chapter 8)

Abbreviations: CNS = central nervous system; DLPFC = dorsolateral prefrontal cortex; DTI = diffusion tensor imaging; EEG = electroencephalography; fMRI = functional magnetic resonance imaging; MDD = major depressive disorder; qEEG = qualitative EEG; SNP = single nucleotide polymorphism; SNRI = serotonin-norepinephrine reuptake inhibitor; SSRI = selective serotonin reuptake inhibitor

Table 5.2 Possible moderators of treatment outcomes unique to particular conditions

Disorder	Parameter	Relevance for treatment outcome
Bipolar disorder	Polarity proneness	Lithium appears more effective in patients who have more manias than depressions; lamotrigine may be more useful when depressive phases outnumber high periods (see Chapter 13)
	Rapid cycling	Antidepressants may worsen longitudinal course in the setting of rapid cycling; acute response to standard antimanic or mood-stabilizing antidepressant agents (e.g., quetiapine) may be diminished in the context of past-year rapid cycling (see Chapter 13)
	Bipolar I vs. II	Antidepressant safety and efficacy may be better in bipolar II than I disorder (see Chapter 13)
	Mixed features	Concomitant manic and depressive symptoms may portend a better acute response to divalproex than lithium as well as a poorer response to adjunctive antidepressants as compared to that seen in "pure" bipolar depression (see Chapter 13)
Schizophrenia/ schizoaffective disorder	Mood incongruence of psychotic symptoms	Mood incongruent features generally are viewed as negative prognostic factors with lesser treatment responsiveness (see Chapter 15)
Major depression	Atypical features; melancholic features	Reversed vegetative signs may portend a better outcome with MAOIs than tricyclic antidepressants; anhedonia and other melancholic features may predict a better response to tricyclic antidepressants than MAOIs (see Chapter 13)
	History of trauma	While not a subtype of depression, a history of childhood trauma has been shown to be a robust negative moderator of recovery in MDD (see Chapter 13)
	Anxiety	Comorbid anxiety symptoms or syndromes tend to confer negative prognostic implications (see Chapter 13)
	Psychosis	Psychotic depressions tend to last longer and in general are harder to treat than nonpsychotic MDEs (see Chapter 13)

6 Complex Regimens and Rationale-Based Combination Drug Therapies

LEARNING OBJECTIVES

- [ ] Understand the three pillars of rational polypharmacy
- [ ] Recognize the signs of serotonin syndrome and its high- versus low-plausibility risks among various serotonergic agents
- [ ] Know when to deprescribe ineffective, redundant, or otherwise inappropriate medications and recognize common obstacles to practicing pharmacological hygiene
- [ ] Recognize medications that have multiple psychotropic properties which can facilitate parsimonious polypharmacy
- [ ] Beware the potential hazards of overaggressive polypharmacy and dosing

Out of intense complexities, intense simplicities emerge.

- Sir Winston Churchill

Many patients with complicated psychiatric disorders – which we will define here as conditions involving multiple comorbidities, atypical or protracted symptoms, persistent functional impairment, and poor treatment response – often find themselves taking multidrug therapy regimens. Sometimes, combination therapies reflect wise, thoughtful, and even elegant amalgams crafted with careful deliberation. Such handiwork might capitalize on pharmacodynamic synergies and complementary, nonredundant mechanisms of action, or specific medications may make unique contributions to an overall regimen (such as drugs thought to exert anti-impulsivity, antisuicide, pro-cognitive, or anxiolytic effects). In a well-devised multidrug treatment plan, each component ideally has a well-defined job description and fills a particular role, much the way each player on a sports team covers a unique position, or every instrument in an orchestra makes its own distinct contribution to form a cohesive whole. In that sense, every drug within a psychopharmacology regimen should serve an identifiable and unambiguous function. While patients and clinicians alike sometimes scoff at the sheer *number* of medications that may be in an extensive treatment regimen, as partners they may neglect to periodically inventory the ensemble drug by drug, reaffirming each component's relevance, purpose, and performance.

Box 6.1

Semantics

The term "polypharmacy" is sometimes used with a pejorative connotation to mean the use of drugs that are nonessential, duplicative, or ineffective. "Complex combination therapy" is sometimes a preferred designation to connote purposeful multidrug regimens.

We would contrast purposeful polypharmacy with more haphazard assemblages of multiple drugs. Given the frankly modest effect sizes for many psychotropic drugs (see Chapter 3, Box 3.6), clinicians may sometimes feel compelled to "throw everything" they can at significant symptoms in hopes of achieving better outcomes, regardless of whether such approaches are evidence-based.

A EXTENSIVE POLYPHARMACY

According to the cross-sectional National Ambulatory Medical Care Survey, prescribing of *three or more* psychotropic drugs occurs in fully one-third of psychiatric outpatient visits seen in US office-based practice settings (Rojtabai and Olfson, 2010). Observed trends from the mid-1990s to the mid-2000s included within-class duplications (e.g., two or more antidepressants, antipsychotics, or sedative-hypnotics), but not mood stabilizer combinations, and a significant rise in antidepressant–antipsychotic combination therapies. A longitudinal study of nearly

3000 bipolar disorder patients found that 21% took four or more psychotropic drugs, a status found more often among patients with psychosis, trauma histories, or comorbid anxiety of borderline personality disorders (Golden et al., 2017). National survey data of children and adolescents from the mid-1990s to the mid-2000s showed a nearly twofold increase in multiclass psychotropic prescribing, particularly in the coprescription of ADHD medications with antipsychotics, and antipsychotics with antidepressants (Comer et al., 2010).

Tip

One in five bipolar patients takes four or more psychotropic drugs.

There has been remarkably little formal study of *very extensive* polypharmacy regimens, and virtually no published systematic observations on the use of four or more coprescribed psychotropic agents. This deficit in the literature stands in contrast to the established and commonplace use of multidrug regimens elsewhere in medicine, such as for treatment-resistant infectious diseases, malignancies, or hypertension. Industry-sponsored clinical trials will likely never have incentive to demonstrate the value or safety of adding competitors' drugs to those they manufacture. Nor is there commercial incentive to study complex combinations simply because they reflect community practices. The use of highly complex and extensive drug regimens in routine practice has far outpaced the evidence base and is among the most glaring of real-world unmet needs within psychiatry.

Box 6.2

Did You Know?

Palliative care patients take an average of 11.5 medications (McNeil et al., 2016); about two-thirds of oncology patients take ≥5 drugs in an antineoplastic regimen (Murphy et al., 2018); in hypertension, monotherapy is effective in only about one-third of cases, making dual or triple pharmacotherapy more common than rare (Frank, 2008).

B DRUG-RELATED PROBLEMS ASSOCIATED WITH COMPLEX REGIMENS

Multidrug regimens arouse concerns because of their potential to create more problems than might be the case when using more parsimonious regimens (see ahead, Table 6.9). The American Society of Hospital Pharmacists (ASHP, 1993) classifies drug-related problems in a number of categories, summarized as follows:

- *Indication without drug/more medication required.* Problematic is that psychiatry abounds with ailments or symptom complexes that lack formal FDA indications – such as borderline and other personality disorders, acute stress disorder, cannabis or cocaine use disorders, psychosis associated with non-Parkinson's dementia, and even the most common of all psychiatric disorders, specific phobias. It has been noted that over 88% of diagnoses listed in DSM-IV-TR lack a drug with regulatory agency approval (Devulapalli and Nasrallah, 2009).
- *Drug without indication/discontinuation of medication required.* In more evidence-based parlance, we would identify this category as "absence of evidence to support the use of a given drug for a particular intended purpose."
- *Wrong drug/inappropriate drug.* Big oops.
- *Overdosage/therapeutic duplication.* We would emphasize the undesirability of duplicative mechanisms of action as contrasted with additive or synergistic effects.
- *Subtherapeutic dosage.* We would emphasize the appropriateness versus inappropriateness of subtherapeutic dosages, based on their pharmacodynamically intended effects. Sometimes in a complex multidrug regimen, concomitant use of multiple agents at lower-than-usual dosages can render synergy while sparing potential dose-related adverse effects.
- *Failure to receive drug/nonadherence.* Many reasons contribute to nonadherence, as discussed below.
- *Adverse drug reaction.* Never desirable, by definition, but adverse effects vary in their severity and medical seriousness versus sheer "nuisance."
- *Potential drug–drug interaction (DDI).* DDIs may occur inadvertently or carelessly or they may be purposeful and strategic (see Tables 6.1 and 6.2)

Drug Interactions: Friend or Foe?

Pharmacokinetic and pharmacodynamic interactions are a reasonable starting point when considering the compatibility of mixing medications. Most clinicians recognize that when a drug is metabolized by a particular catabolic enzyme, its breakdown is delayed by inhibitors and accelerated by inducers of that pathway – due either to pharmacogenetic moderators (see Chapter 8) or the inherent enzyme-inducing or - inhibiting properties of one drug relative to another. Rational or elegant combination therapies often

Box 6.3

Complex Polypharmacotherapy and Treatment Nonadherence

It is often assumed that the use of multiple drugs invariably contributes to (if not drives) nonadherence to psychotropic medications. While this may make intuitive sense, it fails to take into account patients' perceptions of the value of a treatment regimen, however simple or complex it may be. How do the pros and cons of a complex regimen stack up after accounting on the one hand for tangible benefits (e.g., reduction of symptom load or severity, improved psychosocial functioning, better quality of life, antisuicide or other symptom-specific effects) versus detriments (e.g., cost, extent and intensity of adverse effects, frequency of dosing, ease of administration)? Adherence likely declines when patients fail to perceive either efficacy or the *need* for treatment, or when regimens are unduly complex. A well-designed and efficacious but complicated regimen will quickly be abandoned if perceived risks outweigh benefits. Often, patients may under-recognize (or take for granted) meaningful treatment benefits unless the clinician points them out explicitly (e.g., "It's been a long time since you've been plagued by suicidal thoughts," or "Since starting Drug X it seems you've really been doing well at work, you talk a lot about feeling satisfied and secure there, with much less anxiety than before"). Also bearing on the equation between regimen complexity and adherence are patients' and prescribers' assumptions about whether simpler, adequate alternative drug regimen options actually exist, and how realistically each side appraises their viability. "Streamlining" complex regimens simply in order to economize pill counts makes sense only when doing so does not jeopardize meaningful benefits. We encourage clinicians to articulate such risk-benefit analyses as explicitly as possible when counseling patients about treatment options, particularly if they may underappreciate actual (and sometimes elusive or hard-fought) strides made toward recovery.

capitalize on such interactions, while less thoughtful pairings sometimes stumble into treacherous territory.

Common examples of drug pairings that yield *pharmacokinetic* effects that could be either advantageous or deleterious are presented in Tables 6.1–6.3. Potentially advantageous or deleterious *pharmacodynamic* drug interactions are described in Table 6.4.

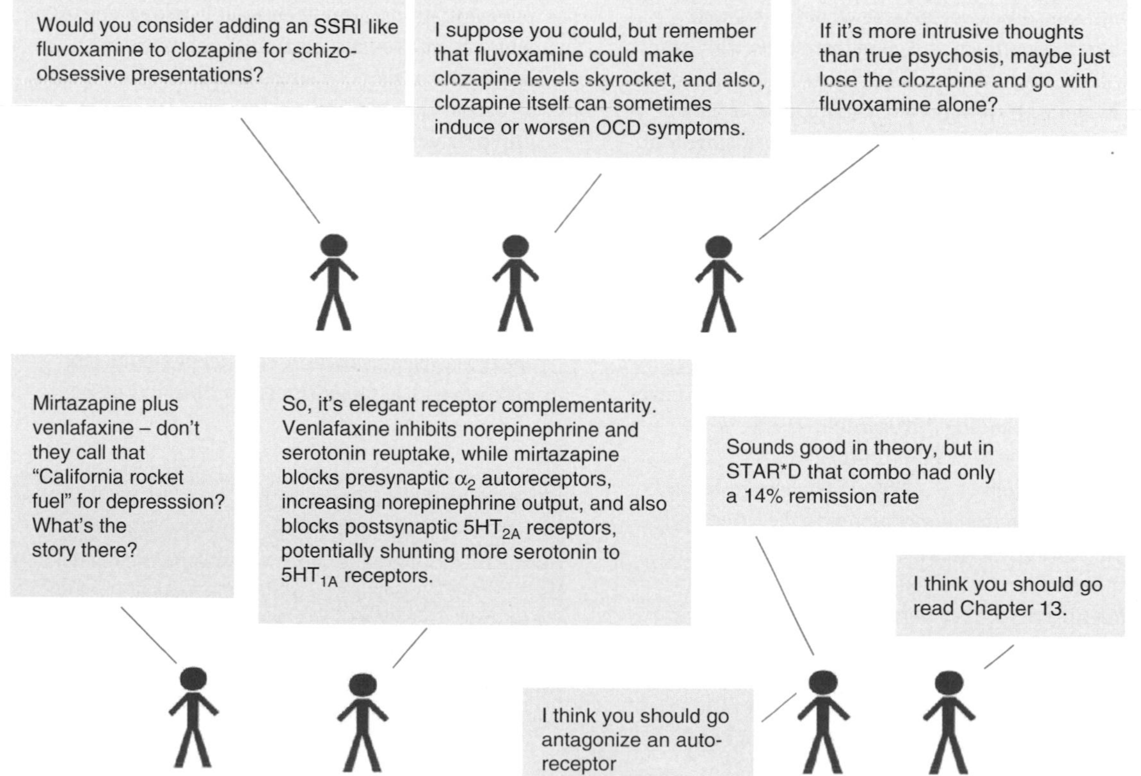

C ODD COUPLES

Some possible combinations of psychotropic drugs are unusual either because of apparent mechanistic redundancies or safety considerations, but nevertheless are sometimes chosen by clinicians, albeit with varying levels of evidence to support safety, efficacy, or in some cases rationales. Examples include the following:

- *Fluvoxamine + clomipramine*. Open trials have been reported with this combination for patients with refractory OCD (Szegedi et al., 1996; Figueroa et al., 1998). Serotonin syndrome is a theoretical (but not reported) complication. Fluvoxamine markedly elevates clomipramine levels, which require monitoring; adverse effects are rare when [clomipramine] <450 ng/dL.
- *SNRI + tricyclic*. There are only so many ways to block the norepinephrine reuptake pump, and mixing an SNRI with any tricyclic is essentially pairing two NE transporter (NET) inhibitors.
- *SNRI + SSRI*. Doubling-up on serotonin transporter reuptake inhibition makes little sense pharmacologically and seems only to invite a higher risk for serotonin syndrome. A handful of case reports exist of depressed patients only partially responsive to optimally dosed venlafaxine who then showed further improvement and good tolerability with low-dose SSRI augmentation (i.e., paroxetine, sertraline, or citalopram) (Gonul et al., 2003). There are also published reports of serotonin syndrome arising from fluoxetine and venlafaxine cotherapy (Bhatara et al., 1998). We cannot think of a good reason to try this approach. For those who may think otherwise, beware adverse *pharmacokinetic* interactions (e.g., fluvoxamine increases duloxetine levels via CYP1A2 inhibition).
- *SSRI + SSRI*. Generally speaking, there is little rationale in combining two drugs having identical mechanisms of action. Small (n ~10) open trials have been reported adding fluvoxamine 50 mg/day (Bondolfi et al., 1996) or fluoxetine 10 mg/day (Bondolfi et al., 2000) to citalopram 40 mg/day after depression nonresponse to the latter. Both augmentations stereoselectively increased S- rather than R-citalopram and led to reduced depression symptom severity, accompanied occasionally by nausea and tremor. Lack of a placebo or other comparison group makes it difficult to interpret these findings as evidence of pharmacodynamic efficacy. *Importantly, fluoxetine or fluvoxamine could each increase citalopram levels via CYP2C19 inhibition (potentially contributing to QTc prolongation on ECG).*
- *SNRI + SNRI*. We can think of no logical reason to combine two SNRIs. Ever. Dissenters should be aware that duloxetine can increase venlafaxine levels via CYP2D6 inhibition.
- *Bupropion + atomoxetine*. Both drugs inhibit NE reuptake (atomoxetine more potently than bupropion) while bupropion also is a weak DA reuptake inhibitor (that is, a blocker of the DAT). As a potent CYP2D6 inhibitor, bupropion will slow atomoxetine metabolism and increase its systemic exposure by about fivefold. There are no published reports of enhanced therapeutic efficacy either in ADD or major depression with this combination.
- *Pregabalin + gabapentin*. Both pregabalin and gabapentin (so-called *gabapentinoids*) target the α2δ subunit of voltage-gated Ca^{++} channels. Both are indirectly GABAergic but neither binds directly to GABA receptors. Reports exist of synergistic analgesic effects in neuropathic pain (Senderovich and Jeyapragasan, 2018); we are aware of no data on their combination for psychotropic purposes (e.g., anxiolysis).
- *Psychostimulant + antipsychotic*. In principle, stimulants and antipsychotics exert diametrically opposing effects: stimulants mainly release dopamine which is an agonist at cortical D_1 receptors and at limbic D_2 receptors, whereas antipsychotics with low D_1 action (e.g., cariprazine, lurasidone, brexpiprazole, aripiprazole) block agonist actions at limbic D_2 receptors but not at cortical D_1 receptors. What is the bottom line? D_1 agonists may exert pro-cognitive effects in the cortex without activating psychosis in the mesolimbic system. Some authors have invoked theories about the so-called "complex dopamine model" of phasic versus tonic DA release to reconcile the ostensible mechanistic conflict of mixing DA agonists with antagonists as described in Box 6.4.

Box 6.4

The Complex Dopamine Model

Grace (1991) put forth the hypothesis that stimulus detection (during attention) involves phasic bursts of prefrontal DA activation, while tonic DA release sets a background level of DA receptor stimulation which, in chronic psychosis (i.e., schizophrenia), becomes downregulated and eventually leads to abnormally high phasic DA release in response to environmental stimuli.

Box 6.5

Examples of Combining Psychostimulants with Antipsychotics

- Lisdexamfetamine (20–70 mg/day; mean dose = 50 mg/day) added to a stable existing SGA regimen (quetiapine, risperidone, olanzapine, paliperidone, or aripiprazole) in stable schizophrenia patients with predominantly negative symptoms showed greater reductions in negative symptoms during a 10-week open-label phase followed by a four-week placebo-controlled phase, with no concomitant worsening of positive symptoms (Lasser et al., 2013)
- Adjunctive risperidone was better than placebo when added to methylphenidate in children with comorbid ADHD and conduct disorder for improving symptoms of both conditions, without worsening of psychopathology (Jahangard et al., 2017)
- Modafinil, which is believed to exert its wakefulness-promoting effects at least in part via DA reuptake inhibition, has been shown to counteract the sedating effects of antihistaminergic antipsychotics with little risk for exacerbating psychosis (Saavedra-Velez et al., 2009)
- A naturalistic Danish study of schizophrenia patients found fewer and shorter hospital admissions as well as lesser total daily doses of antipsychotics among those taking a stimulant (Rohde et al., 2018)

Two equally important considerations when pairing psychotropic agents is their mechanistic or pharmacodynamic rationale alongside the existence of an empirical evidence base demonstrating actual outcomes. Sometimes one condition might be present without the other. The example above in which a stimulant is paired with an antipsychotic offers a useful illustration of this. There is a reasonable empirical literature demonstrating the utility and safety of combining stimulants with antipsychotics, even though their mechanisms of action seem conflictual. Several examples are noted in Box 6.5.

The third pillar of rational polypharmacotherapy, in addition to complementary mechanisms of action and empirical demonstration of favorable outcomes, involves safety. Some potential drug combinations pose *unequivocal* hazards (such as an MAOI + meperidine) or contraindications (such as multiple sympathomimetics in a patient with poorly controlled hypertension). Other combinations pose more relative than absolute contraindications, or may be based solely on theoretical grounds or scattered case reports that are more speculative than definitive in demonstrating causality behind an adverse outcome. Serotonin syndrome represents one such serious outcome for which the potential hazards of various drug combinations are sometimes more urban legend than established reality (Box 6.6).

Tip

Serotonin syndrome is defined by the so-called Hunter criteria, involving: clonus, agitation, diaphoresis, tremor, and hyper-reflexia (Dunkley et al., 2003)

Box 6.6

Serotonin Syndrome: How Real is the Risk?

Serotonin syndrome can arise from very high doses of a single drug that increases serotonergic tone or, at least in theory, from combinations of drugs that upregulate serotonergic function through different receptor mechanisms. We say "at least in theory" because the fact that a drug "affects" serotonin function per se does not necessarily mean it will induce toxicity from "too much" serotonin. An example would be antidepressants whose serotonergic effects solely involve their blocking postsynaptic $5HT_{2A}$ receptors, such as *mirtazapine* or *trazodone* (or, for that matter all SGAs). The literature cautions that serotonin syndrome could possibly result from adding buspirone (a $5HT_{1A}$ presynaptic agonist/postsynaptic partial agonist) to an SSRI but the actual evidence base consists of a single case report (Manos, 2000). *Lithium* increases serotonin synthesis, though it has been identified in a handful of case reports as a possible contributor to serotonin syndrome when combined with an SSRI (e.g., Sobanski et al., 1997) or SNRI (e.g., Adan-Manes et al., 2006; Shahani, 2012). The FDA issued a warning in 2006 that *triptans* added to SSRIs could provoke serotonin syndrome, based on their review of 29 reported cases, although a subsequent electronic health record study of 19 017 patients identified a low incident rate of "definite" or "probable" serotonin syndrome (2.3 cases per 10 000 person-years of exposure) (Orlova et al., 2018). What about

Box 6.6 (Cont.)

tramadol, a weak SNRI analgesic – is there evidence that it could cause serotonin syndrome when paired with a serotonergic antidepressant? Park and colleagues (2014) identified only 10 published case reports of this occurring and concluded that mixing tramadol with an SSRI or SNRI is relatively safe, although combinations with an MAOI may be more hazardous. Risks for serotonin syndrome in general during cotherapies with MAOIs pose a more complex issue and are discussed in their own right below.

MAOIs + TCAs

Single case reports, mostly from the 1960s, identified the combination of an MAOI plus a tricyclic antidepressant (often serotonergic tertiary amines such as PO (by mouth) or IM (intramuscular) imipramine or clomipramine) as causing signs of serotonin syndrome (e.g., hyperthermia and convulsions), or hypertensive crises resulting from increased noradrenergic tone (reviewed by White and Simpson, 1981). Toxicities from adding a TCA to an MAOI have largely been reported in the context of deliberate overdoses, coingestion of barbiturates, or dietary transgressions with tyramine-containing foods. Adding an MAOI to an existing TCA is preferred over the reverse sequence because it is thought that the NET blockade caused by the TCA may minimize or prevent the risk of a hypertensive crisis.

As a rule of thumb:

MAOI added to TCA: **OK**
TCA added to MAOI: **Don't try**

A small literature supports simultaneously starting a secondary amine TCA and an MAOI at low doses and slowly cotitrating dosages upward to about half the maximum usual dose of each agent (White et al., 1982). As discussed more extensively in Chapter 13, MAOIs are a unique antidepressant drug class with robust and often unrivaled efficacy in hard-to-treat forms of depression. However, strategies to devise "heroic" combination drug therapy regimens involving MAOIs are not meant for novice hands and demand a solid understanding of how MAOIs work coupled with a very careful appraisal of likely risks versus benefits. Less than 1% of American psychiatrists prescribe MAOIs and many who do are often only partially familiar with the intricacies of their use, such as those described in Box 6.7.

Tip

Open pilot studies and case reports describe safe and successful MAOI cotherapy with trazodone for insomnia (e.g., Jacobsen, 1990; Nierenberg and Keck, 1989). Mirtazapine could theoretically also *treat* serotonin syndrome (Hoes et al., 1996); in preclinical studies, it has been shown to mitigate hyperthermia induced by fluoxetine plus tranylcypromine (Shioda et al., 2010).

Box 6.7

Essential Knowledge for MAOI Use

- Knowing necessary from unnecessary dietary restrictions based on actual food tyramine content
- Tactics for managing dose-related orthostatic hypotension (see Chapter 10)
- Safe versus unsafe use of high doses
- Differences between comparisons of irreversible versus reversible inhibitors of MAO-A (e.g., moclobemide), the need to overcome MAO-A versus -B isoenzyme selectivity
- Differences between oral versus transdermal selegiline, and in the evidence base between transdermal selegiline and oral irreversible MAOIs
- Last but certainly not least, the safe and rational use or avoidance of relevant pharmacological cotherapies

Key points regarding the last of the issues in Box 6.7 are summarized in Table 6.5, while the former issues are discussed more fully in Chapter 13. There are a number of instances in which the purported riskiness of a combination therapy is based on theoretical concerns but empirically, few or no single case reports exist to substantiate an actual hazard (e.g., adjunctive buspirone or pindolol). Importantly, we must note that the absence of evidence is not evidence of the absence of risk. Fear alone may dissuade clinicians or investigators from undertaking some of the combinations in Table 6.5 (particularly when one recognizes that very few psychiatrists nowadays are comfortable even prescribing MAOIs, much less in combination with other drugs). Ignorance plus inexperience regarding safe and effective MAOI use fosters greater ignorance and more superstition than empirical knowledge about integrating MAOIs in a pharmacotherapy regimen. More about this topic in Chapter 13.

D RATIONALE-BASED POLYPHARMACY: CAN ADJUNCTIVE $5HT_{1A}$ AGONISTS OR PARTIAL AGONISTS KICK-START SSRI RESPONSE IN DEPRESSION?

Before leaving our discussion of complementary versus potentially toxic combined serotonergic pathways, let us briefly consider the unique role of $5HT_{1A}$ agonism and partial agonism. One theory to explain the frequent lag time of at least a few weeks for observing the initial pharmacodynamic effects of an SSRI involves the hypothesis that downregulation of the presynaptic (somatodendritic) $5HT_{1A}$ autoreceptor must occur in order to facilitate increased outflow of presynaptic serotonin.

The presynaptic $5HT_{1A}$ autoreceptor is *the same receptor* found postsynaptically but here functions differently as a kind of gatekeeper of serotonin outflow when blocked. In principle, a presynaptic $5HT_{1A}$ full antagonist (such as pindolol) or postsynaptic partial agonist (such as buspirone) could hasten time until onset of a serotonergic antidepressant, or possibly confer synergy with an SSRI or SNRI in treatment-resistant depression. Combination pharmacotherapies that pair serotonin reuptake inhibition with $5HT_{1A}$ modulation are thus quite rationale-based. How well this strategy actually works in practice is discussed in Chapter 13.

Figure 6.1 The strange world of the pre- and postsynaptic $5HT_{1A}$ receptor

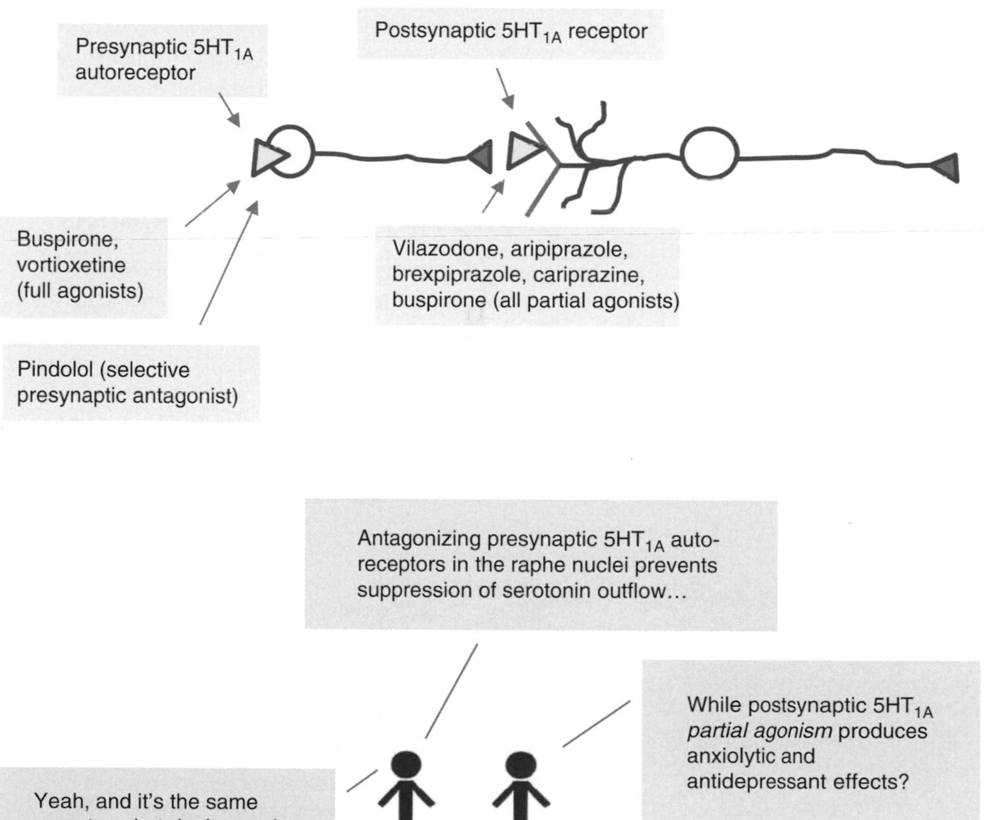

So wait, go back to Figure 6.1. What happens if you combine pindolol *with* buspirone, if pindolol is a $5HT_{1A}$ presynaptic autoreceptor *antagonist* and buspirone an *agonist*?

Ah, great question! Then you get a functional $5HT_{1A}$ *postsynaptic agonist.* In 1997 Pierre Blier and his colleagues in Canada did just that, adding both drugs to an SSRI. They saw depression response occur within a week for most patients.

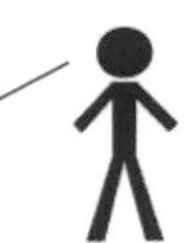

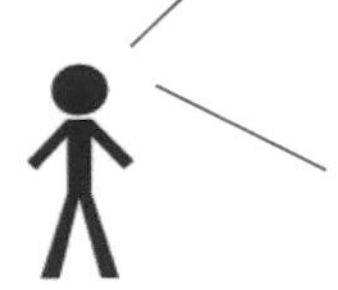

OK, but so then which is more important, the pre- or postsynaptic $5HT_{1A}$ effect?

Both. The autoreceptor is inhibitory – it's a brake preventing presynaptic serotonin release. It eventually desensitizes, permitting more outflow and then postsynaptic agonism has a field day.

E THE BUSINESS OF POLYPHARMACY: MULTIDRUG REGIMENS AS PERSONNEL ROSTERS

It can be useful both to pharmacotherapy decision-making and to the therapeutic alliance for a clinician and patient jointly to undertake a periodic "performance evaluation" of each element within a medication regimen, asking together what each component is bringing to the "organization." This means defining the goals of treatment (see Chapter 1), recognizing unmet needs of unfilled niches (e.g., does the existing regimen adequately and properly address mood, anxiety, sleep, cognition, impulsivity, drive, and motivation?), asking if existing medications are optimally dosed for their intended purposes, whether the composite of medications meshes well without pharmacokinetic or pharmacodynamic conflicts, examining whether drug benefits outweigh risks or adverse effects, and letting the "hiring management team" consider whether there may be a different candidate drug better-suited to the job description.

F PHARMACOLOGICAL HYGIENE: THE ART OF DEPRESCRIBING

The field has only recently begun to consider formal approaches for when, how, and why to stop psychotropic drugs within a complex regimen. Many factors may make clinicians hesitant to discontinue a medication, including those mentioned in Box 6.8.

Box 6.8

Factors Against Deprescribing

- Misperceptions that a patient's clinical status is better than it actually is ("she seemed fine when I saw her last")
- Fear that an ostensibly ineffective drug is in fact delivering partial benefit, leading to further decompensation in its absence
- Hopes that additive effects might show greater benefit at some future point in time
- Disbelief that a previously effective drug could no longer be effective (failure to appreciate tolerance or tachyphylaxis)
- Clinging to an incorrect diagnosis for which a particular drug is appropriate in principle
- Uncertainty about a diagnosis, inspiring the notion that a clinical base is "being covered just in case"
- Falling into the habit of renewing prescriptions in a perfunctory fashion without asking about adverse effects, nonadherence, or perceived lack of benefits
- Lack of firsthand knowledge about the actual effect of a previously introduced drug in a patient who now seems relatively stable (e.g., "the previous psychiatrist felt this could be bipolar disorder so let's just leave the mood stabilizer in place indefinitely")
- Overly speculative ideas about harm reduction ("better to leave him on a benzodiazepine, if I stopped it he might start using opiates and alcohol…")

Deprescribing a drug of questionable relevance can bring about meaningful benefits. For instance, adverse drug effects that could be misperceived as primary psychiatric symptoms (e.g., diminished libido, hypersomnia, restlessness) may be eliminated, overall side effect burden may likely diminish, which could improve both patient morale and treatment adherence, and potentially unrecognized pharmacokinetic inducers of another drug's metabolism could permit better efficacy when the inducer is stopped. On the other hand, when the possible benefits of a drug are ambiguous, its elimination could abruptly reveal previously unappreciated partial efficacy. Careful, systematic, one-drug-at-a-time deprescribing also sometimes can offer a useful (but not entirely risk-free) way for both patient and prescriber to convince themselves about whether a particular drug was or wasn't exerting a meaningful effect (recall the introductory section of Chapter 1 on judging cause-and-effect). A builder wondering whether a wall is load-bearing could simply knock it down and see if the building collapses, but a more gradual and cautious approach is often the safer bet.

Tip

When deprescribing, proceed gradually and cautiously; a drug that was assumed to have no benefit can sometimes quickly make its absence felt in undesired ways.

Basic concepts for deprescribing are relatively straightforward, as summarized in Box 6.9.

Box 6.9

Basics of Deprescribing

- Jointly acknowledge when a member of the drug regimen has failed its periodic performance evaluation
- As when building a regimen, try to deconstruct by changing only one variable at a time
- Phase out presumed dead weight slowly. Favor cross-titrations and slow tapers over abrupt cessations not only to minimize potential discontinuation effects but, moreover, to identify early on an emerging clinical deterioration when the presumed "unnecessary" drug is being phased out
- Be sure an adequate trial (or an insurmountable intolerance) has occurred before relegating a drug to the garbage heap

G PHARMACOLOGICAL PARSIMONY: ONE DRUG, MANY EFFECTS

One obvious aspect of constructing wise and elegant combination regimens is to capitalize whenever possible on the use of single agents that have more than one desired effect. To this end, Tables 6.6–6.8 summarize the diversity of psychotropic effects associated with specific medications broadly classified as anticonvulsants, antidepressants, or antipsychotics. It must be noted, once again, that the absence of evidence does not necessarily reflect evidence of absence. Investigators' and research sponsors' decisions about whether to study (or not study) a particular drug for a particular target domain (such as SSRIs for attention, SNRIs for impulsivity, or lurasidone in acute mania) tend to reflect the commercial interests and priorities of drug manufacturers or other funding sources. Consider, as an example, mirtazapine in anxiety. Preclinical studies suggest its possible anxiolytic effects, mediated through enhanced extracellular hippocampal serotonin transmission. In humans, RCTs have shown efficacy for social anxiety in some studies (Muehlbacher et al., 2005) but not others (Schutters et al., 2010); open trials suggest value in GAD (Gambi et al., 2005), but randomized studies are lacking, and the remaining empirical literature focusing on anxiety is limited to case reports and small open trials. From an evidence-based standpoint, is it fair to consider it as having free-standing anxiolytic properties, or a particular advantage in anxious depression, based mainly on its mechanistic rationale?

One also must consider the problem of so-called pseudospecificity of drug properties (as discussed in Chapter 3) – that is, deciding when a drug's effect on a particular domain (such as insomnia) is merely an epiphenomenon of its treating a broader syndrome (such as depression), as opposed to exerting an effect on a particular domain (such as cognition) independent of its possible effect on a broader syndrome (such as depression, in the case of vortioxetine).

Tip

Quetiapine is by far the most extensively and successfully studied SGA for anxiety.

H PARSIMONIOUS POLYPHARMACY

When one drug can serve more than one useful purpose, pharmacology regimens can become streamlined and simplified. Parsimonious regimens are those that combine multipurpose drugs in complementary fashion, like cross-links in an engineering design. Think of multipurpose tools such as smart phones, chronographic wristwatches, or Swiss army knives. When one drug can accomplish multiple goals, efficiency improves as fewer total separate components are needed.

True parsimony implies true multipurpose efficacy and, as such, differs from products that simply combine two or more separate drugs into one (e.g., an ACE (angiotensin-converting enzyme) inhibitor plus a thiazide diuretic combined into one pill for hypertension; a cold tablet that combines an antihistamine plus decongestant plus antitussive plus analgesic). Baking soda can do more than leaven bread (think sunburn, deodorant, stomach upset, and fire extinguisher). Vinegar is good for a lot more than making salad dressing, dishwashing liquid can also kill weeds and bugs, and WD-40® can do much more than remove rust. Hence, gather together the diverse threads of psychopathology dimensions described in Chapter 2 and imagine constructing parsimonious polypharmacy "solutions" that involve the fewest moves – before encountering the next depressed overweight nonasthmatic smoker with attentional complaints whose comorbid social anxiety and essential tremor failed to improve with SSRIs.[1]

Parsimony

We borrow from economics the term "parsimonious" to connote frugality, or stinginess, in the use of resources – in this case, medications.

Examples of multipurpose psychotropic drugs that lend themselves to "niche" roles, offering the makings for high-efficiency combination regimens, are described in Table 6.9.

Specific evidence-based combination drug regimens are decribed in detail within individual chapters in Part II.

COMBINATIONS OF ANTIPSYCHOTICS

While it is true that the molecular "signatures" of receptor-binding profiles and affinities of antipsychotic drugs are not identical among agents within the class, there are conceptual and practical problems with the all-too-common simultaneous use of multiple antipsychotic drugs. Chief among such concerns is the absence of an evidence base to support the value or safety of using multiple antipsychotics in combination. Nevertheless, in the United States a second antipsychotic drug is prescribed in anywhere from 10–50% of patients who take a first antipsychotic drug on a long-term basis. Schizophrenia patients are about seven times more likely than patients with nonschizophrenia diagnoses to take two or more antipsychotic drugs (Mojtabai and Olfson, 2010). Common reasons, albeit seldom evidence-based, might include those described in Box 6.10.

Box 6.10

Common Reasons for Taking Two or More Antipsychotics

- Patients are in the midst of a cross-taper from one drug to the second and stop either deliberately because of improvement or concern about clinical worsening with further tapering
- Residual symptoms persist during treatment with a first SGA (such as insomnia, anxiety, or agitation) which a clinician thinks would be more responsive to a second (often low-dose, often more antihistaminergic) SGA rather than further optimizing the dose of the first SGA
- There is a basis for thinking the addition of a specific SGA could ameliorate certain adverse effects of the first SGA – such as adding aripiprazole to normalize iatrogenic hyperprolactinemia (Shim et al., 2007) or adding ziprasidone to counter SGA-associated weight gain (Wang et al., 2011)
- Lack of confidence in the efficacy of a first antipsychotic, but reluctance to stop it because of uncertainty about whether its effects may be underappreciated

In the unique case of clozapine – in which no antipsychotic has ever shown superiority to it for treatment-resistant psychotic disorders – there are a handful of controlled trials examining safety and efficacy of augmentation strategies with a second SGA. Findings from these studies are summarized in Chapter 15.

[1] i.e., consider bupropion plus propranolol

Box 6.11

Rationales for Combination Antipsychotics

- When judging tolerability of a newly introduced agent that may be short-lived due to its possible idiosyncratic adverse effects
- When cross-tapering one antipsychotic to another, and "coverage" is sought for both the five half-life time periods of both the new and old drugs being exchanged (to minimize possible discontinuation symptoms and clinical worsening due to absence of a drug that might have been working better than was appreciated)
- When starting a long-acting injectable (LAI) formulation of an antipsychotic, and "coverage" is needed until a minimum therapeutic blood level of the LAI drug is reached
- When specifically targeting hostility and aggression (Morrissette and Stahl, 2014)

There are a number of instances in which combination antipsychotics would be considered rationale- and/or evidence-based, as noted in Box 6.11.

Conceptually, the possible advantages and disadvantages of combining antipsychotics can be summarized as follows:

Advantages:

- Possible unrecognized complementary receptor profiles
- Use of multiple antipsychotics might allow sparing of adverse effects from one drug with lower-than-usual dosing of two or more agents
- The effects of one drug may counter adverse effects of another

Disadvantages:

- Competition for identical receptors; no compelling empirical evidence base for greater efficacy than with any optimized monotherapy
- Even low doses of some antipsychotics may produce significant (and thus additive) adverse effects (e.g., sedation, metabolic dysregulation)
- Greater risk for exacerbation of adverse metabolic effects; additive motor effects (perhaps minimized by favoring so-called "loose" (high Ki) D_2 binders (e.g., quetiapine, clozapine) over "tight" (low Ki) D_2 binders (e.g., risperidone, ziprasidone))

Rules of the road for coprescribing multiple antipsychotic drugs are summarized in Box 6.12:

Box 6.12

Rules for Coprescribing Antipsychotics

- Determine whether, and why, further optimization of a first antipsychotic – or an outright switch to a different antipsychotic – would not be a preferred strategy
- Clearly identify the unmet goals of treatment and intended purpose for the second antipsychotic (e.g., global antipsychotic efficacy? A remedy for insomnia or agitation? Counteracting an adverse effect of the first antipsychotic?)
- Beware of dose-related akathisia and do not mistake it for undertreated psychotic agitation or anxiety
- Monitor for acute dystonia or additive sedation
- Avoid mixing high-potency antipsychotics with "tight" D_2 binding; favor "loose" D_2 binders either in combination (e.g., quetiapine, olanzapine, clozapine) or with one "tight" D_2 binder
- Consider tapering off a first antipsychotic drug if and when its effects seem either negligible or redundant with a second

What About Mixing a D_2 Antagonist with a Partial Agonist or Full Agonist?

The concept behind dopamine partial agonism implies that a molecule will either agonize or antagonize depending on ambient dopaminergic tone. When a D_2 partial agonist (such as aripiprazole, brexpiprazole, or cariprazine) is combined with a full D_2 agonist (such as amphetamine or methylphenidate), the partial agonist functions as a competitive antagonist, producing a net reduction in receptor activity caused by the full agonist. Dopamine agonists have provisionally been examined for specific intended purposes as augmentation strategies to D_2 antagonists. Obvious concerns include the potential for worsening of psychosis with agents such as methylphenidate. The evidence base is limited, and in some instances includes case reports or open trials involving too few subjects to draw meaningful conclusions either for better or worse (e.g., adjunctive bromocriptine or ropinirole).

We can think of several examples of empirically demonstrated robust effects from prescribing a dopamine agonist with an antagonist:

- *Amantadine* has been used as a cognitively sparing alternative to anticholinergic drugs (e.g., benztropine) for antipsychotic-associated parkinsonism. Comparable antiparkinsonian efficacy to benztropine has been shown, but with fewer adverse effects (DiMascio et al., 1976).

- *Amphetamine* may counteract the presumed hypofunctioning of mesocortical and prefrontal D_1 receptor pathways associated with negative symptoms in schizophrenia. In one RCT, lisdexamfetamine (mean dose = 50 mg/day) was significantly better than placebo in reducing PANSS total and subscale scores without exacerbation of psychosis (Lasser et al., 2013).
- *Pramipexole* has been used as an adjunct to haloperidol for resistant schizophrenic negative and positive symptoms; PANSS total scores improved >20% in most patients with no observed clinical worsening (Kasper et al., 1997).

Combining Antipsychotics Plus Mood Stabilizers

There is at least a theoretical rationale for considering a role for GABAergic mood stabilizers (such as divalproex) in the treatment of psychotic disorders, given current understanding about the role of GABA in schizophrenia. Specifically, it is believed that while overactivity of mesolimbic dopaminergic pathways contributes to the pathogenesis of positive symptoms, that event may simply be a "downstream" consequence of corticolimbic glutamate dysfunction. As depicted in Figure 6.2, intact corticolimbic glutamate circuitry provides normal excitatory input to limbic structures which, in turn, regulate dopaminergic pathways. How? Via the parvalbumin class inhibitory GABA interneurons that, when stimulated, suppress mesolimbic dopamine firing. Failure of corticolimbic glutamate pathways to stimulate mesolimbic inhibitory GABA interneurons results in the failure to downregulate dopamine tracts which, when left unsuppressed (by underactivated inhibitory GABA interneurons), leads to dopaminergic overactivity and resultant positive symptoms of psychosis. Put more simply, GABA interneurons are an off-switch to mesolimbic dopamine neurons which should at least in theory help reduce psychotic symptoms (see Figure 6.2). This pathway is discussed further in Chapter 15.

Cortico-brainstem excitatory glutamate tracts regulate mesolimbic DA transmission by stimulating inhibitory GABA interneurons – which, in turn, normally suppress dopamine release; inhibition of GABA interneurons could potentiate psychosis.

Icarus Polypharmacy and Aggressive Dosing

Like the Greek mythological figure whose feather-and-wax wings melted when he stubbornly flew too close to the sun, psychopharmacological aerodynamics often work in an analogous not-too-much but not-too-little fashion. Clinicians who overzealously pursue more and more perfect treatment outcomes through supratherapeutic dosing and/or very aggressive polypharmacy regimens run the risk of scorching the patient. Modest or manageable adverse effects can quickly become lethal when highway drivers become somnolent or have slowed reaction times; hazy thinking attributed to underlying psychopathology can just as easily reflect antihistaminergic or anticholinergic adverse effects; aggressive psychostimulant use (beware their seductively high effect sizes noted in Box 3.6) is literally

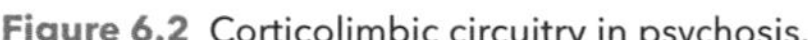

Figure 6.2 Corticolimbic circuitry in psychosis.

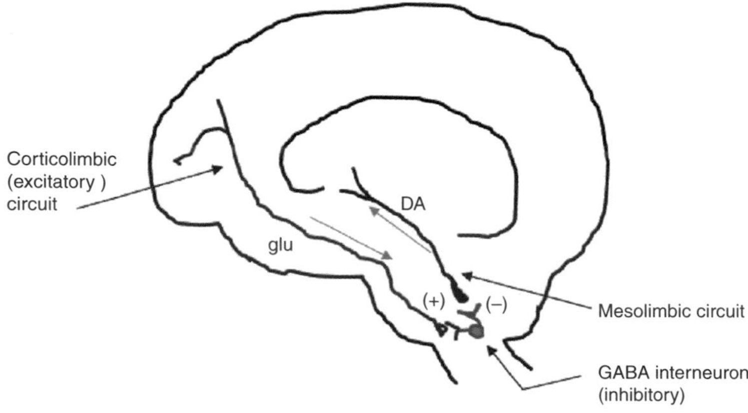

not for the faint of heart (inotropically speaking) and can start to mimic hypomania or induce psychosis in those predisposed. And senseless conglomerations of absurdly or haphazardly constructed overly extensive regimens just create pharmacological anarchy (not to mention, inspire little confidence in the potential value of more thoughtful and synergistically devised complex regimens).

TAKE-HOME POINTS

- Strive to combine individual medications linked to specific intended pharmacodynamic effects.
- Optimize a first drug before contemplating adding a second within-class agent, unless augmentation of a suboptimally dosed drug is intended to spare adverse effects or capitalize on a known pharmacokinetic or pharmacodynamic advantage.
- Devise regimens based on the three pillars of rational polypharmacy: complementary/nonredundant mechanisms, precedent established by empirical observation, and safety.
- Economize via parsimonious drug choices whenever possible.
- Deprescribe "clutter" pharmacotherapies and ineffective drugs that are maintained for no compelling reason; every component of a medication regimen should have a well-defined job description and pass regular performance evaluations at least effortlessly, if not with outright flying colors.

Table 6.1 Examples of potentially advantageous or deleterious *pharmacokinetic* clinically relevant drug-drug interactions: antidepressant combinations

Combination	Catabolic enzyme	Possible advantage	Risk
Bupropion + vortioxetine	Bupropion delays vortioxetine metabolism via CYP2D6 inhibition, elevating vortioxetine levels	Vortioxetine dose should be ≤10 mg/day with bupropion; possible fewer vortioxetine adverse effects with lower dosing; no reported supratherapeutic dose benefit	Supratherapeutic vortioxetine dosing (>10 mg/day with bupropion) could ↑ GI or other adverse effects; no reports of serotonin syndrome
Bupropion + SSRI or SNRI or TCA	Bupropion inhibits CYP2D6, raising serum levels of fluoxetine, paroxetine, venlafaxine, many TCAs	Observed benefits of synergy in cotherapies may be more pharmacodynamic than pharmacokinetic	Possible increased seizure risk, treatment-emergent anxiety with adjunctive bupropion (Mohamed et al., 2017)
SSRI + TCA	Fluoxetine, fluvoxamine, paroxetine and to a lesser extent sertraline (Preskorn et al., 1994) can ↑ TCA levels via CYP2D6 inhibition (Taylor, 1995); fluvoxamine raises imipramine levels via CYP1A2 inhibition	Potentially better antidepressant outcomes with combination therapy than with either monotherapy (Nelson et al., 2004)	Potential for toxic TCA serum levels and more extensive anticholinergic or other adverse effects
SSRI + clomipramine[a]	Increased [clomipramine] can result from cotherapy with fluvoxamine (by CYP1A2 and 2C19 inhibition) or fluoxetine (by CYP2D6 and 2C19 inhibition)	Case reports (only) of better outcomes in refractory OCD when clomipramine has been combined with fluoxetine, fluvoxamine, sertraline or paroxetine; less concern for pharmacokinetic interactions when adding sertraline or paroxetine; see also Table 6.6	Increased serum clomipramine levels can cause cardiac and other anticholinergic adverse effects; theoretical (though unlikely) risk of serotonin syndrome; assure serum [clomipramine] + [desmethylclomipramine] <500 ng/mL
Doxepin + antidepressants or antipsychotics	Doxepin inhibits CYP2D6	Popular nonaddictive sleep aid	Could potentially ↑ levels of many TCAs, fluoxetine, fluvoxamine, atomoxetine, venlafaxine, duloxetine, amphetamine, aripiprazole, risperidone

[a] (SSRI cotherapy with clomipramine is discussed separately from other TCAs due to its more common use in OCD)

Abbreviations: GI = gastrointestinal; OCD = obsessive-compulsive disorder; SNRI = serotonin-norepinephrine reuptake inhibitor; SSRI = selective serotonin reuptake inhibitor; TCA = tricyclic antidepressant

Table 6.2 Examples of potentially advantageous or deleterious *pharmacokinetic* clinically relevant drug-drug interactions: antidepressant or anticonvulsant + SGA or anticonvulsant combinations

Combination	Catabolic enzyme	Possible advantage	Risk
Clozapine + fluoxetine or fluvoxamine	Clozapine metabolism delayed by fluvoxamine (through CYP1A2 and 2C19 inhibition) or fluoxetine (through CYP2C19 inhibition)	Low-dose fluvoxamine (50 mg/day) added to steady-state clozapine (100 mg/day) may achieve serum clozapine levels ≥350 ng/mL without toxicity in nonsmoking schizophrenia patients (Lu et al., 2000) and may also lessen weight gain/metabolic adverse effects (Lu et al., 2004)	Serum clozapine levels must be monitored carefully because their increases can be unpredictable; greater seizure risk and sedative effects
Olanzapine + fluvoxamine	Fluvoxamine inhibition of CYP1A2 increases olanzapine levels up to 112% (Hiemke et al., 2002)	May allow olanzapine dosage reductions (by about 25%, on average) (Albers et al., 2005)	May be well-tolerated but use with caution
Divalproex + sertraline or paroxetine	Sertraline or paroxetine each can ↑ serum [valproate] via CYP2C9 inhibition	Clinicians may sometimes treat bipolar depression with an SSRI + divalproex; serum [valproate] may rise	Monitor for increased serum [valproate] and consequently greater associated adverse effects
Carbamazepine + any other drug	Carbamazepine is among the most potent inducers of Phase I and Phase II enzymes	No known *pharmacokinetic* advantages	Lesser efficacy of any hepatically metabolized coprescribed drugs
Lamotrigine + divalproex	Divalproex delays Phase II metabolism of lamotrigine, increasing serum [lamotrigine]	Possible less prominent depression than with divalproex alone during bipolar maintenance (Bowden et al., 2012)	Increased risk for severe cutaneous reactions

Abbreviations: SGA = second-generation antipsychotic; SSRI = selective serotonin reuptake inhibitor

Table 6.3 Examples of potentially advantageous or deleterious *pharmacokinetic* clinically relevant drug-drug interactions: other substrates

Combination	Catabolic enzyme	Possible advantages	Risk
Tamoxifen + any CYP2D6 inhibitor	CYP2D6 inhibition impairs conversion of tamoxifen to its active metabolite endoxifen	None	Tamoxifen remains a biologically inactive pro-drug in the presence of CYP2D6 inhibitors; avoid such combinations
Dextromethorphan[a] + quinidine	Quinidine, as a P450 2D6 inhibitor, diminishes the degradation of dextromethorphan to dextrorphan	Demonstrated efficacy in pseudobulbar affect	Risk for dose-dependent QTc prolongation
Dextromethorphan[a] + bupropion (AXS-05)	Bupropion, as a P450 2D6 inhibitor, prolongs activity of dextromethorphan	Demonstrated efficacy in MDD	Risk for dose-dependent QTc prolongation
Clozapine + ciprofloxacin or erythromycin	Ciprofloxacin and erythromycin potently inhibit P450 1A2, drastically increasing serum [clozapine]	None	Potential lethality from acute clozapine toxicity (Meyer et al., 2016; Cohen et al., 1996)

[a] Putative pharmacodynamic mechanisms for dextromethorphan are complex and thought to involve NMDA receptor blockade as well as serotonin/norepinephrine reuptake, nicotinic cholinergic receptor antagonism, and sigma-1 receptor agonism (Taylor et al., 2016)

Abbreviations: MDD = major depressive disorder; NMDA = *N*-methyl-D-aspartate; QTc = corrected QT interval

Table 6.4 Examples of potentially advantageous or deleterious *pharmacodynamic* drug-drug interactions

Combination	Rationale	Result
Clozapine + bupropion	Not evidence-based and poor rationale	Additive lowering of seizure threshold
Fluvoxamine + clomipramine	Despite presumed mechanistic redundancy of serotonin reuptake inhibition, may have value in some forms of OCD	Theoretical but unlikely possibility of serotonin syndrome
Lithium + divalproex	Complementary, nonredundant mechanisms may synergize	Better relapse prevention in bipolar disorder than with divalproex monotherapy (BALANCE Investigators and Collaborators, 2010)
Mirtazapine + another antidepressant	Complementary, nonredundant mechanisms that may synergize	Combining mirtazapine with fluoxetine or bupropion or venlafaxine at treatment initiation yielded higher remission rates than seen with fluoxetine alone (Blier et al., 2010)
Bupropion + another antidepressant	Bupropion's pro-catecholaminergic effects, with a relative absence of serotonergic effects, make it a mechanistically attractive cotherapy for many other antidepressants	Meta-analysis of 13 RCTs suggests efficacy for bupropion + SSRIs, SNRIs, or mirtazapine - although most RCTs show comparability to an active comparator rather than a placebo (Patel et al., 2016); in the CO-MED trial, bupropion + escitalopram reduced suicidal ideation better than escitalopram alone or mirtazapine + venlafaxine (Zisook et al., 2011)
Pindolol + SSRI	The beta-blocker pindolol also blocks presynaptic $5HT_{1A}$ autoreceptors, effectively increasing presynaptic serotonin release	Meta-analyses suggest possible faster onset of SSRI antidepressant response and greater likelihood of sustained remission adding pindolol 5 mg PO TID (Portella et al., 2011)
SNRI + TCA	Modest data showing efficacy and safety: one small (n = 11) open trial showed response (in 9/11 subjects) and cardiovascular safety when adding venlafaxine to clomipramine or imipramine after TCA nonresponse (Gómez and Teixidó, 2000)	Mechanistic redundancy, no rationale for synergy, theoretical cardiovascular risks; seldom a favored combination. Remember that duloxetine can ↑ amitriptyline, desipramine, imipramine and clomipramine levels via CYP2D6 inhibition
DORA ± benzodiazepine or benzodiazepine agonist (e.g., zolpidem, eszopiclone) ± antihistaminergic sleep aid (e.g., trazodone, doxepin)	DORA's unique mechanism of action (orexin receptor blockade) makes it a logical (albeit unstudied) adjunctive therapy in hard-to-treat insomnia	Additive sedation

Abbreviations: DORA=dual orexin receptor antagonist (e.g., suvorexant, lemborexant, or daridorexant)"; OCD = obsessive-compulsive disorder; PO TID = oral, three times a day; RCT = randomized controlled trial; SNRI = serotonin-norepinephrine reuptake inhibitor; SSRI = selective serotonin reuptake inhibitor; TCA = tricyclic antidepressent

Table 6.5 MAOI copharmacotherapies: what you need to know

MAOI +	Why frowned upon	Reality
Bupropion	Possible sympathomimetic/pressor effect, could cause a hypertensive crisis	Case reports of successful treatment of refractory depression combining tranylcypromine with bupropion (e.g., Quante and Zeugmann, 2012); must closely monitor blood pressure
Buspirone	As a full agonist at the $5HT_{1A}$ presynaptic inhibitory autoreceptor and a postsynaptic $5HT_{1A}$ partial agonist, buspirone + an MAOI could theoretically cause serotonin syndrome	We are aware of only one published case report of serotonin syndrome (Manos, 2000)
Pindolol	Aside from β-blocking effects, pindolol selectively blocks presynaptic $5HT_{1A}$ autoreceptors; consequent increased presynaptic serotonergic outflow + an MAOI might induce serotonin syndrome	Case reports of safe and successful augmentation of tranylcypromine (Kraus, 1997); we know of no published reports of adverse reactions to pindolol plus an MAOI (see also Figure 6.1)
Carbamazepine	Structural resemblance to TCAs could theoretically increase risk of serotonin syndrome	Open trials of safe and effective coadministration (e.g., Ketter et al., 1995), although no extensive studies
General anesthesia	A handful of case reports of intraoperative hemodynamic instability, hyperpyrexia, or convulsions among MAOI recipients in the 1960s and 1970s led to recommendations that MAOIs be discontinued two weeks prior to elective surgery	No adverse cardiovascular or hemodynamic events and no signs of serotonin syndrome in modern case-control studies (e.g., van Haelst et al., 2012); intraoperative epinephrine poses sympathomimetic risks to MAOI recipients, but modern anesthesiology tends not to eschew MAOI use routinely
Lithium	Putative serotonergic effects of lithium (e.g., via increased postsynaptic $5HT_{1A}$ signaling) could in theory cause serotonin syndrome	Case reports of safe and successful lithium-MAOI cotherapy in refractory depression (e.g., Fein et al., 1988) and rapid improvement when added to phenelzine (Nelson and Byck, 1982)
Psychostimulants	Possible sympathomimetic effects could cause hypertensive crisis and its consequences (e.g., stroke, myocardial ischemia, death)	A review by Feinberg (2004) found no published reports of hypertensive crises or fatalities. We would note that adding a stimulant to an MAOI is nevertheless a very aggressive intervention that should be undertaken with great caution only by well-experienced prescribers
(Ar)modafinil	Theoretical concern that any "stimulant-like" agent combined with an MAOI could cause a hypertensive crisis	(Ar)modafinil shows no sympathomimetic effects and minimal to no cardiovascular or hemodynamic effects in animals. Case reports of safe coadministration with tranylcypromine (Clemons et al., 2004); largely understudied, but in our experience a very rational polypharmacy
Ondansetron, Granisetron	In 2014 the FDA issued a warning that $5HT_3$ antagonists could theoretically cause serotonin syndrome, following a 2012 WHO pharmaceutical newsletter release	$5HT_3$ antagonism does not "increase" serotonin availability or $5HT_{2A}$ or $5HT_{1A}$ agonism, or otherwise lead to toxicity (see critique on the implausibility of this as a mechanism for serotonin syndrome by Rojas-Fernandez, 2014)

Abbreviations: 5HT = serotonin; FDA = US Food and Drug Administration; MAOI = monoamine oxidase inhibitor; WHO = World Health Organization

Table 6.6 Examples of single agents with multiple pharmacodynamic effects: anticonvulsants and lithium

Agent	Depression	Mania	Psychosis	Anxiety	Anti-impulsivity	Affective instability [a]	Hostility-aggression [b]	Neuropathic pain	Trauma/autonomic arousal	Migraine [c]	Insomnia	Binge eating	Attentional processing
Carbamazepine		✓			✓	?	✓						
Divalproex		✓			✓	?	✓			✓			
Gabapentin				✓			?	✓		✓	✓		
Lamotrigine	✓					?	✓						
Oxcarbazepine		?					✓						
Pregabalin				✓			?	✓		✓			
Topiramate					✓		✓		✓	✓		✓	
Lithium	✓	✓			✓	?	✓						

[a] Surprisingly, there has been little to no formal study of medications in this category for targeting moment-to-moment variations in subjective mood states; see Chapter 13

[b] see Cochrane Review, Huband et al., 2010, and Chapter 14

[c] see Cochrane Review, Linde et al., 2013

Blank cells depict instances in which either existing data are predominantly (if not entirely) negative or for which a given use would follow no known rationale; "?" indicates instances where preclinical but not human studies suggest a possible effect, or insufficient human data are available to render an impression about efficacy.

Table 6.7 Examples of single agents with multiple pharmacodynamic effects: monoaminergic antidepressants

Agent	Depression	Mania	Psychosis	Anxiety [a]	Anti-impulsivity [b]	Affective instability [c]	Hostility-aggression [d]	Neuropathic pain [e]	Trauma/autonomic arousal [f]	Migraine	Insomnia	Binge eating/weight loss	Attentional processing [g]
Bupropion	✓											✓	✓
SSRIs:	✓												
(Es)/citalopram	✓			✓	✓	?	✓	?	✓			✓	
Fluoxetine	✓			✓	✓	?	✓	?	✓			✓	
Fluvoxamine	✓		✓ [h]	✓	✓	?	?	?	✓			✓	
Paroxetine	✓			✓	✓	?	?	?	✓			?	
Sertraline	✓			✓	✓	?	✓	?	✓			✓	
SNRIs:	✓			✓									
Duloxetine	✓			✓	✓	?	?	✓	✓	✓		✓ [i]	✓
Levomilnacipran	✓			✓	?	?	?	✓		✓		? [i]	?
(Des)/ Venlafaxine	✓			✓	?	✓	?	✓	✓	? [j]		? [i]	?
TCAs	✓			✓	?	?	?	✓	?	✓	✓		✓ [g]
Mirtazapine	✓			?	?	?	?	?	✓	?	✓		
Nefazodone	✓			?	?	?			✓	?	?		
Vilazodone	✓			✓		?				?	?		
Vortioxetine	✓			✓		?	?	?		?	?		✓

[a] See Chapter 17

[b] See Chapter 14

[c] To our knowledge, "affective instability" or "affective lability" have not been identified as formal secondary outcomes in published RCTs (but see further discussion in Chapter 13)

[d] See Chapter 14; RCT data for antiaggression efficacy of fluvoxamine are limited to use in adults with autism, while data for mirtazapine are nonrandomized and derive mainly from studies in dementia

[e] SSRIs in general have not been extensively studied for treatment of neuropathic pain, although limited data from meta-analyses do report modest overall effects

[f] See Chapter 19

[g] See Chapter 21

[h] Fluvoxamine monotherapy has been reported in open trials to treat delusional depression with response rates up to 84% (Gatti et al., 1996); in general, however, SSRI monotherapy is not considered usual treatment for psychotic depression

[i] Randomized trial data exist with duloxetine while only open-label/case series data exist with levomilnacipran or venlafaxine

[j] Cochrane Review identifies venlafaxine as no better than placebo for migraine based on limited available data; other SNRIs not considered (Banzi et al., 2015)

Blank cells depict instances in which either existing data are predominantly (if not entirely) negative or for which a given use would follow no known rationale; "?" indicates instances where preclinical but not human studies suggest a possible effect, or insufficient human data are available to render an impression about efficacy.

Abbreviations: SSRI = selective serotonin reuptake inhibitor; TCA = tricyclic antidepressant

Table 6.8 Examples of single agents with multiple pharmacodynamic effects: antipsychotics

Agent	Depression [a]	Mania [b]	Psychosis	Anxiety [c]	Anti-impulsivity [d]	Affective instability [e]	Hostility-aggression [f]	Neuropathic pain	Trauma/autonomic arousal [g]	Migraine [h]	Insomnia [i]	Binge eating/weight loss	Attentional processing [j]
Aripiprazole	✓	✓	✓	?		?	✓		✓	?			✓
Asenapine	✓	✓	✓	?	?	✓	✓		?				?
Brexpiprazole	✓	?	✓	?	?	?	✓						?
Cariprazine	✓	✓	✓	?	?	?	✓		?				?
Iloperidone			✓	?	?	?							
Lurasidone	✓	?	✓	✓	?	?	?						✓
Olanzapine	✓	✓	✓	✓	✓	✓	✓		✓	?	✓		✓
Paliperidone			✓	?	✓	?	?						?
Pimavanserin	✓		✓			?	?						?
Quetiapine	✓	✓	✓	✓	✓	?	✓		✓	?	✓		
Risperidone	✓	✓	✓	?	✓	?	✓		?				✓
Ziprasidone		✓	✓			?	?		?	?	✓		?

[a] Aripiprazole has been shown to improve depressive symptoms when added to a traditional antidepressant, but has not demonstrated antidepressant properties as monotherapy in unipolar or bipolar depression; asenapine and lurasidone both have been shown to improve depressive symptoms better than placebo in major depression with mixed features. For full discussion of antidepressant properties of specific SGAs see Chapter 13.

[b] Lurasidone has not been formally studied in acute mania, although it has been shown to reduce mania symptoms during bipolar depressive episodes (McIntyre et al., 2015). Brexpiprazole has two unpublished negative RCTs in mania. Paliperidone was no better than placebo for treating mania (dosed at 3 or 6 mg/day; but successful at 12 mg/day) according to a meta-analysis by Chang et al. (2017).

[c] A Cochrane Database review of SGAs for specific anxiety disorders found no advantages over placebo for olanzapine or risperidone (Depping et al., 2010). However, see fuller discussion of anxiolytic effects of SGAs in Chapter 17.

[d] Impulsivity symptom ratings, within the context of schizophrenia RCTs, improved with brexpiprazole but not aripiprazole (Citrome et al., 2016b). In RCTs of borderline personality disorder, ziprasidone showed no difference from placebo in reducing impulsivity symptoms (Pascual et al., 2008) though impulsive aggression improved more than placebo with risperidone (Rocca et al., 2002) or paliperidone (Bellino et al., 2011).

[e] Positive findings for affective instability derive mainly from RCTs in borderline personality disorder (e.g., Zanarini and Frankenburg, 2001 (olanzapine), Bozzatello et al., 2017 (asenapine)).

[f] In bipolar mania, asenapine reduced hostility and disruptive aggression better than placebo (Citrome et al., 2017b). Brexpiprazole and cariprazine each reduced hostility better than placebo in post hoc analyses in schizophrenia (Citrome et al., 2016a; 2016b). Post hoc analyses from the CATIE schizophrenia trial identified olanzapine as especially useful for hostility (Volavka et al., 2014). In their meta-analysis of antipsychotics for borderline personality disorder, Mercer et al. (2009) note that the effect size of aripiprazole for anger is larger than that of most other antipsychotics. See also Chapter 14.

[g] See Chapter 19.

[h] Preliminary (nonrandomized) data suggest efficacy in migraine and chronic headache with aripiprazole (LaPorta, 2007), olanzapine (Silberstein et al., 2002), quetiapine (Krymchantowski et al., 2010), and ziprasidone (Boeker, 2002).

[i] Low incident rates of somnolence (i.e., high "number needed to harm" (NNH)s) reported in schizophrenia clinical trials with aripiprazole (NNH = 34), asenapine (NNH = 21), brexpiprazole (NNH = 271), cariprazine (NNH = 65), lurasidone (NNH = 20), paliperidone (NNH = 117), and risperidone (NNH = 13) (Citrome et al., 2017a).

[j] See Chapter 21

Blank cells depict instances in which either existing data are predominantly (if not entirely) negative or for which a given use would follow no known rationale; "?" indicates instances where preclinical but not human studies suggest a possible effect, or insufficient human data are available to render an impression about efficacy.

Table 6.9 Pharmacological parsimony and niche roles for individual medications with varied pharmacodynamic properties

	Clinical Domains					
Amphetamine	ADD/slowed attentional processing [a]	Depression	Weight loss/ binge eating	Counteracts iatrogenic sedation		
(Ar)modafinil	Fatigue/daytime sleepiness	Depression	ADD/slowed attentional processing [a]			
Bupropion	Depression	Smoking cessation	Weight loss	ADD/slowed attentional processing [a]		
Carbamazepine	Bipolar disorder (mania > depression, acute > maintenance)	Trigeminal neuralgia	Epilepsy	Diabetic peripheral neuropathy		
Duloxetine (and other SNRIs)	Depression	Anxiety	Neuropathic or musculoskeletal or bone pain	Urinary incontinence	Perimenopausal hot flashes	
Divalproex	Bipolar disorder (mania > depression, acute > maintenance)	Alcoholism in bipolar disorder [b]	Migraine prophylaxis	Impulsive aggression (dementia, borderline personality disorder)	Epilepsy	
Gabapentin	Anxiety	Insomnia (prolongs stage 3/4 sleep)	Neuropathic pain, migraine	Carpal tunnel syndrome	Perimenopausal hot flashes	Epilepsy
Lithium	Bipolar disorder (mania > depression)	Antisuicide effect	Boosts WBC counts (e.g., clozapine cotherapy)	Gout	Cyclical vomiting syndrome	
Propranolol [c]	Tremor	Social anxiety	Hypertension	Akathisia	Agitation [d]	
Topiramate	Migraine	Binge eating/ weight loss	Alcohol misuse	Possibly hyperarousal symptoms of PTSD [e]	Epilepsy	

[a] See Chapter 21
[b] Salloum et al., 2005
[c] One should try to avoid nonselective beta-blockers in asthmatics in order to minimize risk of bronchospasm
[d] Reviewed by Goedhard et al., 2006
[e] See Chapter 19

Abbreviations: ADD = attention deficit disorder; PTSD = post-traumatic stress disorder; SNRI = serotonin-norepinephrine reuptake inhibitor; WBC = white blood cell

7 Laboratory Values and Psychiatric Symptoms: What to Measure, What Not to Measure, and What to Do With The Results

LEARNING OBJECTIVES

- ☐ Know which psychotropic medications do and do not have established therapeutic plasma drug level ranges
- ☐ Recognize which oral medications differ when taken with versus without food on drug absorption, bioavailability, and plasma drug levels
- ☐ Understand evidence-based reasons for when to order a plasma drug level
- ☐ Know when and how to order and interpret plasma drug levels relative to drug half-life and to draws obtained at trough, random, or other times based on convention

Not everything that can be counted counts, and not everything that counts can be counted.

- Albert Einstein

Psychiatrists probably are not so unusual among health care professionals in their desire to measure things. But compared to practitioners in most other areas of medicine, they may be the newest entrants to the world of the quantitative versus qualitative. Measurement-based care (MBC) and laboratory testing have become increasing focal points of clinical practice. Perhaps this comes in response to decades (if not centuries) of an often impressionistic and sometimes sluggishly qualitative way of recording clinical observations; perhaps it is backlash against a psychoanalytic heritage that for too long eschewed quantitative measures and formal outcome tracking; it also reflects the promulgation of research tools (semi-structured interviews, questionnaires, rating scales) into nonresearch clinical settings; and no doubt, MBC has arisen in response to a health care system that has come to link service reimbursement with quantifiable parameters.

Tip

"Therapeutic drug monitoring" (TDM) is a term used to describe the practice of regularly measuring serum drug levels to assure their sufficient concentrations for therapeutic efficacy. It assumes that serum levels correlate with clinical effects.

In this chapter, we will focus on the rationale and relevance (or irrelevance) of laboratory-based measures, end-organ monitoring for drug safety and efficacy, and the role of quantitative symptom tracking and MBC as an adaptation and outgrowth from the research world of RCTs. Let us once again begin with a clinical example (Clinical Vignette 7.1).

CLINICAL VIGNETTE 7.1

Mark is a 34-year-old man with bipolar I disorder that has stably been in remission for over three years. His psychiatrist, Dr. Abbott, prescribes him lithium carbonate 600 mg/day and divalproex sodium 1000 mg/day. His most recent quarterly serum drug levels were [Li^+] = 0.48 mEq/L and [valproic acid] = 42 μg/mL. His serum creatinine at that time was 0.89 mg/dL and his complete blood count (CBC), hepatic enzymes, and thyroid-stimulating hormone (TSH) all were well within their normal ranges. Should his dosages be changed?

Mark has been stable on a fairly simple drug regimen of modestly dosed, diagnosis-appropriate pharmacotherapies for a meaningfully extensive period of time. If his symptoms have been well-controlled for several years, his regimen and dosages have been constant, and his biochemistry markers have been unremarkable, does he really need lab work every three months? The answer largely depends on whom we ask. Some practice guidelines quite conservatively do, for example, advocate indefinite monitoring of serum lithium levels as frequently as every three months. Our perspective is that such blanket recommendations must be interpreted within a particular clinical context. Obvious differences exist among patients who are psychiatrically more or less symptomatic, younger versus older adults, patients with renal disease, those taking thiazide diuretics or ACE inhibitors, those with erratic adherence, those with versus without GI or neurological adverse effects, and those with poorly controlled symptoms. Laboratory monitoring should occur for an intended purpose based on the patient's clinical status.

In the absence of unstable clinical signs or symptoms, there is probably room for more latitude and discretion in deciding on the most appropriate frequency and relevance of Mark's laboratory monitoring. Importantly, from a safety standpoint, we should probably be more concerned with the continued normalcy of Mark's renal and thyroid function than his lithium level (absent symptom or dosing changes), and more with his hepatic function than his valproic acid level. Semi-annual assessment of end-organ laboratory monitoring in this case is likely more than adequate.

A WHEN DOES IT MAKE SENSE TO MEASURE SERUM DRUG LEVELS?

Mark's serum lithium and valproate levels are of secondary importance to his clinical status. One could alter his doses to try to make his numbers conform more closely to the therapeutic ranges described in Table 7.1, but doing that would ignore the established evidence of the clinical stability afforded by his existing regimen. Furthermore, unlike an idealized hypothetical monotherapy patient, Mark takes two medications that may well be clinically synergistic. There is no evidence base from which to presume the necessity of optimized dosing (or serum drug levels) from such a combination therapy regimen. Once again, the patient's own sustained lack of signs or symptoms is irrefutable evidence of his clinical stability. We only impose further evidence-based strategies that could improve his condition when his condition is in need of improvement.

In general, no medical test should be ordered without a reason. In the case of psychotropic drug levels, we can think of several, as summarized in Box 7.1.

Box 7.1

Reasons for Drug Level Tests

- Medication adherence: when pharmacotherapy nonadherence is suspected, an undetectable serum drug level lends credence to speculation.
- Frank toxicity states, or when there are clinical signs suggestive of possible toxicity (coarse tremor, cognitive dulling or sedation, ataxia), it can be useful to determine whether a serum drug level is at or above the upper end of the laboratory reference range. (Note: some drugs, such as lithium, might cause tremor or gastrointestinal upset without such signs necessarily indicating excessive dosing or supratherapeutic serum levels.)
- In a still-symptomatic patient, when an established therapeutic reference range for a particular drug does exist, one might check a serum level to gauge if there is room to increase the dose safely toward the upper end of the reference range.
- When a pharmacokinetic interaction may be pertinent, measuring a level (especially before and after exposure to potential inducing or inhibiting codrug) may help to determine the extent and magnitude of the interaction.
- In treatment-resistant cases where dosing can be guided by plasma drug levels to the point of either tolerability or futility.

As a rule of thumb, one might generally be interested in the extreme values of a drug's laboratory reference range, with especially low levels signaling either poor adherence or ultrarapid metabolism, and unduly high levels suggesting toxicity/overdose, poor metabolism (causing drug build-up), or else the perhaps inadvertent capture of a peak (Cmax) level rather than a trough or steady-state level, as when a specimen is obtained too soon after a last dose. Though clinicians often speak interchangeably

Tip

In TDM, pay attention mainly to the extreme ends of a laboratory reference range; minimal-to-absent levels reflect nonadherence or ultra-rapid metabolism, while levels near or above the upper end of the reference range are consistent with possible toxicity states (depending on a drug's therapeutic index).

about "plasma" and "serum" drug levels, at least in the case of tricyclic antidepressants, plasma blood levels may be significantly higher than corresponding serum levels (Coccaro et al., 1987). Certain specific clinical conditions also are known to alter drug metabolism – for example, as noted in Chapter 12, rising estrogen levels during pregnancy can induce CYP450 enzymes, potentially resulting in reduced serum levels of SSRIs or other P450 substrates; however, routinely measuring serum drug levels for the sake of documenting this event during pregnancy may simply become an academic exercise that merely affirms clinical suspicion.

Definitions

Serum: blood fluid minus clotting factors and red or white blood cells

Plasma: blood fluid containing proteins and blood cells in suspension

In general, if and when measuring serum drug levels, it makes sense to do so after the passage of five half-lives as a reflection of steady-state pharmacokinetics. However, clinically therapeutic effects of a drug may be evident before five half-lives have elapsed, as in the case of very long-half-life drugs with long half-life active metabolites (e.g., fluoxetine, aripiprazole, cariprazine). Unless convention dictates otherwise, meaningfully interpretable levels are usually drawn at trough concentrations (i.e., just before the next dose).

For lithium, the manufacturer's package insert information advises that serum lithium levels be drawn "immediately prior to the next dose when lithium concentrations are relatively stable (i.e., 12 hours after the previous dose)." This, however, presupposes that lithium dosing occurs twice a day, which was the original dosing recommendation made by the manufacturer decades ago when lithium first came to market. Subsequent studies have shown that once rather than multiple daily dosing of lithium appears more protective against nephrotoxicity (Castro et al., 2016). By convention, meaningfully interpretable lithium levels are usually drawn 10–14 hours after the previous dose, although a true "trough" level would refer strictly to levels measured immediately before a next dose (i.e., at Cmin).

Among antidepressants, body weight has not been shown to influence blood levels (Unterecker et al., 2011).

Bioavailability and serum levels are affected by administration with food for some, but not most, psychotropic drugs. Medications that are better absorbed *with* food (possibly leading to higher serum levels), include deutetrabenazine, lithium, lumateperone, lurasidone, nefazodone, paliperidone, quetiapine (modest increase), sertraline (modest increase), vilzodone, and ziprasidone. Those that are better absorbed *without* food (possibly leading to higher serum levels) include asenapine, valbenazine, and zolpidem (modest).

There are a handful of clinical situations in which serum drug levels are decidedly *uninformative* for gauging therapeutic effects. Examples include:

- *Tachyphylaxis*: after prolonged exposure to drugs that can cause physiological tolerance (e.g., benzodiazepines, amphetamines, opiates), a given drug concentration may yield a lesser effect over time;
- *"Hit and run" drugs* that produce an all-or-none effect regardless of dosage. Examples would include antibiotics or irreversible noncompetitive enzyme inhibitors such as MAOIs.

Let us review some basic information about pharmacokinetics, as depicted in Boxes 7.2 and 7.3.

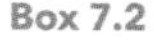

Box 7.2

A Primer on Linear and Nonlinear Pharmacokinetics

Therapeutic Window: refers to the range of dosages of a drug that can produce a therapeutic effect without causing significant adverse effects. Operationally, this is defined as the dosages that fall between the minimum effective concentration and the minimum toxic concentration, illustrated by the following graphic:

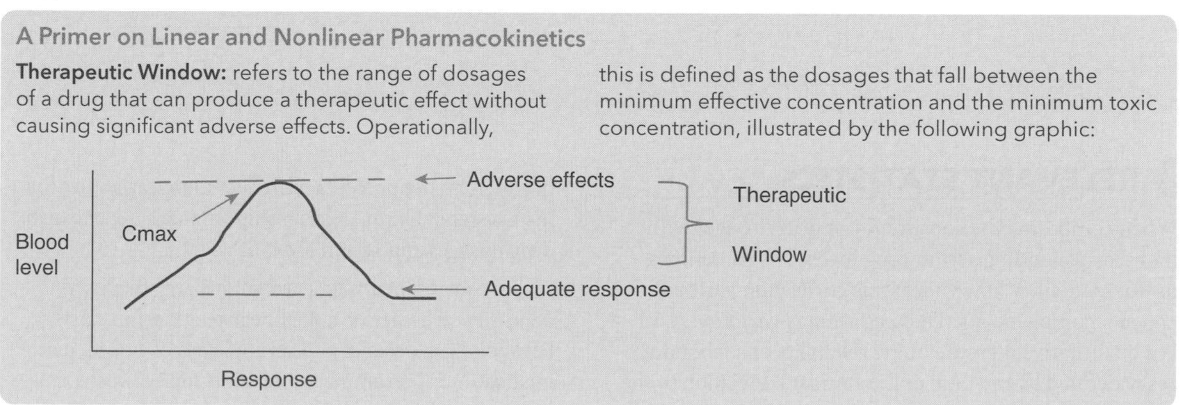

Box 7.2 Cont.

Therapeutic Range: when a defined clinical population (e.g., epilepsy patients, migraine sufferers, panic disorder patients) is exposed to a drug, the range of dosages (or serum levels) that correspond to empirically observed beneficial effects without producing toxicity defines a drug's therapeutic range. Note that the therapeutic range of drug dosages or serum levels for one condition may have no relevance (other than avoiding toxicity) if the same drug is used for a different condition.

Therapeutic Index: refers to the ratio of a drug's median lethal dose (LD_{50}) to its median effective dose (ED_{50}), i.e.:

$$\frac{LD_{50}}{ED_{50}}$$

A large therapeutic index means a safer drug while a narrow one means there is little room for dosing error (e.g., lithium). Drugs with a large therapeutic index sometimes also can produce a more sustained effect that permits once- or twice-daily dosing even if their elimination half-life is relatively short (e.g., beta-blockers).

Box 7.3

Dose-Response Curves

Linear dose-response curve: increases in serum drug levels are directly proportional to drug dosing.

Curvilinear response curve: an optimal effect comes from a dose (or level) that is neither too high nor too low. Notable examples among psychotropic drugs include nortriptyline, imipramine, and amitriptyline.

Logarithmic curve: involves a varying slope that initially shows a steep ascent followed by a plateau or ceiling effect. Examples include inhaled glucocorticoids in asthma.

Sigmoidal curve: follows a roughly linear contour from between 10-20% and 80–90% concentrations, bounded by flatter slope thresholds at lowest and highest dosing levels. Small changes in concentration or blood levels along the steep linear portion of the curve may produce substantial changes in effect. Examples include phenobarbital, lithium, amphetamine, and morphine.

Zero-order (nonlinear) kinetics (aka saturation kinetics): a *constant amount* of a drug is eliminated per unit time, independent of its plasma levels. Half-life and clearance are lower at low serum drug concentrations. Few drugs follow purely zero-order kinetics. Notable examples include ethanol, phenytoin, gabapentin, and high-dose salicylates.

First-order (linear) kinetics: elimination of a drug occurs at *constant fractional rate* per unit time (e.g., along an *exponential decay curve*), proportional to plasma drug levels. Drug clearance and half-life remain constant. Most psychotropic drugs follow first-order elimination, which in general is a much more common phenomenon than zero-order kinetics.

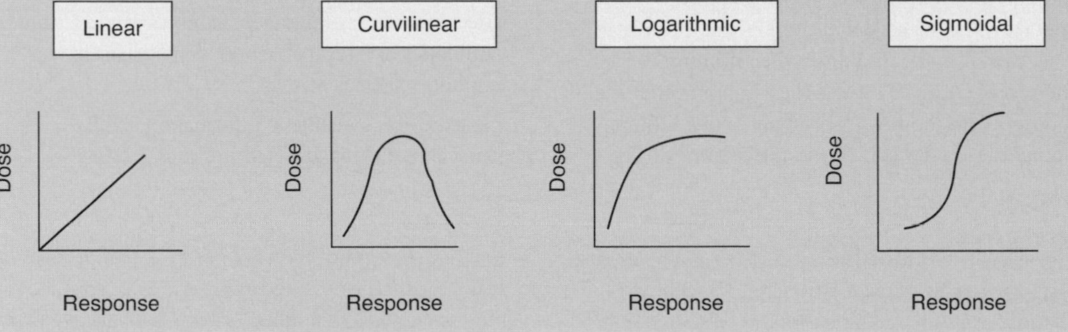

B RELEVANT STATISTICS

When comparing the consistency of drug dosages with their corresponding serum drug levels, it is sometimes useful to identify how widely this correlation varies or appears homogeneous. The *coefficient of variation (CV)* is a quantitative measure of the reliability of a laboratory assay defined by the ratio of the standard deviation to the mean of a population, usually expressed as a percentage, in which higher percentages reflect more variability (or inconsistency) in the relationship (in this case, between drug dosages and serum levels).

Pearson or Spearman correlations are often used to determine whether or not a linear relationship exists between drug dosages and serum levels of a particular medication. To examine the relationship between serum drug levels and therapeutic response, responder and nonresponder groups are usually compared in mean scores of serum drug levels using mean group comparison tests (e.g., t-tests or Mann–Whitney tests). To identify possible "cut-off" or threshold blood levels potentially associated with responder status, receiver operating characteristic (ROC) curves are often examined, as explained earlier in Chapter 3.

One cannot necessarily assume that if and when a therapeutic blood level reference range for a particular drug has been established for one disorder that same range will apply to other disorders for which the drug may be used. Examples of this would include carbamazepine in epilepsy versus bipolar mania, nortriptyline for major depression versus neuropathic pain, bupropion for major depression versus smoking cessation, or divalproex for bipolar mania versus migraine headaches. Preliminary studies would suggest better responses to paroxetine when serum levels are low in the case of panic disorder but high in the case of MDD (see Table 7.2). Many existing studies attempting to assess relationships between drug levels and therapeutic responses are hampered by small sample sizes and nonreplication of findings, as well as a paucity of studies examining whether serum levels remain stable over time in a given patient relative to their clinical response status.

Tables 7.2–7.6 present laboratory reference ranges as reported in the literature for major psychotropic agents, with distinctions drawn for instances in which evidence supports an association between serum levels and therapeutic drug response. In the case of lithium and mood-stabilizing anticonvulsants, it should be noted that some compounds have an evidence base for therapeutic blood levels only in certain illness phases that do not necessarily extrapolate across others (e.g., divalproex in mania but not bipolar depression; lithium in mania or maintenance therapy but not bipolar depression). Trough valproic acid levels are typically obtained 21–24 hours after the last dose of extended-release divalproex; a sample drawn 18–21 hours after the last dose will yield a serum level ~3–13% higher than a trough value, while samples drawn 12–15 hours after a last dose yield a plasma level ~18–25% higher than a true trough level (Reed and Dutta, 2006).

BTW, when should I measure a nortriptyline level in a patient on hemodialysis?

Tricyclics are not dialyzable, so, check a level the same as you would in a nondialysis patient. For dialyzable drugs with relevant serum levels, such as lithium, in a dialysis patient you'd measure a serum level immediately before dialysis.

C NOMOGRAMS AND ORAL LOADING STRATEGIES TO PREDICT OPTIMAL DRUG LEVELS

A nomogram is a graphical method for extrapolating an unknown value based on known parameters. In the early 1970s a nomogram was devised to predict optimal lithium levels (0.6–1.2 mEq/L) for maintenance pharmacotherapy in bipolar disorder following a single test dose of 600 mg, as depicted in Box 7.4 (Cooper et al., 1973).

Several observers who empirically tested this method found that half of more or subjects failed to reach therapeutic serum lithium levels (e.g., Gengo et al., 1980; Kuruvilla and Shaji, 1989). Perry and colleagues (1986) refined this approach by proposing a two-point method (serum lithium measurements at 12- and 36-hour timepoints) that may produce more accurate maintenance levels. Other reports have suggested that additional factors such as age, sex, and weight may further refine the accuracy of predicting a therapeutic lithium level (Zetin et al., 1986). In practice, such methods to achieve rapid therapeutic serum lithium levels have never gained mainstream popularity, perhaps in part because of lingering safety and tolerability concerns posed by lithium's narrow therapeutic index.

Oral loading strategies are another method for achieving rapid therapeutic serum drug levels with agents that have a sufficiently wide therapeutic index to avert toxicity. A small (n = 15) open pilot study of oral lithium loading (20 mg/kg) in hospitalized mania

Box 7.4

"Cooper's Nomogram" for Predicting Maintenance Serum Lithium Levels

Serum [Li+] 24° after initial test dose	Total daily dose
<0.05 mEq/L	3600 mg/day
0.05–0.09 mEq/L	2700 mg/day
0.10–0.14 mEq/L	1800 mg/day
0.15–0.19 mEq/L	1200 mg/day
0.20–0.23 mEq/L	900 mg/day
0.24–0.30 mEq/L	600 mg/day
>0.30 mEq/L	600 mg/day (with caution due to probable decreased clearance)

patients produced serum lithium levels >0.6 mEq/L within one day in all patients, although a majority incurred GI or neurological adverse effects that were judged as "mild" in most instances (Keck et al., 2001). Probably the best-known example of psychotropic oral loading to achieve rapid efficacy is with divalproex in acute mania (dosed at 20–30 mg/kg body weight in acute mania and 15 mg/kg in mild/hypomania, in divided doses for tolerability purposes). Such interventions can safely produce a therapeutic serum valproic acid level within three to five days, with corresponding rapid improvement in affective symptoms (Keck et al., 1993; McElroy et al., 2010a).

D (WHEN) ARE LAMOTRIGINE LEVELS MEANINGFUL IN PSYCHIATRY?

The commercial manufacturer of lamotrigine did not measure serum lamotrigine levels when they undertook FDA registration trials of it for either the acute or maintenance phases of bipolar disorder, making it difficult to surmise whether or not a therapeutic reference range exists correlating lamotrigine mood effects with serum drug levels. In epilepsy, one study of 811 outpatients identified a correlation between serum levels and toxicity (with most toxicity states occurring at [lamotrigine] >20 μg/mL) (Hirsch et al., 2004). In mood-disordered patients, preliminary efforts have been undertaken to explore possible links between therapeutic response and serum [lamotrigine] levels. As noted in Table 7.2, Kagawa and colleagues (2014) used ROC analyses in a study of 34 unipolar and bipolar patients and determined that acute response (>50% reduction from baseline in depressive symptom severity) was significantly associated with achieving a plasma lamotrigine threshold concentration ≥12.7 μmol/L. Subsequently, Nakamura et al. (2016) devised a nomogram for predicting achievement of this minimum threshold [lamotrigine] based on week 2 plasma [lamotrigine]. While this pair of findings from one study group is intriguing, clinicians must recognize their provisional nature and the need for replication in larger samples of well-characterized mood-disordered patients before more definitive conclusions can be drawn.

At present, the one domain in which serum lamotrigine levels hold known clinical relevance is in the case of pregnancy, and possibly also in the setting of cotherapy with estrogen-containing oral contraceptives. Estrogen induces the metabolism of lamotrigine, with clearance rates sometimes becoming up to 250% higher than prepartum, consequently leading to possible diminished serum lamotrigine levels; lamotrigine levels may then rise by a mean of about 150% by 5 weeks postpartum (Clark et al., 2013). Clark and colleagues (2013) advise *routinely* measuring serum lamotrigine levels before conception (or else as early in a pregnancy as possible) followed by serial measurements every four weeks, accompanied by 20–25% upward dosage adjustments based on both symptoms and serum levels. Further management considerations regarding lamotrigine and pregnancy are discussed in Chapter 12.

Estrogen-containing oral contraceptives (aka combination oral contraceptives) can lower serum lamotrigine levels by about 50%. During the "pill-free" week, lamotrigine levels can rise comparably. Some epileptologists advocate measuring serum lamotrigine levels in epileptic women upon beginning or discontinuing a combination oral contraceptive, but there appears to be wide variation in actual clinical practice with little consensus about a standard of care in this area (Privitera et al., 2014). From a practical clinical standpoint in women taking combined oral contraceptives, more relevant than tracking lamotrigine levels is the prescriber's awareness that target symptoms could exacerbate within a week of starting the contraceptive, and dosage adjustments may then consequently become necessary. Similarly, possible adverse effects from lamotrigine (which in general are not much different from placebo) could theoretically worsen when a contraceptive is stopped. It is probably overly fussy to alter lamotrigine dosing during the pill-free week in the absence of significant complaints. Clinicians should not automatically assume that a probable decline of variable magnitude in serum lamotrigine levels will necessarily translate to clinical deterioration. Dosage adjustments should be made based on patients' symptom status, potentially informed (but not dictated) by expectations about nonconstant serum levels.

So, treat the patient, not the number?

Mostly, but keep reading.

E WHEN ARE ANTIDEPRESSANT SERUM LEVELS CLINICALLY RELEVANT?

Among monoaminergic antidepressants, as shown in Tables 7.2–7.6, evidence to support the use of serum trough levels to inform dosing is best established with tricyclics whose levels follow a curvilinear dose–response relationship, suggesting a therapeutic window (i.e., nortriptyline, amitriptyline, and imipramine). Drug and/or metabolite levels for clomipramine and desipramine also can sometimes provide clinically useful information with respect to threshold levels (i.e., still-symptomatic patients whose blood levels fall below the therapeutic range may be more likely to benefit from dosage increases as compared to those whose levels are above the threshold levels described in Tables 7.2–7.6). In studies of fluoxetine, Cain (1992) reported four cases of depressed outpatients who initially responded to fluoxetine 20 mg/day, then relapsed, then responded to drug washout and resumption at a lower dose. That observation prompted the author to speculate that fluoxetine may have a therapeutic window, serum levels above or below which may cause deviation from optimal pharmacodynamic efficacy. While this concept is intriguing, and likely merits further study, we are aware of no other data that empirically support the hypothesis.

There may be value in measuring metabolite levels of bupropion (more reliably than levels of bupropion itself), although this tends not to be done routinely in clinical practice. Among SNRIs, there is modest evidence to support the utility of measuring serum levels of venlafaxine and desvenlafaxine, and possibly duloxetine, but again it is not standard or customary practice routinely to obtain serum drug levels to guide dosing decisions. There is little to no empirical evidence to support therapeutic drug monitoring as a validated means to guide dosing with citalopram, escitalopram, fluoxetine, fluvoxamine, levomilnacipran, MAOIs, mirtazapine, nefazodone, paroxetine, sertraline, vilazodone, or vortioxetine.

F PHARMACOKINETIC EFFECTS OF COTHERAPIES

Certain pharmacokinetic interactions are known to increase serum levels of antidepressants whose metabolism may be inhibited or induced by a coadministered drug (or, in the case of carbamazepine, autoinduction of its own catabolism within about four to six weeks of its initiation, making eventual reductions in serum levels more likely than not). In such instances, measuring a serum drug level can affirm or document a suspected pharmacokinetic event – but once again, the overarching clinical question should be, "Would my clinical management of this patient be different with versus without a laboratory value?" Laboratory confirmation of high or potentially toxic blood levels is of far greater relevance in drugs with a narrow therapeutic index, or to discriminate adverse effects that reflect potentially benign from toxic etiologies (e.g., tremor).

Tables 7.7–7.9 summarize psychotropic drugs that are substrates, inducers, or inhibitors for CYP450 2D6, 2C19, or 3A4, respectively.

CLINICAL VIGNETTE 7.2

Pop Quiz

Ken is a 43-year-old man with schizoaffective disorder recently begun on iloperidone that has been dosed up to 12 mg twice a day, added to existing duloxetine 60 mg/day. He complains of dizziness and sedation. Which one of the following laboratory assessments would be the most immediately relevant?

(a) serum iloperidone level
(b) serum duloxetine level
(c) 12-lead electrocardiogram (ECG)
(d) pharmacogenetic testing of CYP2D6

The correct answer in Clinical Vignette 7.2 is (c). Iloperidone is metabolized by CYP2D6, duloxetine inhibits CYP2D6, and the package insert for iloperidone carries a warning that iloperidone "should be avoided in patients with a known genetic susceptibility to congenital long QT syndrome and in patients with a history of cardiac arrhythmias." The manufacturer of iloperidone advises that dosing should be reduced by half to lessen the risk for QTc when coadministered with drugs that inhibit CYP2D6. While pharmacogenetic testing holds obvious relevance to determine if Ken has a CYP2D6 PM phenotype, the pharmacokinetic horse is already out of the barn; Ken has already begun iloperidone and is now supratherapeutically dosed by virtue of CYP2D6 inhibition from duloxetine cotherapy. Even though his complaints of dizziness and sedation are known and common adverse effects of iloperidone, his maximal dosing in the presence of a CYP2D6 inhibitor merits checking his ECG and/or stopping iloperidone altogether (whichever can happen sooner). The pharmacological "so-what" of Ken's risky regimen is cardiovascular; rather than documenting a high iloperidone level (or even a potentially high duloxetine level if Ken is a CYP2D6 PM, since duloxetine is both an inhibitor and a substrate of that enzyme), prompt determination of a normal QTc interval on ECG is most compelling, given his multiple risks for a specific iloperidone-related arrhythmia.

CLINICAL VIGNETTE 7.3

Another Pop Quiz

Andrea is a 26-year-old anthropology graduate student with a long history of depression and anxiety that has been stably treated with desvenlafaxine 50 mg/day for three years. A change in her health insurance formulary coverage prompted her prescriber to change desvenlafaxine to venlafaxine, which was begun as a direct switchover starting at 75 mg/day. Within several days Andrea began to complain about dizziness, insomnia, and nausea. Suspecting the symptoms represented discontinuation effects of desvenlafaxine her doctor *increased* the dose to 150 mg/day and then again a week later to 225 mg/day, but the dizziness and nausea persisted and intensified. She felt the symptoms were reminiscent of how she felt during previous trials of fluoxetine and paroxetine.

What would be your initial next step in her treatment?

(a) reassure Andrea that she will be fine and encourage her to ride out these symptoms until her body can better accommodate to the changeover
(b) switch her to fluoxetine as a strategy to counteract suspected discontinuation symptoms
(c) measure a serum [o-desmethylvenlafaxine] to assure it is <1000 ng/mL
(d) switch her back to desvenlafaxine 50 mg/day with an urgent appeal to her insurance carrier to cover the previous drug

For this complex scenario, choice (d) would be the most compelling option. Is that simply because she had been stable on desvenlafaxine and her physical distress upon switching to an insurance-mandated alternative mobilizes anger in her prescriber to combat arbitrary third-party intrusion into her treatment? Is it because a placebo benefit was lost, and nocebo artifacts ensued, as psychological (more than pharmacological) ramifications of Andrea's being unduly coerced by a third party to accept desvenlafaxine's dirtier and more unsavory precursor molecule? Perhaps, but consider the pharmacokinetic factors at play. Venlafaxine is metabolized to o-desmethylvenlafaxine by CYP450 2D6 (see Table 7.3) while desvenlafaxine, in turn, is not a CYP450 2D6 substrate (it is primarily metabolized by Phase II UGT isoenzymes and, to a lesser extent, *N*-demethylated via CYP450 3A4). If serotonergic discontinuation effects were the cause of Andrea's symptoms, they should have *improved* (not worsened) with the venlafaxine dosage increase, coupled with the passage of time. But the opposite occurred. Her symptoms are consistent with the known common adverse effects of venlafaxine. We are tipped off in her history to the possibility that she might be a CYP2D6 PM based on her similar previous experiences taking two other CYP2D6 substrates (fluoxetine and paroxetine).

If this were serotonergic discontinuation effects, adding fluoxetine in principle could be helpful, but because discontinuation effects are probably less likely an explanation than impaired conversion of venlafaxine to desvenlafaxine, this would likely not be a helpful intervention – and besides, we know from her history that fluoxetine was poorly tolerated, consistent with a CYP2D6 PM phenotype. Pharmacogenetic testing could confirm our suspicion of the latter – or, we could just play the hunch that the most likely reason she fared better with desvenlafaxine than venlafaxine was that she could not appreciably convert the parent compound to its metabolite. We certainly could measure her o-desmethylvenlafaxine blood level, but if we did that we would be looking not so much to see if it was near-toxic but rather near-zero. Regardless, any such laboratory measures would serve only to affirm, rather than guide, next steps in her proper treatment.

I see really treatment-resistant psychosis patients and sometimes push clozapine blood levels past 1000 ng/mL. What's wrong with that, so long as I'm covering with an anticonvulsant for seizure prophylaxis?

I really would not do that. First, there is no evidence for greater efficacy at serum levels above 1000 ng/mL and second, the risk from clozapine toxicity isn't just seizures, it includes possible anticholinergic delirium, hyperthermia, arrhythmias, miosis, pancreatitis, hepatitis, blood dyscrasias, and death. Shall I continue?

G SECONDARY OUTCOMES

Serum drug levels have preliminarily been studied in relation to clinical phenomena other than the ones we might think of as the primary targets of treatment, such as cognition, or serum BDNF levels. These are summarized in Table 7.10.

H END-ORGAN MONITORING

Perhaps the most critical form of laboratory assessment in psychopharmacology involves knowing relevant end-organ systems that are plausibly affected by a particular medication and the usefulness of specific laboratory monitoring to investigate suspected anomalies. Here again, lab tests should be ordered with a specific question in mind, guided by clinical context. Not everyone taking divalproex needs pancreatic enzyme levels measured, but woe unto the clinician who fails to consider pancreatitis in the differential diagnosis of a patient taking divalproex who develops an acute abdomen. There is really no reason to measure serum prolactin levels in a woman taking a dopamine blocking agent who has normal menstrual periods and no galactorrhea. Table 7.11 summarizes major laboratory parameters for end-organ safety monitoring during psychotropic drug therapy.

Management strategies for identified iatrogenic end-organ abnormalities such as those described above are discussed in Chapter 10.

I ANTIPSYCHOTIC DRUG LEVELS

As noted in a review by Horvitz-Lennon et al. (2017), the evidence base for using antipsychotic plasma levels to gauge drug efficacy is, in general, less well-established than for anticipating problems with tolerability – with the most notable exceptions being haloperidol, perphenazine, and clozapine, and more limited data with olanzapine, risperidone, and aripiprazole. Tables 7.12 and 7.13 summarize findings from empirical trials regarding antipsychotic plasma levels with FGAs and SGAs, respectively.

J EXPERIMENTAL LAB MEASURES THAT BELONG MORE AT THE BENCH THAN THE BEDSIDE

The research world has increasingly devoted energy and resources to measuring serum or other (e.g., urinary) possible biomarkers of psychopathology that, at present, have no established practical relevance outside of investigational laboratory settings. Many if not most candidate biomarkers have enormous inter- and intraindividual variability and are impacted by numerous intrinsic or environmental factors beyond those related to mental health (e.g., age, sex, ethnicity, lifestyle, smoking status, diet, and medical comorbidities, among others). Nevertheless, some practitioners may feel compelled to order and even interpret such tests as if they conveyed meaningful information to guide or even drive treatment. Examples include:

- Serum or urinary neurotransmitter levels
- Serum trophic factors (e.g., brain-derived neurotrophic factor (BDNF)) and the antiapoptotic gene B-cell lymphoma 2 (bcl-2))
- Inflammatory markers (e.g., hs-CRP, TNFα, interleukins (e.g., IL-4, IL-6))
- Telomere length
- *Routine* testing of vitamin and mineral deficiencies
- Serum or salivary cortisol levels
- Serum or salivary melatonin levels
- Serum or salivary gonadal sex steroid hormone levels
- Stool specimen analyses
- Blood pH testing

There may well come a time in the foreseeable future when biomarker tests will acquire the construct validity necessary for them to become meaningfully useful tools within the diagnostic and therapeutic armamentarium. In the meanwhile, standard laboratory measures in psychopharmacology remain secondary affirmations of clinical suspicion that should be used judiciously and purposefully, informed by clinical knowledge of end-organ drug effects with paramount importance placed on the medical maxim *primum non nocere*.

TAKE-HOME POINTS

- Have a specific purpose and question (or hypothesis) in mind when ordering laboratory tests. Use laboratory tests to affirm or refute suspected clinical hypotheses.
- As a rule of thumb, treat the patient rather than the number - unless there is clear evidence of hazard from the number alone. (And remember to recheck rather than automatically embrace abnormal laboratory test results that may be suspect; when in doubt *recheck*.)
- Know which drugs have normed and established therapeutic blood levels and distinguish them from those without established parameters.
- Unexpectedly persistently low serum drug levels, particularly in the setting of relatively high drug dosages, should prompt thinking about poor treatment adherence, ultra-rapid metabolism, or malabsorption syndromes.

Table 7.1 Laboratory drug-level monitoring of lithium and mood-stabilizing anticonvulsant drugs

Medication	Empirical findings regarding serum levels	Relevance of serum drug levels	Caveats
Carbamazepine	4–12 µg/mL in epilepsy	*No demonstrated correlation* between serum [carbamazepine] and clinical response in acute or prophylactic treatment of bipolar disorder (Simhandl et al., 1993; Vasudev et al., 2000)	Autoinduction of carbamazepine often leads to lowered levels several weeks after initiation
Divalproex	*Acute mania*: well-established therapeutic range of 45–125 µg/mL (Bowden et al., 1996); *Bipolar maintenance*: optimal study retention or discontinuation due to a manic or depressive recurrence when serum [valproate] fell between 75 and 99.9 µg/mL (Keck et al., 2005)	Optimal antimanic efficacy when [valproate] >71 µg/mL; highest effect size in mania for [valproate] >94 µg/mL (Allen et al., 2006). No data in bipolar depression.	Free (unbound) [valproate] should be measured (usual range = 6–22 µg/mL) when plasma protein levels may be low (e.g., as in malabsorption or malnutrition/anorexia, or significant hepatic or renal disease)
Lamotrigine	2.5–15.0 µg/mL in epilepsy	There is no established therapeutic serum reference range for purposes other than seizure prevention. One small (n = 34) study combining unipolar and bipolar TRD found significantly greater response when serum [lamotrigine] >2.3 µg/mL (Kagawa et al., 2014)	Estrogen-containing oral contraceptives, as well as pregnancy, can reduce serum lamotrigine levels by up to 50%
Lithium	*Acute mania*: 0.6–1.2 mEq/L is a common convention *Bipolar depression*: no data *Maintenance therapy*: serum levels of 0.8–1.0 mEq/L confer lower relapse risk than levels of 0.4–0.6 mEq/L (Gelenberg et al., 1989)	"Therapeutic" levels in acute mania tend to be higher (closer to 1.0 mEq/L) than during maintenance therapy	Optimum serum lithium levels produce adequate therapeutic benefit at the lowest possible dose, in order to minimize end-organ adverse effects. Also, "established" therapeutic ranges are themselves subject to moderators (e.g., absence of chronicity (Gelenberg et al., 1989)) and mediators (e.g., avoiding abrupt drops in Li^+ levels (Perlis et al., 2002)

Abbreviations: TRM = treatment-resistant depression

Table 7.2 Laboratory drug level monitoring of SSRIs

SSRI	Empirical findings	Relevance and caveats
Citalopram	Serum levels >50 ng/mL are associated with >80% receptor occupancy of serotonin transporter binding sites and greater therapeutic effect (Haji et al., 2011; Hiemke et al., 2018). Extensive inter- and intraindividual variability in serum levels across doses; no established relationship with therapeutic response (Reis et al., 2003). Possible nonlinear (sigmoidal) response curve in OCD (Bareggi et al., 2004)	Therapeutic levels generally considered not well-established although serum [citalopram] >220 ng/mL may be associated with toxicity (Hiemke et al., 2018)
Escitalopram	Preliminary data (one open trial, n = 70) suggest antidepressant response when plasma [escitalopram] >20 ng/mL (Florio et al., 2017). Laboratory reference range = 15–80 ng/mL (Hiemke et al., 2018)	Extensive intra- and interindividual variation between drug doses and serum levels of S-citalopram, S-desmethyl-citalopram, S-didesmethyl-citalopram; no clear threshold of clinical significance (Reis et al., 2007)
Fluoxetine	Laboratory reference range of 125–500 ng/mL (Hiemke et al., 2018) (combined [fluoxetine] + [*N*-desmethyl-fluoxetine])	No correlation between serum [fluoxetine], combined [fluoxetine] + [norfluoxetine], or [fluoxetine]:[norfluoxetine] ratios and response in MDD (Amsterdam et al., 1997) or OCD (Koran et al., 1996). Potential toxicity with [fluoxetine] + [n-desmethylfluoxetine] >1000 ng/mL (Hiemke et al., 2018). Lack of relationship between serum levels and therapeutic response appears well demonstrated
Fluvoxamine	Small 14-day open pilot trial in MDD observed serum [fluvoxamine] range of 23–227 ng/mL; in ROC analysis, responders had serum levels <85 ng/mL (Härtter et al., 1998). In panic disorder, one RCT found remitters usually had serum [fluvoxamine] of 10–100 ng/mL (Sandmann et al., 1998). In OCD, significant correlation observed between serum [fluvoxamine] and change in YBOCS scores among 20 outpatients over six months (Marazziti et al., 2012b)	Serum levels are not well established relative to therapeutic response; toxicity may be associated with serum [fluvoxamine] > 500 ng/mL (Hiemke et al., 2018). Highly variable serum concentrations observed; pilot data findings are nondefinitive
Paroxetine	Some studies report a therapeutic range of 20–60 ng/mL (Tomita et al., 2014) and better and/or faster response with *higher* serum levels in panic disorder and MDD (Gilles et al., 2005; Gex-Fabry et al., 2007); others find better antidepressant response at *low* serum [paroxetine] (Watanabe et al., 2007)	Not well established
Sertraline	Oral dosages from 50–200 mg/day correspond to serum levels ranging from 30–200 ng/mL, but a therapeutic reference range is not well established	Possible toxicity associated with levels >300 ng/mL (Hiemke et al., 2018)

Abbreviations: MDD = major depressive disorder; OCD = obsessive-compulsive disorder; RCT = randomized controlled trial; ROC = receiver operating characteristic; YBOCS = Yale-Brown Obsessive Compulsive Scale

Table 7.3 Laboratory drug level monitoring of SNRIs

SNRI	Empirical findings	Relevance of serum levels and caveats
Desvenlafaxine	Therapeutic response in MDD associated with combined serum [venlafaxine] + [o-desmethyl-venlafaxine] in range of 195–400 ng/mL (Veefkind et al., 2000). Other reports of MDD remission associated with serum [o-des-methylvenlafaxine] >222 ng/mL threshold (Stamm et al., 2014a)	"Wide inter-individual variability of serum concentrations on each dose level" (Reis et al., 2002). Potential toxicity associated with combined levels >1000 ng/mL (Hiemke et al., 2018)
Duloxetine	Laboratory reference range = 30–120 ng/mL (Hiemke et al., 2018). ROC analysis in one study of 103 depressed inpatients showed improvement when serum [duloxetine] >58 ng/mL (Waldschmitt et al., 2009)	Correlation between serum level and therapeutic response *not* well established. Potential toxicity associated with levels >230 ng/mL (Hiemke et al., 2018)
Levomilnacipran	Laboratory reference range = 80–120 ng/mL (Hiemke et al., 2018)	No established correlation between serum levels and therapeutic response. Levels >200 ng/mL may be associated with toxicity (Hiemke et al., 2018).
Venlafaxine	Same as desvenlafaxine	Same as desvenlafaxine

Abbreviations: MDD = major depressive disorder; ROC = receiver operating characteristic

Table 7.4 Laboratory drug level monitoring of tricyclics

Tricyclics	Empirical findings	Relevance and caveats
Amitriptyline	Therapeutic antidepressant response associated with combined serum [amitriptyline] + [nortriptyline] of 93–140 ng/mL (response rate = 50% when within range vs. 30% when outside) (Perry et al., 1994)	Curvilinear relationship. Potential toxicity associated with [amitriptyline] + [nortriptyline] > 300 ng/mL (Hiemke et al., 2018)
Clomipramine	Usual laboratory reference range of 230–450 ng/mL for combined serum [clomipramine] + [*N*-desmethylclomipramine] levels (Hiemke et al., 2018). Ratio of serum [clomipramine] : [*N*-desmethyl-clomipramine] associated with YBOCS improvement in men (Marazziti et al., 2012a)	Toxicity associated with combined serum [clomipramine] + [*N*-desmethylclomipramine] levels >450 ng/mL (Hiemke et al., 2018)
Desipramine	Usual reference range 150–300 ng/mL. Therapeutic response above threshold of 116 ng/mL (response rate above threshold = 51% vs. 15% below threshold) (Perry et al., 1994)	Linear dose-response relationship. Potential toxicity associated with levels >300 ng/mL (Hiemke et al., 2018)
Imipramine	Therapeutic response associated with combined serum [imipramine] + [desipramine] of 175–350 ng/mL (response rate = 67% when within range vs. 39% outside range) (Perry et al., 1994)	Curvilinear relationship. Potential toxicity associated with serum [imipramine] + [desipramine] >300 ng/mL (Hiemke et al., 2018)
Nortriptyline	Therapeutic response associated with serum [nortriptyline] of 58-148 ng/mL (response rate when within range = 66% vs. 26% outside) (Perry et al., 1994)	Curvilinear relationship customarily described for therapeutic window of 50–150 ng/mL. Potential toxicity associated with levels >300 ng/mL (Hiemke et al., 2018)

Abbreviations: YBOCS = Yale-Brown Obsessive Compulsive Scale

Table 7.5. Laboratory drug level monitoring of other monoaminergic antidepressants

Medication	Empirical findings regarding serum levels	Relevance of serum drug levels and caveats
Bupropion	Serum trough [bupropion] of 10-29 ng/mL associated with better response vs. levels >30 ng/mL in a preliminary open study of 23 MDD patients (Goodnick, 1992). Serum [4-hydroxy-bupropion] (bupropion's active metabolite) >860 ng/mL may represent a minimum threshold blood level associated with therapeutic response (Laib et al., 2014)	Curvilinear relationship for serum [bupropion]. Toxicity associated with serum [bupropion] + [4-hydroxybupropion] >2000 ng/mL (Hiemke et al., 2018). Chemical instability of bupropion may favor measurement of its active metabolite 4-hydroxy-bupropion
MAOIs	Poorly established	Therapeutic response depends on inhibition of MAO; as such, drug levels per se do not correlate with pharmacodynamic efficacy
Isocarboxazid	Not established	None
Moclobemide	Laboratory reference range = 300-1000 ng/mL (Hiemke et al., 2018)	No significant correlation with serum concentrations and therapeutic response
Phenelzine	Not established	None
Selegiline	Not established	None
Tranylcypromine	<50 ng/mL (Hiemke et al., 2018)	Upper limit of laboratory reference range pertains to minimizing toxicity
Mirtazapine	Therapeutic oral dosages (15-45 mg/day) found to correspond to serum levels of 5-100 ng/mL but "no concentration-effect relationship could be established" (Timmer et al., 2000). Median observed serum [mirtazapine] = 19.5 ng/mL among 100 depressed outpatients (Shams et al., 2004)	"Wide interindividual variability of serum concentrations on each dose level" (Shams et al., 2004). Toxicity may be associated with serum [mirtazapine] >160 ng/mL (Hiemke et al., 2018). *N*-desmethyl-mirtazapine/mirtazapine ratios >4 associated with more adverse drug effects (Shams et al., 2004)
Nefazodone	Not well-established	None
Vilazodone	Laboratory reference range = 30-70 ng/mL (Hiemke et al., 2018)	No established correlation between serum levels and therapeutic response. Toxicity may be associated with levels >140 ng/mL (Hiemke et al., 2018).
Vortioxetine	Laboratory reference range = 10-40 ng/mL (Hiemke et al., 2018)	No established correlation between serum levels and therapeutic response. Toxicity may be associated with levels >80 ng/mL (Hiemke et al., 2018)

Abbreviations: MAO = monoamine oxidase; MAOI = monoamine oxidase inhibitor; MDD = major depressive disorder;

Table 7.6 Laboratory drug level monitoring of stimulants and stimulant-like agents

Medication	Empirical findings regarding serum levels	Relevance of serum drug levels
Atomoxetine	200–1000 ng/mL (Hiemke et al., 2018)	Unknown
Methylphenidate	13–22 ng/mL Hiemke et al., 2018)	Unknown
Modafinil	1000–1700 ng/mL (Hiemke et al., 2018)	Unknown

Table 7.7 Inducers and inhibitors of CYP450 2D6 psychotropic substrates

Substrates	Inducers	Inhibitors
Amphetamine	Dexamethasone	Bupropion
Dextroamphetamine	Rifampin	Citalopram
Aripiprazole		Doxepin
Atomoxetine		Fluoxetine
Brexpiprazole		Fluvoxamine (weak)
Clomipramine		Imipramine
Deutetrabenazine		Paroxetine
Dextromethorphan		Risperidone
Duloxetine		
Escitalopram		
Fluoxetine		
Fluvoxamine		
Haloperidol		
Iloperidone		
Levomilnacipran		
Mirtazapine		
Nortriptyline		
Paroxetine		
Risperidone		
Valbenazine		
Venlafaxine		
Vortioxetine		

Table 7.8 Inducers and inhibitors of CYP450 2C19 psychotropic substrates

Substrates	Inducers	Inhibitors
Amitriptyline	Barbiturates	Fluoxetine
Aripiprazole	Carbamazepine	Fluvoxamine
Citalopram	Primidone	Moclobemide
Clomipramine	Rifampin	Modafinil
Clozapine		Oxcarbazepine
Desipramine		Topiramate
Diazepam		
Diphenhydramine		
Doxepin		
Escitalopram		
Fluoxetine		
Imipramine		
Levomilnacipran		
Methadone		
Moclobemide		
Nortriptyline		
Olanzapine		
Phenobarbital		

Table 7.9. Inducers and inhibitors of CYP450 3A4 psychotropic substrates

Substrates	Inducers	Inhibitors
Amitriptyline	Carbamazepine	Fluvoxamine
Aripiprazole	Modafinil	Nefazodone
Armodafinil		
Brexpiprazole		
Buspirone		
Carbamazepine		
Cariprazine		
Citalopram		
Eszopiclone		
Iloperidone		
Levomilnacipran		
Lumateperone		
Lurasidone		
Mirtazapine		
Nefazodone		
Nortriptyline		
Pimavanserin		
Quetiapine		
Suvorexant		
Trazodone		
Valbenazine		
Vilazodone		
Ziprasidone		
Zolpidem		

Tables 7.7–7.9 are really important! Nobody ever remembers all the pharmacokinetic drug interactions. Here you can just check them drug by drug, case by case.

You look stuff up?

Table 7.10 Serum drug levels and secondary outcome measures

Outcome	Evidence
Cognition	• In bipolar disorder and schizophrenia patients, serum [venlafaxine] + [o-desmethyl-venlafaxine], but not serum [citalopram] or [escitalopram], correlated with verbal immediate and long-term memory (but not other cognitive domains) (Steen et al., 2015) • Serum [olanzapine] associated with measures of attention; serum [quetiapine] negatively associated with short-term verbal memory, serum [risperidone] negatively associated with verbal fluency (Steen et al., 2017)
Dementia	• Small open trials of citalopram for patients having dementia with behavioral disturbances report higher serum-to-dose ratios of citalopram than in younger patients (Foglia et al., 1997)
Neurotrophic effects	• Serum [paroxetine] correlates with serum [BDNF] (Yasui-Furukori et al., 2011)

Abbreviations: BDNF = brain-derived neurotrophic factor

Table 7.11 End-organ laboratory monitoring

Effects	Relevant psychotropics	Measure what, when?
Serum calcium, parathyroid hormone	Lithium	10–25% of patients taking lithium long term may develop asymptomatic hypercalcemia and hyperparathyroidism; while practice guidelines tend not to advocate regular monitoring of these parameters, we advise annual or semi-annual measurement of PTH and serum Ca^{++}
Electrolytes	Carbamazepine, lithium, oxcarbazepine, serotonergic antidepressants	*Carbamazepine* and *oxcarbazepine*: Monitor for hyponatremia based on clinical concerns and risk factors (e.g., elderly); *lithium* may cause hyponatremia via decreased renal tubular absorption, prompting recommendations to monitor serum electrolyte levels semi-annually; absorption in *SSRIs* and *SNRIs* may cause SIADH, although surveillance monitoring of serum sodium levels is not generally recommended
Glycemic	SGAs	Fasting glucose at baseline, 12 weeks, and every five years thereafter as advised by Consensus Statement from the American Diabetes Association
Hematopoetic	Carbamazepine, clozapine, divalproex	*Carbamazepine*: Baseline (~10% of patients develop a benign, transient leukopenia in first several months); no formal recommendation on surveillance CBCs in absence of clinical concerns about myelosuppression *Clozapine*: Regular CBC monitoring schedule as outlined at www.clozapinerems.com/CpmgClozapineUI/rems/pdf/resources/ANC_Table.pdf *Divalproex*: Potential thrombocytopenia, believed to be dose-related, is usually monitored by CBCs only in the setting of clinical concern (e.g., easy bruising)
Hepatic function	Carbamazepine, disulfiram, divalproex	*All*: Baseline measures are appropriate; subsequent laboratory monitoring typically occurs if and as clinical concerns arise, rather than via a regular or fixed schedule; some experts advocate semi-annual or annual liver enzyme tests when taking divalproex long term
Lipids	SGAs	Lipid panel at baseline, 12 weeks, and every five years thereafter as advised by Consensus Statement from the American Diabetes Association. Notably, US and UK psychiatrists rarely follow baseline and periodic screening recommendations (Mitchell et al., 2012).
Prolactin	Most FGAs and SGAs; dose-related; least risk with aripiprazole > quetiapine> asenpine ≈ olanzapine (see Chapter 10)	Generally, measure serum prolactin levels only when clinically indicated, i.e., in the setting of galactorrhea, amenorrhea, gynecomastia during FGA or SGA use. Clinically relevant hyperprolactinemia usually is >30 ng/mL.
Renal	Lithium	Random serum creatinine semi-annually. Rises above 25% from a previous value may warrant further investigation (e.g., calculation of eGFR via cystatin C rather than creatinine; see Chapter 10).
Thyroid	Lithium	TSH semi-annually; patients with elevated TSH warrant further assessment of thyroid antibodies (i.e., anti-thyroid peroxidase (TPO), anti-thyroglobulin) to discriminate autoimmune from nonautoimmune causes of thyroiditis

Abbreviations: CBC = complete blood count; eGFR = estimated glomerular filtration rate; FGA = first-generation antipsychotic; PTH = parathyroid hormone; SGA = second-generation antipsychotic; SIADH = syndrome of inappropriate antidiuretic hormone secretion; SNRI = serotonin-norepinephrine reuptake inhibitor; SSRI = selective serotonin reuptake inhibitor; TSH = thyroid-stimulating hormone

Table 7.12 Reported relationships between first-generation antipsychotic plasma levels and therapeutic response in psychotic disorders

Agent	Putative therapeutic levels [a]	Comment
Fluphenazine	0.8–1.0 ng/mL (Meyer, 2014)	Serum levels >4 g/mL likely futile (Meyer, 2014)
Haloperidol	5.6–16.9 ng/mL, with maximal effect at 10 ng/mL (Ulrich et al., 1998); clinical benefits decline with levels >26 ng/mL (de Oliveira et al., 1996)	Reported correlations between serum levels and therapeutic response are considered provisional and not routinely measured in clinical practice. Serum levels >30 ng/mL likely futile (Meyer, 2014)
Perphenazine	1.5–3 nmol/L (Hansen et al., 1981)	No significant correlation observed between overall symptom severity scores and serum [perphenazine] or [*N*-dealkylated perphenazine] (Mazure et al., 1990)

[a] "Therapeutic response" in most studies defined as >20% improvement from baseline in BPRS

Abbreviations: BPRS = Brief Psychiatric Rating Scale

Table 7.13 Reported relationships between second-generation antipsychotic plasma levels and therapeutic response in psychotic disorders

Agent	Putative therapeutic levels [a]	Comment
Aripiprazole	Therapeutic response may be more likely if serum [aripiprazole] ≥150 ng/mL (Sparshatt et al., 2010); observed mean 24° [aripiprazole] = 208 ng/mL and [dehydroaripiprazole] = 88 ng/mL at mean dose of 14 mg/day (reviewed by Lopez and Kane, 2013)	Correlations between serum levels and therapeutic responses generally not well established and not routinely measured in clinical practice
Asenapine	Laboratory reference range = 1–5 ng/mL (Hiemke et al., 2018)	Correlations between serum levels and therapeutic response generally not well established and not routinely measured in clinical practice
Cariprazine	Laboratory reference range = 10–20 ng/mL (Hiemke et al., 2018)	Correlations between serum levels and therapeutic response generally not well established and not routinely measured in clinical practice
Clozapine	Therapeutic range >350 ng/mL [b] (Meyer, 2019; VanderZwaag et al., 1996)	Serum levels >838 ng/mL (Remington et al., 2013) to 1000 g/mL (Meyer, 2014) likely futile
Iloperidone	Laboratory reference range = 5–10 ng/mL; potential toxicity if >20 ng/mL (Hiemke et al., 2018)	Correlations between serum levels and therapeutic response generally not well established and not routinely measured in clinical practice
Olanzapine	Reference range: 10–80 ng/mL (Meyer, 2019); therapeutic efficacy associated with serum levels ≥23 ng/mL (mean dose = 12 mg/day) (Perry et al., 2001; Bishara et al., 2013)	Direct linear relationship observed between olanzapine doses and serum drug levels based on meta-regression of 15 studies; men may need higher doses than women (Bishara et al., 2013). Routine measurement is not common in clinical practice. Levels >200 ng/mL likely futile (Meyer, 2014)
Quetiapine	≥100 ng/mL (Hiemke et al., 2018); potential toxicity associated with levels >1000 ng/mL (Hiemke et al., 2018)	Weak correlation between dose and blood level, "not sufficient... to allow determination of a therapeutic plasma level range" (Sparshatt et al., 2011)
Risperidone (Yasui-Furukori et al., 2010)	≥20 ng/mL (= the active moiety, i.e., risperidone + 9-hydroxyrisperidone (Olesen et al, 1998)). The active moiety serum level is approximately 7× the oral dose (de Leon et al., 2010)	Most studies report *no significant correlation* between serum drug or metabolite levels and change in positive and negative symptom severity scores (Lopez and Kane, 2013). Levels of active moiety >112 ng/mL likely futile (Meyer, 2014).
Ziprasidone	Laboratory reference range = 50–200 ng/mL; potential toxicity associated with levels >400 ng/mL (Hiemke et al., 2018)	Large interindividual variation in blood levels. Correlations between serum levels and therapeutic response generally not well-established and not routinely measured.

[a] "Therapeutic response" in most studies defined as >20% improvement from baseline in BPRS

[b] Therapeutic drug monitoring values for clozapine generally focus only on the parent compound (clozapine) rather than clozapine + norclozapine levels

Abbreviations: BPRS = Brief Psychiatric Rating Scale

8 Pharmacogenetics: When Relevant, When Not

AUTHORS' PREFACE

The field of combinatorial pharmacogenomics is fast-evolving. One of the main controversies facing practitioners is understanding how much evidence-based findings from the literature are or are not yet ready for prime-time implementation in routine patient care – or, how much the deliverables remain in the gestational stage, and still belong more at the bench than the bedside. In fact, even experts can find it hard to agree about the distinct role of pharmacogenetics in routine clinical practice. Our main objectives in this chapter are twofold: (1) to help readers acquire a greater sense of literacy for interpreting pharmacogenetics data for themselves, and (2) to make prescribers think more about the neurobiology behind the decisions they make. In the case of pharmacogenetics, that means understanding how to interpret a pharmacogenetics test report, how to separate efficacy and tolerability as distinct drug effects, how to use pharmacogenetics to affirm hypotheses about possible reasons for poor response, and how to integrate pharmacogenetic data alongside other previously discussed moderators and mediators of treatment outcome. We will highlight points where even we, the authors, may differ in our points of view, and the reasons behind divergent perspectives, to help the reader form his or her own conclusions about the evidence base and utility for "bedside" pharmacogenetic testing.

LEARNING OBJECTIVES

- ☐ Define pharmacogenetics, pharmacogenomics, allele, single nucleotide polymorphism (SNP), familiality versus heritability, and complex versus Mendelian traits
- ☐ Understand the difference between safety and efficacy pharmacogenetics, the distinction between pharmacokinetic and pharmacodynamic gene variants, and the relevance of poor metabolizer, extensive metabolizer, and ultra-rapid metabolizer genotypes and phenotypes
- ☐ Know how to interpret the findings of a pharmacogenetics test report and the clinical significance of identified polymorphic variants
- ☐ Understand the strengths and limitations of currently available technology for utilizing pharmacogenetics to inform prescribing decisions in clinical practice

Your genetics is not your destiny.

– *George M. Church*

In Chapter 5, we discussed the growing concept of precision medicine and its forerunner term, "personalized medicine," as the initiative to craft individually tailored treatments. For psychiatry, precision medicine represents the goal of utilizing a given patient's unique clinical and biological profile in order to broker the best fit with a particular drug regimen. That theme is woven throughout this book, as *the means by which* clinicians must interpret large-scale clinical trials and decide whether and how their findings apply to an individual case. In the minds of many psychopharmacologists, pharmacogenetics and pharmacogenomics represent a key component, if not *the* key component, of that endeavor, based on assumptions that everyone's unique genetic architecture must figure critically in how they will respond to a drug – and that without such information, efforts toward devising an

Tip

Pharmacogenetics refers to how the variation in a single gene influences response to one drug. *Pharmacogenomics* more broadly refers to how variation in many genes within the entire genome affects drug response.

appropriate pharmacotherapy regimen are merely trial and error. This chapter will explore the basis for these propositions and critically examine the evidence for if, when, and how pharmacogenetic testing may or may not be useful to personalized psychopharmacology.

A IS DRUG RESPONSE HERITABLE?

A first consideration involves the fundamental question of whether, or how much, drug response is under genetic influence, and if so, how significant its contribution is relative to the myriad other factors that influence pharmacotherapy outcomes. Many clinicians often presume that the effect a particular drug has in a given patient's first-degree relative will, more likely than not, be observed in the patient now before us. Is this an evidence-based concept? The literature answers affirmatively only to a very limited degree. We must first discriminate between familiality and heritability.

Controversy

There is debate and uncertainty about just how much family history informs drug response. There is little formal study of drug response within families. Consequently, clinicians vary in how strongly they perceive drug response to be a true phenotype (meaning that it can run in families, and is strongly under genetic influence).

Whether or not drug response "runs in families" is quite understudied. As noted in Chapter 5, lithium responsivity in bipolar disorder has shown an approximate two-thirds concordance between probands and first-degree relatives, with similar concordance rates in MDD with at least some SSRIs. Beyond these limited data, little to no evidence is available that informs whether or not a family member's response to a psychotropic drug is familial.

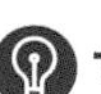

Tip

Familiality refers to whether an observed phenomenon tends to run in families. Examples include speaking the same language, eating turkey instead of lasagna on Thanksgiving, and entering the same profession as one's parents.

The probability that susceptibility to a particular psychiatric disorder (or, a proneness to a particular drug response) runs in families is sometimes confused with the separate issue of how much a particular trait results from the passage of genetic information across generations. Heritability refers only to *how much variability* in a trait (say, a phenomenon like mood or psychosis) within a population is caused solely by variations in genes among members of the population. The term tells us nothing about the likelihood that mood or psychosis per se is *inherited*; only that "high heritability" of mood or psychosis means that its variation from one person to another is heavily influenced by genetic rather than environmental factors. Heritability estimates (h^2) from twin/family studies are high for many psychiatric conditions.

Tip

Heritability refers to how much the variability of a trait within a population comes from genetic as opposed to environmental effects. Examples include eye color, hammertoes, dimples, and freckles.

Note that textbooks and primary literature sources will vary in their reported heritability rates across psychiatric disorders – many sources often cite autism as "*the* most heritable psychiatric disorder" (e.g., Sandin et al., 2014), although absolutes are difficult if not impossible to know with certainty. For exemplary purposes, approximate heritability (h^2) estimates, alongside relative risks (RRs) for disease when present in a first-degree relative, are summarized in Box 8.1.

Box 8.1

Heritabilities of Common Psychiatric Disorders

Disorder	h^2 [a]
Autism spectrum disorders	0.80-0.90
Schizophrenia	0.81
Bipolar disorder	0.75
ADHD	0.75
Alcohol dependence	0.40-0.57
Anorexia nervosa	0.56
Major depressive disorder	0.37
Panic disorder	0.48

[a] As reported by Sullivan et al., 2012

The genetic components of most if not all forms of psychopathology represent complex traits, meaning the coalescence of many genes that each exert small influences on observable phenomena. Unlike

Mendelian genetics, where a single gene can express its dominance in the form of a complete syndrome (e.g., Duchenne's muscular dystrophy, or cystic fibrosis, or Tay Sachs disease), the manifestations of many genes of small effect may contribute to the expression of dimensional phenotypes (such as impulsivity, or attentional processing, or autonomic hyperarousal, or sleep disruptions, or other dimensional characteristics, as described in Chapter 2). In the "cleanest" case, an effective medication is a comprehensive antisyndromal therapy (remember from Chapter 2 the differential diagnosis and treatment of increased abdominal girth); but more often than not, incomplete responses to a particular drug may reflect disparate components of a complex psychiatric syndrome, potentially targeting some but not necessarily all of its elements (such as lithium for impulsivity and suicidal behavior, psychostimulants for slowed attentional processing or low motivation, serotonergic antidepressants for anxiety and depressed mood). Assuming all these elements can fit neatly into a single rubric, then assuming that a single medication will remedy the whole ensemble of features, and then further assuming that the drug's effects are governed in large part by genetic influences, makes for a lot of assuming.

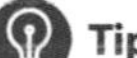

Tip

"Complex traits" refer to heritable phenomena that are governed not by principles of Mendelian genetics but, rather, by multiple genes that are each thought to exert small effects on an overall phenotype. Most if not all heritable psychiatric phenomena involve complex traits.

Controversy

Because psychiatric disorders involve multiple genes having small effects, variants of just one gene are unlikely to exert a large influence over a complex phenotype. Combinatorial pharmacogenetics involves examining a collection of several or more genes, but possibly dozens or even hundreds (from the roughly 20 000–25 000 human genes) may be necessary to understand meaningful effects.

Genetic factors generally are thought to confer diatheses or susceptibilities to psychiatric conditions, rather than to directly cause a condition itself. (Were that not the case, concordance rates among monozygotic twins would be 100%, which is far from the reality of psychiatric genetics.) Analogous to oncogenes and proto-oncogenes, psychiatric genetic predispositions constitute the first "hit" or susceptibility factor, ultimately then activated and expressed by one or more subsequent environmental interactions (second or third or more "hits") that might include exposures such as trauma or abuse, substance misuse, medical illnesses (e.g., strokes, cancer), or poor capacity to manage high-stress life events, among other occurrences.

Before embarking further, let us refresh our knowledge of some fundamental genetics terminology relevant to our further discussion of pharmacogenetics (Box 8.2).

Genetic association studies of complex traits typically focus on one of two approaches:

(a) *Candidate gene studies*: if one suspects that a particular trait might be associated with a specific

Box 8.2

Back to Basics: A Quick Pharmacogenetics Glossary

Allele: A variant or alternative form of a gene located at a specific position (locus) on a chromosome.

Association: Genetic association means that the frequency of a particular genotype (or SNP) is seen more often than would be expected by chance in connection with a particular trait of interest (such as drug response).

Genotype: The combination of alleles for a particular gene or locus.

Haplotype: A set of SNPs that are inherited together (for example, the major histocompatibility complex (MHC)).

Homozygote: A gene that has two identical alleles.

Heterozygote: A genotype having two different alleles.

Hardy-Weinberg equilibrium (HWE): The principle that allele or genotype frequencies within a population remain constant across generations in the absence of disturbing factors (e.g., mutations that introduce new alleles into the population). In candidate gene association studies, it is a quality control measure to show that cases and controls within a population are in HWE. Otherwise, if allele or genotype frequencies deviate significantly from HWE, it means that undetected factors in a population (such as racial or ethnic disparities – called "population structure" or "stratification") are likely present that could account for observed genetic differences. Without demonstrated

Box 8.2 (Cont.)

HWE, reported associations between SNPs and traits could be spurious and invalid.

Linkage disequilibrium (LD): When two separate genes are in LD, it means that alleles at the different loci are associated nonrandomly (i.e., more often than if they were *unlinked*); the genotype at one locus is linked with (not independent of) the genotype at a second locus.

Locus: A fixed position of a gene on a chromosome.

SNP: A single nucleotide polymorphism is a variation in a single base pair within a DNA sequence. Substituting one nucleotide for another (say, T(hymidine) for G(uanine)) results in the transcription of a different amino acid in the gene product encoded by a particular gene. If there is a known physiological consequence for such a variation, the SNP is described as being *functional*.

Variable number of tandem repeat (VNTR): VNTRs are adjacent patterns of nucleotide sequences that repeat within a DNA sequence.

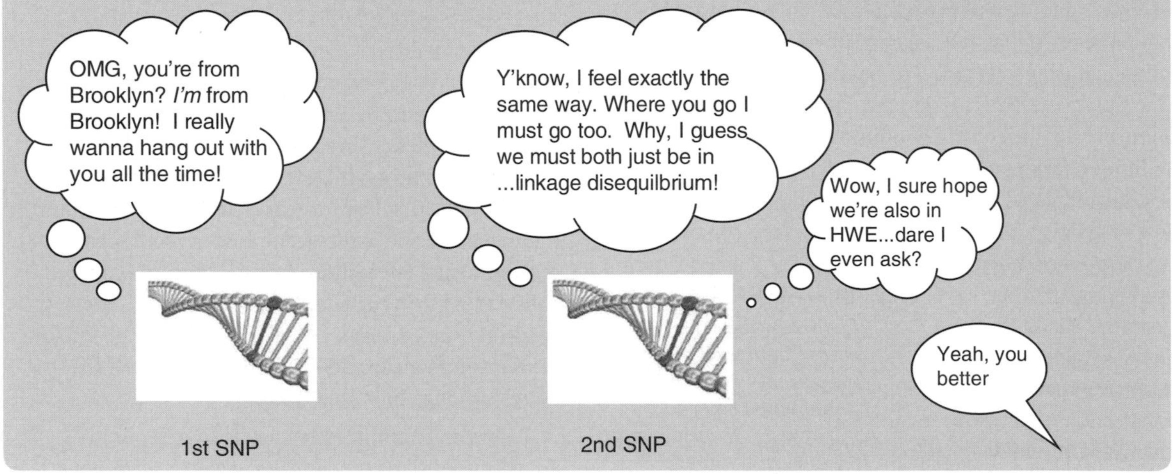

OMG, you're from Brooklyn? *I'm* from Brooklyn! I really wanna hang out with you all the time!

Y'know, I feel exactly the same way. Where you go I must go too. Why, I guess we must both just be in ...linkage disequilbrium!

Wow, I sure hope we're also in HWE...dare I even ask?

Yeah, you better

1st SNP

2nd SNP

enzyme, protein, receptor, or other gene product, that association can be examined or tested when the gene coding for the protein or enzyme of interest has a known, functionally important allelic variant (polymorphism), known as a single nucleotide polymorphism (SNP). For example, the enzyme catechol-*O*-methyltransferase (COMT, which degrades dopamine to its metabolite 3-methoxytyramine), is encoded by a gene (the COMT gene) for which there is a known SNP involving the substitution of a valine for a methionine molecule at position 158 – the so-called *Val*^{158}*Met* polymorphism. When the *Val* amino acid occurs at this position, the resulting COMT product breaks down dopamine up to four times faster than if the *Met* variant occurs at this location. Consequently, a *Met*/*Met* homozygote for the *Val*^{158}*Met* COMT SNP may have increased synaptic availability of dopamine in his or her prefrontal cortex, which in turn may lead to enhanced executive functioning.

> **Tip**
> REMINDER: Val/Val means o<u>v</u>eractive.

SNPs, in general, are often identified by an accession or "rs" number, which denotes their "reference SNP cluster identification." Results from candidate gene studies involving individual SNPs are sometimes hard to replicate because allele frequencies can vary across racial or other ancestral subgroups within a population – a phenomenon called *population stratification*, as noted in Box 8.2. Another substantial limitation of many candidate gene studies is the need for large enough sample sizes to provide sufficient statistical power to detect what are often small effects.

> **Tip**
> A heritable trait that is not *outwardly* visible is called a "hidden" or *endo*phenotype. Examples include verbal fluency and working memory, proneness toward impulsive aggression, and social intuition (sometimes called "theory of mind").

(b) *Genome-wide association studies (or GWAS)*: here, rather than studying the possible association between a given trait (such as disease susceptibility, or

Tip

To learn about the functional importance of any gene, if you know its rs number you can look it up easily at www.snpedia.com.

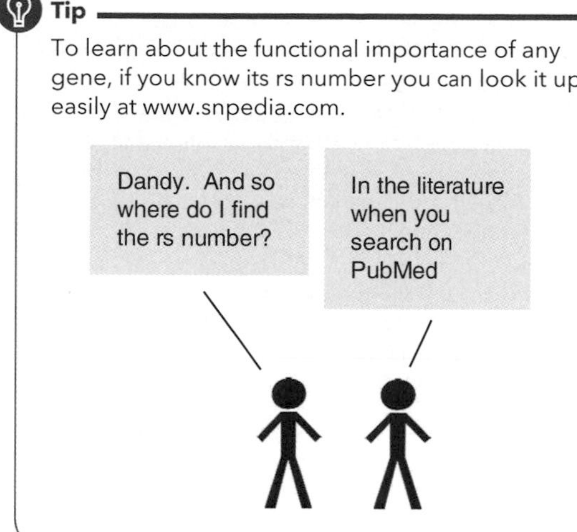

drug response) and SNPs of an *individual* candidate gene of interest, one studies SNPs across the *entire genome* (typically examining over one million SNPs) comparing a group of cases (i.e., the phenotype of interest, such as a clinical diagnosis, or a particular drug response or adverse effect of a drug) with controls (where the phenotype of interest is absent) on allelic frequencies of all SNPs between cases and controls. Odds ratios (ORs) with associated p-values are reported, SNP by SNP, to show whether an allele of interest is over-represented in cases versus controls. However, because so many statistical tests get performed, the α level for significance must be set extremely high – typically at least 5×10^{-8}. That means having a p-value of at least 0.00000005. That means many thousands of subjects in a GWAS to generate enough statistical power to detect a significant association. Consequently, when a signal is detected in a GWAS, the finding often goes unreplicated because the study may be underpowered. Statistical underpowering, along with sample heterogeneity (e.g., population stratification), pose major limitations for declaring existing pharmacogenetic technology as ready for prime-time everyday clinical practice.

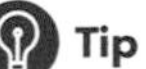

Tip

It takes an *enormous* amount of statistical power (sample size) to detect multiple small effects.

As complex traits, most if not all psychiatric conditions represent an interplay of biological, psychological, developmental, and environmental factors. Similar multideterminate factors are thought to contribute to psychotropic drug response, with genetics being only one of many such contributors. To the surprise and dismay of many clinicians and patients, the present state of pharmacogenetic testing does not provide robust information that tells "what drugs work and what drugs don't" for a given individual. What then is the practical relevance of pharmacogenetics, if not a crystal ball for predicting global treatment outcome?

In the universe of pharmacotherapy outcomes, true phenotypes (that is, phenomena which, by definition, are the product of genetic influences) are traditionally divided into drug effects related to metabolism and adverse effects (usually involving genetic variants of pharmacokinetic enzymes, and termed "safety pharmacogenetics") and drug effects related to intended therapeutic effects (focusing on genetic variants of pharmacodynamic genes, and termed "efficacy pharmacogenetics"). We will consider each of these as separate domains.

B SAFETY PHARMACOGENETICS

It is now well-established that many (but not all) adverse drug effects are more prone to arise in individuals who poorly metabolize drugs that are substrates for catabolic enzymes which, in turn, may vary in their level of activity based on functional genetic variants (SNPs). Note that genetic variants of hepatic catabolic enzymes are irrelevant to medications that are eliminated from the body without first being metabolized (such as lithium or gabapentin). As summarized in Table 8.1, hepatic metabolism is divided into either Phase I (biotransformation usually leading to active metabolites) or Phase II (conjugation of a drug or its Phase I breakdown product with an endogenous compound such as glucuronic acid, usually via transferases, leading to excretable inactive metabolites). Specific examples of known functional SNPs associated with particular Phase I or Phase II catabolic enzymes are summarized in Table 8.2. Let us consider antipsychotic-associated weight gain as a prominent example for which candidate gene studies suggest a possible pharmacogenetic determinant, as described in Box 8.3.

Box 8.3

An Example of Safety Pharmacogenetics: The $5HT_{2C}$ Polymorphism and SGA-associated Weight Gain

The $5HT_{2C}$ receptor (also sometimes referred to as HTR2C) has been implicated in appetite regulation and SGA-associated weight gain. Mice genetically engineered to lack the $5HT_{2C}$ receptor (i.e., "knockouts") show increased feeding behavior and become obese, and SGAs with high liability for causing obesity (such as olanzapine or clozapine) are potent $5HT_{2C}$ antagonists. Schizophrenia patients who possess the "C" rather than "T" allele for the -759 C/T SNP of the $5HT_{2C}$ gene appear significantly more likely to incur substantial weight gain when taking clozapine (Reynolds et al., 2003). Weight gain from olanzapine appears less extensive among "T" carriers at the -759C/T SNP, and "C" carriers at the -697G/C SNP (Goldlewska et al., 2009). Other examples of candidate genes of investigational interest to the pharmacogenetics of SGA-associated weight gain include *LEP* and *LEPR* (variants encoding the satiety-promoting hormone leptin), *HTR2A* (the "T" rather than "C" allele at the T102C SNP has been linked with SGA-associated weight gain (Ujike et al., 2008)), and *MC4R* (the melanocortin 4 receptor; weight gain from SGAs is twice as likely among "A/A" homozygotes than "C/C" homozygotes (Czerwensky et al., 2013)).

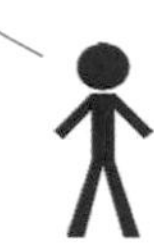

You poor devil of a double-C -759 C/T, double-A MC4R, homozygote you. Let us promptly get you to Chapter 10 without delay.

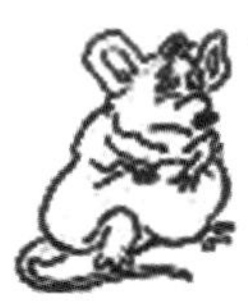

OK, but I really benefit from an SGA.

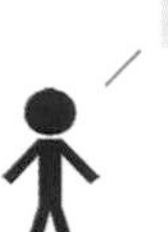

It's Chapters 10, 12 *and* 15 for you, buster. Pronto.

C PHARMACOKINETIC PHARMACOGENETICS

Perhaps the most widely recognized observation from pharmacogenetic testing involves the identification of poor metabolizers (PMs) and ultra-rapid metabolizers (URMs), as distinct from the normal phenotype of extensive metabolizers (EMs) for specific CYP450 isoenzyme SNPs in Phase I metabolism. Obviously, if URMs rapidly degrade their substrates then their pharmacodynamic effects may very well be minimal. Similarly, because PMs catabolize their substrates quite slowly, a little goes a long way and the potential for increased adverse effects due to "substrate buildup" may be considerable. There are several practical implications of the recognition of URMs and PMs:

- URMs may require higher than usual dosages of their relevant substrates in order to generate a discernible pharmacodynamic effect.
- In URMs, it may sometimes be impractical to dose a medication sufficiently above its usual parameters to elicit a therapeutic response, prompting the potential value (when feasible) of choosing a medication that is not metabolized by that catabolic enzyme.
- In PMs, smaller-than-usual doses may help to achieve a therapeutic response, and avert unnecessary adverse effects.
- If PMs are poorly tolerant of a drug metabolized by an affected enzyme, it may be pragmatic to choose a different drug (when feasible) that is metabolized by a different pathway.
- Importantly, PMs of CYP2D6 who take drugs that can prolong the cardiac QT interval may be at increased risk for clinically significant arrhythmias.

There are some additional key points to consider:

- Not all catabolic enzymes have known functional SNPs.
- PMs and URMs are relatively rare genotypes, as shown in Box 8.4.

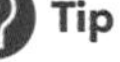
Tip

Poor and ultra-rapid metabolizers of cytochrome P450 substrates comprise a relatively small minority of the patient universe.

In addition to the several recognized CYP450 SNPs, there are a handful of additional SNPs reported more preliminarily in association with distinct adverse drug effects. At present, these associations would be considered provisional and awaiting replication from further studies. Prominent examples are summarized in Table 8.3.

Box 8.4

Prevalence Rates of Poor and Ultra-rapid Cytochrome P450 Metabolizers Across Races

CYP family	Poor metabolizers	Ultra-rapid metabolizers
2D6	Whites: 6–10% Blacks: 2–7% (South African Blacks: 29%) Asians: 0–2% Latinos: 2–6%	Whites: 4% Blacks: 5% (Ethiopians: 29%) Asians: 1% Latinos: 1–2%
1A2	Unknown	Unknown
3A4/5	Whites: 5%	Unknown
2C19	Whites: 3–5% Asians: 15–20%	Unknown

D EFFICACY PHARMACOGENETICS

The prospect that pharmacogenetic test results could point the way toward predicting greater comparative drug efficacy is for many clinicians more exciting than predicting intolerance, and conjures images of psychiatric "precision medicine" at its state-of-the-art best. The dilemmas and limitations for "efficacy pharmacogenetics" begin to unfold only after one acknowledges that there is no simple laboratory test able to bypass the need for complex clinical reasoning or discount the impact of nongenetic factors in influencing drug efficacy.

Pharmacokinetic SNPs can inform drug efficacy in rare specific instances. Most well-recognized is the case of PMs who cannot centrally (hepatically) convert certain pro-drugs to their active metabolites. Common examples include:

- conversion of tamoxifen to endoxifen via CYP2D6-mediated phenyl ring hydroxylation and CYP3A4-mediated *N*-demethylation
- conversion of carbamazepine to carbamazepine-10,11-epoxide via CYP3A4
- conversion of codeine to morphine via CYP2D6-mediated o-demethylation and UGT2B7-mediated glucuronidation
- conversion of hydrocodone to hydromorphone via CYP2D6-mediated o-demethylation and CYP3A4-mediated *N*-demethylation

Additionally, URMs may metabolize a relevant substrate drug so excessively that either a supratherapeutic dose would be needed to achieve meaningful bioavailability or else there occurs an impracticality in attempting to achieve an effect from a drug that essentially never has much of a chance to exert a pharmacodynamic influence. A corollary to URM genotypes would be the coadministration of a potent CYP450 inducer such as carbamazepine, which can substantially reduce the activity of concomitant pharmacotherapies. (For example, in some SGA trials in bipolar mania, cotherapy with carbamazepine yielded poorer efficacy and a reduction of antipsychotic serum levels by about 40% (Yatham et al., 2003).)

Controversy

In November, 2018 the FDA issued a consumer warning about pharmacogenetic testing which stated, "The relationship between DNA variations and the effectiveness of antidepressants has never been established."

The Holy Grail of pharmacogenetic testing is, or in principle would be, identified SNPs that have proven validity to moderate drug efficacy through adequately powered, replicated randomized trials. Commercially sponsored studies have reported findings from studies in which clinicians have been randomized either to receive a comprehensive, commercially produced pharmacogenetics printout based on genotyping for a given patient or treatment-as-usual, touting "better outcomes" for patients treated by the former rather than latter clinician group. The largest of existing pharmacogenetics studies in treatment-resistant MDD patients, the Genomics Used to Improve DEpression Decisions (GUIDED) trial (Greden et al., 2019; Thase et al., 2019a) is discussed in Box 8.5.

Controversy

On April 4, 2019, the FDA sent a warning letter to Inova Genomics Laboratory stating "The relationship between CYP2C19 genotype and drug response to escitalopram and sertraline is not established." The FDA warning letter addressed off-label promotion – but not the actual evidence base.

Counterpoint

The Clinical Pharmacogenetics Implementation Consortium (CPIC) disputes this FDA view and includes CYP2C19 SNPs in its guidelines for SSRI treatment of depression.

Box 8.5

Combinatorial Genetics and TRD Outcome

The GUIDED trial was conducted with an initial (ITT) 1541 treatment-resistant depression (TRD) patients (n = 1398 completers) whose prescribers received either a pharmacogenomics (PGx) report or treatment as usual (TAU). The prespecified primary outcome of the study was relative symptom change on the HAM-D rating scale, which found no significant difference between the PGx and TAU groups. The authors presented secondary outcome measures of "response" and "remission" rates, based on Hamilton Depression Rating Scale scores, as follows:

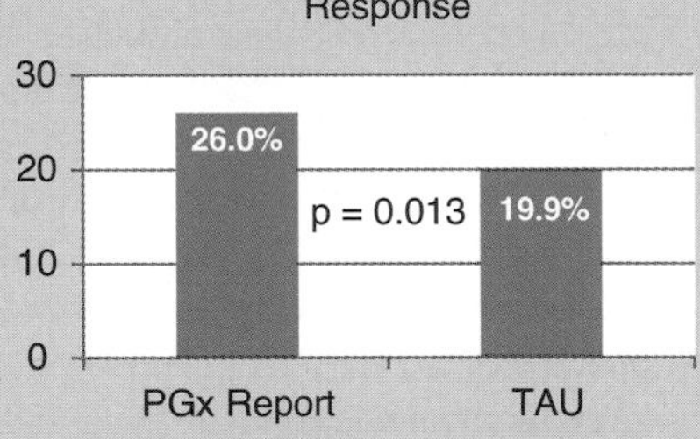

Remission
20
15
10
5
0
15.3%
p = 0.007
10.1%
PGx Report
TAU

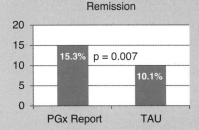

The above secondary outcome differences were reported as statistically significant, but 25 secondary outcome measures were examined with no statistical correction for multiplicity. Bonferroni correction (0.05/25 = p of 0.002) would render the above findings nominal, but even a Bonferroni-corrected alpha level would still be orders of magnitude less powerful to detect a significant difference at a GWAS alpha level of 0.00000005.

Furthermore, the magnitude of the clinical meaningfulness of the findings warrants attention. The results were described as showing that pharmacogenomic testing recipients were "30% more likely to respond to treatment" (that is, there exists a 6% difference in responder rates) and "50% more likely to achieve remission" (that is, a 5% difference in remitter rates). Does this mean much clinically? If we go calculate for ourselves the NNT for response, we find it is 17, with an absolute risk reduction of 5.94%. For remission, our calculations give an NNT of 19, with an absolute risk reduction of 5.34%.

Tip

In epidemiology, the *absolute risk reduction* is the change in risk for an event (such as response or remission) with an intervention relative to control conditions.

Before we can conclude anything about the clinical utility of the intervention, we need to consider the comparison group (that is, the prescribers, not their patients; although, having more detailed information about the patients being treated certainly would not hurt). We don't know how many *prescribers* were randomized, whether they were matched for levels of expertise, or what clinical factors clinicians considered when choosing treatments. We have no way to compare the PGx test to the clinical decision-making methods used during TAU. Without knowing more about the clinical characteristics of the two patient groups (i.e., their nongenetic characteristics that moderate and mediate outcomes), or the expertise of the treaters, it becomes hard to know how much pharmacogenetic testing yielded data above and beyond other information that prescribers might use to make decisions about which medications to use or avoid. What can we conclude from this study? Only that compared to "usual treatment" for TRD, pharmacogenetic testing improved the chances of a patient responding or remitting by about 5–6%. Pharmacogenetic testing could thus be a useful undertaking for about every 17th TRD customer; it upped the doctor's odds of getting a patient better by about 6% irrespective of whatever other information their doctor might use in that effort. Pharmacogenetic testing in the GUIDED study also did not significantly predict either the number of side effects or the proportion of subjects who experienced side effects.

Let us also not forget that TAU can vary greatly depending on the pharmacological savvy and expertise of the treater – such that treatment outcomes guided by pharmacogenetic testing have been shown to be no better than those achieved by highly knowledgeable prescribers, and the avoidance of drugs that undergo oxidative metabolism (Macaluso and Preskorn, 2018).

Controversy

Macaluso and Preskorn (2018) point out that if a prescriber simply avoids drugs that undergo oxidative metabolism, they will arrive at many of the same drug recommendations as in a commercial pharmacogenetics report. Do such tests do more than just flag drugs that are subject to Phase I metabolism?

Another genomics study in depression, known as the Genome-Based Therapeutic Drugs for Depression Project (GENDEP), undertaken as an international joint effort cosupported by European government agencies as well as industry partners, treated 712 MDD patients with escitalopram or nortriptyline for 12 weeks. DNA samples were screened for 610 000 known SNPs, capturing most known common variants in the human genome. None of the a-priori-selected candidate genes showed a statistically significant association with either antidepressant response, but one marker (rs2500535, in a gene that codes for uronyl 2-sulfotransferase) was associated with responder status to nortriptyline at a genome-wide level of significance. Another marker, in the IL-6 gene, was associated with response to escitalopram (Uher et al., 2010) that fell short of genome-wide significance.

What does this mean? The SNPs that were taken as candidates for association with drug response, based on their rationales, ended up being unrelated to treatment outcome, while one never-before-reported SNP out of over 600 000, having little obvious connection to depression or antidepressant mechanisms, unexpectedly came in as the winner. That none of the expected candidate genes yielded significant associations with drug response was a puzzler, but may have been due to inadequate statistical power. Or, it may simply have been a true negative finding. The net–net conclusion of this important study, as stated by the authors, was that "a meta-analysis of several large samples will be needed to establish generalizability of findings reported in the present study."

I notice that desvenlafaxine just about always appears in the "green bin" of favored antidepressants on commercial pharmacogenetics reports. Is that because it's just such a better drug than its parent compound, venlafaxine?

No, not at all! It's only because desvenlafaxine isn't a substrate for any P450 enzymes. It's solely metabolized by Phase II conjugation. Venlafaxine, the parent compound, must be metabolized by CYP2D6 to get to o-desmethyl-venlafaxine, so going straight to the metabolite drug spares any fuss over any P450 gene variants. Nothing to do with better efficacy. Pretty slick, eh?

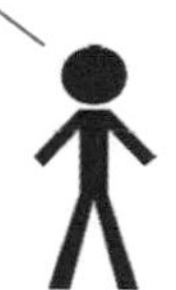

I don't get it, look at all those significant pharmacogenetic predictors of drug response in Tables 8.3 and 8.4. How can I ignore that data?

I never said to ignore the data, I said to interpret it with caution. Most of these studies are underpowered at a GWAS level of significance, haven't been replicated, don't assure the absence of population stratification or don't take into account the many other factors that contribute to drug response besides genetics.

Say, why don't you go re-read Chapter 3?

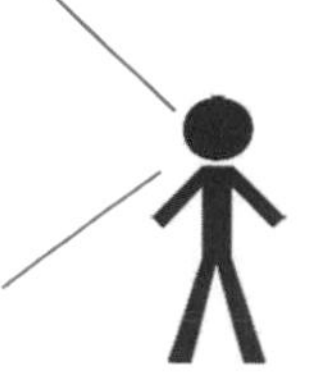

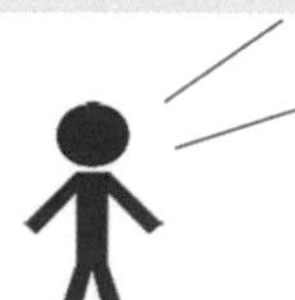

Say, why don't you go karyotype yourself...?

Pharmacogenetic testing, based on candidate gene SNPs, can also lead to clinically misleading guidance. For example, in schizophrenia, Rahman and colleagues (2017) reported the case of a 25-year-old man with highly deteriorated schizophrenia who, on clinical grounds, was deemed a more-than-appropriate candidate for clozapine. A testing protocol of several candidate genes obtained commercially at the behest of his family included the determination of heterozygosity at a SNP encoding the promoter region of the *DRD2* gene, leading the test manufacturer to declare, with no other clinical data, that the patient was unlikely to respond to clozapine (or olanzapine and risperidone). The patient nevertheless was treated with clozapine and had a brisk response, contrary to the expectations set forth by the testing protocol.

The purely psychological impact of pharmacogenetic testing also merits consideration, as in the case of a patient with somatic symptom disorder in search of some external "validation" for the source of their distress, or otherwise somatically preoccupied patients prone to nocebo effects who similarly may think that pharmacogenetics lends "credence" to the physical sensations they perceive.

E ANOTHER PERSPECTIVE: IT'S THE STRATEGY, NOT THE TEST RESULT

So far, therefore, there have been some surprises from pharmacogenomic testing as it enters mental health practice. First, we now know that no single test will tell us what to prescribe or what not to prescribe for a given patient. It is clear that each test result only "biases" us a small amount for or against a given drug choice, and that information must be balanced (i.e., with equipoise) with other personal information from that unique patient. Second, perhaps the most important outcome from pharmacogenomic testing is not necessarily the specific test result, but what this testing leads to that improves outcomes and reduces costs. That is, interpreting pharmacogenomic test results orients the advanced prescriber's thinking along a neurobiological perspective in order to select treatments that are biologically plausible, rather than just utilizing intuition, habit, or trial and error. This appears to have the potential to improve drug selection. Third, we now know that how one utilizes pharmacogenomic test results is not that different from how one utilizes any other personalized clinical information from a given patient. That is, each bit of information from a specific patient, whether clinical or pharmacogenomic testing, contributes at best a very small amount to the variance explaining why someone responds or fails to respond, or tolerates or fails to tolerate a given drug or drug class. Having more information from pharmacogenomic test results provides additional individualized data for a given patient to help weigh the many factors in favor of or against prescribing any given drug. Some skeptics conclude from all of this that no biomarker or genomic test is valuable enough to be part of the standard of psychiatric care, nor useful enough to be reimbursed. Integrating new technologies into clinical practice has always been a messy affair as we learn whether clinical outcomes are better when the test results are utilized than when they are not. Early adopters strive to discover the best utility of new information, while nay-sayers and especially payors remain doubtful. Some practitioners may be more comfortable at the present time using the time-honored classical approach.

On the other hand, early initiators of new technology who study the literature and learn how to properly interpret evolving test results may prefer a more cutting-edge, if controversial, approach. That is not to take a classical trial-and-error approach to selecting treatments, but instead to put the results of pharmacogenomic testing into the decision-making formula by pursuing a genetically informed, neurobiologically empowered, data-oriented, novel, and rational approach to selecting a treatment or combination that is already showing signs of yielding better symptomatic outcomes, better dosing, and reduced cost of treatment in some studies.

Among preliminary findings for specific functional, identified SNPs relevant to efficacy pharmacogenetics, we have the handful of examples listed in Table 8.4.

Table 8.5 summarizes major pharmacokinetic SNPs often found in commercial pharmacogenetics reports – that is, information relevant to the minority of patients who are phenotypically ultra-rapid or poor metabolizers of drugs metabolized by specific substrates of Phase I or Phase II liver enzymes. Tables 8.4 and 8.5 present major pharmacodynamic SNPs typically found in such reports – bearing potential relevance to how a drug might affect the body, rather than how the body affects the drug.

> **Tip**
> *del* means the deletion of a DNA sequence, while *Ins* means its insertion.

F HOW TO INTERPRET A PHARMACOGENETICS REPORT

The readout of a pharmacogenetic test report, as illustrated in Figures 8.1 and 8.2, conveys information that requires interpretation by the clinician, and is not simply a guide for "what to do" – any more than a radiologist's report of a pulmonary infiltrate on a chest X-ray in itself hardly tells the ordering clinician whether to prescribe an antibiotic or order a biopsy. While some manufacturers of pharmacogenetic tests oversimplify the clinical decision-making process by presenting results with colorful columns advising varying levels of encouragement or caution about medication choices, we strongly advise that clinicians make their own interpretations of any pharmacogenetics test they order, alongside other clinical information they possess, no differently than any other laboratory report. Indeed, while pharmacogenetic test results provide information that could be useful for anticipating possible outcomes under certain circumstances for some patients, the vivid color-coding scheme often used to "bin" information about drugs as being safe versus hazardous options plays to an almost Stroop-like effect in the prescriber's DLPFC and anterior cingulate cortex.

Sure, go ahead and prescribe that ...if you really think you know what you're doing...

Commercially available pharmacogenetic testing results that are based on DNA analyses of buccal swab test specimens typically contain three main types of information. The first involves a summary of SNPs deemed relevant to neurotransmitter precursors or receptors involved in the transport and possible pharmacodynamic effects of psychotropic drugs; the second involves SNPs relevant to the synthesis of catabolic enzymes (typically *certain* Phase I cytochrome P450 enzymes or *certain* Phase II glucuronidation enzymes). Think of these two components as the raw data from which practitioners must then draw clinically relevant inferences, similar to findings from a urinalysis, comprehensive metabolic panel, or an imaging study. The third aspect of a commercial test result involves a series of recommendations about which drugs to use or not use. Concerns arise because clinicians (or patients) might be tempted to oversimplify a recommendation as being absolute. Statements such as "use with caution" or "use with increased caution and more frequent monitoring" are merely shorthand regarding the potential for accrual of higher-than-usual plasma levels among PMs.

Tip

The Stroop effect refers to the neuropsychological phenomenon in which cognitive conflict or interference arises between the color versus semantic content of a verbal or visual stimulus, such that the emotional valence associated with the color could over-ride the otherwise emotionally neutral content of the stimulus being presented.

The SNPs reported in Figure 8.1 can be interpreted as follows:

Explanation

1. *SLC6A4*: As noted in Table 8.4, the gene encoding the serotonin reuptake inhibitor has a *s*(hort) and a

Figure 8.1 Representative pharmacogenetic printout: pharmacodynamic genes.

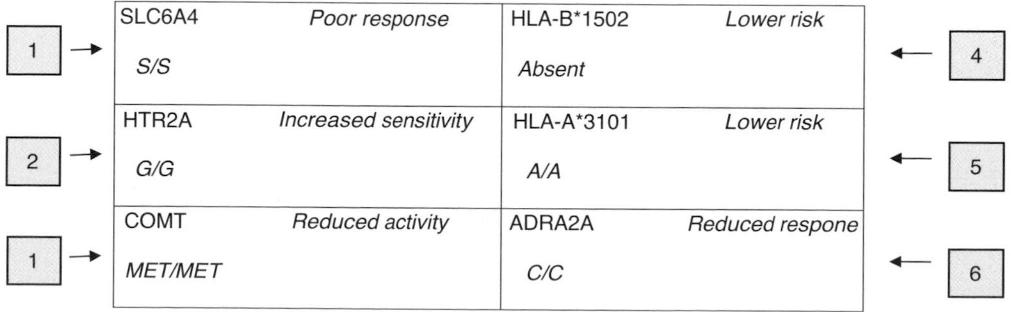

PATIENT GENOTYPES AND PHENOTYPES

PHARMACODYNAMIC GENES

1 →	SLC6A4 *S/S*	*Poor response*	HLA-B*1502 *Absent*	*Lower risk*	← 4
2 →	HTR2A *G/G*	*Increased sensitivity*	HLA-A*3101 *A/A*	*Lower risk*	← 5
1 →	COMT *MET/MET*	*Reduced activity*	ADRA2A *C/C*	*Reduced respone*	← 6

l(ong) allele. Data suggesting poorer antidepressant response derive mainly from a meta-analysis of 16 SSRI RCTs which collectively found that *s*/*s* genotypes were 1.71 times more likely than *l*/*l* genotypes to be SSRI nonresponders ($p = 0.003$) (Porcelli et al., 2012) – however, importantly, readers should note that the associations reported in that study were moderated by sex (women), race (white), age (older), and age at onset (late). In the above testing report, if our hypothetical *s*/*s* genotype patient happened to be an older white female with late-onset depression, that composite might *to some degree* lessen our enthusiasm for using an SSRI over, say, a mainly noradrenergic or dopaminergic agent.

2. *HTR2A*: 5HTR2A G/G homozygosity means that if our patient takes an SSRI or SNRI, he or she may be predisposed to having sexual adverse effects (Table 8.3).
3. *COMT*: The *Met/Met* genotype of the SNP encoding catechol-*O*-methyltransferase (COMT) means a chance of prolonged activity of dopamine (less degradation). This SNP is mainly of interest as a potential biomarker for cognitive function in schizophrenia and other major disorders. From a pharmacogenetics standpoint, concerns about a genetic predisposition to reduced COMT activity would likely be of more immediate concern if our patient should someday find himself or herself in a situation that required his or her taking pressors (such

Figure 8.2 Representative pharmacogenetic printout: pharmacokenetic genes.

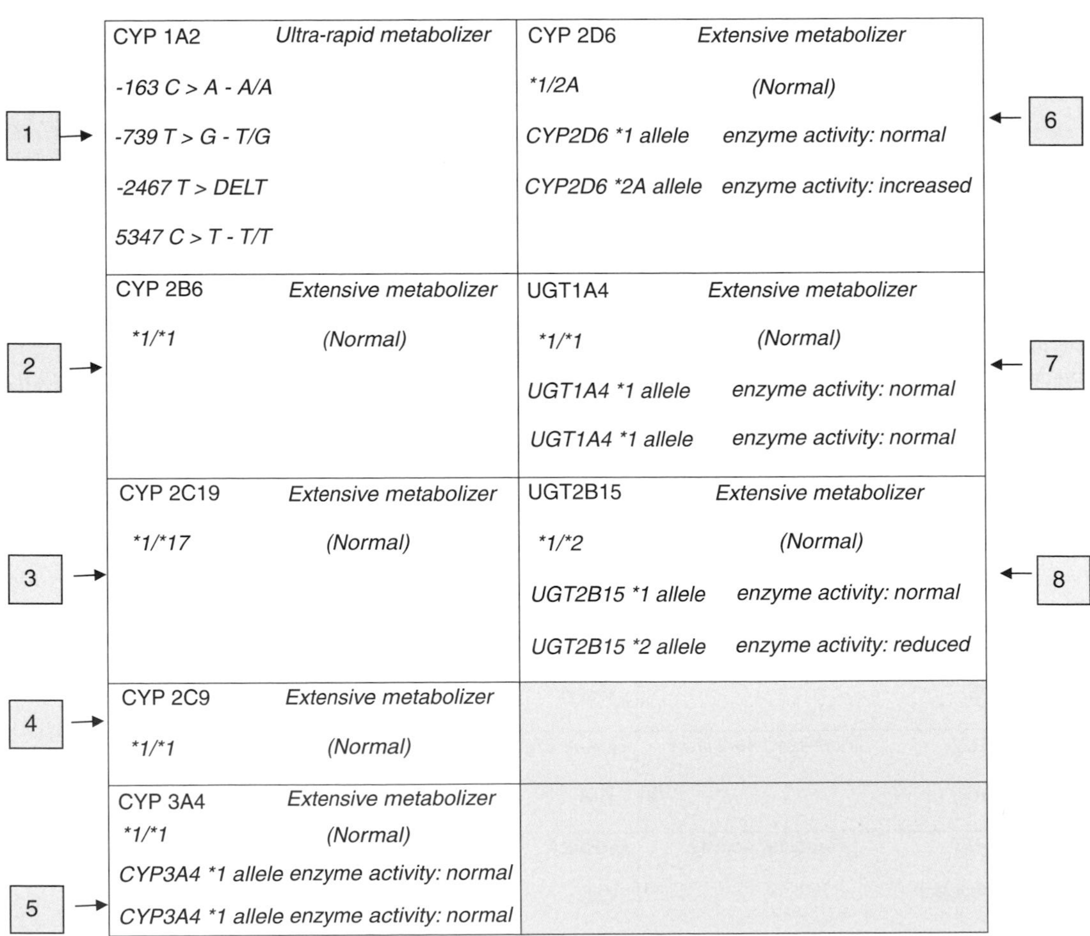

PHARMACOKINETIC GENES

1	CYP 1A2 *Ultra-rapid metabolizer* *-163 C > A - A/A* *-739 T > G - T/G* *-2467 T > DELT* *5347 C > T - T/T*	CYP 2D6 *Extensive metabolizer* **1/2A (Normal)* *CYP2D6 *1 allele enzyme activity: normal* *CYP2D6 *2A allele enzyme activity: increased*	6
2	CYP 2B6 *Extensive metabolizer* **1/*1 (Normal)*	UGT1A4 *Extensive metabolizer* **1/*1 (Normal)* *UGT1A4 *1 allele enzyme activity: normal* *UGT1A4 *1 allele enzyme activity: normal*	7
3	CYP 2C19 *Extensive metabolizer* **1/*17 (Normal)*	UGT2B15 *Extensive metabolizer* **1/*2 (Normal)* *UGT2B15 *1 allele enzyme activity: normal* *UGT2B15 *2 allele enzyme activity: reduced*	8
4	CYP 2C9 *Extensive metabolizer* **1/*1 (Normal)*		
5	CYP 3A4 *Extensive metabolizer* **1/*1 (Normal)* *CYP3A4 *1 allele enzyme activity: normal* *CYP3A4 *1 allele enzyme activity: normal*		

as dobutamine) or an inotropic/chronotropic drug for bradycardia such as isoproterenol – which will likely exert prolonged effects due to slower catabolism of those agents.

4. *HLA-B*1502*: Absence means normal, which means an all-clear signal to give our patient carbamazepine, if he or she needs it, regardless of their possible Han Chinese ancestry, without increased fear of Stevens–Johnson syndrome as an adverse outcome. (Note, while an initial meta-analysis by Zeng et al. (2015) suggested a possible increased risk for SJS or TEN (toxic epidermal necrolysis) from lamotrigine in HLA-B*1502-positive Han Chinese patients, many consider these data inconclusive because of reported unpublished negative findings.)
5. *HLA-A*3101*: A/A homozygosity at this locus means our patient is again free and clear from a genetic predisposition to develop severe cutaneous reactions if they took carbamazepine. Bring on the carb.
6. *ADRA2A*: C/C homozygosity means that if our patient has ADHD or otherwise is a psychostimulant candidate, methylphenidate response may be suboptimal.

The SNPs reported in Figure 8.2 can be interpreted as follows:

G PHARMACOKINETIC GENES

Explanation

1. *CYP 1A2.* The URM genotype for CYP 1A2 means that substrates for this catabolic enzyme may be degraded so rapidly as to negate or else greatly diminish pharmacodynamic effects. All else being equal (which as we know is seldom the case), our hypothetical patient might be better served avoiding drugs that are solely or primarily metabolized by 1A – notably, clozapine or asenapine. Most other 1A2 substrates have additional degradative pathways (e.g., duloxetine is also metabolized by 2D6; mirtazapine is also metabolized by 2D6 and 3A4/5), placing less singular importance on just 1A2 for appropriate catabolism. Cotherapy with a potent 1A2 inhibitor (such as fluvoxamine) might lend interesting though unpredictable counterbalance to an otherwise overactive catabolic system.
2. *CYP 2B6.* The EM genotype means normal function, so go ahead and give our patient as much bupropion as you like, he or she can handle it. (Though, whether or not bupropion will be *helpful* is a separate question…)
3. *CYP 2C19.* A normal (EM) genotype means that we are A-OK giving… well, no common psychotropic drugs are solely or primarily metabolized by 2C19. Perhaps you will exude more confidence if you choose citalopram or escitalopram for this patient, but both of those drugs have collateral metabolic pathways (3A4/5 and 2D6, respectively), so if said patient gets better with either agent, give yourself credit for imparting that much more oomph to the placebo effect without even realizing it.
4. *CYP 2C9.* Ditto to 2C19; 2C9 is just an along-for-the-ride collateral metabolic pathway whenever it is a catabolic enzyme for the handful of psychotropic agents passing through it (e.g., fluoxetine, amitriptyline).
5. *CYP 3A4.* Again with a normal genotype, our patient's liver won't bat an eyelash if we ask it to metabolize one of the psychotropic agents (mostly sleep aids and some antipsychotics) primarily metabolized by 3A4 as a primary substrate (e.g., eszopiclone, lurasidone, quetiapine, suvorexant, trazodone, ziprasidone, zolpidem) – but if he or she were a PM, we would be more leery about giving (or unwittingly overdosing) any of these medications. And we would then also tell him or her to lay off the grapefruit juice.
6. *CYP 2D6.* Once again our patient comes up with a normal genotype, though if he or she were a URM or a PM, we would want to give some extra thought before choosing (or at least dosing) drugs that are primarily 2D6 substrates – such as mixed amphetamine salts, atomoxetine, fluoxetine, or paroxetine.
7. *UGT1A4.* Genotypic normalcy again prevails, so we should feel most confident about giving desvenlafaxine, divalproex, or lamotrigine – at least with respect to metabolism. But we get no information from this test about whether or not any of those drugs will work better than any other … all else, once again, being equal. (*When is that again?*)
8. *UGT2B15.* This Phase II catabolic enzyme is involved mainly in processing toxic xenobiotics. Again a normal genotype, so no worries if our patient slathers on the insect repellant when they go hiking.

Tip

A xenobiotic is a drug that is not naturally produced in the body ("foreign") and often toxic (e.g., insecticides, organic solvents, heavy metals). They can be hard to eliminate and therefore often bioaccumulate.

H WHAT A MTHFR

Methylene Tetrahydrofolate Reductase (MTHFR) Polymorphism

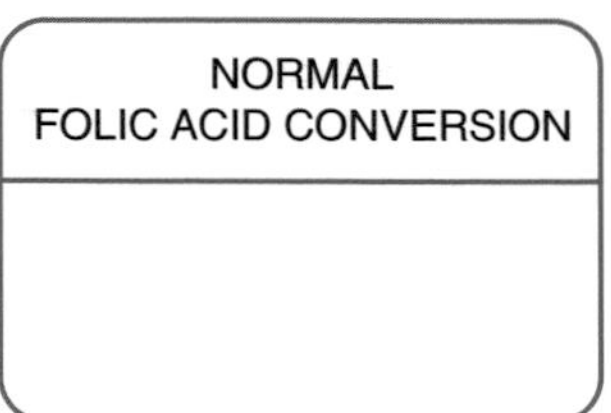

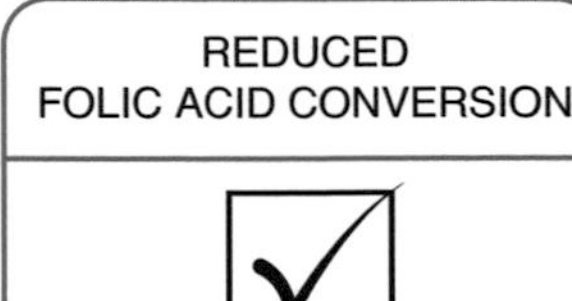

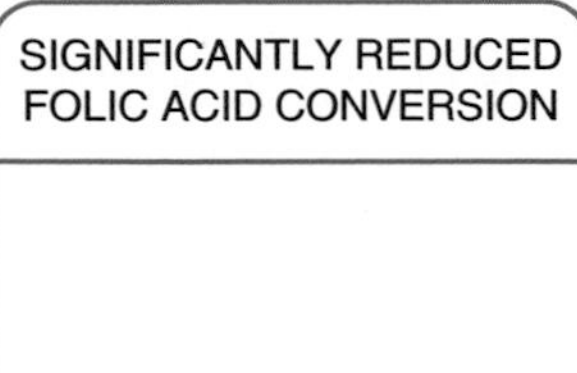

In the case of the MTHFR C677T variant (rs1801133), entire books, websites and support groups have been devoted to "living with the MTHFR mutation." The low-activity variant of the enzyme encoded by the "TT" polymorphism may indeed lead to less conversion of dietary folic acid to L-methylfolate, the form able to cross the blood–brain barrier. That, in turn, could theoretically lead to less bioavailable L-methylfolate for catecholamine and indoleamine synthesis in the brain. C677T "TT" homozygosity is modestly though significantly associated with an increased risk for depression (ORs of about 1.4-fold; Wu et al., 2013). But it remains speculative as to whether or not this means that oral L-methylfolate would more reliably improve depression symptoms in "T" than "C" genotypes, or that "repletion" of L-methylfolate is "indicated" simply on the basis of the presence of two (if not one) C677T "T" alleles on a pharmacogenetics test report. (Or, for that matter, whether oral L-methylfolate supplementation leads to measurably increased catecholamine or indoleamine synthesis or turnover in the mammalian brain.) As tantalizing as this hypothesis may be, evidence on its behalf is scant. One small (N = 75) study found no significant association between C677T genotype (or A1298C genotype) and adjunctive L-methylfolate response (Papakostas et al., 2014).

Aside from uncertainties about the clinical relevance of L-methylfolate supplementation in MTHFR C677T "C" allele carriers, there exists some preliminary work supporting the view that clinically depressed C677T or A1298C "C" allele carriers may benefit from reduced (metabolized) B vitamin supplementation in lowering homocysteine levels in conjunction with improving depressive symptoms (Mech and Farah, 2016). Outside of psychiatry, presence of the "C" allele in the C677T SNP has been shown to increase the risk for toxicity from methotrexate when used for hematological malignancies or rheumatoid arthritis.

Functional significance of the A1298C MTHFR polymorphism (rs1801131) is less well-established than for the C677T SNP.

I BOTTOM LINES

In 2018 the American Psychiatric Association's Council on Research Task Force For Novel Biomarkers and Treatments published its review of existing evidence about the use of pharmacogenetics in clinical practice, concluding "there are insufficient data to support the widespread use of combinatorial pharmacogenetic testing in clinical practice, although there are clinical situations in which the technology may be informative, particularly in predicting side effects" (Zeier et al., 2018).

We recognize that some neuroscientists embrace that impression while others find it totalitarian. There may well be a balance between these extremes. Like any laboratory test, clinicians must interpret the findings. Ideally, tests are ordered purposefully to answer specific questions, rather than with passive reliance that the results will magically reveal an overall best course of action. As the technology of pharmacogenetics testing continues to advance, our hope is that readers will remain current with evolving findings and draw upon such tests as one resource among many to explore formulated hypotheses about patients with treatment-resistant disorders or otherwise atypical responses to traditional pharmacotherapies.

 TAKE-HOME POINTS

- Psychiatric pharmacogenetics is a rapidly evolving field. Present technology allows clinicians to use pharmacogenetics to affirm suspicions about pharmacokinetic variants that may explain sensitivity to adverse effects or inability to convert pro-drugs to necessary active metabolites (poor metabolizers), or repeated nonresponses to drugs that are substrates for a particular metabolic enzyme (suspected ultra-rapid metabolizers). Like all laboratory tests, pharmacogenetics should be ordered when it is believed the results can help to answer a specific question related to tolerability or efficacy.
- Current evidence has linked particular genetic variants with specific adverse effects in definable patient subgroups – notably, risk for severe cutaneous reactions among Southeast Asians carrying particular HLA (human leukocyte antigen) alleles, or risk for cardiac arrhythmias (i.e., QT prolongation) with certain medications metabolized by cytochrome P450 enzymes in poor metabolizer genotypes.
- Interpret and understand the relevance of allelic variants in candidate genes associated with particular phenotypes relevant to distinct pharmacotherapy outcomes – rather than rely passively on pharmacogenetic test results to determine treatment without considering the broader context of clinical moderators and mediators of pharmacotherapy outcome.

Table 8.1 Enzymes involved in Phase I and Phase II hepatic metabolism

Phase I Metabolism	Phase II Metabolism		
	Type of conjugation	Endogenous reactant	Enzyme
Oxidation (e.g., CYP450, isoenzymes, monooxygenases, mixed function oxidases); oxidative reactions include hydroxylation, dealkylation, deamination	Glucuronidation	UDP-glucuronic acid	UDP-glucuronosyl transferase
Reduction (e.g., reductases)	Sulfonation	Sulfate (SO_3^-) (cofactor: PAPS)	Sulfotransferase
Hydrolysis (e.g., esterases, peptidases, amidases)	Amino acid conjugation [a]	gly, cys, glu, taurine, ser, pro, met, asp	Acylsynthetase, acyltransferase
	Glutathione conjugation	GSH	GSH-S-transferase
	Acetylation	Acetyl-CoA	*N*-acetyltransferase
	Methylation	Methyl group (CH_3-) (cofactor: SAMe)	Methyltransferase

[a] Sometimes also referred to as the glycination pathway because gly is the predominant amino acid used in conjugation reactions

Abbreviations: asp = aspartate; cys = cysteine; glu = glutamate; gly = glycine; GSH = glutathione; PAPS = 3′-phosphoadenosine-5′-phosphosulfate; met = methionine; pro = proline; SAMe = *S*-adenosylmethionine; ser = serine; UDP = uridine diphosphate

Table 8.2 Pharmacokinetic SNPs typically reported in commercially available pharmacogenetic test reports

SNP	Mechanistic relevance	Clinical relevance for PMs
ABCB1 (rs10245483G/T, rs2032583C, rs2235040A)	Blood-brain barrier transporter (P-glycoprotein)	↑'d levels of amitriptyline, desvenlafaxine, doxepin, levomilnacipran, nortriptyline, reboxetine, venlafaxine, vilazodone
CYP2D6 Functional: *1, *2 Reduced function: *9, *10, *17, *29, *41 Nonfunctional: *3, *4, *5, *6, *7, *8, *11, *12, *13, *14, *15, *19, *20, *21, *31, *38, *40, *42, *68, *92, *100, *101 Duplication: *1x2, *2x2, *4x2	Catalyzes Phase I oxidative reactions; converts tyramine to dopamine	↑'d levels of aripiprazole,[a] atomoxetine, brexpiprazole,[a] codeine, duloxetine, fluoxetine, iloperidone (↑'d QTc risk), mirtazapine, all TCAs, paroxetine, propranolol, venlafaxine, vortioxetine[a]
CYP2C19 *2, *3, *17	Phase I oxidative reactions	↑'d levels of bupropion, citalopram (↑'d QTc risk), diazepam, escitalopram, moclobemide, omeprazole, plaquenil, primidone, propranolol, 3° amine TCAs
CYP2C9 *2, *3, *5, *6, *7, *8, *9, *11, *13	Phase I oxidative reactions	↑'d levels of amitriptyline, diazepam, fluoxetine, ibuprofen and other NSAIDs, sildenafil, THC, tolbutamide, warfarin
UGT1A1	Phase II glucuronidation reactions; conjugates bilirubin	↑'d levels of desvenlafaxine[b]
UGT1A4	Phase II glucuronidation reactions	↑'d levels of lamotrigine, olanzapine
UGT2B15	Phase II glucuronidation reactions	↑'d levels of lorazepam, oxazepam
N-acetyltransferase	Phase II acetylation reactions	↑'d levels of isoniazid, procainamide, hydralazine
Thiopurine methyltranferase	Phase II methylation of thiopurine compounds	↑'d levels of 6-mercaptopurine or azathioprine

[a] Per manufacturers' labeling, dosing in PMs should be halved

[b] *Note* that while venlafaxine is metabolized by CYP2D6, its own metabolite desvenlafaxine is not, but rather, undergoes Phase II glucuronidation

Asterisks that precede a symbol under the "SNPs" column indicate an allele of a gene, by conventional nomenclature

Abbreviations: NSAID = nonsteroidal anti-inflammatory drug; PM = poor metabolizer; SNP = single nucleotide polymorphism; TCA = tricyclic antidepressant; THC = tetrahydrocannabinol; UGT = UDP-glucuronosyl transferase

Table 8.3 Safety pharmacogenetics: functional SNPs and their reported associations with adverse effects

Phenomenon	SNP	Association
Cutaneous reactions	HLA-B*1502	↑'d risk for SJS in Han Chinese/Malaysians receiving carbamazepine; possibly also lamotrigine (Zeng et al., 2015)
	HLA-A*3101	Possible link with carbamazepine-induced SJS in Japanese/European populations (Mushiroda et al., 2018)
	HLA-B*5801	↑'d risk for SJS with allopurinol
Iatrogenic sialorrhea	DRD2	Association with clozapine-related sialorrhea (Rajagopal et al., 2014)
Hyperprolactinemia	DRD2	Association with prolactin ↑ from antipsychotics in DRD2 Taq1A A1 carriers (Miura et al., 2016)
Antidepressant-associated sexual dysfunction	GRIA3, GRIK2, GRIA1, GRIA2	Variants associated with SSRI-related sexual dysfunction (Perlis et al., 2009)
	5HT2A -1438 G/A	G/G homozygosity linked with SSRI-related sexual dysfunction (Bishop et al., 2006)
Metabolic dysregulation, weight gain	ADRA2, DRD2, HTR2C (aka 5HT2C), MC4 R	Largest effect sizes seen with *ADRA2* (adrenergic receptor β3), *DRD2, HTR2C, MC4 R* (melanocortin 4 receptor) (g = 0.30 to 0.80, OR = 1.47 to 1.96) (reviewed by Zhang et al., 2016)
	Leptin (-2548G/A)	Leptin "G" allele at locus -2548 associated with clozapine-induced weight gain (Zhang et al., 2007a)
	G-protein β3 subunit (GNB3)	GNB3 825 T allele associated with olanzapine-related weight gain (Ujike et al., 2008)
	BDNF (Val^{66}Met)	Low BDNF expression linked with SGA-associated weight gain (Fang et al., 2016)
Antidepressant-associated suicidality	BDNF	BDNF polymorphism associated with antidepressant-related suicidality (Perroud et al., 2009)
	CACNA1C	Exploratory analysis of STAR*D Caucasian subjects, each SNP having an OR~1.3 (nominally significant p-values) (Casamassima et al., 2010)
	Tryptophan hydroxylase 2 (TPH2)	C>T variant associated with antidepressant-related suicidality (Musil et al., 2013)
Tardive dyskinesia	DRD3	Ser→Gly SNP at Exon 1 associated with increased risk for developing tardive dyskinesia during antipsychotic treatment in a pooled sample of 780 patients (OR = 1.52, 95% CI = 1.08–1.68; Lerer et al., 2002)

Abbreviations: BDNF = brain-derived neurotrophic factor; CI = confidence interval; OR = odds ratio; SJS = Stevens–Johnson syndrome; SNP = single nucleotide polymorphism; SSRI = selective serotonin reuptake inhibitor

Table 8.4 Reported SNP associations in efficacy pharmacogenetics

SNP	Association	Comment
CRHBP (corticotropin-releasing hormone binding protein)	"G/G" homozygosity associated with greater response or remission from depression with escitalopram or sertraline, but not venlafaxine XR (O'Connell et al., 2018)	16 SNPs originally were tested in this exploratory study. After controlling for ethnic stratification, findings fell short of Bonferroni-corrected alpha
ADRA2A	In ADHD, "C" allele of the -1291 G>C SNP may *diminish* response to α agonists (e.g., clonidine, guanfacine); methylphenidate response may be better for "G" than "C" allele (Myer et al., 2018)	Postsynaptic α_{2A} receptors regulate prefrontal cortical noradrenergic transmission
ABCB1 gene (encoding p-glycoprotein)	Escitalopram or sertraline response more likely with common than minor allelic variants; minor allele homozygosity predicted response to venlafaxine after Bonferroni correction (Schatzberg et al., 2015)	Increased P-glycoprotein expression (via the minor T allele) could account for enhanced clearance of escitalopram and sertraline
DRD4	VNTR 4 DRD4 may increase methylphenidate responsivity in childhood ADHD (Myer et al., 2018)	Encodes the D2-like receptor targeted by antipsychotic and anti-Parkinson drugs
SLC1A1	Associated with antipsychotic response to risperidone in schizophrenia at a genome-wide significance level (Yu et al., 2018)	Encodes the high-affinity glutamate transporter excitatory amino acid transporter 3 (EAA3)
SLC6A3	A homozygous 10-repeat 40 bp VNTR may lessen methylphenidate efficacy in childhood ADHD (OR = 0.74; 95% CI = 0.60–0.90; Myer et al., 2018)	Encodes the chloride anion exchanger
GRIN2B	C/C genotype associated with better methylphenidate response in ADHD (OR = 9.03, 95% CI = 1.02–79.99; Myer et al., 2018)	Encodes the glutamate ionotropic NMDA receptor subunit 2B
CACNA1C	Associated with antipsychotic response to olanzapine in schizophrenia at a genome-wide significance level (Yu et al., 2018)	Encodes voltage-gated L-type calcium channel
CNTN4 (Contactin 4)	Associated with antipsychotic response to aripiprazole in schizophrenia at a genome-wide significance level (Yu et al., 2018)	Contactin 4 is an immunoglobulin that functions as a cell adhesion molecule
5HTTLPR (SLC6A4)	SLC6A4 has *s*(hort) (low activity) and *l*(ong) (high activity) variants; *l* is further subclassified as a low-activity L_G subvariant and a high-activity L_A subvariant. *s* or L_G alleles transcribe less serotonin transporter. A meta-analysis found a modest association with the "*l*" allele and remission with antidepressants in Caucasians but not Asians (Porcelli et al., 2012); *l/l* associated with higher remission in older adults (Shiroma et al., 2014)	SLC6A4 is among the most widely studied SNPs. Its gene product is a pharmacological target for SSRIs and SNRIs, as well as psychostimulants and the substituted amphetamine MDMA ("Ecstasy")
Tryptophan hydroxylase: TPH1 (TPH1 218A/C); TPH2	TPH1*a allele may be associated with poor response to serotonergic antidepressants; TPH2 A/A genotype correlates with depression severity (Anttila et al., 2009) and SSRI response (Porcelli et al., 2011)	Findings await replication
BDNF	Val^{66}Met SNP identified in one meta-analysis as *the most robust pharmacogenetic predictor* of SSRI response (Niitsu et al., 2013)	Individual studies nonsignificant but pooled findings significant for SSRIs

Abbreviations: ADHD = attention deficit hyperactivity disorder; BDNF = brain-derived neurotrophic factor; bp = base pair; CI = confidence interval; OR = odds ratio; MDMA = 3,4-methylenedioxy-methamphetamine; NMDA = *N*-methyl-D-aspartate; SNP = single nucletide polymorphism; SNRI = serotonin-norepinephrine reuptake inhibitor; SSRI = selective serotonin reuptake inhibitor; VNTR = variable number of tandem repeat

Table 8.5 Pharmacodynamic SNPs typically reported in commercially available pharmacogenetic test reports

SNP	Mechanistic relevance	Clinical relevance
ANK3	Ankyrins are cell motility proteins involved in assembly of voltage-gated Na^+ channels	Associated with general cognitive impairment and cortical thinning
ANKK1 (Taq1A polymorphism)	Originally believed to be a DRD2 SNP, Taq1 is now recognized as encoding ANKK1, controlling DA synthesis	A1 allele associated with a variety of disorders and behaviors related to addiction, impulsivity, and reward
ADRA2A	Presynaptic α_2 adrenergic autoreceptors regulate (inhibit) release of norepinephrine	Associated with CNS noradrenergic function in attention and related cognitive functions
BDNF $Val^{66}Met$	Trophic factor involved in neuronal survival	See Table 8.5
COMT $Val^{158}Met$	Degrades catecholamines (i.e., DA → 3-methoxytyramine; NE →normetanephrine; epinephrine→metanephrine; DOPAC→HVA)	Aggression, possible vulnerability to comorbid panic disorder in bipolar disorder probands; see Table 8.5
DRD2 Taq1A; -141C ins/del	The Taq1A SNP gives rise to the DRD2*A1 allele, while the -141C ins/del SNP encodes the DRD2*A2 allele	Encodes the main receptor target for antipsychotic drugs; poorer antipsychotic response in -141 *del* than *Ins/Ins* (Zhang et al., 2010)
DRD4	See Table 8.4	See Table 8.4
Gβ3, also known as the C825T variant	G-protein β3 subunit	T/T genotype may be associated with antidepressant and sildenafil responsivity (Sperling et al., 2003)
GRIA1, GRIA3 GRIK2	Glutamate receptor proteins (GRIA1 and GRIA3 are AMPA receptors, GRIK2 is a kainate receptor) involved in excitatory neurotransmission	See Table 8.3
$5HT_{2A}$ (102 T/C polymorphism; 1438 G/A polymorphism	5HT2A agonism is associated with the psychedelic effects of LSD and other hallucinogens	"A" allele C/C genotype associated with impulsivity in alcohol dependence (Jakubczyk et al., 2012)
$5HT_{2C}$ (-759 C/T)	5HT2C receptors densely distributed in brain regions regulating mood, feeding behavior, anxiety, and sex drive	See Table 8.3
HLA-B*1502	Class I major histocompatibility complex	See Table 8.3
HLA-B*5801	Class I major histocompatibility complex	See Table 8.3
HRT2A	Excitatory serotonin receptor subtype	In STAR*D, A/A homozygotes had an 18% lesser risk of nonresponse to citalopram (McMahon et al., 2006)
Melanocortin-4 receptor (MC4 R)	The MC4 protein binds α-melanocyte stimulating hormone and appears to be involved in feeding behavior	See Table 8.3
MTHFR C677T ($Ala^{222}Val$)	Involved in homocysteine conversion to methionine (se Figure 11.2, Chapter 11)	C677T: TT genotype (lower activity) may cause less conversion of folic acid to *L*-methylfolate
SCL6A4	See Table 8.4	See Table 8.4
Tryptophan hydroxylase 2 (TPH2)	TPH is the rate-limiting enzyme in the synthesis of serotonin	See Table 8.4

Abbreviations: AMPA = α-amino-3-hydroxy-5-methyl-4-isoxazolepropionic acid; CNS = central nervous system; DA = dopamine; DOPAC = 3,4-dihydroxyphenylacetic acid; HVA = homovanillic acid; LSD = lysergic acid diethylamide; MTHFR = methylene tetrahydrofolate reductase; NE = norepinephrine; SNP = single nucleotide polymorphism; SSL = solute carrier family gene

9 Cross-tapering and the Logistics of Drug Discontinuation

LEARNING OBJECTIVES

- ☐ Recognize clinical situations that warrant stopping an existing psychotropic medication, either abruptly or gradually
- ☐ Identify clinical situations in which it is more appropriate to switch from one drug to another via direct substitution versus cross-tapers, and the pros and cons of each approach
- ☐ Describe risks for rebound effects caused by abrupt cessation of some psychotropic drugs
- ☐ Know how to convert dosages from oral to long-acting injectable antipsychotics, from one benzodiazepine to another, and from one psychostimulant formulation to another
- ☐ Understand the probabilities and timeframes of relapse from randomized drug discontinuation trials in mood and psychotic disorders

It is a bad plan that admits of no modification.

- Publilius Syrus

"Necessary clinical adjustments," as noted in Chapter 1, come with the pharmacological territory for most patients with complex psychiatric disorders – partly because symptoms often can be protean and nonstatic, partly because illness severity can wax and wane, partly because of the impact of cotherapies, and partly from other factors such as pharmacokinetic interactions, treatment nonadherence, loss of efficacy, or other events in the natural evolution of illness. The mechanics and logistics of changing from one pharmacotherapy to another, or deciding when and how to deprescribe an ineffective or otherwise unhelpful medication, are seldom discussed in textbooks or practice guidelines. From an evidence-based perspective, there are few controlled trials designed to compare tolerability and outcomes across various methods and timeframes for stopping and starting or cross-tapering one drug in exchange for another. In this chapter we hope to shed light on how to make decisions about starting, stopping, or replacing drugs within an existing pharmacotherapy regimen safely, effectively, and logically.

Are necessary clinical adjustments really always *necessary?*

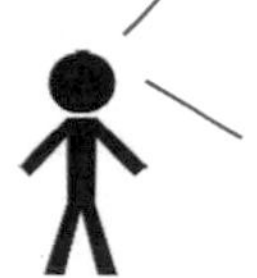

Ah, well, uhm, uh, they ought to be, right? I mean, you wouldn't just tweak dosages or meds around for no good reason, would you?
Or *would* you?

Medications become discontinued for innumerable reasons: deliberately or accidentally, unilaterally or by doctor–patient agreement, because they are inadequately helpful or an alternative agent seems more compelling, or their side effects outweigh benefits, or they are thought to no longer be necessary, or because of acute toxicities, or manufacturing unavailabilities, or cost, or inconvenience, or sheer curiosity about what might happen off medication. We would contrast the mechanics of stopping a drug altogether with replacing it with an alternative agent. There are a handful of scenarios or general situations where a medication is purposefully discontinued without particular thought about its possible future reinitiation or replacement, such as those described in Box 9.1.

A LACK OF EFFICACY

Good pharmacological hygiene, as noted in Chapter 6, means retaining drugs that provide unambiguous benefit while jettisoning those which lack demonstrated efficacy for a given patient. One must obviously assure

Box 9.1

Discontinuation of Medication

- *Pre-pregnancy*: Drugs such as divalproex or carbamazepine have strong relative contraindications in pregnancy (see Chapter 12) and when feasible, taper-offs should be completed by a week before anticipated conception.
- *Toxicity/Overdose*: Particularly for drugs with narrow therapeutic indices, clearance after acute toxicity often necessitates a lengthy period before a drug can safely be reintroduced, if its eventual resumption is deemed appropriate. In the case of lithium, where brain and bone concentrations can remain high after toxicity, long after serum lithium levels are undetectable, many weeks may need to elapse before lithium can be safely reintroduced (guided in part by cognitive and neurological status).
- *Serious or persistent adverse effects*: Adverse drug effects can be benign and annoying or medically hazardous; they are sometimes transient and self-limited (e.g., nausea or headache when starting an SSRI) or manageable by dosage reductions or antidote strategies (see Chapter 10). The latter of these scenarios is especially relevant when few if any viable and effective alternative medication options may exist for a particularly difficult condition (e.g., clozapine for refractory schizophrenia; an MAOI for multidrug-resistant major depression).
- *Hypersensitivity reactions*: Severe reactions may include anaphylaxis (immediate hypersensitivity (Type I) reactions), angioedema, cutaneous reactions such as purpura, vasculitis, or thrombocytopenia, and DRESS syndrome (drug reaction with eosinophilia and systemic symptoms, usually arising in an idiosyncratic fashion two to eight weeks after initiation of the causal agent). Laryngeal angioedema can be life-threatening due to airway obstruction and is a medical emergency managed with antihistamines, possible corticosteroids, and sometimes intubation for airway protection.

that adequate medication trials (adequate dosages for adequate durations for appropriate disorders) have occurred before concluding that a drug is ineffective and should be stopped. Sometimes, particularly if several or more medication trials have yielded no compelling value, one or more stakeholders (patient, clinician, family member) may be inclined to cling to a drug nevertheless, because it "ought" to work (e.g., because it is generally associated with efficacy for a particular diagnosis), even if by all measures it confers no usefulness. Such situations can also foster the idea that, while a patient may remain highly symptomatic despite taking a given medication, their plight might become even worse were they to stop it. Stopping ineffective drugs that "ought" to work for a suspected diagnosis also makes more tangible the possibility that the presumptive diagnosis may simply be wrong. Consider Clinical Vignette 9.1.

More often than not, the intentional decision to continue or stop a medication due to an adverse event becomes a risk–benefit decision without clear or absolute guidelines. Besides the general situations noted above, and apart from judged lack of efficacy after an adequate trial, other specific situations that may necessitate drug discontinuation are summarized in Table 9.1. (See Chapter 10 for further detail on management of adverse effects described.)

CLINICAL VIGNETTE 9.1

Angie was a 27-year-old single female whose "ultra-ultra-rapid cycling bipolar II disorder" failed to respond to multiple adequate trials of lithium, divalproex, lamotrigine, carbamazepine, SSRIs, SNRIs, bupropion, levothyroxine, and several SGAs. Her symptoms consisted mainly of chronic affective instability and easily provoked anger outbursts, as well as chronic insomnia, feelings of boredom and emptiness, low motivation, and low self-worth. During a second-opinion consultation it was noted that her symptoms never coalesced as a distinct constellation to define either hypomania or a major depressive episode, and the psychiatrist wondered if she had been misdiagnosed with bipolar disorder rather than borderline personality disorder. Rather than add more medications, the suggestion was made to consider sequentially removing current medications to gauge their relevance, without replacement, and instead redirect the focus of her care more toward psychotherapy as the cornerstone of her treatment.

B CROSS-TAPERS: THE LOW-DOWN ON THE SLOW-DOWN

As a rule of thumb, there is usually no compelling practical reason to taper off one drug before immediately starting another within the same family, or across families, although in the case of antidepressants some authorities quite conservatively advocate a four-week minimum for tapering off an outgoing antidepressant (e.g., Taylor et al., 2015). Clinicians often worry about a host of theoretical pharmacodynamic adverse effects such as serotonin syndrome from overlapping two serotonergic antidepressants to fears of "rebound" effects when one drug is stopped, or motor dyskinetic effects, or discontinuation phenomena when stopping one antipsychotic and starting another. Psychopharmacologists also are often enamored of counting half-lives and sometimes advise that an optimal "overlap" period from one drug to another might correspond to the passage of five elimination half-lives of both the outgoing and incoming drug. In reality, many of these issues are of more theoretical than practical relevance and generally are unnecessary.

While there is no established standard of care for the logistics of switching from one antidepressant (or antipsychotic, or stimulant, or benzodiazepine) to another, there are three basic strategies one could pursue, each with its own potential advantages and disadvantages:

- *Directly stop one agent, then immediately start another.* This involves immediately discontinuing a first drug without tapering and beginning its replacement the same day or the next. *Advantages* of this approach are that it is simple, involves less risk for medication errors, may be necessary in the setting of toxicity or severe reactions, and minimizes delays in making the switch to a potentially better treatment option. *Disadvantages* are that direct switches may be more difficult when the initial agent is at a high versus low dose; if the outgoing drug and its active metabolites together pose a very long half-life (e.g., fluoxetine, vortioxetine, aripiprazole, cariprazine) then introducing the new drug at a "full" or comparable dose may produce more exaggerated additive adverse effects, and there is also a potential higher risk for relapse until the efficacy of new drug is established.
- *Simultaneous cross-taper both agents.* Logistics of this approach, typically over about a two-week period, involve reducing the dose of the first agent while slowly starting and titrating up the dose of the new agent. *Advantages* of this approach are that it provides more sustained "coverage" from the initial drug while gauging if its replacement is tolerable and effective, it offers a more conservative approach when there is particular concern about relapse or clinical worsening, it may be preferable if the initial drug is at a high dose, and overlap periods are often necessary when converting to or from long-acting injectable antipsychotic formulations. *Disadvantages* involve possible pharmacokinetic interactions and additive pharmacodynamic effects that could be misattributed solely to the new drug, there may be a greater potential for pharmacodynamic redundancies or possible diminished efficacy when drugs compete for binding at the same receptor(s), and there may be a higher potential risk for idiosyncratic toxicities (e.g., serotonin syndrome if overlapping serotonergic effects).
- *Taper off, then taper on.* Logistically, one tapers off the first agent usually over about a week (a little more than five half-lives for most antidepressants or antipsychotics), then begins the second agent as one would ordinarily. *Advantages* of this approach are the minimizing or avoiding of possible drug interactions or additive adverse effects, and it may be necessary when any drug overlap can pose a serious adverse reaction (e.g., pre-MAOI washouts). *Disadvantages* are an increased patient risk window for relapse or further worsening, if the first agent was exerting partial benefit; and it can also be unnecessarily time-consuming, delaying the introduction of a potentially more effective new treatment.

A number of theoretical and practical considerations should bear on decisions about psychotropic cross-tapers versus switches, decided in case-by-case fashion. These are summarized in Box 9.2:

Box 9.2

Cross-Tapers versus Switches

- Outgoing drugs (and their active metabolites) that have a relatively long serum half-life should require little or no taper-off.
- Patients who are known genetically to be poor metabolizers for catabolic enzymes relevant to an outgoing drug (see Chapter 8) should, in principle, require minimal-to-no taper-offs of an existing drug via progressive dosage reductions.
- If an outgoing drug inhibits an enzyme that would delay the metabolism of an incoming drug (e.g., outgoing fluvoxamine with incoming vilazodone), delay initiation of the new drug several days until the metabolic enzyme (e.g., CYP450 3A4) can regenerate.
- Patients who report significant past subjective problems in stopping a psychotropic drug are probably best served with slow cross-tapers and the overlap of "old familiar" with "new and foreign" medications, if for no other reasons than to foster psychological comfort around the unpredictability of change, and to minimize nocebo effects (see Chapter 3).

C PROBLEMS WITH ABRUPT CESSATION OF AN OUTGOING DRUG

Some, but not all, psychotropic drugs pose tolerability problems when stopped abruptly and with no replacement. Types of adverse effects associated with sudden discontinuation are summarized in Box 9.3.

Table 9.2 presents a summary of risks associated with abrupt cessation of varied psychotropic agents and their optimal management strategies.

D ANTIDEPRESSANT DISCONTINUATION SYNDROMES

Antidepressant drugs that affect serotonin function, particularly in the case of drugs with relatively short elimination half-lives, have been recognized as causing diffuse physical complaints upon abrupt cessation – sometimes even after missing only one or two doses. Discontinuation phenomena have been recognized in up to half of antidepressant recipients upon abrupt cessation during RCTs (e.g., randomization from open phases to a placebo arm; study termination) (Fava et al., 2015, 2018a). Discontinuation syndrome features have been prospectively identified in up to two-thirds of MDD patients who abruptly stop an SSRI (Rosenbaum et al., 1998). Features typically persist up to three weeks or longer and, as reported in randomized trials, most often include dizziness (18–29%), nausea (11–29%), nervousness (16–18%), headache (17–18%), insomnia (19%), and abnormal dreams (16%) (Rosenbaum et al., 1998). Some patients also report electrical "jolt" sensations (commonly called "brain zaps"). Kennedy et al. (2016) proposed the mnemonic FINISH to describe common antidepressant discontinuation symptoms (Box 9.4).

The term "discontinuation syndrome" has been criticized by some authors as too euphemistic given the potential severity and intensity of symptoms, with preference for labeling such conditions as "withdrawal syndromes" (Fava et al., 2015, 2018a). However, semanticists would note that "withdrawal" incorrectly reinforces lay misconceptions that antidepressants are

Box 9.3

Adverse Effects of Sudden Discontinuation

- *Cholinergic rebound*: abrupt cessation of anticholinergic drugs (e.g., tricyclics, certain antipsychotic medications) can sometimes precipitate pro-cholinergic effects such as nausea, sweating, diarrhea, and vomiting.
- *Rebound hypertension*: may occur when suddenly stopping α-1 antagonist drugs such as prazosin (popular as a potential treatment for nightmares in PTSD) and terazosin (used sometimes to counteract excessive sweating caused by serotonergic antidepressants) or α-1-agonists (e.g., clonidine used for ADD, opiate withdrawal, or autonomic hyperarousal).
- *Seizure risk*: anticonvulsants raise the seizure threshold and, consequently, their abrupt cessation could at least theoretically provoke an increased risk for seizures – particularly in patients with pre-existing risk factors for seizures, such as epilepsy, significant alcohol use, or cotherapies with medications that lower the seizure threshold (e.g., clozapine and other antipsychotics, stimulants, bupropion). Most manufacturers' product information materials advise discontinuing anticonvulsants over a two-week period for this intended purpose, although the necessity of such tapers in nonepileptic anticonvulsant recipients (e.g., migraine or neuropathic pain sufferers, mood disorders, anxiety and sleep disorders) remains only theoretical, and less pertinent when a new anticonvulsant replaces an outgoing one. Of note, seizure risk is influenced by many factors that are relevant only in epilepsy, such as extent of past seizures, age of first seizure onset, neurological deficits, and developmental delays.
- *Acute withdrawal*: of obvious concern with drugs that may cause physical dependence and tolerance (e.g., benzodiazepines, opiates). Benzodiazepines do cause clinically meaningful dependence, with a potential for withdrawal upon abrupt cessation after only a few weeks of exposure, even to relatively low doses (e.g., alprazolam 0.5 mg/day), although severe manifestations of withdrawal (e.g., seizures, delirium) usually occur from abrupt cessation only after prolonged exposure (months) at high doses (Rosenberg and Chiu, 1985). In patients who take opiates daily, exposure time needed to develop physical dependence can vary greatly, alongside the potential for physiological withdrawal upon abrupt cessation. Usually, unless dosages are inordinately high, use for less than one or two weeks is unlikely to necessitate a gradual taper-off to avoid withdrawal. (And, while opiate withdrawal is not medically hazardous, it can certainly be extremely uncomfortable.)

Box 9.4

The FINISH Mnemonic

Flu-like symptoms
Insomnia
Nausea
Imbalance
Sensory disturbances
Hyperarousal

"addictive" or implies a mechanism related to physiological dependence and tolerance. Closer analogies to "withdrawal" seen with long-term corticosteroid use may be more appropriate. A 1997 consensus panel proposed that somatosensory phenomena related to abrupt antidepressant cessation may reflect sudden reductions of synaptic serotonin availability in the setting of down-regulated serotonin receptors (Schatzberg et al., 1997).

E WHAT ABOUT MONOAMINE OXIDASE INHIBITORS?

MAOIs warrant special attention because of their mechanism of action. The potential concern for adverse drug interactions is not about elimination half-life (as is the case with most other drugs) but, rather, the consequences of having shut down the enzyme MAO, which then does not regenerate for at least two weeks after discontinuation of the inhibitor. This means that if a new antidepressant with serotonergic or pressor effects were to enter the clinical picture, the theoretical risk for serotonin syndrome or a hypertensive crisis persists until the enzyme has regenerated. What about switching from one MAOI to another? In principle, the mechanistic effect is identical (inhibition of MAO), regardless of which specific agent does the honors. In practice, case reports exist of stroke or cerebral hemorrhage, or sudden death following an immediate switch from one MAOI to another (e.g., Bazire, 1986). One case series of eight MDD patients taking an (irreversible) MAOI reported abrupt switching from one such agent to another with generally good tolerability (one case of "withdrawal from tranylcypromine or mild serotonin syndrome") and an antidepressant response in four of the eight switched cases (Szuba et al., 1997). Nevertheless, and despite their apparent rarity, the potential for catastrophic outcomes from converting one MAOI to another without a requisite two-week washout period suggests this approach is unwise and poses an unnecessary potential serious hazard.

Why can't I just switch directly from one MAOI to another? The same enzyme is being blocked regardless of how

Just...don't do it, OK? Just don't. Your patient could stroke.

but...

Just don't!

wimp

F PHARMACOTHERAPY DISCONTINUATIONS PRIOR TO ECT

In nonepileptic patients for whom an anticonvulsant is being tapered down or off prior to starting ECT (where the therapeutic goal is to induce a controlled and monitored seizure), fairly rapid discontinuation is customary and unlikely to pose a hazard. ECT experts often advise that holding just one or two doses of a chronically administered anticonvulsant prior to ECT seldom interferes with obtaining an adequate ECT-induced seizure.

My patient is taking lamotrigine and clonazepam. She can't start ECT till those drugs are tapered off, right?

Not necessarily. Her seizure threshold is higher, that's true, but just reducing the clonazepam and holding the lamotrigine should be adequate. And you could always add chlorpromazine or caffeine pre-ECT to further lower her seizure threshold.

Abrupt cessation of monoaminergic antidepressants before ECT can prolong cortical seizure activity. MAOIs pose no conflict with general anesthesia, contrary to popular misconception (and antiquated stray case reports from a long-ago era) (see el-Ganzouri et al., 1985).

G POTENTIAL ADVANTAGES OF ABRUPT DRUG DISCONTINUATION

There are occasional instances in which abruptly stopping a medication can provide useful practical information about its role within a polypharmacy regimen, particularly when the relevance of a drug is considered dubious, or when trying to tease apart whether symptoms are more likely iatrogenic phenomena versus manifestations of the condition being treated. Consider Clinical Vignettes 9.2 and 9.3.

CLINICAL VIGNETTE 9.2

Phil had been diagnosed with bipolar II disorder and maintained on lithium carbonate 900 mg/day (most recent serum [Li^+] = 0.71 mEq/L) for over one year. During that time he felt persistent depression, lethargy, and low motivation. He wondered if lithium could be causing his depression, while his psychiatrist wondered more if lithium was simply failing to alleviate it. His psychiatrist added lurasidone 20 mg/day as a treatment for bipolar depression. Phil felt decidedly better (less depressed, more motivated) after three weeks, and asked if he could now stop the lithium. His brother, a neurologist, advised a gradual taper of lithium over several weeks to avoid precipitating a relapse, citing well-known literature on the hazards of hastened relapse from abrupt lithium discontinuation in bipolar disorder (Faedda et al., 1993). The psychiatrist politely countered that the literature on relapse after rapid versus gradual lithium cessation pertained to patients who, unlike Phil, were euthymic and unequivocally responsive to lithium monotherapy. She therefore instead favored its deliberate abrupt cessation precisely in order to clarify whether or not lithium was providing a discernible benefit or tangible detriment, or was irrelevant due to presumed lack of efficacy; she reasoned that if lithium had not been helpful prior to its augmentation with lurasidone, the chances of clinical worsening off lithium were low – but that abrupt rather than gradual cessation would better help to clarify whether lithium had been exerting any influence. A rapid loss of improvement if lithium were subtracted from lurasidone would imply a previously unappreciated benefit, an amelioration of lethargy soon after stopping lithium would imply the lethargy was more likely iatrogenic than primary to depression, and a sustained improvement off lithium while remaining only on lurasidone would help to affirm lithium's suspected inconsequentiality to Phil's treatment.

CLINICAL VIGNETTE 9.3

Don was a 20-year-old college student on academic medical leave due to a significant depressive episode that eventually improved with escitalopram 40 mg/day plus quetiapine 100 mg at bedtime. During a second-opinion consultation his parents expressed concern that although Don seemed less sad and was no longer tearful or talking about suicide, he seemed emotionless, apathetic, slow, and in a daze for much of the day. He would sleep more than 13 hours at night and his daytime activity consisted of little more than playing video games in bed, which was inconsistent with his premorbid baseline level of functioning. His current psychiatrist advised further increasing the quetiapine dose to target what he felt were residual anergic depressive symptoms that were hampering his recovery, or else adding a stimulant as an additional antidepressant cotherapy. The consulting psychiatrist was underwhelmed by current depression features and wondered instead about possible adverse motor and cognitive effects from quetiapine's antihistamine properties. He therefore advised *abruptly* stopping the quetiapine with careful monitoring to judge whether Don's affect and energy might brighten in a time frame corresponding to the passage of five elimination half-lives of quetiapine (~7°) plus its active metabolite norquetiapine (~12°) (i.e., about three days).

More often than not, determining relevant pharmacokinetic factors plays a role in deciding when and how to replace one drug with another for the same intended target symptoms. Consider Clinical Vignette 9.4.

CLINICAL VIGNETTE 9.4

Ivan was a 41-year-old man with persistent depressive disorder (formerly termed chronic major depression) and OCD initially treated with fluoxetine up to 60 mg/day, then clomipramine up to 150 mg/day, and now fluvoxamine 200 mg/day plus bupropion SR 200 mg/day. None of these regimens was deemed efficacious and all produced sexual side effects that collectively prompted his interest in changing medications. He is about to begin a new trial of vilazodone. What pharmacokinetic factors bear most directly on how you would choose to switch him to the new regimen?

Figure 9.1 Ivan's terrible pharmacokinetic predicament.

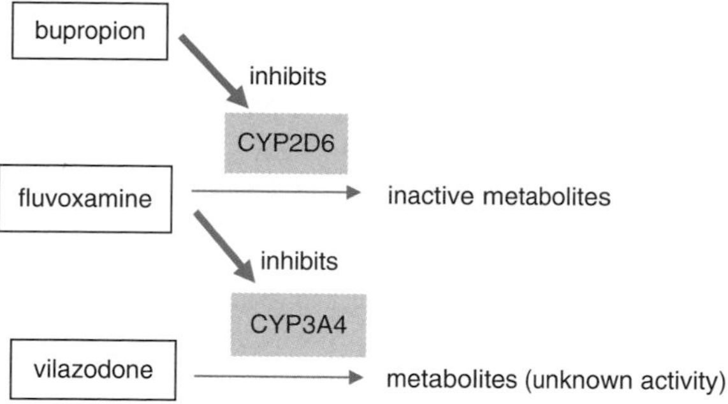

Ivan's pharmacokinetic dilemma involves the potential for fluvoxamine (a CYP3A4 inhibitor) to delay the metabolism of vilazodone (a CYP3A4 substrate) if the latter drug were introduced before the former were fully cleared from his system. Additionally, bupropion's inhibition of CYP2D6 will further prolong the degradation of fluvoxamine (a CYP2D6 substrate). For these specific reasons, it would probably make the most sense to taper off and fully discontinue fluvoxamine before starting vilazodone, especially if one planned to retain the bupropion in the overall mix (Figure 9.1).

H SWITCHING FROM ONE SEROTONERGIC AGENT TO ANOTHER

Although clinicians sometimes favor cross-tapering one serotonergic antidepressant before starting another (or even tapering off the first agent before then starting the second), there is little if any empirical data to support the necessity of this. In reality, drugs that exert comparable serotonergic mechanisms (e.g., serotonin reuptake inhibition) should, in principle, be relatively interchangeable with respect to safety and tolerability – making cross-tapers superfluous. At the same time, abruptly stopping serotonergic drugs that have especially long half-lives (such as vortioxetine, or fluoxetine plus its active metabolite norfluoxetine) should gradually auto-taper but may still pose additive adverse pharmacodynamic effects when a new serotonergic antidepressant is begun – prompting the value of maintaining a low initial dose of the incoming agent.

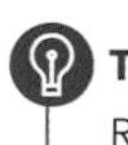

Tip

Remember that $5HT_{2A}$ antagonists (e.g., mirtazapine, trazodone) may help to protect against serotonin syndrome (see Chapter 6, Box 6.6).

I AIN'T BROKE DON'T FIX

Yet another common scenario when considering changes to a longstanding medication regimen is the desire to "update" older for newer medications without regard to the clinical stability of the patient or the acceptability of their existing regimen. There has been little contemporary or systematic study of outcomes from tampering with "drug rituals" in chronic conditions such as schizophrenia or chronic mood or anxiety disorders. Potential concerns would include disruptions to a scheduled routine with established expectations about their strengths, limitations, and ways of compensating for shortcomings. Patients with histories of serious symptomatology in the long-ago past (e.g., suicide attempts, psychosis, markedly poor function) who then achieve and sustain symptomatic remission and recovery for lengthy periods (e.g., years) sometimes invite speculation from both the patient or the clinician as to whether medications are still necessary – or may even invite disbelief or denial about whether serious forms of psychopathology from the remote past ever really in fact existed, with consequent temptation to tinker with a stable drug regimen.

While "newer" medications can sometimes offer specific advantages over older drugs (e.g., sparing of anticholinergic and other cardiovascular side effects with SSRIs or SNRIs over tricyclics), they may not necessarily be more effective, and could involve exchanging one set of adverse effects for another. Inviting a patient to exchange "the devil they know for the devil they don't" means taking such possible outcomes into account with vigilant observation along the way, in contrast to Clinical Vignette 9.5.

CLINICAL VIGNETTE 9.5

Sally was a 63-year-old woman diagnosed in her 20s with schizophrenia. She had stably been maintained on thiothixene 4 mg/day for the past 30 years with no relapses or rehospitalizations. The new psychiatrist she saw doubted that she actually was a stable case of good-prognosis schizophrenia, or schizophrenia of any kind, given her sustained wellness apparently over decades on so low a dose of a medium-potency first-generation antipsychotic and advised its discontinuation. Soon after abruptly stopping thiothixene she began calling the psychiatrist complaining of insomnia and anxiety, for which he prescribed low-dose lorazepam followed by trazodone 50 mg/day without benefit. She continued to "report in" regularly on her waxing and waning anxiety and insomnia, feeling someone might break into her apartment at night, and saying she "just didn't feel right." The psychiatrist added paroxetine 10 mg/day for her anxiety symptoms which persisted even after a dosage increase to 30 mg/day. Buspirone was then added up to 60 mg/day, still with continued complaints of insomnia and "anxiety." Quetiapine 50 mg at bedtime was added, causing excessive daytime sedation but no anxiolytic relief. Hydroxyzine 25 mg twice a day was added for her anxiety and a lamotrigine titration starting at 25 mg/day was begun for her apparent "affective instability." The patient complained that she had gone from being stable on one drug for 30 years to now taking seven new drugs with no relief whatsoever and asked why she couldn't simply just resume low-dose thiothixene, to which her psychiatrist replied that it was "not a good drug" and "hadn't done anything for her," and she "didn't really need it."

We might next consider how to choose the dose of an incoming drug meant to replace an outgoing one.

J CONVERTING FROM ONE DRUG TO ANOTHER: ANTIDEPRESSANT DOSAGE EQUIVALENTS

Perhaps the most practical and immediate question apart from "when and how" to switch from one drug to another is "how much" of a new drug to dose, either to "compensate" for an equivalent amount delivered by the outgoing drug or to otherwise achieve an appropriate, safe, tolerable, and effective strength of the new medication being chosen. There may be more art than science in deducing dosage "equivalents" within broad pharmacotherapy classes, in that data in this area are often extrapolated from comparative reported doses across RCTs that either represent "minimum clinical effective doses" or "mean therapeutic doses."

Figure 9.2 Exponential half-life elimination.

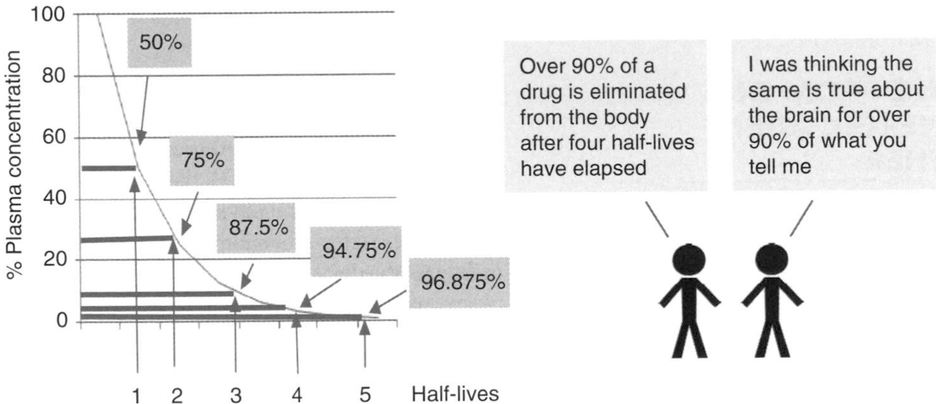

Should a new drug be started at its usual initial dose or higher if it is replacing another drug that has been optimally dosed? And if not, should one try to "approximate" a comparable dose for an incoming drug relative to the dose of the outgoing drug?

There usually is no direct "conversion" formula for gauging the pharmacodynamic potency of one drug over another in dose-by-dose fashion. That said, much depends on how low, medium, or high on the dosing spectrum an outgoing drug has been. As noted above, outgoing drugs with a long terminal elimination half-life may pose a greater risk for additive pharmacodynamic adverse effects until the first few elimination half-lives have elapsed. Bear in mind (as depicted in Figure 9.2) that most of a drug is eliminated from blood circulation by the first two to three half-lives, with the remainder representing increasingly asymptotic remainders of uneliminated drug.

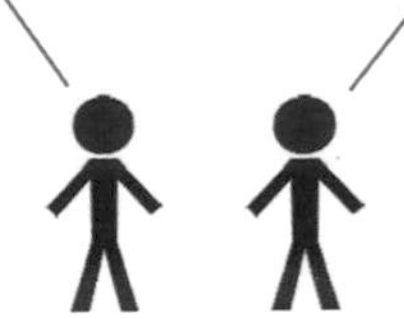

In the case of MDD, Hayasaka and colleagues (2015) reviewed 83 such studies involving 14 131 participants and calculated mean dosage equivalents of antidepressants relative to fluoxetine or paroxetine based on the ratios of means between a target drug and fluoxetine or paroxetine using a fixed-effect statistical model. A summary of the dosage equivalents derived by their estimation appears in Table 9.3.

K DOSING CONVERSIONS AMONG FIRST- AND SECOND-GENERATION ANTIPSYCHOTICS

Efforts to determine dosing equivalents among antipsychotic drugs have traditionally involved either the so-called "classical mean dose" method based on mean dosages used in *flexible-dose* controlled trials (Leucht et al., 2015) or the "minimum effective dose" method (Leucht et al., 2014), in which the minimum (rather than mean final) effective dose relative to placebo is used in *fixed-dose* randomized trials. The former of these methods was first developed by Davis (1974) and for many decades provided a gold standard basis for calculating dosage equivalents using chlorpromazine dosages as a common denominator. The latter of these methods is considered evidence-based for general populations but does not neatly extrapolate to specific subpopulations such as first-episode or multidrug-resistant groups, or provide as much information about low-dose equivalency conversions unless fixed low-dose studies have been conducted. A third strategy is to use expert consensus guidelines for estimating dosing equivalents based on experts' subjective perceptions (e.g., Andreason et al., 2010). Consequently, published or online antipsychotic "dosage equivalents" often vary based on the methodologies used to derive their results.

Tables 9.4 and 9.5 present FGA and SGA dosage equivalents, respectively, rounded to the nearest whole number. Table 9.6 describes how to convert dosing from oral to long-acting injectable forms of FGAs and SGAs.

L CROSS-TAPERING AND CONVERTING AMONG BENZODIAZEPINES

Clinicians often find they must look up benzodiazepine equivalents (e.g., when choosing a longer-acting benzodiazepine as a detoxification strategy from a shorter-acting benzodiazepine), perhaps in part because published or online "conversion tables" can vary and are not definitive. Some longer-acting agents also may have very long half-life active metabolites (e.g., diazepam, chlordiazepoxide, flurazepam). Disparities in the literature may reflect not only variations in measurement techniques but also use in special populations (e.g., healthy controls versus patients with alcohol or sedative-hypnotic use disorder, cigarette smokers, those with hepatic or renal disease, epilepsy, anxiety disorders, obesity, or racial pharmacokinetic differences (e.g., Asians may have higher serum alprazolam levels than Whites)). The data presented in Table 9.7 are based on manufacturers' product label information as well as published empirical studies.

M ANXIOLYTIC ANTICONVULSANTS

Gabapentin and pregabalin are both evidence-based "off-label" pharmacotherapy options for the treatment of varied anxiety disorders (see Chapter 17). While they are structurally unrelated, their pharmacodynamic psychotropic effects can be similar. Based on outcomes from a study of neuropathic pain, Toth (2010) devised the approximate dosing conversion from gabapentin to pregabalin shown in Table 9.8.

N PSYCHOSTIMULANTS

For the purposes of replacing one psychostimulant with another (i.e., variant forms of methylphenidate or amphetamine), approximate dosing equivalents are presented in Tables 9.10 and 9.11. Racemic formulations of amphetamine vary in their ratios of levo- to dextro-enantiomers and dosing equivalents take into account these proportional differences. The dextro-enantiomer of amphetamine binds about three to four times more potently to its CNS molecular targets (meaning that about three-quarters of the dose of dextroamphetamine is more potent and would be comparable to a given dose of mixed amphetamine salts). Levoamphetamine at low doses acts more on NE than DA and in general exerts more peripheral and cardiovascular effects than does amphetamine. Stimulant formulations can differ in potency as well as duration of action, with the latter based not simply on pharmacokinetic half-lives of the active drug (which do not change appreciably across formulations),

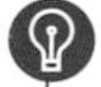
Tip

Amphetamine is about twice as potent as methylphenidate. Therefore 10 mg of amphetamine roughly corresponds to 20 mg of methylphenidate.

but mainly on differences in the delivery systems encasing those active ingredients. For example, lisdexamfetamine is a pro-drug form of amphetamine that liberates active dextroamphetamine when its lysine moiety is hydrolyzed off over time, delivering a measurable effect on attentional processing from about 2–14 hours post ingestion. Evekeo®, a proprietary formulation of amphetamine sulfate, uses a three-beaded system of immediate- and delayed-release phases of drug delivery that collectively afford about 16 hours of pharmacodynamic efficacy. Extended-release (XR) and immediate-release (IR) formulations of amphetamine or methylphenidate do not differ so much in their half-lives (see Tables 9.9 and 9.10) as in the delivery systems that encase their respective active molecules, and may cause a second Tmax to occur several hours after the first, effectively rendering a long-acting preparation of the same fundamental compound.

Chirality

Remember handedness of enantiomers:
levo(rotatory) = left; dextro (rotatory) = right

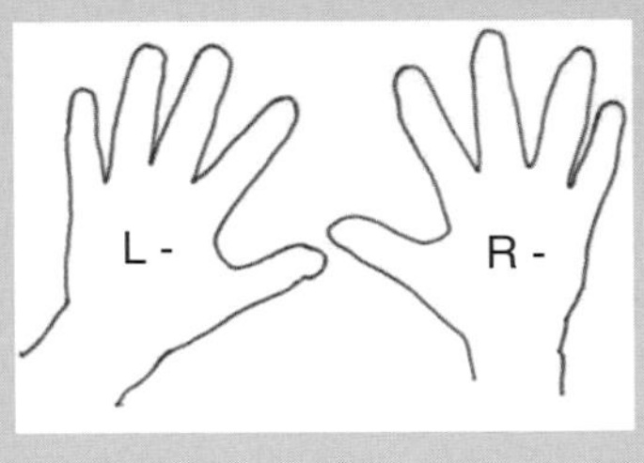

Half-lives

Dextroamphetamine: ~9–11°
Levoamphetamine: ~11–14°
Methylphenidate: ~3°

Conversion of dosing equivalency for lisdexamfetamine to dextroamphetamine or mixed amphetamine salts is complicated by the fact that lisdexamfetamine is a pro-drug that undergoes peripheral conversion to active dextroamphetamine (via hydrolysis in red blood cells) with a conversion factor of 0.2948. Thus, 30 mg of lisdexamfetamine is approximately equivalent to 8.85 mg of dextroamphetamine or 11.8 mg of mixed amphetamine salts.

0 WHEN TO DISCONTINUE MEDICATIONS: REVISITING THE ART OF DEPRESCRIBING

One of the most difficult problems facing psychopharmacologists is the frequent lack of clarity as to when to stop a medication. In Chapter 6 we touched on the concept of deprescribing drugs that appear to exert no discernible benefit after an adequate trial. But what about deciding whether and when to stop an efficacious drug once a response (either partial or full) has been established, and recovery ensues. How long should someone stay on a drug, and are there parameters to spare a patient an indefinite ongoing, open-ended therapy if the optimal medication endpoint need not be "forever" or "until some life event comes along that warrants stopping a drug" or "ghosting" off a drug by arbitrarily not renewing it and dropping out of care.

For many psychiatric conditions, once all parties agree that wellness has been achieved, it is sometimes a reasonable rule of thumb to consider not altering the regimen in any manner for a minimum of four to six months of sustained wellness. Why? In part because this time period is conventionally regarded as the minimum duration to define recovery based on task force consensus views from the American College of Neuropsychopharmacology (Rush et al. 2006a) and the MacArthur Foundation (Frank et al., 1991). Symptoms that re-emerge during the four to six months after initial resolution of an acute psychiatric condition are considered to be a *relapse* – that is, a return of the most recent episode. Achieving four to six months of wellness marks a milestone. Like a driver who has gone 10 years without having an accident and is then rewarded by their insurance company with a safe driver discount, a recovering patient's risk category drops substantially after clearing this hurdle. Symptoms that may then resurface beyond this time are thought to reflect a new episode altogether (termed a *recurrence*, as opposed to a relapse), and new episodes tend to be rarer events than relapses (inasmuch as relapses imply a less complete degree of resolution of that index episode). Sustained wellness tends to predict further sustained wellness, and the farther in time one goes from a last episode or phase of active symptoms, the more durable

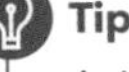

Tip

Axiom

The longer someone remains well, the longer they remain well.

When common receptor targets are shared, must five half-lives routinely elapse after replacing one medication with another before one can assume that the new drug's pharmacodynamic effects are in full force?

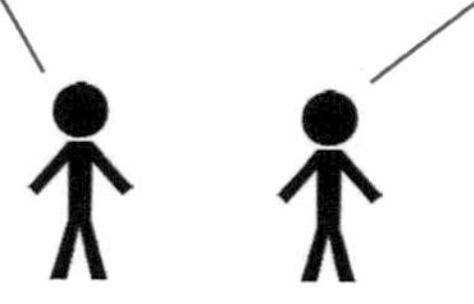

This depends in part on what is meant by "full force." Long half-life drugs can (and do) exert meaningful pharmacodynamic effects before the elapse of five half-lives. Five half-lives is needed to achieve steady-state plasma concentrations (a pharmacokinetic outcome) but pharmacodynamically meaningful clinical effects can often be identified within 1–2 weeks of drug initiation. Consider, for example, SGAs with long terminal elimination half-lives such as aripiprazole (about 75 hours) or cariprazine (whose parent compound's half-life is only 3–6 hours, but its active metabolites (desmethyl cariprazine and didesmethyl cariprazine) can extend that time to up to three weeks (effectively making five half-lives elapse after 12–15 weeks)). Stable response usually is associated with achieving a serum drug level of at least 100 nM, typically reached within the first few weeks of either drug.

Suppose a bipolar patient becomes manic while taking an antidepressant. Should the antidepressant be stopped abruptly or tapered off? And, if the latter, how quickly?

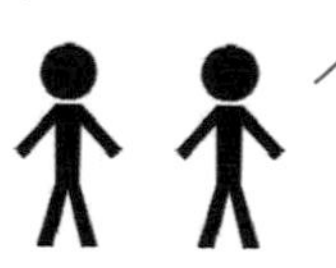

There are reports in the literature to suggest that abruptly stopping antidepressants in someone with bipolar disorder could precipitate mania (Goldstein et al., 1999). Rapidly stopping any short half-life antidepressant, even in the presence of mania, could potentially trigger physiological discontinuation symptoms that then become their own confounding source of agitation and autonomic hyperarousal. For these reasons, while antidepressant elimination is a core principle in treating acute mania (see Chapter 13), some middle ground is often preferable while simultaneously initiating an appropriate antimanic pharmacotherapy.

and even predictable continued wellness becomes. In fact, the longer one accrues consistent "well" time, the more a recurrence becomes an anomaly more than an expectation.

Figure 9.3 illustrates the usual timeframes within which clinical investigators typically divide phases of recurrent disorders into acute, continuation, and maintenance periods of treatment.

Figure 9.3 Phases of treatment.

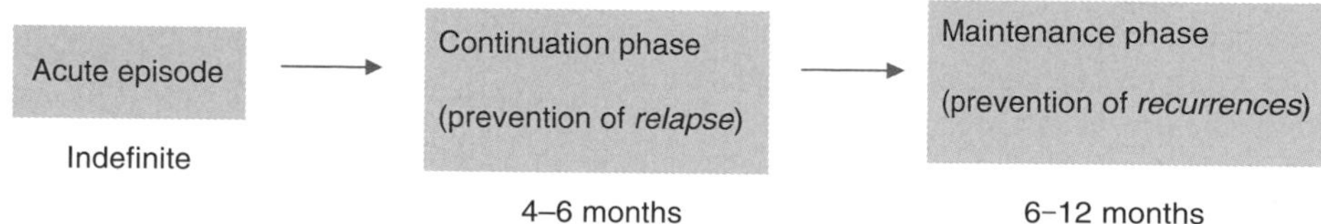

P FOREVER IS A LONG TIME

This brings us to the question of how long continuation and maintenance phases of pharmacotherapy should ideally last. Here the evidence-based literature becomes increasingly scant. On the one hand, it is often pragmatically difficult if not virtually impossible (not to mention ethically challenging) to maintain patients very longterm on an active drug versus a placebo. Though it is true that most relapses and recurrences, by definition, will occur within the first 6–12 months following recovery from their most recent episode, RCTs of longer duration would be needed to determine if there comes a point of diminishing returns for continued pharmacotherapy. Many clinicians think of maintenance pharmacotherapy as involving an indefinite time period, operating as much from the perspective of "ain't broke don't fix" as from any other principle. We might here also reinvoke our *Newtonian First Law of Psychopharmacology* (see Chapter 1) – a clinical system in motion stays in motion unless and until some external force acts on it. Arbitrarily stopping a stable drug or drug regimen unavoidably poses a risk for disrupting equilibrium and homeostasis.

Relapse-prone conditions tend to make clinicians, patients, and their families expect that future occurrences may be almost inevitable, though no one has ever shown in an RCT that such patients kept on a drug forever fare better than those who stay on the same treatment for less than forever. Every psychiatry resident is taught the popular rule of thumb that depressed patients who have had three or more lifetime episodes have over a 90% likelihood of a fourth, and once well they should follow Newtonian psychopharmacology to its fullest and stay on treatment indefinitely. Still, on the other hand, if evidence is lacking to show that indefinite pharmacotherapy truly ups the odds against recurrence beyond, say, some less-than-indefinite prespecified duration of a course of treatment, we run the risk of making decisions based more on lore, superstition, or subjective impressionism rather than empiricism. Blanket recommendations for or against indefinite versus finite durations of maintenance pharmacotherapy also disregard the core concept of patient-specific moderating and mediating factors that might help to individualize treatment and identify clinical profiles for which longer or indefinite pharmacotherapy is likely to mitigate the risk for recurrence (as well as possible profiles of patients who may fare just as well with a more finite course of treatment – or at least, an ability to recognize when indefinite pharmacotherapy may be *unlikely* to forestall future episodes).

As an example of this, consider the following naturalistic findings during five years of maintenance treatment for bipolar disorder reported by the NIMH Collaborative Depression Study (Coryell et al., 1997) (Figure 9.4). The presence rather than absence of lithium was associated with a significantly lower probability of relapse for the first 32 weeks of treatment, however this advantage was no longer evident beyond that time frame (for up to 96 weeks of follow-up).

Does this mean that lithium predictably or expectably will likely cease to confer a benefit against relapse in bipolar disorder if used beyond eight months after an index episode? Of course not. This is one study, it is nonrandomized, and we know nothing about potential confounding by indication with respect to characteristics that may have led some patients to take or not take lithium. However, the study does raise the hypothesis that, in the absence of potentially unidentified confounding factors, lithium's prophylactic effects may be less robust after the first eight months of treatment. So, then, should clinicians stop lithium, or tell their bipolar patients that beyond eight months' time there is insufficient evidence to justify continued use? No again! The study invites us, rather, to recognize the possibility that lithium's prophylactic effects *may* attenuate in some bipolar patients. Okay, then, so what such factors ought clinicians be alert to before writing prescription renewals beyond eight months' duration with an ability to feel secure in the comfort and knowledge that all will remain well. No, again, it is not that simple.

Coryell et al. (1997) did dutifully perform a logistic regression analysis to examine several possible factors that, when controlled for, might help to account for observed differences in when lithium use beyond eight months remained effective. They considered polarity of the index episode (no doubt realizing that lithium works better when manias precede depressions rather than the reverse (Post et al., 1996)) and family history of bipolar disorder, with no discernible differences. Nor did controlling for changes in serum lithium levels over time account for outcome differences in those on versus not on lithium. Without identifiable guideposts for knowing which bipolar patients might bear an inherently greater risk for *early* versus *late* relapse (perhaps not necessarily even unique to lithium so much as to the nature of a given patient's illness), the only firm conclusion to be drawn is, to quote the authors, "patients who survive for 8 months after an episode with neither lithium or a relapse probably will not benefit from lithium begun at that

Figure 9.4 Maintenance pharmacotherapy with lithium for bipolar disorder. (Figure reproduced from: Coryell et al., Lithium and recurrence in a long-term follow-up of bipolar affective disorder, *Psychol Med* 1997; 27: 281-280. Reprinted with permission, Cambridge University Press.)

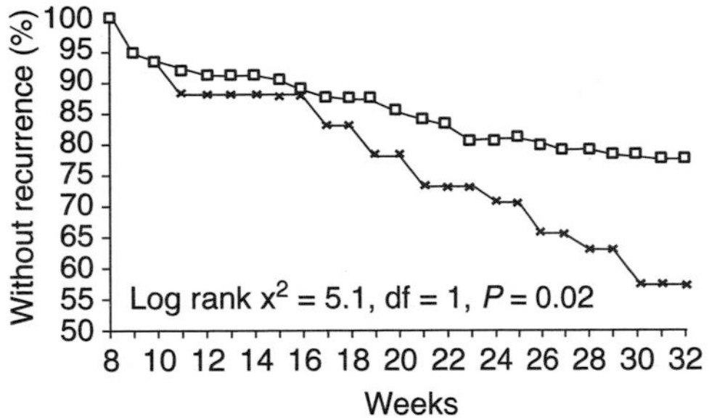

Cumulative probabilities by presence (□, N = 139) or absence (x, N = 42) of lithium prophylaxis: weeks 8–32

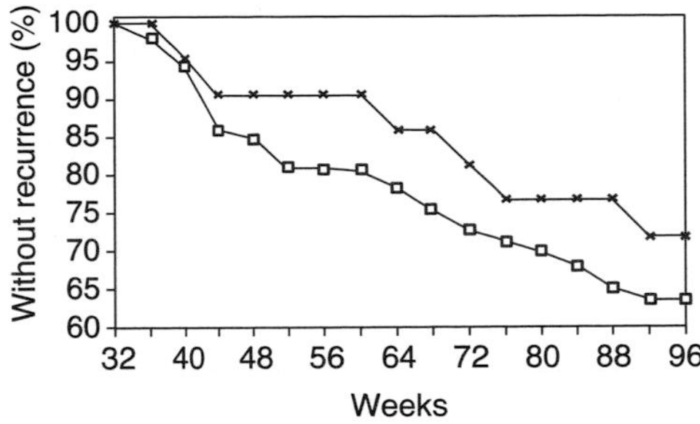

Cumulative probabilities by presence (□, N = 86) or absence (x, N = 22) of lithium prophylaxis: weeks 32–96

point" (Coryell et al., 1997, p. 286). This is a useful point that can help inform clinical decision-making for the unmedicated bipolar patient who presents euthymic nine months after their last episode wondering if it would help reduce their relapse risk to now begin lithium.

Another naturalistic study followed a group of bipolar disorder patients that had been enriched for a longer "lead time" of sustained and established wellness while on lithium (at least two years) who were then either continued or gradually tapered off lithium according to their preference (Biel et al., 2007). Those who opted to remain on lithium after two years of stability had a significantly longer time until recurrence (median survival time = 7.33 years) as compared to those who chose to discontinue lithium after the two-year wellness period (median survival time = 1.33 years). Importantly, after controlling in a Cox regression model for pertinent potential confounders (i.e., age, sex, family history of bipolar disorder, years ill, and number of prior episodes) lithium discontinuation remained associated with a hazard ratio for relapse of 4.85. In another study of bipolar patients who had been stably maintained on lithium for at least five years, a subsequent controlled discontinuation protocol yielded relapse in 62% at one year and 81% after nine years (Yazici et al., 2004). Perhaps these findings collectively once again underscore the above-noted maxim that the longer a patient stays well the longer one might expect them to continue to stay well – and benefit from ongoing maintenance pharmacotherapy.

How about in the world of major depressive disorder? A similar kind of naturalistic (nonrandomized) discontinuation trial was conducted with 87 MDD outpatients who were judged to be "clinically stable" for at least *five years* on SSRI monotherapy (Pundiak et al., 2008). Again according to patient preference, subjects thereafter either continued or stopped their SSRI. Median time to recurrence among those who continued beyond five years was 38 months, as compared to only 10 months among those who discontinued after five years' stability. The resulting hazard ratio (4.9× more likely to relapse off than on continued SSRI) was moderated only by the presence of residual depressive symptoms, but (contrary to expectations) not the prior number of depressive episodes. Again, however, despite controlling for at least some potential confounders, the nonrandomized and self-selected nature of the decision to stop or continue pharmacotherapy after initial success limits our ability to draw inferences about the generalizability of observed outcomes.

Similar naturalistic findings in panic disorder also suggest that longer is better when it comes to duration of pharmacotherapy for relapse prevention. Adult outpatients with panic disorder that had been stable for at least three years with varied drug regimens (including tricyclics, SSRIs, and/or benzodiazepines) were invited to stop or continue their existing pharmacotherapy as per their preference and were followed for up to eight years (Choy et al., 2007). Time to relapse was significantly longer among those who continued treatment (median survival time = 5.67 years) than in those who stopped (median survival time = 1.17 years), with time to relapse once again moderated by the presence of baseline residual symptoms. A pooled meta-analysis of 28 relapse-prevention trials using antidepressants for up to one year across varied anxiety disorders (including OCD and PTSD) broadly found about a threefold increased likelihood for remaining relapse-free among those who continued antidepressants (16.4% summary relapse rate) versus those randomized to placebo (36.4% summary relapse rate) (Batelaan et al., 2017); however, the variable timeframes of follow-up (ranging from 8 weeks to 52 weeks), collapsing of diagnostic categories, and lack of controls for confounding variables (e.g., baseline severity, residual symptoms, chronicity, episode number) limits extrapolation of the findings to specific patient profiles.

The best way to know empirically whether there exists an optimal duration for continued pharmacotherapy, beyond which further advantages to continued therapy diminish, is to conduct a randomized discontinuation trial. Far too few such studies exist in the literature, probably in no small part because there is little commercial incentive for pharmaceutical manufacturers to conduct studies to determine when their products become unnecessary and to help clinicians recognize when to stop prescribing them. The handful of notable exceptions to this scarcity of research is summarized in Table 9.11.

The above constraints notwithstanding, clinicians need some broad guidance or principles for deciding whether and when to eventually discontinue a pharmacotherapy, apart from obvious determinants such as drug intolerances, serious adverse events, or patients' refusal to continue. Table 9.12 provides a summary of such recommendations as culled from practice guidelines, the available RCT literature, and our own collective experience.

TAKE-HOME POINTS

- Decisions about when and how to cross-taper versus stop-and-start medications are often individualized and should depend on factors such as dosages, half-lives, pharmacokinetic interactions, tolerability, past experiences, risks for rebound or discontinuation effects, and duplicative or redundant mechanisms of action. As always, it is important to have a nonarbitrary rationale for decisions about the logistics of making changes to a medication regimen.
- Recognize medical emergencies that mandate abrupt medication cessation (e.g., serotonin syndrome, neuroleptic malignant syndrome, Stevens–Johnson syndrome, hypersensitivity syndromes, etc.).
- Recognize high- versus low-risk windows for relapse in the setting of chronic or recurrent disorders, and consider appropriate timing when planning drug discontinuations.
- Plan ahead of time for treatment options and courses of action to pursue in the event that a medication change leads to deterioration. Like a good scout, always be prepared.

Table 9.1 When to stop a medication

Drug class	Event	Comment
Anticonvulsants	Hypersensitivity/ severe cutaneous reactions	Abruptly stop. In principle, sudden discontinuation can lower the seizure threshold, increasing seizure risk; in practice this is unlikely unless there is an existing seizure disorder
	Hepatic dysfunction	Major increases in liver enzymes (AST, ALT>3–4× the upper limit of normal) warrant drug cessation
	Myelosuppression	Generally discontinue if WBCs fall to <3000 mm^3 or ANC <1500 mm^3, if persistent or accompanied by infection, or in thrombocytopenia when platelet counts are <100 000 per mm^3
Antidepressants	Emergence of mania/hypomania	As a rule, antidepressants should be stopped in the setting of acute mania or hypomania, although, as noted in Chapter 13, this is often easier said than done; short half-life antidepressants may require modified tapers to minimize discontinuation effects
	Hyponatremia/ SIADH	Serotonergic antidepressants should be discontinued when hyponatremia/ SIADH occurs without other more likely causes; mirtazapine and tricyclics may be less risky (De Picker et al., 2014)
	Serotonin syndrome	Characterized by clonus, tremor, hyper-reflexia (see Chapter 6), usually within 24 hours of starting or raising the dose of a serotonergic agent. $5HT_{2A}$ antagonists may be protective
	Worsening of suicidal features	Assess overall clinical picture to gauge likelihood that exacerbations of suicidal thoughts or behaviors reflect iatrogenic causes versus worsening of an underlying disorder
Antipsychotics	Neuroleptic malignant syndrome	Abruptly stop; most often occurs in first 10–14 days after start of treatment; case reports of cautious rechallenges with alternative antipsychotics more than five days after symptom resolution, although recurrence rates up to 40% (Caroff and Mann, 1993); mortality=5%
	Myelosuppression	FGAs or SGAs other than clozapine carry a class warning for rarely causing leukopenia, neutropenia, or agranulocytosis; specific criteria for monitoring or drug discontinuation are not established but discontinuation would seem logical in the setting of apparent infection or if WBCs fall to <3000 mm^3 or ANC <1500 mm^3
	Myocarditis (clozapine)	Abruptly stop and generally do not rechallenge, due to high chance for recurrence
	QTc prolongation on ECG	Not an absolute contraindication to continued antipsychotic use; must consider magnitude of QTc, underlying correctable factors, concomitant medications, overall risk-benefit analysis
	Tardive dyskinesia	Do not discontinue antipsychotic if benefit exceeds risk, particularly given option of VMAT2 inhibitors (see Chapter 10)
Lithium	Acute toxicity	Abruptly stop. After significant toxicity (e.g., serum $[Li^+]$ >1.5 mEq/L; renal consequences; mental status changes) do not reinstitute (even when serum levels are zero) until mental status changes clear and neurological exam is nonfocal
	Unacceptable ↓ renal function	Typically reduce lithium dose, dose once daily, re-estimate eGFR via cystatin C (Shlipak et al., 2013), increase frequency of renal function monitoring (e.g., every three months); anticipate and attempt eventual need to cross-taper to an alternative agent when feasible
Stimulants	Tolerance; misuse	Can be abruptly stopped without adverse physiological effects

Abbreviations: ALT = alanine transaminase; ANC = absolute neutrophil count; AST = aspartate aminotransferase; ECG = electrocardiogram; eGFR = estimated glomerular filtration rate; FGA = first-generation antipsychotic; SGA = second-generation antipsychotic; SIADH = syndrome of inappropriate antidiuretic hormone secretion; VMAT2 = vesicular monoamine transporter 2; WBC = white blood cell

Table 9.2 Risks and management strategies associated with abrupt psychotropic drug cessation

Agent	Recommendations for discontinuation
α_1 antagonists (e.g., prazosin, terazosin) or α agonists (e.g., clonidine)	Abrupt cessation may lead to rebound hypertension
Clozapine	Abrupt cessation is necessary when WBCs <2000/mm^3 and ANC <1000/mm^3 or if ANC ≤500/mm^3, successful rechallenges are rare after discontinuation due to severe neutropenia
Lamotrigine	Formal recommendation from the manufacturer is to reinitiate dosing titration from the beginning in patients who have been off medication for more than five days (i.e., five half-lives). In our experience, because serious rashes are extremely unlikely to occur after the first few months of initial treatment, a more liberal approach to resuming a usual maintenance dose may be appropriate in some patients who have been taking lamotrigine for more than a year
Lithium	Abrupt lithium cessation (i.e., over less than a two-week period) has been reported to increase the risk for rapid relapse in patients with bipolar disorder, and may also be associated with poorer treatment response upon subsequent rechallenge
MAOIs	Case reports exist of psychosis developing upon abrupt discontinuation
SSRIs	Fluoxetine and its active metabolite norfluoxetine together take up to five weeks to be eliminated
Non-SSRI serotonergic antidepressants	Vilazodone, with a half-life of 66 hours, typically can be safely stopped from a dose of 10 mg/day without the need for further tapering

Abbreviations: ANC = absolute neutrophil count; MAOI = monoamine oxidase inhibitor; SSRI = selective serotonin reuptake inhibitor; WBC = white blood cell

Table 9.3 Approximate mean dose equivalents among antidepressants[a]

Antidepressant	Dosage equivalent
Amitriptyline	122.3 mg/day
Bupropion	348.5 mg/day
Clomipramine	116.1 mg/day
Desipramine	196.3 mg/day
Doxepin	140.1 mg/day
Escitalopram	18.0 mg/day
Fluvoxamine	143.3 mg/day
Imipramine	137.2 mg/day
Mirtazapine	50.9 mg/day
Moclobemide	575.2 mg/day
Nefazodone	535.2 mg/day
Nortriptyline	100.9 mg/day
Reboxetine	11.5 mg/day
Sertraline	98.5 mg/day
Trazodone	401.4 mg/day
Venlafaxine	149.4 mg/day

[a] based on dose equivalence to 40mg fluoxetine; findings as reported by Hayasaka et al., 2015

Table 9.4 Dosage equivalents among first-generation antipsychotics [a]

Agent	Dosage equivalents
Chlorpromazine	100 mg
Fluphenazine	2 mg
Haloperidol	2 mg
Loxapine	10 mg
Perphenazine	8 mg
Pimozide	2 mg
Prochlorperazine	15 mg
Trifluoperazine	2–5 mg
Thioridazine	100 mg
Thiothixene	4 mg

[a] Based on dose–response curves and a random-effects dose–response meta-analysis conducted by Leucht et al. (2020)

Table 9.5 Dosage equivalents among second-generation antipsychotics [a]

Agent	Dosage equivalents
Amisulpride	85.8 mg
Aripiprazole	1.8 mg
Asenapine	2.4 mg
Brexpiprazole	0.54 mg
Cariprazine	Not established
Clozapine	100 mg
Iloperidone	3.2 mg
Lurasidone	23.5 mg
Olanzapine	2.4 mg
Paliperidone	2.1 mg
Quetiapine	77 mg
Risperidone	1 mg
Ziprasidone	30 mg

[a] Based on dose-response curves and a random-effects dose-response meta-analysis conducted by Leucht et al. (2020)

Table 9.6 Converting from oral to long-acting injectable antipsychotics (LAIs)

Agent	Conversion to long-acting injectable
First generation	
Fluphenazine	20 mg/day of oral fluphenazine hydrochloride is approximately equivalent to 25 mg (1 mL) fluphenazine decanoate IM administered every three weeks; antipsychotic efficacy is generally noted within 96 hours of administration
Haloperidol	Haloperidol decanoate is available in dosages of 50 mg (1 mL) or 100 mg (2 mL), typically administered once monthly. In patients deemed to be stable on oral haloperidol, a decanoate dose of 10–15× the oral dose is recommended both initially and for ongoing monthly injections (maximum equivalent to 10 mg/day of oral haloperidol, i.e., 150 mg (3 mL) of decanoate). In less stable patients, decanoate dosing may begin at 20× the oral dose with subsequent monthly injections of 10–15× the oral dose
Second generation	
Aripiprazole	Tolerability must initially be established to oral aripiprazole over two weeks. Two LAI forms of aripiprazole are available: aripiprazole extended-release injectable (brand name: Abilify Maintena®, marketed for bipolar disorder) and aripiprazole lauroxil (brand name: Aristada®, marketed for schizophrenia). The extended-release injectable is typically begun with a single injection of 400 mg IM and continued monthly thereafter. The lauroxil formulation is begun as a single initial injection of 675 mg IM (Aristada Initio®, corresponding to a dose of 459 mg of aripiprazole), via either deltoid or gluteal injection, taken in combination with one dose of oral aripiprazole 30 mg. Subsequent administration of aripiprazole lauroxil can then occur either the same day (in a different muscle) or up to 10 days later. Dosing is flexible and can occur monthly (either 441 mg or 662 mg or 882 mg) or every six weeks (882 mg) or every eight weeks (1064 mg IM, gluteal)
Olanzapine pamoate (Zyprexa Relprevv®) [a]	Targeted *oral dose of 10 mg/day* converts to *starting dose* of 210 mg IM every two weeks or 405 mg IM every four weeks and *maintenance dose* of 150 mg IM every two weeks or 300 mg IM every four weeks; Targeted *oral dose of 15 mg/day* converts to *starting dose* of 300 mg IM every two weeks and *maintenance dose* of 210 mg IM every two weeks or 405 mg IM every four weeks; Targeted *oral dose of 20 mg/day* converts to *starting dose* of 300 mg IM every two weeks and *maintenance dose* of 300 mg IM every two weeks. Injections must be gluteal using a 19 gauge 1.5″ or 2″ needle. Steady-state pharmacokinetics are achieved by about eight weeks
Paliperidone (Invega Sustenna®)	Dosing typically begun at 234 mg IM (deltoid) on Day 1 then 117 mg IM once monthly (can be modified if/as needed from 39–234 mg/month)
Risperidone (Risperdal Consta®)	Assure stabilization and tolerability to oral risperidone. Then, in patients taking ≤4 mg oral risperidone, administer Risperdal Consta® 25 mg IM (deltoid or gluteal) and repeat every two weeks. Continue oral risperidone for three weeks after initial injection, then usually can abruptly discontinue oral formulation. May increase the LAI dose to 37.5 or 50 mg IM every two weeks if inadequate response. Higher doses have no known value.

[a] Note that in order to minimize the risk for postinjection delirium/sedation syndrome (PDSS) from olanzapine LAI, patients must be observed for at least three hours following administration; additionally, prescribers must undergo an online training program (www.zyprexarelprevvprogram.com/PDF/ZYPREXA%20RELPREVV%20REMS%20HCP%20Training.pdf) and the prescriber, health care facility, patient, and dispensing pharmacy must all register with the Zyprexa Relprevv Patient Care Program. PDSS events involve sedation, delirium, confusion, and agitation without cardiovascular or respiratory changes, and are thought to be related to excessive plasma olanzapine concentrations. They are estimated to occur in about 1 in 1400 administrations.

Table 9.7 Dosing equivalents of benzodiazepines

Agent	Approximate oral dose equivalent	Half-life [active metabolite]	Time until onset after oral administration
Alprazolam	0.5 mg	~11 hours	15-30 minutes (extended-release formulation shows similar time to peak onset but longer duration (mean 11.3 hours vs. 5.1 hours) than immediate release (Sheehan et al., 2007))
Chlordiazepoxide	25 mg	5-30 hours	15-30 minutes
Clonazepam	0.5 mg	18-50 hours	15-30 minutes
Clorazepate	15 mg	36-200 hours	≤1 hour
Diazepam	10 mg	20-100 hours [26-200]	15 minutes
Estazolam	1-2 mg	10-24 hours	≤1 hour
Flurazepam	30 mg	40-250 hours	15-30 minutes
Lorazepam	1 mg	12-15 hours	15-30 minutes
Oxazepam	20 mg	4-15 hours	1-3 hours
Temazepam	20 mg	8-22 hours	0.5-1 hour
Triazolam	0.5 mg	2 hours	15-30 minutes

Table 9.8 Approximate dosing conversion from gabapentin to pregabalin

Gabapentin dose (mg/day)	Pregabalin dose (mg/day)
0-900	150
901-1500	225
1501-2100	300
2101-2700	450
>2700	600

Table 9.9 Dosing equivalents of amphetamine formulations

Agent	Dextro:levo ratio	Brand names	Dose equivalence	Tmax	Half-life
Amphetamine sulfate (racemic)	1:1	Evekeo®	Not established	3-3.5 hours	Dextroamphetamine = 10–11 hours; *L*-amphetamine = 12–14 hours
Dextroamphetamine	1:0	Dexedrine®	7.5 mg	3 hours	12 hours
Dextroamphetamine sulfate	1:0	Zenzedi®	Not established	8 hours	12 hours
Lisdexamfetamine	1:0	Vyvanse®	25 mg	Lisdexamfetamine = 1 hour; Dextroamphetamine = 3.5 hours	Lisdexamfetamine <1 hour; Dextroamphetamine = 12 hours
Mixed salts of a single-entity amphetamine product capsule (dextroamphetamine sulfate, amphetamine sulfate, dextroamphetamine saccharate, amphetamine aspartate monohydrate)	3:1	Mydais®	15 mg	7–12 hours	*D*-amphetamine = 10–11 hours; *L*-amphetamine = 12–14 hours
Mixed amphetamine salts (dextroamphetamine saccharate, amphetamine aspartate, dextroamphetamine sulfate, amphetamine sulfate)	3:1	Adderall ® Adderall XR ®	10 mg 10 mg	3 hours 7 hours	*D*-amphetamine = 10–11 hours; *L*-amphetamine = 12–14 hours

Table 9.10 Dosing equivalents of methylphenidate formulations

Agent	Brand names	Dose equivalence	Tmax	Half-life
Methylphenidate (*d*- and *l*-*threo*-methylphenidate) (racemic)	Ritalin®	10 mg	2.5–3 hours	1–3 hours
Methylphenidate transdermal patch	Daytrana®	10 mg @ 12.5 cm^2	8–10 hours	*d*-methylphenidate = 4-5 hours; *l*-methylphenidate = 1.5–3 hours
Dexmethylphenidate	Focalin®	5 mg	1–3 hours	2.2 hours
Methylphenidate ER (OROS methylpenidate)	Concerta®	12 mg*	6.8 hours	3.6 hours

* OROS methylphenidate dosages of 18 mg, 36 mg, 54 mg and 72 mg are equivalent to respective methylpenidate dosages of 15 mg, 30 mg, 45 mg and 60 mg.

Table 9.11 Randomized discontinuation trials in psychopharmacology

Clinical situation	Design	Outcome
Bipolar disorder		
Adjunctive risperidone or olanzapine for bipolar relapse prevention	52-week RCT of lithium or divalproex + continued risperidone or olanzapine versus placebo substitution after an index mania stabilized on the combination (Yatham et al., 2016)	Longer time to relapse with combination than monotherapy for 24 weeks; no further advantage for relapse prevention with continued risperidone beyond that time; continued adjunctive olanzapine up to 52 weeks yielded longer survival (but more weight gain) than mood stabilizer monotherapy
Lithium or divalproex + olanzapine or + placebo after acute mania response to the combination	Acute mania remitters after six weeks of combination therapy randomized for up to 18 months of the continued combination versus lithium or divalproex + placebo (Tohen et al., 2004)	Significantly longer time until symptomatic relapse with combination (median 163 days) than mood stabilizer alone (median 42 days), but no differences in time until syndromal relapse
Bipolar depression relapse prevention	- After acute response to mood stabilizer + antidepressant, randomized adjunctive antidepressant continuation vs. discontinuation for up to one year (Altshuler et al., 2003)	Higher one-year depression relapse rates after antidepressant discontinuation (70%) than continuation (36%) with no higher risk for switch to mania/hypomania; better depression relapse prevention with continued antidepressant if robust acute response
	- Acute response to antidepressant + mood stabilizer, sustained euthymia × two months before randomized discontinuation to mood stabilizer alone vs. sustained combination therapy for up to one year (Ghaemi et al., 2010)	The continued combination regimen prolonged time until depressive relapse > mood stabilizer alone (HR = 2.13), without increased manic symptom. However, past-year rapid cyclers who remained on an antidepressant had more subsequent depressive episodes than those who continued only on a mood stabilizer
Major depression		
Fluoxetine + olanzapine or fluoxetine + placebo for relapse prevention (Brunner et al., 2014)	27-week RCT of olanzapine/fluoxetine combination or fluoxetine alone after stabilization on open-label combination drug for six–eight weeks	Longer time to relapse with continued combination than with fluoxetine minus olanzapine, but more weight gain
Recurrent MDD patients stabilized for three years on imipramine ± interpersonal psychotherapy (Kupfer et al., 1992)	Randomization to continued imipramine (± interpersonal psychotherapy) vs. placebo for an additional two years	Longer time until relapse with additional two years of imipramine (mean survival = 99.4 weeks) than placebo (mean survival = 54.0 weeks)
Social anxiety disorder		
Randomized continuation vs. discontinuation of paroxetine after initial stabilization	Patients stabilized after 11 weeks of open-label paroxetine then randomized to additional 12 weeks of paroxetine or placebo (Stein et al., 1996)	Higher relapse rate among discontinuers than continuers

Abbreviations: HR = hazard ratio; MDD = major depressive disorder; RCT = randomized controlled trial

Table 9.12 Guiding concepts for continuing or discontinuing pharmacotherapies

Situation	Usual recommended duration	Reasons for discontinuing
Major depression	1st episode: most guidelines advise continued pharmacotherapy for four–nine months once remission is achieved; in recurrent MDD Kupfer et al. (1992) findings argue for at least five years of continued pharmacotherapy in those initially stabilized. The CANMAT guidelines usefully advise continued treatment for >2 years (possibly indefinite) when there exist repeated episodes that are frequent, chronic, severe, recurrent, comorbid, difficult-to-treat, and/or with residual symptoms (Kennedy et al., 2016)	First lifetime uncomplicated major depressive episode, single episode treated to full remission, no antecedent subthreshold depression, no residual depression (especially if an abrupt/noninsidious onset and negative family history)
Bipolar disorder	1st lifetime mania/hypomania: treat for a minimum of six months; may consider stopping treatment and observing if full recovery and if the index episode was not of high severity 2nd (or beyond) lifetime mania/hypomania: most experts advise open-ended, indefinite pharmacotherapy for relapse prevention	Episode was nonpsychotic, of only mild/moderate severity, full remission without residual symptoms, no antecedent psychopathology (especially if negative family history, and no comorbid psychopathology or substance use disorder)
Anxiety disorders	The World Council of Anxiety (WCA) (Pollack et al., 2003) and the International Consensus Group on Depression and Anxiety (ICGDA) (Ballenger et al., 1998) both advise maintenance treatment for at least 12–24 months ("and in some cases indefinitely" (Pollack et al., 2003))	Consider medication discontinuation in patients who have achieved and sustained full remission for at least 6–12 months. Some studies suggest comparable relapse rates regardless of whether pharmacotherapy is discontinued at 6 or up to 30 months following response – but that residual symptoms may moderate relapse risk more than duration of treatment (Mavissakalian and Perel, 2002)
Schizophrenia and other nonaffective psychoses	Meta-analyses indicate that continuous, indefinite treatment consistently outperforms intermittent pharmacotherapy for relapse prevention (three- to sixfold OR) (De Hert et al., 2015). Naturalistic studies collectively suggest a recurrence rate of 77% at one year and >90% at two years (Zipursky et al., 2014), even after full initial recovery (Mayoral-van Son et al., 2016); higher risk with comorbid cannabis abuse (Bowtell et al., 2018)	Practice guidelines advise discontinuing antipsychotics after patients are symptom-free for one year or more (Lehman et al., 2014). Those remaining relapse-free for 6–10 months after stopping antipsychotics appear at low risk for later relapse (the so-called "discontinuation paradox") (Harrow and Jobe, 2013). Naturalistic studies suggest up to 30% of schizophrenia patients at 10-year follow-up may function well medication-free (Wils et al., 2017).

Abbreviations: CANMAT = Canadian Network for Mood and Anxiety Treatments; MDD = major depressive disorder; OR = odds ratio

10 Managing Major Adverse Drug Effects: When to Avoid, Switch, or Treat Through

LEARNING OBJECTIVES

- ☐ Understand ways to establish likely cause-and-effect relationships for suspected adverse drug effects
- ☐ Understand the phenomenology of the nocebo effect
- ☐ Differentiate relative degrees of binding affinity for psychotropic drugs at key receptor sites associated with clinically significant adverse drug effects
- ☐ Recognize comparative psychotropic and other risk factors for QTc prolongation
- ☐ Identify viable pharmacological antidote strategies for managing common nonhazardous adverse psychotropic drug effects

The remedy is worse than the disease.

- Sir Francis Bacon

We hope that things have changed for the better since the time of Sir Francis Bacon's seventeenth-century appraisal of medical treatment risks and benefits. Drugs themselves may not know the differences between the beneficial versus adverse effects they may exert, but prescribers should. All substances, even placebos, can cause negative effects in the minds and bodies of those who consume them, depending on expectations (e.g., past experiences, perceptions of help versus harm), underlying psychopathology (e.g., anxiety, somatization, paranoia), psychological dimensions (e.g., an external locus of control, suggestibility) as well as pharmacokinetics (e.g., delayed metabolic clearance) and, last but not least, pharmacodynamics. Paradoxical drug reactions (such as worsening of psychosis after starting an antidopaminergic drug, or intensified suicidal thoughts or urges after beginning an antidepressant) pose especially challenging dilemmas, as clinicians must try to determine when, faced with a clinical effect opposite to the one expected, there exists a truly iatrogenic effect versus the natural course of illness with mere lack of efficacy (at least thus far) of the chosen intended remedy.

Tip

Adverse effects due to placebos are termed *nocebo effects*. These most often (>10% of patients) include dizziness, headache, nausea, diarrhea, sedation, insomnia, anorexia, nervousness, and anxiety.

In establishing likely causal connections between a potential medication and a suspected adverse effect, it can be useful to consider the items in Box 10.1.

Particularly given the varied cognitive, emotional, and perceptual disruptions to information processing

Box 10.1

Considerations for Adverse Effects

- Is there a plausible (versus contradictory) mechanism (e.g., anticholinergic drugs are unlikely to cause sialorrhea) and time course (e.g., drug rashes are unlikely to occur years after having begun a drug)
- How far in time did the suspected adverse effect arise relative to the last change made in a drug regimen?
- How confident is the clinician that the suspected adverse effect is not simply a manifestation of the underlying psychiatric condition being treated (e.g., worsening suicidal thoughts in a depressed patient, or nonspecific symptoms in a patient with somatic symptom disorder)
- Is the suspected adverse effect likely common and transient (e.g., headache or nausea upon starting an SSRI or SNRI) and prone to resolve spontaneously?
- Is the suspected adverse effect annoying (e.g., yawning from SSRIs, mild weight gain, benign rashes), potentially hazardous (e.g., metabolic dysregulation, impaired balance) or serious and potentially life-threatening (e.g., Stevens–Johnson syndrome, anaphylaxis)?

that are inherent to psychiatric (as compared to most nonpsychiatric) disorders, care must be taken to evaluate complaints of adverse effects beyond their superficial face value. In RCTs of depression, reported adverse drug effects occur in about two-thirds of subjects taking placebo, and 5% may drop out prematurely specifically due to perceived adverse effects during placebo treatment (Dodd et al., 2015). Termed *nocebo effects* by Barsky and colleagues (2002), they may be more likely to arise in patients with high levels of neuroticism, phobic-obsessive traits, suggestibility, alexithymia, and excessive or elaborate expectations about treatment outcomes (Goldberg and Ernst, 2019).

A comprehensive review and discussion of all adverse effects associated with psychotropic drugs is beyond the scope of this chapter, although for a more detailed discussion the reader is invited to see Goldberg and Ernst (2019). In the current chapter, our focus will be directed more toward a concise summary of major adverse effects and the psychotropic drugs likely to cause them, along with practical recommendations about their assessment and management.

Tip

Countless obscure complaints are sometimes attributed to medications as side effects. *Rare* possible side effects can occur with any drug, but cause-and-effect relationships may be hard to infer. In such instances it can be useful to tell patients (or colleagues) that the chance of a certain drug causing a particular side effect is no greater than is the case with a placebo.

A ACNE

Acne can result from (or become exacerbated by) use of lithium, possibly because of increased neutrophil chemotaxis, stimulation of lysosomal enzyme release, and induced follicular hyperkeratosis (Yeung and Chan, 2004). Topical benzoyl peroxide, retinoids (e.g., retinoic acid cream or gel), and antibiotics (clindamycin, erythromycin, tetracycline) remain the usual preferred management strategies. Notably, acne caused or exacerbated by lithium can be notoriously difficult to treat and tends to respond more poorly to traditional acne regimens than in the absence of lithium. Spironolactone, which is often prescribed for women with adult acne and hirsutism because of its putative antiandrogenic effects at the site of sebaceous glands, can increase lithium levels and is sometimes advised with careful monitoring of lithium levels.

B ALOPECIA

Reports of varying frequencies (usually <15%) exist linking alopecia with anticonvulsants (carbamazepine, divalproex, topiramate), monoaminergic antidepressants (SSRIs, SNRIs, TCAs) and psychostimulants, arising at any point in treatment, usually not dose-related. Patient-specific risk factors have not been identified. When drug continuation is favored over cessation or finding a suitable alternative, symptomatic management may include oral biotin 10 000 μg/day and topical minoxidil. Some authorities advocate oral supplemental zinc and selenium, based mainly on observed links between alopecia areata and low serum levels of these trace elements (Jin et al., 2017), plus observations that zinc may function as a 5-α- reductase inhibitor (inhibiting the

Can escitalopram cause laryngospasm?

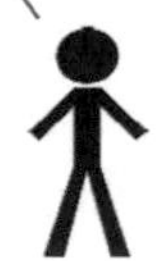

I read on the internet that brexpiprazole can cause appendicitis.

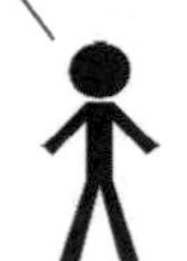

Then it must be true.

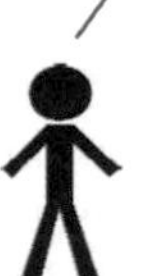

My patient got hemorrhoids after taking N-acetylcysteine.

Extraordinary. What's the mechanism? Is it related to glutathione function on rectal epithelium?

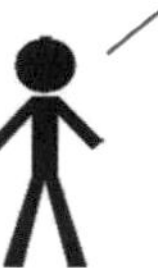

transformation of testosterone to dihydrotestosterone, which in turn can cause hair loss). While generally safe at doses found within standard multivitamins, RCTs have not demonstrated benefit for countering iatrogenic alopecia in the absence of baseline serum deficiencies.

C BLEEDING

Serotonergic antidepressants have been associated with decreased platelet aggregation and the potential for impaired hemostasis. A meta-analysis of 11 cohort studies (n = 187 956 patients) identified an increased bleeding risk of 36% during SSRI therapy (Laporte et al., 2017), although the absolute risk appears low, with a crude estimate of one upper GI bleeding event per 8000 SSRI prescriptions. It is difficult to account for additional factors that may increase or decrease propensity on an individual case level. The most salient diathesis for bleeding during SSRI or SNRI therapy appears to be a history of GI bleeding, especially in patients taking aspirin or nonsteroidal anti-inflammatory drugs (Andrade et al., 2010), which raises the odds ratio for GI bleeding from the range of 1.16–2.36 upwards to 3.7–10.9 (Bixby et al., 2019). Use of concomitant proton pump inhibitors may help lessen this risk by about 60% (Targownik et al., 2009). Some authors advise favoring antidepressants with little or no binding affinity for the serotonin transporter (i.e., bupropion or mirtazapine) as preferred options in patients with a bleeding diathesis (Bixby et al., 2019).

Epidemiological studies also identify a rare increased risk of intracerebral or intracranial hemorrhage associated with SSRI exposure history (more short than long term) – translating to an incidence of 24.6 per 100 000 person-years, or one additional event per 10 000 persons treated for one year (Hackam and Mrkobrada, 2012). (Similarly, amid controversy about whether to withhold SSRIs preoperatively because of a potential increased risk for peri- or postoperative bleeding, Mrkobrada and Hackam (2013) note the great rarity of only a 1 in 1000 hazard from propensity-matched analyses, arguing against broad or absolute preoperative contraindications.)

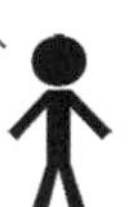

Just tell me if I should tell the surgeon to stop SSRIs before surgery.

I'm afraid it's again not that black and white and must be a case-by-case decision. Bleeding is a very rare event. So consider the relative risks: how long is the SSRI half-life? How likely would antidepressant withdrawal be if it were stopped? How extensive is the expected blood loss from the procedure? Stuff like that.

Existing studies are mostly observational rather than randomized, making it difficult to account for potential confounding factors (remember Chapter 3) that may predispose to bleeding. Risk for impaired hemostasis with serotonergic antidepressants is in general a relative rather than an absolute consideration, and depends on cumulative patient-specific clinical factors within a risk–benefit paradigm. Consider the example in Clinical Vignette 10.1.

CLINICAL VIGNETTE 10.1

Norman is a 71-year-old man who two years ago underwent successful coronary artery stenting for dual vessel atherosclerotic coronary artery disease, and has since been maintained on apixaban 5 mg twice daily. His body weight and serum creatinine are within normal limits (75 kg and 1.1 μmol/L, respectively) and he has mild congestive heart failure (CHF). There is no history of gastritis, ulcerative disease, or diverticuli. He now presents with moderately severe symptoms of a second lifetime nonpsychotic major depression. His prior episode occurred with no obvious psychosocial antecedents at age 58 and fully remitted with sertraline 100 mg/day, which was discontinued after nine months with no recurrence until now.

In Norman's case, should sertraline be resumed on the grounds of Norman's personal history of an excellent response, coupled perhaps with the known safety and efficacy of sertraline (fortuitously) in patients with coronary heart disease (Glassman et al., 2002), even in the setting of CHF (O'Connor et al., 2010)? Or, does his existing anticoagulant treatment pose a relative contraindication to his taking an SSRI? If an SSRI is resumed, can we quantify the risk for abnormal bleeding, assuming he remains on apixaban? For the latter question, there is no known quantifiable *absolute* risk above and beyond the baseline use of an SSRI. In Norman's case, the absence of a history of GI bleeding or intracranial hemorrhage bodes more favorably for the safety of restarting sertraline than had either of those conditions been part of his history. (There is also little to no harm in "covering" Norman for prophylaxis of a GI bleed with a proton pump inhibitor.) Nevertheless, if one were still especially concerned about Norman's bleeding risk, one could consider favoring bupropion or mirtazapine instead of an SSRI or SNRI – although Norman's prior good outcome with sertraline must be weighed against the uncertainty of using untried alternative pharmacotherapies, each with their own unknown potential risks.

D BLOOD DYSCRASIAS

Suppression of white blood cells (WBCs), red blood cells (RBCs), or platelets can occur from a variety of psychotropic drugs with varying risk factors, time courses, and levels of severity, as outlined for anticonvulsants in Table 10.1. Note as well that all antipsychotic drugs can be associated with leukopenia.

Notably, lithium is often underappreciated for its hematopoetic value to increase WBC production via stem cell mobilization and direct stimulation of granulocyte colony stimulating factor (G-CSF) – a property ripe for potential exploitation as an adjunctive therapy in patients taking clozapine, carbamazepine, or other psychotropics that may be associated with leukopenia (Focosi et al., 2009).

E BRUXISM

Night-time teeth-grinding, known also as bruxism, may result at any time from SSRIs, SNRIs, buspirone, FGAs, SGAs, atomoxetine, stimulants, or dopamine agonists such as pramipexole. It does not necessarily appear to be dose-related, and may be somewhat more likely to arise in older patients, women, and smokers. Non-pliable dental appliances are considered the most effective remedy for persistent bruxing. For iatrogenic bruxism most available pharmacological antidote strategies are more anecdotal (e.g., case report) than evidence-based, but may include: clonazepam 1 mg PO qHS (every night at bedtime), propranolol 60–160 mg PO qHS, cyclobenzaprine 2.5–5 mg PO qHS, buspirone 10 mg PO BID-TID, *l*-dopa 100 mg PO qHS, trazodone 150–200 mg PO qHS, divalproex 500 mg PO qHS, topiramate 25–100 mg PO qHS, hydroxyzine 10–25 mg PO qHS, metoclopramide 10–15 mg PO qHS, or gabapentin 300 mg PO qHS.

F CARDIOVASCULAR EFFECTS

Bradycardia: May infrequently be associated with SSRIs, typically benign requiring no intervention.

Myocarditis: Rare (<0.2% incidence) consequence of clozapine, usually arising within the first four to eight weeks of treatment, potentially dose-related, and associated with unduly rapid dose titration; treated by immediate drug cessation and possible use of beta-blockers, ACE inhibitors, and/or diuretics. Although case series have reported that up to two-thirds of patients may have successful outcomes when later rechallenged after resolution of myocarditis (Manu et al., 2018), sample sizes are relatively small and the risk for relapse is significant.

Orthostatic Hypotension: Orthostatic hypotension is conventionally defined by a drop in systolic blood pressure of ≥20 mmHg or diastolic blood pressure of ≥10 mmHg within three minutes of standing. Common iatrogenic psychotropic causes include α-1 antagonists (i.e., both FGAs and SGAs, TCAs, terazosin, prazosin, selegiline, MAOIs (may be dose-related), and trazodone). Compression stockings or abdominal binders can be helpful, although forced oral hydration or increased salt intake may be less useful in the absence of hypovolemia (although dehydration can be an exacerbating factor). When significant and persistent, oral fludrocortisone 0.1–0.2 mg/day (maximum 0.4–0.6 mg/day) or midrodine 0.5 mg PO TID may remedy the problem.

Orthostatic hypotension is closely linked pharmacodynamically with α-1 receptor antagonism. Box 10.1 summarizes the relative α_1 receptor binding affinities across SGAs. Iloperidone, for example, having the tightest binding affinity at α_1 receptors, is strongly associated with dizziness and orthostatic hypotension.

Box 10.1

Relative α_1-Receptor Binding Affinities Across SGAs

SGA	Ki (nM)
Iloperidone	0.36
Clozapine	1.62
Paliperidone	2.5
Brexpiprazole	3.8
Asenapine	8.9
Ziprasidone	18
Quetiapine	22
Aripiprazole	25.9
Lurasidone	47.9
Lumateperone	<100
Olanzapine	109-115
Cariprazine	155

QTc Prolongation: Prolongation of the QTc interval on ECG can result from a wide range of both psychotropic and nonpsychotropic drugs; clinicians must recognize cumulative pharmacological as well as other risk factors, as summarized in Box 10.2.

The FDA considers drugs that increase the QTc interval to be clinically meaningful ("definite concern") when it rises more than 20 ms. However, it is important for clinicians to appreciate that the issue of whether or not a particular medication may increase the QTc interval is not an absolute/all-or-none phenomenon, and depends heavily on more comprehensive aspects of a given patient's clinical circumstances. A drug that may prolong the QTc by 20 ms probably matters less in a patient whose baseline QTc is 345 ms than 485 ms. Moreover, even though the risk for *torsade de pointes* (and possible consequent ventricular fibrillation) is considered to be of greatest concern when the QTc exceeds 500 ms, that arrhythmia remains a rare event and not likely a highly probable consequence in most patients whose QTc exceeds that threshold.

Box 10.2

Risk Factors for QTc Prolongation

Nonpharmacological	Nonpsychotropic medications	Psychotropic medications
Older age	Antifungal agents (ketoconazole, fluconazole)	Citalopram >40 mg/day
Female sex	Cyclobenzaprine	Fluoxetine (case reports)
Significant alcohol use	Ondansetron	Chlorpromazine
Congenital risk	Tetrabenazine, valbenazine	Thioridazine
Congestive heart failure	Solefenacin	SGAs
Thyroid abnormalities	Vardenafil	Trazodone
Hepatic dysfunction	Fluoroquinolone antibiotics (e.g., ciprofloxacin, levofloxacin, ofloxacin)	TCAs
Hypokalemia	Macrolide antibiotics (erythromycin, clarithromycin)	Methadone
Hypomagnesemia	Antimalarials (mefloquine, chloroquine)	Pimavanserin
	Class I antiarrhythmics (quinidine, disopyramide, procainamide) and Class II antiarrhythmics (amiodarone, sotalol, dofetilide)	

Among SGAs, Huhn and colleagues (2019) updated a prior meta-analysis of risk for QTc prolongation with antipsychotics (Leucht et al., 2013a), identifying a hierarchical relative risk across 15 agents ranging from lowest (lurasidone) to highest (sertindole); this updated (2019) meta-analysis included 51 controlled trials with 15 467 subjects (see Figure 10.1). Note that (a) CIs crossing zero are not statistically significantly different from placebo in risk for QTc prolongation and (b) no drugs studied are *safer* than placebo.

Tachycardia: psychostimulants, noradrenergic drugs, and anticholinergic drugs can all increase resting heart rate, usually in benign fashion.

G CHRONIC KIDNEY DISEASE

Lithium is perhaps the most notorious among psychotropic drugs for its potential to cause nephrotoxicity, either acutely in the aftermath of an overdose or gradually due to progressive glomerulosclerosis with an accompanying steady decline in glomerular filtration rate (GFR). Nephrologists tend to demarcate a clinically significant decline or impairment in renal functioning when a patient's estimated GFR falls below 60 mL/min (corresponding to Stage 3 chronic kidney disease). While up to half of bipolar patients who take lithium for over 20 years may show at least some degree of GFR reduction higher than would be expected for normal aging (Bocchetta et al., 2015), the incidence of moderately decreased GFR or greater (Stage 3 chronic kidney disease as classified by the National Kidney Foundation) is less than 20% (Lepkifiker et al., 2004). Once-daily dosing of lithium may help reduce the risk for eventually developing glomerulosclerosis (Castro et al., 2016).

A sudden rise in serum creatinine, or a progressive increase over time, signals the need for further evaluation, including urinalysis to determine the presence or absence of proteinuria and hematuria. "Limited elevation in serum creatinine" is considered an increase ≤30% from usual baseline, while "acute renal failure" describes rises from baseline serum creatinine of >0.5 mg/dL. Some authorities advise measuring serum cystatin C, either as an alternative or additional marker for calculating eGFR that provides a more sensitive estimate for developing end-stage renal

Figure 10.1 Comparative rates of QTc prolongation among antipsychotics in RCTs. Illustration based on mean scores with accompanying 95% CIs, as reported by Huhn et al. (2019).

Antipsychotic	Mean Difference (95% CI)
Lurasidone	−2.21 (−4.54 to 0.15)
Brexpiprazole	−1.46 (−4.71 to 1.81)
Cariprazine	−1.45 (−6.20 to 3.20)
Aripiprazole	−0.43 (−3.62 to 2.77)
Placebo	0.00 (0.00 to 0.00)
Paliperidone	1.21 (−2.89 to 5.31)
Haloperidol	1.69 (−0.23 to 3.64)
Quetiapine	3.43 (0.94 to 6.00)
Olanzapine	4.29 (1.91 to 6.68)
Risperidone	4.77 (2.68 to 6.87)
Asenapine	5.60 (−0.94 to12.00)
Iloperidone	6.93 (4.49 to 9.36)
Ziprasidone	9.70 (7.43 to 12.04)
Amisulpride	14.10 (7.71 to 20.45)
Sertindole	23.90 (20.56 to 27.33)

disease and all-cause mortality (Shlipak et al., 2013). Work-up of possible chronic kidney disease includes considering nonpharmacological/noniatrogenic etiologies, such as vasculitis, systemic lupus erythematosus, diabetic nephropathy, hypertension, urinary tract obstruction, or intrinsic kidney disease (e.g., polycystic kidney disease, glomerulonephritis, interstitial nephritis, or vesicoureteral reflux), among other causes. In patients taking lithium who develop elevated serum creatinine levels, there is no universal determinant for if and when lithium should be discontinued, and decisions once again depend on a patient-specific risk–benefit analysis.

More Terminology

The term "*protopathic bias*" (also called "*reverse causality*") is sometimes used to describe situations where a suspected adverse event (say, dementia) is misattributed to treatment (say, benzodiazepines) when the event is actually a sign of the disorder itself (e.g., anxiety or agitation in a patient with prodromal features of dementia). It differs from *confounding by indication* (also called "*indication bias*"), in which a treatment is prescribed (or avoided) based on an outcome of interest (say, avoiding benzodiazepines in older adults for fear they cause dementia, and then looking back to see if indeed benzodiazepine-avoiders seldom developed dementia).

H DEMENTIA

Several observational studies have reported associations between anticholinergic drug use or benzodiazepine use and the development of dementia. The largest of those focusing on anticholinergic drugs involved a nested case control study of 58 769 patients with dementia and 225 574 controls matched for age (>55), sex, exposure window, and other factors, reporting a 1.49-fold increase in the likelihood of dementia arising in those who took anticholinergic drugs for three or more years (OR = 1.49, 95% CI = 1.44–1.54) (Coupland et al., 2019). In the case of benzodiazepines, a meta-analysis of 11 891 dementia cases and 45 391 controls found a 1.49-fold increased risk for the diagnosis of dementia among subjects who ever (versus never) took a benzodiazepine (Zhong et al., 2015). Problematic with all such observational reports, despite their very large sample sizes, is their noncontrolled, nonrandomized design, precluding the ability to draw causal inferences. The potential for *confounding by indication* is of particular concern: for example, depression, anxiety, and sleep disturbances all may represent prodromal elements of eventual dementia that can arise ≥10 years before the diagnosis of dementia is evident (Amieva et al., 2008). Anticholinergic drugs obviously can have adverse cognitive effects in the short term; while it is certainly possible that these drug classes could exert enduring adverse cognitive effects, reverse-causality is equally plausible (patients at risk for dementia may be more likely to receive anticholinergic drugs or benzodiazepines). We therefore advise case-by-case assessment of the relative risks and benefits of these medications, particularly in patients with established risk factors for dementia (e.g., poorly controlled hypertension, smoking), rather than all-or-none admonitions about their safe use.

I DISCONTINUATION SYNDROMES

As noted in Chapter 9, gradual tapers of short half-life serotonergic antidepressants help to minimize the chances of discontinuation syndromes that might otherwise occur in up to two-thirds of SSRI or SNRI recipients. Taper-offs are likely unnecessary when an outgoing drug is immediately replaced with an alternative agent that binds to the serotonin reuptake receptor. If discontinuation symptoms are especially difficult to manage with conservative measures (e.g., reassurance and education, slow tapers, adjunctive antinausea drugs such as trimethobenzamide 300 mg orally every six hours as needed; meclizine 25 mg orally every six hours as needed for dizziness or vertigo, hydration), substitution of a short-acting SSRI or SNRI with a longer-acting agent (such as fluoxetine or vortioxetine) should promptly overcome most if not all target symptoms (Zajecka et al., 1997).

J DRUG-INDUCED LUPUS ERYTHEMATOSUS

Arthralgias, myalgias, fever, serositis, and rash raise concerns about possible autoimmune disease. Drug-induced lupus is a relatively rare phenomenon that typically occurs months to years after exposure to a causal agent. The list of medications traditionally associated with drug-induced lupus is relatively short (see Box 10.3) – although stray one-off case reports possibly linking the phenomenon with dozens of other (low or very low probability) drugs appear in the literature. The number of psychotropic drugs associated with drug-induced lupus is quite short.

Box 10.3

Medications Associated with Drug-induced Lupus Erythematosus	
Acebutol	Minocycline
Anticonvulsants (e.g., carbamazepine, divalproex, phenytoin)	Penacillamine
Calcium channel blockers	Procainamide
Chlorpromazine	Proton pump inhibitors
Hydralazine	Quinidine
Hydrochlorothiazide	Statins
Isoniazid	Sulfasalazine
Methyldopa	TNF-α inhibitors

Diagnosis is confirmed by laboratory measures (antinuclear antibody (ANA), anti-single-stranded (ss) DNA antibodies, increased ESR (erythrocyte sedimentation rate), and perinuclear antineutrophil cytoplasmic antibodies (pANCA). Symptoms typically resolve within days to weeks of discontinuing the causal agent.

K DRY MOUTH (XEROSTOMIA)

Xerostomia can result from anticholinergic drugs or lithium. It can lead to poor dentition if chronic and unaddressed. Conservative treatment approaches include glycerin-based oral lubrication solutions, lipid-based oxygenated glycerol triester (OGT) oral sprays, cevimeline 30 mg PO qDay (once daily), pilocarpine 2.5–10 mg PO 1–3× qDay, or bethanechol 25 mg PO TID.

L GASTROINTESTINAL UPSET

Nausea and GI upset are among the most ubiquitous adverse effects seen across classes of psychotropic medications, including placebo. Serotonergic drugs that indiscriminately agonize postsynaptic $5HT_3$ receptors are thought to induce nausea (treatable, if necessary, by $5HT_3$ antagonists such as ondansetron, granisetron, or high-dose metoclopramide, or, conceivably, by $5HT_3$-blocking antidepressants such as mirtazapine or SGAs such as olanzapine or quetiapine).

Vortioxetine poses a special case inasmuch as it commonly causes nausea *despite* its potent $5HT_3$ antagonism (Ki = 3.7 nM); therefore, adding a(nother) $5HT_3$ antagonist such as ondansetron or mirtazapine as an antinausea/antiemetic countermeasure would make little sense. Mechanistically, it is thought that nausea from vortioxetine stems from its $5HT_{1A}$ full agonism, similar to aripiprazole, or cariprazine, or buspirone (see Chapter 17, Table 17.6). Antihistaminergic antinausea drugs (e.g., trimethobenzamide, promethazine) may be more efficacious and rationale-based strategies if and when antinausea antidotes for such drugs are needed.

M HEPATIC DYSFUNCTION

Drug-induced hepatitis is a rare complication of all drugs, including most psychotropic agents. Antidepressants as a class have been associated with up to a 3% incidence of benign, asymptomatic transaminitis, usually independent of dosage (Voican et al., 2014). Frank and potentially

So, cannabidiol is thought to treat nausea by allosteric inhibition of the $5HT_3$ receptor, mediated through $5HT_{1A}$ partial agonism. Can I get medical marijuana if, say, an SSRI makes me queasy?

LOL. Why don't you instead just try adding cyproheptadine, if the thing you're looking for is $5HT_{1A}$ *antagonism*?

lethal hepatotoxicity is a still rarer phenomenon that most often arises within the first 6 months of drug exposure and may be less evident with SSRIs (notably, citalopram, escitalopram, paroxetine, fluvoxamine) than other monoaminergic antidepressants (Voican et al., 2014). Divalproex and nefazodone carry FDA boxed warnings regarding the potential for fatal hepatotoxicity. Semi-annual monitoring of hepatic function is sometimes recommended for patients taking divalproex long term (see Chapter 7, Table 7.11), but otherwise, because onset may be sudden, routine surveillance monitoring of liver enzymes with other psychotropics is generally not recommended in the absence of clinical signs of liver disease.

In patients with pre-existing liver disease (e.g., cirrhosis, chronic hepatitis) or malnutrition, beware of hypoalbuminemia with resultant loss of carrying capacity for protein-bound drugs. (Measure free (unbound) drug fractions in such instances; see Chapter 7, Table 7.1).

N HYPERHIDROSIS

Excessive sweating is an uncommon adverse effect associated with most SSRIs, potentially occurring at any time point and not clearly in a dose-related fashion. Pharmacological antidotes may include terazosin 1–2 mg/day, clonidine 0.1 mg/day, glycopyrrolate 1 mg PO qDay or BID, and oxybutynin 5–10 mg PO qD-TID. The topical anticholinergic agent glycopyrronium 2.4% solution, formulated as a cloth wipe, also may be of value for excessive axillary sweating.

O HYPERPARATHYROIDISM (WITH OR WITHOUT HYPERCALCEMIA)

Lithium can cause increased parathyroid hormone (PTH) release by (1) antagonizing the calcium sensing receptor (CaSR) on parathyroid cells and (2) inhibiting renal excretion of calcium, potentially resulting in parathyroid hyperplasia and potential hypercalcemia in about 10–25% of patients taking lithium (Shapiro and Davis, 2015). Differences between hyperparathyroidism associated versus unassociated with lithium are summarized in Box 10.4.

If periodic monitoring of serum PTH and calcium levels reveals hyperparathyroidism, imaging to determine the presence of single- or multiglandular disease is generally advised, often followed by bone mineral densitometry to gauge the presence and extent of osteopenia. Cessation of lithium (even when feasible psychiatrically) may not necessarily reverse iatrogenic hyperparathyroidism. When symptomatic (e.g., serum calcium >1 mg/dL, CrCl <60 mL/min, bone density T-score <2.5 SD), surgical parathyroidectomy is often recommended but not always curative. Calcimimetic agents such as cinacalcet are sometimes recommended by endocrinologists for symptomatic patients who are not surgical candidates or for whom parathyroidectomy fails to normalize serum Ca^{++} levels.

Tip

Bone mineral density (BMD) T-scores are expressed in standard deviations (SDs) relative to the young adult mean. Negative numbers reflect low BMD. Normal BMD is within ± 1 SD of the young adult mean; T-scores from -1 to -2.5 SD reflect low bone mass; scores of -2.5 SD or lower indicate osteoporosis, while scores lower than -2.5 SD with a history of bone fractures reflect severe osteoporosis.

P HYPERPROLACTINEMIA

Most FGAs and SGAs can increase serum prolactin levels in a dose-related fashion by blocking tonic dopaminergic inhibition of prolactin release from the posterior pituitary within the tuberoinfundibular pathway. Besides dopamine-blocking drugs, hyperprolactinemia may less commonly result from use of ramelteon, opiates, TCAs, fluoxetine, paroxetine, and venlafaxine. Medications that raise prolactin are especially undesirable in women with histories of estrogen-receptor-positive breast cancer due

Box 10.4

Lithium-induced versus Primary Hyperparathyroidism

Lithium-induced hyperparathyroidism	Primary hyperparathyroidism (unrelated to lithium)
↑ serum Ca^{++}	↑ serum Ca^{++}
↓ urine Ca^{++}	↑ urine Ca^{++}
Normal serum phosphate	↓ serum phosphate
↑ serum Mg^{++}	Normal serum Mg^{++}

to potential trophic effects from prolactin. D_2/D_3 partial agonists (i.e., aripiprazole, brexpiprazole, cariprazine) are among the least likely of SGAs to elevate serum prolactin and may even normalize high baseline levels. Normal serum prolactin levels tend to be <20 ng/mL. The relative magnitude of hyperprolactinemia secondary to dopamine-blocking drugs tends to be <100 ng/mL, whereas pituitary adenomas often will cause serum prolactin levels to exceed 100–150 ng/mL.

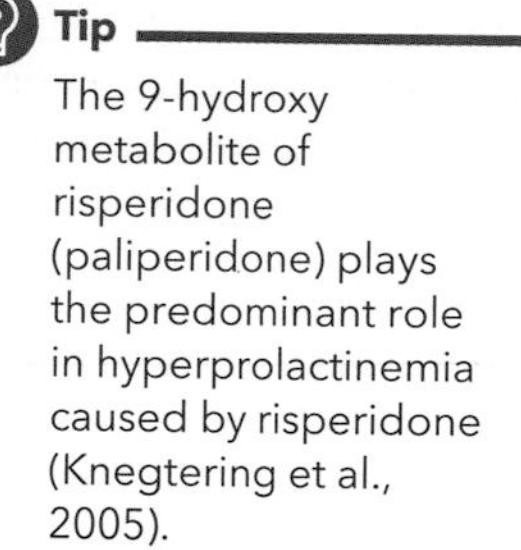

Tip
The 9-hydroxy metabolite of risperidone (paliperidone) plays the predominant role in hyperprolactinemia caused by risperidone (Knegtering et al., 2005).

A comparative analysis (predating the latter two of these drugs) examining changes from baseline prolactin seen across trials of FGAs and SGAs is presented in Figure 10.2, with clozapine and aripiprazole emerging as among the agents least likely to offend, and paliperidone, risperidone, and haloperidol being among those most likely to increase serum prolactin levels.

Serum prolactin levels are usually not measured routinely in patients taking dopamine receptor-blocking drugs but, rather, based on suggestive clinical features (e.g., amenorrhea, galactorrhea, gynecomastia). Apart from favoring psychotropic agents that exert minimal effects on prolactin release (as described in Figure 10.2), countermeasures that may remedy iatrogenic hyperprolactinemia include the use of adjunctive aripiprazole (e.g., Chen et al., 2015) or dopamine agonists (e.g., bromocriptine 2.5–10 mg/day, amantadine 100–300 mg/day, pramipexole ≤1 mg/day, or ropinirole 0.75–3 mg/day).

Figure 10.2 Comparative rates of hyperprolactinemia among antipsychotics in RCTs. Illustration based on mean scores with accompanying 95% CIs, as reported by Huhn et al., 2019. EPS = extrapyramidal symptoms.

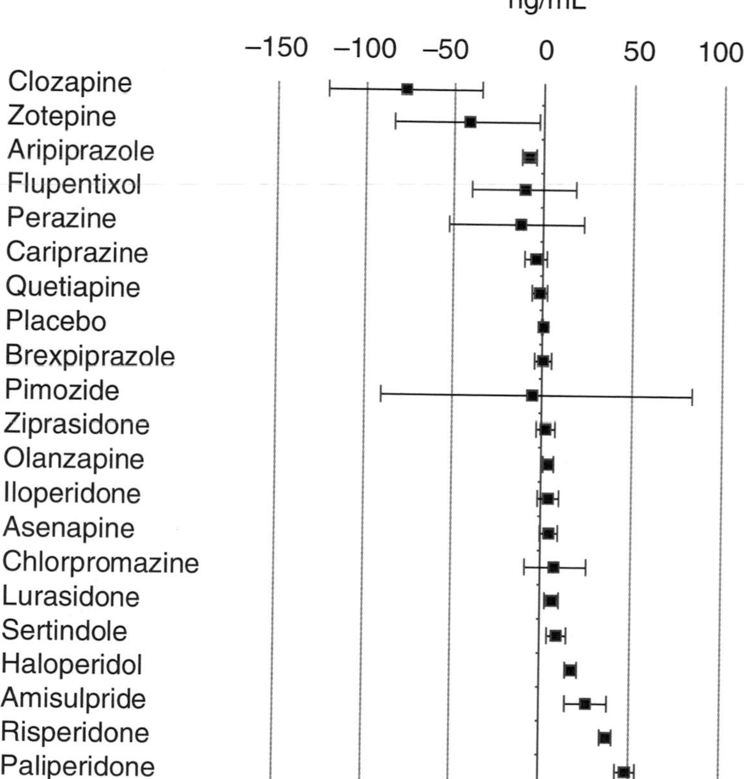

Q NEPHROGENIC DIABETES INSIPIDUS

Nephrogenic diabetes insipidus (NDI) refers to kidney unresponsiveness to the effects of antidiuretic hormone, resulting in excessive thirst, polyuria, and dilute urine (specific gravity <1.005, urine osmolality <200 mOsm/kg). Noniatrogenic causes must be ruled out (e.g., hypokalemia, hypercalcemia, Cushing's disease, sickle cell trait), as well as nonpsychotropic drug-induced causes (e.g., diuretics, colchicine) and central/neurogenic causes of diabetes insipidus due to lack of antidiuretic production in the brain. Routine laboratory assessment of suspected NDI includes:

- 24° urine collection for total volume, urine specific gravity, and urine osmolality
- Serum osmolality
- Serum electrolytes and glucose
- Serum antidiuretic hormone level

NDI secondary to lithium does not in itself require drug cessation, and is often managed with amiloride 5 mg PO BID (along with monitoring of serum K^+).

R NEUROLEPTIC MALIGNANT SYNDROME

Neuroleptic malignant syndrome (NMS) is conventionally defined by body temperature >38 °C, extreme muscle rigidity, possible elevated serum creatine kinase (CK; often in excess of 1000 IU/L), possible hyper-reflexia, labile blood pressure, tachypnea, and diaphoresis. Symptoms often occur within one week of beginning an FGA or SGA or increasing its dose. It may be a dose-related phenomenon. Treatment involves rapid diagnosis and discontinuation of dopamine-blocking drugs accompanied by hydration and supportive measures (e.g., cooling blankets). Parenteral dantrolene is typically begun if fever and autonomic instability persist despite the above measures.

S EXTRAPYRAMIDAL SIDE EFFECTS

"Extrapyramidal side effects" (EPS) broadly encompass a range of phenomena including akathisia, dystonias, dyskinesias, akinesia, and parkinsonism that result from the use of FGAs or SGAs. We will focus in this section on akathisia, parkinsonism, and acute dystonias. Tardive dyskinesia will be described separately.

All FGAs and SGAs have the potential to cause EPS to varying degrees. Low-potency agents have built-in anticholinergic properties and therefore may pose a somewhat lesser EPS hazard than high-potency antipsychotics or SGAs with relatively loose binding affinities to the D_2 dopamine receptor. Figure 10.3 summarizes comparative findings from a meta-analysis of incident rates of EPS across antipsychotics.

Akathisia may occur not only from FGAs and SGAs, but reportedly also from lithium, some SSRIs, or mirtazapine. It is often dose-related and may occur either soon after starting a causal drug or later in treatment (tardive akathisia). Risk factors in addition to medication dosage may include older age, female sex, negative symptoms in schizophrenia, presence of affective symptoms, cognitive dysfunction, iron deficiency, and use of two or more antipsychotic drugs. Apart from dosage reductions, management involves the use of beta-blockers (e.g., propranolol 30–90 mg/day) or benzodiazepines. (The former strategy bears on the proposed mechanism of akathisia involving low dopaminergic tone from the midbrain to the ventral striatum with compensatory noradrenergic upregulation from the locus coeruleus to the shell of the nucleus accumbens and prefrontal cortex (Loonen and Stahl, 2011)). Other viable evidence-based strategies may include amantadine 100–200 mg/day and gabapentin 300–1200 mg/day. Anticholinergics are not considered to be useful for akathisia.

Parkinsonism specifically describes the presence of a bilateral and symmetric rhythmic rest tremor with increased motor tone, bradykinesia, a festinating gait, and potential cogwheel rigidity; it must be differentiated from other forms of EPS or other abnormal motor movements altogether (e.g., neurotoxicity, essential tremor, motor tics, stereotypies), for which antidote strategies may be different. Dopaminergic projections in the striatum tonically inhibit the release of acetylcholine; antidopaminergic drugs disinhibit the release of striatal acetylcholine, producing subcortical movements that resemble Parkinson's disease. Anticholinergic drugs (benztropine, trihexyphenidyl) remain the mainstay of treatment for parkinsonism induced by FGAs or SGAs, but are generally begun if and when needed, at the lowest effective doses, rather than prophylactically. The dopamine agonist amantadine 100–300 mg/day is an alternative strategy for managing iatrogenic parkinsonism, with the advantage of sparing adverse cognitive and other CNS effects of anticholinergic drugs.

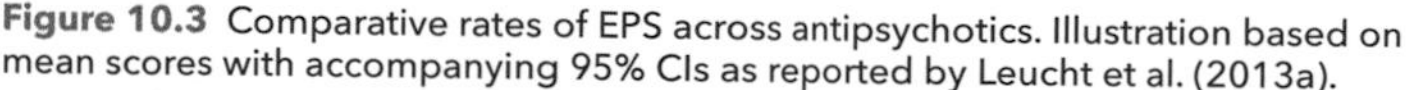

Figure 10.3 Comparative rates of EPS across antipsychotics. Illustration based on mean scores with accompanying 95% CIs as reported by Leucht et al. (2013a).

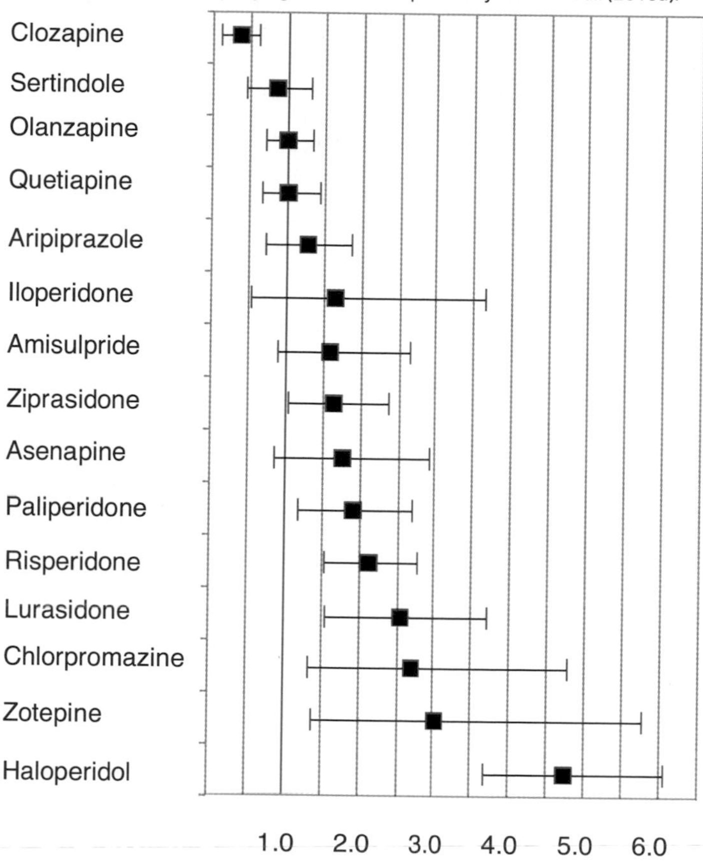

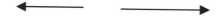

Acute dystonic reactions are more common in men than women and younger than older patients. Reactions may include cervical dystonia (torticollis, or unilateral pulling of the neck), oculogyric crises, blepharospasm (uncontrollable and excessive blinking), laryngospasm, trismus (lockjaw), and opisthotonos (severe spasm and hyperextension of the extremities). They usually occur soon after treatment initiation or dosage increases, but may also arise months or years after taking a dopamine receptor-blocking drug, and in such instances are often permanent (tardive dystonia). In all instances, rapid diagnosis is essential and treatment involves the prompt administration of (preferably parenteral) anticholinergics or antihistamines, i.e., benztropine 1–2 mg IM q15–30 minutes (up to 8 mg), diphenhydramine 50 mg IM q15–30 minutes (up to 200 mg), trihexyphenidyl 5 mg IM q15–30 minutes (up to 20 mg), or biperiden 1–5 mg IM q15–30 min (up to 16 mg). Diazepam 5–10 mg IM is sometimes also identified as a potential treatment strategy for acute dystonias, but benzodiazepines can also rarely *cause* acute dystonias.

Box 10.5 summarizes comparative receptor binding affinities at D2 receptors across SGAs.

Box 10.5

Relative D_2 Receptor Binding Affinities of Second-generation Antipsychotics

Looser → Tighter

SGA	Ki (nM)
Quetiapine	245
Clozapine	157
Lumateperone	32
Asenapine	8.9
Iloperidone	6.3
Olanzapine	3.0–106
Ziprasidone	4.8
Risperidone	3.57
Cariprazine	0.49–0.69
Aripiprazole	0.34
Brexpiprazole	0.30

Might I want to favor high Ki SGAs in, say, patients with Parkinson's disease who need an SGA?

Indeed you might. You might also want to read Chapter 12.

I might indeed

I don't understand this dopamine partial agonism business. The three existing D_2/D_3 partial agonists, aripiprazole, cariprazine, and brexpiprazole, all have tight binding affinities at the D_2 receptor, but as partial agonists, shouldn't they entirely spare the nigrostriatal pathway and not cause EPS or akathisia or dystonia unless there is underlying hypodopaminergic tone in that circuitry?

What a great question! You'd think all brain dopamine pathways should be equally subject to the effects of a partial agonist depending on their ambient dopamine tone, but that may not be the case. Animal models raise several possible explanations: there could be regional selectivity, meaning that overactive mesolimbic circuitry is easier to modulate than nigrostriatal. That theory is supported by observations that *presynaptic* mesolimbic dopamine function is elevated in schizophrenia (Howes et al., 2012) – so maybe dopamine partial agonists exert different effects outside of mesolimbic tracts, or dopamine partial agonists may really function as presynaptic agonists and postsynaptic antagonists, and with more postsynaptic than presynaptic receptor density, it's easier to tone down mesolimbic hyperactivity; or, maybe there's some kind of window or threshold effect that either spares or antagonizes nigrostriatal versus mesolimbic pathways.

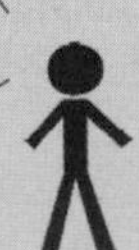
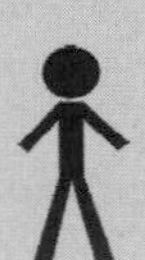

So basically, you don't know

I don't think anybody knows for sure. It's complicated and we can only make educated guesses.

T SEDATION AND SOMNOLENCE

Antihistaminergic drugs, α_1 agonists (e.g., clonidine) and some GABAergic agents (e.g., benzodiazepines, gabapentin) commonly produce sedation or somnolence, often in dose-related fashion. Some but not all patients accommodate with prolonged exposure or dosage reductions if necessary. Antihistaminergic effects account for both sedation and weight gain caused by many SGAs and other compounds. (However, a drug such as lumateperone has minimal H_1 antagonism or α_1 agonism yet still may produce significant sedation, presumably via its potent $5HT_{2A}$ antagonism.) A summary of H_1 receptor binding affinities across SGAs and related serotonergic compounds is presented in Box 10.6. When clinically appropriate, use of psychostimulants or (ar)modafinil may safely and effectively counteract sedation when it persists, drug benefits outweigh risks, and there are no psychiatric or physiological contraindications.

Tip

Remember that modafinil and armodafinil induce CYP1A2 (as well as 3A4 and 2B6, and inhibit 2C9 and 2C19). Levels of coadministered clozapine may decline.

Box 10.6

Relative H_1 Histamine Receptor Binding Affinities Across SGAs and Serotonergic Antidepressants/Related Compounds

SGA	Ki (nM)	Function
Mirtazapine	0.14–1.6	Antagonist
Olanzapine	0.65–0.49	Inverse agonist
Asenapine	1.0	Antagonist
Clozapine	1.13	Antagonist
Quetiapine	2.2–11	Antagonist
Ziprasidone	15–130	Antagonist
Brexpiprazole	19	Antagonist
Paliperidone	19	Antagonist
Risperidone	20.1	Inverse agonist
Cariprazine	23.2	Antagonist
Aripiprazole	27.9-61	No data
Lumateperone	>100	Antagonist
Trazodone	220–1100	Antagonist
Citalopram	283	Antagonist
Iloperidone	437	Antagonist
Lurasidone	>1000	Unknown
Escitalopram	2000	Antagonist
Fluoxetine	3250	Antagonist
Paroxetine	>10 000	Antagonist
Sertraline	24 000	Antagonist

U SEIZURES

Antipsychotic drugs, tricyclics, and bupropion are all associated to varying degrees with dose-dependent lowering of the seizure threshold. Clinicians should be aware of the cumulative seizure risks for a given patient (including history of head trauma, past seizures, infection, alcohol, or benzodiazepine or illicit substance use, and spotty medication adherence and dosing of prescribed drugs that could have pro-convulsant effects), rather than thinking in all-or-none absolute terms about whether any one drug is "safe" to use from the standpoint of seizure risk.

V SEROTONIN SYNDROME

Defined traditionally by "Hunter's triad" of autonomic dysfunction, neuromuscular excitation (e.g., tremor, clonus) and an altered mental status, serotonin syndrome is a potentially fatal consequence of drug interactions that effectively lead to serotonin toxicity. Common examples include combining MAOIs with an SSRI or SNRI or dextromethorphan or meperidine. A host of other serotonergic drugs have been described in the literature that, at least in theory, could also cause serotonin toxicity, including combinations of SSRIs or SNRIs plus buspirone (a $5HT_{1A}$ partial agonist) or lithium (mildly serotonergic) or tramadol (a weak SNRI) or triptans (controversially identified in a 2006 FDA warning as potential contributor when mixed with a serotonergic antidepressant, but an electronic health records database of 19 017 triptan recipients who were coprescribed antidepressants revealed only two definite cases (Orlova et al., 2018)).

It is sometimes difficult to distinguish from anticholinergic toxicity, neuroleptic malignant syndrome, malignant hyperthermia, or encephalitis.

W SEXUAL DYSFUNCTION

Sexual dysfunction remains among the most common and vexing adverse effects across psychotropic drugs, particularly antidepressants and antipsychotics. SSRI-associated anorgasmia or delayed ejaculation generally tends to be a dose-related phenomenon, although large-scale systematic studies examining dose relationships across medications are neither extensive nor definitive. Sexual dysfunction associated with antidopaminergic drugs is thought to be less common among more prolactin-sparing agents, although true incident rates from RCTs are often underestimated due to nonsystematic prospective assessment. Evidence-based pharmacological antidotes to iatrogenic sexual dysfunction tend to exert modest and variable efficacy, but nevertheless represent viable strategies worth undertaking when the benefits of continuing an offending agent outweigh the risks of discontinuing. Pertinent information is summarized in Table 10.2.

X SIALORRHEA

Hypersalivation can occur from clozapine and a number of other SGAs (rather paradoxically, in light of the inherent anticholinergic effects of clozapine and many other SGAs). Clinicians should assure that hypersalivation is not an indication of laryngeal dystonia in patients taking dopamine-blocking drugs. Otherwise benign sialorrhea can often be effectively managed symptomatically by appropriating an anticholinergic solution (e.g., ipratropium bromide 0.03% nasal spray, or atropine sulfate 1% ophthalmic solution) for sublingual administration (one to two drops before bedtime). Other oral remedies vary in their effectiveness as well as their potential for producing systemic adverse effects of their own (e.g., glycopyrrolate 1 mg PO BID, hyoscine (scopolamine) 0.3 mg/day, biperiden 2 mg PO qDay or BID, metoclopramide 10–30 mg PO qDay).

Y SUICIDALITY

Treatment-emergent suicidal thoughts or behaviors are an important and compelling example of the ambiguity when judging whether symptoms are iatrogenic rather than reflective of the underlying ailment being (unsatisfactorily) treated.

Antidepressants: In October, 2004 the FDA issued a boxed warning that all drugs classified as "antidepressants" could increase the risk for suicidal thoughts or behaviors in people aged 24 and under. That conclusion derived from an FDA review of 25 RCTs (16 in MDD) involving approximately 4000 children and adolescents in which 109 postmarketing events were reported as "possibly suicide related" (but none involved suicide completions).

Anticonvulsants: In 2008 the FDA issued a class warning that anticonvulsant drugs could increase the risk for suicidal thoughts or behaviors, based on their meta-analysis of 199 placebo-controlled trials involving 11 medications. Subsequent authors critical of this warning have pointed out the failure of the FDA meta-analysis to account for moderating factors (such as the presence of a psychiatric diagnosis, or a past suicide attempt) as influencing suicide risk irrespective of anticonvulsant use; they also note that epilepsy itself is a known risk factor for suicide (Hesdorrfer et al., 2010).

Isotretinoin: Since 2005 isotretinoin has carried a warning in its manufacturer's product label that it "may cause depression, psychosis and, rarely, suicidal ideation, suicide attempts, suicide, and aggressive and/or violent behaviors." As an isomer of retinoic acid, the active form of vitamin A, some authors propose that isotretinoin may induce suicidal or other psychiatric symptoms by causing hypervitaminosis A (Bremner et al., 2012). Those authors also cite 41 reports to the FDA of isotretinoin challenge/dechallenge/rechallenge (two-thirds of cases having no prior psychiatric history), with resolution of depressive features off drug and re-emergence upon re-exposure. A retrospective 20-year review of cases reported to the FDA since 1997 identified 2278 instances of suicidal ideation, 602 reported suicide attempts, and 368 completions; reports of depression and anxiety occurred mostly in patients aged 10–19, and this study deduced an overall suicide completion rate of 8.4 per 100 000 in 2009 and 5.6 per 100 000 in 2010 (Singer et al., 2019). The authors remarked that factors such as emotional distress from acne may contribute more directly to depression and suicidality among isotretinoin recipients than does drug exposure, and posit that successful acne treatment with isotretinoin may consequently actually *diminish* suicide risk as compared to the general population. Problematic with this report is its observational design; because it is not a controlled study, one cannot know the risk for suicidal events among young adults whose acne remains untreated, or treated by alternative means, or whose dermatological results are unsatisfying. Pretty much nobody notifies the FDA MedWatch program of uneventful outcomes. An NNH cannot be calculated without a comparison group. Therefore, our own approach is to assure that depressed patients who are considering isotretinoin are properly counseled as to the possibility that depressive or suicidal features could intensify and that this risk must be properly and systematically monitored.

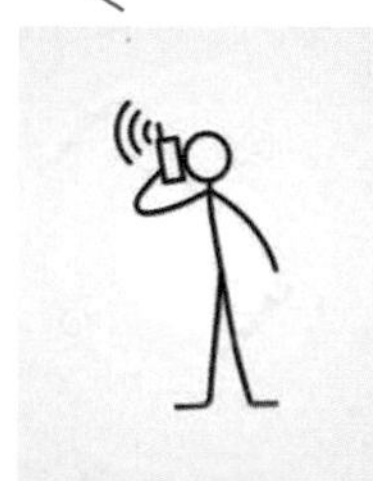

Hello, FDA? I hear you need denominators. I'm calling to tell you about all my patients who took a medication and had no serious adverse effects.

Z SYNDROME OF INAPPROPRIATE ANTIDIURETIC HORMONE SECRETION

All antidepressants, as well as carbamazepine and oxcarbazepine, rarely may cause SIADH, defined biochemically by a low serum Na^+ (usually <130 mmol/L) accompanied by the so-called Bartter–Schwartz criteria, as summarized in Box 10.7.

> **Tip**
> Measure urine electrolytes and urine osmolality in suspected SIADH. Dilute urine (urine Na^+ <20 mmol/L) is more suggestive of psychogenic polydipsia.

In the absence of other recognized etiologies (e.g., paraneoplastic syndrome, infection, hypothyroidism, meningitis), one is generally obliged to stop all antidepressants and serially monitor serum sodium levels, typically alongside fluid restriction to 1 L/day. Some authors have observed possibly lesser risks for SIADH with mirtazapine, bupropion, or tricyclic antidepressants than with other antidepressants, although the literature in this area is far from definitive.

Box 10.7

Bartter-Schwartz Criteria for SIADH

- Decreased serum osmolality <275 mOsm/kg
- Concentrated urine (urine osmolality >100 Osm/kg)
- Increased urine Na^+ (>20 mEq/L)
- Euvolemic
- Euthyroid

AA TARDIVE DYSKINESIA

SGAs were initially hailed as carrying a substantially lesser risk than FGAs for causing adverse motor effects, including tardive dyskinesia (TD). While the overall risk appears somewhat lower, it remains far from nil. A meta-analysis of 41 studies found a 20.7% prevalence of TD in SGA recipients as compared to 30.0% among patients taking only FGAs (Carbon et al., 2017). Contemporary studies estimate an annual TD incidence risk of 5.4% in adults over age 54 who take an SGA (Correll et al., 2004). On a practical level, cumulative lifetime exposure to any and all dopamine-blocking drugs collectively adds to overall risk for TD, often making it difficult to know "which" one of many cumulative agents is most blameworthy if and when TD symptoms arise. Case reports exist of TD-like syndromes arising after exposure to drugs that do not block DA receptors (e.g., SSRIs, tricyclics) but such occurrences are rare and thought to occur from an unmasking effect after "priming" by exposure to DA-blocking agents (D'Abreu and Friedman, 2018). Lithium also has not been proven to cause (or treat) TD. Discontinuing antipsychotics or lowering dosages does not necessarily improve signs of tardive dyskinesia, even if and when doing so were psychiatrically feasible (Soares-Weiser and Rathbone, 2006).

> **Tip**
> TD movements disappear during sleep.

> **Tip**
> TD risk factors include older age, duration of antipsychotic exposure, high dosages, and psychiatric illness duration; female sex and the diagnosis of an affective disorder may also increase TD risk.

Management of TD fundamentally changed in 2017 with the emergence of two novel drugs that are molecular variations of tetrabenazine: valbenazine (begun at 40 mg PO qDay and increased after one week to 80 mg PO qDay) and deutetrabenazine (typically begun at 6 mg PO BID; may increase at weekly intervals of 6 mg/day as needed to a maximum of 24 mg PO BID). Both agents can symptomatically reduce (but fundamentally not eradicate) hyperkinetic movements by reversibly depleting catecholamines at the synaptic cleft – specifically, by inhibiting vesicular monoamine transporter type II (VMAT2), in turn reducing the availability of presynaptic

Figure 10.4 VMAT2 inhibition and dopamine supersensitivity in tardive dyskinesia. Reprinted from Stahl, 2018, with permission, Cambridge University Press.

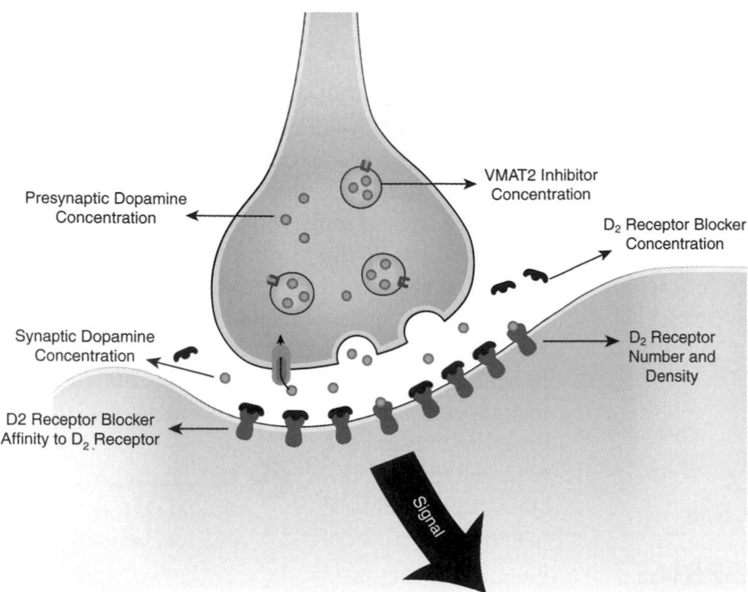

DA release and thus decreasing postsynaptic striatal DA receptor stimulation (see Figure 10.4). Unlike tetrabenazine for treatment of movement disorders, valbenazine and deutetrabenazine both have longer half-lives that permit less frequent dosing schedules and serum fluctuations and also spare tetrabenazine's risk for inducing or exacerbating depression and suicidality. Comparative TD outcome differences between valbenazine and tetrabenazine have not been made but a comparison of both agents is summarized in Box 10.8. Both exert clinically large effects (valbenazine NNT = 4 (Solmi et al., 2018); deutetrabenazine NNT = 7 (Solmi et al., 2018)). VMAT2 inhibitors also may cause or worsen parkinsonian symptoms.

Anticholinergic drugs generally worsen TD (Alphs and Davis, 1982), although challenges can arise in the case of complex movement disorders in which patients taking dopamine-blocking drugs might manifest signs of TD, parkinsonism, and akathisia – all of which may require separate pharmacological interventions (VMAT2 inhibitors, amantadine preferred over anticholinergics in the setting of TD, and beta-blockers, respectively).

Box 10.8

Comparison of Valbenazine and Deutetrabenazine

Valbenazine	Deutetrabenazine
Metabolized to the (+) α dihydro- isomer of tetrabenazine	Deuterated racemic tetrabenazine, metabolized to four isomers
Selective inhibition of VMAT2	May target not only VMAT2 but also $5HT_7$ and D_2 receptors
Longer half-life (15–20 hours), once-daily dosing	Shorter half-life (9–20 hours), twice-daily dosing
Narrow dosing range (40 or 80 mg/day)	Greater dosing range (6 mg PO BID up to 24 mg PO BID) allows titration for more varying degrees of VMAT2 occupancy

While VMAT2 inhibitors are now considered first-line treatments for TD, a (much more) limited earlier database exists using vitamin E 800–1600 IU/day ("no clear difference … from placebo" in a 2018 Cochrane review of 13 RCTs, although "more deterioration" was subsequently observed with placebo than Vitamin E; Soares-Weiser et al., 2018), vitamin B6 1200 mg PO qDay, amantadine 100 mg PO BID, biperiden 2 mg PO

BID, melatonin 6 mg PO qDay, insulin 10 U SC/day, α-methyldopa 750–1500 mg PO qDay, levetiracetam 500–3000 mg PO qDay, and clozapine 300–400 mg PO qDay (collectively reviewed in Goldberg and Ernst, 2019).

CLINICAL VIGNETTE 10.2

A Pharmacological Puzzle

Martin is a 44-year-old man with schizoaffective disorder successfully maintained on quetiapine 300 mg/day and divalproex 1000 mg/day. He has had mild-to-moderate TD which has also successfully been managed for the past six months with valbenazine 80 mg/day. In response to complaints of excessive daytime sedation, armodafinil 150 mg/day was added which led to a rapid improvement in wakefulness and alertness. After several days he also began to report a worsening of involuntary tongue movements and grimacing. Why?

The example in Clinical Vignette 10.2 prompts thinking about both pharmacokinetic and pharmacodynamic drug interactions. Modafinil and its enantiomer armodafinil are both believed to function as DA reuptake inhibitors and, as such, could exacerbate TD. Adding armodafinil to a VMAT2 inhibitor could therefore potentially worsen TD via a pharmacodynamic effect, making a reduction of armodafinil dose (e.g., from 150 to 75 mg/day) the most logical first step. At the same time, consider that modafinil and armodafinil both induce the metabolism of CYP3A4 substrates. (They also inhibit the metabolism of CYP2C19 substrates, such as phenytoin, clomipramine, diazepam, omeprazole, and propranolol.) Valbenazine is metabolized primarily by CYP3A4 and, as such, it could theoretically have undergone more rapid metabolism and elimination when armodafinil was added to Martin's regimen, leading to lesser efficacy for TD.

Should Martin's valbenazine dose be increased beyond the maximum FDA-approved dose that he already takes? (The manufacturer's product labeling for valbenazine technically discourages its use in combination with a potent CYP3A4 inducer, although the chronology of medication exposures in this case is unusual.) Should a valbenazine serum level be measured to determine if the level is, indeed, low due to hastened metabolism? (Problematic with the latter strategy is the lack of a normed serum therapeutic range for valbenazine.) Should valbenazine be switched to the alternative VMAT2 inhibitor deutetrabenazine, because the latter is primarily a substrate for CYP2D6 (and, to a lesser extent, CYP3A4 and CYP1A2) – presumably allowing for greater compatibility with armodafil coadministration?

The remedy in Martin's case was hardly complex. His armodafinil dose was reduced by half, which was sufficient to overcome his daytime sedation and simultaneously led to improvement in his TD symptoms, presumably via less interference with the VMAT2 inhibitory effects of valbenazine. Clinical Vignette 10.3 looks at Martin's brother.

Clinical Vignette 10.3

Another Pharmacological Puzzle

Martin's fraternal twin, Marvin, also diagnosed with schizoaffective disorder, had developed TD likely from years of exposure to various SGAs that eventually markedly improved with valbenazine 80 mg/day. About two months later, pre-existing desvenlafaxine was successfully replaced by the combination of olanzapine (5 mg/day) plus fluoxetine (40 mg/day) for treatment-resistant depression. About a month later, Marvin began to complain of worsening anxiety that was deemed to be akathisia. Olanzapine dosing was reduced to 2.5 mg/day and then 1.25 mg/day with no improvement in motor restlessness and only modest relief from clonazepam 2 mg/day and propranolol 20 mg three times daily. He then developed new parkinsonism. Both adverse effects still persisted several weeks after the olanzapine was stopped altogether. What is going on?

Akathisia is often confused phenomenologically with anxiety (see also Chapter 17); the former usually improves with dosage reductions and/or benzodiazepines and/or propranolol, but not in Marvin's case. The persistence of akathisia coupled with the emergence of parkinsonism even after cessation of the antipsychotic seemed hard to explain, much less treat. His complete lack of improvement in EPS despite all of the above interventions lessened enthusiasm for further raising the dose of either his clonazepam or propranolol. Instead, valbenazine dosing was reduced from 80 to 40 mg/day. Akathisia and parkinsonism then markedly improved within two to three weeks.

VMAT2 inhibitors can, rarely, cause both akathisia and parkinsonism (as noted by a 2019 FDA drug safety labeling change for valbenazine), although such motor symptoms are thought more likely to be elicited in individuals with pre-existing known basal ganglia disease (which was not the case for Marvin). VMAT2 inhibitor dosage reductions or else outright drug elimination unfortunately may become necessary in instances such as this.

AB TICS

Motor tics can be caused or exacerbated by psychostimulants and, more rarely, bupropion, SSRIs, imipramine, lamotrigine, and carbamazepine. They are not necessarily a dose-related phenomenon. The RCT literature on managing tics is based mainly on treatment of tics associated with Tourette syndrome, rather than on iatrogenic tics. If discontinuing the causal agent is not feasible, significantly greater effects than placebo (extrapolating from the adult and/or child Tourette syndrome literature) have been observed with clonidine 0.1–0.3 mg PO qDay, guanfacine 1.5–3.0 mg PO qDay (divided as BID dosing) and aripiprazole 2–10 mg PO qDay, all showing medium effect sizes. More provisional data support the use of haloperidol (2–10 mg PO qDay) or risperidone 0.5–4 mg PO qDay. Pimozide (dosed from 1–12 mg PO qDay) appears better than placebo, but somewhat less efficacious than haloperidol (Pringsheim and Marris, 2009). Atomoxetine appears not to worsen tics in children with comorbid ADHD. There are insufficient or negative RCT data using baclofen, levetiracetam, *N*-acetylcysteine, omega-3 fatty acids, topiramate, ziprasidone, or tetrahydrocannabinol (collectively reviewed by Pringsheim et al., 2019).

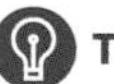

Tip

Pharmacological parsimony would favor α agonists for tics in the setting of autonomic hyperarousal, inattention, or insomnia, and aripiprazole or risperidone for tics in patients with OCD, psychosis, or mood disorders.

AC TREMOR

Tremor requires careful assessment to discern the presence of medication-related neurotoxicity versus non-toxic states (e.g., as can occur with drugs such as lithium, divalproex or bupropion) versus primary movement disorders (e.g., benign essential tremor, Parkinson's disease) versus acute withdrawal from alcohol or benzodiazepines. Drug-induced tremors tend to be postural (i.e., evident when arms are fully extended against gravity without external support), coarse rather than fine, nonrhythmic, and evident both at rest and upon action. Tremor as a sign of neurotoxicity demands broader attention to the potential hazards of overdose, particularly with medications that have narrow therapeutic indices (such as lithium) that may require active interventions beyond dosage reductions or cessation (e.g., hydration and ECG monitoring when serum lithium levels exceed 1.5 mEq/L). When tremor is not deemed to be a sign of neurotoxicity, symptomatic management apart from dosage reductions as feasible customarily includes use of propranolol 10–20 mg PO BID or TID (maximum 320 mg/day) or primidone 50–100 mg/day (may increase in 50 mg increments up to 500 mg/day; be aware of the potential for significant and dramatic induction of CYP450 3A4 and 1A2 isoenzymes, with consequent hastened metabolism of those catabolic enzyme substrates).

AD WEIGHT GAIN AND METABOLIC DYSREGULATION

Weight gain and obesity (the latter operationally defined as a BMI >30 kg/m^2) remains one of the most common and vexing adverse effects associated with almost all classes of psychotropic drugs. Common mechanisms associated with weight gain include direct appetite stimulation (e.g., through hypothalamic serotonergic (e.g., $5HT_{2C}$ blockade) effects), antihistamine effects, and (in the case of some SGAs) promotion of insulin resistance. Hypothalamic $5HT_{2C}$ receptor binding mediates levels of the circulating anorexigenic hormone leptin, in turn affecting satiety (Reynolds et al., 2006); preclinical studies show that $5HT_{2C}$ agonism is pro-anorectic, and $5HT_{2C}$ knockout mice overeat and become obese. Recall from Chapter 8 that in the case of weight gain resulting from drugs that *block* $5HT_{2C}$, pharmacogenetic studies suggest that the $5HT_{2C}$ *C/C* variant may predispose to weight gain with SGAs that block $5HT_{2C}$. Newer serotonergic antidepressants such as vortioxetine and vilazodone have no appreciable binding affinities at $5HT_{2C}$, which may partly account for their relative weight neutrality.

Boxes 10.6 and 10.9 summarize relative receptor binding affinities for $5HT_{2C}$ and for H_1 targets of SGAs and serotonergic antidepressants. However, $5HT_{2C}$ or H_1 receptor Kis alone may not in themselves be so informative about weight gain potential in the absence of other contributing factors (such as genetic predispositions) or other relevant receptor systems (such as antihistaminergic drug effects). Bear in mind as well the varying pharmacodynamic functions at receptor sites for the agents described; inverse agonists function essentially as antagonists.

Among monoaminergic antidepressants, paroxetine has been shown across RCTs to be more likely than other SSRIs to cause weight gain (Fava, 2000), although the mechanism for this remains speculative inasmuch as paroxetine is not highly antihistaminergic (see Box 10.6) nor is its $5HT_{2C}$ binding affinity very high (Ki = 9000 nM). Fluoxetine may be the least likely traditional SSRI to cause weight gain.

When considering risk–benefit analyses for psychotropic drugs with potential high liability for weight gain or other adverse metabolic effects (e.g., clozapine, olanzapine), it is often useful for clinicians to take into consideration broad atherosclerotic cardiovascular disease (ASCVD) risk (e.g., using an online risk estimator to calculate a given patient's pooled cohort equation (e.g., https://clincalc.com/cardiology/ascvd/pooledcohort.aspx) to gauge the 10-year likelihood for developing ASCVD). Medications with lower metabolic liability are obviously ideally more desirable in patients at higher risk for ASCVD, but depending on the level of psychiatric symptom severity, risk–benefit analyses for treatment options may not always permit the sparing of psychiatrically high-potency drugs that increase weight, lipids, or glycemic parameters.

Among SGAs, a comparative meta-analysis by Huhn and colleagues (2019) found a hierarchical risk for iatrogenic weight gain, but note that confidence intervals overlap for the reported standardized mean differences (SMDs) of many of the agents studied. (True between-drug differences exist only where CIs do not overlap.) As shown in Figure 10.5, most agents studied have the potential to cause weight gain, although in this meta-analysis, only ziprasidone, aripiprazole, and lurasidone had CIs that overlapped with weight changes seen with placebo.

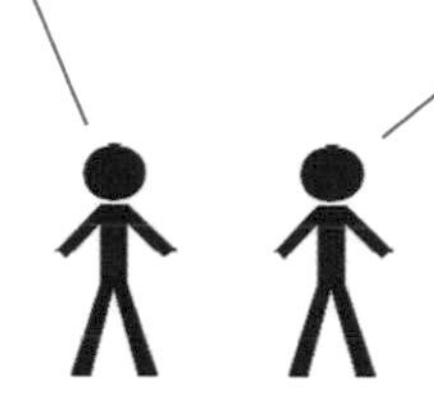
So I'd bet a $5HT_{2C}$ receptor agonist could help promote satiety and weight loss. Are there any?
Now you're thinking like a neuropsychopharmacologist! Not many $5HT_{2C}$ agonists exist. The only real one out there was lorcaserin, a potent and selective $5HT_{2C}$ agonist that was officially used as a weight loss drug.* Buspirone has $5HT_{2C}$ agonism but only with very weak binding affinity.

* Lorcaserin was voluntarily withdrawn from the US market by its manufacturer in 2020 following concerns about increased risk for pancreatic, colorectal, and lung cancers over a five-year period.

OK so now wait, suppose I went and got pharmacogenetic testing, even though you told me never to do that...
I never said never to order...
...and then suppose the test protocol results for $5HT_{2C}$ genotyping came back as homozygous C/C. Would that make the patient a more ideal candidate to take lorcaserin?
OMG, you are *SO* thinking like a neuropsychopharmacologist! That's stupendous! What a penetrating insight! Now, if you go look on Index Medicus, you'll see there are no studies of this...yet. Nobody seems to have taken your clever idea and asked the question in a research setting whether $5HT_{2C}$ C/C homozygotes preferentially respond to a $5HT_{2C}$ agonist for iatrogenic weight loss, but what a great research study that would make. You wanna write up a grant proposal...?
Nah I'm good, thanks. But you go ahead.

Box 10.9

Relative $5HT_{2C}$ Receptor Binding Affinities Across SGAs and Serotonergic Antidepressants

SGA	Ki (nM)	Function
Ziprasidone	0.72–13	Partial agonist
Olanzapine	6.4–29	Inverse agonist
Mirtazapine	8.9–39	Antagonist
Clozapine	9.44	Inverse agonist
Asenapine	10.5	Antagonist
Brexpiprazole	12–34	Partial agonist
Risperidone	12.0	Inverse agonist
Aripiprazole	15–180	Partial agonist
Paliperidone	48	Unknown
Nefazodone	72	Antagonist
Fluoxetine	72.6	Antagonist
Flibanserin	88.3	Antagonist

SGA	Ki (nM)	Function
Cariprazine	134	Inverse agonist
Lumateperone	173	Antagonist
Lurasidone	415	Unknown
Buspirone	490	Agonist
Citalopram	617	Antagonist
Duloxetine	916	Antagonist
Venlafaxine	2004	Antagonist
Sertraline	2298	Antagonist
Escitalopram	2500	Antagonist
Quetiapine	2502	Antagonist
Fluvoxamine	5786	Antagonist
Paroxetine	9000	Antagonist

Lifestyle modification represents a fundamental cornerstone of managing metabolic risk, including nutritional counseling, physical activity and aerobic exercise, treating potential sleep apnea, management of hypertension, and addressing smoking cessation and alcohol intake. In patients taking polypharmacy drug regimens, the streamlining of possible redundant drug classes that each carry metabolic (e.g., antihistaminergic) risk can be helpful. Pharmacological "antidote" strategies to counteract iatrogenic weight gain, as described in Tables 10.3 and 10.4, have gained increasing interest among both patients and practitioners, and are often advisable and necessary, but they come with caveats, as noted in Box 10.10.

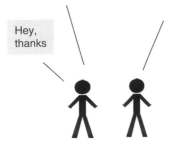

Oh wow, look, mirtazapine is a really potent antihistamine. Bet that could make it a good sleep aid, huh?

Hey, thanks

Box 10.10

Caveats to "Antidote" Strategies

- Drugs that promote weight loss tend to have relatively modest impact on weight reduction relative to the potential magnitude of weight gain caused by some psychotropics
- The effects of weight loss drugs usually eventually plateau and their benefits may reverse if and when the "antidote" drug is eventually stopped
- All medicines, including those meant as antidotes, can have their own adverse effects, and weight-loss drugs are no exception

Box 10.11 presents a rank ordering of relative liabilities across metabolic parameters among FGAs and SGAs, based on analyses by Pillinger et al. (2020). Relative rankings, called p-scores, are based on Bayesian probabilities according to surface under the cumulative ranking curve (SUCRA; see Chapter 3) that compared point estimates across a meta-analysis of 100 trials involving 25,952 participants with schizophrenia. So, for example, lurasidone emerges as the drug with least glycemic liability, haloperidol and ziprasidone both have the least adverse impact on weight and body mass index (BMI), and cariprazine has the least rank-

Figure 10.5 Comparative weight gain SMDs across antipsychotics in RCTs. Ilustration based on weighted mean differences with accompanying 95% CIs as reported by Huhn et al. (2019).

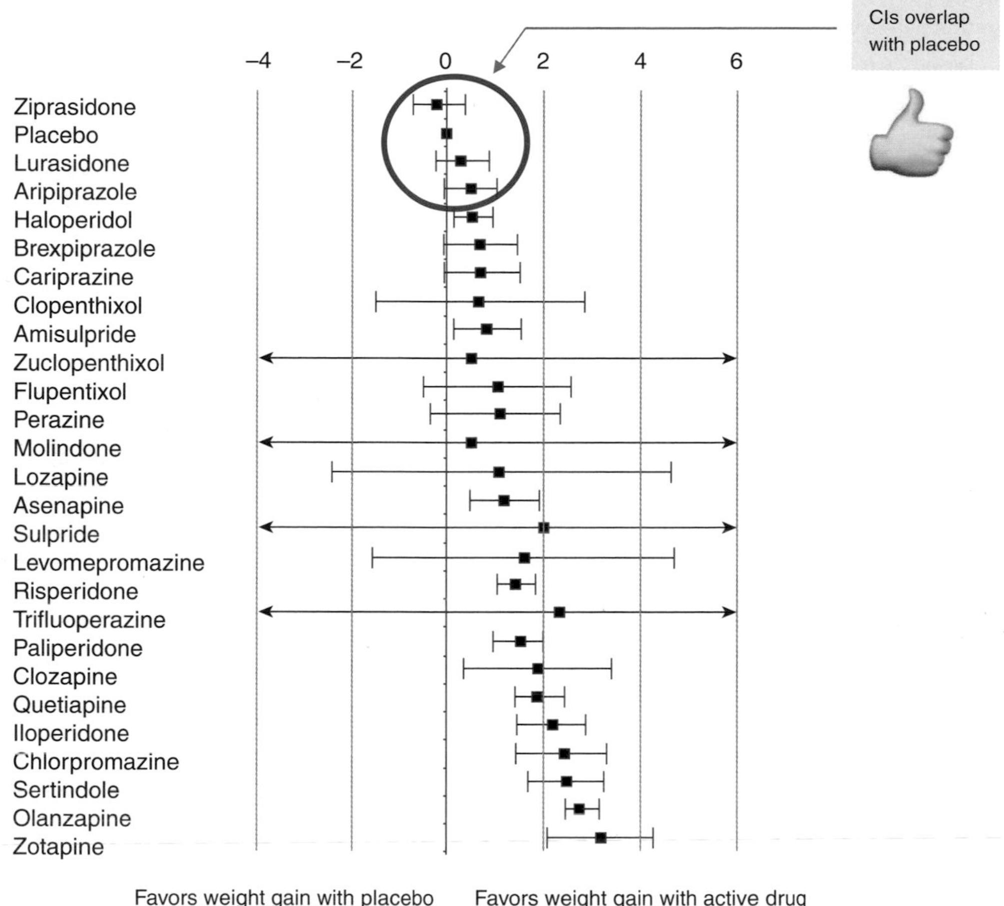

ordered risk for aggravating LDL-cholesterol or total cholesterol.

As a final note regarding weight management strategies, we would emphasize that it is far easier to avoid iatrogenic weight gain than to reverse it once it has occurred. That is the principle (and main observation) when combining olanzapine with amantadine from the outset of treatment (as noted in Table 10.3). The novel μ-opioid receptor antagonist samidorphan is under development as a potential similar weight-mitigator when coprescribed with olanzapine (Silverman et al., 2018), suggesting a possible role of modulation of the opiate system in regulating perhaps both appetite and energy metabolism.

AE SUMMARY

Virtually all psychotropic drugs pose the risk for adverse effects and in most instances prescribing decisions must be made according to a risk–benefit analysis that can vary from patient to patient, depending on the clinical circumstances, illness presentation and severity, alternative treatment options, and viable antidote strategies that may exist for adverse effects that are manageable and medically not hazardous. A summary of strategies to optimize drug tolerability across major psychotropic drug classes is presented in Tables 10.5–10.7.

Box 10.11 Relative Rankings[1] of Metabolic Liability Across Antipsychotics[2]

A summary of ordered rankings of metabolic liability parameters across antipsychotics - thus, ziprasidone, aripiprazole and lurasidone are among the lowest risk for weight, glycemic and lipid changes.

Antipsychotic	Weight	BMI	Glucose	LDL-c	TC	HDL-c	TG
Haloperidol	0.10	0.08	0.59		0.59		0.63
Ziprasidone	0.10		0.42	0.12	0.25	0.24	0.33
Aripiprazole	0.26	0.11	0.55	0.48	0.50	0.26	0.33
Lurasidone	0.32	0.37	0.09	0.27	0.27	0.45	0.26
Cariprazine	0.37		0.70	0.07	0.16	0.47	0.28
Fluphenazine	0.38						
Amisulpride	0.41		0.14		0.64	0.83	0.42
Brexpiprazole	0.45		0.40	0.66	0.52	0.18	0.23
Flupenthixol	0.44						
Asenapine	0.56		0.22				
Risperidone and Paliperidone	0.58	0.56	0.46	0.54	0.55	0.51	0.39
Quetiapine	0.65	0.68	0.47	0.91	0.82	0.59	0.71
Iloperidone	0.70		0.73		0.19		0.63
Sertindole	0.81	0.72	0.36		0.26		0.29
Zotepine	0.88		0.94				0.94
Clozapine	0.90	0.85	0.97		0.97		0.97
Olanzapine	0.92	0.93	0.67	0.96	0.91	0.76	0.83

[1] Numbers are p-scores (ranging from 0 to 1), in which higher values reflect a greater degree of metabolic dysregulation – except in the case of HDL-c, where higher scores reflect lesser metabolic risk

[2] Based on findings reported by Pillinger et al., 2020

Abbreviations: BMI=body mass index; HDL-c= high density lipoprotein cholesterol; LDL-c=low density lipoprotein cholesterol; TC=total cholesterol; TG=triglycerides

TAKE-HOME POINTS

- Pay careful attention to plausibility and Hill criteria when judging the likelihood that a particular symptom is iatrogenic rather than simply a persistence of worsening manifestation of the condition being treated.
- Differentiate benign (though annoying) from medically serious adverse effects, and those which tend to be transient or persistent and dose-related versus dose-independent.
- Remember that all treatments, including placebos, can cause side effects. Every clinical decision involves a risk-benefit analysis that must take into consideration the severity of the ailment under treatment alongside the viability of alternative treatment options.
- Recognize when pharmacological antidote strategies are feasible and available that can safely counteract an adverse drug effect. Engage patients in a shared decision-making process when considering the options of treating-through an adverse effect (particularly if alternative treatment options are limited, or a marked treatment response has occurred) versus changing regimens altogether in hopes of finding comparably effective and better tolerated alternatives. Point out relevant uncertainties with respect to both efficacy and tolerability, and favor a collaborative partnership approach to maximize satisfaction with treatment outcomes.

Table 10.1 Blood dyscrasias associated with anticonvulsants and their management

Blood dyscrasia	Description	Management strategy
Leukopenia		
Carbamazepine	Benign leukopenia occurs transiently in about 10% of patients during the first three months and in ~2% persistently (Sobotka et al., 1990). Frank aplastic anemia occurs in ≤1 in 200 000 exposures. Thrombocytopenia resulting from carbamazepine has been described in case reports. Note that oxcarbazepine is not associated with blood dyscrasias	Monitor based on clinical judgment (e.g., signs of infection); typically requires no intervention. Discontinue if WBCs drop to <3000 per mm^3 or ANC <1500 per mm^3. Adjunctive lithium may stimulate WBC production if necessary
Divalproex	Rare idiosyncratic reports, potentially arising even years after treatment initiation	Often asymptomatic and reversible either via dosage reductions or cessation
Other FGAs, SGAs	Leukopenia in nonclozapine antipsychotic recipients for more than six months reported in up to 18% of schizophrenia patients (Rettenbacher et al., 2010), presumably immune-mediated, possibly dose-dependent at least in some instances (Sood, 2017); risk may be higher in first month after starting therapy (Stübner et al., 2004)	Routine CBC monitoring is not indicated in the absence of clinical signs (e.g., infection). Unlike clozapine, no formal recommendations or criteria exist for stopping a suspected causal drug or managing leukopenia
Thrombocytopenia		
Carbamazepine	Case reports without known incident rate	Discontinue if platelets counts drop to <100 000 per mm^3
Divalproex	Case reports; defined usually by serum platelets <140 000 × 10^9 per L	Thought to reflect a dose-related toxicity state, usually remits with dosage reductions without need for drug discontinuation

Abbreviations: ANC = absolute neutrophil count; CBC = complete blood count; FGA = first-generation antipsychotics; SGA = second-generation antipsychotics; WBC = white blood cell

Table 10.2 Pharmacological strategies to counteract psychotropic-induced sexual dysfunction

Agent	Rationale	Clinical findings
Amantadine 50–100 mg PO qDay	Dopamine agonist	Favorable case reports overcoming SSRI-associated anorgasmia; though negative small placebo-controlled trials (Michelson et al., 2000)
Bupropion 150–300 mg PO qDay	Pro-dopaminergic, noradrenergic agent	One positive and two negative placebo-controlled trials added to SSRIs in remitted depressed patients (reviewed by Goldberg and Ernst, 2019)
Buspirone 20–60 mg PO qDay	$5HT_{1A}$ partial agonist	One positive and one negative placebo-controlled trial as adjuncts to SSRIs; low dosing may have underestimated potential magnitude of effect
Cyproheptadine 4–12 mg PO 1–2 hours before sexual activity	Serotonin antagonist	Open trials added to SSRIs show improved ejaculation delay in men; no RCTs (reviewed by Goldberg and Ernst, 2019)
Mirtazapine 15–30 mg PO qDay	$5HT_{2A}$ antagonist	Favorable open trial data as adjunct to SSRIs in remitted depressed patients (Ozmenler et al., 2008) but RCT data no different from placebo (Michelson et al., 2002)
Sildenafil 50–100 mg/day	PDE inhibitor	Two positive RCTs in men, one positive RCT in women (reviewed by Goldberg and Ernst, 2019), but may be a cumbersome long-term strategy
Trazodone 50–100 mg PO qDay	$5HT_{2A}$ antagonist	Favorable open trial data added to SSRIs in remitted depressed men and women (reviewed by Goldberg and Ernst, 2019)
Yohimbine 6 g PO qDay	Presynaptic α_2 antagonist, increases noradrenergic tone	Favorable effects shown mostly in open trials added to SSRIs; potential for significant hypertension, tachycardia, anxiety, psychosis (reviewed by Goldberg and Ernst, 2019)

Abbreviations: PO = by mouth; qDay = once daily; PDE = phosphodiesterase; RCT = randomized controlled trial; SSRI = selective serotonin reuptake inhibitor

Table 10.3 Pharmacological strategies to counter iatrogenic weight gain; appetite suppressants

Agent	Clinical context	Findings
Amantadine 300 mg PO qDay	Shown to help delay or prevent (more than reverse) iatrogenic weight gain when coprescribed with olanzapine (and may also help cognition, negative symptoms, pseudoparkinsonism)	Meta-analysis of five RCTs (mean of eight weeks) showed greater mean weight loss (–2.22 kg) than with placebo (Zheng et al., 2017a)
Bupropion 150–300 mg PO qDay (± naltrexone)	Prior to its incarnation as an antidepressant, bupropion was originally developed as a weight loss drug. Its weight loss effects can synergize with naltrexone (dosed from 100–300 mg/day) to create do-it-yourself Contrave®. Has not formally been studied as a potential antidote to psychotropic-induced weight gain. (Parsimony beckons its use for depressed overweight smokers who binge drink alcohol.)	In otherwise healthy obese adults, 55% taking bupropion + naltrexone lost >5% of their initial weight; mean weight loss at one year ~5 kg more than with placebo (Khera et al., 2016)
Phentermine 37.5 mg PO qAM	Most modern studies focus on the combination of phentermine + topiramate rather than phentermine monotherapy for weight loss in obese but otherwise healthy adults. No RCTs specifically to counteract iatrogenic weight gain. Despite its sympathomimetic properties as an amphetamine analogue, phentermine has *not* been shown to increase heart rate or blood pressure (Hendricks et al., 2011)	Recognized as monotherapy by the FDA only for short-term (12 weeks) use, although RCT data are available up to 36 weeks and open data report outcomes up to 104 weeks (Hendricks et al., 2011)
Topiramate 100–200 mg PO qDay	The mechanism by which topiramate can cause appetite suppression and weight loss is unknown. May be combined with phentermine to create do-it-yourself Qsymia®	Over 44 weeks, obese adults lost ~15% of their initial body weight (Astrup et al., 2004). Combined with phentermine for one year, mean weight loss = 8.8 kg (Khera et al., 2016). The combination of topiramate + phentermine is among the most likely of pharmacological strategies to achieve loss of ≥5% of initial body weight (Khera et al., 2016)
Zonisamide 200–400 mg PO qday	Anticonvulsant drug that has shown greater efficacy than placebo for weight loss in healthy adults as well as schizophrenia patients taking SGAs	One-year RCT in obese adults: zomisamide dosed at 400 mg/day produced significantly more weight loss (7.3 kg) than did placebo + diet and lifestyle counseling (Gadde et al., 2012). Ten-week RCT in schizophrenia yielded greater weight loss than placebo (mean difference = –0.8 kg) during SGA treatment (Ghanizadeh et al., 2013)

Abbreviations: FDA = US Food and Drug Administration; PO = by mouth; qAM = once daily in the morning; qDay = once daily; RCT = randomized controlled trial; SGA = second-generation antipsychotic

Table 10.4 Pharmacological strategies to counter iatrogenic weight gain: putative metabolic regulators

Agent	Clinical Context	Findings
Liraglutide titrated to 3 mg SC qDay	Classified as an incretin mimetic or glucagon-like peptide 1 (GLP-1) receptor agonist, liraglutide has been studied in placebo-controlled trials to counteract weight gain and metabolic dysregulation from clozapine or olanzapine in schizophrenia patients	Added to olanzapine or clozapine over 16 weeks, body weight decreased significantly more than placebo (mean difference = 5.3 kg) as did glucose intolerance, waist circumference, systolic blood pressure, visceral fat and low density lipoprotein (LDL) cholesterol (Larsen et al., 2017); adverse effects were mainly gastrointestinal
Metformin (usually dosed 500 mg PO BID to 1000 mg PO TID)	Oral hypoglycemic that decreases insulin sensitivity, may help promote weight loss from SGAs by helping to overcome iatrogenic insulin resistance (e.g., when weight gain occurs despite awareness of any appetite stimulation)	Meta-analysis of 12 RCTs versus placebo for SGA-related weight gain revealed mean weight loss of −3.27 kg and diminished insulin resistance (de Silva et al., 2016)
Orlistat 360 mg PO qDay	A gastric and pancreatic lipase inhibitor that blocks intestinal fat absorption, studied for up to 16 weeks in both open and randomized placebo-controlled trials to counteract olanzapine- or clozapine-associated weight gain	Approximate 1–2 kg weight loss, men > women. For noniatrogenic weight gain, observed mean weight loss of 2.6 kg (pooled RCT data) after one year (Khera et al., 2016). May cause bloating, steatorrhea, anal leakage

Abbreviations: BID = twice a day; PO = by mouth; qDay = once daily; RCT = randomized controlled trial; SC = subcutaneous; SGA = second-generation antipsychotic; TID = three times a day

Table 10.5 Strategies to optimize psychotropic drug tolerability: anticonvulsants and lithium

Agent	Optimal management of adverse effects
Carbamazepine	- ~10% develop benign leukopenia in first three months; aplastic anemia is exceedingly rare (1 in 200 000 exposures); some experts favor measuring a CBC at baseline and then periodically for the first few months, but no standard of care has been established - Remember potent induction of P450 substrates, Phase II metabolism substrates, and autoinduction
Divalproex	- Serum valproate levels >90–100 g/mL tend to confer no psychotropic benefit but mainly cause nausea, sedation, and tremor - There is no reason to monitor serum ammonia levels in the absence of a clinical indication. High ammonia levels (e.g., >130 µg/dL) in symptomatic patients (lethargy, mental slowing) can usually be countered with *l*-carnitine 1000 mg PO BID - Thrombocytopenia may occur in up to 10–20% of patients taking divalproex and is thought to reflect a dose-related toxicity; dosage reductions should rectify identified casehood - If tremor, assure nontoxic serum level; can treat with propranolol (if no asthma and no cardiac contraindication) or primidone (but beware of induction of P450 substrates) - Pancreatitis is a rare adverse effect but laboratory assessment (serum lipase, amylase) should occur for patients who develop acute abdominal symptoms
Gabapentin	- Sedation is common (favor the majority of dosing at night) - Small bowel drug absorption via the amino acid transport system is saturable and likely unable to absorb more than 5000 mg/24 hours
Lamotrigine	- Risk for serious rash is greatest in weeks 2-8; watch for systemic symptoms and oropharyngeal blistering-like lesions; treat obviously benign rashes with topical steroid creams, antihistamines; if uncertain etiology, stop lamotrigine. Manufacturer advises restarting of titration schedule if patients have been off drug for more than five days - Rechallenge after benign rash using low dosing and rash precautions often yields outcomes with favorable tolerability, provided less than three associated signs of rash seriousness (e.g., exfoliation, blistering/tenderness, mucous membrane involvement, lymphadenopathy, fever/malaise/arthralgias, leukocytosis, transaminitis) (Aiken and Orr, 2010) - Remember to halve dose if coadministered with divalproex and double dose if used in conjunction with carbamazepine - Serum lamotrigine levels are normed for epilepsy and generally not informative about psychotropic efficacy
Lithium	- Once-daily dosing minimizes potential renal toxicity - If tremor, assure nontoxic serum level; can treat with propranolol (if no asthma and no cardiac contraindication) or primidone (mindful of induced metabolism of cotherapies that are P450 substrates) - Can treat urinary frequency or nephrogenic diabetes insipidus with amiloride 5 mg PO BID - reduce dose by 20% if NSAIDs are coadministered; monitor levels closely also with coadministered thiazide diuretics
Pregabalin	- Sedation and dizziness are most common adverse effects, may be dose-related or require slower titrations to accommodate
Topiramate	- Adverse cognitive effects may be dose-related and occur in a *minority* of patients - Beware ~1/100 risk for nephrolithiasis, watch for low back pain and dysuria, or appearance of calcium oxalate crystals on urinalysis (discontinue drug)

Abbreviations: BID = twice daily; CBC = complete blood count; NSAID = nonsteroidal anti-inflammatory; PO = by mouth

Table 10.6 Strategies to optimize psychotropic drug tolerability: monoaminergic antidepressants

MAOIs	- Suspected hypertensive crises (e.g., headache) should be assessed by prompt blood pressure monitoring and referred to the emergency department if significant; once-popular home use of oral or sublingual nifedipine in such settings is no longer considered safe or appropriate (Grossman et al., 1996) - Orthostatic hypotension is dose-related and, if not improved through hydration and oral salt supplementation, may be manageable by adding fludrocortisone 0.1–0.2 mg/day (watch for hypokalemia) or midrodine 5 mg PO TID
SSRIs	- Sexual dysfunction may be manageable with adjunctive buspirone (>40 mg/day) or buspirone (300 mg/day), cyproheptadine (4–12 mg 1–2 hours before sexual activity) or adding a phosphodiesterase inhibitor for either men or women (e.g., sildenafil); otherwise switching to vilazodone, mirtazapine, nefazodone, or bupropion are the most evidence- (or rationale-) based alternatives
SNRIs	Mild, dose-related diastolic hypertension (<5 mmHg) is rarer with desvenlafaxine (~1% incidence) or venlafaxine XR (≤3% incidence) than venlafaxine IR (3–13%); favor non-noradrenergic antidepressants in the setting of baseline poorly controlled hypertension - No good data on whether SNRIs are more or less likely than SSRIs to cause adverse sexual effects. Management strategy options are similar to those for SSRIs
Tricyclics	- Anticholinergic effects (dry mouth, sedation, constipation) are usually manageable with conservative/over-the-counter remedies. Case reports describe successful treatment of severe anticholinergic-induced constipation with the muscarinic agonist bethanechol (10–25 mg PO TID).

Abbreviations: IR = immediate release; MAOI = monoamine oxidase inhibitor; PO = by mouth; SNRI = serotonin-norepinephrine reuptake inhibitor; SSRI = selective serotonin reuptake inhibitor; TID = three times a day; XR = extended release

Table 10.7 Strategies to optimize psychotropic drug tolerability: antipsychotics

SGAs	- Can treat clozapine-associated sialorrhea with sublingual ipratropium bromide 0.03% nasal spray, or atropine sulfate 1% ophthalmic solution - antipsychotic-associated sedation can often be managed by favoring less antihistaminergic agents when feasible (e.g., lurasidone, iloperidone, aripiprazole), dosing the majority of drug at bed time, minimizing sedating cotherapies (e.g., benzodiazepines) or augmenting with (ar)modafinil; adjunctive amphetamine or methylphenidate should be used cautiously with attention to possible exacerbations of psychosis - Can potentially minimize SGA-associated weight gain with amantadine 100–300 mg/day; most potent and evidence-based pharmacotherapies to counter iatrogenic weight gain include metformin, liraglutide, topiramate, sibutramine - Track weight, fasting glucose or hemoglobin A1c, lipids, and intervene sooner than later if anomalies become evident - Monitor regularly for abnormal involuntary movements (e.g., formal AIMS assessment every six months (every three months for patients >age 50)) - Differentiate akathisia from anxiety/agitation; manage with antipsychotic dosage reductions when feasible or else adjunctive benzodiazepines or beta-blockers (not anticholinergics)

Abbreviations: AIMS = Abnormal Involuntary Movement Scale; SGA = second-generation antipsychotic

11 Novel Drug Therapeutics: Nutraceuticals, Steroids, Probiotics, and Other Dietary Supplements

LEARNING OBJECTIVES

- ☐ Understand safety concerns for patients who take nutraceutical products, from both a pharmacokinetic and a pharmacodynamic perspective
- ☐ Recognize the distinction between repletion versus supplementation of dietary vitamins or other nutritional supplements
- ☐ Appreciate the highly variable evidence base for claims of psychotropic efficacy for specific nutritional supplements

Let not thy food be confused with thy medicine.

- Diane Cardenas, on misquotation attributed to Hippocrates

The relationship between food products and pharmacodynamically active agents traces at least to antiquity, even if Hippocrates never actually did say "let food be thy medicine and medicine be thy food" (Cardenas, 2013). In modern times the relationship between dietary supplements and medicine has come to pose a rather peculiar dichotomy between what might be called "legitimate" or "mainstream" medicine and nonstandard or "alternative" medicine. Interventions in the latter category suffer from issues of credibility due to an often less rigorous RCT database, at times poorly established rationales and/or mechanisms of action, and lack of regulatory agency product oversight for quality assurance purposes. Many patients obtain information about herbal products or dietary supplements simply from internet searches with little awareness of the scientific rigor or credibility behind advertising claims or consumer postings and testimonials, or cognizance of potential pharmacokinetic interactions.

Proponents of nutritional supplements sometimes conflate "natural" with "safe," despite the plethora of poisonous natural substances (e.g., hemlock, arsenic, cyanide, strychnine, mercury, and tetrodotoxin) devoid of therapeutic value except perhaps as defenses against predators. A study of 121 Ayurvedic or Chinese herbal natural health products found that most contained measurable levels of toxic elements (notably, lead, mercury, cadmium, arsenic, and aluminum), though fewer than 10% of products tested had levels exceeding the established daily limit of toxicant exposure (Genuis et al., 2012). Safety and efficacy command equal importance throughout medicine, no more nor less for psychopharmacology in particular, regardless of whether a compound is "natural" or synthetic. And while even placebos can have adverse effects, and sometimes exert astonishing potency (see Chapter 4), products that are entirely harmless still pose the hazard of being ineffective as compared to those that are better (and have large effect sizes) relative to placebo.

Ancient Cures

In the eighteenth century, tobacco smoke enemas were considered state-of-the-art remedies for both epilepsy and respiratory failure; fried pigeon dung was a first-line treatment for dyspepsia; white lead was used to stop hemorrhaging or diarrhea; and dried toad was believed to cure asthma. Such practices have long been abandoned by traditional medicine without the necessity of RCTs to establish their lack of efficacy.

When little or no data exist to guide treatment decisions, practitioners are more vulnerable to clinical impressionism or other low-tier levels of evidence (see Chapter 1, Figure 1.1). Many nutraceutical products that predate modern practices have garnered popularity because their perceived pharmacodynamic effects have been reinforced by cultural lore (e.g., "used for centuries" by ancient civilizations) or anecdote, sometimes underscored by dramatic endorsements from sufferers or practitioners. Certainly, there are times when the potential value of an intervention is so intuitively obvious and compelling that RCTs appear unnecessary – as in the utility of parachutes during airplane jumps. (But, consider that comparative trials would still be needed to judge how well parachutes fare in comparison to, say, jet packs, or knowing when two or three parachutes may produce a better effect than just one or two, or deciding when dome-canopy versus annular or ram-air designs deliver a better result, or whether nylon versus silk versus terylene construction tends to land jumpers more safely and soundly.) Lead – albeit a natural substance – probably makes a parachute less useful than having none at all.

Finer Point on the Need for Placebo-controlled Trials

When leaping from an airplane (recall from Chapter 1), note that altitude is a critical moderator of response to parachute efficacy; parachutes have been shown not to reduce death or major trauma when deployed from stationary aircraft on the ground (Yeh et al., 2018).

Psychotropic drugs are parachutes for when mental health enters into free fall. Marketers of dietary supplements often tout nonspecific and/or nebulous mental health benefits such as "relief of nervous tension or stress," "improves mental and physical performance," "enhances overall vitality," or "body cleansers" – variables that are difficult to quantify or translate into tangible targets when treating psychopathology. In this chapter, we will direct our focus on the existing evidence base for the relative safety and psychotropic efficacy of nutritional or dietary supplements, examining specific intended targets of mental health treatment.

A DEFINING TERMINOLOGY: DIETARY SUPPLEMENTS

Exact terminology varies across countries, but broadly speaking, food products that may have pharmacodynamic effects have been referred to as dietary supplements, nutraceuticals, functional foods, phytochemicals, biochemopreventatives, or designer foods. In Japan, such products are called foods for special health use (FOSHU). "Natural health products" is the preferred category descriptor in Canada (where a government database maintains up-to-date information on product safety and efficacy (www.canada.ca/en/health-canada/services/drugs-health-products/natural-non-prescription/applications-submissions/product-licensing/licensed-natural-health-products-database.html)). The term *nutraceutical* was coined in 1989 by Stephen DeFelice of the Foundation of Innovative Medicine and encompasses dietary supplements, isolated nutrients, and herbal products. Under the Dietary Supplement Health and Education Act, "dietary ingredients" found in dietary supplements may include "vitamins, minerals, herbs, amino acids, enzymes, organ tissues, glandulars, and metabolites."

The National Institute of Health's Center for Complementary and Integrative Health estimates that about 59 million Americans annually spend over $30 billion out of pocket on dietary health supplements (https://nccih.nih.gov/research/statistics/NHIS/2012).

DSHEA

The Dietary Supplement Health and Education Act (DSHEA) of 1984 defined "dietary supplements" as food exempt from FDA oversight or regulation. There is no federal scrutiny over the safety or efficacy of dietary supplements or their promotional marketing, although regulation 21 CFR part 111 requires "good manufacturing practice conditions" for US-made dietary supplements.

B SAFETY CONCERNS

One concern about product quality control, in the absence of regulatory agency oversight, involves the potential for high variability in the actual content of marketed products. For example, one study of 31 over-the-counter melatonin products in Canada found that actual melatonin content (relative to the amount claimed to be in the product) varied from −83% to +478% (Erland et al., 2017). Pharmacokinetic (as well as adverse additive pharmacodynamic) interactions also rank high on the list of safety concerns and have garnered formal study through pharmacokinetic investigations only fairly recently.

Table 11.1 summarizes pharmacokinetic effects, as well as examples of pharmacodynamic adverse effects, related to common nutraceuticals.

In a comprehensive review of pharmacokinetic (PK) interactions with "natural products," Sprouse and van Breemen (2016) found no evidence of adverse PK effects associated with acai (*Euterpe oleracea*), cinnamon (*Cinnamomum* spp.), elderberry (*Sambucus nigra*), flax seed (*Linum usitatissimum*), ginger (*Zingiber officinale*), horny goat weed (*Epimedium spp*), or maca (Lepidium *meyenii*), among others.

C "REPLETION"

The concept of repletion, or replenishment, pertains to compensating for deficiencies of an endogenous compound that has caused (or could cause) a pathological state. Common examples in medicine include the intravenous repletion of fluids or electrolytes after intractable vomiting, or replenishment of packed red blood cells after hemorrhage. Gross deficiencies of essential[1] vitamins and minerals lead to well-recognized disease states (e.g., rickets from vitamin D deficiency; scurvy from vitamin C deficiency; osteomalacia from calcium deficiency). Less well-established in clinical psychopharmacology is the concept of "repleting" dietary nutrients in the absence of known or obvious deficiencies, with the hope of resultant psychiatric benefits. (Recall from Chapter 8 the lack of demonstrated empirical evidence for "repleting" *L*-methylfolate specifically in depressed patients with the MTHFR low activity polymorphism.) In the absence of nutritional deficiencies, the psychotropic value of administering vitamins and trace minerals remains a matter of debate. One relevant consideration involves the expected presence of more systemic phenomena resulting from the suspected clinically meaningful deficiency of an essential vitamin or trace mineral. Tables 11.2 and 11.4 summarize medical and psychiatric manifestations of deficient levels of fat-soluble and non-fat-soluble vitamins, respectively, as well as potential adverse effects of excessive dosing.

D WHEN DID VITAMIN D BECOME A CELEBRITY?

Purported links between vitamin D deficiency and a host of medical conditions, including depression, have received tremendous attention in the popular media. However, according to the US Preventative Services Task Force, *proactive screening and oral supplementation yield no conclusive health benefits outside of high risk populations* (i.e., those with low dietary intake, malabsorption, inflammatory bowel disease, a history of gastric bypass, dark skin pigmentation, and restricted or minimal sunlight exposure) (www .uspreventiveservicestaskforce.org/Page/Document/

CLINICAL VIGNETTE 11.1

Devin was a 25-year-old man with chronic schizophrenia, multiple hospitalizations, persistent psychosis, and persistently poor functioning despite multiple adequate trials of SGAs including olanzapine up to 40 mg/day and clozapine up to 400 mg/day. His spouse asked his primary care doctor to measure Devin's 25-OH-D3 level and when it came back low at 19 ng/mL she wondered if this was at long last the "missing link" that could finally now explain his condition. She exhorted Devin's psychiatrist to "replenish" his vitamin D with 50 000 IU cholecalciferol weekly. The psychiatrist was happy to add vitamin D but expressed skepticism about the likelihood that the low vitamin D level was causing his schizophrenia (and suggested that a more likely scenario was that his social isolation and limited exposure to sunlight was probably more its result than cause) and instead suggested that consideration might be given to ECT as a heroic measure for refractory multidrug-resistant psychosis. Rejecting his suggestion, the spouse ended Devin's treatment with the psychiatrist in order to find a different doctor who would be "more open minded" about treating the nutritional deficiencies she believed were causing Devin's psychiatric problems.

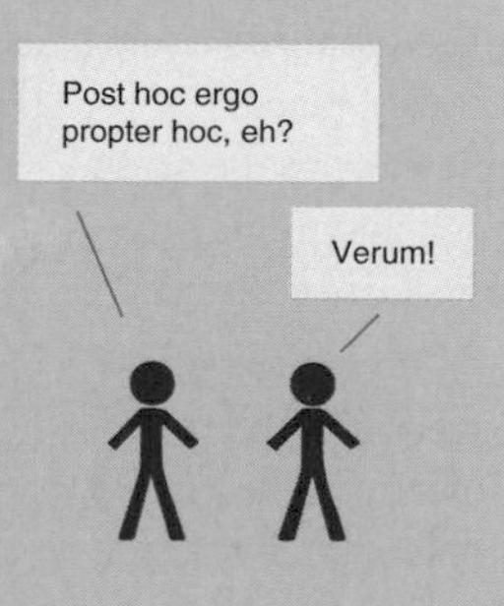
Post hoc ergo propter hoc, eh?
Verum!

1 "Essential" vitamins or other nutrients are thusly named because the body cannot synthesize them.

Box 11.1

Treatment of Low Serum Vitamin D

The treatment of low vitamin D levels depends in part on how low measured serum levels actually are. Very low levels (i.e., <12 ng/mL) likely warrant a medical workup to assess osteomalacia. Repletion usually involves a loading dose of cholecalciferol (vitamin D3) 50 000 IU orally once weekly for 6–8 weeks or three times per week for one month, and then rechecking serum 25-(OH)D levels. Baseline serum levels of 12–20 ng/mL usually can be managed with over-the-counter ergocalciferol (vitamin D2) 1000 IU daily with rechecking of labwork after about two months. Serum levels of 20–30 ng/mL can usually be effectively treated with vitamin D2 600–800 IU daily and a reassessment of labwork after several months. Maintenance/prevention oral daily dosing of 800–2000 IU is often then recommended if risk factors for recurrent deficiency remain (Kennel et al., 2010).

RecommendationStatementFinal/vitamin-d-deficiency-screening#Pod4). "Low" serum levels of 25-hydroxy-vitamin D (25-OH-D) are generally defined as <20–30 ng/mL. Associations have been reported between clinical depression and low vitamin D levels (e.g., Anglin et al., 2013; Ju et al., 2013), but causality remains poorly demonstrated (i.e., do low vitamin D levels lead to depression or does depression tend to limit sunlight exposure and appropriate dietary intake?). Existing studies are mainly cross-sectional (Ju et al., 2013) and do not account for possible confounding factors in the relationship (such as previous depressive episodes or lifestyle factors). The perils of emotional overinvestment in low vitamin D levels as explaining the pathogenesis of severe psychopathology are illustrated in Clinical Vignette 11.1. Once-held theories about other vitamin deficiencies as the supposed etiology of major psychiatric disorders (notably, niacin deficiency as the cause of schizophrenia) are described in Box 11.2.

Tip

The Centers for Disease Control estimates that only about 30% of Whites and 5% of African Americans have sufficient vitamin D levels (defined as >30 ng/mL) (Ginde et al., 2009).

With respect to treatment, as shown in Table 11.1, supplemental vitamin D (administered orally as 50 000 IU cholecalciferol/week for anywhere from 8–52 weeks or 1500 IU vitamin D PO qDay or a single dose of 300 000/150 000 IU cholecalciferol IM) may be associated with antidepressant efficacy in depressed patients – but existing studies are few, do not account for baseline vitamin D deficiencies relative to depression severity, and await more definitive replication. Parameters for the treatment of vitamin D deficiency are further described in Box 11.1.

Other theories of historical interest linking vitamin deficiencies with major form of psychopathology include links between niacin (vitamin B3) deficiency and schizophrenia, as described in Box 11.2.

Information about the rationale and evidence base for taking supplemental vitamins for psychiatric purposes is summarized in Tables 11.3 and 11.5.

Box 11.2

The Adrenochrome Hypothesis of Schizophrenia

In the 1950s, Canadian psychiatrist Dr. Abram Hoffer proposed that niacin deficiency could cause schizophrenia. He reasoned that adrenochrome (an oxidative metabolite of epinephrine) induced psychosis and suspected that schizophrenia resulted from "leakage of adrenochrome and its derivatives into the blood and into the brain" (Hoffer, 1994) and was therefore remediable by high-dose niacin with vitamin C. This etiopathological model was bolstered slightly by observations that schizophrenia patients may have an attenuated "skin flush" response to niacin, and suggestions that impaired skin flush response to niacin may be an endophenotypic marker found in unaffected siblings of schizophrenic probands (Chang et al., 2009).

Despite being one of the first studies to draw attention to antioxidant defense systems in the pathogenesis and treatment of severe psychopathology, the concept that schizophrenia arises from the hallucinogenic effects of stress hormone metabolites has fallen out of favor, taking with it the putative antipsychotic value of vitamin B3 – largely due to the failure of RCTs to demonstrate efficacy of high-dose niacin as impacting any domains of psychiatric symptoms or psychosocial functioning in schizophrenia (e.g., Wittenborn et al., 1973).

E MACRO- AND TRACE MINERALS

The potential importance of macro-minerals (such as calcium and magnesium) and trace elements (such as zinc, selenium, copper, iron, and manganese) has gained growing attention in studies of the pathophysiology of depression, schizophrenia, autism, dementia, and a host of other psychiatric and nonpsychiatric maladies. Once again, random internet searches open the door into a Wild West of information that is often sensationalist, scientifically unmonitored, and virtually impossible to navigate for technical accuracy and medical credibility, even by mental health professionals, much less by intelligent lay people. Advocates of evidence-based medicine are, as always, encouraged to search Index Medicus and the medically peer-reviewed literature in order to obtain reliable information.

Table 11.6 summarizes basic knowledge about the known physiological effects and psychiatric relevance of essential minerals, and the rationales and evidence base (if any) for exceeding US recommended dietary allowance (RDA) recommendations when known deficiencies are absent. In some instances, *relative* intake bears on traditional health recommendations – for example, zinc:copper ratios (ideally 1:8 according to the National Academy of Sciences) are thought to be more important than the measurement of either of these metals alone, or zinc supplements may decrease GI chromium absorption. Lithium orotate is another example of an elemental "nutrient" with supposed health benefits – and popular misperception as a viable alternative to prescription lithium carbonate or lithium citrate – as described in Box 11.3.

F DO NUTRACEUTICALS CROSS THE BLOOD–BRAIN BARRIER? OR, WHEN YOU CAN'T GET THERE FROM HERE

Among dietary supplements that are herbal products or intended precursors for neurotransmitter synthesis, a key concern involves whether it is possible to "boost" neurotransmitter precursors in order to increase the physiological availability or function of their CNS end products. Related to this issue is the question of whether dietary neurotransmitter supplements cross the blood–brain barrier (BBB). Most circulatory amino acids require a facilitative transport system to traverse the BBB but even when such transport mechanisms exist, entry is usually not in appreciable quantities. Hence, BBB entry remains the subject of debate in the case of orally consumed GABA (at least in humans (Boonstra et al., 2015)) and glutamate (Hawkins, 2009). Serotonin does not cross the BBB but its precursors,

Box 11.3

What is Lithium Orotate and Does it Work?

Elemental lithium must be noncovalently bound to an anion in order for its safe bioavailability from dietary ingestion. Carbonic acid or citric acid are the most widely used compounds for this purpose (lithium chloride was briefly popularized in the 1940s as a viable alternative form of table salt to sodium chloride with possibly less adverse impact of cardiovascular health - until its renal and thyroid toxicity became apparent). Orotic acid combined with elemental lithium creates lithium orotate, which contains 3.83 mg elemental lithium per 100 mg (by contrast, lithium carbonate contains 18.8 mg per 100 mg). This means that lithium orotate would need to be dosed about three times higher than lithium carbonate to achieve comparable brain levels. A 120 mg tablet of lithium orotate contains about 5 mg of elemental lithium, in contrast to a 300 mg tablet of lithium carbonate containing about 56 mg of elemental lithium.

There has been very little empirical study of the safety and efficacy of lithium orotate in humans, and no published RCTs for its use in the treatment of bipolar disorder. Proponents have anecdotally claimed value for its use in the possible prevention of dementia and the effects of aging. Human clinical trials are limited to a small open-label case series describing its potential value dosed at 150 mg PO qDay in alcoholism (Sartori, 1986). Animal studies have raised concern about substantial nephrotoxicity at doses comparable to those of lithium carbonate (Smith and Schou, 1979). In the absence of more extensive data on both safety and efficacy, the possible psychiatric benefits of lithium orotate would not at present be considered evidence-based.

Figure 11.1 Serotonin synthesis.

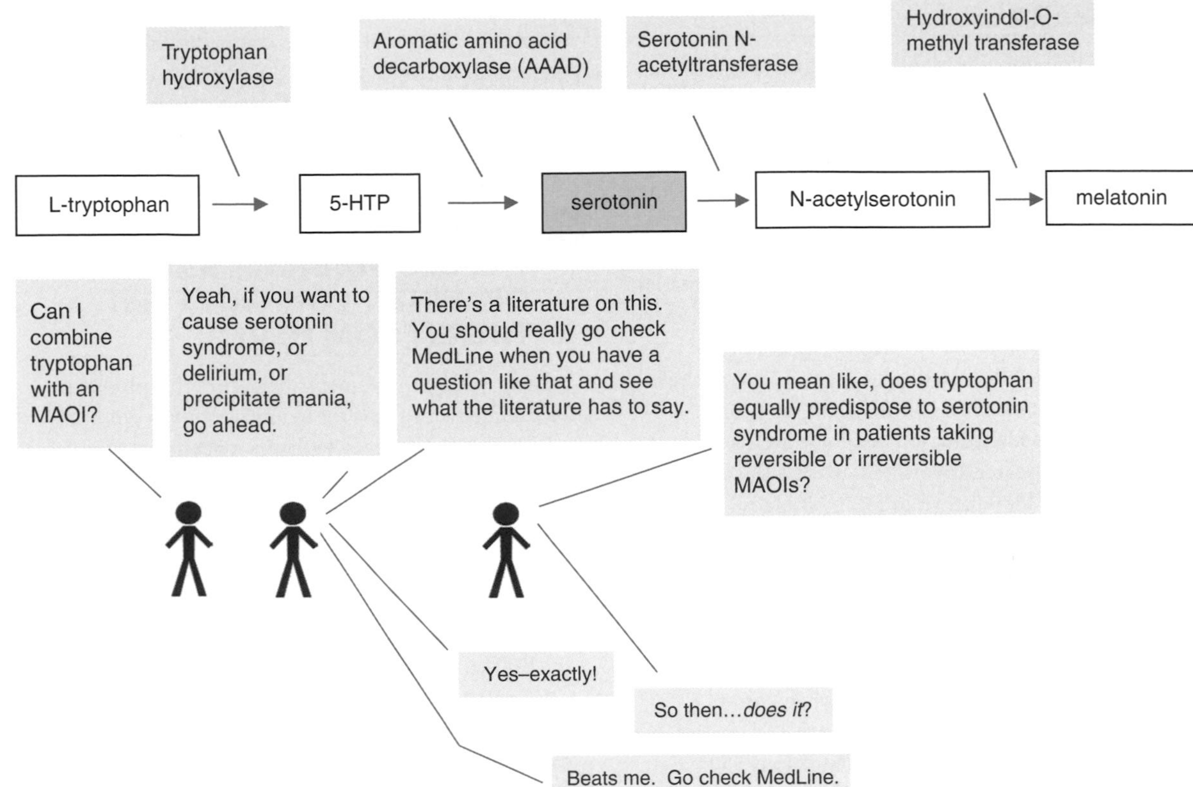

5-hydroxytryptophan (5HTP) and *l*-tryptophan (see Figure 11.1), both do so readily.

Tables 11.7–11.0, respectively, summarize information about the possible psychotropic relevance of nonprescription supplemental neurotransmitters (e.g., GABA, 5HTP, taurine), steroids (e.g., DHEA, melatonin, pregnenolone), herbs (e.g., *Ginkgo biloba*, St. John's wort, kava), and other compounds (e.g., amino acids, enzymes, cofactors) alongside their potential risks.

Box 11.4

What About Cannabidiol?

Derived from the glandular trichomes (plant hairs) of *Cannabis sativa*, cannabidiol (CBD) is a phytocannabinoid that is technically considered to be nonpsychoactive, but has gained increasing interest for its putative anticonvulsant, anxiolytic, sedative-hypnotic, neurotrophic, anti-inflammatory, antioxidant, analgesic, and possible antipsychotic properties, coupled with low observed toxicity or abuse potential in human and animal studies. Unlike tetrahydrocannabinoid (Δ9-THC), CBD has low binding affinity to cannabinoid receptors (CBD1 and CBD2) but may function as a CBD2 inverse agonist (Thomas et al., 2007). Its reputed anxiolytic effects (in contrast to the more common *anxiogenic* effects of Δ9-THC) are known mainly from preclinical studies (reviewed by Scuderi et al., 2009). Among drug-abstinent adults with heroin use disorder, an RCT of CBD dosed at 400 or 800 mg/day for three days significantly reduced cue-induced craving and anxiety better than placebo (Hurd et al., 2019). An exploratory six-week RCT of CBD 1000 mg/day or placebo added to antipsychotic medications in 88 schizophrenia patients revealed greater improvement in positive symptoms and global improvement (McGuire et al., 2018). Blessing et al. (2015) advise oral dosing from 300–600 mg/day as useful for anxiety disorders. Broader controlled trials of CBD for anxiolytic, antipsychotic, or other possible psychotropic effects in humans are needed, alongside long-term studies, before a more generalizable evidence base can be established. Additionally, quality assurance remains a concern with the production of nonregulated over-the-counter formulations, particularly vaporization liquid and CBD oil; one study found 43% of online cannabidiol products had less actual CBD content while 31% had higher content than their labels advertised (Bonn-Miller et al., 2017).

In 2018 cannabidiol was approved under the brand name Epidiolex® for the treatment of seizures in two developmental forms of childhood epilepsy (Lennox-Gastaut syndrome and Dravet syndrome). Somnolence, fatigue, diarrhea, and GI distress may occur as adverse effects. For more on the possible anxiolytic properties of CBD, see Chapter 17.

Definitions

Phytocannabinoids are exogenous, naturally occurring cannabinoids, in contrast to endogenous (endocannabinoids) or synthetic cannabinoids.

Hemp refers to the fiber of the *Cannabis sativa* plant. It contains <0.3% Δ9-THC.

Cannabis indica tends to have lower Δ9-THC and higher CBD content than does *Cannabis sativa*, although hybrid strains often make their distinction difficult. Aficionados often describe *indica* as more likely to produce relaxation, anxiolysis, and antinociceptive effects while *sativa* tends to be more associated with euphoria, energy, and psychedelic effects.

Speaking of herbs, let us give special consideration to cannabidiol (CBD), as discussed in Box 11.4.

G ONE-CARBON NUTRACEUTICALS, S-ADENOSYLMETHIONINE, AND DEPRESSION

In amino acid metabolism, folic acid, vitamin B2, vitamin B6, and vitamin B12 are all involved as coenzymes in the transfer of one-carbon donor molecules (usually from serine or glycine) to tetrahydrofolate. One-carbon transfer reactions are needed to convert homocysteine to methionine to S-adenosylmethionine, in turn methylating downstream targets (e.g., DNA, as a way to modify its function). As shown in Figure 11.2, B vitamins

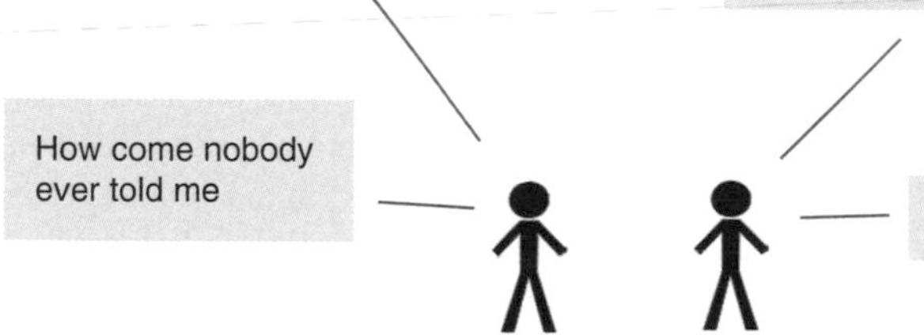

Figure 11.2 Simplified depiction of one-carbon transfer. Abbreviations: MTHFR = methylenetetrahydrofolate reductase; SAH = S-adenosylhomocysteine; SAMe = S-adenosylmethionine

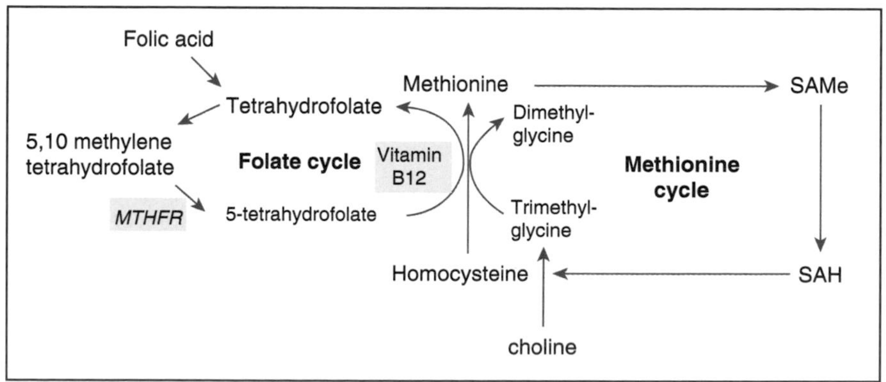

and reduced homocysteine are necessary cofactors for the synthesis of CNS monoamines. Vitamin B12 deficiency causes elevation of serum homocysteine levels, while folic acid is necessary for the synthesis of tetrahydrofolate and maintenance of the folate cycle.

There has been much interest in the potential psychotropic effects of dietary supplementation with components of one-carbon transfer biochemical processes because of their ultimate necessity for the synthesis of dopamine, serotonin, and acetylcholine. Conceptually, it is also worth noting that:

- Folic acid must be methylated in order to cross the BBB (*L*-methylfolate), for which intact MTHFR activity (and vitamin B12 availability) is necessary.
- Dietary supplementation with SAMe "bypasses" this step altogether.

Does dietary supplementation with one-carbon metabolism components actually translate to observable improvement in depression symptoms? Sarris and colleagues (2016) examined 15 datasets involving SAMe (800–1600 mg/day), folic acid (0.5–10 mg/day), methylfolate (15–30 mg/day), vitamin B6, and vitamin B12 in the treatment of depression. In their meta-analysis, no significant differences were found in depression outcomes between folic acid and placebo (Hedge's g = 0.487, p = 0.233). In contrast, four open-label or placebo-controlled trials of SAMe in TRD revealed significant improvement compared to placebo.

In major depressive disorder, Mech and Farah (2016) found superiority to placebo using a monotherapy proprietary combination of reduced B9 vitamins plus micronutrients.[2]

H SHOULD I USE *L*-METHYLFOLATE, AND IF SO, WHEN?

Folic acid must undergo methylation in order to cross the BBB. *L*-methylfolate, a necessary cofactor for monoamine synthesis, is a nutritional supplement that could allow for greater bioavailability of folic acid deliverable to the CNS. RCTs of *L*-methylfolate in depression have yielded mixed results: when added to an ineffective SSRI (held at constant dose), initial *L*-methylfolate dosing of 7.5 mg/day for one month followed by 15 mg/day dosing for one month was no better than placebo; however adjunctive dosing of 15 mg/day throughout a 60-day period improved depressive symptoms better than SSRI plus placebo (Papakostas et al., 2012a). As noted in Chapter 8, contrary to expectations, the MTHFR genotype has *not* been shown to predict *L*-methylfolate response in MDD. *L*-methylfolate appears to be a safe option in MDD, but further studies are needed to render more definitive information about which patients have a greater or lesser likelihood for benefit.

In schizophrenia, a meta-analysis of RCTs involving folate or *L*-methylfolate added to dopamine-blocking drugs demonstrated a significant advantage over placebo for improving negative symptoms, although the effect size was small ($d = -0.20$) (Sakuma et al., 2018).

I SLEEP AIDS

A systematic review of herbal remedies for insomnia, examining 14 RCTs involving 1602 subjects, found no significant differences from placebo or from an active control among subjects who received valerian, chamomile, kava, or wuling (Leach and Page, 2015). (See also Table 11.9.)

J ADAPTOGENS

The term "adaptogen" was coined in the 1940s and more formally defined in the 1960s to describe substances that were "nontoxic" and helped to "increase… the resistance of the organism to a broad spectrum of adverse biological, chemical, and physical factors" (Brekhman and Dardymov, 1969). Their putative effect is to reduce stress reactions and diminish exhaustion by strengthening physiological adaptations to stress. Preclinical studies suggest they may exert effects on neuropeptide Y, stress-activated protein kinase (SAPK/JNK), phosphorylated kinase (p-SAPK/p-JNK), cortisol, and nitric oxide (NO), among other targets. Most studies' agents are geographically specific variants of ginseng, as described in Table 11.11, with varied results, as noted across clinical and nonclinical (but "stressed" or "aesthenic,") otherwise healthy participants.

Tip

"Asethenia" means physical weakness, low energy and loss of strength.

[2] Including citrated folic acid 1 mg + folinic acid 2.5 mg + *L*-methylfolate 7 mg + thiamine pyrophosphate 25 µg + flavin adenine dinucleotide 25 µg + pyridoxal 5'-phosphate 25 µg + adenosylcobalamin 50 µg + nicotinamide adenine dinucleotide (NADH) 25 µg + trimethylglycine 500 µg + AminoFerr 1.5 mg + zinc ascorbate 1 mg + magnesium ascorbate 1 mg + *l*-threonic acid magnesium 1 mg + phosphatidylserine-omega-3 conjugated.

Ⓚ THE MICROBIOME: BRAIN–GUT INTERACTIONS

In recent years there has been growing interest in possible two-way interactions between brain and gut. Gut microbiome flora of MDD patients differ from that of healthy controls. For example, stool samples from MDD patients have shown relative deficiencies of *Faecalibacterium* (Jiang et al., 2015) as well as *Coprococcus* and *Dialister* (Valles-Colomer et al., 2019), and an overabundance of *Enterobacteriaceae*, *Alstipes*, and *Flaviofractor* (Jiang et al., 2015). Most gut microflora produce neurotransmitters such as serotonin and dopamine, while others (such as *Coprococcus* and *Faecalibacterium*) produce inflammatory agents such as butyrate. Possible directional causal relationships remain speculative (does depression alter the gut microbiome or does an altered gut microbiome lead to depression?) but it is thought that gut→brain input could derive from vagal nerve afferent communication. Alteration of the gut microbiome may therefore represent a viable novel target for treatment of depression and potentially other psychiatric disorders.

Among SSRI or tricyclic recipients for MDD, cotherapy with oral *Lactobacillus helveticus* or supplemental *Bifidobacterium longum* supplementation over two months led to significantly better improvement on Beck Depression Inventory scores, as compared to a control group given the prebiotic galactooligosaccharide or a placebo (Kazemi et al., 2019). Larger effects were associated with increasing sample sizes and study durations, and for studies of clinical rather than community participants. That report was consistent with positive findings from a prior meta-analysis of 23 RCTs focusing on probiotics in depression (see Table 11.12). A related meta-analysis of 22 RCTs by the same authors, focusing on probiotics for the treatment of anxiety, similarly identified a small but significant overall probiotic effect.

Definitions

Probiotic: live beneficial bacteria

Prebiotic: nondigestible food product (e.g., fiber) whose fermentation in the colon fosters growth of desirable gut bacteria

Ⓛ SO, (WHEN) SHOULD PROBIOTICS BE PRESCRIBED FOR PSYCHOTROPIC REASONS?

Insofar as probiotics are generally safe, the risk–benefit ratio for including them as an option for adjunctive treatment of depression is likely neutral at worst. At present, none would be considered an evidence-based monotherapy for any psychiatric disorder, and in our estimation there are insufficient replicated data to advise the inclusion of any specific bacterial strain as being a critical component of any commercially available probiotic combination.

Ⓜ FINAL CONSIDERATIONS

In our experience, patients who convey a predilection for pursuing unconventional or unusual therapies in lieu of more established treatments may be somewhat more likely to espouse unusual or odd beliefs, magical thinking, or sometimes veiled signs of psychosis. In patients who express more than a casual interest or curiosity about natural products, or who may even seem steeped in excessive or peculiar concerns about how the body works, gentle probing about unusual health beliefs can sometimes net diagnostically useful information, as illustrated in Clinical Vignette 11.2.

CLINICAL VIGNETTE 11.2

Helena, a 54-year-old single unemployed woman, came for an initial psychiatric consultation with extensive concerns about the toxicity of "synthetic" medicines. She brought with her reams of information about adverse drug effects that she downloaded from the internet, along with a shopping bag full of over-the-counter nutraceutical products that included Quercetin, Bio-B Complex, E-mulsion 200, Neurosol, Flax Seed/Borage Oil, Parabiotic Plus, Bioprotect, Thyrosol, Biotin, Platinum Plus Essential Amino Acid, Ginger Root, CoQ Select, Lipogen, Huperazine A, Bio-D-Multion Forte Drops, Gastro Select, Plasmanex 1 BFP8, Biodoph 7 Plus, Rhodiola Extract, Formula 416-Protease with Calcium, ginseng, Green T-Max, *Ginkgo biloba*, Nervia Softgels, Adrenal Energy Formula, and Enhanced Sex for Women 50+. Though she conveyed a global sense of paranoia about being "harmed" by purveyors of Western medicine, no formal delusions or hallucinations could be elicited. A working diagnosis of schizotypal personality disorder was made based on her extreme social anxiety, lack of emotional responsivity, rambling speech, and preoccupations with mysticism and the occult. Whether or not any of her symptoms might be iatrogenic from the collection of compounds that she carried with her remained a point of speculation.

TAKE-HOME POINTS

- There is an ever-growing array of nutraceutical products relevant to a wide range of psychiatric conditions, supported by a highly variable evidence base. Redirect patient attention to the available evidence base when considering the possible utility and safety of nutraceutical products. Clarify common patient misconceptions between "natural" and "safe and effective."
- Recognize instances in which bioavailability or passage across the blood brain-barrier for certain nutraceuticals may not be well established.
- Beware of pertinent pharmacokinetic interactions between nutraceutical products and prescription medications (e.g., St. John's wort and induction of cytochrome P450 enzymes).
- Gently educate patients when there is an absence of evidence that vitamin, mineral, or other nutrient supplementation is likely to produce psychiatric benefits in the absence of known metabolic deficiencies.

Table 11.1 Potential pharmacokinetic safety concerns with nutraceuticals

Nutraceutical	Popular health uses	Known CYP450 enzyme effects				
		2D6	3A4	2C9	2C19	1A2
Celery root extract	Structurally similar to estrogen, believed helpful in menopause	INH? [a]	–	–	–	–
Black cohosh (*Actaea racemosa*)	Perimenopausal hot flashes, menstrual cramps	–	INH	–	–	–
Cranberry (*Vaccinium macrocarpon*)	Antioxidant; perceived cognitive benefits	–	INH [b]	–	–	–
Echinacea purpurea	Perceived anxiolytic effects	–	INH	–	–	?
Evening primrose	Possible effects for premenstrual dysphoria, atopic dermatitis	–	INH	–	–	–
Gingko biloba [c]	Perceived cognitive benefits	?	?	–	–	–
Ginseng [d]	Perceived cognitive benefits	–	?	–	–	?
Green tea (*Camellia sinesis*) (contains l-theanine)	Weight loss; possible benefits for mood and positive and negative symptoms of schizophrenia	–	INH [e]	INH	–	INH
Himalayan goji juice	"Body cleanser"	–	–	INH [f]	–	–
Kava (*Piper methysticum*)	Perceived anxiolytic effects; may pose hepatotoxic risk	?	–	INH	INH	?
Milk thistle (*Silybum marianum*)	Antioxidant and anti-inflammatory, possible cognitive and hepatic benefits	–	INH	–	–	–
Saw palmetto (*Serenoa repens*)	Anti-inflammatory, possible anti-androgen (inhibits 5α-reductase) in managing BPH and alopecia	INH	INH	INH	–	–
St John's wort (*Hypericum perforatum*)	Used for mild-moderate depression	–	IND [g]	–	–	–
Valerian (*Valeriana officinalis*)	Perceived anxiolytic, sedative-hypnotic effects	INH	INH	–	–	–

[a] Case reports of mania induction when added to venlafaxine plus St John's wort (Awortwe et al., 2018)
[b] Has been shown to amplify effects of midazolam
[c] In HIV+ patients, reports of increased viral load when taken with efavirenz (Awortwe et al., 2018)
[d] Also inhibits CYP450 2A6 as well as UGT2B7 (reports of DRESS syndrome among patients taking lamotrigine) (Awortwe et al., 2018)
[e] Reports of transaminitis when used with simvastatin (Awortwe et al., 2018)
[f] Could potentiate effects of warfarin (increased bleeding risk (Awortwe et al., 2018)); co-therapy may lessen efficacy of clozapine (Awortwe et al., 2018)
[g] Case reports of upper GI bleeding among patients taking warfarin, possibly due to additive clotting effect (Awortwe et al., 2018)

Abbreviations: DRESS = drug reaction with eosinophilia and systemic symptoms; GI = gastrointestinal; HIV = human immunodeficiency virus; IND = inducer; INH = inhibitor

Table 11.2 Psychiatric and other medical features associated with vitamin deficiencies: fat-soluble

Vitamin	Deficiencies may present psychiatrically with...	...But would expectably also be accompanied by...	...In the setting of identifiable risk factors...	Potential adverse consequences of excessive dosing
A	None known	Visual problems, acne, poor wound healing	Excessive alcohol use, restrictive eating disorders	Toxicity with chronic doses >50 000 IU; blurry vision, ↓'d appetite, hypercalcemia, hepatotoxicity, dry skin, oropharyngeal ulcers
D	Depression	Osteoporosis, muscle twitches	Older adults, those with limited sun exposure, individuals with dark skin pigmentations	Chronic doses >4000 IU may cause GI upset, arthralgias, hypercalcemia, vascular calcifications, fractures, pancreatic/ prostate cancers
E	Possible depression	Muscle weakness, neuropathy, ataxia, visual problems	Poor dietary fat absorption, cholestatic liver disease	Possible bleeding/coagulopathy, GI upset, fatigue, blurry vision
K	Depression	Bruising, osteopenia	Low dietary intake	Hypoglycemia

Table 11.3 Fat-soluble vitamins

Vitamin	Normal physiological role	Potential psychiatric utility of supplementation
A	Maintaining vision and normal immune system functioning	None known
D	Regulates calcium homeostasis and bone health; may also regulate neurotrophic factors and broadly promote neuroprotection	- In MDD, meta-analysis of four RCTs (n = 938) compared to placebo, no treatment, or fluoxetine monotherapy revealed a pooled effect size of *d* = 0.58 (Vellekkatt and Menon, 2019) - One negative RCT (800 IU PO qDay) in women over the age of 70 with winter depression (Dumville et al., 2006) - In schizophrenia patients with baseline vitamin D levels <75 ng/mL, adjunctive vitamin D 14 000 IU/week added to clozapine for eight weeks was no better than placebo for improving psychosis or depression (Krivoy et al., 2017) - In autism spectrum children with low baseline 25-OH-D levels <30 ng/mL, open trial data using vitamin D3 (300–5000 IU PO qDay) improved stereotypy, eye contact, and attention span (Saad et al., 2016) [a]
E	Antioxidant, helps prevent platelet hyper-aggregation (e.g., atherosclerosis and thromboemboli)	- Limited evidence to suggest possible slowing of progression of tardive dyskinesia up to 1600 IU PO qDay (RR = 0.23, 95% CI = 0.07–0.76) (Soares-Weiser et al., 2018) - Dosing of 1000 IU twice daily may help reduce mortality in patients with Alzheimer's dementia (Pavlik et al., 2009)
K	Primary roles in hemostasis and promoting bone calcification. Also involved in sphingolipid biosynthesis; low dietary intake may be associated with more severe subjective memory complaints in older adults (Soutif-Veillon et al., 2016)	Unsubstantiated claims that supplementation may help to prevent Alzheimer's dementia

[a] A subsequent placebo-controlled RCT from the same study group was retracted by journal editors based on lack of confidence in the findings (*J Child Psychol Psychiatry*. 2019 Jun;60(6):711. doi: 0.1111/jcpp.13076. Epub 2019 May 6)

Abbreviations: CI = confidence interval; IU = international unit; MDD = major depressive disorder; PO = by mouth; qDay = once a day; RCT = randomized controlled trial; RR = relative risk

Table 11.4 Psychiatric and other medical features associated with vitamin deficiencies: water-soluble

Vitamin	Deficiencies may present psychiatrically with...	...But would expectably also be accompanied by...	...In the setting of identifiable risk factors...	Potential adverse consequences of excessive dosing
B1 (thiamine)	Wernicke's encephalopathy	Fatigue, hyporeflexia, paresthesias, muscle weakness, blurry vision	Excessive alcohol use, diabetics, older adults, patient with malabsorption syndromes	Generally nontoxic
B2 (riboflavin)	None known	Cracked lips, fatigue, pharyngitis, conjunctivitis, photophobia	Older adult, heavy alcohol users, low dietary intake of animal/dairy products	Generally nontoxic
B3 (niacin)	Dementia in pellagra, depression, memory deficits	Fatigue, canker sores, GI upset/vomiting	Heavy alcohol users, malabsorption syndromes; prolonged use of isoniazid	Flushing; gastritis; hepatotoxicity with doses >1000 mg/day; may interfere with anticoagulants, statins
B6 (pyridoxine)	Depression	Dermatitis, headache	Older adults, oral contraceptive or heavy alcohol users	Neuropathy (Levine and Saltzman, 2004), paresthesias, gait disturbances
B9 (folate)	Weakness, appetite loss	Appetite/weight loss, weakness, megaloblastic anemia	Pregnancy, heavy alcohol users, patients with liver dysfunction	GI distress, cognitive disturbances; controversy whether high folic acid levels may be carcinogenic
B12 (cobalamin)	Depression, fatigue, lethargy, agitation/irritability, psychosis, cognitive impairment, dementia	Paresthesias, dyspnea, weakness, gait disturbance, pallor, atrophic glossitis, cold intolerance, megaloblastic anemia	Older adults with atrophic gastritis, vegetarians and vegans, those with malabsorption syndromes (e.g., Crohn's disease, gastric bypass surgery)	Dizziness, headache, anxiety, nausea, vomiting
C	Irritability, appetite/weight loss	Fatigue, anemia, joint pain	Smokers, patients with malabsorption syndromes or dietary citrus deficiencies	GI upset; possible renal calculi (dosing >1000 mg/day)

Table 11.5 Dosing recommendations: non-fat soluble vitamins

Vitamin	Normal physiological role	US recommended daily dosing	Potential psychiatric utility of supplementation in absence of deficiencies
B1 (thiamine)	ATP production; energy/metabolism	Men: 1.2 mg/day; women: 1.1 mg/day	None known
B2 (riboflavin)	Antioxidant; energy/metabolism	Men: 1.3 mg/day; women: 1.1 mg/day	Component (400 mg riboflavin) of Migravent® or Dolovent® treatment for migraine headaches (Gaul et al., 2015)
B3 (niacin)	Energy and metabolism	Men: 16 mg/day; women: 14 mg/day	Anecdotal reports for treating depression
B5 (pantothenic acid)	Energy/metabolism, fatty acid and cholesterol metabolism	No established US RDA. Adequate intake for men or women: 5 mg/day	None known
B6 (pyridoxine)	Involved in neurotransmitter synthesis; gluconeogenesis and glycogenolysis	Men or women aged 19–50: 1.3 mg/day; men age >50: 1.7 mg/day; women age >50: 1.5 mg/day	Anecdotal reports of reduced psychotic symptoms in schizophrenia but negative RCTs (e.g., Lerner et al., 2002); short-term (four-week) RCT data suggest possible benefit for tardive dyskinesia (Lerner et al., 2001)
B9 (folate)	Necessary for red blood cell synthesis, DNA and RNA synthesis and repair, neural tube development	Men or women: 400 μg/day	In MDD: meta-analysis of four RCTs showed no significant difference from placebo (Sarris et al., 2016)
B12 (cobalamin)	Neuronal growth and development; facilitates conversion of homocysteine to methionine (see Figure 11.2)	Men or women: 2.4 μg/day	In MDD: one positive six-week RCT of adjunctive vitamin B12 (1000 μg IM) versus TCA or SSRI alone (reviewed by Sarris et al., 2016)
C (ascorbic acid)	Antioxidant; synthesis of collagen, connective tissue, neurotransmitters and adrenal steroids; intestinal iron absorption	Men: 90 mg/day; women: 75 mg/day	In MDD: one positive six-month RCT (dosed 1 g PO qDay) added to fluoxetine, one negative eight-week RCT (dosed 1 g PO qDay) added to citalopram (Sarris et al., 2016)

Abbreviations: ATP = adenosine triphosphate; DNA = deoxyribonucleic acid; PO = by mouth; qDay = once daily; RCT = randomized controlled trial; RDA = recommended dietary allowance; RNA = ribonucleic acid; SSRI = selective serotonin reuptake inhibitor; TCA = tricyclic antidepressant

Table 11.6 Macro- and trace minerals

Mineral	Potential psychiatric utility of supplementation	Potential hazards of excessive dosing
Calcium	Calcium carbonate 600 mg PO BID reduced premenstrual dysphoria symptoms better than placebo (Thys-Jacobs et al., 1998)	Renal calculi, GI distress
Chromium	In atypical depression, 600 μg/day PO may improve hyperphagia and carbohydrate craving better than placebo (Docherty et al., 2005).	Renal failure, hepatotoxicity, anemia, thrombocytopenia
Copper	No established benefit	Hepato- and nephrotoxicity; nausea, vomiting, coma
Iodine	No established benefit	Ingestion of elemental *iodine* causes chemical burns and can be lethal
Iron	Dietary iron supplementation can sometimes help to treat pica	Liver and intestinal damage, death
Magnesium	- In MDD: one open 12-week crossover trial of magnesium chloride (248 mg of elemental Mg^{++}) demonstrated significant improvement from baseline in depression and anxiety scores (Tarleton et al., 2017); magnesium oxide 500 mg PO qDay × eight weeks improved depression better than placebo (Rajizadeh et al., 2017); negative small RCT using magnesium aspartate (Ryszewska-Pokraśniewicz et al., 2018) - Component (600 mg magnesium) of Migravent® or Dolovent® treatment for migraine headaches (Gaul et al., 2015)	Excessive use may cause diarrhea and GI upset; potentially hazardous in chronic kidney disease or cardiac arrhythmias
Manganese	Low levels associated with depression and anxiety; no evidence that dietary supplementation confers a psychiatric benefit	Neurotoxicity (psychosis, parkinsonism), pulmonary and hepatic toxicities
Potassium	No established benefit	Hyperkalemia can be arrhythmogenic
Selenium	Case-control reports linking low dietary selenium with MDD (OR ~threefold) (Pasco et al., 2012); no established psychiatric benefit for dietary supplementation	Diarrhea/GI upset, dermatological changes (hair loss, nail discoloration/brittleness), neuropathy
Sodium	No established benefit (but, in those taking lithium, low dietary sodium can elevate lithium levels via excessive renal absorption)	Fluid retention, hypertension, pulmonary edema, kidney failure, seizures
Zinc	- In anorexia nervosa, zinc gluconate 100 mg/day increased BMI better than did placebo (Birmingham et al., 1994) - In MDD: one positive 12-week placebo-controlled trial (dosed 25 mg/day) added to SSRIs, one negative RCT added to imipramine (reviewed by Sarris et al., 2016)	Daily dosages >25 mg can lead to copper deficiency; may decrease chromium absorption

Abbreviations: BID = twice daily; BMI = body mass index; GI = gastrointestinal; MDD = major depressive disorder; OR = odds ratio; PO = by mouth; qDay = once daily; RCT = randomized controlled trial; SSRI = selective serotonin reuptake inhibitor

Table 11.7 Neurotransmitters

Neurotransmitter	Potential psychotropic relevance	Typical supplement dosing
GABA	May hasten sleep onset (Yamatsu et al., 2015)	100 mg/day
Glutamate	No known psychiatric benefit	No established dosing
Glutamine	No established psychotropic benefit	Dosing of 20–30 g as an exercise supplement (Gleeson, 2008); 40 g PO qDay used in HIV wasting
5HTP (5-hydroxytryptophan)	In MDD: one positive four-week RCT vs. placebo added to clomipramine (reviewed by Sarris et al., 2016); long-term use may deplete monoamines and worsen depression (Hinz et al., 2012); anecdotal reports claim value for fibromyalgia, binge eating disorder, insomnia, headaches	300 mg/day
l-Arginine plus *l*-Lysine	Small RCTs mainly in healthy volunteers have shown greater reductions in trait anxiety than with placebo (Lakhan and Vieira, 2010)	3 g PO qDay
l-Theanine	- Eight-week open-label l-theanine added to antidepressants significantly improved depression symptoms as well as verbal memory and executive function from baseline (Hidese et al., 2017) - In schizophrenia or schizoaffective disorder: l-theanine 400 mg/day added to antidopaminergic drugs improved anxiety and positive symptoms better than did placebo (Ritsner et al., 2011)	250 mg PO qDay
Taurine	In first-episode psychosis, taurine was superior to placebo (added to antidopaminergics) in reducing BPRS and depression scores and improving global functioning; no observed cognitive benefit (O'Donnell et al., 2016)	4 g PO qDay

Abbreviations: BPRS = Brief Psychiatric Rating Scale; GABA = gamma aminobutyric acid; HIV = human immunodeficiency virus; MDD = major depressive disorder; PO = by mouth; qDay = once daily; RCT = randomized controlled trial

Table 11.8 Steroids

Steroid	Potential psychotropic relevance	Main known risks
Dehydroepiandrosterone (DHEA)	- Touted as an antiaging remedy, antiobesity, pro-cognitive, antidepressant effects; may ↑ sexual function - Improves dysthymia/minor depression in HIV-positive men and women (mean dosages = 386 mg/day and 243 mg/day, respectively (Rabkin et al., 2006)); in mid-life MDD or minor depression, DHEA (90 mg/day or 450 mg/day) superior to placebo (Wolkowitz et al., 1999; Bloch et al., 1999; Schmidt et al., 2005)	Case reports of new onset mania or psychosis at doses of 150–300 mg/day
Dessicated thyroid extract	None; sometimes recommended over synthetic T_4 or T_3. One grain = 38 μg of T_4 and 9 μg of T_3.	Exact ratios of T_4 to T_3 as relevant for humans can be inconsistent
Estrogen	In perimenopausal depressed women, a meta-analysis of 26 studies found an effect size of 0.68 (Zweifel and O'Brien, 1997)	Potential increased risk for endometrial cancer, thrombus formation
Human growth hormone (hGH)	Oral: likely to produce minimal or no effects (due to gastric degradation) vs IM preparations	Insulin resistance, heart disease, joint pain, edema
Mifepristone (aka RU-486)	Preliminary studies in psychotic depression (dosed from 50–1200 mg/day) or chronic depression (200 mg/day), and bipolar depression (600 mg/day); reverses psychosis in Cushing's syndrome (Gallagher and Young, 2006)	Possible adrenal insufficiency, rash, fatigue
Melatonin	Primarily used as sleep aid at doses of 1–3 mg/day (equating to 1–20× physiologic levels)	Although synthesized from serotonin (see Figure 11.1), no evidence that excessive dietary melatonin can cause serotonin syndrome
Pregnenolone	- In schizophrenia, pregnenolone 50 mg/day + SGAs reduced positive and negative symptoms better than placebo (d = 0.79) (Ritsner et al., 2014); may improve attention and executive functioning vs. placebo (Kreinin et al., 2017) - May protect against cannabis intoxication (Vallée et al., 2014)	No known risks
Progesterone	May induce depression (Holst et al., 1989), increase risk of postpartum depression (Dennis et al., 2008). However, allopregnanolone may have antidepressant, anxiolytic, and pro-cognitive effects (see Chapter 12)	Nausea, fatigue, breast tenderness, GI distress, mood worsening
Raloxifene	In women with schizophrenia, raloxifene 120 mg/day was superior to placebo in PANSS total scores; no effect on positive symptoms, mood, or cognition (Kulkarni et al., 2016)	Hot flashes, sweating, dizziness
Testosterone	Meta-analysis of 27 RCTs in depressed men showed greater improvement than placebo but small effect (g = 0.21) at doses ≥0.5 g/week (Walther et al., 2019)	Acne, hirsutism, ↓'d libido, mood changes, adverse cardiovascular/pro-thrombotic effects

Abbreviations: GI = gastrointestinal; HIV = human immunodeficiency virus; IM = intramuscular; MDD = major depressive disorder; PANSS = Positive and Negative Syndrome Scale; RCT = randomized controlled trial; SGA = second-generation antipsychotic

Table 11.9 Herbs

Herb	Evidence	Main known risks
Bacopa monnier (Brahmi)	One 12-week RCT of 300 mg/day found greater anxiolytic effects and better visual processing speed and learning and memory consolidation than with placebo (Stough et al., 2001)	None known
Centella asiatica (Gotu kola)	Open trial data (500 mg PO BID) over two months revealed significant reductions from baseline anxiety and depression (Jana et al., 2010)	None known
Citrus aurantium	Nine RCTs in anxious surgical patients showed improvement vs. placebo (Mannucci et al., 2018)	None known
Matricaria chamomilla (Chamomile)	Chamomile extract capsules (begun as 220 mg/day and increased to 1100 mg/day) reduced anxiety and depressive symptoms better than placebo over eight weeks in GAD (Amsterdam et al., 2009); a subsequent 26-week placebo-controlled relapse prevention trial (dosed at 500 mg PO TID) among acute responders to open-label chamomile found greater anxiety symptom reduction but not lower relapse rates (Mao et al., 2016)	May potentiate the effects of anticoagulants
Crocus sativus (Saffron)	Review of six RCTs (three antidepressant-comparator, three placebo), 30–50 mg/day, found comparability to antidepressants and superiority to placebo, with large effect size (Sarris, 2018)	Reports of dry mouth, dizziness, headache, nausea, anxiety
Curcuma longa (Curcumin)	Meta-analysis of six acute MDD RCTs (500 mg PO BID) found greater efficacy than with placebo (Ng et al., 2017)	Considered safe at oral doses <12 000 mg/day; may cause iron-deficient anemia (case reports of severe allergic reactions or death when administered parenterally)
Free and Easy Wanderer Plus (FEWP) (Xiao yao yan)	12-week RCT: FEWP (36 mg PO qDay) > placebo added to carbamazepine for bipolar depression symptoms ($p = 0.032$) (Zhang et al., 2007c); greater improvement than with placebo in MDD ($p < 0.001$) (Zhang et al., 2007b)	None
Ginkgo biloba (Ginkgo)	- In elderly adults a six-year RCT (dosed 120 mg PO BID) found no advantage for *Ginkgo biloba* over placebo in forestalling dementia, regardless of the presence or absence of baseline minimal cognitive impairment (DeKosky et al., 2008) - Four-week RCT (dosed at 240 or 480 mg PO qDay) in GAD patients reduced anxiety better than placebo (Woelk et al., 2007)	Induces CYP2C19. May increase bleeding risk or diminish the efficacy of anticoagulants; GI distress
Galphimia glauca (Galphimia)	- Four-week RCT in GAD patients given 320 mg PO BID versus lorazepam 1 mg PO BID found no significant differences in anxiety scores; a 15-week follow-up found greater anxiolysis with Galphimia than lorazepam (reviewed by Sarris, 2018)	None known

Table 11.9 Cont.

Herb	Evidence	Main known risks
Hypericum perforatum (St. John's wort)	Meta-analysis of 18 RCTs in MDD favored SJW over placebo; later data suggest possible value in severe as well as mild-to-moderate depression based on studies (dosed up to 900 mg/day) showing superiority to some SSRIs (Sarris, 2018)	Dermatological and GI adverse effects; generally safe and well-tolerated; weak MAOI
Piper methysticum (kava or kava kava)	Possible anxiolytic and sedative (meta-analysis of seven RCTs, dosing of 60–280 mg/day) revealed significant difference in anxiety scores, though small effect sizes (Pittler and Ernst, 2003)	Fulminant hepatic failure (50–100 reported cases; may present with jaundice within two weeks of exposure)
Lavandula spp. (lavender)	Potential synergy with imipramine or citalopram in MDD (reviewed by Sarris, 2018)	None known
Lepidium meneyii (maca, or Peruvian ginseng)	In a meta-analysis of four RCTs, two found improved sexual functioning (1.5–3 g PO qDay) over placebo, one found no difference, and a fourth found improved male erectile dysfunction (Shin et al., 2010)	None known (but not well-studied)
Passiflora incarnata (passion flower)	Comparable anxiolytic efficacy to oxazepam 30 mg/day in GAD; and superiority to placebo for preoperative anxiety in psychiatrically healthy surgical subjects (Sarris, 2018)	None known
Valeriana officinalis (valerian)	Promoted as possible sleep aid and "mild sedative." A review of nine RCTs for insomnia (dose range 400–900 mg PO qDay) deemed results inconclusive (Stevinson and Ernst, 2000)	Avoid in the setting of liver disease or pregnancy

Abbreviations: BID = twice daily; GAD = generalized anxiety disorder; GI = gastrointestinal; MAOI = monoamine oxidase inhibitor; MDD = major depressive disorder; PO = by mouth; qDay = once daily; RCT = randomized controlled trial; SJW = St John's wort; TID three times daily

Table 11.10 Other Compounds

Agent	Potential psychotropic relevance	Typical dosing	Main known risks
Agmatine	Case reports demonstrate antidepressant efficacy separable from effects on serotonin	2-3 mg/day	None known
Biotin	None known; popular as a potential antidote for alopecia secondary to divalproex	US RDA: men and women: 30 μg/day	None known
Choline	Pilot open trial of choline 3-8 g PO qDay added to lithium with improved manic and depressive symptoms in four of six refractory rapid cycling bipolar patients (Stoll et al., 1996)	US RDA: men: 550 mg/day; women: 425 mg/day	Abdominal cramps, GI upset
Citicoline	Preliminary data suggest potential value to reduce cocaine use in people with bipolar disorder (Brown et al., 2015) and possibly negative symptoms in schizophrenia (Ghajar et al., 2018a)	2000-2500 mg/day	None known
Coenzyme Q (ubiquinone)	- In bipolar depression, one eight-week RCT added 200 mg/day to existing pharmacotherapy and found greater improvement in depressive symptoms than with placebo (d = 0.87) (Mehyrpooya et al., 2018) - In older adult bipolar depression, one positive open trial added 800 mg/day to existing pharmacotherapy (Forester et al., 2015) - Component (150 mg CoQ) of Migravent® or Dolovent® treatment for migraine headaches (Gaul et al., 2015) - Endogenous CoQ levels are reduced in Parkinson's disease; however exogenous supplementation has not been shown to improve motor dysfunction (Zhu et al., 2017)	200-800 mg/day (acceptable daily intake = 12 mg/kg/day; Hidaka et al., 2008)	GI upset; may decrease the anticoagulant efficacy of warfarin
Creatine	- In MDD, one positive eight-week RCT of adjunctive creatine added to escitalopram was superior to placebo (Lyoo et al., 2012) - May improve memory, attention, reaction time better than placebo in healthy volunteers (Ling et al., 2009); effects on executive function, reaction time and verbal fluency less apparent (Avgerinos et al., 2018)	5 mg PO qDay	Possible nephrotoxicity if combined with NSAIDs
Myoinositol	In MDD: small proof-of-concept studies but two negative placebo-controlled trials (reviewed by Sarris et al., 2016)	12 g PO qDay	GI upset

Agent	Potential psychotropic relevance	Typical dosing	Main known risks
N-acetyl-cysteine (NAC)	12-week RCT of NAC or placebo + usual treatment, then 16-week follow-up: no significant improvement in 1° outcome but some benefit in 2° outcome measures (Berk et al., 2014)	1200–2400 mg PO qDay	GI, musculoskeletal adverse effects
Omega-3 fatty acids (eicosopentanoic acid)	Meta-analysis of 11 RCTs in MDD revealed a significant overall effect (g = 0.608, p = 0.009) (Sarris et al., 2016)	Commonly 1–2 g PO qDay but can vary from 930 mg to 4.4 g PO qDay	Potential dose-related increased risk for bleeding/hemorrhagic stroke
Quercetin	Anecdotal reports of improved social interactions in patients with autism	No established dose	None known
Tryptophan	In MDD, four of seven RCTs positive (reviewed by Sarris et al., 2016)	Variable across RCTs from 3–18 g PO qDay	*d*-isomer less effective than *l*- or *dl*-racemic mixture; a 1989 epidemic of eosinophilia-myalgia syndrome traced to a single source led to FDA banning of *l*-tryptophan until 2005

Abbreviations: CoQ = coenzyme Q; GI = gastrotintestinal; MDD = major depressive disorder; NSAID = nonsteroidal anti-inflammatory drug; PO = by mouth; qDay = once daily; RCT = randomized controlled trial; RDA = recommended dietary allowance

Tip

N-acetylcysteine poorly crosses the blood-brain barrier. Coadministration with probenecid (dosed at 500 mg PO BID), which prevents efflux of glutathione (Hagos et al., 2017), may increase its CNS bioavailability.

Table 11.11 Adaptogens

Compound	Known effects
Eleutherococcus senticosus (Siberian ginseng) root extract	No significant difference in cognitive performance, fatigue, mood, sleep or stress measures as compared to two days' intensive stress management training in a group of subjects with "aesthenia" (physical weakness) (Schaffler et al., 2013)
Panax ginseng (Asian ginseng)	Review of 65 trials found possible benefit for improving glucose metabolism and immune response modulation; no specific psychiatric benefits (Shergis et al., 2013)
Panax quinquefolius (aka American ginseng)	Randomized crossover trial in 32 healthy volunteers found significant improvement in working memory (dose = 100 mg/day) (Scholey et al., 2010)
Rhodiola rosea	- 28-day RCT of 60 participants identified with "stress-related fatigue" who were prescribed standardized extract of roots of *Rhodiola rosea* (576 mg/day) scored better at study end than those given placebo on measures of "burnout" and attention (continuous performance task), as well as morning cortisol levels (Olsson et al., 2009) - Six-week RCT in mild-to-moderate depression of *Rhodiola rosea*, doses of 340 mg/day or 680 mg/day both improved HAM-D scores better than placebo (Darbinyan et al., 2007)
Schisandra chinensis berry extract	Preliminary RCT data (784 mg/day dose) suggest superiority to placebo for treating hot flashes, sweating, and heart palpitations in perimenopausal women (Park and Kim, 2016)
Withania somnifera (aka ashwaganda or Indian ginseng)	- Review of five 6–16 week RCTs, dosing from 125–1200 mg PO qDay, in healthy stressed controls revealed better stress outcomes (Pratte et al., 2014) - 500 mg/day over eight weeks may improve cognitive functioning better than placebo in bipolar disorder patients (Chengappa et al., 2013) - Adjunctive treatment (1000 mg PO qDay) with antidopaminergic drugs in schizophrenia over 12 weeks may improve positive and negative symptoms better than adjunctive placebo (Chengappa et al., 2018)

Abbreviations: HAM-D = Hamilton Ratings Scale for Depression; PO = by mouth; qDay = once daily; RCT = randomized controlled trial

Table 11.12 Summary of findings involving probiotics across psychiatric disorders

Disorder	Evidence base	Main findings
Anxiety	Meta-analysis of 22 RCTs involving *Lactobacilli*, *Bifidobacterium longum* or *Bacillus coagulans* lasting from eight days to 45 weeks (Liu et al., 2019b)	Small but significant overall effect for probiotics over placebo (d = -0.10, 95% CI = -0.19 to -0.01, p = 0.03)
Autism	Review of two RCTs and three open trials involving *Lactobacilli*, *Bifidobacterium longum*, or *Bifidobacterium abifidum* (Liu et al., 2019a)	Modest observed behavioral improvements but small effect sizes, small sample sizes, brief study periods
MDD	Review of 23 RCTs involving great variation in study samples (clinical versus community, subjects with versus without irritable bowel syndrome) and sizes (Liu et al., 2019b)	Small but significant overall effects observed (d = -0.24, 95% CI = -0.36 to -0.12, p <0.01). Negative as well as positive RCTs exist with some strains (e.g., *Bifiderobacterium longum*)
Schizophrenia	Meta-analysis of three RCTs involving *L. rhamnosus* strain GG, *Bifidobacterium animalis* subspecies *lactis* strain Bb12 for 12–14 weeks (Ng et al., 2019)	No significant differences found between probiotics and placebo (d =-0.09, 95% CI = -0.380 to 0.204, p = 0.551)

Abbreviations: CI = confidence interval; RCT = randomized controlled trial

12 Human Diversity and Considerations in Special Populations

LEARNING OBJECTIVES

- [ ] Appreciate known pharmacokinetic and pharmacodynamic differences in psychotropic drug response across sexual, racial/ethnic, age-based, and other distinct patient subgroups such as those who smoke cigarettes or significantly drink alcohol
- [ ] Recognize psychotropic drug safety concerns during pregnancy, lactation, and the postpartum period
- [ ] Recognize associations between mood disorders and menstrual dysregulation, and appropriate pharmacotherapies
- [ ] Understand the complexities of treating (and distinguishing iatrogenic from primary illness symptoms in) patients with somatic symptom disorder
- [ ] Understand the implications of major medical conditions for prescribing psychotropic medications
- [ ] Know the impact of diminished hepatic or renal function on drug metabolism and clearance

Today you are You, that is truer than true. There is no one alive who is Youer than You.

- Dr. Seuss

All patient subpopulations are inherently "special" based on their unique constellations of clinical and demographic features that moderate and mediate treatment outcomes. This chapter will focus on diversity across distinct clinical subpopulations for which moderating or mediating factors do not simply provide information about the likelihood of a favorable drug response, but more specifically identify the need to adjust medication dosages or regimens, or favor certain medications over others based on evidence for safe and effective use in a particular patient group. Chronological age and biological sex assignment rarely in themselves signal the need for dosage adjustments, although associated features (e.g., diminished hepatic or renal function; pregnancy, premenstrual mood disturbances) may bear on a select evidence base for a given subpopulation. Metabolic (e.g., CYP450) enzymes also can vary by race, gender, age, and genetic polymorphisms, as noted in Chapter 8.

For all medications with any FDA approval, manufacturers' product information sheets routinely discuss use in "specific populations" in Section 8. More specifically, Sections 8.1 and 8.2 focus on pregnancy and lactation, respectively; Sections 8.4 and 8.5 discuss

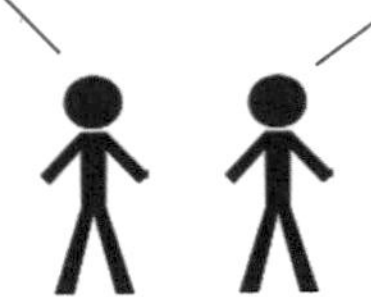
I have many overweight depressed patients. Should I give them higher than usual antidepressant doses?
Uh, no, adult dosing adjustments depend more on hepatic function for metabolized drugs, renal function for renally cleared drugs, and volume of distribution – not weight per se. See Unterecker et al., 2011.

pediatric and geriatric uses, respectively; and Sections 8.6 and 8.7 typically discuss patients with hepatic and renal impairment, respectively. Note that the product labels for relatively older medications (e.g., bupropion) are sometimes less explicit than for newer medications in the language they use to specify dosage modifications in special populations (e.g., bupropion in renal impairment).

This chapter is subdivided into two main sections: populations stratified by: (a) clinically definable

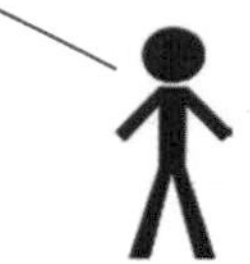
I like to read drug manufacturers' product information sheets from start to finish on a regular basis

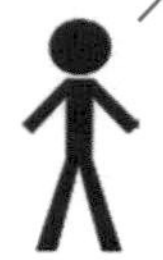
Yeah, I think that's mentioned in the sections on managing insomnia

subgroups (including racial–ethnic–ancestral groups, sex differences, children/adolescents, geriatric/older adult patients, pregnancy/lactation, smokers, substance use disorders, and patients prone to somatization) and (b) those with clinically significant medical comorbidities or chronic medical conditions. Among the latter, rather than attempt to recapitulate the vast material contained in textbooks devoted to the topic of consultation-liaison (C-L) psychiatry, we have chosen instead to focus on a select number of commonly encountered medical conditions that bear directly on pharmacological decision-making for practitioners without formal subspecialty training in C-L psychiatry.

Box 12.1

Terminology

Ethnicity refers to cultural factors such as language, ancestry, religion, heritage, and customs. Ethnic influences might, for example, foster shunning the use of medication for depression, or pursuing spiritual rather than medical solutions to mental health problems.

Race is meant to classify groups based on shared physical attributes such as skin color, bone structure, eye color, and hair color and texture. Suspected racial predispositions to pharmacokinetic and pharmacodynamic outcomes may be confounded by ethnic, socioeconomic, geographic, or other nonbiological factors. Increasingly, race has been criticized in both the scientific and lay literature as a purely social, scientifically artificial construct that has no basis in genetics or any other biological framework.

Ancestry has become an increasingly preferred term to describe allelic variation based on someone's geographic origins. (The term "Caucasian," for example, emanates from an eighteenth-century racial taxonomy which proposed that Whites descended from ancestry in the Caucasus mountain region spanning Europe and Asia.) Ancestry, more than race, may more accurately describe one's genetic composition and consequent predisposition to particular health conditions (e.g., sickle cell anemia may be more prevalent among individuals who hail from sub-Saharan Africa, rather than among those with any particular skin color).

A CLINICAL AND DEMOGRAPHIC SUBGROUPS

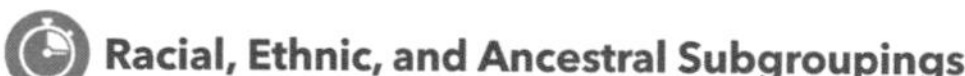

Racial, Ethnic, and Ancestral Subgroupings

Ethnic and racial diversity remains a controversial topic regarding psychiatric diagnosis and treatment in general, and pharmacotherapy in particular. In part, there is much debate as to whether race constitutes a biologically valid differentiator for parsing disease susceptibility factors and treatment parameters or pharmacodynamic outcomes. Box 12.1 provides distinguishing definitions for key concepts in this area.

The psychopharmacological (and other psychiatric) literature broadly addressing "race" as a construct relevant to pharmacokinetics and pharmacodynamics has only recently begun to draw formal distinctions between racial, ethnic, and geographic-ancestral groupings. More specifically, psychopharmacologists are interested in how best to recognize population stratification by differentiable allelic frequencies across groups (e.g., consider the known variations in allelic frequencies for CYP450 isoenzymes described in Box 8.4 in Chapter 8). Existing literature on race or ethnicity in psychopharmacology usefully identifies racial-ethnic disparities in prescribing patterns (e.g., after the 2004 FDA boxed warning regarding suicidality and antidepressant use in youth, antidepressant prescribing in the United States declined more precipitously for Whites than for Blacks or Latinos (DePetris and Cook, 2013)). Elsewhere, the literature offers descriptive observations about "race" that may be cruder than intended, without accounting for geographic, ancestral, or cultural confounders. See Box 12.2 for examples.

Historically, RCTs have tended to enroll more White than non-White participants, thereby generating more unknowns about the generalizability of treatment outcomes to more diverse populations. Other relevant considerations to psychopharmacology outcomes include:

- Ethnic–racial groups that vary in baseline rates of underlying medical vulnerabilities (e.g., diabetes, hypertension) or lifestyle (e.g., smoking) may be more

Box 12.2

Examples of Observations About Race/Ethnicity in the Literature

- As compared to White patients, African Americans with psychotic disorders tend to receive higher doses of antipsychotics, more frequent depot antipsychotics, longer overall exposure durations, and more frequent cotherapy with multiple antipsychotics (Chaudhry et al., 2008)
- Asian and Latino patients appear more prone to antipsychotic extrapyramidal adverse effects than African Americans or Whites (Binder and Levy, 1981) and respond to lower antipsychotic doses as compared to Whites (Ruiz et al., 1999)
- Latino women are more likely than White women to report side effects when taking tricyclic antidepressants (Sramek and Pi, 1996)

or less predisposed to certain adverse drug effects (e.g., metabolic dysregulation)

- Ethnic–racial–ancestral differences in pharmacokinetics and pharmacodynamics may influence the presentation and treatment of certain psychiatric disorders: for example, relatively underactive forms of *aldehyde dehydrogenase* among individuals with Japanese and other Asian ancestry tend to diminish the risk for alcoholism; meanwhile, low activity variants of *alcohol dehydrogenase* appear to be over-represented among people with Native American ancestry, in turn raising vulnerability to heavier alcohol consumption (Peng et al., 2014) (see Box 12.3)
- Higher rates of benign ethnic neutropenia (BEN) among people of African or Middle Eastern descent (as high as 25–50%; Haddy et al., 1999) differentially impacts the hematological safety profile for clozapine
- People of Asian (Ng et al., 2005) or Korean descent (Matsuda et al., 1996) may require lower mean oral clozapine dosages than do Whites to achieve comparable serum clozapine levels
- Ethnic rather than racial differences might account for phenomena such as the substantially higher age-adjusted suicide rates among Native Americans/Alaska natives (22.15 per 100 000) than among Asian/Pacific islanders (6.75 per 100 000)
- Ethnic differences in diet and nutrition, access to health care, primary prevention, smoking status, attitudes toward psychoactive substances, and preferences for nutraceutical products
- Cross-cultural differences in attitudes about mental illness, pharmacotherapy in general, and treatment adherence

My people heavily consume cabbage, broccoli and brussel sprouts, and we savor the polyaromatic hydro-carbons found in over cooked meats

Well then we'd better not give your people any P450 1A2 substrates like imipramine, clozapine or propranolol, since their metabolism will be inhibited. Care to change your habits?

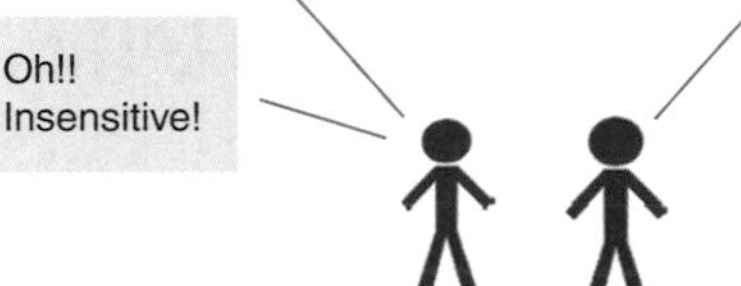

Box 12.3

Metabolic Pathway of Alcohol

BIOCHEMICAL PATHWAY REMINDER:

Alcohol → (*Alcohol dehydrogenase*) → Acetaldehyde → (*Aldehyde dehydrogenase*) → Acetic acid → $CO_2 + H_2O$

Alcohol dehydrogenase: Low activity = fosters high alcohol reinforcing effects

Aldehyde dehydrogenase: Low activity = may help protect against alcohol reinforcing effects

- Increasing racial diversity and inter-racial marriage, coupled with ever-increasing geographic mobility, tends to blur categorically defined racial or ethnic group affiliations. Expanding rates of individuals with mixed racial, geographic, and ethnic ancestries introduce further layers of population stratification that go well beyond the five standard racial categories specified by the US Office of Management and Budget (1997).

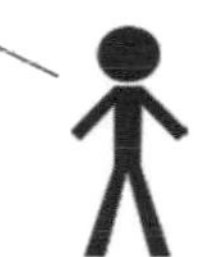

I'm part Portuguese, Irish, Chinese, Native Hawaiian, Jewish and Afro-Caribbean. What antidepressant can I take?

Oh man, you don't also eat a lot of broccoli, do you?

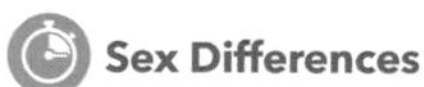

Sex Differences

In general, there are relatively few robust differences in pharmacotherapy dosing and pharmacodynamic outcomes based strictly on sex. Pharmacokinetic sex differences can arise based on drug bioavailability (e.g., women have lower gastric acid secretion and slower gastric emptying than men) and metabolism/excretion (e.g., estrogen induces P450 enzymes). Longer drug elimination half-lives in women versus men have been observed with mirtazapine (37 hours versus 26 hours), zolpidem (45% higher C_{max} and AUC, hence the manufacturer's recommendation for 5 mg per night standard dosing in women versus 10 mg/HS in men) and olanzapine (30% reduced clearance in women than men). Women have demonstrably higher serum concentrations than men receiving comparable doses of amitriptyline, nortriptyline, doxepin, citalopram, and mirtazapine (Unterecker et al., 2013). Women also tend to have lower-activity forms of gastric and hepatic alcohol dehydrogenase as compared to men, leading to the potential for higher blood alcohol levels and reduced tolerance to the effects of alcohol in women than men.

In the case of depression, women tend to manifest more atypical depressive features (i.e., hypersomnia, hyperphagia, anergia) than do men, as well as more extensive anxiety comorbidity, suicide attempts, and seasonal mood variation patterns. Whether or not antidepressant treatment outcomes differ in women versus men remains an open question. One oft-cited study in chronic depression (Kornstein et al., 2000), involving a post hoc analysis of sex differences on treatment outcomes with sertraline versus imipramine, found that women responded better to sertraline while men responded better to imipramine, and postmenopausal women had comparable response rates to both antidepressant classes. That study also prompted interest in the hypothesis that SSRIs may work better in the presence of estrogen, a hypothesis further supported by a short-term (four-week) study showing better antidepressant efficacy in perimenopausal women taking estradiol (17 β-estradiol (100 micro g/day)) than placebo (Cohen et al., 2003). However, numerous subsequent prospective studies and meta-analyses have failed to replicate the finding of a sex difference in antidepressant responses with other SSRIs or SNRIs (Sramek et al., 2016).

Factoid

Antidepressant adherence has been shown to be better in men than women during youth (ages 20–40), but in women more than men during middle and older age (ages 50–70) (i.e., adherence is better in older women than older men (Krivoy et al., 2015)).

When prescribing FGAs or SGAs to women, clinicians should remember that agents with high risk for causing hyperprolactinemia are relatively contraindicated in patients with a history of estrogen receptor (ER)-positive breast cancer, due to the potential trophic effects of prolactin on ER-positive malignant tissue. Prolactin-sparing SGAs such as aripiprazole remain a preferred agent in such instances. Hyperprolactinemia caused by SGAs in general tends to be somewhat higher in women than men, and for women in particular may more often lead to osteoporosis (as well as more common galactorrhea than in men).

Transsexual, Transgender, and Gender-Nonconforming Psychopharmacology

Little has been written about possible unique psychopharmacotherapy issues in transgender individuals. Among individuals diagnosed with gender dysphoria, incident rates of depression, suicidal thinking, and self-harm/nonsuicidal self-injury are disproportionately elevated as compared to the general population, often within the context of interpersonal problems, issues involving low self-esteem, and poor perceived social support (Claes et al., 2015; Witcomb et al., 2018).

Nearly 70% of male-to-female (MtF) or female-to-male (FtM) adults with gender dysphoria have an identifiable current or lifetime psychiatric disorder, most often affective and anxiety disorders, while rates of personality disorders appear comparable to those seen in the general population (Heylens et al., 2014). Social anxiety disorder, in particular, was noted in nearly one-third of a cohort of 210 subjects prior to biological sex reassignment interventions, who were studied as part of a specialized transgender unit within a university hospital in Spain (Bergero-Miguel et al., 2016).

With respect to further diagnostic issues, some authors have noted that primary psychotic disorders such as schizophrenia can involve "*pseudo*transsexualism" (Borras et al., 2007) or delusions related to the idea of sex reassignment that may attenuate with appropriate antipsychotic treatment – noting that transgender concerns are difficult to evaluate as bona fide phenomena when they may be secondary to untreated psychosis in patients who manifest signs of schizophrenia or other psychotic disorders.

We are aware of no formal trials of any pharmacotherapies specifically among transgender individuals. At least on theoretical grounds, clinicians should be mindful of the potential impact of gonadal steroid treatment on mood and thinking, in addition to pharmacokinetics. In FtM persons, high-dose testosterone has been shown to increase serotonin transporter binding in limbic structures and the dorsal striatum – although potential links with these observations and depression symptoms or serotonergic antidepressant response remain purely speculative (Kranz et al., 2015).

Children and Adolescents

Rather than embark on any diluted attempt to address the vast topic of evidence-based pharmacotherapies in children and adolescents, we wish instead here to draw attention to known differences in pharmacotherapy safety and efficacy in youth versus adulthood across major domains of psychopathology. Main findings across broadly defined drug classes are presented in Tables 12.1–12.7.

Geriatric Psychopharmacology

Safety concerns with psychotropic drugs in the elderly are summarized in a consensus panel statement by the American Geriatrics Society known as the Beers Criteria® for potentially inappropriate medication (PIM) use (2019 American Geriatrics Society Beers Criteria® Update Expert Panel), a document that undergoes updates approximately every three years. Among the key recommendations regarding psychotropic use in older adults within the 2019 guidelines are the following:

- Avoid coprescribing opiates with benzodiazepines or gabapentinoids (i.e., gabapentin, gabapentin enacarbol, or pregabalin) (see Box 12.4)

Box 12.4

What's Wrong with Gabapentinoids?

A large (n = 191 973) Swedish registry study found a hazard ratio of 1.26 for suicidal behavior, 1.24 for unintentional overdoses, 1.22 for head/body injuries, and 1.13 for motor vehicle accidents among gabapentin or (especially) pregabalin recipients (Molero et al., 2019). While that study controlled for age, sex and several other potential confounders, its nonrandomized design precludes assessing for possible confounding by indication in possible higher-risk subgroups within the population. Other observational reports identify increased misuse/abuse (Chiappini and Schifano, 2016) as well as a sharp rise in the use of gabapentinoids in age-associated intentional drug overdoses since 2007 (Daly et al., 2018a).

- Prior recommendations to avoid H_2 blockers in older adults based on concerns that they can cause dementia were removed, because evidence to support such a correlation is weak – although H_2 blockers are considered a risk for causing or worsening delirium and should be avoided in that setting
- Dextromethorphan/quinidine can increase the risk for falls and drug–drug interactions and lacks value in dementia unless pseudobulbar affect is clearly present (See Box 12.5)
- In the setting of Parkinson's disease, avoid all anti-dopaminergic antipsychotics other than quetiapine or clozapine (presumably based on relatively low risk for adverse motor effects or nigrostriatal DA blockade, due to less potent D_2 receptor binding; see also Chapter 10, Box 10.5)

Box 12.5

What is Pseudobulbar Affect (PBA)?

PBA is a neurological phenomenon that involves uncontrollable fits of crying or laughing, most often resulting from traumatic brain injury, stroke, dementia, multiple sclerosis, amyotrophic lateral sclerosis, or Parkinson's disease. It is sometimes treated with dextromethorphan/quinidine.

Other psychotropic medications considered "inappropriate" for older adults according to the Beers Criteria®, identified as "strong" recommendations, are shown in Box 12.6.

Box 12.6

Inappropriate Medications for Older Adults*

- *Anticholinergics*: diphenhydramine, hydroxyzine
- *Antiparkinsonian*: benztropine, trihexyphenidyl
- *Cardiovascular*: prazosin, terazosin
- *Antidepressants*: amitriptyline, amoxapine, clomipramine, desipramine, doxepin >6 mg/day, imipramine, nortriptyline, paroxetine, protriptyline, trimipramine
- *Antipsychotics*: "avoid, except in schizophrenia or bipolar disorder" [1]
- *Barbiturates*: all, due to "high rate of physical dependence, tolerance to sleep benefits, greater risk of overdose at low doses"
- *Benzodiazepines*: all, due to "increased risk for cognitive impairment, delirium, falls, fractures, motor vehicle crashes"
- *Nonbenzodiazepine benzodiazepine receptor agonist hypnotics* ("Z-drugs"): eszopiclone, zaleplon, zolpidem (similar concerns as with benzodiazepines)

* As per the Beers Criteria®

Is There a Favored Sleep Aid in Older Adult Patients?

Given the concerns with benzodiazepines and "Z-drugs" noted in the Beers Criteria® recommendations, alternative preferred sleep aids would include ramelteon and suvorexant. Are they evidence-based, or just lesser evils? In a study of 829 elderly patients with chronic insomnia, 4 or 8 mg/HS of ramelteon improved sleep latency and total sleep time, with mild-to-moderate nausea and headache being the most common associated adverse effects (Roth et al., 2006). Similar findings showing improved sleep latency with good tolerability were found over five weeks among 157 older adults (mean age 72.3 years) taking ramelteon 8 mg/HS (Mini et al., 2007). Suvorexant and lemborexant have a novel mechanism of action involving orexin receptor blockade that spares antihistaminergic or anticholinergic pathways. A pooled analysis of three-month data with suvorexant involving 319 adults over the age of 65 with chronic insomnia showed efficacy and good tolerability as compared to placebo in improving sleep latency and continuity; daytime somnolence occurred in 5–9% of subjects, with no evidence of adverse cardiovascular effects (Herring et al., 2017). FDA registration trials for suvorexant also included 159 patients aged 75 or over, again with observed good tolerability.

The *combination* of ramelteon plus suvorexant has been shown to safely and effectively improve sleep quality as well as reduce the risk for poststroke delirium as compared to GABAergic drugs (Kawada et al., 2019). Notable as well are randomized data showing a significantly reduced risk for developing intensive care unit (ICU) delirium with suvorexant (15–20 mg/HS) than seen with conventional sedative-hypnotics (Azuma et al., 2018).

Other Pharmacological Safety Considerations in Older Adults

Risk for hyponatremia and SIADH with antidepressant use is higher in older adults. Some primary care physicians therefore advise checking serum Na^+ levels about a month after starting a serotonergic antidepressant (Frank, 2014); the Beers Criteria® advise "close monitoring" of serum Na^+ levels in older adults taking SSRIs, SNRIs, mirtazapine, tricyclics, carbamazepine, or oxcarbazepine.

Because of increased falls risk in the elderly, α_1-blocking agents (with a resultant risk for orthostatic hypotension), alongside anticholinergic drugs (and their potential for adverse cognitive effects) are generally discouraged.

[1] Manufacturers' product inserts for all antipsychotics carry a boxed warning of an increased risk for all-cause mortality when used for dementia-related psychosis. The Beers Criteria® support this perspective "unless nonpharmacological options (e.g., behavioral interventions) have failed or are not possible and the older adult is threatening substantial harm to self or others."

Coadministration of lithium with ACE inhibitors or loop diuretics is also discouraged (by Beers Criteria®) due to a risk for lithium toxicity (or, otherwise, in our view very close monitoring of serum lithium levels is advisable if benefits are thought to outweigh risks).

Tip

For patients taking lithium who also require treatment with a nonsteroidal anti-inflammatory, lower the dose of lithium by at least 20% for the duration of cotherapy and for five days after NSAID discontinuation, while following lithium levels to assure absence of toxicity.

Geriatric Depression: Is There a Favored Antidepressant?

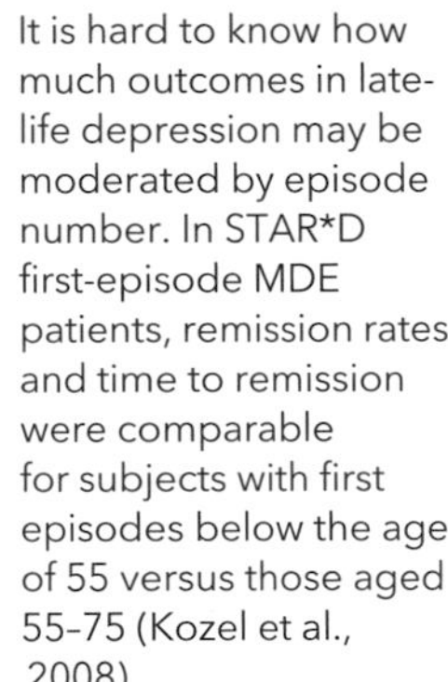

Tip

It is hard to know how much outcomes in late-life depression may be moderated by episode number. In STAR*D first-episode MDE patients, remission rates and time to remission were comparable for subjects with first episodes below the age of 55 versus those aged 55-75 (Kozel et al., 2008).

Antidepressant response rates in older adults are notoriously lower than in younger populations. In a meta-analysis of 10 acute (6–12 week) placebo-controlled antidepressant trials in late-life depression, Nelson and colleagues (2008) found a pooled response rate with antidepressants (44.4%) that was only modestly better than placebo (34.7%), with a somewhat higher probability of response during longer trials (10–12 weeks; OR = 1.73) than shorter trials (6–8 weeks; OR = 1.22). A moderator analysis involving 7 of these 10 trials found that *duration of illness* (especially >10 years) and *higher baseline depression symptom severity* were the two most robust predictors of antidepressant response; in other words, antidepressants had little to no difference versus placebo when late-life depression was of short duration and only mild-to-moderate severity (Nelson et al., 2013).

A later meta-analysis involving 15 RCTs examined older as well as newer-generation antidepressants for MDD patients aged 55 and older (Tedeschini et al., 2011). Overall antidepressant response among MDD patients aged over 65 was found to be no better than with placebo (p = 0.265; NNT for this group was 21), while placebo response rates in themselves were similar in older and younger adult MDD groups. Observed risk ratios for response across RCTs in that meta-analysis are presented in Table 12.8.

Finally, another network analysis of 15 RCTs examined partial response relative to all-cause dropout (i.e., effectiveness) and found the strongest evidence for effectiveness (i.e., efficacy balanced against all-cause dropout) with sertraline (RR for partial response = 1.28), paroxetine (RR for partial response = 1.48) or duloxetine (RR for partial response = 1.62) relative to placebo, with less robust effectiveness seen with citalopram, escitalopram, venlafaxine, or fluoxetine (Thorlund et al., 2015). Among adverse effects, dizziness was least common with sertraline (RR = 1.14) or duloxetine (RR = 1.31) and most severe with duloxetine (RR = 3.18) or venlafaxine (RR = 2.94).

In addition to the above findings are the following:

- Vortioxetine dosed at 5 mg/day was superior to placebo, and well tolerated, in a dedicated placebo-controlled trial for late-life depression (Katona et al., 2012).
- Two RCTs of duloxetine in late-life depression subsequent to the Tedeschini et al. (2011) meta-analysis yielded conflicting results: in the above-noted placebo-controlled trial of vortioxetine (Katona et al., 2012), duloxetine as an active comparator showed efficacy versus placebo, but another 24-week trial found no difference from placebo in depression outcomes (although pain scores improved more with duloxetine); about a quarter of depression nonremitters to a 60 mg/day dose by week 12 went on to subsequent remission after dosing was increased up to 120 mg/day (Robinson et al., 2014).

Tip

In older adult patients beware the risk of acute urinary retention with SNRIs.

- A post hoc analysis of nine pooled desvenlafaxine MDD RCTs revealed no significant moderating effect of age from 18–40 versus 41–54 versus 55–64; too few subjects precluded assessment of those aged 65 or over; a higher incidence of orthostatic hypotension than seen in younger adult populations was noted (Mosca et al., 2017). No RCTs of desvenlafaxine for MDD in adults aged over 65 are available.
- FDA registration trials of vilazodone enrolled 2.2% (n = 65) of subjects aged over 65, although no separate analyses examined treatment outcomes in that subpopulation. No specific dosing adjustments are advised in the elderly.
- In FDA registration trials of levomilnacipran for MDD, 2.8% of enrolled subjects were aged over 65, but no separate analyses of efficacy and tolerability have thus far been reported.

From a safety standpoint, although anticholinergic antidepressants are shunned by the Beers Criteria®, it is noteworthy that placebo-controlled trials support the safety/tolerability and efficacy of low-dose paroxetine CR for MDD in adults over 60, as noted in Table 12.3; as well as secondary amine tricyclics such as nortriptyline (especially for older adult depression with melancholic features, where it outperformed fluoxetine; Roose et al., 1994). In a large Medicare database of new SSRI users in a nursing-home setting (n = 19 952), incident rates of newly diagnosed dementia over a two-year period were no higher among those who took paroxetine than other SSRIs (Bali et al., 2015).

In the 2001 Expert Consensus Guideline Series on the pharmacotherapy of depression in older adult depression (Alexopoulos et al., 2001), lower dosages and slower titration periods were a maxim described in most instances; the expert panel advocated making no changes to a low-dose drug regimen for two to four weeks if little or no response is evident, and waiting three to five weeks in the case of a partial response. In patients able to tolerate higher doses, three to six weeks is considered an adequate trial if no response is evident, while four to seven weeks is recommended if a partial response is detected. After response or remission to a first episode, the experts collectively advise continuation pharmacotherapy for one year; for a second lifetime episode, most experts advised continuation therapy for two years (39%) or three or more years (37%), with a minority advising shorter durations. Nearly all (98%) advocated continued therapy for longer than three years in patients with more than three lifetime episodes.

Adjunctive Strategies in Older Adult MDD

In depressed venlafaxine (up to 300 mg/day) nonresponders over the age of 60 (n = 181), adjunctive aripiprazole (2–15 mg/day) for 12 weeks yielded a higher remission rate than did adjunctive placebo (44% versus 29%, respectively; OR for remission = 2.0, NNT = 6.6); parkinsonism was a notable adverse event arising in 17% of those taking active drug (Lenze et al., 2015). A post hoc analysis of that study found that response was moderated by unimpaired baseline set-shifting (measured by Trail-Making task condition 4 versus 5) on neurocognitive testing (Kaneriya et al., 2016). Brexpiprazole[2] (1–3 mg/day) has been studied in open-label fashion over 26 weeks as an adjunct to monoaminergic antidepressants, with outcomes complicated most often by fatigue and restlessness (18% withdrew due to adverse events) (Lepola et al., 2018). In a dedicated late-life MDD trial, quetiapine XR monotherapy dosed from 50–300 mg/day (mean dose = 158 mg/day) over nine weeks in 166 MDD patients aged 66 or over yielded a greater reduction in depressive symptoms than seen with placebo (n = 172); the most commonly seen adverse events were dizziness, somnolence, and headache (Katila et al., 2013). A post hoc analysis from that study found efficacy for quetiapine XR over placebo regardless of the presence or absence of baseline anxiety, high or low sleep disturbances, and pain scores (Montgomery et al., 2014).

Psychostimulants have long been of interest in the treatment of anergic depression both in younger- and older-adult MDD. An RCT of methylphenidate dosed from 5–40 mg/day (mean dose = 16 mg/day) or placebo added to citalopram (dosed from 20–60 mg/day, mean dose = 32 mg/day) showed faster and more extensive improvement with combination therapy; cognitive outcomes and adverse effects were similar for both treatment groups (Lavretsky et al., 2015). That study affirmed and extended findings from a previous small (n = 16) 10-week pilot RCT of adjunctive

Does modafinil or armodafinil pose any cardiac safety issues in older adults?

In healthy volunteers, a 400 mg one-time dose of modafinil raised systolic blood pressure an average of 7 mmHg, diastolic 5 mmHg, and heart rate 9 beats/minute. However, pooled cardiovascular safety data from 7 RCTs found no significant differences from placebo in changes from baseline in blood pressure or heart rate (Sackner-Berstein et al., 2004).

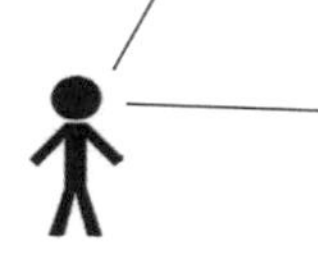

So is that a "yes" or a "no"?

It's a "maybe." Probably much less of a concern for adrenergic tone than a traditional stimulant, and not an absolute no-no, but I'd be watchful in someone with a pre-existing arrhythmia or poorly controlled hypertension.

[2] On the other hand, studies elsewhere have shown that baseline neurocognitive performance *did not* influence response versus nonresponse to short-term open-label trials of an SSRI or SNRI with subsequent SGA augmentation in late-life depression (Koenig et al., 2014).

methylphenidate (Lavretsky et al., 2006). Clinical trials are lacking in late-life MDD with amphetamine formulations, modafinil/armodafinil, or solriamfetol, although each of these compounds has a rationale particularly in anergic, nonagitated, or hypersomnic presentations of MDD.

Older Adult Anxiety

Anxiolytic pharmacotherapy in older adults involves similar concerns as for depression regarding pharmacotherapy safety and tolerability, although the hazards of sedative-hypnotics pose particular limitations. A meta-analysis of 32 RCTs assessing psychosocial interventions as well as pharmacotherapies (benzodiazepines, SSRIs, SNRIs, SGAs, TCAs, and other drugs, including buspirone, nefazodone, and carbamazepine) found overall greater improvement resulting from pharmacotherapy than psychosocial interventions alone, with no single preferred agent identified (Pinquart and Duberstein, 2007).

SGA Use in Older Adults

Limited RCT data address the safety and efficacy of SGAs in patients over 65, across varied indications, either relative to placebo or in head-to-head comparisons between active agents. Generally, manufacturers' product labeling does not advise dosing adjustments in older adults unless factors that directly impede metabolism or drug clearance (i.e., renal or hepatic impairment) are known to be present. In schizophrenia, one meta-analysis of 18 RCTs involving 1225 participants found mainly that olanzapine was superior to haloperidol in treating overall and negative symptoms, incurred less use of antiparkinsonian drugs, and had fewer dropouts than did risperidone (Krause et al., 2018b). Insufficient data precluded a network meta-analysis. SGAs whose FDA registration trials enrolled sufficient numbers of adults over the age of 65 to determine that *age alone* did not impair tolerability include quetiapine (n = 232), olanzapine (n = 263), and paliperidone (n = 125 schizophrenia patients aged 65 or over (n = 22 aged 75 or over), as well as an additional 114 in a dedicated six-week trial in schizophrenia patients aged 65 or over). Each of these databases suggest no inherent differences in tolerability or efficacy among older versus younger patients based on age alone.

Pharmacotherapy Considerations in Smokers

Tobacco smoke induces CYP450 1A1, 1A2 and 2E1. Accordingly, with respect to monoaminergic antidepressants, cigarette smokers would be expected to have decreased serum concentrations of duloxetine (metabolized by CYP 1A2 and 2D6; bioavailability (AUC) is reduced by about one-third), fluvoxamine (metabolized by CYP 1A2 and 2D6), and mirtazapine (metabolized by CYP 1A2, 2D6, and 3A4). Serum trazodone levels also were found to be lower among smokers than nonsmokers, even though its metabolism is only via CYP 3A4 (reviewed by Oliveira et al., 2017). Metabolic clearance of olanzapine (primarily a CYP 1A2 substrate) is ~40% higher in smokers than nonsmokers. Although asenapine is predominantly a CYP 1A2 substrate, smokers have not been shown to differ from nonsmokers in clearance. Smoking has not been shown to affect serum levels of fluoxetine but may raise levels of its metabolite norfluoxetine.

Ok, so, I get it that benzodiazepines are problematic in older adults because of adverse cognitive effects and falls risk, that the beer vendors don't like SGAs outside of psychosis, and even gabapentinoids are frowned on – really?! – But the fact is that I have a lot of anxious older adults already on SSRIs who are still anxious, so what pharmacotherapy options are there?

It's the Beers Criteria®, not the beer vendors. Look, there are no easy answers here. Everything is a risk–benefit analysis and you have to use your best judgment and follow a rationale. If someone clearly has benefitted from a low-dose SGA and their QTc interval is OK, or trazodone isn't overly sedating and you're tracking their cognitive status, or a low-dose secondary amine tricyclic and their ECG is OK, just spell out your rationale. That's the most anyone can do.

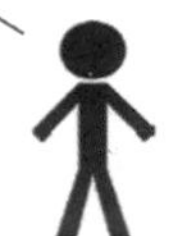

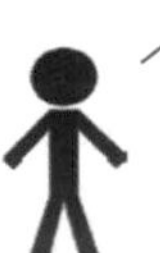

Do e-cigarettes increase CYP450 induction?

No, it's the combustion of nicotine that liberates polycyclic aromatic hydrocarbons in tobacco smoke, which in turn is thought to cause induction of CYP P450 1A2

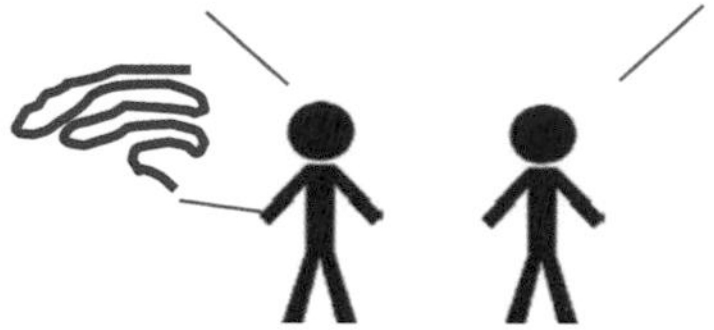

Patients with Alcohol Use Disorders

All psychotropic drugs carry manufacturers' warnings against concomitant use of any alcohol. Why? There are several reasons. First, from the standpoint of absorption and bioavailability, gastric emptying is accelerated by consuming low-content alcohol beverages (<15%; e.g., beer and wine) and delayed via high-alcohol-content beverages. Acute alcohol use also delays gastric emptying and small bowel transit time, while chronic use more likely accelerates gastric emptying and transit time in the small intestines. These factors could result in relatively higher or lower absorption and bioavailability of contemporaneously ingested psychotropic compounds. Second, pharmacokinetically, alcohol induces CYP450 enzymes, in turn accelerating the metabolism of hepatically cleared medications. First-pass metabolism is also thought to be lower in people who regularly drink significant amounts of alcohol, especially in women or people who take H_2 blockers, due to decreased activity of alcohol dehydrogenase (Oneta et al., 1998). Alcohol in combination with opiates or benzodiazepines at sufficient quantities poses a significant risk for respiratory suppression and cardiovascular collapse. Finally, the CNS depressant effects of alcohol (and its eventual withdrawal) are at pharmacodynamic cross purposes with the intended effects of most psychotropic medications, very likely negating their intended benefits.

B REPRODUCTIVE PSYCHOPHARMACOLOGY

Peri- and Postpartum Mood Disorders

Depression during pregnancy (antepartum) has been estimated to arise in 7–25% of women with stratification higher among low- and middle-income nations (Gelaye et al., 2016). Its known risk factors are summarized in Box 12.7.

Box 12.7

Risk Factors for Depression During Pregnancy

- Four or more depressive episodes prepregnancy (Yonkers et al., 2011)
- Prior postpartum depression(s) (Altemus et al., 2012; Viguera et al., 2011)
- Psychosocial stressors (Altemus et al., 2012)
- Younger age at onset (Viguera et al., 2011)
- Fewer years of illness (Viguera et al., 2011)
- Fewer children (Viguera et al., 2011)
- Race/ancestry is a correlate in some studies (i.e., Black (HR = 3.69) or Latino (HR = 2.33) (Yonkers et al., 2011)) but not others (i.e., Guitivano et al., 2018)

Epidemiologically, 15–20% of women develop a major depressive episode postpartum. Postpartum depression is formally identified as occurring in the month following delivery, although most clinicians more broadly interpret the construct to bear on the first year after the end of a pregnancy. One study found that 94% of postpartum MDEs arose in the first four months after delivery (Altemus et al., 2012). MDEs arising during pregnancy have been shown to occur with equal risk across trimesters except for a higher first-trimester risk in women who discontinued a stable antidepressant in the previous year (Altemus et al., 2012). However, some reports suggest that in women with a history of depression, continued use versus cessation of antidepressants during pregnancy was *not* found to predict perinatal depression (Yonkers et al., 2011). Obsessive-compulsive and psychotic symptoms are more common in MDEs arising postpartum than during pregnancy (Altemus et al., 2012). Overall risk for mood episodes is approximately 3.5 times higher postpartum than during pregnancy (Viguera et al., 2011).

Postpartum mood episodes, especially depressions, may represent a genetic subtype of mood disorder, carrying an approximate two to fivefold increased likelihood in the first-degree relatives of bipolar (Payne et al., 2008) or unipolar (Kimmel et al., 2015) probands with postpartum mood episodes. A history of bipolar disorder confers a 50% increased risk per pregnancy for perinatal depression, but risk also remains high in women with a history of unipolar depression (Di Florio et al., 2013). Women with bipolar disorder collectively tend to have a higher risk for postpartum mood episodes than do women with a history of unipolar depression; however, postpartum mood disorders should not be construed as necessarily being synonymous with a more likely bipolar than unipolar underlying diagnosis.

Robertson and colleagues (2004) undertook two meta-analyses of risk factors for postpartum depression, involving over 24 000 pregnant cases. The main findings, presented in descending order based on relative effect sizes, are presented in Box 12.8.

Box 12.8

Clinical and Demographic Predictors of Postpartum Depression

Predictor variable	Effect size (Cohen's *d*)
Depression during pregnancy	0.75
Anxiety during pregnancy	0.68
Stressful life events	0.61
Poor social supports	-0.64
Previous history of depression	0.58
Neuroticism	0.39
Poor marital relationship	0.39
Low socioeconomic status	-0.14
Obstetrical complications (e.g., pre-eclampsia, fetal distress, preterm delivery, unplanned caesarean section, excessive intrapartum bleeding)	0.26

Obsessive-compulsive disorder (Altemus et al., 2012) or obsessive-compulsive personality traits (van Broekhoven et al., 2019) may represent additional risk factors for postpartum mood disorders.

Pharmacotherapy During Pregnancy and Lactation

Pharmacokinetic changes in pregnancy can result from rising estrogen levels during the third trimester (which can induce CYP450 hepatic enzymes 3A4, 2D6, and 2C9[3] as well as UGT1A4 and UGTA1/9), resulting in more extensive drug metabolism, and also from diminished bioavailability because the volume of distribution (Vd) of a given drug changes as plasma volume increases by >40%. Albumin levels also decrease up to 13% by 32 weeks' gestation, reducing the carrying capacity for protein-bound drugs. GFR increases by up to 50% in the first trimester of pregnancy and continues thereafter (Davison and Dunlop, 1980).

There are several basic concepts worth noting regarding psychopharmacology during pregnancy. Relatively few medications have "absolute" known teratogenic risks, though most if not all can pose "unknown" risks. As a rule of thumb, it is advisable to minimize the number of exposures to multiple agents in order to keep to a minimum as best as possible the number of "unknown" unknowns. Most organogenesis occurs in the first trimester, meaning that many women exposed to psychotropic medications may not be aware that they are pregnant until much of this time window has already elapsed.

Tip

The safety of IV or IN (es)ketamine during pregnancy has not been established. Animal studies suggest that intrauterine exposure may impair fetal synaptic plasticity and cause neurobehavioural deficits in newborns.

It can be difficult to parse the potential impact of medication exposures from the effects of undertreated psychopathology on fetal development and obstetrical outcomes. Severe mood or psychotic disorders have in themselves been associated with low birth weight and preterm delivery, as well as increased risks for miscarriage and intrapartum bleeding (Bonari et al., 2004).

Baseline rates for major congenital malformations range from 2–5.5% (Egbe et al., 2015) and vary considerably based on socioeconomic and other demographic factors. Findings on the risk for congenital malformations among infants with intrauterine exposure to psychotropic drugs are presented in Table 12.9. Statistics are based on network meta-analyses where available, such as a review of 96 published trials involving

[3] CYP 2C19 and CYP1A2 activities decrease during pregnancy

Box 12.9

A Word on Opiates in Pregnancy

Generally speaking, it is undesirable for a pregnant woman to withdraw from opiates due to added physiological stress on the developing fetus. Methadone maintenance is widely considered to be the safest and most efficacious treatment of choice for managing opiate dependence during pregnancy. A small but growing database also suggests safety and efficacy for use of buprenorphine during pregnancy; a meta-analysis of 3 RCTs and 15 observational cohort studies showed a significantly reduced risk for preterm birth, greater birth weight, and larger head circumference in newborns exposed to buprenorphine born to mothers with opiate use disorders, with no statistically significant increased risk for fetal demise (Zedler et al., 2016).

58 461 pregnant patients taking anticonvulsant drugs by Veroniki et al. (2017). The management of opioid physiological dependence during pregnancy is discussed in Box 12.9.

Psychopharmacology and Lactation

Most psychotropic drugs are excreted in breast milk, although in most instances there are no known adverse clinical consequences to a nursing infant. Highly protein-bound drugs are less likely readily to enter the milk compartment (see Table 12.10). Manufacturers' product labels typically include language stating that in such instances a medication should be used only if the benefits outweigh the potential risk to the child. Large-scale studies are essentially nonexistent, and estimates of maternal milk to plasma (M/P) ratios (i.e., a measure of drug transfer into breast milk) or relative infant dose (RID; calculated as daily infant dose (mg/kg/day) ÷ daily maternal dose (mg/kg/day) × 100) are based largely on case reports or small open trials. *M/P ratios >1 suggest that a drug is detectable in breast milk at high concentrations.*

Tip

Nortriptyline, paroxetine, and sertraline appear to be the least likely antidepressants to have appreciably detectable levels in breast milk.

Postpartum Mood Disorders

The postpartum period is among the highest of all risk periods for relapse of mood disorders. Relapse concerns specific to women with bipolar disorder are described in Box 12.10.

Among traditional antidepressants for *preventing* postpartum depression (PPD), a review of four RCTs ranging in duration from 6–20 weeks found no significant advantage for nortriptyline or single-dose IV ketamine versus placebo, but sertraline, trazodone, and diphenhydramine were each better than placebo at preventing PPD (Frieder et al., 2019).

I thought lithium was a no-no in breastfeeding.

Not necessarily. In a woman who is an excellent lithium responder without compelling alternatives, the benefits may outweigh the potential risks.

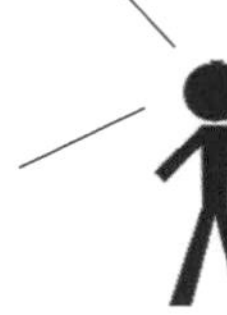

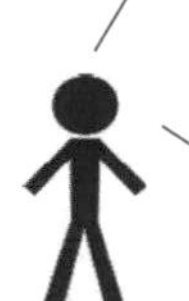

And just what are those potential risks?

About 20% of breastfed infants of mothers taking lithium will have *transient* short-term adverse effects such as renal or thyroid abnormalities. If hypotonia, weight loss or dehydration occur they usually reflect toxicity. Monitor maternal and infant lithium levels at delivery and at 48 hours and then 10 days postpartum. No need to continue monitoring both if infant levels are <0.30 mEq/L.

Box 12.10

Bipolar Postpartum Relapse: Watch the Time

In a prospective study of women with bipolar disorder who discontinued lithium within six days of conception, no significant differences in mood disorder relapse rates were evident as compared to a matched sample of nonpregnant women who discontinued lithium for the first 40 weeks (Viguera et al., 2000). However, promptly thereafter, recurrences happened dramatically faster and were three times more in postpartum than nonpregnant women (70% versus 24%) – meaning that the immediate days and weeks following delivery pose an especially high-risk time window for affective relapse in bipolar women.

Brexanolone

Brexanolone, an analogue of the endogenous neurosteroid and progesterone metabolite allopregnanolone (formerly known as SAGE-547), acts as a positive allosteric modulator of $GABA_A$ receptors that gained attention (and FDA approval) in 2019 for the treatment of postpartum depression (Kanes et al., 2017). Due to poor oral bioavailability, brexanolone is administered intravenously over 60 hours with a resulting significant improvement in depression symptom severity as compared to placebo by completion of the infusion, with a large effect size ($d = 1.2$). Its manufacturer's product label includes a boxed warning concerning the risk for excessive sedation and loss of consciousness, and its administration must occur under a Risk Evaluation and Mitigation Strategy (REMS) protocol.

C PREMENSTRUAL DEPRESSION, OR PREMENSTRUAL DYSPHORIC DISORDER (PMDD)

In PMDD, so-called *luteal-phase dosing* (begun on Day 14 of the menstrual cycle and discontinued within a few days after menstruation begins) of SSRIs (notably, clomipramine or sertraline) has been described as an effective and viable strategy with results comparable to full-cycle dosing (Freeman et al., 1999). As noted in Chapter 11, calcium carbonate 600 mg PO BID has been shown in preliminary studies to be a possible evidence-based treatment option for PMDD. Later efforts to replicate those initial findings did observe greater depressive symptom reduction with calcium carbonate than placebo but with a small effect size ($d = 0.10$–0.44 across outcome measures), while a comparison treatment arm of fluoxetine 20 mg PO qDay also yielded significantly greater improvement than placebo but with larger effect sizes ($d = 0.80$–2.08) (Yonkers et al., 2013). SSRI discontinuation symptoms have not been reported following abrupt cessation of short half-life SSRIs such as sertraline when used only for luteal phase dosing (Yonkers et al., 2015).

Terminology

PMS (premenstrual syndrome) refers to both emotional and physical symptoms (e.g., bloating, fatigue, breast tenderness) occurring one to two weeks before menstruation.

PMDD (premenstrual dysphoric disorder) is considered a more severe subtype of PMS that involves mainly more prominent mood symptoms.

So how is it that in Chapter 11, progesterone was a *pro*-depressant – and, after all, a 2008 Cochrane Database Review cautioned against using synthetic progestogens postpartum because they can increase the risk of depression – but now, progesterone's "analogue," allopregnanolone, works as a fancy new-fangled *anti*-depressant?

So, allopregnanolone, aka brexanolone, is a neurosteroid that acts as an allosteric modulator at the $GABA_A$ receptor. Progesterone is not a neurosteroid and doesn't modulate GABA. Preclinical data suggest that in depression, enzymatic conversion of progesterone to allopregnanolone may be downregulated, and that mechanism may at least partly account for postpartum depression. Infusion of IV brexanolone rapidly brings allopregnanolone levels to about the same level we would expect to see at the end of a pregnancy that was not complicated by depression.

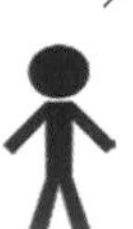

In contrast to PMDD, where depressive symptoms are largely confined to the time between ovulation and menstruation, late luteal phase exacerbations of (full cycle) MDD anecdotally have not been reported to respond simply to luteal phase SSRI pulse-dosing, although no formal RCTs of pulsed dosing versus through-the-month dosage increases have been published.

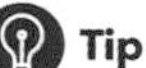

Tip

In PMDD without major depression, consider pulsed/luteal phase antidepressant dosing. In MDD with premenstrual exacerbations of depression, consider increased dosing through the month.

What is the role, if any, for oral contraceptives in the treatment of premenstrual depression? A 2012 Cochrane Database review examined five RCTs with 1920 subjects taking placebo or progestin/low-estrogen dose oral contraceptives to treat PMDD and found that drospirenone 3 mg plus ethinyl estradiol 20 µg (brand names Gianvi®, Loryna®, Nikki®, Yasmin® or Yaz®) improved depression and other related PMS symptoms better than placebo (Lopez et al., 2012). PMDD symptom data for levonorgestrel 150 µg plus ethinyl estradiol 30 µg (brand names Amethyst®, Aviane®, Lybel®) were inconclusive. Outcomes for desogestrel 150 µg plus ethinyl estradiol 30 µg (brand names Apri®, Caziant®, Desogen®) were similar to those seen with drospirenone plus ethinyl estradiol.

One cannot discuss the relationship between mood disorders and dysregulation of the menstrual cycle without considering possible iatrogenic moderating factors. Notably, in the 1990s, concerns arose about a potential association between divalproex and polycystic ovarian syndrome, both in women with epilepsy and bipolar disorder. These complexities are discussed in Box 12.11.

Box 12.11

Divalproex and Polycystic Ovarian Syndrome

Polycystic ovarian syndrome (PCOS; also known as Stein–Leventhal syndrome) is defined as hyperandrogenism and chronic anovulation or oligomenorrhea or amenorrhea. An early report linked use of divalproex with PCOS in women with epilepsy (Isojärvi et al., 1993), but controversy ensued regarding potential confounding factors such as the impact of associated obesity, hyperinsulinemia causing hyperandrogenism, and epilepsy itself on reproductive hormone function (Ernst and Goldberg, 2002). A prospective study in women with bipolar disorder, controlling for effects of pharmacotherapy, found an incident rate of 7.5% (95% CI = 1.7 to 34.1, p = 0.002) for new-onset oligomenorrhea and hyperandrogenism associated with divalproex use over at least a 12-month period (Joffe et al., 2006). Since then, the general recommendation has been to monitor clinically for menstrual cycle irregularities and signs of hyperandrogenism (e.g., acne, hirsutism) in women of reproductive age who begin taking divalproex.

Are oral contraceptives evidence-based just for PMDD or also for premenstrual exacerbations of major depression?

Interesting you ask. So, there was an open trial of ethinyl estradiol plus drospirenone added to existing antidepressants for two cycles which showed improvement in depression (Joffe et al., 2007), followed by a later placebo-controlled trial where the difference just missed statistical significance (Peters et al., 2017). What does that tell you?

Was the study underpowered?

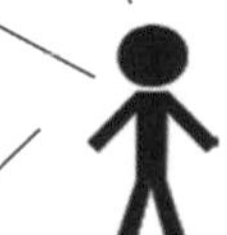

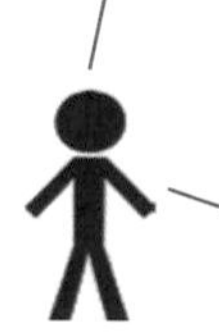

The sample size was 25 completers – about half each on drug or placebo. What does that tell you?

It tells me either the effect size was probably too small for that study to pick up, or else that you want me to go write a grant for a larger study.

D SOMATIC SYMPTOM DISORDER AND PRONENESS TO SOMATIZATION

DSM-5 has reorganized the construct of somatization disorders, and somatoform pain disorders, under the rubric of somatic symptom disorder. For the current purposes we will use interchangeably the terms "somatization," "somatic symptoms," and "medically unexplained physical symptoms (MUPS)." We consider as a "special population" patients with excessive preoccupations and distress related to somatic symptoms because pharmacotherapy can often pose unique complications. Generally speaking, structured forms of psychotherapy offer a more evidence-based treatment approach for the distress arising from MUPS. Pharmacotherapy, if and when useful, tends to provide a decidedly ancillary role, accompanied by modest expectations about their helpfulness. One 30-year literature review found that serotonergic antidepressants may offer greater value for targeting "obsessional" rather than somatic or pain-based features (Fallon, 2004). A Cochrane Database Review of 26 RCTs involving 2159 participants found no significant outcome differences between tricyclics and placebo (SMD = –0.13, 95% CI = –0.39 to 0.13) (Kleinstäuber et al., 2014). Newer-generation antidepressants (SSRIs (paroxetine, citalopram, sertraline) or SNRIs (venlafaxine, milnacipran)) exerted a large, significant effect size (SMD = –0.91, 95% CI = –1.36 to –0.46) based on three studies lasting 8–12 weeks that all were considered to be of "very low" quality. (Secondary analyses showed significant reductions in anxiety and depressive symptoms but not dysfunctional cognitions.) Two studies of natural products (e.g., St John's wort) also found a fairly large effect (SMD = –0.74, 95% CI = –0.97 to –0.51) of "low" quality evidence for reducing the intensity of MUPS, with secondary analyses again showing significant reductions in anxiety and depression. Two RCTs suggest that an SGA (specifically, quetiapine or paliperidone) plus an SSRI (specifically, citalopram or paroxetine) outperform SSRI monotherapy (SMD = 0.77, 95% CI = 0.32 to 1.22; evidence deemed "low quality").

Reminder

Confidence intervals that cross zero are nonsignificant.

E CLINICALLY SIGNIFICANT COMORBID OR CHRONIC MEDICAL CONDITIONS

Cardiac

Depression After Acute Myocardial Infarction

Depression in the aftermath of a myocardial infarction inherently constitutes an increased risk for mortality. A primary treatment concern involves the hazard of post-MI arrhythmias.

Sertraline represents the best-studied pharmacotherapy for post-MI depression, as shown in a 24-week flexibly dosed RCT versus placebo in 369 MDD patients hospitalized for an acute MI or unstable angina (Glassman et al., 2002). Response rates were significantly greater with sertraline than placebo, especially in those with a prior history of depression and those with higher baseline severity. Importantly, sertraline had no adverse effects on left ventricular ejection fraction, ventricular premature complexes (VPCs), or changes in QTc duration. Other RCTs have shown that use of *any* SSRI for MDD post MI reduces all-cause mortality as well as risk for a recurrent MI (Taylor et al., 2005).

QTc Prolongation

As touched on earlier in Chapter 10 (Figure 10.1), sudden cardiac death due to ventricular arrhythmias is a concern associated with all antipsychotic drugs, which overall confer an approximate twofold adjusted incidence-rate ratio (Ray et al., 2009).

Cerebrovascular

Poststroke Depression

There is a remarkably sparse controlled trial literature for treating poststroke depression. A meta-analysis by Sun and colleagues (2017) found from among 12 RCTs involving 707 subjects, reboxetine had the highest cumulative probability of *efficacy* (100%), followed by paroxetine (87.5%), then doxepin (83.2%), then duloxetine (62.4%). Rankings for *acceptability* favored paroxetine (92.4%), followed by placebo (63.5%), then sertraline (57.3%), then nortriptyline (56.3%). Paroxetine and reboxetine overall each demonstrated among the best combinations of efficacy and acceptability, as depicted in Figure 12.1.

Figure 12.1 Clustered ranking plot for efficacy and acceptability of pharmacotherapies for poststroke depression. Adapted from Sun et al., 2017.

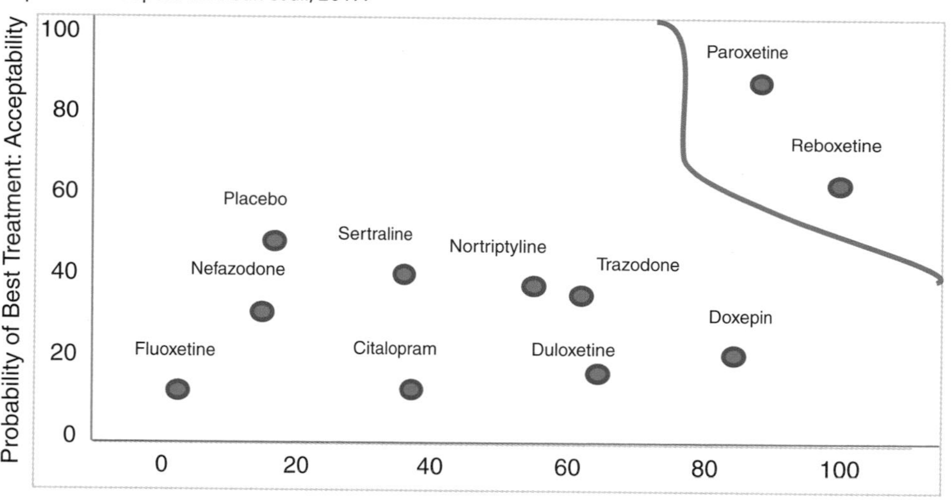

A Bayesian network meta-analysis involving 23 antidepressant RCTs for poststroke depression found better response rates with placebo than with tricyclic antidepressants (OR = 8.01, 95% CI = 4.16–15.42), SSRIs (OR = 3.55, 95% CI = 1.98–6.46), or the Chinese herbal medicine Free and Easy Wanderer Plus (FEWP) (OR = 3.48, 95% CI = 1.62–7.89); hierarchically, the observed mean differences in Hamilton Ratings Scale for Depression scores favored paroxetine > imipramine > reboxetine > nortriptyline > duloxetine > citalopram > sertraline > FEWP > fluoxetine > clomipramine > venlafaxine (Deng et al., 2017).

In studies focused on *prevention* of poststroke depression in initially nondepressed stroke patients, escitalopram was superior to both placebo and to structured psychotherapy, while controlling for relevant confounders (e.g., history of mood disorder, severity of impairment, demographic characteristics) (Robinson et al., 2008); prophylactic escitalopram post stroke also improved cognitive function better than placebo or psychotherapy (Jorge et al., 2010).

In open trials using stimulants (either methylphenidate or dextroamphetamine), improvement in depressive symptoms has been reported in up to 70–80% of recipients with good tolerability (Masand et al., 1991; Lazarus et al., 1992), although findings are based on small sample sizes using open-label study designs. Antidepressant response to methylphenidate in poststroke depression may be faster (less than three days) than seen with nortriptyline, based on retrospective data (Lazarus et al., 1994). In studies of poststroke fatigue, modafinil dosed at 200 mg/day has demonstrated both positive (Bivard et al., 2017) and negative (Poulson et al., 2015) effects.

In hemorrhagic strokes, serotonergic antidepressants arguably might be worth avoiding at least within the first 30 days of an acute bleed. In contrast, concerns about bleeding diatheses do not bear similarly on ischemic strokes. In fact, the safety of SSRIs after ischemic stroke has been well demonstrated in the Fluoxetine for Motor Recovery After Acute Ischemic Stroke (FLAME) study, in which fluoxetine 20 mg/day or placebo was begun within 5–10 days after an ischemic stroke in 113 nondepressed patients (Chollet et al., 2011). That study did not evaluate the prevention of poststroke depression, but instead focused on (and demonstrated) improvement of hemiparesis or hemiplegia, based on hypotheses that an SSRI might enhance neuronal recovery.

Chronic Obstructive Pulmonary Disease (COPD)

A Cochrane Database Review of pharmacotherapy for depression in COPD (four RCTs, n = 201 subjects) found short-term (12-week) greater improvement in depressive symptoms with nortriptyline than placebo but no improvement in quality of life or dyspnea measures (Pollok et al., 2018). Two RCTs involving SSRIs (paroxetine (20 mg/day) or low-dose sertraline (50 mg/day)) revealed no significant difference in change in depression symptom scores as compared to placebo. Notably, sample sizes were small (<30 subjects per arm in the paroxetine trials, for example), and in one of the trials nearly 30% of paroxetine recipients dropped out prematurely due to drug intolerance. On the other hand, exercise tolerance (a secondary outcome) at study end was better with SSRIs than placebo.

Perhaps even more importantly than depression, the safe and effective management of anxiety disorders or symptoms in COPD patients warrants consideration, given the potential for benzodiazepines to suppress central respiratory drive. So-called "Z-drugs" (zolpidem, zaleplon, eszopiclone) bind less potently at $GABA_A$ benzodiazepine sites and are considered less hazardous in patients with sleep apnea. Paroxetine, while undistinguished for its antidepressant effects in COPD, as noted above, has elsewhere been shown to reduce anxiety symptoms (dosed at 20 mg/day) better than placebo (Usmani et al., 2018). Buspirone, from a mainly older literature, has not been shown to improve anxiety in COPD patients (Singh et al., 1993) but according to some reports may nevertheless improve exercise tolerance (Argyropoulou et al., 1993). Most of the literature on managing anxiety in asthma or other COPD patients has focused more on behavioral strategies (e.g., cognitive-behavioral therapy, mindfulness-based stress reduction or meditation, yoga, Tai Chi) than pharmacotherapies. We would note anecdotally that novel anxiolytics such as gabapentin or pregabalin, while not (yet) formally studied in COPD patients, may warrant consideration based on their relatively favorable safety profiles and database for efficacy across several anxiety disorders in general (see Chapter 17).

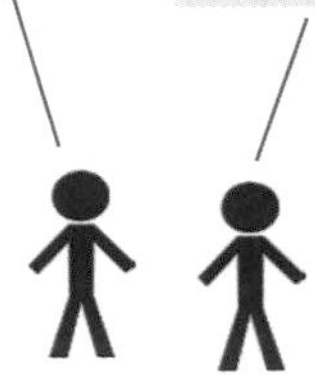

So should I not use SSRIs in depressed COPD patients?
It's not that black and white. We can say that paroxetine and sertraline haven't been shown to be especially helpful, but that doesn't negate the possibility SSRIs can help. Dosing in those studies may have been too low. Other SSRIs might work better. So it really just means the limited database can't definitively guide us.

With respect to antipsychotic use in COPD patients, a population-based study of 5032 Taiwanese patients with acute respiratory failure found a dose-dependent relationship with antipsychotic use (2.16-fold overall adjusted increased risk; 1.52-fold for low-dose daily use and 3.74-fold for high-dose daily use) (Wang and colleagues, 2017b). While those authors interpreted their findings as the basis for caution against regularly using high-dose antipsychotics in COPD patients, we would note the potential methodological confounds of descriptive (nonrandomized) population-based studies such as this – notably, that high-dose daily SGA use might also *indirectly* account for respiratory failure if it serves as a marker for more proximal causes of respiratory failure such as obesity, high BMI, smoking, or concomitant sleep apnea.

Dementia

Dementia poses unique challenges for pharmacotherapy in light of the increased risk for all-cause mortality associated with antipsychotic use set against modest efficacy with most studied compounds. In the Clinical Antipsychotic Trials of Intervention Effectiveness-Alzheimer's Disease study (CATIE-AD), SGAs were found to worsen cognition more than placebo (Vigen et al., 2011). Agitation and aggression in Alzheimer's dementia patients has been shown to improve significantly more with citalopram (dosed from 10–30 mg/day in a large (n = 186) multisite trial; Porsteinsson et al., 2014) or with dextromethorphan-quinidine (Cummings et al., 2015). Among SSRIs other than citalopram, sertraline, but not fluoxetine, also has preliminarily shown efficacy versus placebo for reducing agitation symptoms in dementia

Tip

When serum drug levels of medications that are transported by carrier proteins (e.g., divalproex) are unexpectedly low, assure serum albumin levels are also not low (as may occur in patients with celiac disease or when malabsorption and malnutrition are concerns); then measure free (unbound) drug fractions.

(Seitz et al., 2011). Neither trazodone (Martinon-Torres et al., 2004) nor divalproex (studied across five RCTs, n = 475, dosed from 480–1000 mg/day; Baillon et al., 2018) has shown a benefit relative to placebo for agitation symptoms of dementia.

 Gastrointestinal Disorders

Celiac Disease

Obvious concerns for psychopharmacology in the setting of celiac disease involve the potential for drug malabsorption as well as the potential for decreased albumin production (due to possible malnutrition) as a drug carrier protein.

Gastric Bypass

Patients who have undergone a Roux-en-Y gastric bypass procedure are generally unable to absorb extended-release formulations of medication. In general, SSRI and SNRI serum levels have been shown to decrease by about 50% one month after a Roux-en-Y procedure but usually return to baseline within six months (Lloret-Linares et al., 2015).

Irritable Bowel Syndrome

A meta-analysis of 17 placebo-controlled antidepressant trials for irritable bowel syndrome (IBS) found a significant advantage for antidepressants (either SSRIs or TCAs) relative to placebo (RR = 0.66, 95% CI = 0.56–0.76), with an associated NNT of 4.5 (Ford et al., 2019). The RR and NNT for symptom improvement overall were similar between TCAs and SSRIs. It has often been noted in the literature that TCAs may be a preferred treatment option in diarrhea-predominant IBS (because they slow gut transit time) while SSRIs may be more beneficial in constipation-prone cases, although formal randomized studies testing these hypotheses are lacking. Linaclotide (typically dosed at 290 mcg orally, at least 30 minutes before a first daily meal) represents another option for IBS with constipation, increasing gut water and chloride transport to soften stools.

Another meta-analysis of 12 RCTs found a pooled RR for improvement of 1.36 with TCAs (95% CI = 1.07–1.71) as compared to a nonsignificant RR = 1.38 (95% CI = 0.83–2.28) with SSRIs (Xie et al., 2015). Specifically, significant improvement was seen in global symptoms as well as abdominal pain. Other literature suggests that fluoxetine may be more beneficial than placebo to treat bloating and abdominal discomfort specifically in constipation-prone manifestations of IBS (Vahedi et al., 2005).

SSRI trials in IBS tend to use doses comparable to those used to treat MDD while TCA doses tend to be somewhat lower than in MDD. Efficacy for IBS symptoms appears *not* to be contingent on significant changes in concomitant depression symptom rating scales.

 Hepatic Impairment

In addition to consulting manufacturers' package insert product information about the use of specific medications in the setting of hepatic impairment, clinicians can obtain up-to-date drug information about hepatotoxicity online at https://livertox.nih.gov. Patients with significant hepatic dysfunction typically have difficulty catabolizing drugs that must undergo Phase I or Phase II metabolism, making it preferable to favor the use of hepatically metabolized drugs whose terminal elimination half-lives are relatively short (e.g., oxazepam, flurazepam, temazepam, alprazolam) rather than long (e.g., clonazepam, diazepam, chlordiazepoxide). Additionally, in the setting of severe liver disease, patients may have markedly reduced production of albumin and α-1 acid glycoprotein, which bears on their capacity to transport drugs that are highly protein-bound (i.e., >80–85%; see summary depicted as those drugs in the dark-shaded region of Box 12.12). Keep in mind that both psychotropic and nonpsychotropic drugs that compete for protein binding sites (e.g., coumadin) run the risk of displacing coadministered competitor agents, potentially leading to greater variation in bioavailability and therefore more unpredictable pharmacodynamic effects. Tables 12.11 to 12.16 summarize information about use and dosing modifications of psychotropic drugs in patients with hepatic impairment (and see also individual product manufacturers' product information, typically Sections 8.6 or 8.7).

 Glaucoma

Patients with narrow-angle glaucoma incur the risk of angle-closure attacks in response to medications that trigger pupillary dilatation (e.g., many antidepressants) if

Box 12.12

Protein Binding Across Psychotropic Medications

% Protein Binding	Agents
>99%	Aripiprazole, brexpiprazole, suvorexant, valbenazine
98-99%	Sertraline, nefazodone, vortioxetine
96-99%	Amitriptyline, clozapine, lumateperone, vilazodone
95%	Iloperidone, pimavanserin
94-95%	Fluoxetine, lemborexant
93%	Olanzapine
92%	Nortriptyline, zolpidem
91%	Desipramine
89-95%	Trazodone
85-94%	Divalproex
86%	Imipramine
85%	Mirtazapine
84%	Bupropion
80%	Citalopram, fluvoxamine
75-80%	Carbamazepine, doxepin
74%	Paliperidone
60-68%	Deutetrabenazine, modafinil
60%	Zaleplon
56%	Escitalopram
55%	Lamotrigine
52-59%	Eszopiclone
30%	Desvenlafaxine, venlafaxine
22%	Levomilnacipran
15-40%	Amphetamine
13-17%	Methylphenidate, pramipexole, solriamfetol, topiramate
<3%	Gabapentin
<1%	Pregabalin

What's the safest sleep aid to give to my patient with severe liver disease?
What's the least protein bound? See Box 12.12. And the least hepatically metabolized? See Table 12.14. And the shortest half-life? Does the patient also have renal impairment? If so, see Table 12.20. What about any anticholinergic or arrhythmogenic concerns? See Box 16.2 and Figure 10.1.
OK, OK, I get it!

a given patient does not have a patent iridectomy. Other medications that can cause pupillary dilatation and pose this risk include benzodiazepines, anticholinergics, and stimulants.

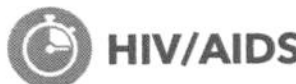

HIV/AIDS

The emergence of highly active antiretroviral therapy (HAART) in the mid–late 1990s has largely transformed HIV/AIDS from a lethal illness to a chronic, manageable condition. Of general concern for psychopharmacologists is the potential for pharmacokinetic interactions caused by protease inhibitors and nonnucleoside reverse transcriptase inhibitors, as shown in Box 12.13.

In the pharmacotherapy of depression in HIV+ patients, the following basic observations are noteworthy:

Box 12.13

Pharmacokinetic Effects of Protease Inhibitors and Non-nucleoside Reverse Transcriptase Inhibitors

CYP34 Inducers	CYP3A4 Inhibitors	CYP2D6 Inhibitors	CYP12 Inducer
Efavirenz	Delavirdine	Ritonavir	Ritonavir
Nevirapine	Saquinivir		
	Indinavir		

- In treating *depression* in HIV+/AIDS patients, double-blind trials support the efficacy and tolerability of imipramine, fluoxetine, and paroxetine (all yielding single-digit NNTs) (reviewed by Ferrando and Freyberg, 2008) as well as DHEA (dosed from 100–400 mg/day; NNT = 4; Rabkin et al., 2006). Open trial data have shown value with citalopram, which may hold particular appeal because its hepatic metabolism (CYP 1A2) poses no pharmacokinetic conflicts with protease inhibitors. Small open trials also support the use of mirtazapine (potentially especially useful when insomnia and anorexia are present), nefazodone (which remains an available, though less popular, antidepressant since concerns about its 2003 FDA warning for rare (1 in 250 000) risk for fulminant hepatic failure), and bupropion SR (reviewed by Ferrando, 2009). Effective pharmacotherapy for depression in HIV+ patients has been shown to improve HAART adherence (Yun et al., 2005). Psychostimulants and related compounds have been reported to improve depressed mood and fatigue in HIV+ patients, particularly with use of dextroamphetamine up to 40 mg/day (Wagner and Rabkin, 2000), modafinil 50–400 mg/day (mean dose among responders = 135 mg/day; Rabkin et al., 2004), and methylphenidate up to 60 mg/day (Breitbart et al., 2001).
- With respect to *mood stabilizers* and other antimanic pharmacotherapies, it is worth noting that although valproic acid has been shown to increase HIV viral replication in vitro, there is no evidence of it worsening viral load in vivo; lithium remains an appropriate pharmacotherapy, although HIV+ patients may be especially sensitive to its dose-related potential adverse neurologic effects. Its neuroprotective properties have made lithium an attractive candidate treatment in dementia, although no formal studies have as yet demonstrated its effects in patients with AIDS dementia.
- For treatment of *anxiety* symptoms and disorders, SSRIs represent the most appropriate first-line pharmacotherapy, although the evidence base to support their efficacy in HIV+ patients is largely anecdotal. Benzodiazepines pose particular risks for excessive sedation and cognitive impairment, as well as abuse potential. Other safe and potentially useful anxiolytics include hydroxyzine, trazodone, and buspirone. Gabapentin has demonstrated safety and tolerability in treating neuropathic pain in AIDS patients but has not been formally studied for its possible anxiolytic efficacy.
- *Antipsychotics* have received remarkably little study in patients with HIV+/AIDS, and much of the existing literature has focused on FGAs (e.g., chlorpromazine, haloperidol) in the treatment of delirium. The literature regarding SGA use is limited mainly to case reports. In general, low dosing with slow titration schedules is advisable due to an increased susceptibility for EPS in HIV+ patients coupled with viral concentrations being especially high in the CNS reservoir.

Tip

Renal disease decreases protein binding of medications. Drugs that are more highly protein bound (see Box 12.12) generally require renal dosing because of potential toxicity from the unbound drug fraction.

Kidney Disease

Notably, few dedicated RCTs have focused on treating psychopathology in patients with severe chronic kidney disease (CKD). One such large RCT, comparing flexibly dosed sertraline (n = 102) versus placebo (n = 99) for MDD over 12 weeks in patients with stages 3, 4 or 5 non-dialysis-dependent CKD, found no greater improvement over placebo, but significantly more nausea, vomiting, and diarrhea (Hedayati et al., 2017). According to a Cochrane Database Review, demonstrated efficacy for any specific antidepressant to guide MDD treatment decisions in the setting of severe CKD is lacking (Palmer et al., 2016).

Box 12.14

Pharmacological Terminology Relevant to Patients with Hepatic or Renal Impairment

Bound and *unbound drug fractions*: only the free portion or fraction of a drug (i.e., unbound to plasma proteins) is available to exert pharmacodynamic effects or to be excreted in urine

Fraction excreted unchanged (fe): the proportion of a drug that is renally cleared and excreted unchanged in the urine; medications with an fe > 0.50 generally should be given at a lower dose in patients with clinically significant kidney disease

Intrinsic clearance (Cl_{int}): refers to the ability to metabolize (remove) unbound drug from circulation (independent of its protein binding)

Extraction ratio: refers to the percentage of a compound that enters the kidney and is ultimately excreted in urine

Volume of distribution (Vd): the volume that a drug theoretically would occupy if it were uniformly distributed throughout the body

Patients with reduced eGFR eliminate renally cleared drugs more slowly than those with normal kidney function. Renal dosing is usually appropriate for drugs that undergo at least 50% elimination via renal clearance (or, said differently, renal dosing should occur for drugs whose *fraction excreted unchanged* (fe) is ≥0.50). In such instances, dosing should be reduced proportionally to the degree of reduced renal clearance as follows:

$$\text{Renal dose} = \text{usual dose} \times ((1 - \text{fe}) + \text{fe} \times (\text{eGFR}/\text{normal eGFR}))$$

Specific dosing modifications for drugs that require renal dosing are summarized in Tables 12.17–12.22 (and, in manufacturers' product information, typically see Sections 8.7 or 8.8).

Drugs that *require* renal dosing are shaded. More detailed information about drug-specific renal dosing modifications can also be found at https://globalrph.com/drugs/renal-dosing-database/.

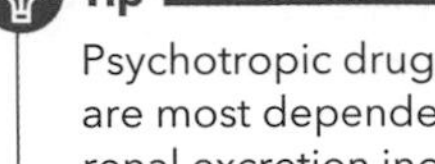

Tip

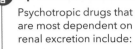

Psychotropic drugs that are most dependent on renal excretion include:

- gabapentin
- topiramate
- lithium
- pregabalin
- paliperidone

Parkinson's Disease

Clinicians should keep in mind that VMAT2 inhibitors (i.e., valbenazine, deutetrabenazine) used to treat tardive dyskinesia may cause or exacerbate parkinsonian symptoms. In a meta-analysis of all-cause mortality among antipsychotic recipients (68 trials, over 4.8 million participants), as history of Parkinson's disease and age 65+ were identified as significant moderating factors (Yang et al., 2018). Quetiapine and clozapine are both often thought to be better tolerated than most other antipsychotics in patients with parkinsonism or Parkinson's disease; however antipsychotic efficacy for either compound appears no better than placebo based on a separate meta-analysis (seven RCTs, 17 615 participants) (Chen et al., 2019a). Pimavaserin is generally considered to be the treatment of choice for psychosis in patients with Parkinson's disease.

Sleep Apnea

Of particular concern in patients with either central or obstructive sleep apnea is the risk of medications that can

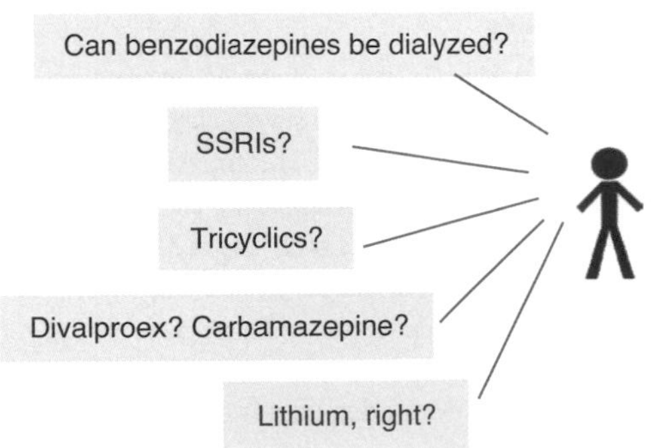

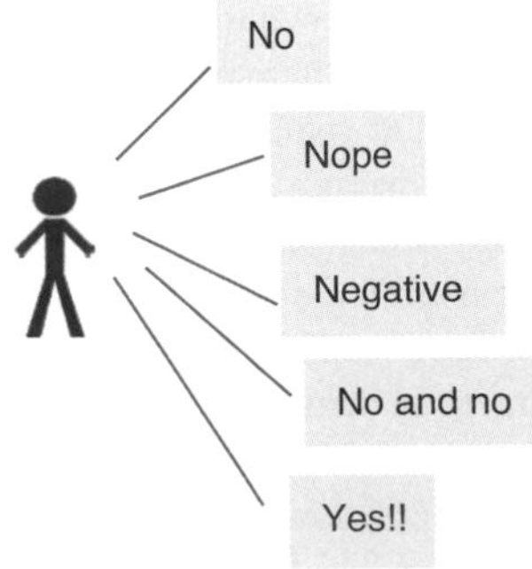

suppress central respiratory drive (notably, opiates and benzodiazepines). Among sleep aids, FDA registration trials of suvorexant enrolled 26 patients with mild-to-moderate obstructive sleep apnea with minimal observed impact on an apnea–hypopnea index. A Cochrane Database review of sedative-hypnotic use in sleep apnea patients found no significant disruptions in oxygen desaturation or apnea/hypopnea events with eszopiclone 3 mg/HS or sodium oxybate (both of which actually *decreased* apnea/hypopnea events significantly more than placebo), or with zolpidem, flurazepam, or triazolam (Mason et al., 2015).

TAKE-HOME POINTS

- Important clinical subpopulations exist that may pose a source of stratification for pharmacological treatment outcomes. Understand ways in which pharmacotherapy effects may differ across particular groups based on race/ethnicity, sex, age, pregnancy/postpartum, comorbidities, and underlying medical conditions.
- Somatically preoccupied patients can pose special challenges for discriminating iatrogenic/adverse drug effects from underlying heightened concerns about physical complaints and sensations. In such instances, pharmacotherapy efforts often must become subservient to psychotherapeutic interventions as the primary focus of treatment.

Table 12.1 Pharmacological safety considerations in children and adolescents: antidepressants

Broad drug classification	Key findings
Antidepressants	- Class warning for increased risk of suicidal thoughts or behaviors in youth <age 24 - A review of 36 RCTs of SSRIs and SNRIs in children and adolescents identified a small effect size in depressive disorders (*g* = 0.21 with SSRIs, *g* = 0.16 with SNRIs), reflecting a large placebo response rate (Locher et al., 2017). Most extensively studied SSRIs for childhood depression include fluoxetine > paroxetine > sertraline > citalopram or escitalopram. Two placebo-controlled trials each examined venlafaxine or duloxetine. Within-drug group analyses revealed the largest response with duloxetine (*g* = 1.95) and the smallest for fluvoxamine (g = 1.22). SSRIs and SNRIs collectively exerted a larger effect in RCTs for anxiety disorders (across seven SSRI RCTs, *g* = 0.71; across four SNRI RCTs, *g* = 0.41) or OCD (nine SSRI RCTs; *g* = 0.39). One SSRI RCT in PTSD (sertraline) yielded a small effect size (*g* = 0.16).

Abbreviations: PTSD = post-traumatic stress disorder; RCT = randomized controlled trial; SNRI = serotonin-norepinephrine reuptake inhibitor; SSRI = selective serotonin reuptake inhibitor

Table 12.2 Pharmacological safety considerations in children and adolescents: SGAs

Drug class	Key findings
SGAs	- Magnitude of iatrogenic cardiometabolic risk appears higher in children and adolescents than in adults; over a mean of 10.8 weeks, aripiprazole may have a somewhat lower risk for inducing dyslipidemias than olanzapine or risperidone (Correll et al., 2009) - In a review of de novo movement disorders across 10 SGA RCTs in children and adolescents, Correll and Kane (2007) reported an annualized TD rate of 0.42%

Abbreviations: RCT = randomized controlled trial; SGA = second-generation antipsychotic; TD = tardive dyskinesia

Table 12.3 Pharmacological safety considerations in children and adolescents: lithium

Drug class	Key findings
Lithium	- A meta-analysis of 12 (mostly short-term) RCTs in pediatric bipolar disorder reported efficacy in up to 50% of patients with no reported instances of kidney injury and rare hypothyroidism; most common adverse effects across trials were GI upset, polyuria, and headache (Amerio et al., 2018); appetite increase and weight gain have been reported across short-term trials (~10% incidence) but not significantly different from that of placebo - A task force report from the International Society for Bipolar Disorders-International Group for the Study of Lithium Treated Patients (ISBD-IGSLi) that examined lithium use in childhood mania concluded that lithium was superior to placebo (SMD = -0.42), comparable to divalproex (SMD = -0.07), and less effective than risperidone in the setting of protracted mania and comorbid ADHD (SMD = 0.85) (Duffy et al., 2018) - The usual recommended target dose in pediatric mania is 30 mg/kg, aiming to achieve a therapeutic serum level comparable to that sought in adults (0.6–1.2 mEq/L) - A small open pilot trial in manic or mixed bipolar youth (mean age 11.4 years) reported an effect size of 1.63 (Kowatch et al., 2000)

Abbreviations: ADHD = attention deficit hyperactivity disorder; RCT = randomized controlled trial; SMD = standard mean difference

Table 12.4 Pharmacological safety considerations in children and adolescents: anticonvulsants

Agents	Key findings
Carbamazepine	- Limited noncontrolled trials/retrospective chart reviews (e.g., Ginsberg, 2006) and open trials (e.g., Findling and Ginsberg, 2014) in pediatric bipolar manic or mixed episodes (modal dose ~1200 mg/day); common adverse effects across trials include somnolence, fatigue, nausea, headache, dizziness, rash - A small open pilot trial in bipolar manic or mixed bipolar youth (mean age 11.4 years) reported an effect size of 1.00 (Kowatch et al., 2000)
Divalproex	- The side-effect profile of divalproex in adolescent bipolar disorder appears relatively similar to that seen in adults (Redden et al., 2009) - A small open pilot trial in manic or mixed bipolar youth (mean age 11.4 years) reported an effect size of 1.63 (Kowatch et al., 2000) - Limited noncontrolled trials/retrospective chart reviews (e.g., Ginsberg, 2006) open trials (e.g., Findling and Ginsberg, 2014) in pediatric bipolar manic or mixed episodes (modal dose ~1200 mg/day); common adverse effects across trials include somnolence, fatigue, nausea, headache, dizziness, rash - A small open pilot trial in bipolar manic or mixed bipolar youth (mean age 11.4 years) reported an effect size of 1.00 (Kowatch et al., 2000)
Gabapentin	- Pediatric safety data limited to epilepsy and neuropathic pain; no RCTs assessing possible anxiolytic or other psychotropic effects
Lamotrigine	- No large-scale RCTs - Age <18 is one factor linking lamotrigine with an increased risk for serious skin rashes, requiring a slower dosing titration schedule than occurs in adults - One small (n = 19) eight-week open label flexibly dosed trial (mean dose = 131.6 mg/day) in adolescent acute bipolar depression yielded 84% response rate with good tolerability, no incidence of rash (Chang et al., 2006) - Another small (n = 39) 12-week open-label flexibly dosed monotherapy trial (mean dose = 160.7 mg/day) in adolescent acute mania yielded significant improvement from baseline in manic, depressive, attentional, and psychotic symptoms; several rashes occurred, none serious, all resolved with drug discontinuation (Biederman et al., 2010) - One 36-week randomized bipolar relapse prevention study (after acute open-label stabilization) found no overall advantage versus placebo on primary time-to-event outcome (Findling et al., 2015)
Oxcarbazepine	- In children and adolescents with epilepsy, most common adverse events were headache (33%), somnolence (32%), nausea or vomiting (1–28%), dizziness (23%), rash (3%), and fatigue (1.6%) (Bourgeois and D'Souza, 2005). In the sole published RCT of oxcarbazepine in pediatric mania, no differences in efficacy versus placebo were observed over six weeks; nausea was the most common adverse event; weight gain was significantly greater with oxcarbazepine (+0.83 kg) than placebo (-0.13 kg); no observed hyponatremia (Wagner et al., 2006)
Pregabalin	- No data on safety or efficacy for psychotropic use in children and adolescents
Topiramate	- RCTs for psychiatric uses in children and adolescents are limited to Tourette's syndrome, suggesting only modest benefit for tic control; common adverse effects include drowsiness (up to 16%), appetite loss (up to 17%), cognitive dysfunction (up to 13%), and weight loss (up to 11%) (Yang et al., 2013)

Abbreviations: RCT = randomized controlled trial

Table 12.5 Pharmacological safety considerations in children and adolescents: anxiolytics

Agent	Key findings
Benzodiazepines, buspirone, hydroxyzine, or sedative hypnotics	- No published RCTs in pediatric GAD - One small (n = 30), likely underpowered RCT of alprazolam for DSM-III "overanxious and avoidant disorders" found no significant differences from placebo (Simeon et al., 1992)

Abbreviations: GAD = generalized anxiety disorder; RCT = randomized controlled trial

Table 12.6 Pharmacological safety considerations in children and adolescents: ADHD treatments

Agent	Key findings
Psychostimulants and other treatments for ADD/ADHD	Table 12.7 presents a summary of relative efficacies (ORs for treatment response, with 95% CIs) pairwise between ADHD pharmacotherapies and placebo or as comparisons between pairs of active drugs based on random-effects Bayesian network meta-analyses involving 171 RCTs with 22 961 patients (Catalá-López et al., 2017). Main findings from these network meta-analyses included the following: • Amphetamine exerted the largest magnitude of effect versus placebo • Methylphenidate, amphetamine, atomoxetine, guanfacine, clonidine, and modafinil were more efficacious than placebo (but weaker quality of studies with clonidine and modafinil) • Methylphenidate or amphetamine were each more efficacious than atomoxetine or guanfacine • Amphetamine produced more weight loss and insomnia than did methylphenidate, though methylphenidate produced more insomnia than did atomoxetine

Abbreviations: ADD = attention deficit disorder; ADHD = attention deficit hyperactivity disorder; CI = confidence interval; OR = odds ratio; RCT = randomized controlled trial

Table 12.7 Comparative efficacy and acceptability across pharmacotherapies for ADD/ADHD in children and adolescents (OR (95% CI))

Placebo	**0.59 (0.46-0.75)**	0.78 (0.52-1.18)	0.85 (0.68-1.07)	**0.40 (0.20-0.78)**	0.79 (0.54-1.14)	0.67 (0.37-1.24)	1.54 (0.39-6.76)
5.26 (4.09-6.82)	**Methylphenidate**	1.33 (0.85-2.08)	**1.45 (1.09-1.91)**	0.68 (0.33-1.35)	1.34 (0.86-2.07)	1.14 (0.61-2.19)	2.60 (0.66-11.64)
7.45 (5.10-11.09)	1.42 (0.92-2.20)	**Amphetamine**	1.09 (0.71-1.66)	0.51 (0.23-1.11)	1.01 (0.58-1.72)	0.86 (0.42-1.79)	1.96 0(0.47-9.21)
3.63 (2.81-4.73)	**0.69 (0.52-0.92)**	**0.49 (0.32-0.74)**	**Atomoxetine**	**0.47 (0.22-0.94)**	0.92 (0.61-1.41)	0.79 (0.42-1.52)	1.80 (0.45-8.03)
3.96 (1.89-8.41)	0.75 (0.36-1.58)	0.53 (0.23-1.22)	1.09 (0.50-2.39)	**Clonidine**	1.99 (0.91-4.33)	1.69 (0.70-4.33)	3.88 (0.82-20.02)
3.29 (2.27-4.82)	**0.62 (0.40-0.98)**	**0.44 (0.26-0.75)**	0.91 (0.58-1.41)	0.83 (0.36-1 92)	**Guanfacine**	0.86 (0.42-1.76)	1.95 (0.47-8.84)
5.51 (3.04-10.32)	1.05 (0.56-2.00)	0.74 (0.36-1.54)	1.52 (0.79-2.94)	1.41 (0.53-3 66)	1.68 (0.82-3.45)	**Modafinil**	2.28 (0.52-11.33)
2.41 (0.48-11.63)	0.46 (0.09-2.21)	0.32 (0.06-1.65)	0.67 (0.13-3.29)	0.61 (0.10-3 36)	0.74 (0.14-3.72)	0.44 (0.08-2.36)	**Bupropion**

Data below the diagonal (clear cells) represent *efficacy* (odds ratios for treatment response); data above the diagonal (shaded cells) represent *acceptability* (odds ratios for all-cause discontinuation). Note that ORs <1.00 reflect a lower probability of an event while ORs >1.00 indicate increased probability of an event. Statistically significant ORs (with 95% CIs) are bolded.

Findings are based on data reported by Catalá-López et al., 2017.

Table 12.8 Relative risk for response with antidepressants in late-life depression[a]

Antidepressant	N	Dosing range	RR for response
Nortriptyline			
Georgotas et al., 1986	25	25–125 mg/day	4.692
Nair et al., 1995	38	25–75 mg/day	1.105
Phenelzine			
Georgotas et al., 1986	22	15–75 mg/day	4.692
Fluoxetine			
Tollefson et al., 1995	335	20 mg/day	2.150
Schatzberg and Roose, 2006	100	20–60 mg/day	0.875
Kasper et al., 2005	164	20 mg/day	0.787
Trazodone			
Gerner et al., 1980	19	100–400 mg/day	2.142
Halakis, 1995	48	40–280 mg/day	1.171
Duloxetine			
Raskin et al., 2007	207	60 mg/day	2.000
Mirtazapine			
Halakis, 1995	49	5–35 mg/day	1.457
Paroxetine CR			
Rapaport et al., 2009	177	25 mg/day	1.450
Rapaport et al., 2003	104	12.5–50 mg/day	1.319
Rapaport et al., 2009	168	12.5 mg/day	1.300
Sertraline			
Schneider et al., 2003	371	50–100 mg/day	1.346
Bupropion XR			
Hewett et al., 2010	211	150–300 mg/day	1.232
Escitalopram [b]			
Bose et al., 2008	130	10–20 mg/day	1.210
Kasper et al., 2005	173	10 mg/day	0.978
Imipramine			
Gerner et al., 1980	21	50–200 mg/day	1.809
Schweizer et al., 1998	60	50–150 mg/day	1.722
Paroxetine			
Rapaport et al., 2003	106	10–40 mg/day	1.191
Venlafaxine			
Schatzberg and Roose, 2006	104	75–225 mg/day	1.050
Citalopram			
Roose et al., 2004	84	10–40 mg/day	1.081
Moclobemide			
Nair et al., 1995	36	100–400 mg/day	0.921

[a] Based on findings reported in meta-analysis by Tedeschini et al., 2011

[b] The two RCTs of escitalopram for acute late-life depression noted here did not show a difference from placebo; however, elsewhere, escitalopram was superior to placebo for depression relapse prevention after acute open-label remission (Gorwood et al., 2007)

Table 12.9 Psychotropic drug safety in pregnancy

Agent	Main findings for pregnancy outcomes and congenital risks
Anticonvulsants	Collectively, an increased risk for adverse pregnancy outcomes (placenta-mediated complications or preterm birth) with the use of anticonvulsants (i.e., carbamazepine, oxcarbazepine, lamotrigine, topiramate, or divalproex) or lithium dissipated after controlling for confounding factors (Cohen et al., 2019)
Carbamazepine	RR = 1.37, 95% CI = 1.10–1.71 for major malformations (Veroniki et al., 2017); may be associated with neural tube defects, urinary tract malformations, orofacial cleft and craniofacial malformations, fingernail hypoplasia, and possible neurodevelopmental delays (e.g., low IQ) (reviewed by Albertini et al., 2019)
Divalproex	RR = 2.93, 95% CI = 2.36–3.69 for major malformations (boxed warning for neural tube defects) (Veroniki et al., 2017), including craniofacial, cardiac, genital, and skeletal or limb abnormalities (possibly dose-related) in up to 15% of exposed infants (Jentink et al., 2010) A population-based study in Denmark involving 665 615 children, including 508 exposed intrauterine to divalproex, identified an absolute risk of 4.42% (HR = 2.9, 95% CI = 1.7–4.9) for developing autism spectrum disorders (Christensen et al., 2013); boxed warning for causing low IQ and neurodevelopmental disorders
Gabapentin	No apparent increased risk for major malformations but associations with preterm birth and low birth weight among neuropathic pain or epilepsy recipients (Fujii et al., 2013)
Lamotrigine	RR = 0.96, 95% CI = 0.72–1.95 (Veroniki et al., 2017)
Topiramate	RR = 1.90, 95% CI = 1.17–2.97 (Veroniki et al., 2017) In utero exposure associated with cleft lip/palate and hypospadias
Antidepressants	A Nordic database registry from 1996–2010 examining major congenital malformation and studying 36 772 infants with first-trimester exposure to SSRIs or venlafaxine, reported incidence of 3.7% as compared to 3.1% among unexposed infants (covariate adjusted OR = 1.13, 95% CI = 1.06–1.20) (Furu et al., 2015) Early reports linking in utero antidepressant exposure with an increased risk for autism spectrum disorders (ASDs) likely confounded by maternal mental illness (Andrade, 2017) Findings from one investigative group (Chambers et al., 2006) that paroxetine exposure after gestational week 20 could increase the risk for persistent pulmonary hypertension in the newborn (PPHN) led to a 2006 FDA public health advisory, rescinded in 2011 amid subsequent conflicting reports and acknowledgment of confounding contributors to PPHN (notably, maternal obesity and smoking)
Antipsychotics	Modest, nonsignificant increased risk for major malformations in exposed versus unexposed infants (OR = 1.25, 95% CI = 0.13–12.19) (Cohen et al., 2016). Initial findings of low birth weight, preterm birth, or neonatal complications from pregnancy registration databases are often unadjusted for confounders such as concomitant medications, substance abuse, and prepregnancy diabetes or hypertension (Khan et al., 2016)
Lithium	Dose-related risk for cardiac valve malformations (RR = 1.65; 95% CI = 1.02–2.68), but magnitude of risk is less than originally thought (Patorno et al., 2017) Polyhydramnios, floppy baby syndrome, premature delivery, potential for arrhythmias (T-wave flattening, S-A node dysfunction) and nephrogenic diabetes insipidus
Sedative-hypnotics	A meta-analysis of eight studies found no increased risk for major malformations after benzodiazepine in utero exposure (OR = 1.13, 95% CI = 0.99–1.30) (Grigoriadis et al., 2019); diazepam and chlordiazepoxide are the most extensively studied and therefore may be preferred agents within-class (e.g., Bellatuono et al., 2013)
Stimulants	Small increased risk for pre-eclampsia (RR = 1.29) and preterm birth RR = 1.06); "women with significant ADHD should not be counseled to suspend their ADHD treatment based on these findings" (Cohen et al., 2017); possible increased risk for spontaneous abortion with methylphenidate (Bro et al., 2015)

Abbreviations: ADHD = attention deficit hyperactivity disorder; CI = confidence interval; FDA = US Food and Drug Administration; HR = hazard ratio; IQ = intelligence quotient; OR = odds ratio; RR = relative risk; SSRI = selective serotonin reuptake inhibitor

Table 12.10 Psychotropic medications and lactation

Drug class, broadly defined	Measurable drug levels in breast milk
Anticonvulsants	A review of lactation data with anticonvulsant drugs reported the following M/P ratios: (Davanzano et al. (2013)): Carbamazepine: M/P = 0.69 Divalproex: M/P = 0.42 Gabapentin: M/P = 0.7–1.3 Lamotrigine: M/P = 0.057–1.47 Oxcarbazepine: M/P = 0.5 Topiramate: M/P = 0.86–1.1
Antidepressants	A pooled analysis of 57 published trials found that nortriptyline, paroxetine, and sertraline produced undetectable infant blood levels, while fluoxetine produced the highest (22%) followed by citalopram (17%) (Weissman et al., 2004)
Antipsychotics	Uguz (2016) calculated the relative infant dose (RID)[a] of several SGAs based on pooled data: Olanzapine: RID = 1.59%; M/P ratio = 0.57 Risperidone: RID = 3.59%; M/P ratio = 0.45 Clozapine: M/P ratio = 2.79 (with risk for leukopenia in infant)
Anxiolytics	No evidence of excessive sedation or other adverse outcomes in nursing newborns (Kelly et al., 2012)
Lithium	M/P = 0.49 (Imaz et al., 2019)
Stimulants	No evidence of adverse growth, behavioral or developmental effects in nursing newborns

[a] RID calculated as daily infant dose (mg/kg/day) ÷ daily maternal dose (mg/kg/day) × 100

Abbreviations: M/P ratio = maternal milk to plasma ratio; SGA = second-generation antipsychotic

Table 12.11 Psychotropic use in patients with hepatic impairment: anticonvulsants

Agent	Comments/necessary dosing adjustments
Carbamazepine	Usually benign transaminitis occurs in up to one-fifth of patients; elevation of GGT usually reflects benign hepatic enzyme induction. Hepatotoxicity is a rare phenomenon usually related to drug rash with eosinophilia and systemic symptoms (DRESS) syndrome. No specific dosing recommendations other than warning "may cause hepatic failure"
Divalproex	Contraindicated in severe hepatic dysfunction; generally considered appropriate at usual dosing if liver enzymes remain less than three times upper limit of the normal laboratory reference range
Gabapentin	Not hepatically metabolized. May therefore be an especially attractive option for hepatically impaired patients with anxiety or insomnia
Lamotrigine	In moderate or severe impairment without ascites: reduce dose by ~25%; in severe impairment with ascites: reduce dose by ~50%
Oxcarbazepine	No adjustment if mild or moderate hepatic impairment; not evaluated in severe impairment
Pregabalin	No adjustment if mild to severe hepatic impairment
Topiramate	"Use with caution"[a] in moderate to severe hepatic impairment

[a] Language from manufacturer's product information materials

Abbreviations: GGT = gamma-glutamyl transpeptidase

Table 12.12 Psychotropic use in patients with hepatic impairment: antidepressants

Agent	Comments/necessary dosing adjustments
Esketamine	"Patients with moderate hepatic impairment may need to be monitored for adverse reactions for a longer period of time"
MAOIs	No specific recommendations other than "dose with caution"[a]
Mirtazapine	Oral clearance is reduced by ~30% in hepatically impaired patients
SNRIs	- Duloxetine: avoid use in patients with chronic liver disease or cirrhosis - Levomilnacipran: no adjustment if mild to severe hepatic impairment - Venlafaxine: halve dose if moderate or severe impairment
SSRIs	- Citalopram: maximum dose = 20 mg/day in patients with any hepatic impairment - Escitalopram: 10 mg/day is recommended dose in patients with mild or moderate impairment; use not recommended in severe impairment - Fluoxetine: "caution is advised" regarding dosing in patients with hepatic impairment and "a lower or less frequent dose… should be used in patients with cirrhosis" - Fluvoxamine: clearance is decreased by ~30%; "it may be appropriate to modify the initial dose and the subsequent dose titration" - Paroxetine: "initial dosage should… be reduced in patients with severe… impairment" - Sertraline: halve dose in mild impairment; avoid in moderate or severe
Tricyclics	In severe hepatic impairment: "use with caution"
Vortioxetine	No adjustment if mild to severe impairment

[a] Language from manufacturer's product information materials

Abbreviations: MAOI = monoamine oxidase inhibitor: SNRI = serotonin-norepinephrine reuptake inhibitor; SSRI = selective serotonin reuptake inhibitor

Table 12.13 Psychotropic use in patients with hepatic impairment: SGAs

Agent	Comments/necessary dosing adjustments
Aripiprazole	No dosage adjustment needed if mild, moderate or severe impairment
Asenapine	No dosage adjustments needed if mild impairment; use not recommended if moderate or severe
Brexpiprazole	"Reduce the maximum recommended dose"* in moderate to severe impairment
Cariprazine	No dosage adjustments needed if mild to moderate impairment
Clozapine	In severe hepatic impairment "dose reduction may be necessary"[a]
Iloperidone	Use not recommended in patients with hepatic impairment
Lumateperone	No dosage adjustments needed if mild impairment; use not recommended if moderate or severe
Olanzapine	Mild, often transient and reversible transaminitis may occur in 10–50% of patients taking olanzapine long term
Paliperidone	No dosage adjustment is required in patients with mild to moderate hepatic impairment
Pimavanserin	"Not recommended in patients with hepatic impairment"[a]
Quetiapine	Initiate dosing at 25 mg/day, increase by 25–50 mg/day based on response and tolerability
Risperidone	In severe hepatic impairment, "the recommended initial dose is 0.5 mg twice daily … Dosage increases in these patients should be in increments of no more than 0.5 mg twice daily. Increases to dosages above 1.5 mg twice daily should generally occur at intervals of at least 1 week. In some patients, slower titration may be medically appropriate" [a]
Ziprasidone	AUC increases by 13% in patients with "severe" and 34% in those with "moderately severe" hepatic impairment, with nearly a 50% increase in elimination half-life. No specific dosing modifications advised by manufacturer

[a] Language from manufacturer's product information materials

Abbreviations: AUC = area under curve; SGA = second-generation antipsychotic

Table 12.14 Psychotropic use in patients with hepatic impairment: sedative-hypnotics

Agent	Comments/necessary dosing adjustments
Doxepin	Initiate at 3 mg/day "and monitor closely for adverse daytime effects"
Eszopiclone	Maximum dosage 2 mg/HS in patients with severe hepatic impairment
Lemborexant	Maximum dosage 5 mg/HS in patients with moderate hepatic impairment; use not recommended in severe impairment
Ramelteon	"Use with caution"[a] in moderate impairment; no data in mild impairment and use is not recommended in severe impairment
Suvorexant	No dosage adjustments necessary in the setting of renal impairment
Zaleplon	In mild to moderate hepatic impairment, dosing is 5 mg/day; not recommended for use in the setting of severe impairment
Zolpidem	Maximum dose 5 mg PO qHS in the setting of mild to moderate hepatic impairment

[a] Language from manufacturer's product information materials

Abbreviations: PO = by mouth; qHS = every night

Table 12.15 Psychotropic use in patients with hepatic impairment: stimulants and related compounds

Agent	Comments/necessary dosing adjustments
Amphetamine	"Administer with caution"[a] in the setting of hepatic impairment
(Ar)modafinil	Halve the usual dose in the setting of hepatic impairment
Methylphenidate	No adjustment if mild to severe hepatic impairment
Solriamfetol	No specific recommendations but minimally metabolized before excretion

[a] Language from manufacturer's product information materials

Table 12.16 Psychotropic use in patients with hepatic impairment: pro-cognitive agents

Agent	Comments/necessary dosing adjustments
Amantadine	"Use with caution"[a]
Donepezil	No specific recommendations
Galantamine	Dosing should not exceed 16 mg/day in setting of moderate impairment; use is not recommended in patients with severe hepatic impairment
Memantine	No adjustment if mild or moderate impairment; "use with caution"[a] in severe impairment
Rivastigmine	"The dose may need to be lowered" in mild or moderate hepatic impairment

[a] Language from manufacturer's product information materials

Table 12.17 Psychotropic use in patients with renal impairment: anticonvulsants and lithium

Medication	Renal recommendations
Carbamazepine	- No specific dosing adjustments
Divalproex	- No specific dosing adjustments
Gabapentin	- If CrCl >60: normal dosing - If CrCl = 30–59 mL/min: halve the total daily dose - If CrCl = 15–29 mL/min: dosing range = 200–700 mg/day administered in once-daily dose - If CrCl <15 mL/min: dosing range =100–300 mg/day; "reduce daily dose in proportion to creatinine clearance"[a]
Lamotrigine	- "reduced maintenance doses may be effective for patients with significant renal impairment"[a]
Oxcarbazepine	- If CrCl <30 mL/min, halve the usual dose
Pregabalin	- If CrCl = 30–60 mL/min: *halve* the usual dose (BID or TID) - If CrCl =15–30 mL/min: *quarter* the usual dose (BID or TID) - If CrCl <15 mL/min: reduce dose by 1/6 to 1/12 of usual dose (i.e., a usual dose of 150 mg/day→25 mg/day; 300 mg/day→25–50 mg/day; 450 mg/day→ 50–75 mg/day; 600 mg/day→75 mg/day) (BID or qDay) - Following hemodialysis, a supplemental dose may be necessary
Topiramate	- If CrCl <70 mL/min, halve the usual dose
Lithium	- If CrCl = 30–89 mL/min: "begin with lower doses and titrate slowly"[a] - If CrCl >30 mL/min: "not recommended"

Drugs that require renal dosing are shaded

[a] Language from manufacturer's product information materials

Abbreviations: BID = twice daily; CrCl = creatinine clearance; qDay = once daily; TID = three times a day

Table 12.18 Psychotropic use in patients with renal impairment: antidepressants

Antidepressants	Renal recommendations
Bupropion	- "Use with caution"[a] (reduced dosing or frequency) in patients with renal impairment
Citalopram	- No dosage adjustment in mild to moderate kidney disease - If CrCl = 30-59 mL/min "use with caution"[a] and titrate slowly
Desvenlafaxine	- If CrCl = 30-59 mL/min, dose no higher than 50 mg/day - If CrCl <30 mL/min, dose no higher than 50 mg qOD
Duloxetine	- No dosage adjustment necessary in mild to moderate kidney disease; do not use if CrCl <30 mL/min (because its active metabolites are measurably elevated in patients with ESRD)
Escitalopram	- No dosage adjustment in mild to moderate kidney disease - No data available in severe renal impairment or ESRD
Esketamine	- No specific recommendations
Fluoxetine	- No dosage adjustments necessary
Fluvoxamine	- No data
Levomilnacipran	- Renal dosing unnecessary if CrCl ≥60 mL/min - If CrCl = 30-59: maximum dose is 80 mg/day - If CrCl = 15-29 mL/min, maximum dose is 40 mg/day
MAOIs	- No specific recommendations other than "dose with caution"[a]
Mirtazapine	- Clearance is reduced by ~30 if CrCl = 11-39 mL/min and by ~50% if CrCl ≤10; "caution is indicated in administering mirtazapine to patients with compromised renal function"[a]
Paroxetine	- No dosage adjustment in mild to moderate kidney disease - If CrCl <30 mL/min, initiate at 10 mg/day, maximum dose = 40 mg/day
Sertraline	- No dosage adjustments necessary
Tricyclics	- No specific dosage adjustment are provided in manufacturers' product information other than to use "care" or "caution" in patients with renal impairment
Venlafaxine	- If CrCl = 10-70 mL/min, reduce dose by 25-50% - In ESRD patients undergoing hemodialysis, reduce dose by 50% and withhold until completion of dialysis
Vilazodone	- No dosage adjustment needed if CrCl is 15-90 mL/min

Drugs that require renal dosing are shaded

[a] Language from manufacturer's product information materials

Abbreviations: CrCl = creatinine clearance; ESRD = end-stage renal disease; qOD = every other day

Table 12.19 Psychotropic use in patients with renal impairment: SGAs

SGAs	Renal recommendations
Aripiprazole	- No dosage adjustment needed if CrCl is 15-90 mL/min (primarily excreted unchanged in feces)
Asenapine	- No dosage adjustment needed if CrCl is 15-90 mL/min
Brexpiprazole	- "Reduce the maximum recommended dosage in patients with moderate, severe, or end-stage renal impairment (CrCl <60 mL/minute)"[a]
Cariprazine	- No dosage adjustment needed if CrCl ≥30 mL/min; use not recommended (unstudied) if CrCl <30 mL/min
Clozapine	- In severe renal disease "dose reduction may be necessary"[a]
Iloperidone	- No dosage adjustment needed if CrCl is ≥30 mL/min; use not recommended (unstudied) if CrCl <30 mL/min
Lumateperone	- Not reported
Lurasidone	- If CrCl = 30–59 mL/min, initial dosing is 20 mg/day, maximum is 80 mg/day
Olanzapine	- No specific dosing adjustments are recommended
Paliperidone[b]	- If CrCl = 50–80 mL/min, initial dosing is 3 mg/day, may increase to 6 mg/day based on response and tolerability - If CrCl =10–49 mL/min initiate dosing at 1.5 mg/day, maximum dose of 3 mg/day - Use not recommended in end stage renal disease
Pimavaserin	- No dosage adjustment needed if CrCl is ≥30 mL/min
Quetiapine	- No dosage adjustments are necessary
Risperidone	- In severe renal impairment initial dose is 0.5 mg twice daily, then increase by increments of ≤0.5 mg twice daily. At dosages >1.5 mg twice daily, further dosage increases should occur no faster than ≥1 week.
Ziprasidone	- No specific recommendations; "renal impairment alone is unlikely to have a major impact on the pharmacokinetics of ziprasidone"[a] (primarily excreted unchanged in feces)

Drugs that require renal dosing are shaded

[a] Language from manufacturer's product information materials

[b] Note: Paliperidone is *the one SGA* for which use is discouraged in ESRD ← TIP

Abbreviations: CrCl = creatinine clearance; ESRD = end-stage renal disease

Table 12.20 Psychotropic use in patients with renal impairment: sedative-hypnotics

Agent	Renal recommendations
Sedative-hypnotics	- No dosing adjustments are necessary in mild or moderate renal dysfunction with eszopiclone, ramelteon, suvorexant, zaleplon, or zolpidem - No specific recommendations for doxepin in patients with renal impairment - Lemborexant and suvorexant requires no dosage adjustment in mild through severe renal impairment

Table 12.21 Psychotropic use in patients with renal impairment: stimulants and related compounds

Agent	Renal recommendations
Amphetamine	- No specific manufacturer recommendations
(Ar)modafinil	- "There is inadequate information to determine safety and efficacy of dosing in patients with severe renal impairment"[a]
Methylphenidate	- No specific manufacturer recommendations
Solriamfetol	- If CrCl = 30-59 mL/min: begin dosing at 37.5 mg/day, may increase to 75 mg/day after seven days, if tolerated - If CrCl =15-29 mL/min: begin and remain at 37.5 mg/day - If CrCl <15 mL/min: use is not recommended

[a] Language from manufacturer's product information materials

Abbreviations: CrCl = creatinine clearance

Table 12.22 Psychotropic use in patients with renal impairment: pro-cognitive agents

Agent	Renal recommendations
Amantadine	- If CrCl >50: normal dosing - If CrCl = 30-50 mL/min: 200 mg × 1 then 100 mg q 24 hours - If CrCl = 15-29 mL/min: 200 mg × 1 then 100 mg q 48 hours - If CrCl <15 mL/min: 200 mg q seven days - If hemodialysis: 200 mg q seven days
Donepezil	- No specific recommendations
Galantamine	- If CrCl = 9-59 mL/min, maximum daily dose should not exceed 16 mg. Use not recommended in patients with severe renal impairment
Memantine	- No dosage adjustment if CrCl = 30-80 mL/min; if CrCl <30 mL/min, dose at 5 mg PO BID (immediate release) or 14 mg/day (extended release)
Rivastigmine	"The dose may need to be lowered" in setting of mild or moderate renal impairment"[a]; no data in severe renal impairment

[a] Language from manufacturer's product information materials

Abbreviations: CrCl = creatinine clearance; BID = twice daily; PO = by mouth; q = once every

PART II Targets of Pharmacotherapy

13 Disordered Mood and Affect

LEARNING OBJECTIVES

- ☐ Understand how dimensions of mood disorders, such as polarity, psychosis, chronicity, recurrence, and comorbidites are moderators of pharmacotherapy outcome
- ☐ Know the evidence base for use of antidepressants in adjustment disorders
- ☐ Describe the relative efficacy of monoaminergic antidepressants for major depressive episodes
- ☐ Understand the interplay between medication dose, duration, illness chronicity, and speed of pharmacodynamic onset
- ☐ Know plausible rationales for switching versus augmenting pharmacotherapies for mood disorders after an initial inadequate response
- ☐ Understand the evidence base and dosing strategies for pharmacotherapies in treatment-resistant depression
- ☐ Describe evidence-based treatments for depression with comorbid anxiety and other psychiatric conditions
- ☐ Identify evidence-based pharmacotherapies for depression relapse prevention after ECT
- ☐ Recognize clinical candidacy criteria for using antidepressants, lithium, and particular anticonvulsants, SGAs or other psychotropic agents across phases of bipolar disorder

The world breaks everyone and afterward many are strong at the broken places.

–Ernest Hemingway

Younger readers may not appreciate that prior to DSM-IV, the phenomena that we today call "mood disorders" were identified more precisely as *affective* disorders, denoting a fundamental distinction between disturbances of mood (the subjective experience of emotion) and affect (the objective behavioral expression of mood). Given that problems with "mood" are ubiquitous throughout virtually all aspects of psychopathology, links between the signs and symptoms of "mood problems" are critical both to nosological classification and to identifying targets of pharmacotherapy interventions. Features associated with *affective* disorders encompass problems with energy, the sleep–wake cycle, thinking and perception, impulse control, cognition (e.g., attentional processing, problem-solving), motivation/arousal, and eating behaviors, among others.

In this chapter, we present information about the treatment of mood/affective disorders as a broad overarching category, with subdistinctions (such as polarity) highlighted as clinical descriptors, rather than as fundamentally different illnesses. This may trouble some readers. Yet, one could slice the affective pie innumerable ways. Box 13.1 summarizes at least 20. Arguably, each of these dimensions could constitute its own illness, as opposed to instead representing (in our view) distinct moderators of treatment outcome. Additionally, one could classify affective disorders based on specific drug responsivity (analogous to how one classifies some infectious diseases based on their being antibiotic-responsive or -resistant), or perhaps some day, based on biomarker corroborators (remember DST nonsuppressive depression? If not, read on). In keeping with the spirit of *practical* psychopharmacology, and fostering a more dimensional than categorical approach to diagnosis and treatment, we will focus on dimensions of affective disorders rather than attempt to tackle 20 or more nosologically "unique" categories of mood problems.

Some of the terminology noted in Box 13.1 has become antiquated in modern parlance (e.g., DSM-5 subsumes

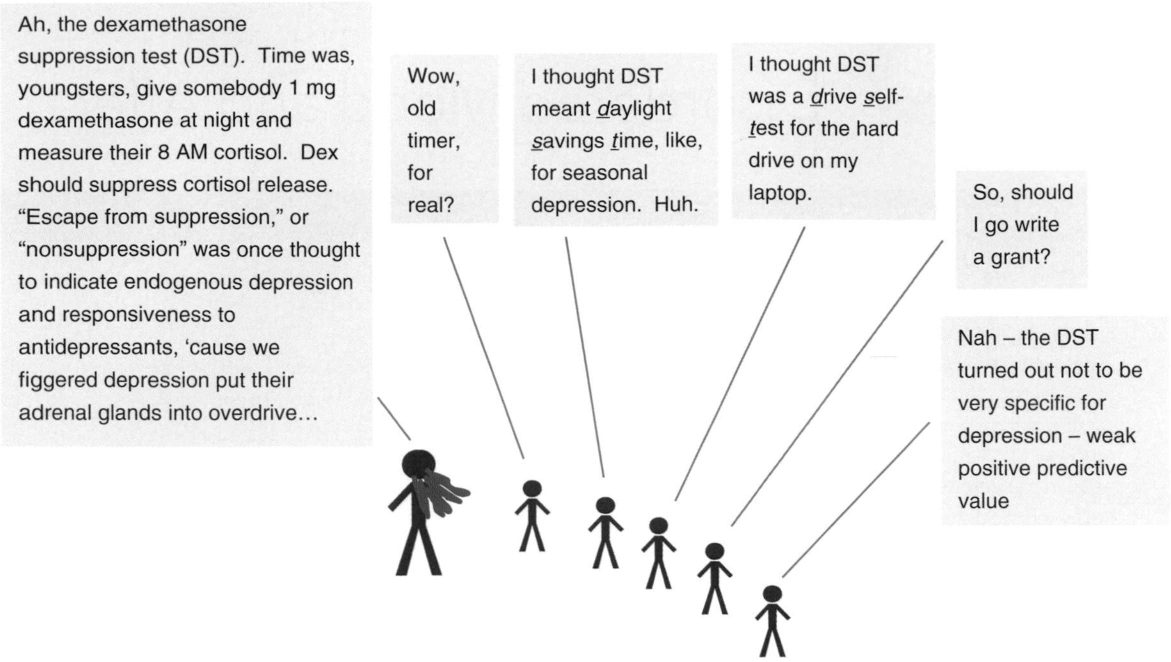

Ah, the dexamethasone suppression test (DST). Time was, youngsters, give somebody 1 mg dexamethasone at night and measure their 8 AM cortisol. Dex should suppress cortisol release. "Escape from suppression," or "nonsuppression" was once thought to indicate endogenous depression and responsiveness to antidepressants, 'cause we figgered depression put their adrenal glands into overdrive…
Wow, old timer, for real?
I thought DST meant daylight savings time, like, for seasonal depression. Huh.
I thought DST was a drive self-test for the hard drive on my laptop.
So, should I go write a grant?
Nah – the DST turned out not to be very specific for depression – weak positive predictive value

Box 13.1

Dimensions of Affective Disorders

- Polarity (uni- versus bi-)
- Persistent (dysthymic/chronic)
- Highly recurrent versus nonrecurrent
- Psychotic versus nonpsychotic (and therein: mood congruent versus incongruent)
- Endogenous versus reactive (formerly "neurotic")
- Catatonic
- Typical versus atypical
- Anxious versus nonanxious
- Agitated versus anergic
- Noradrenergic symptom cluster
- High versus low severity
- Early versus late onset
- Late-life versus younger adult versus pediatric
- Seasonal versus nonseasonal
- Treatment-resistant versus nonresistant
- Medically comorbidly ill
- Primary versus secondary to other medical conditions/substance use
- Pregnant or postpartum
- Inflammatory versus noninflammatory

"dysthymic disorder" with chronic major depression under the broad heading of "persistent depressive disorders," and the terms "endogenous" and "neurotic" are no longer recognized). Nevertheless, many clinicians still draw on at least some of the concepts behind these elements when they formulate a clinical presentation and consider pharmacotherapy decisions. As discussed in Chapter 5, most real-world patients manifest various combinations of features such as those listed in Box 13.1, generating a unique clinical profile for every patient as an individual. Certain symptom clusters – such as anhedonia, indecisiveness, and diminished activity – may hold particular negative prognostic importance above and beyond moderators such as baseline severity (Uher et al., 2012). And even affective polarity – considered by some as a sacrosanct dichotomy in mood disorders

– really represents just one of many moderating factors that influence course and outcome. To classify someone's ailment based solely on one moderating characteristic to the exclusion of others oversimplifies the complexity of mood disorders and can unwittingly set the stage for poor outcome to an ostensibly appropriate treatment for a given disorder.

A WHEN IS PHARMACOTHERAPY FOR DEPRESSION INDICATED?

The American Psychiatric Association Practice Guideline for the Treatment of Major Depressive Disorder, 3rd Edition (2010) states that "An antidepressant medication is recommended as an initial treatment choice for patients with mild to moderate major depressive disorder and definitely should be provided for those with severe major depressive disorder unless ECT is planned." More specific, additional relevant considerations should rightfully include *high severity, melancholic features, suicidality, psychosis, functional impairment,* and *chronicity.* It is worthwhile to assess a patient's attitudes and expectations about what medications can and cannot do, and to gauge outcomes from past psychotherapy or other nonprescription interventions (e.g., exercise, light therapy, nutraceuticals). Equally important is forecasting the likelihood of medication responsivity: Is there an *a priori* reason to think someone might not benefit from a traditional monoaminergic antidepressant? A history of complete nonresponses to numerous prior adequate antidepressant trials certainly does not contraindicate more antidepressant trials, but demands considerable reflection, lest one continue to do the same thing over and over again and expect different results (consider, for example, the ever-increasing likelihood of remission after multiple iterative antidepressant trials, as illustrated in Box 13.6, below). Is there an untreated medical, psychiatric or substance-use comorbidity that requires hierarchically more immediate attention? Or, does a depressive episode entail mixed (manic or hypomanic) features, which could be worsened by traditional antidepressants (Frye et al., 2009)? Has psychosis been missed? Has treatment adherence been poor?

Consider also whether another psychiatric condition may be present for which "depression" may be a chief complaint but syndromal criteria for an MDE are absent, and the presenting symptoms could be mimicking depression (e.g., negative symptoms of schizophrenia, abstinence or withdrawal symptoms of alcohol or an illicit substance, mania which the patient incorrectly identifies as depression, frank psychosis (for which an antipsychotic is likely a more core treatment than an antidepressant) or an adjustment disorder with depressed mood for which syndromal criteria of a major depression are absent.

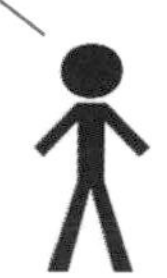

My depressed patient's TSH is 71 mU/L. What antidepressant should I give him?

It's called levothyroxine.

Are Antidepressants Inappropriate for Adjustment Disorders?

Clinicians generally presume that adjustment disorders with depressed mood (historically also referred to as "situational" depressions) are self-limited psychological phenomena that either do not require or otherwise do not empirically benefit from antidepressant pharmacotherapy. (At the same time, some experts think that adjustment disorders may be *form fruste* presentations that confer a higher risk for eventual development of a full depressive syndrome.) From an evidence-based standpoint, this is actually a very interesting and largely unstudied question with only limited empirical data. Preliminary, small open trials have examined bereavement (normal grief) in the absence of a syndromal MDE and suggested possible benefit from bupropion (150–300 mg/day for eight weeks), showing improvement from baseline depression symptom severity (HAM-D scores) as well as grief intensity ratings (Zisook et al., 2001). More recently, an RCT of a structured psychotherapy (complicated grief treatment (CGT)) plus citalopram significantly improved associated subthreshold depressive symptoms more than CGT alone, but overall outcome was no better with CGT + citalopram than with CGT alone (Shear et al., 2016). Patients who present solely with depressed mood in the context of a devastating interpersonal or other adverse life event that might also evolve into an MDE should be screened for a personal and family history of significant affective illness, and should be monitored for clinical worsening and the potential future role for pharmacotherapy in the event that psychotherapy and/or the natural course of time alone fails to avert progression and worsening of the condition.

B MONOAMINERGIC ANTIDEPRESSANTS

Antidepressants are among the most widely prescribed drugs in the United States, and fully one-quarter of people who take an antidepressant do so for at least 10 years (www.dcd.gov/nchs/data/databriefs/db283.pdf). According to the Centers for Disease Control, antidepressant use increased by 65% from 1999–2014. Some experts credit this increase with destigmatization efforts alongside greater public awareness and screening for depression. At the same time, though, depression is often as much a symptom in search of a diagnosis as it is a unifying diagnosis unto itself, and the sharp rise in antidepressant use over the past two decades does not necessarily reflect diagnostic refinement or greater recognition of the many psychiatric, medical, or substance-related problems for which depressed mood may just be one manifestation of a more complex or insidious condition.

C WHICH ANTIDEPRESSANTS ARE MOST EFFECTIVE *AND* WELL-TOLERATED?

Cipriani and colleagues (2018) conducted a meta-analysis of 21 antidepressants across 522 RCTs involving 116 477 subjects. As depicted in the forest plot shown in Figure 13.1, the most efficacious antidepressants in MDD with respect to probability (odds ratio) of response (i.e., ≥50% improvement from baseline severity) were amitriptyline (OR = 2.13), mirtazapine (OR = 1.89), duloxetine (OR = 1.85), and venlafaxine (OR = 1.85), while the *lowest* odds of response were seen with trazodone (OR = 1.51), clomipramine or desvenlafaxine (both having an OR = 1.49), or reboxetine[1] (OR = 1.37). It should be noted, however, that there was substantial overlap of credible intervals (CrIs) flanking individual ORs, meaning that actual probabilities for response across most agents were not substantially different from one another. Figure 13.1 also depicts the relative effect sizes (noted as SMDs) for

Figure 13.1 Relative efficacy across antidepressants. Data based on meta-analysis reported by Cipriani et al. (2018). An asterisk indicates the drug is not available in the USA.

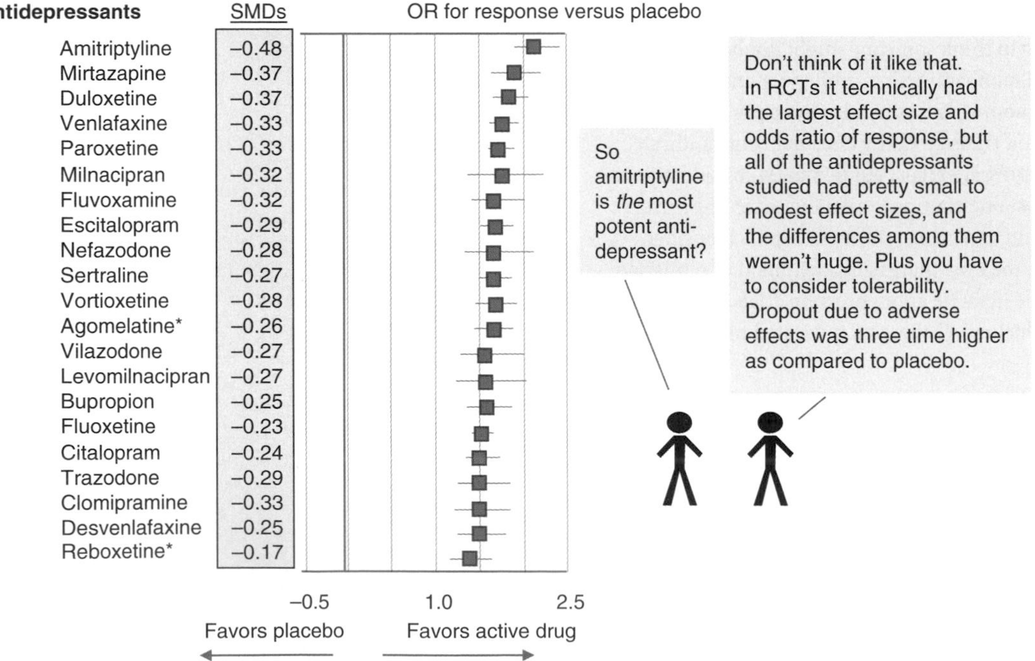

each antidepressant, which closely parallel the response ORs. Note that the overall SMD for antidepressants was a very modest 0.30 (and a narrow 95% CrI of 0.26–0.34, meaning not much variance), and, apart from amitriptyline, none had even a near-medium effect size.

As shown in Figure 13.2, antidepressant acceptability (all-cause dropout relative to placebo) was best with agomelatine[2] (OR = 0.84) and fluoxetine (OR = 0.88) and poorest with clomipramine; for all other agents studied, CrIs included 1 (making them not significantly different from placebo).

With respect to dropout specifically due to adverse effects, probabilities were *most favorable* with agomelatine (OR = 1.21), vortioxetine or milnacipran (both with OR = 1.64), desvenlafaxine (OR = 1.66), escitalopram (OR = 1.72), and fluoxetine (OR = 1.82); least favorable probabilities for avoiding dropout due to adverse effects were associated with clomipramine (OR = 4.44), amitriptyline (OR = 3.11), trazodone (OR = 3.07), and venlafaxine (OR = 2.95). Collectively, when response, remission and improvement in depressive symptoms were considered among head-to-head

Figure 13.2 Relative tolerability/dropout across antidepressants. Data based on meta-analysis by Cipriani et al., 2018. An asterisk indicates the drug is not available in the USA.

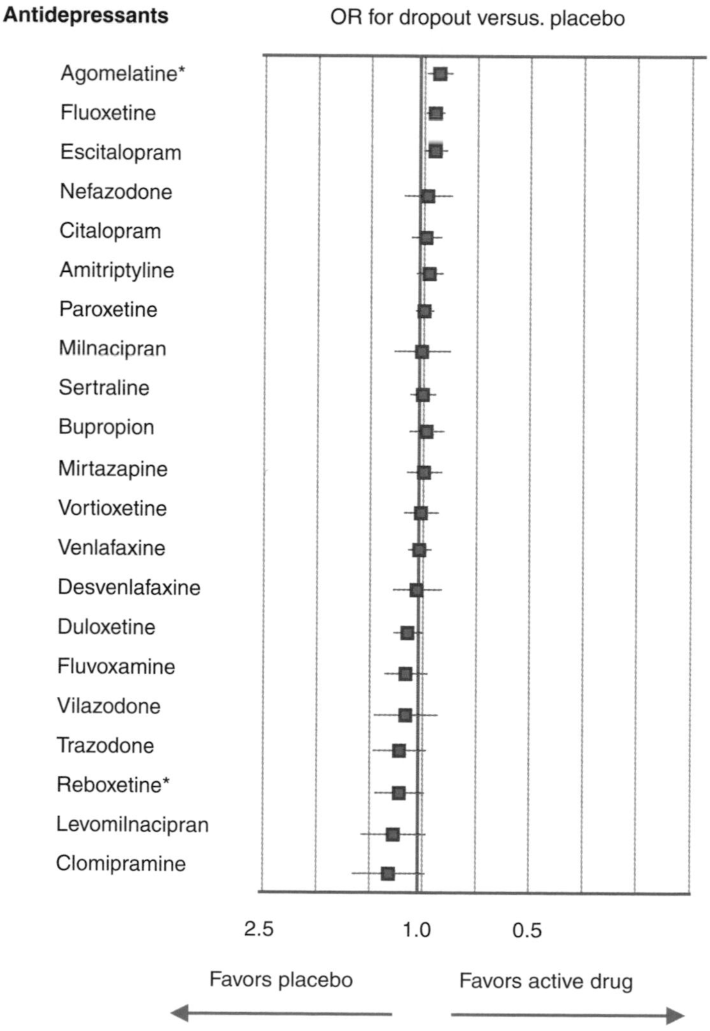

Antidepressants OR for dropout versus. placebo

Agomelatine*
Fluoxetine
Escitalopram
Nefazodone
Citalopram
Amitriptyline
Paroxetine
Milnacipran
Sertraline
Bupropion
Mirtazapine
Vortioxetine
Venlafaxine
Desvenlafaxine
Duloxetine
Fluvoxamine
Vilazodone
Trazodone
Reboxetine*
Levomilnacipran
Clomipramine

2.5 1.0 0.5

Favors placebo ← → Favors active drug

antidepressant (rather than placebo) comparisons, escitalopram, vortioxetine, amitriptyline, and bupropion emerged as being most favorable, while reboxetine, trazodone, fluoxetine, and citalopram ranked least favorably.

D HOW TO CHOOSE FROM AMONG MONOAMINERGIC ANTIDEPRESSANTS FOR DEPRESSION

On the whole, differences among monoaminergic antidepressants are nuanced and bear more on their relative tolerabilities than their efficacy versus placebo. Some have more of an evidence base in distinct populations because they were studied in those populations (e.g., bupropion in seasonal depression, fluoxetine or sertraline in bipolar II depression) or demonstrated utility for particular comorbidities (e.g., norepinephrine reuptake inhibitors (NERIs) for neuropathic pain, bupropion for smoking cessation, fluoxetine for bulimia) or a subcomponent of depression (e.g., vortioxetine for cognitive dysfunction) or related characteristic (e.g., serotonergic agents for anxiety). Some also lend themselves more than others to potential pharmacodynamic synergy in combination with other agents and therefore are often thought of more as "sidekick" agents (e.g., bupropion, mirtazapine), despite their stand-alone data in MDD.

Tables 13.1–13.6 summarize information about clinical characteristics that might help guide choosing from among monoaminergic antidepressants, as well as usual dosing parameters and strategies to optimize response.

What is Bupropion Hydrobromide?

Bupropion originally was formulated as a hydrochloride salt. In 2008 it was formulated as a hydrobromide salt (brand name Aplenzin®) with different dosing strengths (174 mg, 348 mg, and 522 mg). Both the hydrochloride and hydrobromide formulations are efficacious antidepressants that exert comparable effects to one another. There is no specific pharmacoequivalent dosing between bupropion HCL and bupropion HBr. There are fundamentally no known pharmacodynamic differences between the two agents; the choice of one over the other is merely a matter of a prescriber's personal preference.

E MORE ON SUPRATHERAPEUTIC DOSING

Legend has it that a renowned psychiatrist once remarked that a "psychopharmacologist" was someone who used higher medication dosages than did other clinicians. There is general lore that higher-than-usual doses are essential to overcome hard-to-treat forms of depression and other psychiatric problems. Whether or not this idea is evidence-based remains hotly debated. Particularly in a health care climate of intense treatment oversight by third-party payers, a growing challenge in the treatment of mood disorders involves parsing the effects of drug dose escalation versus time-on-drug as impacting outcomes.

In some studies, antidepressant dosage increases beyond a minimum therapeutic dose for MDD in general have not been shown to drive ultimate treatment

I work on an acute inpatient unit with severely depressed patients and simply don't have the time to wait for an antidepressant "adequate trial" to occur. What's wrong with cranking to higher antidepressant doses from the get-go?

Nothing except it's completely unscientific and quite likely unnecessary. There's just no way to make time go faster, and allowing enough time becomes a critical and possibly inescapable variable for judging antidepressant effect. Keep reading.

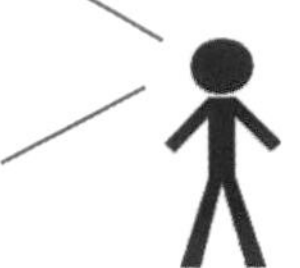

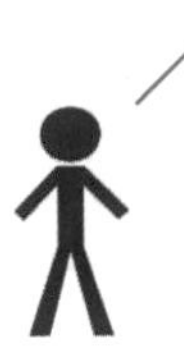

Yeah, OK, fine, just tell me how fast I can go up on drug doses.

responsivity. One meta-analysis of seven acute MDD RCTs involving 1208 participants (randomized to fluoxetine, sertraline, paroxetine, duloxetine, or maprotiline) found that dose escalation was *not* more effective than maintaining standard dosing to reduce depressive symptoms ($g = -0.04$, 95% CI = −0.20 to 0.12, p = 0.63), although all-cause dropout was higher among subjects who underwent dose escalation than continued standard dosing (Dold et al. 2017). Another meta-analysis focusing on SSRIs (including 40 RCTs with 10 039 participants) found a small but statistically significant correlation between SSRI dose and efficacy, offset by more dropouts due to intolerances (Jakubovski et al., 2016). Among nonresponders to an appropriately dosed SSRI, yet another meta-analysis found that subsequent dosage increases yielded negligible further improvement in depressive symptoms (Rink et al., 2018).

So, do antidepressant dose–response curves – at least in the case of SSRIs for MDD – really become flat much sooner than one might think? The answer may vary depending on study methodologies. Using patient-level data, Hieronymous and colleagues (2016) conducted a post hoc "mega-analysis" of 11 industry-sponsored fixed-dose SSRI trials (citalopram, sertraline, paroxetine), comparing doses above versus below a minimum effective threshold (i.e., citalopram 10–20 mg/day, sertraline 50 mg/day, paroxetine 10 mg/day), and focusing solely on the "sad mood" item (#1) of the Hamilton Depression Scale as a more sensitive outcome measure. They identified significant differences in optimal- versus low-dose citalopram (60 mg versus 20 mg: ES = 0.41, p = 0.003), sertraline (100 mg versus 50 mg: ES = 0.35, p = 0.004), and paroxetine (20 mg versus 10 mg: ES = 0.27, p = 0.005).

However, supratherapeutic doses (e.g., sertraline dosed at 400 mg/day) were not more efficacious beyond the above thresholds for a minimum effective dose.

The key question about supratherapeutic antidepressant dosing for MDD may be less about *whether* to press beyond a minimum effective dose before changing strategies as opposed to *when*, and with *which* antidepressants, and in patients with *what kinds of moderating factors*. In *chronic* MDD, for example, simply imposing lengthier time on same-dose sertraline or imipramine (16 weeks beyond an initial 12-week acute treatment phase) converted 40% of partial remitters to full remitters – although with no placebo arm, it is difficult to distinguish drug effects from the natural course of illness

So then if there's even a *chance* that higher-than-usual antidepressant doses may work better, why shouldn't I titrate as fast as possible to as high a dose as tolerable?

Tolerable is the key word. If there is a greater benefit, it's likely not huge, but intolerance causing dropout can be huge. Also, some studies find that dose escalations above standard doses are only effective after four weeks, and not sooner (Ruhé et al., 2006a).

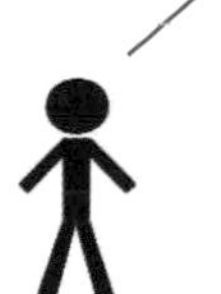

Cranking the oven up to 1000 degrees doesn't make the cake rise any faster.

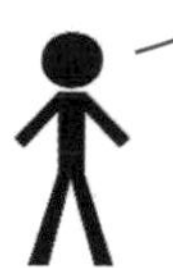

What about that business from Chapter 1, "if there hasn't been a 20% improvement by two weeks" then crank up the dose?

We're talking here about *supratherapeutic dosing*, not optimizing within the *usual* dosing range. So, yes, as mentioned in Chapter 1, if there has been less than a 20% improvement in the first two weeks, continue to optimize the dose as tolerated. But whether or not *very high doses* produce better antidepressant effects than lower doses as a general rule is more of an uncertainty.

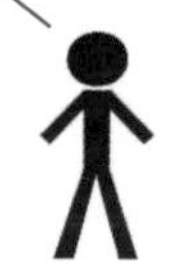

(Koran et al., 2001). In this same vein, a meta-analysis of nine studies of antidepressant trials in 3466 major depression patients found that about 1 in 5 nonresponders by week 4 will go on to demonstrate an antidepressant response by weeks 5–8 (NNT = 11 after four weeks), and about 1 in 10 will begin to respond only after week 9 (NNT = 17 after week 8) (Henssler et al., 2018).

Some antidepressants engage different receptor targets only at higher doses. For instance, paroxetine exerts moderate dose-related binding affinity for the NET at serum concentrations ≥100 ng/mL, corresponding to oral dosing of ≥40 mg/day (Gilmor et al., 2002); venlafaxine dosed at 75 mg/day acts mainly as an SSRI, while doses at or above 225 mg/day exert both 5HT and NE reuptake inhibition (Debonnel et al., 2007). Lore has arisen that mirtazapine at high doses exerts more noradrenergic effects that may "over-ride" the sedation caused by its antihistaminergic effects, but contrary to urban legend, empirical trials have failed to support the hypothesis of greater "activation" at high versus low doses (Shuman et al., 2019).

Most existing RCTs have not specifically rerandomized nonresponders to usual versus supratherapeutically dosed regimens, making the evidence base not as informative as we might hope on this issue. Possible ceiling effects as to what constitutes "supratherapeutic" dosing also remain highly uncertain, and prone to anecdotal evidence where patient-specific moderators are unknown. Consider, for example, a small MAOI case series among MDD patients unresponsive to a mean of eight prior antidepressants, where full responses with adequate tolerability were reported in five of seven patients given very-high dose tranylcypromine (up to 170 mg/day; mean dose among responders = 112 mg/day) (Amsterdam and Berwish, 1989). This is a highly refractory patient subgroup, for whom heroic dosing such as this may be justifiable, but it remains a highly experimental approach.

A practice survey of the American Society of Clinical Psychopharmacology membership assessed high-dose prescribing habits in the treatment of depression, with findings summarized in Table 13.7.

F SWITCH OR AUGMENT?

The pharmacological rule-of-thumb has long favored augmentation of partial responses and switching for nonresponses, although in the post-STAR*D era – where no particular augmentation or switching strategy produced an outcome superior to any other – some experts have come to favor switching rather than augmenting after an inadequate response, in part to minimize extensive polypharmaceutical "clutter" and potential mechanistic redundancies, as well as additive adverse effects. Still others point out that there is no body of data to support switching versus augmenting as an overall preferred "next step," and between-class switches have not been shown to yield better results than within-class switches (Ruhé et al., 2006b).

Are "broader spectrum" monoaminergic antidepressants associated with more robust efficacy than "narrower" spectrum drugs (such as SSRIs)? In an exhaustive meta-analysis of 93 RCTs involving 17 036 subjects, Papakostas and colleagues (2007) showed that "broadening the spectrum" from an SSRI to an SNRI yielded a meager 5.9% increased likelihood for achieving response. Said differently, switching to venlafaxine after an SSRI nonresponse yielded a modest NNT of 13 (95% CI = 9.1–25.0) (Ruhé et al., 2006a). However, as compared to SSRIs, SNRIs may have a somewhat faster onset of action.

G AUGMENTATION STRATEGIES

If switching from a single to a dual monoaminergic antidepressant yields only minimal benefit after

Box 13.3

Why Did "Later-Level" Interventions in STAR*D Perform so Miserably?

The NIMH-sponsored multisite STAR*D study sought to identify next-best interventions after nonresponse to an SSRI (citalopram) in MDD. As noted in earlier sections, response and remission probabilities declined precipitously after the first two intervention rounds. While STAR*D showed that no particular next step achieved substantial benefits, the remarkably low success rates observed with several "big gun" third- and fourth-round-level interventions was striking – specifically, the combination of mirtazapine and venlafaxine (response rate = 13.7%; McGrath et al., 2006a), adjunctive lithium (response rate = 15.9%; Nierenberg et al., 2006), and even tranylcypromine (response rate = 6.9%; McGrath et al., 2006a). Some observers would point out that while the STAR*D study group was meant to be representative of real-world patients, it was comprised of a particularly chronic and severely ill cohort (80% had chronic MDD, most subjects had six or more previous episodes, most had multiple psychiatric comorbidities) – enriching for poor response at the outset. Others would note that some of the more "aggressive" interventions (such as tranylcypromine) were in fact not used all that aggressively (i.e., tranylcypromine mean dose was a rather modest 36.9 mg/day; lithium mean dose was only 859.9 mg/day). And by the time persistently depressed subjects reached the third and fourth levels of intervention, dropout from the initial cohort further enriched the remaining study group for those with the poorest prognoses. Fully one-third of those who eventually responded to any 12–14-week medication trial in STAR*D only did so after six weeks (again pointing to time as an inescapable variable in treatment outcome). While observers can and will continue to debate issues of dosing and time, the sobering fact remains that monoaminergic antidepressants are limited in the size of their effect and breadth of spectrum in difficult-to-treat forms of depression.

nonresponse to an SSRI, and if STAR*D points to no specific preferred strategy from among SSRI augmentations with bupropion, buspirone, lithium, or triiodothyronine, how can clinicians best draw from the available evidence base while integrating rationales for complex combination therapies (as discussed in detail in Chapter 6)? Let us consider the evidence base, starting with the most commonly used adjunctive pharmacotherapy class: SGAs.

Can Moderators Guide Next Steps?

Among MDD nonresponders to ≥1 antidepressant, *age* >65 and *mixed features* together favored better outcomes from adding aripiprazole rather than switching to bupropion (see Zisook et al., 2019)

H SECOND-GENERATION ANTIPSYCHOTICS

SGAs constitute the most widely studied (and, hence, perhaps the most popular) augmentation strategy after an incomplete response to a monoaminergic antidepressant – a role accorded to lithium in the "tricyclic and MAOI generation," and to bupropion (Zisook et al., 2006) in the "SSRI and SNRI generation." Does their extensive database mean they are an inherently *better* choice than other possible adjunctive options? Certainly not; they are just better studied. Why is that? Well, one must concede the enormous commercial impetus for the pharmaceutical industry to study SGAs as viable antidepressant adjuncts given the long-range proprietary status of many such agents beginning in the mid-1990s. In those days (and since then), nonproprietary adjunctive treatment options such as lithium, tricyclics, bupropion, and the like offered no commercial incentive for innovative industry study as compared to proprietary compounds. And with no fundamentally new mechanistic strategies (other than monoamines) to treat depression into the second decade of the twenty-first century, proprietary SGAs – for better or worse – offered the only real commercial prospect for industry pursuit. The results tell us that many (but not all) SGAs added to a monoaminergic antidepressant can further improve depression symptoms after an initial incomplete response.

Tip

When reading published RCTs in MDD, pay attention to how much global improvement is explainable by effects on *core mood symptoms* (e.g., sadness, anhedonia) versus physical symptoms (e.g., agitation, insomnia, or appetite loss). Review individual items on the rating scale used and ask if an adjunctive SGA has leveraged improvement by virtue of both or just one of these domains.

Meta-analyses show that SGAs collectively yield about a 1.7-fold greater likelihood for response (and about a twofold greater likelihood for remission), as compared to placebo, when added to a traditional antidepressant (Nelson et al. 2009). However, individual SGAs vary greatly in their evidence base (or lack thereof) for adjunctive therapy of depression – as summarized in Table 13.8.

I WHAT IS THE RATIONALE FOR USING SGAs TO TREAT DEPRESSION?

While precise mechanisms to explain observable psychotropic effects of many psychiatric drugs remain speculative, there are putative rationales and hypotheses worth considering. FGAs, though anxiolytic, have been associated with *induction* of depression. In contrast, in the case of SGAs as putative antidepressants

The clock's still ticking on my depressed patient's length of stay. Why not just start every severely depressed patient on an adjunctive SGA to improve their chances of a faster response?

No one's ever shown you'll necessarily achieve a faster response – just that, after incomplete response to a monoaminergic antidepressant, the chances of further improvement are greater with SGA augmentation. And be careful: not all SGAs have been studied for that purpose, and some – like ziprasidone – have been shown to be no better than placebo, so don't go making unjustified class overgeneralizations.

Actually, that's not all *entirely* true. Yargic et al. (2004) showed that paroxetine plus quetiapine (up to 200 mg/day) *from the outset* yielded a better response than did paroxetine alone in anxious MDD patients who had *not* already failed paroxetine alone. So at least adjunctive quetiapine might hasten paroxetine response.

Yeah well if you're gonna go there let's also acknowledge the Garakani et al. (2008) study showing that quetiapine added to fluoxetine did nothing to speed onset of response. So much for generalizability.

(at least in some instances), a first consideration involves their relative blockade of postsynaptic $5HT_{2A}$ receptors – analogous to the presumed serotonergic antidepressant effects of mirtazapine (Ki = 6.3–69 nM) or nefazodone (Ki = 26 nM). (Here, pimavanserin and perhaps lumateperone (see Chapter 15) become especially promising candidate antidepressants at least on theoretical grounds.) Box 13.4 summarizes relative $5HT_{2A}$ binding affinities across SGAs. Noteworthy is their variability; quetiapine, one of the more potent antidepressant SGAs, is among the weakest of all $5HT_{2A}$ binders from among the agents listed. Clozapine – a drug with minimal, if any, known antidepressant effects – has high $5HT_{2A}$ occupancy (up to 94%); and furthermore, even some FGAs have relatively high $5HT_{2A}$ binding affinities (e.g., loxapine Ki = 6.6 nM; perphenazine Ki = 5.6 nM), at least in vitro. Additional monoaminergic targets are only somewhat helpful when considering SGA antidepressant properties. For example, many SGAs have Ki values well above 1000 nM at the serotonin transporter protein (SERT) (e.g., olanzapine, lurasidone, aripiprazole, quetiapine) or the norepinephrine transporter (NET) (e.g., olanzapine, aripiprazole). Ziprasidone binds with greater affinity than most other SGAs at both the SERT (Ki = 112 nM) and the NET (Ki = 44 nM), yet RCTs have failed to demonstrate antidepressant properties (Table 13.3).

Box 13.4

$5HT_{2A}$ Binding Affinities of SGAs

Agent	$5HT_{2A}$ Ki (nM)	Action
Asenapine	0.06	Antagonist
Ziprasidone	0.08–1.4	Antagonist
Pimavanserin	0.087	Inverse agonist/ antagonist
Risperidone	0.17	Inverse agonist
Brexpiprazole	0.47	Antagonist
Lumateperone	0.54	Antagonist
Paliperidone	1.1	Unknown
Olanzapine	1.32-24.2	Inverse agonist
Lurasidone	2.03	Antagonist
Aripiprazole	3.4-35	Antagonist
Iloperidone	5.6	Antagonist
Clozapine	9.15	Antagonist
Cariprazine	18.8	Antagonist
Quetiapine	96-101	Antagonist

Based partly on data from Eison and Mullins, 1996

Once again, putative drug mechanisms remain a point of speculation and theoretical interest, but from a pragmatic standpoint, empirically demonstrated

Reminder

An inverse agonist binds to the same receptor site as does an agonist on constitutively active receptors, but induces the opposite effect of an agonist; like a dimmer switch, it causes a decrease in basal signaling. An antagonist, by contrast, acts more like an "off" switch that blocks any receptor activity other than constitutive (basal) activity.

pharmacodynamic effects remain the fundamental consideration, regardless of putative compelling (or elusive) mechanisms of action.

Box 13.5

More on $5HT_{2A}$ and Depression

Some monoaminergic antidepressants are thought to exert their antidepressant effects primarily via $5HT_{2A}$ antagonism – perhaps most notably, mirtazapine (with Ki = 6.3–69 nM). You might wonder about the novel $5HT_{2A}$ antagonist *pimavanserin* (officially regarded as an FDA-approved treatment for psychosis in patients with Parkinson's disease, where any D_2 antagonism would only make things worse), given its tight $5HT_{2A}$ binding affinity (Table 13.4). In fact, a preliminary Phase II 10-week RCT, dosed at 34 mg/day in SSRI- or SNRI-nonresponsive MDD, showed separation from placebo on $HAM\text{-}D_{17}$ scores (ES = 0.497) as well as a number of secondary outcome measures (www.acadia-pharm.com/pipeline/pimavanserin-major-depressive-disorder).

You might now ask, well, if $5HT_{2A}$ *antagonism* is thought to produce an antidepressant effect, how could hallucinogenic $5HT_{2A}$ *agonists* such as *psilocybin* or *lysergic acid dethylamide (LSD)* also be reported to have antidepressant properties in (mostly open-label) experimental trials (e.g., Carhart-Harris et al., 2018)? This is a complex apparent paradox for which a definitive answer remains speculative. Plausible hypotheses would likely include differences in the ways these drugs may ultimately impact other circuitry, such as pyramidal glutamate neurons and GABA interneurons, and possible differential effect on a complex cortical–subcortical circuitry region known as the *default mode network*, largely responsible for self-reflection, autobiographical memory, and mind-wandering.

J ADJUNCTIVE BUSPIRONE

As noted in earlier sections (e.g., Chapter 6, Figure 6.1), buspirone has a highly conceptually appealing mechanism that in principle should make it a powerhouse augmentation for any serotonergic antidepressant – downregulating the presynaptic autoreceptor that ultimately releases more serotonin, while "steering" more post-synaptic serotonin quanta to bind to the $5HT_{1A}$ receptor. And yet, by general reputation buspirone is often considered a weak psychotropic drug, and in STAR*D it remained undistinguished as an add-on to citalopram. Buspirone has a relatively weak binding affinity to the $5HT_{1A}$ receptor (see Chapter 17, Box 17.6). Elsewhere, only slightly more impressive data exist with its adjunctive use with SSRIs; Appelberg and colleagues (2001), for example, showed that adjunctive buspirone *sped up onset* of response to SSRIs, though it ultimately did not yield greater overall antidepressant efficacy. Whether or not other $5HT_{1A}$ partial agonists (such as brexpiprazole or vilazodone) hold particular value for hastening or amplifying antidepressant response through a comparable mechanism remains a point of speculation.

Doesn't pindolol, a $5HT_{1A}$ full antagonist, speed SSRI onset? Since it downregulates the autoreceptor?

Early reports hinted at that but a meta-analysis of five RCTs found no advantage (Liu et al., 2015).

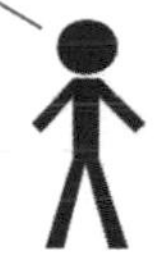
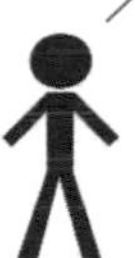

K ADJUNCTIVE LITHIUM

Lithium stands as a time-honored antidepressant augmentation strategy in both unipolar and bipolar depression, though with the exception of STAR*D (where response after two prior antidepressant failures was a mere 15.9% over a mean of 9.6 weeks; Nierenberg et al., 2006), most RCTs are of pre-twenty-first-century vintage. A 2014 meta-analysis of nine RCTs, adding lithium to TCAs, trazodone, phenelzine, SSRIs or mianserin,[3] ranging from 2–42 days, found a "response" OR of 2.80 (95% CI = 1.40–5.59) when added to TCAs and OR = 3.06 (95% CI = 1.19–7.88) when added to SSRIs or other second-generation antidepressants (Nelson et al., 2014). There are no robust data that identify predictors of response as an antidepressant adjuvant, nor has a relationship been established between antidepressant response and serum blood levels.

3 Not available in the USA.

L ADJUNCTIVE LAMOTRIGINE

Limited data exist on the use of lamotrigine added to antidepressants in MDD patients with no history of mania or hypomania. We are aware of benefits reported only in a handful of small open trials (n <20). Eight-week RCTs adding lamotrigine to an antidepressant have failed to show differences in efficacy versus placebo (e.g., Barbee et al., 2011).

M ADJUNCTIVE MIRTAZAPINE

The conceptual appeal of adding mirtzapine to almost any antidepressant comes from its novel mechanism, compatible and nonredundant with most other drugs. Its clinical profile favors use in anxious/agitated (rather than anergic/hypersomnic) patients and those with appetite loss. Its adjunctive use at the outset with an SSRI, SNRI, or bupropion may hasten overall antidepressant response (Blier et al., 2010). However, as noted earlier, its use in conjunction with venlafaxine in STAR*D produced only modest efficacy after several previous treatment nonresponses. A later, large (n = 480) RCT in MDD patients treated in a primary care setting found no advantage for its augmentation to an SSRI or SNRI after initial nonresponse (Kessler et al., 2018).

N ADJUNCTIVE THYROID HORMONE

Exogenous thyroid hormone is believed to exert trophic effects and increase serotonin signaling in prefrontal brain regions, collectively providing a rationale for its use as an antidepressant adjunct. For such purposes, oral triiodothyronine (T_3) dosing typically is 25–50 µg/day; dosages >62.5 µg/day may be more prone to cause toxicity. In the treatment of primary hypothyroidism, most available evidence suggests there is no advantage for combining synthetic T_3 plus levothyroxine over levothyroxine monotherapy (Clyde et al., 2003). Mood improvements do not account for subjective preference for combination over monotherapy among hypothyroid patients (Appelhof et al., 2005).

> **Tip**
>
> 20% of T_3 is secreted directly by the thyroid gland; 80% is derived from peripheral deiodination of thyroxine (T_4) to T_3. "Low T_3 syndrome" describes depressed patients with normal T_4 and normal TSH but low T_3 due to diminished conversion of T_4 to T_3, potentially evident in ~6% of clinically depressed patients (Premachandra et al., 2006).

In patients with primary diagnoses of MDD, studies of adjunctive thyroid hormone as a psychotropic agent mainly address the utility of adding T_3 (typically 25–50 µg/dL) to a monoaminergic antidepressant (e.g., sertraline; Cooper-Karaz et al., 2007), although the onset of antidepressant effect does not appear to be faster with this approach (Garlow et al., 2012). A meta-analysis of four RCTs found no overall difference between SSRI monotherapy and adjunctive T_3 (Papakostas et al., 2009), although the limited database in this area leaves open the question of whether certain depressed patient subgroups (e.g., those with atypical features, or in women more than men (Altshuler et al., 2001)) might nevertheless benefit from adjunctive T_3.

The STAR*D study found a 24.7% remission rate when T_3 was added to existing treatments for depression after two failed prior trials, which was statistically no different from adjunctive lithium (15.9% remission rate) (Nierenberg et al., 2006). A network meta-analysis

If I successfully treat a non-hypothyroid patient with adjunctive thyroid hormone, how long should I continue it once they are better?

Good question, and since there are neither long-term studies nor randomized discontinuation trials to guide us, I'll give you my opinion, which is to stop thyroid hormone in a euthymic, euthyroid patient who has no intrinsic hypothyroidism within 6-12 months of remission or possibly sooner, depending on their risk for osteoporosis or cardiac arrhythmias.

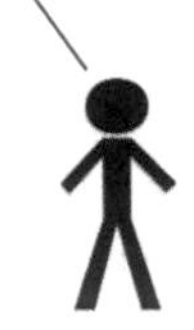
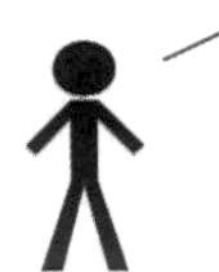

of adjunctive pharmacotherapies for depression found an OR of 1.84 (CrI = 1.06–3.56) for response to thyroid hormone relative to placebo (Zhou et al., 2015), while an earlier meta-analysis pointed out that, when considering only RCTs, the likelihood of response from adding T_3 to TCAs was nonsignificant (OR = 1.53, 95% CI = 0.70–3.35, NNT = 12.5; Aronson et al., 1996). A review of six trials (mostly RCTs, some open label) of T_3 augmentation specifically of SSRIs yielded mixed findings notable for small study group sizes, nonoptimized dosing of existing SSRIs, and difficulty forming generalizable conclusions due to varying methodologies (Touma et al., 2017).

O PSYCHOSTIMULANTS AS ANTIDEPRESSANT ADJUNCTS

Psychostimulants have enjoyed a longstanding, albeit often anecdotal, tradition as adjunctive pharmacotherapies for depression, particularly in the context of anergic/amotivational presentations, comorbidities involving frank ADD or features of inattention and executive dysfunction, or reverse neurovegetative symptoms (notably, hypersomnia and hyperphagia). Stimulants are generally thought of as fast-acting and, as noted in Box 3.6 in Chapter 3, they can exert relatively large effect sizes. McIntyre and colleagues (2016) conducted a meta-analysis of 21 acute RCTs in MDD (n = 1900 participants randomized to active treatment and 1823 to placebo) involving amphetamine, dextroamphetamine, lisdexamfetamine, or methylphenidate, as well as modafinil or armodafinil, yielding a pooled response rate (OR) of 1.41 relative to placebo (95% CI = 1.13–1.78). As those authors note, some of the included studies involved small sample sizes (e.g., n = 22 for dextroamphetamine) and short study periods (e.g., two weeks), limiting the confidence with which definitive conclusions about both efficacy and safety can be drawn. Also notably, a separate (albeit small; n = 4 RCTs) meta-analysis of lisdexamfetamine as augmentation to antidepressants in TRD found only a small effect (g = 0.126, 95% CI = −0.040 to 0.291), with an OR for remission of only 1.206 (95% CI = 0.745 to 1.954, p = 0.446) (Giacobbe et al., 2018).

Modafanil (and it enantiomer armodafinil), sometimes perceived as a "safer" stimulant-like alternative to traditional Schedule II agents, has been examined separately in a meta-analysis of six RCTs involving 910 MDD or bipolar depression patients; an OR of 1.61 for remission (versus placebo) emerged, as did a modest (small-to-medium) effect size (g = 0.35), and comparable outcomes with respect to efficacy and tolerability in both unipolar and bipolar depression (Goss et al., 2013). However, the extent to which adjunctive (ar)modafinil impacts major depression by virtue of an effect on core psychological dimensions (e.g., sad mood, anhedonia, low self-worth, guilt) versus physical symptoms (e.g., anergia, lethargy, poor concentration) remains a point of speculation.

P WHAT ABOUT MUSCARINIC PROCHOLINERGICS IN DEPRESSION?

In the 1970s, the so-called "cholinergic–adrenergic balance" hypothesis of depression derived from observations that the cholinomimetic drug physostigmine appeared to counteract mania and potentially cause depression (Janowsky et al., 1972). Interest then turned to the question of whether anticholinergic drugs could exert antidepressant properties. Most notably, in the modern era, scopolamine administered experimentally as a 4 μg/kg IV infusion has been associated with 34–56% remission rates within three days, with a larger effect in women than men, and in both unipolar and bipolar depression (Drevets et al., 2013).

Q TRUE TREATMENT RESISTANCE

The term "treatment resistance" is often invoked by both clinicians and patients in reference to poor outcomes after multiple treatment efforts, although it is important for clinicians to differentiate true lack of (or inadequate) response to appropriately dosed pharmacotherapies for sufficient durations versus inappropriate medications, underdosed/insufficient trials, or prematurely aborted trials due to poor adherence or intolerances. Nonresponse to one or more adequate trials of traditional monoaminergic antidepressants should prompt a review of pertinent moderators (i.e., severity, polarity, psychosis, comorbidities) and mediators (i.e., adherence, P–K interactions) that could account for *pseudo*-resistance.

Efforts to quantify degrees of treatment resistance suggest that the probability of response or remission decreases with every subsequent failed adequate medication trial for a given episode. In the STAR*D major depression trial, for example, the likelihood of response after initial nonresponse to an SSRI (citalopram) declined from 37% to 31%; a third trial carried a 14% likelihood of response, while a fourth trial held a 13% overall response rate (Rush et al., 2006b). An empirical staging method for treatment resistance in MDD, developed at the Massachusetts General Hospital (MGH), accords one "point" for each nonresponse to an adequately dosed antidepressant trial lasting six or more weeks; dosing optimization or augmentation adds 0.5 point per trial and nonresponse to ECT increases a total score by 3 (Petersen et al., 2005). This rating system, as depicted in Box 13.6, suggests that the probability of achieving remission after five failed adequate antidepressant trials (or two nonoptimized/nonaugmented trials plus failed ECT) is approximately zero.

Box 13.6

MGH Staging Model for TRD

Score	Remitters	Nonremitters
0	100%	0%
1	67%	33%
1.5	33%	67%
2	27%	73%
2.5	22%	78%
3	17%	83%
4	13%	87%
5	0	100%

While it is anathema to imagine declaring out loud a "zero" probability of remission with pharmacotherapy plus or minus ECT, it is important to adopt a realistic perspective on the likelihood of remission, or a reconfiguring of treatment goals and reasonable expectations, based on past outcomes of appropriate treatments. Reconfiguration of treatment goals may mean focusing on improving specific target symptoms (e.g., suicidality, insomnia) rather than full syndromes (see Chapter 1, on "Defining the Goals of Treatment"); it may also mean adopting a stronger stance when recommending treatments that may be considered more "heroic" and carry greater safety risks (e.g., MAOIs, especially at high doses), novel strategies (e.g., ketamine), device-based therapies (e.g., ECT, repetitive transcranial magnetic stimulation (rTMS), vagal nerve stimulation (VNS)), or experimental therapies.

While there exists a considerable literature on "treatment-resistant depression," surprisingly few controlled trials have focused specifically on patients who have not responded to *numerous* agents. In patients with *highly* treatment-resistant depression the formal evidence base is remarkably limited and, apart from ketamine,[4] includes what we will call The Big Three: traditional *MAOIs, olanzapine/fluoxetine combination*, and *pramipexole* (see Boxes 13.7–13.9).

Box 13.7

MAOIs

Open-label retrospective data preliminarily suggest safety and efficacy (~80% response) after adding tranylcypromine to amitriptyline in ECT-nonresponsive depression with no observed adverse cardiovascular events (Ferreira-Garcia et al., 2018). Tranylcypromine in very high doses (see Table 13.1) or in conjunction with dextroamphetamine (though technically contraindicated due to risk for hypertensive crisis) has been reported in case fashion with success (and no adverse cardiovascular or cerebrovascular outcomes) in highly treatment-resistant depression (Stewart et al., 2014). As noted earlier, the relatively low mean dose of tranylcypromine used in STAR*D may account for the surprisingly low response rate observed in that TRD trial. Many experts believe that irreversible inhibition of MAO-A provides a markedly more potent antidepressant strategy than can occur with reversible MAO-A inhibitors (e.g., moclobemide).

What sort of informed consent do you obtain before adding a stimulant to an MAOI?
I try to be completely transparent.

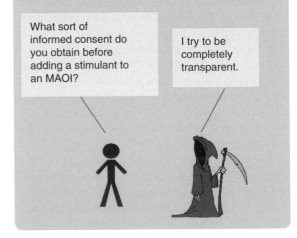

[4] Note: in FDA registration trials of intranasal esketamine, subjects failed two or more but no more than five monoaminergic antidepressants in their current episode.

Box 13.8

Olanzapine/Fluoxetine Combination (OFC)

One of only two drugs FDA-approved for TRD (the other being esketamine), the database with OFC is impressive in that, in the initial study, more than half of fluoxetine (mean dose 52.0 mg/day) nonresponders converted to responders with olanzapine augmentation (mean dose 13.5 mg/day), with separation from placebo (i.e., continued fluoxetine alone) evident after one week (Shelton et al., 2001). Enrollees had not responded to at least two prior antidepressants from different classes. While a later, larger multisite eight-week RCT failed to show separation from placebo on primary endpoint (change in MADRS at study end), a post hoc moderator analysis showed significantly greater improvement in the previously SSRI-nonresponsive (but not nortriptyline-nonresponsive) subgroup (Shelton et al., 2005). Cumulative data from across all industry-sponsored OFC trials (n = 1146) using MMRM analyses showed a significantly greater remission rate with OFC (25.5%) than continued fluoxetine alone (17.3%) (NNT = 8.7) (Trivedi et al., 2009).

Box 13.9

Pramipexole

Mostly small proof-of-concept trials have examined this D_2/D_3 agonist in TRD in both unipolar and bipolar patients. Notably, Fawcett et al. (2016) published a case series of 42 outpatients with MDD or bipolar depression who failed to respond to at least four adequate antidepressant trials (mean = 6.0 ± 1.5) in the current episode who were treated with open-label high-dose pramipexole (up to 5 mg/day; mean dose among responders/remitters = 2.5 + 1.1 mg/day), among whom 76% had a persistent response or remission with minimal adverse effects (initial transient nausea and rare agitation/irritability). That study makes pramipexole one of the very few agents that has been evaluated in depressed patients unresponsive to more than three interventions in the current episode. Tolerability concerns mainly involve sedation and nausea. Rare reports exist of new-onset impulse control problems (e.g., gambling) or narcolepsy-like sleep attacks.

"BIG GUN" ANTIDEPRESSANTS

More on MAOIs: Logistics

Described by some experts as the "secret weapon" of depression psychopharmacology, MAOIs can be enormously effective in TRD and other depression subtypes but are widely shunned by most psychiatrists mainly because of lack of familiarity with their safe use. Their common adverse effects are not dramatically different from those of other monoaminergic antidepressants with the unique exceptions of the risks for: (a) serotonin syndrome when coadministered with other serotonergic agents, or (b) hypertensive crises when coadministered with foods with high tyramine content (see Box 13.11) or sympathomimetic drugs (e.g., pseudoephedrine, psychostimulants).

MAO exists as two isoenzymes, each having differing substrates and found in different parts of the body (see Box 13.10).

Traditional MAOIs (isocarboxazid, phenelzine, tranylcypromine) *irreversibly* inhibit MAO-A. *Reversible* inhibitors of MAO-A ("RIMAs") such as moclobemide (available outside of the United States) do not carry restrictions against dietary tyramine – although the magnitude of their effect may be less robust than seen with irreversible MAO-A inhibition. Inhibitors of MAO-B (e.g., selegiline) have no CNS activity and, therefore, CNS-active MAOIs must overcome the nonselectivity of the A and B isoezymes in order to exert psychotropic effects. Oral selegiline can be dosed at supratherapeutic levels to over-ride this isoenzyme selectivity, as noted in Table 13.3, although transdermal selegiline more feasibly overcomes MAO-B selectivity to enable MAO-A irreversible

Tip

Because it takes two weeks for the body to regenerate MAO upon cessation of an MAOI, a two-week washout period is generally needed after stopping an MAOI and beginning a different serotonergic (or sympathomimetic) agent.

Box 13.10

Isoezymes of MAO

Isoenzyme	Substrates	Found in
MAO-A	Serotonin, dopamine, norepinephrine, melatonin	Neurons, glia, gut, liver, pulmonary vascular endothelium, placenta
MAO-B	Phenylephrine, dopamine	Neurons, glia, platelets

inhibition relevant for depression. MAOI dosing is described in Table 13.3 at the end of this chapter. MAO metabolizes dietary tyramine, leading to its buildup (with consequent hypertension) when MAO is inhibited. Tyramine-"rich" foods contain >6 g/serving (Walker et al., 1996); those that do (and do not) need to be avoided when taking an irreversible MAOA inhibitor are summarized in Box 13.11.

Why aren't you supposed to use carbamazepine with MAOIs? There's no pressor effect or known serotonergic effect.

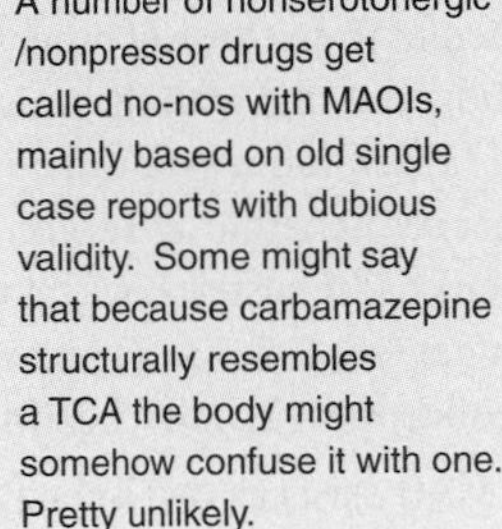

A number of nonserotonergic /nonpressor drugs get called no-nos with MAOIs, mainly based on old single case reports with dubious validity. Some might say that because carbamazepine structurally resembles a TCA the body might somehow confuse it with one. Pretty unlikely.

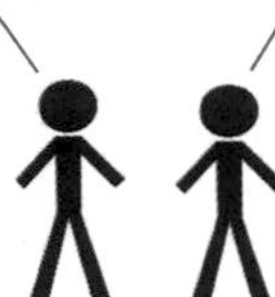

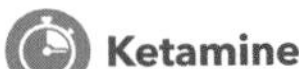

Ketamine

Ketamine is a complex drug with multiple receptor targets. Based on findings reported by Newport et al., 2015, these are believed to include:

- NMDA receptor antagonism
- μ-opioid antagonism
- σ_1 or σ_2 agonism
- D_2 agonism
- serotonin reuptake inhibition
- NET reuptake inhibitor
- DAT reuptake inhibition
- Cholinesterase inhibition
- α_7 nicotinic antagonist
- Muscarinic M1, M2, M3 antagonism

Tip

The σ receptors, once thought to be related to opioid receptors, constitute their own family and interact with a wide range of ligands that include phencyclidine, cocaine, dextromethorphan, and neurosteroids such as DHEA and pregnenolone, among other compounds. CNS effects include regulation of mood, but the full extent of their physiological functions within the CNS remain not fully understood.

Ketamine thus defies categorization by any single all-encompassing mechanism. Its diverse pharmacodynamic effects are dose-related and range from anesthesia induction to dissociation to antinociception to antidepressant efficacy. One must keep in mind that mechanisms of action identified from in vitro studies may not necessarily translate to in vivo effects in humans. Likely, different mechanisms of action or combinations of mechanisms contribute to ketamine's varying pharmacodynamic effects, both mood-related and unrelated.

Depending on how it is delivered, ketamine causes a rapid burst of synaptic glutamate release, increased GABA concentrations, and changes in neuronal architecture within hours of its administration that are thought to lead to neuroprotective effects, such as increased transcription of BDNF. However, while ketamine is often

Box 13.11

MAOI Dietary Restrictions

Food	Must avoid	Unnecessary to avoid
Cheeses	Aged cheeses (e.g., cheddar, Swiss, blue, stilton, brie) – think rind and/or holes within	Fresh mozzarella, cream cheese, farmer cheese, commercial pizzas, feta, processed fresh cheese slices
Meats and fish	Any aged/nonfresh, including air-dried sausage	Fresh-sliced meats (bologna, pastrami, ham), non-aged sausage, pepperoni
Alcohol	Tap beer	Bottled beer, chianti wine (in moderation)
Soy sauce	More than three tablespoons	≤1 mg tyramine in three tablespoons
Other	Overly ripe bananas, sauerkraut, fava beans or broad-bean pods, non-fresh tofu, yeast extract	Chocolate, yogurt, fresh tofu, avocados, Worcestershire sauce, raspberries, bananas (unless over-ripe), soy milk

Based on Gardner et al., 1996; Walker et al., 1996; Shulman et al., 1989; Shulman and Walker, 1999 primarily identified as an NMDA receptor antagonist, it is not so clear whether the mechanism of NMDA receptor blockade confers a class effect for antidepressant properties. There are now many negative RCTs in MDD using other NMDA receptor antagonists, such as *rapastinel* (a positive NMDA receptor modulator), *riluzole* (Na^+ channel-blocker and NMDA receptor antagonist commonly used in demyelinating disorders), *memantine* (which possesses weak NMDA receptor antagonist properties), *traxoprodil* (aka CP101-606, which binds to the NMDA receptor allosteric site on GluN2B subunit), *lanicemine* (a "low-trapping" NMDA receptor antagonist), and *MK-0657* (aka CERC-301, which binds to the NMDA receptor at an allosteric site of the GluN2B subunit). Further suggestions that mechanisms other than NMDA receptor blockade likely account for (or at least contribute to) ketamine's antidepressant effect come from two additional lines of evidence:

- Preclinical studies show that ketamine's active metabolite, hydroxynorketamine, depends on signaling via AMPA (and not NMDA) receptor activation (Zanos et al., 2016)
- Pretreatment with the opiate antagonist naltrexone was shown in a preliminary trial of 12 MDD subjects to block the antidepressant effects of subsequent ketamine infusion (Williams et al., 2018). This latter observation prompted a flurry of editorial exchanges disputing the interpretation that ketamine's antidepressant properties could be mediated primarily if not solely via the opioid system.

Before we further discuss ketamine, see Box 13.12 for a quick review of the different kinds of glutamate receptors.

Box 13.12

Ionotropic and Metabotropic Glutamate Receptors

Glutamate transmission between neurons occurs through two types of receptors: *ionotropic* and *metabotropic*. Ionotropic glutamate receptors affect synaptic transmission via ion channels and currents and come in three known forms: the *N*-methyl-D-aspartate (*NMDA*) receptor, the α-amino-3-hydroxy-5-methyl-4-isoxazolepropionic (*AMPA*) receptor, and the *kainate* receptor. Metabotropic glutamate receptors (abbreviated mGluR) cause signaling to occur via second messengers and G-protein coupled receptors; there are eight types (mGluR1→mGluR8) and three groups: *Group 1* (mGluR1→mGluR5) are mainly postsynaptic, may ↑ NMDA activity, and are involved in *increasing excitotoxicity*; *Group 2* (mGluR2 and mGluR3) are mainly presynaptic, may ↓ NMDA receptor activity, and contribute to *decreasing excitotoxicity*; and *Group 3* (mGluR4, mGluR6→mGluR8), which are mainly presynaptic, may ↓ NMDA receptor activity and are involved in *decreasing excitotoxicity*. Mood disorders research has focused heavily on drugs believed to modulate ionotropic (mostly NMDA or AMPA) receptors rather than mGluRs, although the latter category modulates other receptors, protects neurons from excitotoxicity, plays a key role in learning and memory, and may hold importance for understanding disease states such as psychosis, anxiety, dementia, Parkinson's disease, and other psychopathological conditions.

I hear you're not supposed to coadminister lamotrigine with ketamine for depression. Why's that?

Complicated question. Some years ago, a study found that administering lamotrigine prior to ketamine infusion in 16 healthy subjects blocked ketamine's dissociative effects (Anand et al., 2000). That study's design was based on the premise that lamotrigine's inhibition of presynaptic glutamate release might thwart ketamine's putative glutamate burst. There is the same concern with benzodiazepines, BTW. The idea that such a mechanism could diminish ketamine's antidepressant efficacy is relevant, but purely theoretical and has not been demonstrated empirically. To the contrary, a single 300 mg oral lamotrigine dose administered two hours prior to ketamine infusion in MDD patients was shown *not* to diminish ketamine's antidepressant efficacy (Mathew et al., 2010). *If* someone is having a clear benefit from lamotrigine there's no compelling reason to stop or alter it prior to giving them ketamine.

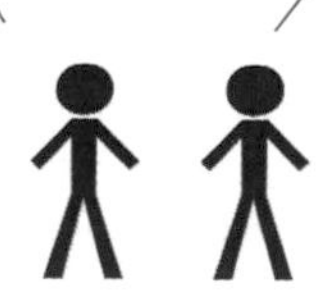

Studies of intravenous ketamine delivered at 0.5 mg/kg over about 40 minutes collectively show that about 50–70% of MDD or bipolar depressed patients will have a marked improvement in depressive symptoms within a day, but only about one-third will retain their improvement by one week and about 10% after two weeks (Newport et al., 2015). In 2019, enantiomeric esketamine received FDA approval as an intranasal (IN) option for TRD as an add-on to a newly begun monoaminergic antidepressant. Per the manufacturer's study protocol, dosing is divided into an initial induction phase (twice a week for four weeks, begun as 56 mg and then may be titrated upward to 84 mg or down to 28 mg at the discretion of the clinician) followed by a maintenance phase (once a week or once every two weeks). Adverse effects with short-term administration of either racemic or enantiomeric ketamine are modest and limited mainly to transient dissociative phenomena as well as the potential for transient hypertension in about one-third of patients. (Consequently, patients who take pressor agents such as stimulants are generally advised to skip their dose on days they receive ketamine.) A minimum two-hour monitoring period after administration is necessary to observe blood pressure[5] as well as the resolution of any treatment-emergent dissociative phenomena.

Apart from the above-noted uncertainties about its mechanism of action, there are several important unresolved questions about the practical use of ketamine:

Tip

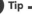

Assure patients are normotensive before administering ketamine or esketamine; wise to defer treatment if resting BP >140/90 mmHg.

- *Relative Potency*: Esketamine has about a three to four times greater binding affinity at the NMDA receptor than the *R*-enantiomer, but IN administration has only about 45–50% bioavailability as compared to 100% bioavailability via parenteral administration. Does this come out as comparable efficacy? While both IV ketamine and IN esketamine are significantly more effective than placebo for depression, the effect size of the former technically is greater than the effect size of the latter (see Chapter 3, Box 3.6) – although one must keep in mind that the data with esketamine in MDD are adjunctive to a newly begun antidepressant, while the comparator arm represents antidepressant monotherapy rather than a placebo.
- *Time to Judging Responder Status*: Impressions from initial IV ketamine studies have been that patients who have failed to show any signs of a discernible response (say, 20% improvement from baseline) by three treatments are unlikely to go on to convert to robust responders. However, in the case of IN esketamine, where the "induction" phase entails eight treatments over four weeks, primary outcome (reduction in MADRS depression scores, rather than "responder" status) was judged at Day 28. Data on visit-wise responder status across successive insufflations over four weeks (based on a pooled analysis of FDA registration trials for esketamine in MDD) revealed the results shown in Figure 13.3. Notably, slightly more than half of esketamine recipients who were not responders by Day 2 or Day 8 went on to achieve responder status by Day 28.
- *Dosing*: Ketamine produces different pharmacodynamic effects at different doses. IV ketamine for depression typically is dosed at 0.5 mg/kg. Higher doses have not suggested a signal for greater efficacy for depression, although subanesthetic analgesia typically occurs at doses from 0.35–1 mg/kg, and intraoperative anesthesia may occur with a 0.6 mg/kg infusion (Schwenk et al., 2018).
- *Number of Treatments to Sustain a Benefit*: Perhaps the most vexing problem that confronts ketamine-responsive patients is what to do next. No controlled trials have ever identified a best pharmacological course of action to sustain benefits after an acute antidepressant response to IV ketamine (in contrast, see section below regarding pharmacotherapy for relapse prevention following acute response to ECT). In intramural NIMH studies, only about 13% of unipolar or bipolar TRD patients who responded to a single IV ketamine infusion remained well after two weeks – a phenomenon best predicted by a higher degree of dissociation during the treatment as well as a family history of alcohol use disorders (Pennybaker et al., 2017). A relapse prevention trial of IN esketamine (56 mg or 84 mg at clinician's discretion, administered either weekly or biweekly) added to a monoaminergic antidepressant found an approximate 50% reduced relapse risk among initial remitters (n = 176; NNT = 6) and ~70% reduced

[5] Blood pressure peaks ~40 minutes after insufflation; mean overall change in systolic blood pressure (SBP) or diastolic blood pressure (DBP) is <10 mmHg but in ~15% of patients DBP may rise >25 mmHg or SBP may rise >40 mmHg.

Figure 13.3 IN esketamine in MDD: visit-wise responder status. Based on data from Turkoz et al., 2021.

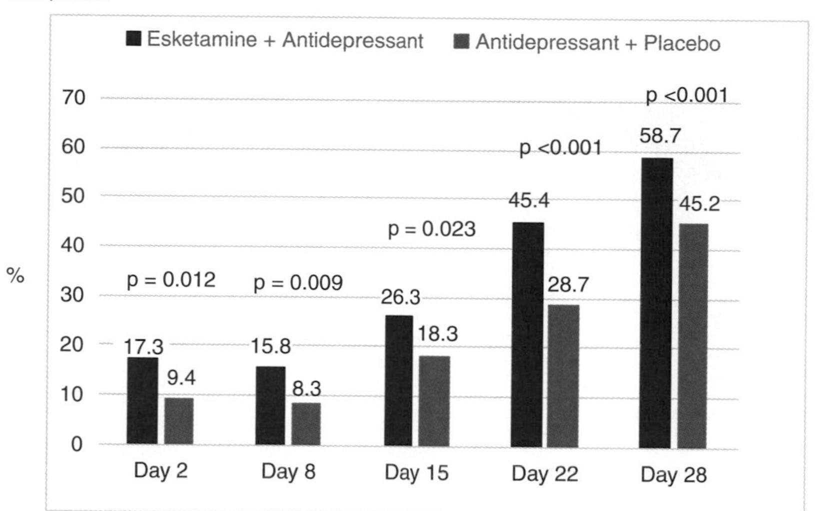

relapse risk among initial responders (n = 121; NNT = 4) (Daly et al., 2019).

- *Other What-Next Strategies for Relapse Prevention*: Studies of other NMDA receptor antagonists (notably, riluzole) have been shown in RCTs not to sustain mood improvement better than placebo after ketamine response (Mathew et al., 2010). Lithium was not better than placebo to prevent depression relapse after ketamine response (Costi et al., 2019). There are also one-off case reports in the literature with memantine after ketamine response. Otherwise, given the absence of evidence (or data), the most intuitive strategy is repeated IV ketamine infusions – albeit with little long-term safety or efficacy data for relapse prevention. The literature contains reports of up to six IV ketamine infusions over 12 days with median times to relapse ranging from 18 days (Murrough et al., 2013) to 41 days (Albott et al., 2018). An RCT of six IV ketamine infusions or placebo over three weeks in 26 severe TRD patients with *chronic* suicidal ideation found no benefit (Ionescu et al., 2019). Long-term potential risks of chronic ketamine use include ulcerative cystitis and possibly irreversible deficits in episodic and semantic memory and attentional functioning (Morgan et al., 2004).

Key points regarding the use of ketamine as an antidepressant are summarized in Box 13.13. A summary of findings from clinical trials with its intranasally administered enantiomer esketamine for depression appears in Table 13.9 at the end of this chapter.

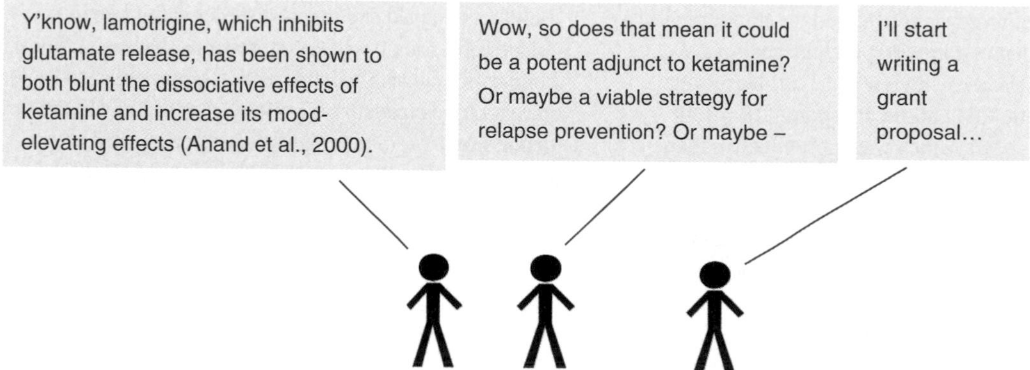

Box 13.13

Ketamine: Key Points

- Exact antidepressant MOA is unknown; may involve glutamate, other transmitter systems
- There is a rapid antidepressant effect in about 50% of depressed patients, both unipolar and bipolar
- About one-third of responders sustain benefits up to one week
- Ketamine and esketamine appear to exert a distinct and rapid reduction in suicidal ideation
- Likelihood of response greatly diminishes if there is no effect after several treatments (though response-by-treatment-number is unknown in the case of IN esketamine)
- Esketamine is about three to four times more potent than *R*-ketamine but IN bioavailability is about half that of IV ketamine
- Oral ketamine has about 20% bioavailability. A review of 13 published studies (mixture of retrospective and prospective trials and case reports) observed significant improvement in depressive symptoms only after two to six weeks of treatment, with oral dosages of 1–2 mg/kg every one to three days, and no significant adverse effects (Rosenblat et al., 2019)
- Dissociation is common and transient; hypertension may occur in about one-third of subjects given IV ketamine and about 10% of those given intranasal esketamine
- It can be administered in older adults but a dedicated IN esketamine trial in MDD patients aged over 65 failed to show benefit over placebo
- There are no systematic data on safety and efficacy of long-term administration for purposes of preventing relapse after acute IV administration, and no established optimal schedule for repeated IV administrations

Say, can I use IV ketamine for anesthesia purposes when I administer ECT for depression, and get a two-fer?

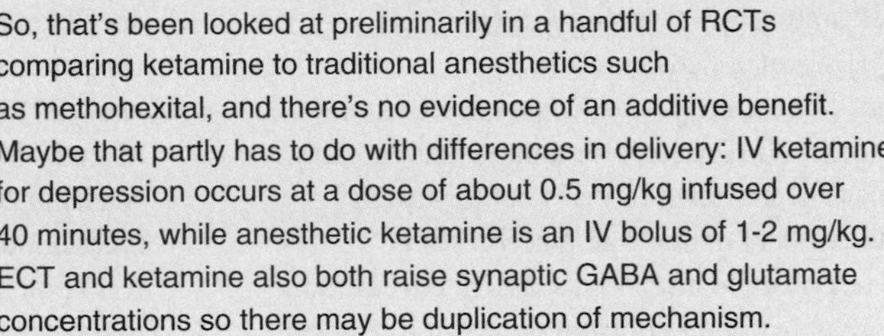

So, that's been looked at preliminarily in a handful of RCTs comparing ketamine to traditional anesthetics such as methohexital, and there's no evidence of an additive benefit. Maybe that partly has to do with differences in delivery: IV ketamine for depression occurs at a dose of about 0.5 mg/kg infused over 40 minutes, while anesthetic ketamine is an IV bolus of 1-2 mg/kg. ECT and ketamine also both raise synaptic GABA and glutamate concentrations so there may be duplication of mechanism.

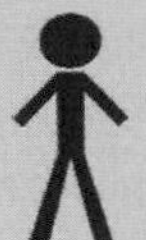

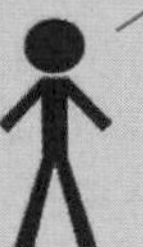

S PSYCHOTIC DEPRESSION

Short of undertaking ECT, antidepressant plus antipsychotic cotherapy is considered the standard of care for major depression with psychotic features. A 2015 Cochrane Database review of 12 antidepressant plus antipsychotic RCTs found a response RR = 1.49 (95% CI = 1.12–1.98), which was more effective than antipsychotic monotherapy or placebo (Wijkstra et al., 2015). Studied antidepressants include amitriptyline, imipramine, nortriptyline, fluvoxamine, fluoxetine, sertraline, paroxetine, mirtazapine, and venlafaxine; studied antipsychotics include olanzapine, quetiapine, and perphenazine. The existing database does not permit meaningful between-drug comparisons for judging relative efficacy.

T CHRONIC/PERSISTENT DEPRESSION

DSM-5 subsumed dysthymic disorder with chronic major depression based on impressions that their clinical similarities outweighed differences. Most published RCTs have focused on dysthymic disorder (or so-called "double depression," i.e., major depression superimposed on pre-existing dysthymia). A meta-analysis by von Wolff and colleagues (2013) found an overall significantly greater response with SSRIs than placebo (benefit ratio = 1.49, 95% CI = 1.29–1.72; NNT = 6 for "response" and 7 for "remission") or TCAs than placebo (benefit ratio = 1.74, 95% CI = 1.50–2.02, NNT = 4 for "response" and 7 for "remission"). More dropout due to adverse drug effects was observed with TCAs than SSRIs.

U CATATONIA

Once considered mainly a subtype of schizophrenia, catatonia is now viewed as a nonpathognomonic complex syndrome with an unclear pathophysiology that can arise in a number of psychiatric conditions, including mood disorders. Key characteristics, in addition to mutism, excitement, or posturing (e.g., waxy flexibility), may include extreme negativism, echolalia, or echopraxia. Lorazepam (6–20 mg/day; dosing may occur as often as every 20–30 minutes based on response) or ECT remain the treatments of choice. Manic delirium often involves catatonic features. (Some authors conceptualize it specifically as a severe form of catatonia.) If inadequately managed it may progress to a malignant form involving autonomic instability, rigidity, and hyperthermia. FGAs are contraindicated because of their risk for neuroleptic malignant syndrome (though some authors believe that certain SGAs – notably clozapine or quetiapine – may be acceptable (albeit nonrapid) treatment options). Anticholinergics are similarly eschewed because they could lead to a worsening of mental status.

V DEPRESSION WITH ATYPICAL FEATURES

The constellation of hypersomnia, hyperphagia, mood reactivity, rejection sensitivity, and markedly low energy ("leaden paralysis") gained attention in the 1970s as a possible moderator for depression that favored response to MAOIs over TCAs. DSM-IV also differentiated "atypical" from "melancholic" or catatonic depression, and DSM-5 notes that seasonal MDEs often entail hypersomnia, hyperphagia/weight gain, and carbohydrate craving. Though phenomenologically tantalizing, the construct is beleaguered by its many confounding factors (such as early age at onset, traumatic or other adverse early life experiences, interpersonal sensitivity trait, comorbid personality, or anxiety disorders (particularly social anxiety disorder), bipolarity, and seasonality, among others).

In a comparison of atypical, melancholic or anxious-depressive subtypes, only 39% of 1008 MDD patients in the iSPOT-D trial had a pure form of only one subtype, as did 4% of those in STAR*D; 36% of iSPOT-D MDD subjects met criteria for two or more subtypes, as did 26% of STAR*D enrollees, while 25% in iSPOT-D met no subtype definition, as did 33% in STAR*D. In neither study did depression subtype moderate response to any particular antidepressant (Arnow et al., 2015).

W AGITATION

The construct of "agitated depression," while absent from all editions of the DSM, was first described in the late nineteenth century. Its operational definition became formalized in the Research Diagnostic Criteria (RDC), a forerunner to DSM-III. Its original (RDC) definition entailed psychomotor agitation, inner tension, and "crowded thoughts." Some authors have postulated that agitated depression is a variant psychotic depression, while still others have wondered whether it reflects a variant of bipolar mixed states. Such speculations aside, the RCT literature, though modest, supports the use of antipsychotics combined with antidepressants – e.g., quetiapine added to venlafaxine (Dannlowski et al., 2008). Separately, in early fluoxetine monotherapy trials, post hoc analyses found better outcomes with active drug (or with a TCA comparator) than placebo despite the presence of baseline agitation, although dropout due to intolerance was higher with a TCA than fluoxetine (Tollefson et al., 1994). Open trials and case reports also suggest value in combining other SGAs with a serotonergic antidepressant. However, so long as "agitated depression" remains a construct outside of the DSM, it is unlikely that large-scale prospective trials will address its optimal pharmacotherapy.

X ANXIETY

Anxiety (both syndromal and symptomatic) is a common, often underappreciated, and certainly understudied co-occurring phenomenon among mood-disorder patients regardless of polarity. In both unipolar and bipolar depression, epidemiological studies point to comorbid anxiety disorders (not to mention subdiagnostic symptoms) in half or more of community samples.

In the NIMH STAR*D trial, comorbid anxiety disorders accounted substantially for poor treatment response to antidepressants (Fava et al., 2008). The diagnostic construct of "mixed anxiety and depression" was vetted in previous editions of the DSM but ultimately rejected as a construct distinguishable from major depression with a discernible comorbid anxiety disorder.

Serotonergic antidepressants are widely considered the first-line treatment of both depression and anxiety. Yet, when both conditions co-occur, outcomes are notably poorer. SNRIs have not demonstrated clearly better results for anxious depression, although some carry specific FDA indications for generalized anxiety disorder.

Box 13.14

FDA-Approved Monoaminergic Antidepressants for Anxiety Disorders

Agent	Generalized anxiety disorder	Social anxiety disorder	Panic disorder	PTSD [a]
Duloxetine	✓			
Escitalopram	✓			
Fluoxetine			✓	
Paroxetine	✓	✓	✓	✓
Sertraline		✓	✓	✓
Venlafaxine	✓	✓		

[a] No longer classified as a subtype of anxiety disorder in DSM-5

Accordingly, for purely informational purposes, we will momentarily break from our deliberate avoidance of FDA approval status as an organizing principle of this book (as opposed to the evidence- and rationale-based approach) in order to consider those monoaminergic antidepressants that carry FDA indications for specific anxiety disorders (Box 13.14).

Post hoc analyses of nefazodone in MDD with comorbid anxiety symptoms have shown greater improvement in both mood and anxiety symptoms as compared to placebo (Zajecka, 1996). Mirtazapine (15–45 mg/day) monotherapy was shown in small open trials to improve both depression and GAD symptoms (Goodnick et al., 1999) and, anecdotally, is often regarded as especially beneficial in the context of concomitant anxiety and depression. An older literature spoke to the value of TCAs on both depression and anxiety disorders such as panic disorder as separate entities, more so than conducting RCTs in comorbid presentations.

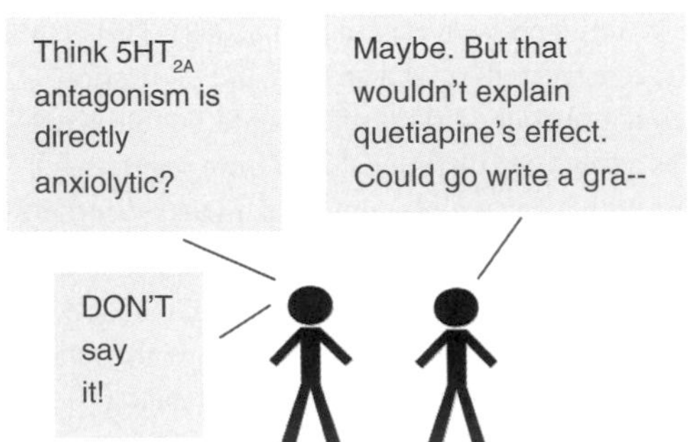

Think $5HT_{2A}$ antagonism is directly anxiolytic?
Maybe. But that wouldn't explain quetiapine's effect. Could go write a gra--
DON'T say it!

At least some adjunctive SGAs may hold value in particular for presentations involving the admixture of significant depression and anxiety. Quetiapine, in particular, added to an existing monoaminergic antidepressant, has been preliminarily shown to further improve both depressive and anxiety symptoms better than continued SSRI or venlafaxine alone at a mean quetiapine dosing range of 150–200 mg/day (McIntyre et al., 2007; Li et al., 2016). In the world of bipolar depression (see more in the later section on "Bipolar Disorder" in this chapter), all four FDA-approved pharmacotherapies (i.e., OFC, quetiapine, cariprazine, and lurasidone) reduced concomitant anxiety symptoms better than did placebo.

Concurrent benzodiazepines are nonideal for long-term management of anxiety in depression. Anxiolytic anticonvulsants such as gabapentin or pregabalin have not been formally studied as adjuncts to antidepressants for mixed anxiety-depression presentations but may represent an intriguing option to consider.

Noradrenergic Symptom Cluster

Some authors have identified key symptoms of depression thought to be associated with suboptimal functioning of noradrenergic brain circuitry – in particular, apathy, fatigue, indifference, low energy, and decreased cognitive function. Linked with this construct is the idea that pro-noradrenergic agents increase tonic NE activity and diminish phasic NE reactivity (thereby leading to reductions in anxiety, as observed in RCTs of SNRIs such as duloxetine or levomilnacipran).

Y ATTENTIONAL PROBLEMS ASSOCIATED WITH DEPRESSION

Related to the broader noradrenergic symptom cluster of depression, depressive presentations that involve slowed attentional processing or diminished associative fluency lead one to consider the potential value of pro-noradrenergic or pro-dopaminergic agents such as NERIs, SNRIs, bupropion, and stimulants. As a NET reuptake inhibitor, atomoxetine would seem to be a logical adjunctive treatment to a serotonergic antidepressant (akin to the rationale for adjunctive bupropion), particularly in the setting of comorbid ADHD. Rather surprisingly, however, randomized trials have shown no greater benefit with it than placebo when used in children with ADHD plus comorbid MDD or in adults with MDD when added to optimally dosed sertraline. However, atomoxetine has not been extensively studied for its possible antidepressant properties, and the sole randomized trial for MDD in adults was an industry-sponsored study which may not generalize to augmentation with non-noradrenergic antidepressants as a class.

Vortioxetine has garnered interest for its possible unique value to address cognitive symptoms in depression by virtue of its $5HT_7$ antagonism. Using the Digit Symbol Substitution Task (DSST; a broad measure of attentional processing and psychomotor function), McIntyre and colleagues (2016) found significantly greater improvement in cognitive functioning with vortioxetine than placebo while controlling for changes in depression symptom severity over eight weeks – an effect not seen with duloxetine as a comparator – though with a small effect size ($d = 0.24$).

Z INFLAMMATORY AND NONINFLAMMATORY DEPRESSION

Growing interest has coalesced about the presence of elevated serum inflammatory markers (such as interleukins and inflammatory cytokines) in the setting of depression. The bidirectionality of this association remains poorly understood, in that it is not well-established whether clinical depression leads to the elevation of systemic inflammatory markers or if people with high baseline inflammation (from a variety of possible etiologies) may be at greater risk to develop depression. High inflammatory states coincident with depression have been cited as possible contributors to increased medical comorbidity and excess mortality from cardiovascular and other nonsuicide-related causes. Treatment implications, at present, remain provisional, although one RCT found that in MDD patients with baseline C-reactive protein (CRP) >1 mg/L, antidepressant outcomes were better with nortriptyline than escitalopram, while in low-inflammatory-state depressions (CRP <1 mg/L), escitalopram out-performed nortriptyline (Uher et al., 2014). Rather than think of "inflammation" as an obligate corollary to mood disorders, one might instead consider the possibility that there may be a pro-inflammatory subtype of depression which could have unique treatment implications.

Should I be measuring CRPs in my depressed patients?

If you're doing a research study maybe, otherwise, no established value as yet.

Can anti-inflammatory drugs treat depression? Findings from a meta-analysis of 14 RCTs found a modest benefit with NSAIDs ($d = 0.34$ overall; slightly less with celecoxib specifically: $d = 0.29$); no adverse GI or cardiovascular events were noted (Köhler et al., 2014). A separate meta-analysis focusing solely on celecoxib (five RCTs) added to antidepressants in MDD or bipolar depression found a significant difference in reducing Hamilton Ratings Scale for Depression scores, with a higher overall response rate (pooled OR = 6.6, 95% CI = 2.5 to 17.0, p <0.0001) and remission rate (pooled OR = 6.6, 95% CI = 2.7 to 15.9, p <0.0001) than with placebo (Faridhosseini et al., 2014).

Additionally, the antibiotic *minocycline* possesses anti-inflammatory as well as neuroprotective and anti-glutamatergic effects: a meta-analysis of three RCTs revealed a significant difference from placebo with a large effect size ($d = 0.78$) (Rosenblat and McIntyre, 2018); while promising, the preliminary nature of these initial studies requires replication with larger sample sizes.

AA PSYCHEDELICS AND DEPRESSION

Serotonergic psychedelic drugs, notably, LSD, psilocybin, and ayahuasca, were traditionally considered potential adjuvants to psychotherapy until their broad prohibitions by mainstream medicine in the 1960s and 1970s. Latter-day investigators have begun to reapproach this drug class with renewed interest in depression (the literature has focused largely on the use of psilocybin in terminally ill cancer patients). A review of 19 RCTs by Rucker et al. (2016) found that nearly 80% of clinicians perceived benefit (improved mood symptoms) following psychedelic treatment. Additionally, a single-dose RCT of ayahuasca or placebo in 29 TRD outpatients showed greater antidepressant benefits than seen with placebo over seven days ($d = 1.49$ for change in MADRS; Palhano-Fontes et al., 2019).

AB PHARMACOTHERAPIES TO PREVENT RELAPSE AFTER ELECTROCONVULSIVE THERAPY

A significant limitation of ECT for mood disorders is the very high likelihood of affective relapse (>80%) within three to six months after a treatment course has concluded (Sackeim et al., 2001), unless a preventative intervention is in place. Degree of treatment resistance (i.e., number of previous failed antidepressant trials) has been associated with a higher likelihood of relapse during pharmacotherapy after ECT in some studies, but not others (Prudic et al., 2013). Table 13.10 at the end of this chapter summarizes current evidence on pharmacotherapies for preventing depression relapse after ECT.

Prudic and colleagues (2013) found no significant advantage for delaying depressive relapse after ECT when pharmacotherapy was begun during versus after completion of ECT – although the magnitude of ECT efficacy in the short term appears somewhat greater (by ~15%) when ECT is coadministered with antidepressant pharmacotherapy.

AC LONG-TERM ISSUES

What is the optimal duration of ongoing or maintenance-phase pharmacotherapy to prevent relapses after initial remission? Practice guidelines tend to advise ongoing pharmacotherapy for anywhere from four months to one year after resolution of an initial depressive episode, with longer durations in patients with one or more prior episodes. After three or more prior episodes, where the risk of relapse is thought to be >90%, indefinite ongoing therapy after a remission is regarded by many experts as the usual preferred recommendation. A dilemma for evidence-based decision-making is that very few RCTs extend beyond one year's duration – often for obvious and insurmountable reasons, such as the ethical and practical challenges of keeping high-risk patients on placebo for long periods of time, the inevitability of dropout and consequent loss of statistical power to detect between-group differences, the cost of conducting very long-term studies, and the likelihood that if a depressive recurrence is going to occur, it is most often going to happen in the first year after recovery.

Tolerance, or a resurgence of symptoms following an initial improvement, has been described with MAOIs and SSRIs in MDD patients without a clear consensus on its mechanism (i.e., is it true pharmacological tachyphylaxis

So then. How do I go about picking an antidepressant from the many that are out there?

Well, it's a thought exercise really. First decide if you're facing an ailment for which you have reason to think an antidepressant would be helpful. And then, go through all these moderating characteristics beyond categorical diagnosis – chronicity, multiepisode, degree of treatment resistance, anxiety or other comorbidities, polarity, psychosis, past treatments and adherence...any acute medical issues...past side-effect sensitivities... opportunities for parsimony with comorbidities or capitalizing on side-effect profiles...then get familiar with what's been studied in clinical trials for a given clinical profile, then consider pro's and con's of the viable options and discuss it all with the patient. Makes sense?

Got it. Just start with an SSRI.

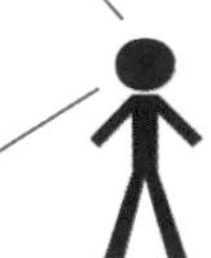

or cycling as part of the natural course of illness?). Some authors believe that SSRI "poopout" is actually the loss of an initial placebo response, occurring within the first few months of ostensible improvement (Stewart et al., 1998). Dosage increases (Fava et al., 1995) or augmentation with bupropion or possibly other pro-dopaminergic agents have been described as viable strategies that may help to recapture an initially lost initial drug response. Drug holidays have also been described as a potential means by which presumably to restore receptor sensitivity.

BIPOLAR DISORDER

Some authors have proposed expanding the notion of the so-called "bipolar spectrum" to include a broader swath of affective disturbances than traditionally recognized. While there is theoretical interest in considering features such as early age at onset or family history as possible diagnostic corroborators, "bipolarity" as an evidence-based construct still requires the occurrence of at least one lifetime mania or hypomania – syndromes that involve a constellation of signs and symptoms reflecting high mood and energy, enduring for at least several days, and constituting a meaningful change from one's usual baseline. It can be risky to extrapolate from the treatment literature on bipolar disorder to other more ill-defined free-standing phenomena (such as mood dysregulation, irritability, problems with impulse control, poor distress tolerance, high recurrence, or simply "antidepressant resistance") because one cannot necessarily assume expectable outcomes. Accordingly, in the case of evidence-based pharmacotherapies for bipolar disorder, we would emphasize that conclusions about drug efficacy or safety drawn from studies of patients with unequivocal bipolar I or II episodes may not necessarily translate to those with *form fruste* ("not otherwise specified," or "not elsewhere classified") presentations.

Our goals in this section are to provide a pragmatic and concise overview of key issues in treating distinct affective poles and the "switch" process itself, and to address points of popular controversy such as evidence-based treatments for depression in people who have a history of mania or hypomania. We will demur on the DSM-5 construct of major depression with mixed features other than to touch on its potential longitudinal diagnostic relevance and issues surrounding the use of antidepressants in the setting of depression with low-grade hypomania symptoms, regardless of an "overarching" affective diagnosis.

Choosing an Antimanic Drug

Treating mania means more than slowing down a whirling dervish, or subduing affective lability. Mania and hypomania both involve constellations of signs and symptoms that involve high energy, a reduced need for sleep, fast thoughts, fast speech, risk-taking, and an expansive accrual of ideas, projects, and tasks that defy contemplative reflection. The ideal antimanic drug addresses all of these components without causing excessive sedation, inducing depression, or producing intolerable adverse effects. Antimanic mood stabilizers should realign mood and energy toward euthymia, rather than bludgeon away drive, initiative, and spirit. They should temper impulsivity without quashing spontaneity. Mania often impairs insight about whether anything is even awry (at times verging on frank anosognosia), and imposes a kind of cognitive rigidity and defiant circularity of thinking. Sometimes, in order to treat entrenched and extreme cognitive and behavioral inflexibility, the use of drugs that can be highly sedating may be unavoidable. Cognitive rigidity reaches its peak when abject psychosis is present (as can happen in about half of patients with severe mania), and a loss of filter in speech and behavior gives way to raw and unfiltered primary process thinking.

A meta-analysis of RCTs in acute mania (Yildiz et al., 2011a) found striking consistency in outcomes across trials of SGAs, with no evidence of significant antimanic efficacy using anticonvulsants other than divalproex or carbamazepine (i.e., lamotrigine or topiramate) (see Figure 13.4).

Should Antipsychotic Drugs Always Be Used in Mania?

An expanding database using SGAs for phases of bipolar disorder other than acute mania has sparked interest in their broadened role, both short and long term. The magnitude of reduction in mania symptoms is roughly comparable across most if not all adequately dosed SGAs that have been studied in bipolar I mania (meaning that mean reductions in mania symptoms from baseline are similar, and confidence intervals across studies tend to overlap).

Notably, two as yet unpublished RCTs of brexpiprasole in bipolar mania found no significant difference from placebo in reducing mania symptom severity. Across FDA registration trials in bipolar mania, adding an SGA to lithium or divalproex tends to improve overall response rates by about 25% (as compared to lithium or divalproex alone). Studied agents specifically include risperidone (Sachs et al., 2002; Yatham et al., 2003), olanzapine

Figure 13.4 Meta-analysis of antimanic efficacy across pharmacotherapies for bipolar mania. Based on findings reported by Yildiz et al., 2011a.

	g (95% CI)
Tamoxifen	2.32 (1.67 to 2.96)
Risperidone	0.66 (0.45 to 0.88)
Carbamazepine	0.61 (0.32 to 0.89)
Haloperidol	0.54 (0.35 to 0.73)
Cariprazine	0.51 (0.13 to 0.89)
Olanzapine	0.46 (0.29 to 0.62)
Ziprasidone	0.42 (0.19 to 0.66)
Asenapine	0.40 (0.13 to 0.66)
Quetiapine	0.40 (0.20 to 0.59)
Lithium	0.39 (0.22 to 0.55)
Paliperidone	0.30 (0.11 to 0.49)
Divalproex	0.28 (0.09 to 0.47)
Aripiprazole	0.26 (0.10 to 0.41)
Licarbazepine	0.09 (–0.27 to 0.45)
Verapamil	–0.02 (–0.86 to 0.83)
Lamotrigine	–0.02 (–0.43 to 0.39)
Topiramate	–0.06 (–0.25 to 0.13)

−1.25 0 1.25 2.50

Favors placebo ← → Favors active drug

(Tohen et al., 2002), quetiapine (Sachs et al., 2004), and aripiprazole (Vieta et al., 2008b) – but *no differences* from lithium or divalproex alone were seen in registration trials for adjunctive ziprasidone (Sachs et al., 2012). Practical differences among agents therefore depend more on their relative tolerabilities and specific end-organ effects (such as metabolic dysregulation, sedative effects, or iatrogenic motor dysfunction), or on data from clinical trials that span both acute illness phases and relapse prevention, or efficacy for both manic and depressive episodes.

Antipsychotics typically have fast onsets, wide therapeutic indexes, low risk for mortality in overdose, and pharmacodynamic compatibility with virtually all other psychotropic classes used in mood-disorder patients.

Mood Stabilizers

The term "mood stabilizer" is something of a misnomer in that the drugs commonly included within this category have been studied primarily to treat or prevent *syndromes* of mania or depression lasting for days or weeks at a time in people with bipolar disorder – rather than targeting day-to-day or moment-to-moment vicissitudes of mood per se. NbN focuses on a drug's mechanism of action rather than its anticipated pharmacodynamic effect, although in neither case is there a clear overarching framework to apply broadly. The NbN glossary identifies some "mood stabilizers" based on their putative glutamatergic mechanisms (e.g., voltage-gated Na^+ channel blockers (as in the case of lamotrigine)) or both Na^+ and Ca^{++} channel blockers (as in the case of carbamazepine); divalproex lacks an NbN classification while lithium's mode of action involves "enzyme interactions" (https://www.nbn2.com/). Both lithium and divalproex are protein kinase C inhibitors (as is tamoxifen), but not all protein kinase C inhibitors have been shown to treat mania (e.g., verapamil, omega-3 fatty acids). Apart from putative mechanisms of action, from a more practical standpoint, one might think of a "mood stabilizer" as any intervention that can achieve and/or sustain euthymia, and more specifically, a compound may be said to exert its mood-stabilizing properties mainly by virtue of its relative antimanic versus antidepressant effects.

A related concept relevant to the term *mood stabilizer* bears on a drug's "anti-cycling" effect – that is, its ability to prevent recurrences per se, irrespective of polarity changes.

When mapping the history of someone with multiple affective episodes, one is concerned as much with the switch process itself (i.e., how often they go from one pole to the other) as with the particular symptoms of either given polarity. For patients, the analogy of crossing the equator from one hemisphere to the other may be useful. The goal to reduce "equator-crossings" is a key focus of pharmacotherapy, often more so than pharmacologically chasing the illness from one pole to the other. Much as repeated trips from Brazil to the Bahamas are fraught with the nautical hazards of traversing the Bermuda Triangle, so too might frequent switches between depression and mania pose a risk to a patient's fundamental and consistent emotional stability. Mixed features (blending aspects of both poles at the same time) thus pose an especially chaotic challenge both conceptually and pragmatically, as the target of treatment involves all of the above elements simultaneously.

The "anti-switch" properties of a drug might be thought of as those meant to prevent or reduce equator crossings, while "anti-recurrence" interventions are those that reduce frequent episodes, regardless of polarity. Some agents are more efficacious against "north-to-south" excursions, while others may hold more value for the opposite emotional-geographic dilemma. Lithium, for example, exerts a more substantial effect against manic than depressive recurrences (having about a 38% versus 28% relative risk against each respective pole; Geddes et al., 2004) while lamotrigine may be the "prototype" antidepressant mood-stabilizing agent. Truly "bimodal" mood-stabilizing efficacy would reflect comparable effect

Figure 13.5. Anti-switch versus anti-recurrence targeting of therapy.

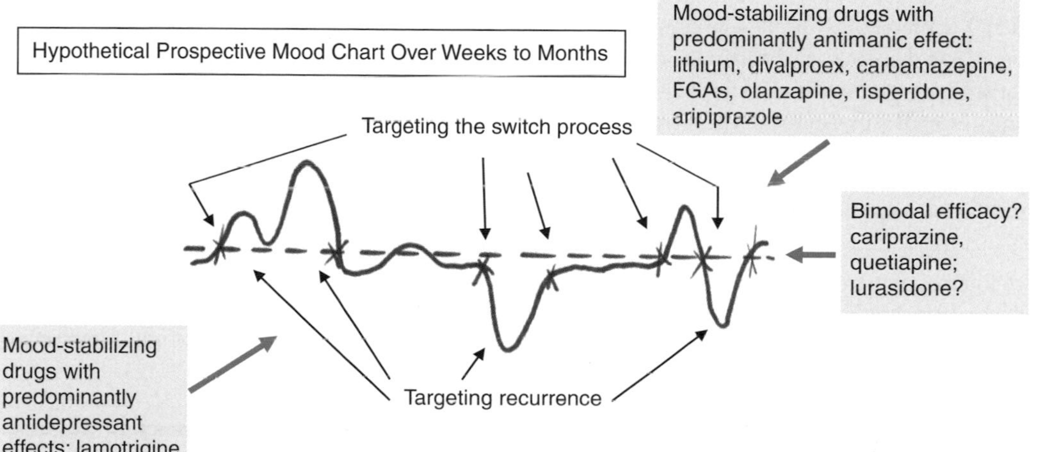

So, my manic patient is better on the combination of an SGA plus an antimanic mood stabilizer. How long should I continue both?

So, the answer to that question isn't arbitrary and comes from randomized discontinuation trials. One such study found that after stabilizing from mania on lithium or divalproex plus either risperidone or olanzapine, patients remained relapse-free longer on the mood stabilizer/SGA combo for the first 24 weeks but thereafter the chance of relapse was no better at 52 weeks than at 24 weeks (Yatham et al., 2016). Then, another similar study looking only at the randomized discontinuation of adjunctive olanzapine found that after acute mania stabilized on combination therapy, time until symptomatic relapse was significantly longer with continuing olanzapine plus lithium or divalproex (median time = 163 days) than with the mood stabilizer alone (median time = 42 days) (Tohen et al., 2004). So, I'd say, don't touch a successful regimen for *at least* six months unless there's a very compelling reason to tinker.

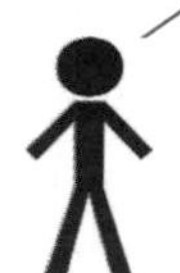

My bipolar disorder patient has had multiple episodes. Should I put him on a long-acting injectable SGA the way the pharma ads say to?

Perhaps – and please don't make medical decisions based just on advertisements – but, to your question, it all depends. If his relapses are more mania- than depression-prone, the data with aripiprazole or risperidone LAI preparations are more compelling to prevent manias than depressions. Does he relapse due to poor adherence, or is it just lack of efficacy? What do you think the moderating factors are? Any comorbidities? Adequate trials?

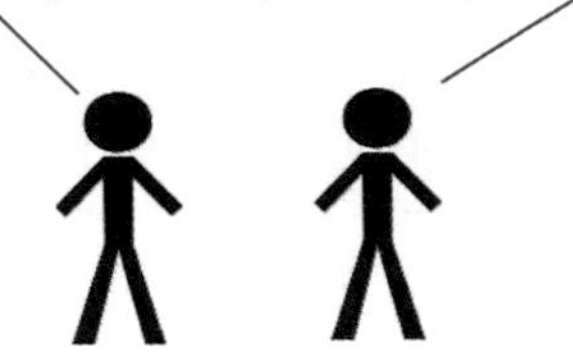

sizes against both poles of the illness. Arguably few agents have demonstrated this property in RCTs – quetiapine, cariprazine, and ECT at present may be the sole examples, although membership in this category is partly an artifact of whether or not an agent has been studied formally across illness states – a endeavor usually driven more by commercial than scientific interests.

What About Affective Instability?

Emotional lability or affective instability is a broad construct that cuts across numerous categorical psychiatric diagnoses and should not be misconstrued as a sine qua non feature of bipolar disorder. In fact, moment-to-moment shifts in mood have never formally been recognized in the operational criteria for defining bipolar disorder. The concept of cyclothymia perhaps comes closest to the time scale of measuring mood changes on a day-to-day (rather than week-to-week or month-to-month or longer) basis, but mood changes within a single day – whatever their origin – have never been the primary subject of rigorous pharmacotherapy trials. One practical issue involves how best to operationally define and then prospectively measure affective instability. Daily prospective mood charting offers one such strategy for tracking daily deviations from euthymia. Among bipolar disorder patients with past-year rapid cycling, Goldberg and colleagues (2008) used prospective mood charting to show that lamotrigine over six months was associated with nearly a twofold increased likelihood over placebo for achieving a mood rating of "euthymic" at least once per week over six months, incurring 0.69 more days per week with euthymia as compared to subjects taking placebo.

Cyclothymic Disorder

The concept of cyclothymic disorder describes numerous periods of hypomania and/or depression that never achieve syndromal status by virtue either of the number of requisite symptoms and/or their duration. It is thought to be within the so-called bipolar spectrum, although there remains debate about the extent to which it represents more of a temperamental and psychological (best treated with a structured psychotherapy such as CBT) rather than biological phenomenon responsive to mood stabilizers or other pharmacotherapies (Baldessarini et al., 2011). The evidence base for its pharmacological treatment is unfortunately scant and limited to open-label, nonrandomized studies with lithium (Peselow et al., 1982) or quetiapine (Bisol and Lara, 2001), with less robust value seen with lamotrigine (Montes et al., 2005).

When and How Did "Bipolar Depression" Become a Thing?

Prior to the work of nosologists Karl Kleist, Edda Neele, and Karl Leonhard in the 1930s, *polarity* distinctions involving major depression were less fundamental than other descriptors (such as "hypochondriacal depression," "self-tortured depression," "apathetic depression," or "suspicious depression"). In 1980, DSM-III renamed manic-depressive illness "bipolar disorder" and the fundamental role of polarity began to assume greater importance in both the descriptive classification and treatment of depressive disorders. In the late 1980s, intramural NIMH studies began to draw attention to the potential for tricyclics to induce mania or accelerate cycling frequency in some bipolar patients. Those studies were mostly observational (nonrandomized) and/or based on small study groups of on/off/on treatment exposures. This in turn prompted growing concern that antidepressants (possibly TCAs more than then-newer SSRIs) might incur risk for mood destabilization – a hypothesis that rather quickly became embraced with only limited testing from any large RCTs. Papers began to emerge espousing concerns about diagnostic misclassification and proposing that bipolar depression might differ in fundamental ways from unipolar depression. At the same time, a swell of commercial interests in developing broadened uses for newer anticonvulsants and SGAs began to tap "bipolar" depression as a distinct market.

Antidepressants in Bipolar Disorder: Good, Bad, Neither or Both?

Where does the foregoing bring us? Many clinicians and patients have come to embrace as dogma the proposition that antidepressants commonly trigger mania or rapid cycling, or possibly even cause bipolar disorder to arise de novo. Practice guidelines and influential editorials amplified the hypothesis to create ideological entrenchment that antidepressants are detrimental.

What does the evidence here actually show? The largest meta-analysis examining treatment-emergent affective switch (TEAS) to date, encompassing 51 trials with 10 098 bipolar subjects, identified an overall risk of 18.8% (95% CI = 14.7–23.7%) for TEAS events following antidepressant exposure; 12 prospectively designed RCTs (free from retrospective recall bias) revealed a still lower risk of 11.8% (95% CI = 8.4–16.3%) (Fornaro et al., 2018). However, with no placebo comparator group, it becomes hard to differentiate TEAS risk attributable to antidepressant exposure versus the natural course of illness.

The empirical literature as well as expert consensus suggest that the greatest risk of using antidepressants in people with bipolar disorder involves their relative lack of demonstrated efficacy (NNTs ~30 based on meta-analyses of randomized trials) (Sidor and MacQueen, 2011); in contrast, the risk of TEAS (regarded by some authors as the greater short- or long-term hazard of antidepressant use) appears to be a far less common event than was once presumed (NNHs ~200 according to current meta-analyses) (Sidor and MacQueen, 2011). The natural course of a bipolar depressive episode, regardless of any specific treatment, is about 15 weeks (Solomon et al., 2010), and given that about 15–20% of bipolar disorder patients experience four or more affective episodes per year, it can sometimes be hard to distinguish drug effects (both good and bad) from the natural course of illness. There should be a logical time frame within which to judge whether symptom improvement or worsening is reasonably attributable to pharmacodynamic effects. Some authorities propose that beyond 12–16 weeks after starting an antidepressant or increasing its dose, it becomes difficult to parse new mania symptoms as "resulting" from the antidepressant versus the natural course of illness (Tohen et al., 2009).

Collectively, findings from large RCTs suggest that about half of bipolar II disorder patients seem to benefit acutely from adjunctive agents such as some SSRIs (i.e., sertraline or fluoxetine), bupropion, or venlafaxine added to antimanic mood stabilizers such as lithium or divalproex. Guidelines often vigorously warn not to use antidepressants unless first combined with an antimanic mood stabilizer, but it is not well-established that concomitant mood stabilizers lessen the risk for TEAS. Strikingly, no antidepressants developed after 1999 (i.e., mirtazapine, desvenlafaxine, levomilnacipran, vilazodone, and vortioxetine) have ever been formally studied in bipolar depression. Generalizability about the safety and efficacy of "antidepressants" as a class is thus limited to a somewhat older literature regarding mainly TCAs, early SSRIs, tranylcypromine, and bupropion.

Returning to the concept of sample enrichment, and moderators and mediators of outcome (as discussed in Chapter 5), the evidence base would argue not that antidepressants either do or do not induce mania as if it were a simple dichotomy, but rather, that certain patient-specific characteristics may predispose at-risk patients for mood destabilization with antidepressants (while the absence of those factors may be protective). Known factors shown most robustly to increase the hazard for antidepressant-associated mania or hypomania are summarized in Table 13.11 at the end of this chapter.

The characteristics described in Table 13.11 at the end of this chapter form the basis for the flow diagram presented in Figure 13.6 for determining candidacy for antidepressant use in bipolar depression.

Do Antimanic Drugs Protect Against TEAS?

While regarded by many clinicians as a simple truism, the database empirically addressing the "necessity" of antimanic cotherapy with an antidepressant drug in bipolar disorder is remarkably scant. A meta-analysis by Tondo and colleagues (2010) of 109 trials involving 114 521 subjects found that the likelihood for TEAS events during antidepressant therapy in bipolar disorder was not substantially different when it occurred in the presence (15.9% incidence) or absence (13.8%) of an antimanic mood stabilizer. A smaller observational retrospective study (n = 158) over an unspecified exposure period reported a significantly lower risk for TEAS during antimanic cotherapy with an

Figure 13.6 Flow diagram for treatment decisions in treating bipolar depression. Reprinted from Goldberg JF. Determining patient candidacy for antidepressant use in bipolar disorder. *Psychiatr Ann* 2019; 49: 386–391, with permission from SLACK Incorporated.

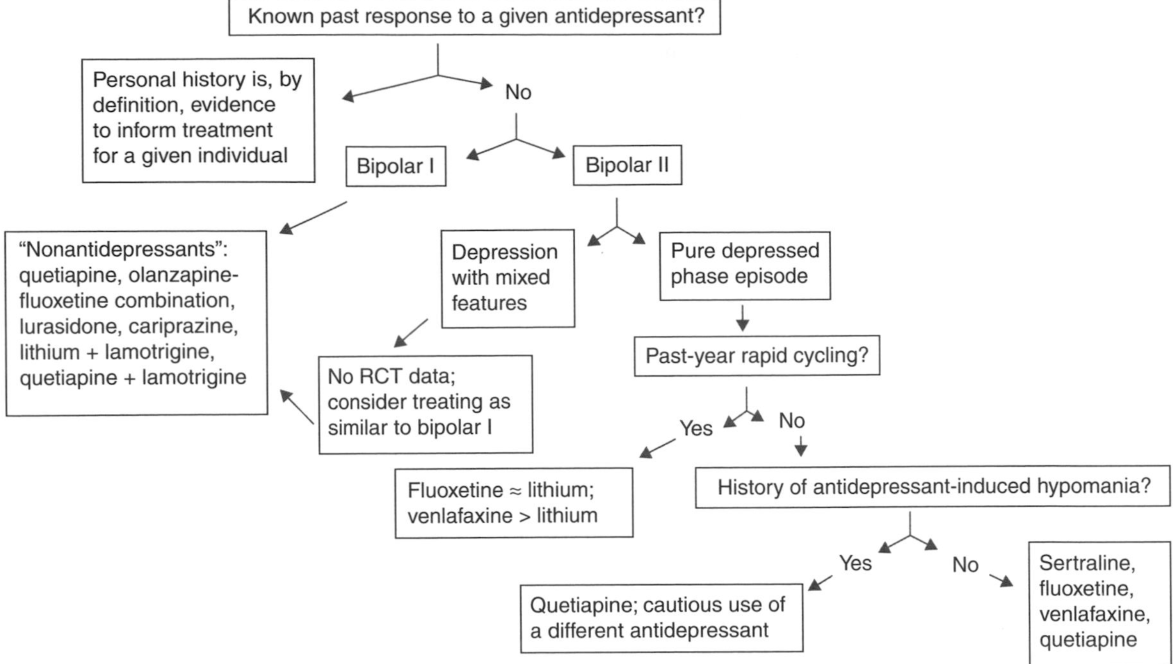

antidepressant (OR = 0.30, 95% CI = 0.13–0.69; Bottlender et al., 2001); however, the nonrandomized, retrospective design of this latter study allowed no consideration for confounding (moderating) contributors to TEAS (such as those identified in Table 13.11), and the lack of a placebo arm makes it impossible to distinguish possible drug-induced effects from the natural course of illness. On balance, "fear" about using antidepressants in bipolar depression rightfully should reflect concerns about the meager effect of the handful of agents studied more so than the risk of TEAS or cycle acceleration as differentiable from the natural course of illness.

The previously acknowledged four FDA-approved pharmacotherapies for bipolar depression (OFC, quetiapine, cariprazine, and lurasidone) share mechanisms involving dopamine modulation, but all nevertheless have distinct molecular signatures, and as noted earlier, not all SGAs possess antidepressant properties. Standard dosing information about commonly used mood-stabilizing drugs for bipolar depression is presented in Table 13.12 at the end of this chapter.

Selle and colleagues (2014) provided a useful meta-analysis broadly examining mood stabilizers with antidepressant properties as well as other evidence-based treatments for bipolar depression. Findings from that study are summarized in Figure 13.7.

A meta-analysis of five RCTs with IV ketamine for acute bipolar depression produced a strikingly large SMD of 1.01 (95% CI = 0.69–1.43) (Lee et al., 2015).

Combination Pharmacotherapy for Bipolar Disorder

Cross-sectional studies show that about 20–40% of bipolar patients routinely take four or more psychotropic medications (Goldberg et al., 2009; Weinstock et al., 2014; Golden et al., 2017). Extensive drug therapy regimens among bipolar patients tend to be more common in White women over age 50 with a history of psychosis, high depressive illness burden, comorbid PTSD, anxiety, borderline personality disorder, low levels of extraversion and conscientiousness, and those with a history of suicide attempts (Goldberg, 2019). As noted in Chapter 6, optimal multidrug regimens involve thoughtful, nonredundant medication combinations that capitalize on pharmacokinetic and pharmacodynamic synergies with distinct symptom targets. Such a treatment approach becomes readily comprehensible given that bipolar disorder tends to involve multiple comorbidities (about one-quarter of patients have more than three comorbid psychiatric and/or substance-use comorbidities; McElroy et al., 2001). In fact, one might imagine that complex polypharmacotherapy

Figure 13.7 Random effects meta-analysis of drug-placebo differences in bipolar depression. Based on data in Selle et al., 2014.

Agent	NNT (95% CI)
OFC	1.8 (2.7 to 7.2)
Divalproex	4.4 (2.7 to 12.0)
Quetiapine	5.9 (4.7 to 7.8)
Lurasidone	4.6 (3.3 to 7.8)
Carbamazepine	3.4 (1.9 to 19.0)
Olanzapine	5.9 (4.7 to 7.8)
Lithium	15 (5.4 to 20.0)
Lamotrigine	10 (6.1 to 32.0)
Ziprasidone	87 (14 to ∞)
Aripiprazole	100 (58 to ∞)

g (95% CI)

−0.4 −0.2 0.0 0.2 0.4 0.6 0.8

regimens would logically reflect ancillary treatment goals (e.g., anxiolysis, anti-impulsivity, and anticraving drug targets). While this certainly occurs (e.g., adjunctive lisdexamfetamine for bipolar disorder with ADD/ADHD; adjunctive divalproex for bipolar disorder with alcoholism), the literature on add-on pharmacotherapies for comorbid presentations tends more often to involve open trials and provisional case series. Formal RCTs of complex combination pharmacotherapy that do exist mostly involve comparing two drugs versus one or, at most, three drugs versus two, and instead tend to focus more on specific mood states (e.g., treatment-resistant bipolar depression) or highly relapsing illness subtypes (e.g., rapid cycling). Table 13.13 at the end of this chapter presents a summary of complex combination pharmacotherapy in bipolar disorder alongside targeted symptom complexes and rationales (negative studies are shaded).

Given the very high reported rates of comorbid psychopathology in bipolar disorder, one would think that studies would abound involving logical combination drug therapies meant to target associated symptoms such as anxiety, substance misuse, and attentional processing. There are in fact surprisingly few – nevertheless, Table 13.14 at the end of this chapter presents clinical combinations that have at least theoretical rationales, if not proof-of-concept preliminary evidence from clinical trials.

Clinicians often wonder if SSRIs "should" be used to treat prominent anxiety in patients with bipolar disorder, discounting the wrinkle that, to date, no controlled trials have examined the efficacy or safety of SSRIs for anxiolytic purposes in bipolar disorder. A possible exception comes from a secondary analysis of paroxetine (used as an active comparator in an FDA registration trial of quetiapine for bipolar depression), in which it was found to improve HAM-A scores significantly better than placebo, although it did not improve depression symptoms (McElroy et al., 2010a). Randomized trials of lurasidone, quetiapine, olanzapine/fluoxetine combination, and divalproex each included secondary analyses that showed reductions of anxiety symptoms specifically in the context of treating acute episodes of bipolar depression (in patients without current comorbid anxiety disorders). In some of those studies, the magnitude of anxiolytic effects was even greater than that seen for treating depressive symptoms (e.g., Davis et al., 2005). Notably, each of those studies measured anxiety symptoms using the HAM-A, which attaches considerable importance to physical anxiety symptoms that may not as fully capture elements of psychic anxiety (such as worry and apprehension).

Tip

It is hard to legitimately interpret a positive secondary analysis from a study in which the primary analysis was negative.

In the manufacturer's RCTs of lamotrigine in the acute or maintenance treatment of bipolar disorder, baseline anxiety was not predictive of successful outcomes. It has been hypothesized that lamotrigine may possess minimal anxiolytic properties based on its relative lack of GABAergic effects, as opposed to its more prominent antiglutamatergic effects.

The anxiolytic anticonvulsants gabapentin and pregabalin each have demonstrated efficacy as compared to placebo in RCTs of generalized anxiety disorder or social anxiety disorder (see Chapter 17), but have been studied less formally in treating anxiety symptoms in mood-disorder patients. However, their putative mechanisms of action and clinical profiles nevertheless make them attractive, rationale-based treatments for at least some instances of prominent anxiety in mood-disorder patients.

What About Adding Stimulants in Bipolar Disorder?

For all the apprehension many clinicians voice about possible safety (and efficacy) concerns with the use of stimulants in bipolar disorder, it is worth noting that the existing empirical database, while not extensive, appears more favorable than not. In acute mania, many would presume that stimulants (as theoretically mania-inducing) are anathema; however, the literature is surprisingly contrarian: based on the "vigilance regulation model of mania," Hegerl and colleagues (2018) found in a multicenter RCT that a brief (2.5-day) treatment with methylphenidate 20–40 mg/day posed no hazards for worsening existing mania, although the ultra-brief initial exposure did not significantly improve mania symptoms. Elsewhere, using a Swedish national registry naturalistic database, methylphenidate use was associated with a 6.7-fold increased likelihood of a manic episode occurring within three months of initiation, although that risk was mitigated by concomitant use of mood stabilizers (Viktorin et al., 2017). In acute bipolar depression, a small (n = 25) RCT of lisdexamfetamine found significant improvement of depressive symptoms as well as daytime fatigue, binge eating, and metabolic laboratory parameters, with no signs of mania induction (McElroy et al., 2015). Another small (n = 45) open trial of flexibly dosed adjunctive lisdexamfetamine (30–70 mg/day), targeting comorbid ADHD in bipolar outpatients, found significant improvement in self-reported ADHD symptoms, depression symptom severity, body weight, and lipid (but not glycemic) parameters (McIntyre et al., 2013).

What about (armodafinil) in bipolar depression? A meta-analysis of five RCTs (n = 795 drug, 790 placebo) revealed a significantly greater likelihood of response (RR = 1.18, 95% CI = 1.01–1.37, p = 0.03) or remission (RR = 1.38, 95% CI = 1.10–1.73, p = 0.005) with no increased risk for mood polarity switches or suicide attempts (Nunez et al., 2020).

On the whole, the database with stimulants suggests more safety than harm, provided they are used in conjunction with an antimanic mood stabilizer, and that efficacy may be evident with respect to bipolar depressive symptoms, attentional complaints, and possible features related to binge eating, weight loss, and hyperlipidemia. Likely, one would be less enthusiastic about using stimulants in the setting of psychosis, agitation, or active substance misuse, and data are insufficient or otherwise lacking regarding their sustained use during mania or over long-term periods.

Why Lamotrigine Isn't Considered an Antidepressant, and Why a-mood-stabilizer-is-not-a-mood-stabilizer-is-not-a-mood-stabilizer

The clinical trials base for lamotrigine tells an interesting story behind the evolution of a molecule whose psychotropic properties have become rather ill-defined relative to its evidence base. Lamotrigine was first studied as a monotherapy for acute bipolar depression in a seven-week industry-sponsored multisite randomized trial that found a numerical, but statistically nonsignificant, reduction in depression symptoms (dosed either at 50 mg/day or 200 mg/day) as compared to placebo on the designated primary outcome measure (the 17-item Hamilton Rating Scale for Depression; HAM-D_{17}) using LOCF analyses. When using an analysis of *observed cases*, both lamotrigine doses were significantly better than placebo.

What if we try using a different rating scale than the one that was specified a priori as the primary outcome measure? Lo and behold, as shown in Figure 13.8, a statistically significant advantage for lamotrigine dosed at 200 mg/day was now observed versus placebo when using a secondary measure of depressive symptoms, the Montgomery-Åsberg Depression Rating Scale (MADRS) (Calabrese et al., 1999).

Tip

Remember, "observed cases" analyses ignore noncompleters and therefore tend to overestimate within-group changes from baseline.

If only the MADRS had been chosen instead

Ketter's Hypothesis

Terence Ketter and colleagues (1999) proposed that GABAergic anticonvulsants (such as divalproex or carbamazepine) were more impactful for psychomotorically activated states such as mania, while predominantly antiglutamatergic drugs such as lamotrigine were more efficacious for depression.

Figure 13.8 Antidepressant efficacy of lamotrigine in bipolar I depression. Based on findings by Calabrese et al., 1999.

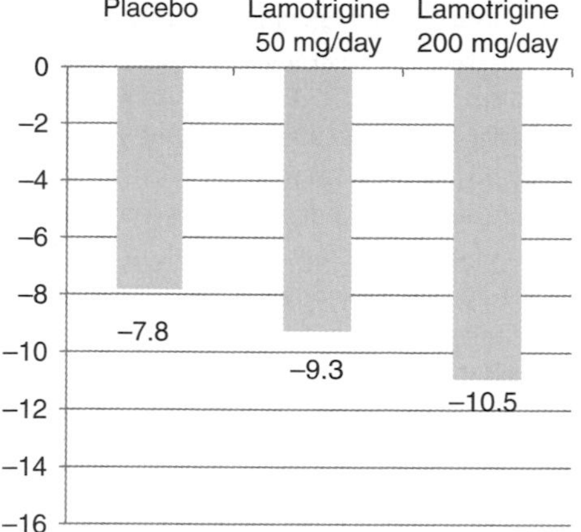

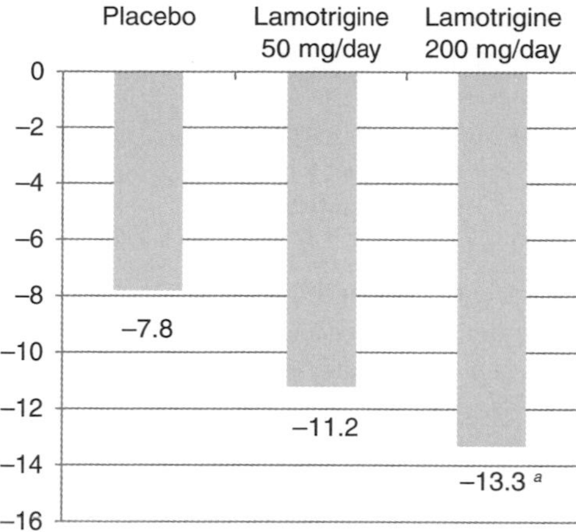

of the HAM-D$_{17}$ as the primary outcome measure! Was the MADRS a *better* scale to use for bipolar depression than the HAM-D$_{17}$? That's what the authors of that study wondered in the Discussion section of their paper, noting that the HAM-D$_{17}$ scale is weighted heavily toward somatic symptoms, unlike the MADRS. Did the chosen measurement scale "fail" to detect what may be a drug effect that is truly significantly different from placebo, or was this initial pivotal study simply negative? Further complicating our understanding of the possible acute antidepressant effects of lamotrigine is its dosing schedule; later studies that focused on relapse prevention in bipolar I disorder found that either 200 or 400 mg/day was superior to placebo while 50 mg/day dosing was perceived to be subtherapeutic (see Box 13.15).

The pattern and magnitude of differences in depressive symptom reduction were similar for the two rating scales, but technically the study was deemed negative because of the failure to achieve statistical significance on the primary outcome measure (the HAM-D$_{17}$). As noted in Chapter 5, and as shown

Tip

Use caution when judging efficacy if combining lamotrigine with folic acid. In the "CEQUEL" study of lamotrigine plus quetiapine in bipolar depression (Geddes et al, 2016), adjunctive folic acid eliminated the benefit of lamotrigine – *presumably* because lamotrigine inhibits dihydrofolate reductase, reducing the conversion of dihydrofolate to tetrahydrofolate, in turn reducing the availability of *L*-methylfolate.

Box 13.15

Is There an Ideal Lamogrigine Dose for Bipolar Depression?

The generally recognized target dose for lamotrigine is 200mg/day, based mainly on relapse prevention studies and acute augmentation trials. Are lamotrigine dosages above 200mg/day more effective, either acutely or prophylactically? Empirically, we do not know. The two FDA registration lamotrigine maintenance trial designs used either: (a) flexible dosing from 100–400mg/day (precluding the opportunity to make comparisons between fixed doses, and no mean final dose was reported in the manuscript) (Bowden et al., 2003) or (b) a combined subject group that lumped together those who were originally enrolled in separate 200 or 400 mg/day arms into a single study arm, due to slow enrollment (Calabrese et al., 2003). In the latter study, no exploratory analyses comparing 200 vs. 400 mg/day outcomes were examined. A separate NIMH intramural acute crossover study of treatment-resistant unipolar and bipolar disorder patients using flexibly dosed lamogritine (mean dose = 274±128 mg/day) reported significantly greater overall "response" with lamotrigine then either placebo or gabapentin using CGI scores - but did not report outcomes with symptom-specific rating scales; CGI subcomponent ratings for mania or depression were not statistically significant (Frye et al., 2000). Our subjective overall impression: lamotrigine doses >200 mg/day (sans carbamazepine cotherapy) may sometimes fine tune a partial response, or recapture a euthymia fading into depression during maintenance therapy, but higher doses are unlikely to convert an outright nonresponse to a response. Higher doses may also incur more nonspecific CNS adverse effects (e.g., dizziness, lightheadedness, headache).

by Geddes et al. (2009) for the industry-based acute bipolar depression trials with lamotrigine, high baseline severity was found to moderate treatment outcomes (i.e., suppress placebo responsivity and increase drug–placebo differences) (depicted in Box 13.16). Note from Box 13.16 that lamotrigine response rates were similar for patients with either moderate or high baseline severity; placebo response was much lower when baseline severity was high, allowing for statistically significant separation from active drug.

In our experience, lamotrigine does indeed possess acute antidepressant properties, both alone and with other agents. The "ideal patient candidate" for lamotrigine is described in Box 13.17.

As a final consideration regarding the evidence base for lamotrigine in bipolar disorder, we would point out that the manufacturer's pivotal trials in acute depression consistently found better efficacy (i.e., separation from placebo) in bipolar I than bipolar II subjects (perhaps reflecting higher placebo responsivity in the latter than the former group). While some practitioners may feel compelled to initially treat bipolar II patients with lamotrigine as a maintenance therapy, the data to support this use is scant and based mainly on open-label trials (e.g., Terao et al., 2017).

Box 13.16

Acute Bipolar Antidepressant Response: Lamotrigine or Placebo

	Moderate baseline severity	High baseline severity
Lamotrigine response rate	48%	45%
Placebo response rate	45%	30%

Box 13.17

When to Use Lamotrigine

- Relapse prevention (depression > mania) in bipolar I disorder
- No established value in mania/hypomania though no evidence for induction of mania (Goldberg et al., 2009)
- Minimal baseline anxiety
- Absence of mixed features (no data)
- Adjunct to lithium (target dose 200 mg/day) in acute bipolar depression (Van der Loos et al., 2009)
- As an adjunct to quetiapine (Geddes et al., 2016)

Rapid Cycling

The term rapid cycling was originally coined by Dunner and Fieve (1974) as a descriptor of poor response to prophylactic lithium, defined operationally as more than four episodes per year. The term should not be confused with mixed features within a single episode, or with sheer affective instability; many patients and practitioners alike mistakenly invoke the term to mean fluctuating mood states, irrespective of the nonmood psychomotor (e.g., sleep/energy) manifestations of a manic or hypomanic episode. While the original descriptive studies linked rapid cycling with lithium nonresponse, later studies broadened its prognostic relevance in showing comparable prophylactic effects with either lithium or divalproex (Calabrese et al., 2005). A history of rapid cycling in the preceding year generally is considered a poor prognostic feature, and a factor that should discourage antidepressant use. One should also keep in mind that a true study of "rapid cycling" focuses not on any acute phase of illness but rather on at least a one-year time period in order to discern whether an intervention is able to reduce the frequency of recurrences (as opposed to ameliorating the symptoms of a single acute episode).

Interest has grown regarding the use of lamotrigine in rapid-cycling bipolar patients. What is the evidence base for this? A six-month industry trial examining lamotrigine versus placebo for relapse prevention in bipolar I or II patients with rapid cycling (Calabrese et al., 2000) took as its primary outcome Time until the need for Intervention for an emerging Mood Episode (TiME; that is, the point at which a clinician would logically feel compelled to alter the existing treatment due to impending or worsening signs of mania or depression). TiME was not significantly longer with lamotrigine than placebo. However, "survival in the study" was longer with lamotrigine than placebo in the bipolar II subgroup; this meant that patients on lamotrigine were *less likely to drop out of the study prematurely*, as compared to those taking placebo. To further complicate the story, a study of adding lamotrigine versus placebo onto an existing stable combination of lithium plus divalproex failed to alleviate ongoing depression symptoms in a group of bipolar patients with rapid cycling (Kemp et al., 2012); however, the apparent negative findings from that study were hard to interpret

Tip

Triple-mood-stabilizer therapy, while conceptually appealing in rapid cycling, has not shown superiority to double-mood-stabilizer treatment in controlled trials.

because of high dropout of subjects due to adverse effects and poor adherence to the study protocol, rendering the study itself underpowered to show (or not show) efficacy, and standing as testament to the practical and logistical challenges of conducting long-term randomized trials in patients with hard-to-treat bipolar disorder.

Other evidence-based treatment options targeting the reduction of episode frequency in rapid cycling are unfortunately few in number (summarized in Table 13.15).

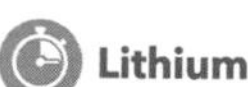

Lithium

Though often referred to by some as the "gold standard" mood stabilizer, lithium carbonate actually has a relatively narrow breadth of spectrum in its efficacy across subtypes of bipolar disorder, making it in some ways more the "penicillin" than "vancomycin" of mood stabilizers. Rather than think of its utility in an all-or-none fashion, as with most psychotropics it would be more precise to identify specific clinical situations in which lithium is appropriate. A judged "excellent response" to lithium with complete and sustained remissions occurs in only a minority of individuals with bipolar disorder, evident in only about 5–10% of bipolar disorder patients according to some large-scale data registry studies. Partial or nonresponses to lithium may be more the norm. Lithium responsivity may in fact be a heritable trait or endophenotype of the illness, with concordance rates of about 65% between an affected individual and their lithium-treated first-degree relative with bipolar disorder (Grof et al., 2002). Other factors that may portend a more favorable response to lithium are summarized in Box 13.18.

Box 13.18

When to Use Lithium

- Better outcomes when introduced within the first few episodes
- Mania rather than depression as the dominant episode polarity
- Manias precede depressions followed by an intermorbid period ("M-D-I")
- Absence of four or more episodes/year
- "Pure" euphoric manias with an absence of mixed features
- (+) Family history of lithium-responsive bipolar disorder
- Absence of comorbid substance use disorders

Cognitive Impact of Lithium

Reports of adverse cognitive effects from lithium (such as decreased short-term memory) are in some ways at variance with lithium's neuroprotective effects, as established from both preclinical and clinical studies. Lithium has been shown to help prevent neuronal death by increasing expression of antiapoptotic genes such as bcl-2, while increasing neurotrophic factors such as BDNF. It can also reduce the area of neuronal damage after laboratory-induced cerebral infarcts in rodents, and can increase total volume of both cortical and subcortical (e.g., hippocampal, amygdala, thalamus) brain regions. However, it remains to be demonstrated whether or not those effects necessarily translate into functional cognitive benefits. Multiple affective episodes in themselves may pose a risk factor for cognitive decline and possible dementia, although at least some observational studies report a correlation between lithium use and a decreased incident rate of dementia in bipolar disorder patients. (It is difficult to infer causality or directionality in this possible relationship because enrichment or confounding by indication may go undetected; the decision to prescribe and continue lithium may itself simply be a

My bipolar patient who takes lithium is going hiking in the Himalayas. Should I change her lithium dose?

High altitude increases RBC production within a day and lithium binds strongly to RBCs. Lithium's half-life and its volume of distribution both increase and total clearance decreases by about 40% in response to chronic exposure to high altitude. So, I'd say, if her dose is on the high end (say, levels ≤0.7-0.8 mEq/L) and she'll be there more than a few days, it wouldn't hurt to lower her lithium dose by a third to even a half. If her dose is lower you can probably leave it alone but make sure she doesn't get dehydrated or salt-depleted.

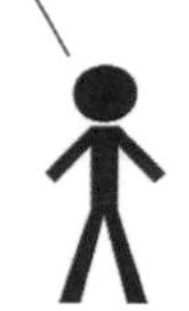

proxy for good prognosis, low recurrence risk, absence of comorbidities, or other factors that could self-select against the risk for dementia.)

 Low-dose Lithium

There has long been interest and speculation that some mood disorder patients of either polarity might benefit from low-dose adjunctive lithium (i.e., at serum levels below or even much below the generally accepted therapeutic reference range). The basis for such a perspective is largely anecdotal, especially since comparative effectiveness studies have found no advantage in reducing affective symptoms over six months when "optimized personalized treatment" included adjunctive placebo versus adjunctive moderate-dose lithium (defined as dosages begun at 600 mg/day initially for two months, then modified based on symptoms, yielding serum lithium levels in the range of 0.4–0.5 mEq/L) (Nierenberg et al., 2013). Some studies also report lower incident rates of suicide completions in geographic regions with higher lithium levels in drinking water, although such findings appear to be less robust when lithium levels are less than 31 µg/L. Practical considerations when using lithium are summarized in Table 13.16 at the end of this chapter.

 Carbamazepine

Clinical trials with carbamazepine in bipolar mania emerged in the 1980s, largely as an alternative or adjunct in lithium nonresponders. Initial efforts undertaken intramurally at NIMH often involved small crossover trials with on-off-on designs (rather than separate comparison groups receiving a placebo). Acute mania trials designed for FDA registration purposes occurred in the early 2000s using extended-release carbamazepine (mean dose 642 mg/day) (Weisler et al., 2005). Systematic relapse prevention studies have not, as yet, been undertaken. Box 13.19 provides a summary of clinical "profile" characteristics when judging individual patient candidacy for carbamazepine in bipolar disorder.

 **Tip**

Remember that carbamazepine also induces its own metabolism (autoinduction) after several weeks.

Box 13.19

When to Use Carbamazepine

- Manic or mixed episodes
- As part of a treatment regimen for rapid cycling with other mood stabilizers or SGAs
- Minimal practical concerns about hepatic enzyme induction or pharmacokinetic interactions with other hepatically metabolized drugs
- Among the few relatively weight-neutral antimanic agents

 Divalproex

Trials with divalproex in acute manic or mixed episodes emerged in the early 1990s. Together with carbamazepine, divalproex ushered in an era in which anticonvulsants were perceived as having a mood stabilizing class effect, and offering a viable alternative to lithium. (Perhaps ironically, neither carbamazepine nor divalproex has an established evidence base for relapse prevention in bipolar disorder – a property that some would argue represents a critical component of "mood stabilization" over the longitudinal course of bipolar disorder.) Features describing an ideal clinical profile for judging patient candidacy for divalproex appear in Box 13.20.

Box 13.20

When to Use Divalproex

- Need for rapid mania symptom control via oral loading at 20–30 mg/kg
- Manic or mixed episodes > depression-predominance
- Multiepisode presentations
- Comorbid alcohol/substance use disorders (provided that liver enzymes remain three times the upper limit of normal or less)
- Not a sexually active woman of child-bearing potential
- Absence of irregular menstrual cycle
- Impulsive aggression

 What About Other Anticonvulsants?

The evidence base for all anticonvulsants other than lamotrigine, divalproex, and carbamazepine is meager for addressing mood stabilization, but as shown in Table 13.17, appears quite varied with respect to psychotropic properties other than mood regulation. Please do not refer to anticonvulsants that are not divalproex, carbamazepine, or lamotrigine as "mood stabilizers," because there is no evidence base from which to support their reliable efficacy to treat mood symptoms in any phase of bipolar disorder.

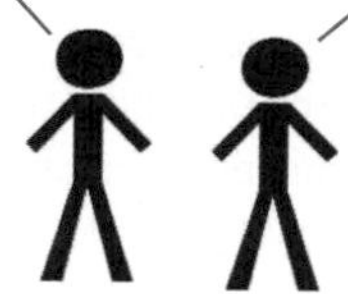

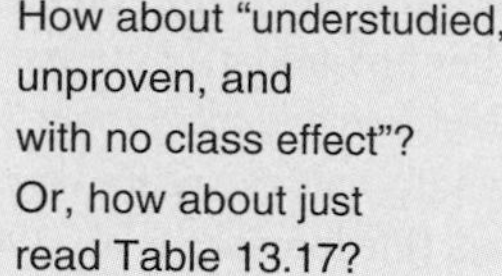

How about "understudied,
unproven, and
with no class effect"?
Or, how about just
read Table 13.17?

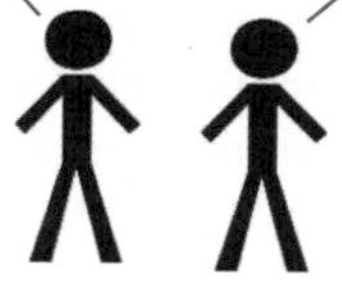

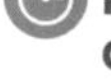 SGAs and Bipolar Depression

As of this writing, only four SGAs carry FDA indications for acute bipolar depression (quetiapine, lurasidone, cariprazine, and olanzapine/fluoxetine combination). An industry-sponsored meta-analysis of SGAs in bipolar depression found no differences in change in MADRS between lurasidone and olanzapine or quetiapine, although weight gain was less with lurasidone than either agent (Ostacher et al., 2018). The many negative SGA RCTs in bipolar depression (see Tables 13.18 and 13.19 for summary; negative trials or conditions with no data are again shaded) raise questions about possible idiosyncratic differences among compounds, with no clearer evidence of a broad class effect here than with anticonvulsants broadly describable as mood stabilizers.

Pharmacotherapy of Bipolar Disorder With Comorbid Conditions

OCD

There are few systematic studies devoted to the treatment of bipolar disorder with comorbid OCD. Pooled data estimate the lifetime prevalence of such dual-diagnosis presentations at about 17% (Amerio et al., 2015). Some authors hold the view that "true" OCD is rare in bipolar disorder, and that for many patients the phenomena identified as OCD are really artifacts of mania that expectably respond to lithium or other antimanic mood stabilizers. In our experience, the presence of frank obsessions and compulsions demarcates a more severe overall form of illness that responds more poorly to any single pharmacotherapy. Studies of adjunctive SSRIs or clomipramine – mainstay treatments for OCD without comorbidity – are limited mainly to small open trials and case reports, from which it is difficult to estimate reliable rates of response or treatment-emergent mania/hypomania. The modest RCTs database that does exist supports the efficacy of aripiprazole added to lithium for both mania and OCD symptoms (Saharian et al., 2018). Other SGAs such as olanzapine or risperidone have less extensive data, and there are also reports of clozapine or other SGAs paradoxically causing or exacerbating OCD symptoms.

Anxiety Disorders

Dual-diagnosis anxiety disorders have been reported to occur in up to 45% of adults with bipolar disorder (Pavlova et al., 2015), yet dedicated systematic studies of such patients are scarce. In FDA RCTs in acute bipolar depression using quetiapine, olanzapine/fluoxetine combination, lurasidone, or cariprazine, secondary analyses found that each of these agents demonstrated greater improvement in overall anxiety symptoms as compared to placebo. Of note, post hoc analyses involving cariprazine for acute bipolar depression have shown significant reductions in anxiety symptoms when dosed at 1.5 mg/day but not higher. Clinicians often assume that SSRIs or other serotonergic agents are "necessary" (i.e., reliably efficacious) to target anxiety symptoms arising in patients with bipolar disorder, but this assumption is hard to justify in the absence of formal studies of dual-diagnosis patients. As noted earlier in this chapter, in an RCT of quetiapine for acute bipolar depression, paroxetine was an active comparator and while it failed to separate from placebo on improvement in depression symptoms (the primary outcome), anxiety symptoms did improve better than with placebo on a secondary outcome analysis (McElroy et al., 2010b). Secondary analyses of RCTs involving divalproex for acute bipolar depression also demonstrate greater reduction in concomitant anxiety symptoms with active drug than placebo (Davis et al., 2005; Ghaemi et al., 2007).

Because of the complexity of addictions and conceptual overlaps with mood disorders, impulsivity, and dysfunction of the reward pathway, we separately present information on treatment of bipolar disorder with comorbid substance use disorders in Chapter 18.

Major Depressive Disorder with Mixed Features: Is it a Thing?

Since the DSM-5 establishment of major depression with mixed features (MDD-MF), questions linger regarding the construct validity of the diagnosis, its longitudinal stability (is it a harbinger of eventual full mania or hypomania?), and appropriate pharmacotherapy. Two placebo-controlled trials presently exist: one found efficacy with ziprasidone (mean dose = 130 mg/day) for reducing depression symptoms (NNT = 4 for response, NNT = 3 for remission) but no significant change in mania symptoms (Patkar et al., 2012). Another larger placebo-controlled RCT of lurasidone monotherapy (mean dose = 36.2 mg/day) found a significant reduction in both manic and depressive symptoms ($d = 0.80$) (Suppes et al., 2016). The construct of MDD-MF remains sufficiently nascent to preclude definitive, empirically based forecasts on the likelihood of this condition representing a "prebipolar" state; follow-up studies preliminarily suggest that a minority of such identified patients (about 20%) will over time meet syndromal criteria for developing bipolar I or II disorders (Fiedorowicz et al., 2011). An expert consensus panel identified lurasidone as the sole psychotropic having favorable RCT data for acute treatment of MDD-MF, noting the paucity of both phenomenology and treatment studies of this clinical entity in general (Stahl et al., 2017).

TAKE-HOME POINTS

- Mood disorders involve complex symptom constellations involving affective, behavioral, psychomotor, interpersonal, cognitive and other psychiatric phenomena, often in a chronic or recurrent pattern.
- It can be useful to conceptualize mood disorders based on factors beyond polarity, including psychosis, comorbidity, chronicity, recurrence, and degree of treatment-resistance.
- Most depressed patients have an inadequate response to first-line treatments, particularly if presentations involve high severity, chronicity, comorbidity, or illness complexity.
- Chronic or persistent depression often requires longer trial durations than is customary in nonchronic depression.
- After poor responses to adequate trials of appropriate pharmacotherapies, decisions about augmentation versus class-switching must be individually based and depend largely on symptom profiles, degree of partial response, drug tolerability, and viability of alternative agents.
- Rationales for complex combination regimens should involve agents with nonredundant (and ideally, synergistic) mechanisms of action.
- Mixed features, involving elements of both mania/hypomania and depression, are often more common than "pure" polarity presentations among complex mood disorder patients; "pure" polarity divisions may be diagnostically and phenomenologically more rare than customary for many patients.
- Constructs around "mood stabilization" should take into consideration factors such as polarity proneness, degree of affective switch (versus persistence of a single mood state), and long-term drug acceptability and tolerability.

Table 13.1 Usual and maximally studied dosing ranges for antidepressants: SSRIs

Agent	Clinical profile	Usual dosing	"Tricks of the trade" and heroic maneuvers for inadequate responses
SSRIs	- Anxiolytic as well as antidepressant efficacy - Obsessive-compulsive features - Bulimia - Sertraline and fluoxetine are both relatively well-studied in bipolar II depression (as noted in the main text)	*Fluoxetine*: Usually begun at 20 mg/day (or 10 mg/day if concerns about sensitivity to adverse effects), dosed typically qAM; may increase by 20 mg/day every several weeks to maximum of 80 mg/day *Paroxetine*: IR dosing usually begun at 20 mg/day (or 10 mg/day if concerns about sensitivity to adverse effects); may increase by 10 mg/day increments up to 50 mg/day. CR dosing begun at 25 mg/day, may increase by 12.5 mg/day increments once a week to maximum of 62.5 mg/day *Sertraline*: Usually begun at 50 mg/day (25 mg/day for panic disorder), can be adjusted upward weekly to maximum of 200 mg/day *Fluvoxamine*: Usually begun at 50 mg PO qHS, may increase in 50 mg/day increments every 4–7 days to target range of 100–300 mg/day. While the manufacturer advises BID dosing above 100 mg/day, fluvoxamine's 16-hour half-life likely accommodates qHS dosing *Citalopram*: Usually begun at 20 mg/day, may increase to 30 or 40 mg/day after one week at the discretion of the prescriber. Higher doses have not shown greater antidepressant efficacy in RCTs *Escitalopram*: Usually begun at 10 mg/day; may increase to 20 mg/day but RCTs show no superiority of 20 mg over 10 mg/day	Literature on the safety and efficacy of supratherapeutically dosed SSRIs tends to focus more on treatment of OCD than MDD

Abbreviations: BID = twice a day; CR = controlled release; IR = immediate release; MDD = major depressive disorder; OCD = obsessive-compulsive disorder; PO = by mouth; qAM = every morning; qHS = every night at bedtime ;SSRI = selective serotonin reuptake inhibitor;

Table 13.2 Usual and maximally studied dosing ranges for antidepressants: SNRIs

Agent	Clinical profile	Usual dosing	"Tricks of the trade" and heroic maneuvers for inadequate responses
SNRIs	- Anxious depression - Only about a 6% greater response rate than SSRIs (Papakostas et al., 2007) - Neuropathic pain - Perimenopausal hot flashes	*Venlafaxine*: XR formulation begun at 75 mg/day, titrated by 75 mg/day no sooner than every four days to maximum of 375 mg/day; in GAD or panic disorder, maximum dose 225 mg/day; in social anxiety disorder, maximum dose 75 mg/day *Desvenlafaxine*: 50 mg/day is considered therapeutic; higher doses have not shown clear added benefit. Longer half-life (~12°) than venlafaxine (~5°), with less risk of discontinuation symptoms *Duloxetine*: Begun at 20 mg PO BID or 30 mg PO qDay; after one week may increase daily dose by 20–30 mg/day to 60 mg/day; dosages >60 mg/day have not shown clear added benefit for depression or pain (though maximum 120 mg/day customary in GAD) *Levomilnacipran*: Begun at 20 mg PO BID for two days then 40 mg/day; may increase by 40 mg/day every two days to maximum of 120 mg/day	- SNRI + mirtazapine ± bupropion or stimulant (monitor blood pressure); compatible with SGAs, thyroid hormone, buspirone - Optimally dosed duloxetine (60 mg PO BID) outperformed escitalopram in treating core emotional symptoms (energy/fatigue, concentration/decision-making, loss of interest, sad mood, feelings of worthlessness) when comparing distinct symptom cluster improvements across antidepressants (Chekroud et al., 2017)

Abbreviations: BID = twice a day; BP = blood pressure; GAD = generalized anxiety disorder; PO = by mouth; qDay = once a day; SGA = second-generation antipsychotic; SNRI = serotonin-norepinephrine reuptake inhibitor; XR = extended release

Table 13.3 Usual and maximally studied dosing ranges for antidepressants: MAOIs

Agent	Clinical profile	Usual dosing	"Tricks of the trade" and heroic maneuvers for inadequate responses
Irreversible MAOIs	- Anxious or anergic depression - Highly mood reactive depression - Depression in borderline personality disorder - TRD	*Isocarboxazide*: Begun at 10 mg PO BID, increased by 10 mg/day every two to four days to 40 mg after one week; further increase by 20 mg/week to maximum of 60 mg/day in BID or QID dosing *Phenelzine*: Begun at 15 mg PO TID, rapidly increase to 60 mg/day up to 90 mg/day; maintenance dose may be 15 mg/day or every other day *Tranylcypromine*: Begun at 30 mg/day in divided doses, may increase by 10 mg/day every one to three weeks to a maximum of 60 mg/day *Selegiline*: *Transdermal* selegiline begun at 6 mg per 24 hours. Dosing may increase by 3 mg per 24 hours every two weeks to a maximum of 12 mg per 24 hours. Dietary tyramine restrictions are considered necessary only at doses >6 mg. *Oral* selegiline must be dosed high enough to overcome MAO nonselectivity to exert antidepressant efficacy (~30 mg/day; see Mann et al., 1989)	- Supratherapeutic dosing: tranylcypromine 90–130 mg/day (Amsterdam and Berwish 1989) - Cotherapy with bupropion or a stimulant is aggressive and risky from a cardio- and cerebrovascular standpoint and requires fastidious blood pressure monitoring, but can be done with great caution (Stewart et al., 2014); (ar)modafinil may be less autonomically hazardous - Should be compatible with mirtazapine without fear of serotonin syndrome (see Chapter 6, Box 6.1)
Reversible inhibitors of MAO-A (RIMAs) (many are no longer marketed, such as caroxazone or minaprine) or were discontinued during development (e.g., brofaromine)	- Averts need for tyramine-free diet - Social phobia - Possibly less weight gain than with irreversible MAOIs - Regarded by some experts as less potent than irreversible MAOIs	*Moclobemide*: Begun at 150 mg PO BID, may increase to 600 mg/day (divided) after four days	Combinations with other serotonergic antidepressants are not evidence-based and still pose risk for serotonin syndrome. Moclobemide levels are increased by coadministered CYP 2C19 inhibitors (e.g., modafinil, topiramate, oxcarbazepine) - Compatible with SGAs, thyroid hormone

Abbreviations: BID = twice a day; MAO = monoamine oxidase; MAO-A = monoamine oxidase A; MAOI = monoamine oxidase inhibitor; PO = by mouth; QID = four times a day; SGA = second-generation antipsychotic; TID = three times a day; TRD = treatment-resistant depression

Table 13.4 Usual and maximally studied dosing ranges for antidepressants: Tricyclics

Agent	Clinical profile	Usual dosing	"Tricks of the trade" and heroic maneuvers for inadequate responses
Tricyclics	- Melancholic features (Roose et al., 2004) - Neuropathic pain; secondary amines (nortriptyline, desipramine) tend to be better tolerated than tertiary amines (amitriptyline, imipramine, clomipramine) - Tertiary amines (e.g., amitriptyline, doxepin) useful for insomnia	*Amitriptyline*: Usually begun at 75 mg in divided doses *or* 50–100 mg qHS, dosed up to 150–200 mg/day, rarely *up to 300 mg/day* *Desipramine*: Usually begun at 25–50 mg/day either in divided doses or one-nightly and gradually increased to 100–200 mg/day, *maximum 300 mg/day* *Clomipramine*: Usually begun at 25 mg/day, may gradually increase to 100 mg/day over first two weeks, *maximum 250 mg/day*. Divided dosing with meals is advised during titration but thereafter dosing is usually once daily at bedtime *Doxepin*: Usually begun at 75 mg PO qHS (or as low as 25–50 mg/day in mild depression) *Imipramine*: Usually begun at 75–100 mg/day, gradually increased to 200 mg/day as necessary; may increase to *maximum of 250–300 mg/day* after two weeks if inadequate response; usual maintenance dose 50–150 mg/day dosed at bedtime *Nortriptyline*: Usually begun at 75–100 mg/day (some practitioners prefer 25–50 mg/day) in divided dosing or once daily, may increase as needed to *maximum of 150 mg/day;* monitor serum levels for doses >100 mg/day *Protriptyline*: Usually begun at 15–40 mg/day in three to four divided doses, *maximum of 60 mg/day*	- Can combine TCA with SSRI but beware increased levels via CYP 450 inhibition from fluoxetine (2D6, 2C19), fluvoxamine (2D6, 1A2, 3A4, 2C19), or paroxetine (2D6) - An MAOI can be (cautiously) added to a TCA, with less risk of a hypertensive crisis than adding a TCA to an MAOI (see Chapter 6) **Tip** Protriptyline is unique among TCAs because it is activating rather than sedating.

Abbreviations: MAOI = monoamine oxidase inhibitor; qHS = every night at bedtime; SSRI = selective serotonin reuptake inhibitor; TCA = tricyclic antidepressant

Table 13.5 Usual and maximally studied dosing ranges for antidepressants: novel serotonergic agents

Agent	Clinical profile	Usual dosing	"Tricks of the trade" and heroic maneuvers for inadequate responses
Vilazodone	- Anxious depression or comorbid GAD (Durgam et al., 2016c)	Usually begun at 10 mg PO qDay with food for seven days then increase to 20 mg PO qDay with food. The manufacturer advises optionally increasing to 40 mg/day if inadequate response though in our experience a dose of 30 mg/day is often useful	- Can combine with bupropion, mirtazapine, secondary amine TCAs, SGAs, stimulants, thyroid hormone - As a $5HT_{1A}$ partial agonist, would be redundant with buspirone
Vortioxetine	- Low incidence of iatrogenic sexual dysfunction - May have particular anxiolytic value due to $5HT_{1A}$ agonism - Demonstrated cognitive benefits independent of effects on mood (McIntyre et al., 2016)	Usually begun at 10 mg/day then increased to 20 mg/day as tolerated. Across the six FDA registration trials in MDD, 20 mg/day dosing arms were consistently superior to placebo, whereas all lower doses studied (5 mg, 10 mg, 15 mg) had both significant and nonsignificant treatment outcomes	- If combined with bupropion, manufacturer advises maximum dosing at 10 mg/day due to CYP 2D6 inhibition. However, in our experience, vortioxetine dosed to 20 mg/day is well-tolerated and efficacious in conjunction with bupropion
Mirtazapine	- Anxious depression - Anorectic depression - Depression with insomnia - Late-life depression - May counteract akathisia (Hieber et al., 2008)	Begun at 15 mg qHS, may increase by 15 mg q1-2 weeks to maximum of 45 mg/day	- Co-therapy hastens onset with SSRI, SNRI (Blier et al., 2010) - Anxiolytic properties - Mixes safely, and often effectively, with virtually any psychotropic - $5HT_{2A}$ antagonism makes risk for serotonin syndrome highly unlikely (see Chapter 6, Box 6.1)
Nefazodone	- Low incidence of iatrogenic sexual dysfunction - Open trial data support use in GAD, social anxiety disorder	Usually begun at 100 mg PO BID then increased by increments of 100-200 mg/day once per week to a target range of 300-600 mg/day in divided doses (half-life 2-4 hours)	- Can combine with bupropion, secondary amine TCAs, SGA, stimulants, thyroid hormone, buspirone

Abbreviations: BID = twice a day; FDA = US Food and Drug Administration; GAD = generalized anxiety disorder; MDD = major depressive disorder; PO = by mouth; qDay = once a day; SGA = second-generation antipsychotic; TCA = tricyclic antidepressant

Table 13.6 Usual and maximally studied dosing ranges for antidepressants: bupropion

Agent	Clinical profile	Usual dosing	"Tricks of the trade" and heroic maneuvers for inadequate responses
Bupropion	- May be more useful in anergic than anxious/ agitated depression - Minimal to no sexual side effects - May promote weight loss - Useful for smoking cessation - Seasonal depression	IR formulation dosing begun at 100 mg PO BID, may increase to 100 mg PO TID after three days, maximum dose 450 mg/day; SR formulation dosing begun at 100–150 mg PO qDay, may increase after three days to target dose of 300 mg/day (divided); XL formulation dosing begun at 150 mg PO qAM, may increase after four days to 300 mg PO qAM, with a maximum dose of 450 mg/day	Doses >450 mg/day substantially increase seizure risk (~10-fold) without clearly greater efficacy; bupropion potently inhibits CYP 2D6, delaying the metabolism of some SSRIs or SNRIs. Beware of coadministered CYP 2B6 inducers (e.g., carbamazepine, antiretroviral drugs) that may hasten metabolism

Abbreviations: BID = twice a day; IR = immediate release; PO = by mouth; qAM = every morning; qDay = every day; TID = three times a day; SR = slow release; SNRI = serotonin-norepinephrine reuptake inhibitor; SSRI = selective serotonin reuptake inhibitor; XL = extended release

Table 13.7 High-dose antidepressant prescribing habits reported among clinicians

Antidepressant	Mean (SD) maximum dose (mg/day)	Percentage of clinicians who report prescribing above manufacturers' maximum recommended dosages
Bupropion	430.5 (131.0)	9% prescribed >450 mg/day
Citalopram	53.2 (20.5)	53% prescribed >40 mg/day
Desvenlafaxine	99.8 (88.9)	29% prescribed >100 mg/day
Escitalopram	34.2 (15.5)	70% prescribed >20 mg/day
Mirtazapine	52.6 (21.1)	12% prescribed >60 mg/day
Sertraline	232.7 (72.3)	40% prescribed >200 mg/day
Venlafaxine	356.1 (138.0)	83% prescribed >225 mg/day

Data based on findings reported by Goldberg et al., 2015

Table 13.8 SGA RCTs in MDD

SGA	Evidence base
Aripiprazole	- Four positive placebo-controlled acute RCTs (mean dose = 11.8 mg/day in Berman et al., 2007; mean dose = 10.7 mg/day in Berman et al., 2009; mean dose = 11.0 mg/day in Marcus et al., 2008; mean dose = 9.8 mg/day in Kamijima et al., 2013) - One negative low dose (2 mg/day) acute (60-day) RCT (Fava et al., 2012)
Brexpiprazole	- Four positive placebo-controlled acute RCTs, dosages from 2–3 mg/day; effect size of *d* = 0.33 (reviewed by Thase et al., 2019b)
Cariprazine	- One positive RCT: cariprazine 2–4.5 mg/day (n = 276) (but not 1–2 mg/day; n = 274) was superior to placebo (n = 269) added to an antidepressant in MDD (Durgam et al., 2016a) - Two *negative* RCTs: (i) a large (n = 530) 18–19 week RCT as adjunct (1.5–4.5 mg/day) to antidepressant (Earley et al., 2018), and (ii) a 19-week augmentation of antidepressants with low-dose (0.1–0.3 or 1–2 mg/day) cariprazine (Fava et al., 2018b)
Clozapine	Single case reports
Lurasidone	One positive RCT as monotherapy in MDD with mixed features (Suppes et al., 2016); no data as adjunct to monoaminergic antidepressants in MDD
Olanzapine	- Two parallel eight-week acute RCTs in TRD comparing olanzapine 6 mg/day + fluoxetine 50 mg/day combination (OFC) versus fluoxetine 50 mg/day or olanzapine 6 mg/day; no significant between-group differences in Study 1 but OFC improved depression symptoms significantly more than did fluoxetine or olanzapine in study 2; pooled OFC response rate from both trials = 27% (Thase et al., 2007) - After SSRI nonresponse, olanzapine + fluoxetine showed more rapid onset but ultimately no difference from fluoxetine alone or nortriptyline alone (Shelton et al., 2005) - Olanzapine+fluoxetine > olanzapine monotherapy (but not fluoxetine or venlafaxine monotherapy) (Corya et al., 2006) - Studies of olanzapine combined with antidepressants other than fluoxetine for MDD (notably, citalopram, venlafaxine, mirtazapine, or sertraline) are limited to small open trials that fail to show an accelerated onset of antidepressant effect (Parker et al., 2005)
Paliperidone	Single case reports
Pimavanserin	One positive unpublished preliminary monotherapy 10-week RCT in TRD (www.acadia-pharm.com/pipeline/pimavanserin-major-depressive-disorder/)
Quetiapine	- Eight positive placebo-controlled acute RCTs, dosages from 50–300 mg/day (Yargic et al., 2004; McIntyre et al., 2007; El-Khalili et al., 2010; Bauer et al., 2009; Cutler et al., 2009; Weisler et al., 2009; Bortnick et al., 2011; Katila et al., 2013) - One positive six-week comparison to adjunctive lithium (Bauer et al., 2013) - One positive unpublished 52-week maintenance monotherapy trial (AstraZeneca, 2008) - One negative RCT (quetiapine augmentation of fluoxetine did not hasten acute response as compared to fluoxetine alone; Garakani et al., 2008) - One unpublished failed RCT (neither quetiapine nor escitalopram was better than placebo; AstraZeneca, 2007)
Risperidone	- Three positive placebo-controlled RCTs, dosage <2 mg/day (Mahmoud et al., 2007; Reeves et al., 2008; Keitner et al., 2009) - Two negative relapse prevention trials for depression (Alexopoulos et al., 2008; Rapaport et al., 2006)
Ziprasidone	No different from placebo in two RCTs (dosed up to 160 mg/day for 12 weeks in a study by Papakostas et al., 2012b; dosed at 80 mg/day or 160 mg/day as augmentation of sertraline in study by Dunner et al., 2007)

No studies of case reports with asenapine or iloperidone
Abbreviations: MDD = major depressive disorder; RCT = randomized controlled trial; SGA = second-generation antipsychotic; TRD = treatment-resistant depression

Table 13.9 IN esketamine acute RCTs in MDD

Authors	Design	Outcome
Canuso et al., 2018	Esketamine 84 mg/day versus placebo for four weeks	Depression symptoms improved significantly more with esketamine > placebo at four hours (*d* = 0.61) and 24 hours (*d* = 0.65) *but not Day 25* (*d* = 0.35); suicidal thinking better only at 24 hours
Daly et al., 2018b	Esketamine 28, 56, or 84 mg/day or placebo twice a week, with rerandomization of placebo nonresponders, then open-label once-weekly then bi-weekly	All esketamine doses > placebo (ascending dose-response relationship); response sustained for two months during maintenance low-dose open-label phase
Fedgchin et al., 2019	Esketamine 56 mg or 84 mg or placebo	No difference from placebo with 84 mg dose; 56 mg/day could not be formally tested
Popova et al., 2019	Esketamine flexibly dosed at 56 mg or 84 mg versus placebo for 28 days	Overall significant advantage for esketamine > placebo at Day 28. NNT for response = 6, NNT for remission = 5. ES for change in MADRS score = 0.30

Table 13.10 Pharmacotherapy strategies for depression relapse prevention after ECT

Strategy	Observed outcomes	Comment
Nortriptyline monotherapy	~60% relapse rate at six months (Sackeim et al., 2001)	Inferior to the combination of lithium + nortriptyline (Sackeim et al., 2001)
Lithium (dosed to target serum [lithium] = 0.5–0.7 mEq/L) + nortriptyline (dosed to target serum [nortriptyline] = 100–120 ng/mL)	~32% (Kellner et al., 2006) to 39% (Sackeim et al., 2001) relapse rate at 6 months	Comparable efficacy to venlafaxine + lithium (Prudic et al., 2013); higher relapse risk associated with younger age (Prudic et al., 2013)
Venlafaxine (target dose 300 mg/day) + nortriptyline or lithium	Comparable relapse rates and tolerability (Prudic et al., 2013)	Higher relapse risk associated with younger age (Prudic et al., 2013)

Table 13.11 Factors influencing antidepressant outcomes in bipolar depression

Favors antidepressant use	Discourages antidepressant use	Why?
BP II depression	BP I depression	Higher risk for TEAS in BP I than BP II (Altshuler et al., 2006); no evidence of adjunctive antidepressant superiority to placebo in BP I depression (McGirr et al., 2016)
No mixed features/ concomitant subthreshold hypomania	Any mixed features/ concomitant subthreshold hypomania	Even low-grade mixed features may increase risk for TEAS (Frye et al., 2009)
No past-year rapid cycling	Four or more episodes in past year	Ongoing antidepressant use among rapid cyclers increases risk for further relapses, particularly depressions (El-Mallakh et al., 2015)
Absence of mania in past few months	Manic or hypomanic episode in past few months	Better outcomes observed when antidepressants are used for depression following euthymia than for depression following mania/hypomania (MacQueen et al., 2002)
Absence of comorbid alcohol/substance use disorders	Presence of comorbid alcohol/ substance use disorders	Two observational studies have linked a history of alcohol or substance use disorders with an increased risk for TEAS during antidepressant therapy, with reported odds ratios ranging from 5.1 (95% CI = 1.31–19.64; Manwani et al., 2006) to 7.0 (95% CI = 1.6–32.3; Goldberg and Whiteside, 2002)
Prior favorable and robust antidepressant response	Past antidepressant nonresponse or incomplete response	In their prospective RCT, magnitude of initial antidepressant response significantly influenced likelihood of sustained wellness with long-term (one year) antidepressant continuation (Altshuler et al., 2009)
No personal history of antidepressant-associated mania/ hypomania	A personal history of antidepressant-associated mania/ hypomania	Recidivism suggests a patient-specific diathesis to TEAS; in a retrospective STEP-BD study, a history of previous TEAS increased the likelihood of future TEAS with other agents (Truman et al., 2007)
SLC6A4 homozygous *l/l* genotype	SLC6A4 homozygous *s/s* genotype	Modest increased risk for TEAS among "s" allele carriers (RR = 1.35, 95% CI = 1.04–1.76) (Daray et al., 2010)

Abbreviations: BP = bipolar disorder; CI = confidence interval; TEAS = treatment-emergent affective switch

Note that wide OIs mean less precise actual ORs

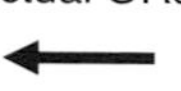

Table 13.12 Dosing of evidence-based treatments for bipolar depression

Agent	Dosing
Cariprazine	1.5–3 mg/day was most robustly associated with acute antidepressant efficacy in bipolar depression
Lumateperone	42 mg/day
Lurasidone	In flexible-dose monotherapy studies, low- (20–60 mg/day) and high- (80–120 mg/day) dose ranges produced identical effect sizes (*d* = 0.51). The eventual mean dose was seldom much higher than the starting dose in both the low-dose range (32 mg/day) and high-dose range (82 mg/day) (Loebel et al., 2014a)
OFC	Fixed-dose schedules examined olanzapine dosed at 6 or 12 mg/day paired with fluoxetine at 25 or 50 mg/day
Quetiapine	A target dose of 300 mg/day was used throughout acute RCTs in bipolar depression
Lamotrigine	The "target" dose of 200 mg/day was established from trials in relapse prevention (not acute treatment) of bipolar I disorder (Calabrese et al., 1999). Nevertheless, 200 mg/day has come to be viewed as a reasonable target dose in acute bipolar depression, despite the absence of an extensive evidence base. Anecdotally, higher doses (up to 400 mg/day) may sometimes help to fine tune a partial response

Abbreviations: OFC = olanzapine/fluoxetine combination

Table 13.13 Combination pharmacotherapy regimens studied in bipolar disorder

Medication combination	Targeted illness state	Outcome
SGA + mood stabilizer		
Olanzapine or placebo + lithium or divalproex (Tohen et al., 2004)	Relapse prevention over 18 months	Adjunctive olanzapine (n = 51, mean dose = 8.6 mg/day) > placebo (n = 48) for symptomatic (but not syndromal) relapse for either polarity. More weight gain, less insomnia with olanzapine than placebo
Aripiprazole or placebo + lithium or divalproex (Marcus et al., 2011)	Relapse prevention over 52 weeks	Adjunctive aripiprazole (n = 168, mean dose = 15.8–16.9 mg/day) > placebo (n = 169) for mania but not depression relapse
Olanzapine, risperidone or placebo + lithium or divalproex (Yatham et al., 2016)	Relapse prevention over 52 weeks	Either adjunctive SGA (n = 52) produced longer time until relapse than did adjunctive placebo up to 24 weeks but not significant advantage over placebo at 52 weeks
Ziprasidone or placebo + lithium or divalproex (Bowden et al., 2010)	Eight-week open-label stabilization, 16 weeks continuation	Ziprasidone (n = 127, stratified doses of 80, 119 or, 160 mg/day) more effective than placebo in time until any mood episode of either polarity
Multiple mood stabilizers		
Lithium + divalproex versus either monotherapy (BALANCE) (BALANCE Investigators and Collaborators, 2010)	Relapse prevention for 24 months	Lithium + divalproex (n = 110) > divalproex (n = 110) but not lithium (n = 110) monotherapies; comparable tolerability
Oxcarbazepine versus placebo + lithium (Vieta et al., 2008a)	Relapse prevention over 52 weeks	Oxcarbazepine (n = 26, mean dose = 1200 mg/day) no better than placebo

Negative trials or conditions with no data are shaded
Abbreviations: SGA = second-generation antipsychotic

Table 13.14 Common complex clinical and comorbid presentations in bipolar disorder

Comorbid condition	Treatment regimen
Bipolar disorder + alcohol use disorders	- TAU + divalproex > TAU + placebo in alcohol use/heavy drinking (but no better than TAU to improve mood symptoms) (Salloum et al., 2005) - Adjunctive topiramate (based on RCTs for alcohol use disorders independent of bipolar disorder; see Chapter 18)
Bipolar disorder + binge eating	- Adjunctive lisdexamfetamine (small (n = 25) eight-week preliminary RCT versus placebo in context of bipolar depression; McElroy et al., 2015)
Bipolar disorder + anxiety	- Adjunctive gabapentin (may improve anxiety and alcohol symptoms in bipolar patients based on open-label data) (Perugi et al., 2002)
Bipolar disorder + ADD/ attentional processing problems	- Adjunctive lisdexamfetamine (mean dose = 60 mg/day) over four weeks in affectively stable bipolar adult outpatients improved ADD symptoms, mood, weight, and lipid parameters (McIntyre et al., 2013) - Observational (nonrandomized) studies suggest that adjunctive methylphenidate when added after antimanic mood-stabilizing agents are in place appears safe and effective (Viktorin et al., 2017)

Abbreviations: ADD = attention deficit disorder; RCT = randomized controlled trial; TAU = treatment as usual

Table 13.15 Evidence-based treatments for reducing relapse risk in rapid cycling

Intervention	Outcome
Lamotrigine	Possible advantage for time until relapse in BP II > BP I disorder (Calabrese et al., 2000)
Lithium + divalproex	The likelihood of achieving an acute response appears greater with the combination than either monotherapy (Calabrese et al., 2005)
Nimodipine	Small proof-of-concept (on-off-on design, n = 12) in ultra-rapid-cycling bipolar patients (Pazzaglia et al., 1993) Isradipine, another *l*-type dihydropyridine, has been observed less systematically to exert similar effects
Suprametabolic thyroid hormone	Following early preliminary observational data citing "clear-cut response" in 10/11 rapid-cycling bipolar patients (Bauer and Whybrow, 1990), a later RCT of adjunctive levothyroxine (but not triiodothyronine) significantly reduced amount of time spent depressed or mixed, and increased the amount of time spent euthymic (Walshaw et al., 2018)

Abbreviations: BP = bipolar disorder; RCT = randomized controlled trial

Table 13.16 Practical considerations using lithium

Consideration	Comment
Timing and interpretation of serum lithium levels	Although "trough" levels refer to measurements made immediately before a next dose, by convention serum lithium levels are drawn and interpreted based on levels obtained 10–14 hours after a last dose. As noted in Chapter 7, serum levels are established for acute mania and maintenance treatment, but not in relation to judging efficacy in acute depressive episodes
Coadministration with other agents	NSAIDs inhibit prostaglandins, thereby constricting renal artery blood flow, decreasing lithium clearance, and potentially increasing serum lithium levels by ~20% ACE inhibitors can ↑ serum lithium levels by ~36% Spironolactone can ↑ serum lithium levels by ~16% Thiazide diuretics can ↑ serum lithium levels due to reabsorption in the proximal tubule
ECG concerns	Sick sinus syndrome, T-wave flattening or inversion
Abrupt cessation	Discontinuation faster than over two weeks has been shown to hasten time until a next affective episode (either polarity (mania HR = 2.8, depression HR = 5.4) (Faedda et al., 1993)
Minimizing renal impairment	Once-daily dosing may reduce nephrotoxicity by reducing the number of Cmax events per day
Thyroid considerations	About 5% of patients who take lithium will develop hypothyroidism; those with autoantibodies are predisposed

Abbreviations: ACE = angiotensin-converting enzyme; ECG = electrocardiogram; HR = hazard ratio; NSAIDs = nonsteroidal anti-inflammatory drugs

Table 13.17 Psychotropic profiles of anticonvulsants

Agent	Mania	Depression	Anxiety	Neuropathic pain	Insomnia	Binge eating
Carbamazepine	✓	3 RCTs [a]	No RCTs	✓ (trigeminal neuralgia)	No RCTs	No RCTs
Divalproex	✓	3 (+) RCTs	? [h]	✓ (migraine)	No RCTs	No RCTs
Eslicarbazepine	1 (+) RCT [b]	No RCTs	No RCTs	No RCTs	No RCTs	No RCTs
Gabapentin	2 (–) RCTs [c,d]	No RCTs	✓	✓	✓	No RCTs
Lamotrigine	2 (–) RCTs [e]	✓	No RCTs	No RCTs	No RCTs	No RCTs
Oxcarbazepine	1 (–) RCT [f]	?	No RCTs	No RCTs	No RCTs	No RCTs
Tiagabine	No RCTs	No RCTs	No RCTs	No RCTs	No RCTs	No RCTs
Topiramate	4 (–) RCTs [g]	No RCTs	No RCTs	No RCTs	No RCTs	✓

✓ indicates a well-established clinical niche with multiple (+) RCTs
[a] Mostly on/off/on designs with ambiguous results (reviewed by Reinares et al., 2013)
[b] Grunze et al., 2015
[c] Pande et al., 2000a
[d] Frye et al., 2000
[e] Unpublished industry trials
[f] Wagner et al., 2006
[g] Kushner et al., 2006
[h] Secondary analyses of RCTs for bipolar depression demonstrate significant reductions in Hamilton Anxiety scores
Abbreviations: RCT = randomized controlled trials

Table 13.18 Compare and contrast: SGAs in bipolar disorder – D_2/D_3 partial agonists

Agent	Mania	Depression	Relapse prevention
Aripiprazole	Two (+) RCTs (FDA registration)	Two (–) RCTs (Thase et al., 2008). However, initial separation from placebo lost in the final week of each trial	Two (+) RCTs for prevention of mania but not depression (oral; Keck et al., 2007 or LAI (Calabrese et al., 2017b)) – although index episode of mania enriches design for mania rather than depression prevention
Brexpiprazole	Two (-) RCTs (https://investor.lundbeck.com/news-releases/news-release-details/lundbeck-and-otsuka-report-phase-iii-data-evaluating)	No data	No data
Cariprazine	Three (+) RCTs (Calabrese et al., 2015; Durgam et al., 2015; Sachs et al., 2015)	Two (+) RCTs (FDA registration)	No data

Abbreviations: FDA = US Food and Drug Administration; LAI = long-acting injectable; RCT = randomized controlled trial; SGA = second-generation antipsychotic

Table 13.19 Compare and contrast: SGAs in bipolar disorder - D_2 antagonists

Agent	Mania	Depression	Relapse prevention
Asenapine	Two (+) acute (three-week) RCTs, mean dose = 18.3 mg/day, composite *g* = 0.42 (Vita et al., 2013); and improvement of depressive symptoms during mania (Szegedi et al., 2011)	No data	One (+) RCT, prevention of both manic and depressive episodes (Szegedi et al., 2018)
Iloperidone	No data	No data	No data
Lumateperone	No data	One (+) six-week RCT (Durgam et al., 2019)	No data
Lurasidone	No data, although post hoc analyses in bipolar depression show improvement of mixed subthreshold mania symptoms (McIntyre et al., 2015)	Two (+) RCTs (monotherapy (Loebel et al., 2014a); augmentation of lithium or divalproex (Loebel et al., 2014b), flexibly dosed; identical effect sizes (*d* = 0.51) at low dose (mean 32 mg/day) or high dose (mean 82 mg/day) monotherapy	One (-) RCT as augmentation (20–80 mg/day) of lithium or divalproex (Calabrese et al., 2017a)
Olanzapine	Two (+) RCTs (FDA registration)	Two (+) RCT (Tohen et al., 2013) [a]	Two (+) RCTs (FDA registration)
Paliperidone	Two (+) three-week RCTs (Vieta et al., 2010; Berwaerts et al., 2012b); one (-) RCT + lithium or divalproex (Berwaerts et al., 2011)	No data	One (+) RCT after treatment of acute mania; significantly longer median time to recurrence with paliperidone (558 days) than placebo (283 days) (Berwaerts et al., 2012a)
Quetiapine	Two (+) RCTs	Two (+) RCTs	One (+) adjunctive RCT
Risperidone	Two (+) RCTs	No data	One (-) RCT (LAI)
Ziprasidone	Two (+) acute monotherapy RCTs (Potkin et al., 2005; Keck et al., 2003); one (-) adjunctive trial added to lithium or divalproex (Sachs et al., 2012)	Two (-) RCTs (Lombardo et al., 2012; Sachs et al., 2011); NNT = 144	One (+) six-month maintenance trial; longer median time to intervention for a mood episode with adjunctive ziprasidone (43 days) versus mood stabilizer alone (26.5 days) (Bowden et al., 2010)

Is 16.5 days longer so clinically meaning-ful?

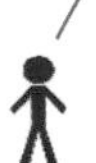

[a] In post hoc analyses, olanzapine monotherapy (without adjunctive fluoxetine) improved all MADRS depression symptom items better than placebo except for suicidal thinking and concentration problems; baseline melancholic features were predictive of antidepressant response to olanzapine monotherapy (Tohen et al., 2013)

Abbreviations: FDA = US Food and Drug Administration; LAI = long-acting injectable; NNT = number needed to treat; RCT = randomized controlled trial; SGA = second-generation antipsychotic

14 Disorders of Impulsivity, Compulsivity, and Aggression

LEARNING OBJECTIVES

- ☐ Understand features of impulsivity, compulsivity, and impulsive aggression as manifestations of dysregulated cortico-limbic ("top-down") and limbo-cortical ("bottom-up") circuitry
- ☐ Define the cognitive construct of *salience*
- ☐ Describe the evidence base for serotonergic antidepressants, lithium, anticonvulsants, FGAs and SGAs in treating disorders of impulsivity, compulsivity, and impulsive aggression
- ☐ Describe evidence-based pharmacotherapy options for treatment of aggression in the setting of psychosis
- ☐ Describe the strengths and limitations of evidence-based pharmacotherapies studied for nonsuicidal self-injurious forms of behavior

It is hard to fight against impulsive desire; whatever it wants it will buy at the cost of the soul.

- Heraclitus

In this chapter we will focus on dimensional constructs of impulsive versus compulsive behaviors and their interface with aggression in relation to pharmacotherapy. Like so many other psychopathological states, impulsivity and compulsivity are not pathognomonic of any particular categorical diagnostic entity and may fit within the broader constellation of numerous conditions that affect mood, development, personality, addiction, cognition, and perception. Particular issues arise when considering trait versus state features of psychopathology and environmental factors that may exacerbate or otherwise contribute to an underlying diathesis.

We will begin with some definitions, followed by a quick review of pertinent neural circuitry that bears on relevant psychopathology and psychopharmacology (Box 14.1).

Tip

A hallmark distinction between obsessions and delusions is that people with obsessive thoughts usually recognize the content as peculiar, unreasonable, senseless, or excessive; delusions, by definition, involve poor reality testing and their content may often seem plausible and rational.

Box 14.1

- ***Impulses*** are irresistible urges to perform an action; little if any planning and forethought bear influence over the desirability, acceptability, and consequences of the action, making deliberation relatively absent from the mental process.
- ***Obsessions*** are persistent and disturbing preoccupations which maintain someone's attention mainly because of anxiety related to the content of thought, rather than because of its validity or objective importance to an individual. Obsessions may thus take the form of *intrusive thoughts* (e.g., an uncontrollable and distressing urge to jump in front of a moving train even though one has no wish to die). Obsessions can be contrasted with *ruminations*, which are repetitive and perseverative thoughts involving negative content, usually leading to amplified emotional distress. They tend not to be "senseless" the way obsessions usually are.
- ***Compulsions*** are behaviors that typically arise in response to the impulse to perform an action, usually in an effort to relieve anxiety or distress. In that sense their driving force may reflect underlying circuitry based more on anxiolysis than the pursuit of reward. Anxiety relief from compulsive behaviors may be transient, and may involve associated feelings of shame, guilt, or isolation.

In order to tie together obsessive or ruminative thoughts with impulses toward actions aimed to alleviate distress, and then turn toward their relevant pharmacotherapies, let us consider the neural circuitry involved in logical planning, reasoning, and deliberation as balanced with more primordial drives and urges.

> **Who's Who**
>
> ***DLPFC***: the dorsolateral prefrontal cortex, involved in motivation and executive function
>
> ***ACC***: The anterior cingulate cortex, regulating affect, selective attention, social interactions
>
> ***Limbic system***: Comprised of the amygdala, hippocampus, and maybe sometimes additional structures as described in Box 14.1 (and see also Figure 15.1 in Chapter 15).

A TOP-DOWN (COLD) AND BOTTOM-UP (HOT) COGNITION

Prefrontal cortical structures that govern executive functioning (planning, organizing, problem-solving, deliberative reasoning) maintain a balance with subcortical limbic regions that drive urges and emotional reactivity to environmental threats or other stimuli – an all-important circuit often referred to as the *corticolimbic loop*, depicted in Figure 14.1. Ordinarily there exists an equilibrium such that prefrontal (specifically, orbitofrontal and anterior cingulate) rational and deliberative "cold" processes temper or regulate (from the "top down") more evolutionarily primitive "hot" emotional urges and impulses driven by limbic structures (from the "bottom up"). Derangement of this balance impacts numerous forms of psychopathology in ways that are easy enough to envision. Put in the language of dialectical behavior therapy (DBT), the rational "wise mind" exerts prefrontal control over more limbic and paralimbic "emotional mind" structures, creating a dialectic or kind of metaphysical contradiction that needs vigilant oversight (mindfulness) to maintain a sense of psychic balance.

B MORE ON THE PFC, ACC, AND LIMBIC/PARALIMBIC CIRCUITRY

The schematic in Figure 14.1 is greatly oversimplified in several respects. For one, there is some debate over what structures besides the *amygdala* and *hippocampus* technically hold unequivocal membership in the limbic system. The limbic system is where subcortical and cortical structures relevant to emotional processing meet. The term "paralimbic" is sometimes used to identify structures in relevant border zones.

Like a rock band whose classic lineup is occasionally augmented by session musicians or players from other bands, certain anatomical structures that are not universally regarded as "official" components of the limbic system have at times nevertheless been associated with limbic functions. The *hypothalamus* and *mammillary bodies* often serve as touring members,

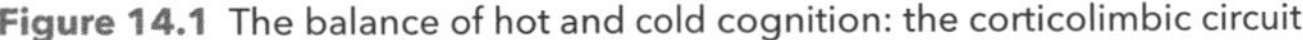

Figure 14.1 The balance of hot and cold cognition: the corticolimbic circuit.

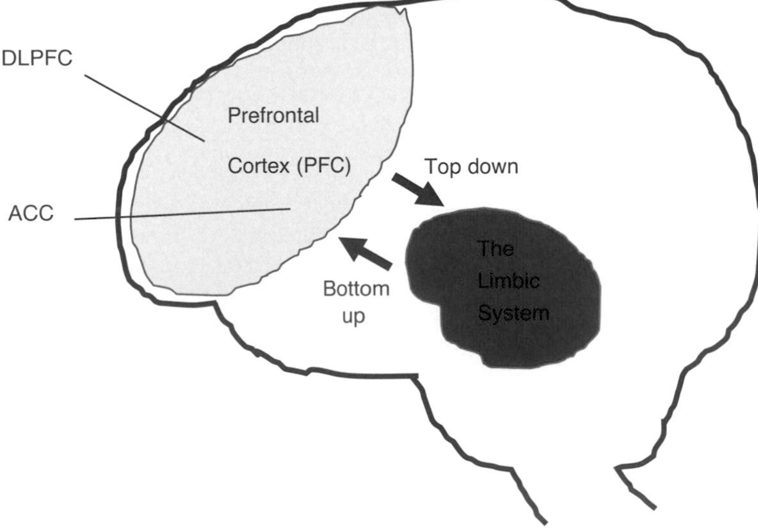

accompanied sometimes by the *anterior nuclei of the thalamus*. Additionally, the *insula* (aka the anterior insular cortex; a cortical structure embedded within the lateral sulcus) and the *fornix* (a C-shaped fiber bundle that conveys output from the hippocampus) are also often considered elements of the limbic system.

Paralimbic structures from the border zone include the *orbitofrontal cortex* (OFC, involved in decision-making, inhibition, and social cognition) and parts of the *ACC*. The ACC has a dorsal component (involved in cognitive processing) and a ventral component (more directly linked to emotional processing). Therefore, the ventral ACC is often identified as a limbic band member, while the dorsal ACC sits in the control booth in a more monitoring/production role (appraising threat, maintaining attention, and tending to working memory).

The *reward pathway* (comprised of the *ventral tegmentum* and *nucleus accumbens*), viewed as synonymous with the mesolimbic pathway, figures prominently in incentive-based behavior.

And finally, what about the PFC – the wise mind, in DBT language? We can divide that into three subcomponents:

- *DLPFC*: The dorsolateral prefrontal cortex is involved in higher cognitive functions such as shifting attention, working memory, and response inhibition.
- *VMPFC*: The ventromedial prefrontal cortex is anatomically synonymous with the OFC.
- *VLPFC*: The ventrolateral prefrontal cortex plays a role in response inhibition, particularly involving motor activity.

Box 14.2 defines core terminology related to cortico-limbic system function and dysfunction.

Box 14.2

Key Terminology Related to Limbic System Function and Dysfunction

Working Memory

Working memory is an executive function that refers to one's short-term memory capacity to "hold things in mind," such as a set of instructions, or remembering contingency plans (e.g., if the store has no skim milk then buy 1% but make sure to get organic). A reduced working memory capacity may be associated with increased trait impulsivity, although the directionality of this relationship is uncertain (Gunn and Finn, 2013).

Salience Network

"Salience" means that a given stimulus stands out as distinct from others. The salience network, involving the dorsal anterior cingulate cortex and the anterior insula, is relevant to gauging motivation to pursue (incentive/reward) or avoid (aversive) particular stimuli. In psychosis, aberrant salience may become assigned to distorted internal representations of external stimuli. Attention that is driven by salient stimuli is largely a bottom-up cognitive process. More on this later.

Somatic Marker Hypothesis

The proposition that conscious decision-making is guided in part by awareness of visceral sensations that help someone appraise a stimulus as likely having a positive versus negative outcome (thought to be processed through the VMPFC).

So, I might use an antipsychotic drug to modulate the fear circuitry involved when my psychotic patient assigns abnormal salience to benign stimuli in the environment, and his bottom-up limbic activity overdrives his capacity to make more rational judgments about perceived threats, 'cause his faulty working memory and executive dysfunction can't exert adequate top-down regulation in order to maintain homeostasis?

Mainly that's correct except we don't know for sure if bottom-up limbic activity is really overdriving things in schizophrenia or if it's more just the loss of top-down regulation. You could speculate about other conditions though in which the dynamic interplay of hot and cold cognition becomes lost and impairment of both top-down and bottom-up processes causes trouble.

Trauma maybe? Addictions? Severe personality disorders?

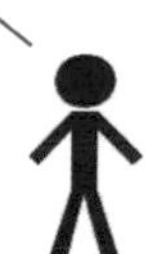

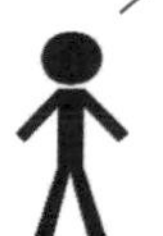

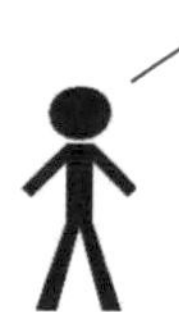

C DISORDERS OF IMPULSE CONTROL

Intact top-down regulation of hot cognitive processes holds impulses and urges in check. One can imagine a variety of psychopathological states in which disinhibition stands as a hallmark feature, whether overdriven from below (e.g., via reward circuitry, autonomic hyperarousal and fear circuitry, inappropriate assignment of salience, or anxious apprehension and relief from emotional distress,) or underdriven from above (e.g., impaired attentional processing or executive functioning). Consider these neural functions when conceptualizing psychiatric phenomena (such as psychosis, anxiety, or cognitive complaints) and contemplating the role of psychotropic medications to target subjective complaints and objective signs.

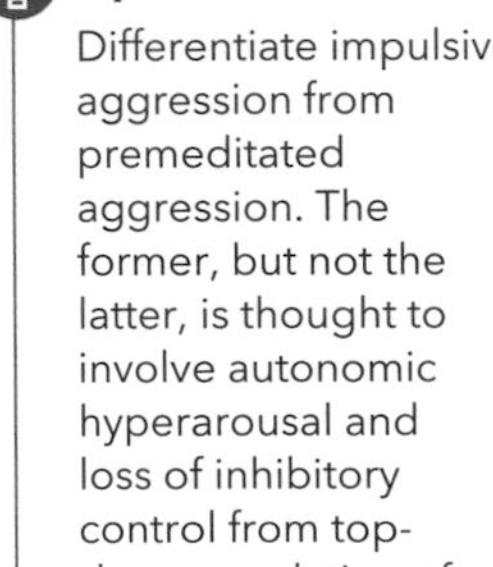

Tip

Differentiate impulsive aggression from premeditated aggression. The former, but not the latter, is thought to involve autonomic hyperarousal and loss of inhibitory control from top-down regulation of corticolimbic circuitry.

D IMPULSIVITY AND AGGRESSION

A wide range of psychiatric conditions may result from the common starting point of an impaired executive capacity to over-ride impulses, including personality disorders, mood disorders (both unipolar and bipolar), anxiety disorders, post-traumatic stress disorder, dissociative disorders, addictions and substance use disorders, dementias, traumatic brain injury, developmental disabilities, and conditions secondary to other medical conditions (e.g., malignancy, stroke).

From a pharmacotherapeutic standpoint, no single medication realistically treats all of impulsivity and aggression for all comers irrespective of the clinical context. For instance, impulsivity and impulsive aggression may present uniquely in mood-disordered versus dementia patients versus addictions. We might therefore consider both the phenomenology and pharmacotherapy of impulsivity and aggression across key subtypes of psychopathology, starting with mood disorders.

E IRRITABILITY AND ANGER IN AFFECTIVE AND PSYCHOTIC DISORDERS

While some clinicians believe that prominent irritability is in itself a robust differentiator of polarity in mood disorders, the evidence base points instead to irritability as a polarity-independent phenomenon that may simply capture other broad aspects of affective disturbance. Notably, in the STAR*D MDD trials, 40% of MDD patients reported feelings of irritability more than half the time, arising especially in women, younger patients, those who were unemployed, and those with a history of one or more suicide attempts (Perlis et al., 2005). Relatedly, a series of studies by Fava and Rosenbaum (1998) examined the phenomenology of anger attacks in the course of clinical depression. In these studies, anger attacks were likened to panic attacks with respect to suddenness of onset and their association with autonomic signs (e.g., tachycardia, sweating, chest-tightness). In related placebo-controlled trials, the frequency of anger attacks was reduced with the use of sertraline (by 53%) or imipramine (by 57%) (Fava et al., 1997).

In bipolar disorder, anger and irritability are considered to be more state-dependent phenomena that arise in the context of other psychomotor and affective signs of a discrete syndrome. Impulsivity per se, however, has been shown to be a persistent trait phenomenon that is independent of mood states in adults with bipolar disorder (Swann et al., 2001). Persistent, trait-based features of anger and irritability are more characteristic of chronic, nonepisodic conditions such as borderline and other personality disorders, dementia, developmental disabilities, traumatic brain injury, and substance use disorders (related to intoxication/withdrawal states).

In people with schizophrenia and other primary psychotic disorders, an increased risk for impulsive aggression has been linked with cognitive deficits and negative emotionality (Ahmed et al., 2018a). It can also arise from psychotic misperception, impulsive reactions, and deliberately intimidating behavior (Volavka and Citrome, 2011) and is thought to involve orbitofrontal and temporal lobe dysfunction (Soyka, 2011). FGAs and SGAs have collectively shown value in reducing impulsive-aggressive behavior in schizophrenia, as discussed further later in this chapter.

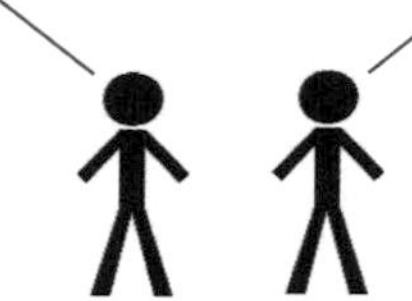

You're quite the biological reductionist. Can't there just be some people who are temperamentally predisposed, for whatever reasons, to rash behavior, hasty thinking, and a tendency to be gruff?
I couldn't agree more, which is why we want to determine if there is evidence of psychopathology accompanying those kinds of features. Remember from Chapter 2, we're looking for constellations of signs and symptoms that point to a clinical syndrome, before assuming that psychopharmacology is appropriate or likely to be helpful – not to address a symptom in isolation, but as the tell-tale indicator of a broader condition.

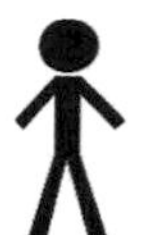

Yeah, like what about plain old psychopathy?

That's premeditated aggression, not impulsive aggression, you nitwit! Pay attention! And don't make me get angry at you.

Serotonergic Antidepressants

Serotonergic circuitry has long been implicated in the neurobiology of hostility and impulsive aggression. Correspondingly, SSRIs have a well-established database for treatment of impulsive aggression, particularly in the setting of borderline personality disorder. In clinical practice, the question often arises about how best to gauge the likelihood that "agitation" and irritability in a patient with depression symptoms would likely improve or worsen, if agitation and irritability were construed as reflecting possible mania or hypomania (which monoaminergic antidepressants could potentially exacerbate, as discussed in Chapter 13). Table 14.1 presents a summary of empirical trial findings using serotonergic antidepressants targeting impulsive aggression.

F LITHIUM AND IMPULSIVE AGGRESSION

Despite common perception that lithium exerts a distinct anti-impulsivity/antiaggressivity effect in people (some experts think that lithium's antisuicide effect mainly reflects its anti-impulsivity properties, putting a "brake" on the impulse to act on suicidal thoughts), formal literature examining this specific domain is scant, impressionistic, and rather dated. Sheard and colleagues (1976), studying 66 young (ages 16–24) prison inmates with "chronic impulsive aggressive behavior," reported "significant reductions in aggressive behavior" as judged by "decreased infractions involving violence." Another early study, in children with "sporadic unprovoked physical aggression," reported "a substantial reduction in unprovoked aggressive outbursts" while taking lithium over three months, although quantitative outcome measures were not included (Siassi, 1982).

Formal studies of lithium targeting aggressive behavior in children and adolescents with conduct disorder have produced mixed findings. One retrospective study of 60 youths with conduct disorder found that lithium led to a significant reduction in overaggressive behavior, with effect sizes across submeasures >0.80, over an approximate eight-month study period (Masi et al., 2009). In hospitalized children aged under 13 with aggressive conduct disorder (n = 61), lithium and haloperidol both were superior to placebo in reducing aggressive behavior, although adverse effects were more extensive with haloperidol (Campbell et al., 1984). A later four-week RCT in hospitalized children with conduct disorder found significantly greater reductions in overt aggression with lithium than placebo (Malone et al., 2000), although another two-week placebo-controlled trial of lithium in a similar inpatient study group found *no benefit* for reducing aggressive behaviors (Rifkin et al., 1997). Another six-week RCT of lithium (mean dose 1248 mg/day, mean serum [lithium] 1.12 mEq/L) versus placebo in children with conduct disorder "hospitalized for treatment-refractory severe aggressiveness and explosiveness" found a significant but only modest effect of lithium, varying based on the outcome measure used (Campbell et al., 1995). Interpretation of these findings may involve the extent to which aggressive behavior in children with conduct disorder is reliably impulsive versus intentional and deliberate.

Use of lithium for behavioral control problems in children or adults with autism or other developmental disorders is supported by a more modest empirical literature. One small (n = 14) retrospective study reported improvement in 73.7% of those for whom lithium was added to an existing regimen, with anecdotal impressions of a more robust effect in those with comorbid ADHD (Mintz and Hollenberg, 2019).

G ANTICONVULSANTS FOR IMPULSIVE AGGRESSION

As a class, anticonvulsant drugs have long garnered interest as possible remedies for impulsive aggression based on hypotheses that enhanced GABAergic tone might confer antiexcitatory/pro-inhibitory CNS effects. Anticonvulsants actually vary substantially across their individual psychotropic properties, including those related to impulsive aggression. Collectively, data appear to be strongest for the targeted use of divalproex and for topiramate; Table 14.2 provides a summary of the evidence base for their use across clinical populations with impulsive aggression.

H FGAs AND SGAs FOR AGGRESSION IN PSYCHOTIC DISORDERS

In their systematic review of eight RCTs of FGAs or SGAs targeting the treatment of impulsive aggression across several psychiatric disorders (schizophrenia, borderline personality disorder, and PTSD), Goedhard and colleagues (2006) concluded that the overall antiaggressive efficacy for antipsychotics was modest, noting relatively short study durations, small sample sizes, and outcome measures that do not necessarily capture incident-based behaviors. On the other hand, a retrospective review of naturalistic treatment outcomes for autistic youth (mean age 15.1 years) taking two or more antipsychotics found significant improvement in agitation/irritability, physical aggression, and self-injury (Wink et al., 2017). A review by Victoroff et al. (2014) determined that clozapine managed overt aggression better than haloperidol or chlorpromazine, and was more effective than olanzapine or haloperidol for managing aggression in physically assaultive inpatients; that meta-analysis concluded that overall, paliperidone-XR was the most effective and most evidence-based option for managing hostility among schizophrenia inpatients.

Findings from antipsychotic RCTs targeting impulsive aggression are summarized in Table 14.3.

A meta-analysis across RCTs of antipsychotics or benzodiazepines targeting acute agitation and aggression compared agents across PANSS-excitement components (EC) subscale changes from baseline and relative to placebo, with findings as summarized in Figure 14.2. Note that largest effects, depicted as weighted mean changes, are seen with olanzapine, risperidone, or haloperidol plus promethazine.

Tip

Contrary to popular belief, beta-blockers have *not* been shown to commonly cause depression, according to a meta-analysis of 15 RCTs involving >35 000 subjects – in which the absolute annual risk was calculated as 6 per 1000 patients (Ko et al., 2002)

Why don't psychiatrists use much phenytoin, or even think of it very often, for things like impulsive aggression?

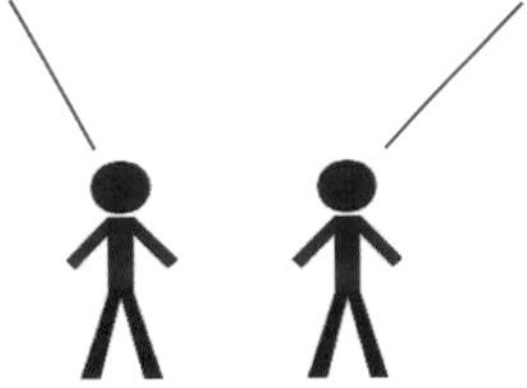

So, you know from Chapter 13 that, contrary to popular legend, the psychotropic effects of anticonvulsants vary greatly and most have *not* been shown to help regulate mood. Phenytoin has been studied more for aggressive behavior than mood symptoms per se, although there actually are small pilot studies suggesting its possible value for mania and relapse prevention in bipolar patients (see, e.g., Bersudsky, 2006). Mainly, its extensive side effects and drug interactions limited enthusiasm for its further exploration and development of its psychotropic profile.

Figure 14.2 PANSS-EC weighted mean changes across antipsychotics and benzodiazepine RCTs. Adapted from Bak et al., 2019.

Benzodiazepine RCTs

Placebo	ZIP	LEV	HAL	RIS + CLON	LOR	RIS + LOR	HAL +	ARI	OLZ	RIS	HAL + PRO
5 RCTs n = 261	1 RCT n = 79	2 RCTs n = 62	5 RCTs n = 205	1 RCT n = 104	2 RCTs n = 117	1 RCT n = 83	2 RCTs n = 109	2 RCTs n = 40	13 RCTs n = 612	1 RCT n = 14	1 RCT n = 27

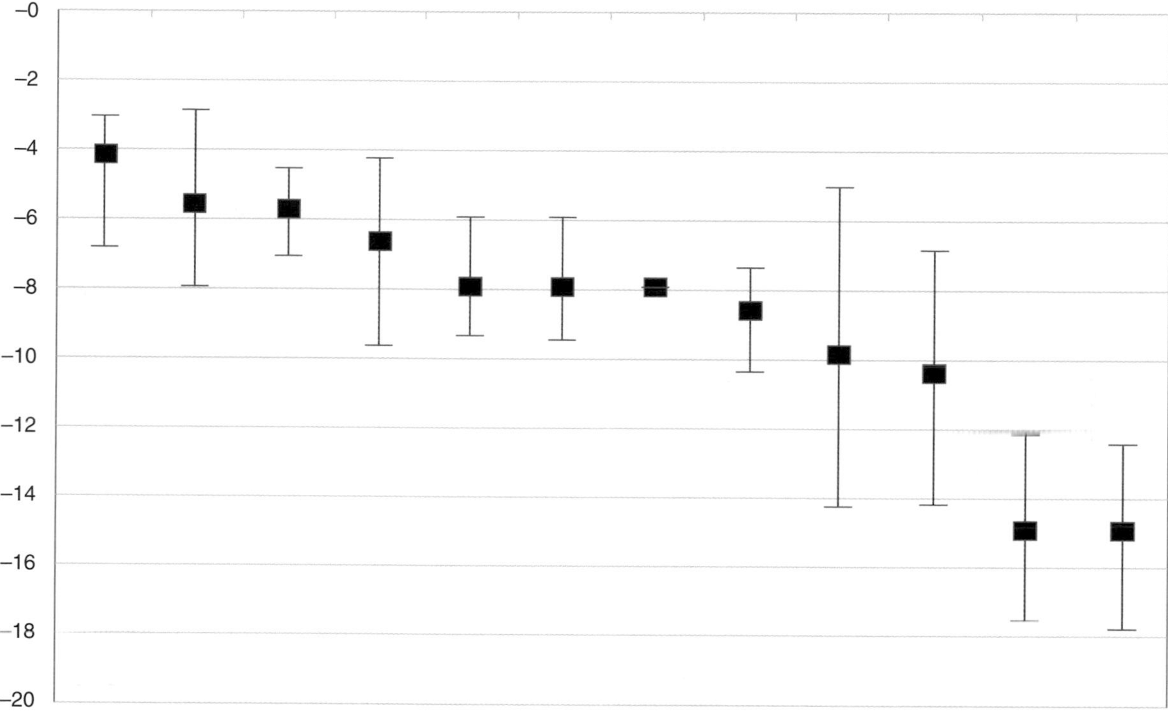

Abbreviations: ZIP = ziprasidone; LEV = levopromazine; HAL = haloperidol; RIS = risperidone; CLON = clonazepam; LOR = lorazepam; ARI = aripiprazole; OLZ = olanzapine; PRO = promethazine

So there I am in the ER with an impulsive aggressive patient who's threatening me and everyone else around him. No time for differential diagnosis or reading review papers. How should I manage the situation pharmacologically?

It certainly helps to know what the underlying ailment is. Agitation in someone with frontal lobe disease won't likely get better with benzodiazepines, and psychotic agitation from phencyclidine isn't so wise to treat with antipsychotics. A toxic delirium can probably be managed reasonably well with any antipsychotic – except, manic delirium is better treated with benzodiazepines, the same as catatonic excitement. Or, someone who's combative because they're in alcohol withdrawal needs benzodiazepines. You really do need to clarify the nature of the underlying problem, I'm afraid.

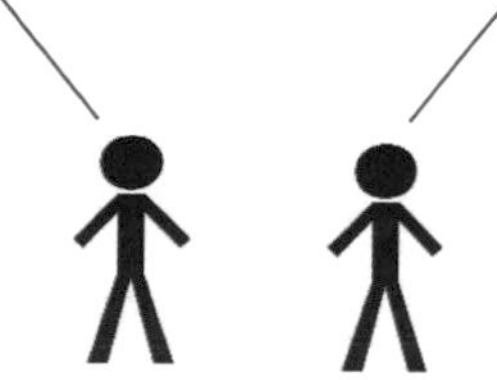

Consider the following case (Clinical Vignette 14.1):

CLINICAL VIGNETTE 14.1

Izzy was a 24-year-old man with nonverbal autism whose problems with impulse control and low frustration tolerance were easily set off by the slightest of variations in his daily routine. In addition to a behavior management plan implemented by the group home in which he lived, divalproex 1500 mg/day (serum [valproate] = 74 μg/mL) had been used with partial success in reducing incidents of "anger-out" explosive rage (punching, hitting) in response to frustrations. During a routine physical exam he was noted on laboratory testing to have a low white blood cell (WBC) count of 3.1 per μL with an absolute neutrophil count (ANC) of 1.7 × 10^9/L (normal reference range = 1.5–8.0 × 10^9/L). Concern was raised about whether divalproex was causing his mild leukopenia. No thrombocytopenia was evident nor were other blood cell lines abnormal. Previous complete blood counts (CBCs) were unavailable for comparison. There was no history of infections. Izzy's mother shared that she too had often been told by doctors that she had "low WBCs." Izzy's ancestry was neither African nor Middle Eastern, to the best of his parents' knowledge, Making the diagnosis of benign ethnic neutropenia possible but less compelling. After divalproex was lowered to 1000 mg/day Izzy's counsellors noted a worsening of his anger outbursts and asked if his usual higher divalproex dose could be resumed. His repeat CBC values on less divalproex were not appreciably better and the primary care doctor advised stopping the divalproex and having Izzy see a hematologist. A consultant advised replacing the divalproex with an SGA but his psychiatrist was less eager to do that after having read Goedhard et al.'s (2006) underwhelming review of antipsychotics for chronic impulsive aggression. Instead, the psychiatrist opted to add lithium to the divalproex, both for its potential value for impulsive aggression as well as its hematopoetic potential to counter leukopenia, as discussed in Chapter 10.

I BETA-BLOCKERS AND IMPULSIVE AGGRESSION

Interest in, and evidence for, using beta-blockers to treat impulsive aggression comes originally from an older (and largely case-based) literature for conditions ranging from traumatic brain injury to developmental disorders, dementia, and other neurological conditions (e.g., Huntington's disease). Most extensively studied has been *propranolol* (dosed up to 200 mg/day), or the long-acting peripheral beta-blocker *nadolol* (dosed to 80 mg/day). Studies with propranolol in patients with rage attacks associated with head trauma or chronic neuropsychiatric conditions (e.g., Wilson's disease, epilepsy, or developmental disorders) have mostly involved case reports and open trials, with dosing as high as 520 mg/day (Yudofsky et al., 1981). Two favorable placebo-controlled trials of nadolol in forensic populations (violent inpatients) include: (a) a three-week trial of 80 or 120 mg/day in 30 diverse inpatients, yielding improvement in BPRS "hostility" and "activation" factors (Alpert et al., 1990) and (b) a 17-week RCT in 41 chronic inpatients with aggressive outbursts (fewer aggressive outbursts were prospectively observed over the 17-week period) (Ratey et al., 1992). Another placebo-controlled trial of nadolol 120 mg/day in 24 male schizophrenia inpatients revealed initial improvement but ultimately no difference from placebo, regardless of the presence or absence of akathisia (Allan et al., 1996). Of note, a small crossover study found benefit with pindolol (both a nonselective beta-blocker and a $5HT_{1A}$ autoreceptor antagonist, as described in Chapter 6, Figure 6.1) in 11 patients with "impulsive/explosive behaviors" secondary to CNS injury (Greendyke and Kanter, 1986).

While the mechanism by which beta-blockers may help manage impulsive aggression remains uncertain, the effects of *peripheral* NE blockade (as occurs with nadolol) raise speculation about diminishing autonomic stimulation, as described in the somatic marker hypothesis (see Box 14.2).

J INTERMITTENT EXPLOSIVE DISORDER

Intermittent explosive disorder (IED) is sometimes considered a diagnosis of exclusion for people with sudden rage attacks (particularly in young men) that are not better accounted for by other psychiatric conditions that impair control over aggressive impulses. The diagnosis carries some degree of controversy when issues related to social accountability or legal consequences arise in the aftermath of violent behaviors. The pharmacotherapy literature on IED is small, largely unreplicated, and focused mainly on the potential utility of SSRIs such as fluoxetine, as described earlier in Table 14.1. The question sometimes arises as to whether an antimanic mood stabilizer such as lithium or divalproex would be preferable to a serotonergic antidepressant based on concerns that IED symptoms could, for some patients, reflect a bipolar diathesis. In the absence of

This is all very interesting, but, in what kind of patients, if any, should I consider actually using beta-blockers to treat impulsive aggression? They're not so mainstream. And should that be propranolol or nadolol or another one?

Either of those beta-blockers would be a viable and evidence-based option to consider in any impulsively aggressive patient with TBI, conduct disorder, or a psychotic disorder whose aggression is inadequately responsive to other more first-line treatments, and assuming there are no cardiac or other systemic contraindications to beta-blockers.

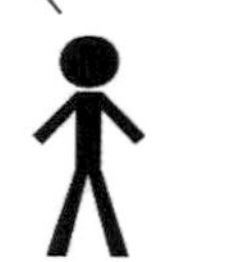

One more thing. How do we know whether a beta-blocker added to an antipsychotic is really treating agitated aggression or just akathisia?

Excellent question. Nadolol is a peripheral (noncentral) beta-blocker, and noncentrally acting beta-blockers like it (or metoprolol or atenolol) show little efficacy in akathisia (Dupuis et al., 1987; Dumon et al., 1992) – arguing against akathisia as being the underlying mechanism behind its efficacy for agitated aggression.

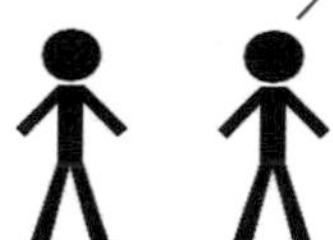

One more thing. I should avoid using a beta-blocker for agitation in an asthmatic patient, right?

Nadolol has been shown not to precipitate or exacerbate mild asthma (Hanania et al., 2008). Betaxolol is β_1 specific, so it spares the bronchioles, but there are no studies of it for impulsive aggression. If you want, you could write a grant to study that...

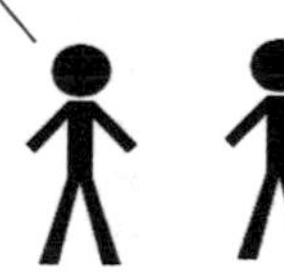

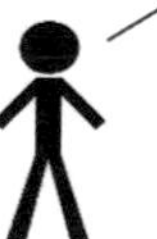

any comparative RCTs of an antimanic mood stabilizer versus an SSRI, outcomes for one strategy versus another remain purely speculative. We would encourage clinicians to screen for a history of mania, hypomania, or depression in all patients with prominent affective dysregulation and impulsive aggression, but not to equate impulsive aggression per se with the diagnosis of a mood disorder (of any polarity) as if the two were synonymous, unless associated signs and symptoms of a manic/hypomanic or depressive syndrome are also present.

K OBSESSIVE-COMPULSIVE PHENOMENA

The DSM-5 opted to remove obsessive-compulsive disorder (OCD) from its previous designation as a subtype of anxiety disorder and instead classify it as its own unique condition. Genuinely obsessional thinking (as contrasted with either ruminations or delusions) and impulsive/compulsive behaviors obviously both entail phenomena related to anxiety, but the neural circuitry underlying these phenomena differ from the

If disorders of *impulsivity* involve poorly controlled bottom-up processing, then what happens in disorders of *compulsivity*?

Both kinds of psychopathology are thought to reflect dysfunction of bottom-up processing, but involving different pathway subcomponents. To understand that, we need to revisit the salience network and consider cortico–striatal–thalamo–cortical loops...

kinds of autonomic hyperarousal states we typically associate with, say, phobias, panic, or even generalized anxiety.

Let us now further consider the neural circuitry involved in attentional salience and its interplay with impulse regulation, as discussed in Box 14.3.

Serotonergic antidepressants remain the mainstay of treatment for OCD, although their impact tends to be modest and at least half of SSRI-treated patients show poor responses. A 2008 Cochrane Database review of 17 studies of SSRIs over 6–13 weeks identified a weighted mean difference of 3.21 versus placebo, but no statistically significant differences between any specific SSRIs (Soomro et al., 2008). A later network meta-analysis involving 53 RCTs with 6652 participants also found that SSRIs exerted a large class effect as compared to placebo (mean difference = –3.49, 95% CrI = –5.12 to –1.81), adding that the efficacy of clomipramine appeared to be

Box 14.3

Why Psychopharmacologists Should Care About Dysfunctional Cortico-Striatal-Thalamo-Cortical Circuitry

Earlier we mentioned an aspect of attention called salience - how we recognize a stimulus as standing out from among others in the background, and the ways in which we decide to accord importance to one stimulus over another as being *worthy* of attention. Paying attention to salient stimuli requires our brains to inhibit attention to nonsalient stimuli. The circuitry involved in salience is called the salience network and within that network is a particular regulatory circuit known as the cortico-striatal-thalamo-cortical (CSTC) loop. That loop has a ventral and a dorsal component.

Functional neuroimaging studies tell us that patients with impulse control disorders (e.g., pathological gambling) have lower bottom-up connectivity in the dorsal circuit and greater bottom-up connectivity in the *ventral circuit* - in contrast to high-compulsivity patients (e.g., OCD) having lower bottom-up connectivity in the *dorsal circuit* (Parkes et al., 2019). In other words, both impulsivity and compulsivity may involve impaired bottom-up processing, but in ways that involve different components of corticolimbic circuitry.

Additionally, hyperconnected orbitofrontal cortex (OFC)-basal ganglia circuitry also appears to play a key role in the pathophysiology of OCD (Beucke et al., 2013). The OFC receives dense serotonergic innervation from the dorsal raphe nucleus, suggesting a possible rationale for the use of SSRIs or other serotonergic agents (Roberts, 2011).

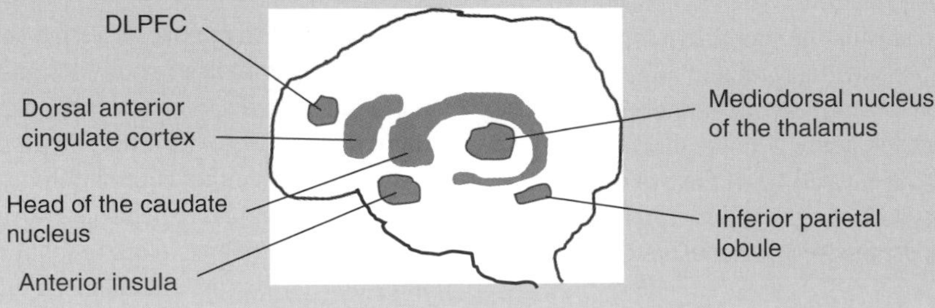

As riveting as the information in Box 14.3 is, I must still ask, from a *practical* standpoint, how does this help me decide what medicine to use in my patients?

Think of the relevance around circuitry more in possible etiologic ways. Someone with socially objectionable behavior – say, frequent anger outbursts – likely has a different underlying substrate when it occurs in an impulsive versus premeditated or intentional fashion. Psychotropic medications don't do as much to alleviate such behaviors if they are deliberate as opposed to impulsive. This brings us back to issues raised in Chapter 1 regarding speculations about etiologies of mental illness. You would treat shortness of breath differently if you thought it was caused by a respiratory infection versus a pulmonary embolism versus a foreign body obstruction. Analogously, omnipresent anger outbursts related to loss of top-down regulation might be exacerbated by the disinhibiting effects of a benzodiazepine but improved by, say, a beta-blocker or perhaps divalproex.

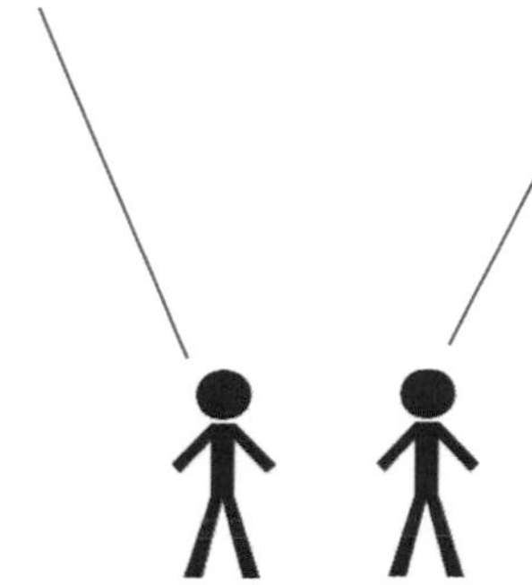

no better than that of SSRIs (mean difference −1.23, 95% CrI = −3.41 to 0.94) (Skapinakis et al., 2016). The latter finding contrasts with that of a previous meta-analysis done 20 years earlier which found clomipramine to be more effective than fluoxetine (Stein et al., 1995a). In general, the effect sizes for pharmacotherapies for OCD are smaller ($g \sim 0.20$) than those seen with behavioral therapies (such as exposure therapy with response prevention; $g \sim 0.40$); effect sizes tend to be higher with SSRI + behavioral therapy combination, as compared to SSRI pharmacotherapy alone, although not to behavioral therapy alone (Romanelli et al., 2014). SSRI dosing tends to be higher in OCD than in MDD or anxiety disorders in general (e.g., escitalopram up to 60 mg/day with good effect and no evidence of cardiac arrythmias (Rabinowitz et al., 2008)). Intravenous citalopram (administered daily, initially at 20 mg and increased to a maximum of 80 mg) also has been reported to be efficacious in OCD that is unresponsive to oral SSRIs (response rates near 60% after three weeks of open-label treatment) (Pallanti et al., 2002).

What are evidence-based strategies for OCD that incompletely responds to an optimally dosed SSRI? Probably the most widely studied and utilized next intervention is augmentation with an SGA; however, broad class effects with respect to efficacy for OCD are not well-established (probably because of true within-class drug differences, rather than insufficient study of the different available agents). A meta-analysis of 14 RCTs in which an SGA was added after at least 8–12 weeks of SSRI treatment identified a small-to-medium overall effect size ($d = 0.40$), corresponding to about a 10% reduction in total YBOCS score (Veale et al., 2014). Aripiprazole was associated with the largest effect (two RCTs, $d = 1.11$), followed by risperidone (five RCTs, $d = 0.53$), while neither quetiapine nor olanzapine differed significantly from placebo (see Table 14.4).

Combinations of clomipramine with an SSRI are somewhat controversial, as noted in Chapter 6 (Table 6.2), because of the theoretical risk for serotonin syndrome as well as the potential pharmacokinetic inhibition of clomipramine's metabolism that requires vigilant monitoring of serum clomipramine levels. That said, from an evidence-based standpoint in SSRI-nonresponsive OCD:

- Adjunctive clomipramine (25–75 mg/day) plus fluoxetine was well-tolerated and superior to quetiapine plus fluoxetine (Dinz et al., 2011)
- Clomipramine plus citalopram was superior to citalopram alone over 90 days in 16 adult outpatients with treatment-resistant OCD (and, note that citalopram, which inhibits CYP2D6 but no other P450 isoenzymes, does not alter clomipramine levels because clomipramine is not metabolized by CYP2D6) (Pallanti et al., 1999)
- An open-label case series (n = 7) in which clomipramine was added to fluvoxamine, paroxetine, or sertraline in youths with OCD over 5–22 months

described clinical efficacy but identified two instances of QTc prolongation on ECG (Figueroa et al., 1998).

Other strategies in treatment-resistant OCD that have been described in RCTs include the following:

Adjunctive gabapentin. An initial small, open case series in five partial responders to fluoxetine for OCD described significant improvement after augmentation with gabapentin (mean dose = 2520 mg/day by six weeks) (Corá-Locatelli et al., 1998). However, a later large (n = 99) RCT found no advantage for adding gabapentin over placebo to existing fluoxetine in treatment-resistant OCD (Farnia et al., 2018).

Adjunctive lamotrigine. In a 16-week double-blind add-on trial, lamotrigine (n = 33) was better than placebo in reducing total symptoms as well as YBOCS ("obsessive" and "compulsive" subscales (Bruno et al., 2012).

Adjunctive topiramate. A 12-week placebo-controlled augmentation of SSRIs (mean topiramate dose 177.8 mg/day) produced a significant reduction in compulsions but not obsessions (Berlin et al., 2011).

Mirtazapine. In a 12-week open trial begun at 30 mg/day and increased as tolerated to 60 mg/day, 16/30 (53.3%) acutely responded; subsequent randomization to eight weeks' continuation therapy showed significantly greater deterioration with placebo than mirtazapine (Koran et al., 2005).

Reminder

Keep in mind that individual proof-of-concept studies, especially from a single site, require replication before their findings can be embraced as generalizable or anything more than provisional.

Adjunctive memantine. Typically dosed at 20 mg/day, efficacy with adjunctive memantine as compared to placebo was associated with a 3.6-fold increased likelihood of response, and a mean 11.7-point reduction in YBOCS scores, with a resultant NNT = 1.6, according to a meta-analysis of eight studies (four RCTs) (n = 125) (Modaressi et al., 2019). All were conducted in Iran, and await replication from subjects drawn from elsewhere in the world.

Adjunctive riluzole. Another putative antiglutamatergic agent (though one that disappointingly failed in RCTs of TRD, as noted in Chapter 13), riluzole (dosed at 50 mg twice daily) was found to be superior to placebo when added to fluvoxamine 200 mg/day in a group of 50 Iranian OCD patients (Emamzadehfard et al., 2016).

Adjunctive $5HT_3$ antagonists. Ondansetron 8 mg/day was superior to placebo in a group of 46 Iranian OCD patients unresponsive to fluvoxamine 200 mg/day (Heidari et al., 2014), while granisetron 1 mg twice daily was superior to placebo in 42 Iranian OCD patients over eight weeks, with remission occurring in a strikingly great majority (90%) of subjects, and improvement evident in both obsessive and compulsive YBOCS subscales (Askari et al., 2012).

Adjunctive amantadine. Adding the DA agonist amantadine (dosed at 100 mg/day) to fluvoxamine 200 mg/day in a 12-week RCT with 100 Iranian OCD patients led to significantly greater YBOCS total and "obsession" subscale scores as compared to placebo (Naderi et al., 2019).

Dextroamphetamine. Following positive findings from a small (n = 12) crossover trial (Insel et al., 1983) and a small (n = 11) randomized comparison to placebo (and with greater efficacy than seen with methylphenidate 40 mg/day) (Joffe et al., 1991), response rates in a somewhat larger (n = 24) RCT of dextroamphetamine (30 mg/day) after SSRI or SNRI nonresponse were no different from those seen with caffeine 300 mg/day (50% and 58%, respectively) (Koran et al., 2009).

What's the rationale for *d*-amphetamine as an anti-OCD strategy?

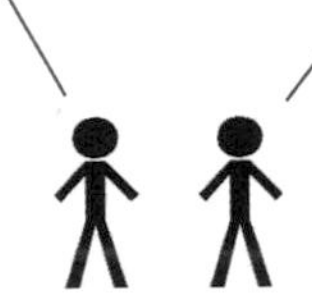

Possibly increased PFC D_1-receptor stimulation leading to increased attention and working memory, with better set-shifting away from intrusive thoughts.

L SKIN EXCORIATION

Deliberate, pathological skin excoriation is also referred to as skin-picking disorder or psychogenic excoriation. It may include scratching, picking, gouging, or squeezing. Studies tend to measure outcome using modified YBOCS scales, conceptualizing skin picking behavior as primarily a compulsion. A summary of findings from the clinical trials literature appears in Table 14.4. Notably, a meta-analysis of SSRI trials did find a collective significant improvement with a large effect size ($g = 0.98$) (Schumer et al., 2016). Another meta-analysis of nine clinical trials similarly reported a large effect size for all treatments collectively ($g = 1.19$), particularly with SSRIs ($g = 1.09$) or lamotrigine ($g = 0.98$) (Selles et al., 2016).

M TRICHOTILLOMANIA

SSRIs or clomipramine are considered the first-line treatments for compulsive hair-pulling, which has been conceptualized by some authors as a variant of OCD and by others as a non-OCD repetitive-type behavior involving stereotyped movements. However, the empirical pharmacotherapy database is not extensive, and from the existing literature actual data are more compelling for clomipramine than for SSRIs or predominantly noradrenergic TCAs (such as desipramine). Two small RCTs studying clomipramine (n = 13, mean dose 180.8 mg/day, and n=14, mean dose=120 mg/day, respectively) reported significantly greater reductions in hair-pulling behavior than with desipramine (mean dose 173.1 mg/day and 135 mg/day, respectively) (Swedo et al., 1989; Leonard et al., 1991). A third RCT of somewhat low-dose clomipramine (mean dose = 116.7 mg/day) found comparable improvements to those seen with cognitive behavior therapy (Ninan et al., 2000b). Two small, separate randomized crossover design trials (each n <20) of fluoxetine dosed up to 80 mg/day found no difference from placebo in hair-pulling behavior (Christenson et al., 1991; Streichenwein and Thornby, 1995).

Among the stronger of RCTs of nonserotonergic agents for trichotillomania is a 12-week placebo-controlled trial of NAC (1200–2400 mg/day), which resulted in significantly greater reductions in hair-pulling behavior than seen with placebo ("very much" or "much improved" status was seen in 56% of NAC recipients versus 16% of placebo recipients) (Grant et al., 2009a). A negative RCT was reported with use of naltrexone, although cognitive flexibility was shown to improve more with drug than placebo (Grant et al., 2014). Pilot trial data also suggest potential value for olanzapine or dronabinol (the latter based on the premise of a putative antiglutamatergic effect) (Grant et al., 2011). A review by Sani et al. (2019) also identified proof-of-concept individual trials with inositol, lamotrigine, and olanzapine.

N NONSUICIDAL SELF-INJURY (NSSI) AND SELF-INJURIOUS BEHAVIOR (SIB)

Deliberate, self-inflicted damage to skin or body tissues without the intent to die represents a complex form of psychopathology that transcends diagnostic boundaries. Self-injurious behaviors may include cutting, hitting, scratching, burning, and head-banging. Seldom does NSSI simply represent a component element within the definable constellation of a broader psychiatric syndrome (like cough in pneumonia, or insomnia in depression) for which comprehensive treatment of the broader syndrome expectably renders relief of ancillary symptoms. NSSI is often encountered in autism and related developmental disorders, the phenomenon has been described in bulimia patients, and individuals with trauma histories are more prone to self-harm – in particular, NSSI and SIBs are often viewed as efforts to self-soothe emotional distress in people with borderline personality disorder. Cognitive-behavioral approaches to managing self-destructive urges are often considered a mainstay of treatment, with pharmacotherapy representing a more subsidiary function.

NSSI and SIBs are together perhaps as compelling an example as any that exists of psychiatric phenomena for which there is virtually no systematic pharmacotherapy database. Most of the literature in this area involves small open trials or case reports from which really no generalizable conclusions about therapeutic strategies can be drawn. With that caveat, existing data involving the rationale and use of particular psychotropic agents for NSSI or SIBs are summarized in Table 14.5.

O OTHER DISORDERS OF IMPULSE CONTROL

Compulsive shopping (also called oniomania), along with compulsive sexual behaviors and kleptomania, were collectively considered for inclusion in DSM-5 as behavioral addictions but ultimately were not included as such. There is an obvious nosological interface between compulsive behaviors and addictions, where the concepts of *reward*-based versus *relief*-based motivations hold particular importance as organizing principles for understanding behavior. These issues (along with other behavioral addictions, such as pathological gambling) will be explored more fully in Chapter 18. Here, let us consider the role of pharmacotherapies for the specific examples of compulsive shopping, hoarding, and kleptomania.

Compulsive Shopping Disorder

Also known as compulsive buying behavior, this phenomenon remains diagnostically homeless in formal psychiatric nosology, but is nevertheless considered a definable clinical entity related to impaired impulsivity/compulsivity with motivation thought to be driven by relief-seeking from problems with mood, stress, and self-esteem (Lejoyeux and Weinstein, 2010). A seven-week open trial of citalopram (dosed up to 60 mg/day) followed by a nine-week randomized placebo-controlled discontinuation phase in 24 subjects found a significant initial improvement using an adapted YBOCS scoring system (63% met "responder" criteria) and subsequently significantly fewer relapses with continued citalopram than placebo (Koran et al., 2003). In contrast, two small placebo-controlled trials in compulsive shopping examining fluvoxamine (dosed up to 300 mg/day) found no differences from placebo: a first nine-week RCT in 23 subjects with a mean dose of 220 mg/day (Black et al., 2000) and a second 13-week RCT in 37 subjects with a mean dose of 215 mg/day (Ninan et al., 2000a).

Compulsive Hoarding

Though viewed as conceptually distinct from OCD (or, possibly, a variant of OCD), pharmacotherapy studies of compulsive or pathological hoarding behavior have largely focused on the utility of serotonergic antidepressants, mostly in OCD patients with prominent hoarding features. An open trial of paroxetine (mean dose = 41.6 mg/day) in 79 OCD patients (among whom 32 had compulsive hoarding) showed significant improvement irrespective of the presence or absence of hoarding behavior, but with poor overall tolerability (Saxena et al., 2007). Dedicated trials devoted to pathological hoarding irrespective of the diagnosis of OCD are limited to small open-label studies. First, a small (n = 4) case series examined methylphenidate-XR (mean dose = 50 mg/day) based on hypotheses that hoarding behavior reflected inattention; three of four subjects showed improved attention (based on a continuous performance task) but only modest reductions in hoarding symptoms (Rodriguez et al., 2013). A second study, examining venlafaxine-XR in 24 subjects (mean dose 204 mg/day) reported a significant improvement from baseline (by 32–36%) across several self-reported hoarding scale measures (Saxena and Sumner, 2014).

Kleptomania

There is often a fine line between impulsive versus premeditated aggressive acts; stealing is a good example. Picture someone who steals things because they feel entitled to rewards that are not rightfully theirs and feel no remorse about harming the victim but, instead, a sense of social defiance. Contrast that with someone overcome by an irresistible urge to take something that is not theirs, even if they do not necessarily want or need it, and are consumed afterward with a sense of shame and guilt. In the middle ground may lie instances in which someone contemplates taking things that do not belong to them but only acts on the impulse at whatever time the opportunity presents itself to do so. Kleptomania is a complex disorder of impulse control, reward behavior, and frequent comorbidity with mood disorders, personality disorders, and addictions, for which no standard pharmacotherapy has well-established efficacy. Pilot studies suggest potential value with the use of naltrexone: an eight-week RCT using doses up to 150 mg/day (mean dose 116.7 mg/day) revealed significantly greater reductions in stealing urges and behaviors as compared to placebo, with good tolerability (Grant et al., 2009b). Serotonergic antidepressants also suggest themselves for possible value when construing kleptomania as an impulse control disorder, although their clinical trials database is scant: escitalopram dosed from 10–20 mg/day showed a high response rate during initial open-label treatment but then no difference from placebo over a subsequent 17-week randomized relapse prevention phase (Koran et al., 2007).

TAKE-HOME POINTS

- Impulsivity and compulsivity are sometimes, but not always, opposite sides of the same coin (meaning, they often are evident in the same patient) and can manifest themselves across a wide range of psychiatric conditions.
- Problems with impulsivity/compulsivity can be core elements of psychopathology (e.g., OCD and intermittent explosive disorder) but at other times they may represent dimensions or elements of other, broader psychiatric disorders, such as anxiety disorders, mood disorders, addictions, dementia, and personality disorders.
- Aggressivity may or may not color the presentation of impulse control problems. Differential pharmacotherapies depend on recognizing when an overarching condition exists for which impulsivity/compulsivity/aggressivity are mainly subcomponent features of a broader constellation (e.g., antipsychotics for psychosis or mania, propranolol or nadolol for impulsive aggression in TBI or schizophrenia, lamotrigine or divalproex in borderline personality disorder, aripiprazole augmentation of SSRIs for treatment-resistant OCD).
- Impulsivity/compulsivity/aggressivity can be stand-alone phenomena for which symptom-targeted treatments are appropriate (e.g., beta-blockers, *N*-acetylcysteine in trichotillomania, naltrexone in kleptomania).
- Structured psychotherapies (and other nonpharmacological interventions, such as biofeedback and mindfulness meditation), which have not been reviewed here, also represent an important approach to behavioral management of impulse control disorders and associated autonomic hyperarousal, with findings that may synergize with pharmacotherapy.

Table 14.1 Use of serotonergic antidepressants for impulsive aggression

Agent	Study group	Findings
Citalopram	Hostility in adults with no Axis I psychiatric diagnosis	After two months of open-label citalopram 40 mg/day, significant reductions from baseline in state anger and hostile affect (Kamarck et al., 2009)
	Cluster B personality disorders	Eight-week open trial of citalopram 20–60 mg/day (mean dose = 45.5 mg/day) yielded significant reductions from baseline in ratings of overt aggression and irritability, and subjective irritability (Reist et al., 2003)
Duloxetine	Borderline personality disorder	12-week open trial (60 mg/day) in 14 patients was associated with significant reductions from baseline in Borderline Personality Disorder Severity Index total score and items reflecting "impulsivity," "outbursts of anger," and "affective instability" (Bellino et al., 2010)
Fluoxetine	Intermittent explosive disorder	Double-blind placebo-controlled trial of fluoxetine (up to 60 mg/day) for 12 weeks associated with significant improvement in overt aggression, independent of effects on depression or anxiety (Coccaro et al., 2009)
	(All) personality disorders	Double-blind controlled trial of fluoxetine (20–60 mg/day) for three months; significantly greater reductions in overt aggression (mainly verbal aggression and aggression against objects) with fluoxetine than placebo (Coccaro and Kavoussi, 1997)
Fluvoxamine	Adults with autism	12-week RCT (mean dose = 276.7 mg/day) found significantly greater reductions in aggression (as well as maladaptive behavior, social relatedness, and repetitive thoughts and behavior), as compared to placebo (McDougle et al., 1996)
Mirtazapine	Agitation in patients with Alzheimer's disease	12-week open trial (n = 16; dosing range 15-30 mg/day) associated with significant reduction in clinician-rated agitation (Cakir and Kulaksizoglu, 2008)
Sertraline	(All) personality disorders	Small (n = 12) eight-week open trial of sertraline produced significant improvements in irritability and overt aggression (Kavoussi et al., 1994)

Abbreviations: RCT = randomized controlled trial

Table 14.2 Summary of findings on anticonvulsants for impulsive aggression

Agent	Findings relative to placebo
Carbamazepine	Superior for self-injurious aggression seen in women with borderline personality disorder (mean dose = 820 mg/day) but not for aggression in youth with conduct disorder (mean dosing from 450–683 mg/day) (Cochrane Database review by Huband et al., 2010)
Divalproex	Dosed at ≥750 mg/day, superior for men with impulsive aggression, impulsively aggressive adults with Cluster "B" personality disorders, and youths with conduct disorder; not for impulsive aggression in youths with pervasive developmental disorder (Cochrane Database review by Huband et al., 2010); additionally, a multisite RCT of divalproex in outpatients with Cluster "B" personality disorders, intermittent explosive disorder, or PTSD found no overall effect across groups, but within personality disorder subjects benefit was observed in verbal aggression, irritability, and assault against objects (Hollander et al., 2003b).
Lamotrigine	- An eight-week RCT in 25 female outpatients with borderline personality disorder found significant improvement in state-trait anger scores with lamotrigine (mean dose = 200 mg/day) than placebo (Tritt et al., 2005) - In nondepressed temporal-lobe epilepsy patients, a 10-week open trial of lamotrigine (mean dose = 135 mg/day) added to existing anticonvulsants (mostly carbamazepine and topiramate) significantly reduced symptoms of physical aggression and anger (but not verbal aggression or hostility) (Kato et al., 2011); single case reports also describe improved overt aggression in patients with borderline personality disorder and body dysmorphic disorder (dosing of 200 mg/day) (Pavlovic, 2008)
Oxcarbazepine	Superior for verbal aggression and aggression against objects in adult outpatients (mean dose = 1500 mg/day; Cochrane Database review by Huband et al., 2010)
Phenytoin	- Superior for impulsive (but not premeditated) aggressive acts within a prison population and male outpatients with personality disorders (Cochrane Database review by Huband et al., 2010) - A meta-analysis of five placebo-controlled trials in male prisoners with impulsive aggression or formal diagnoses of intermittent explosive disorder found significant reductions in frequency and intensity of aggressive acts (mean dose ~300 mg/day) (Jones et al., 2011)
Topiramate	- An eight-week RCT in 29 women with borderline personality disorder found significantly greater reductions across measures of anger (except for inwardly directed anger) with topiramate (titrated to 250 mg/day by six weeks) than placebo (Nickel et al., 2004) - An eight-week RCT in 42 male outpatients with borderline personality disorder found greater improvement with topiramate (titrated to 250 mg/day by six weeks) than placebo on state-trait anger measures (Nickel et al., 2005)

Abbreviations: PTSD = post-traumatic stress disorder; RCT = randomized controlled trial

Table 14.3 Use of antipsychotics for treatment of impulsive aggression

Agent	Study focus and design	Main findings
Aripiprazole (IM)	Cochrane review of three RCTs involving 707 subjects (Ostinelli et al., 2018)	Better control over agitation within two hours, and less need for additional injections, as compared to placebo
Asenapine	12-week adjunctive open trial in 50 nonsyndromal bipolar I outpatients (& % with comorbid borderline peronality disorder) (Aguglia et al., 2018)	Significant and comparable improvement in aggression and impulsiveness rating scle scores for bipolar patients with comorbid borderline personality disorder (mean dose = 14.8 mg/day or without comorbid borderline personality disorder (mean dose = 15.3 mg/day)
Brexpiprazole	Six-week RCT of adjunctive brexpiprazole (3 mg/day) or placebo after antidepressant nonresponse in MDD (Fava et al., 2016)	Significantly greater improvement than with placebo on irritability and anger-hostility within the context of treating MDD
Cariprazine	Pooled post hoc analyses involving three RCTs in schizophrenia (Citrome et al., 2016a)	Significantly greater improvement in PANSS hostility item with cariprazine than placebo
Clozapine	14-week randomized comparison versus olanzapine, risperidone, or haloperidol in 157 schizophrenia or schizoaffective disorder patients (Citrome et al., 2001)	Clozapine superior to other treatments in reducing PANSS hostility scores
Iloperidone	Crossover study in 13 MDD outpatients incompletely responsive to SSRIs augmented with iloperidone for four weeks (Ionescu et al., 2016a)	No significant difference from placebo on anger-hostility measures
Olanzapine	- Six-month RCT versus placebo in 28 women with borderline personality disorder (Zanarini and Frankenburg, 2001)	Olanzapine (mean dose = 5.3 mg/day) was significantly better in reducing anger-hostility
	- Rapid initial dose escalation of olanzapine (40 mg PO on Days 1 and 2, 30 mg PO on Day 3, then 5–20 mg PO qDay) in acutely agitated schizophrenia or bipolar mania patients (Baker et al., 2003)	Greater reduction in PANSS excitation score at 24 hours and in all agitation measures by study end as compared to usual care
Paliperidone	Six-month open label flexibly dosed trial (target dose 6 mg/day; range 3–12 mg/day) in 199 Thai schizophrenia patients (Jarivavilas et al., 2017)	Significant improvement from baseline in PANSS hostility subscale
Risperidone	- Eight-week RCT versus placebo in 1362 schizophrenia patients (Peuskens, 1995)	Greater improvement with risperidone (4 or 8 mg/day fixed doses) on PANSS hostility subscale
	- Six-week RCT versus placebo in 15 combat veterans with PTSD (Monnelly et al., 2003)	Greater improvement in irritability with risperidone (0.2–2 mg/day)
	- Five-week RCT versus placebo or haloperidol in 513 chronic schizophrenia patients (Marder et al., 1997)	Greater improvement in PANSS hostility ratings with risperidone (6–16 mg/day) than haloperidol or placebo
	- Nine-week RCT versus placebo or haloperidol in 139 schizophrenia patients (Czobor et al., 1995)	Greater improvement in PANSS hostility ratings with risperidone (6, 10, or 16 mg/day) than haloperidol or placebo

Abbreviations: IM = intramuscular; MDD = major depressive disorder; PANSS = Positive and Negative Syndrome Scale; PO = by mouth; PTSD = post-traumatic stress disorder; qDay = every day; RCT = randomized controlled trial

Table 14.4 Pharmacotherapy evidence base for skin excoriation

Medication	Study designs	Findings
SSRIs		
Escitalopram	18-week open trial (n = 29), mean maximal dose 25 mg/day (Keuthen et al., 2007)	Significantly reduced skin-picking behaviors from baseline
Fluoxetine	Small (n = 21) 10-week placebo-controlled trial, mean dose = 55 mg/day (Simeon et al., 1997)	Greater reductions in skin-picking behavior with fluoxetine than placebo
	Small (n = 15) six-week open trial then six-week placebo-randomized continuation trial (target dose 60 mg/day) (Bloch et al., 2001)	8/15 initially responded to open label; all those randomized to continuation fluoxetine retained their improvement
Fluvoxamine	12-week small (n = 14) open trial (Arnold et al., 1999)	All subjects had improved "presence of skin sensations, skin appearance and lesions, behaviors involving the skin, control over skin behavior, and global assessment"
Sertaline	Open trial in 28 patients, mean dose = 95 mg/day (Kalivas et al., 1996)	19/28 (68%) had significant reduction in open skin lesions
***N*-acetyl cysteine (NAC)**	12-week, two-site placebo-controlled trial (n = 66, mean dose = 1200–3000 mg/day) (Grant et al., 2016)	Significantly greater reductions in modified YBOCS and global impressions scale with NAC than placebo
Anticonvulsants		
Lamotrigine	One small (n = 24) open trial (Grant et al., 2007); one 12-week RCT in 32 adults (dosing 12.5–300 mg/day) (Grant et al., 2010)	Significant improvement in open trial but no significant difference from placebo in RCT – although post hoc exploratory analyses suggested possible benefit in patients with poor cognitive flexibility
Topiramate	Small (n = 10) open trial, dosing from 25–200 mg/day (Jafferany and Osuagwu, 2017)	Significant reductions from baseline in time spent skin-picking, anxiety, depression
Opioid antagonists	Single case reports using naltrexone dosed at 50 mg/day	Clinical improvement reported as a qualitative outcome for single cases

Abbreviations: RCT = randomized controlled trial; YBOCS = Yale Brown OCD Scale

Table 14.5 Pharmacotherapy strategies for nonsuicidal self-injury and self-injurious behavior

Pharmacotherapy	Rationale	Evidence base
Opioid antagonists (naltrexone) or partial agonists (e.g., buprenorphine)	Putative dysregulation of the endogenous opiate system (e.g., NSSI patients demonstrate low CSF beta-endorphin and met-enkephalin levels (Stanley et al., 2010)	Open case series with naltrexone (n = 5, dosed at 50 or 100 mg/day) with "reduced daily frequency of self-injurious thoughts" over three weeks (Sonne et al., 1996) and in a case report of a woman with borderline personality disorder in whom "cutting" behavior previously had not improved with multiple various psychotropics (Agarwal et al., 2011)
SGAs	Serotonergic and dopaminergic dysfunction may contribute to impulsive aggression	- Aripiprazole: eight-week RCT (15 mg/day) - greater reduction in state-trait anger expression but no difference from placebo in frequency of NSSI events (Nickel et al., 2006) - Anecdotal case reports and small open trials (n <10) suggest possible value with ziprasidone (dosed from 40–80 mg/day), risperidone, clozapine (up to 800 mg/day), and olanzapine (up to 22 mg/day) (reviewed by Wollweber et al., 2015). Other reports suggest that use of SGAs in intellectually disabled adults more successfully improves aggression but not SIBs (Ruedrich et al., 2008)
SSRIs	Mostly indirect extrapolation about central serotonergic dysfunction from collective findings on trait impulsivity, aggression, and suicidality	- Fluoxetine 20–40 mg/day for more than three months in 21 profoundly mentally retarded adults led to marked improvement in SIBs in about two-thirds (Markowitz, 1992) - Open-label fluoxetine dosed up to 80 mg/day in 12 self-mutilating patients with borderline or schizotypal personality disorder over 12 weeks produced significantly reduced cutting behavior in 10/12 subjects (a nearly 75% reduction occurred in the number of self-mutilation episodes) (Markovitz et al., 1991) - One-year open-label high-dose sertraline (mean dose = 322 mg/day) significantly reduced the number of self-injury events per week (Markovitz, 1995)
Anticonvulsants	GABAergic inhibition over aberrant neuronal excitation	Oxcarbazepine dosed from 1200–1500 mg/day was reported in two open cases of bulimic patients with improvement in headbanging, self-punching, self-burning, and self-mutilation (Cordás et el., 2006)

Abbreviations: CSF = cerebrospinal fluid; NSSI = nonsuicidal self-injury; RCT = randomized controlled trial; SGA = second-generation antipsychotic; SIB = self-injurious behavior; SSRI = selective serotonin reuptake inhibitor

15 Psychosis

LEARNING OBJECTIVES

- ☐ Understand the relationship between specific dopamine tracts and positive or negative symptoms in patients with psychosis, and their "higher" regulation by cortical glutamatergic circuitry
- ☐ Understand the interplay between $5HT_{2A}$ and DA circuitry relevant to the pharmacotherapy of psychosis
- ☐ Discuss the potential utility of antipsychotic medications for cognitive rigidity, impaired set-shifting, and related components of executive dysfunction
- ☐ Describe the evidence base, and possible risks versus benefits, for using high-dose antipsychotic drugs
- ☐ Understand the use and logistics of short- and long-acting IM injectable antipsychotics
- ☐ Identify evidence-based augmentation strategies for antipsychotics and the database to inform pros and cons of combining multiple antipsychotic drugs
- ☐ Describe challenges in the pharmacotherapy of cognitive dysfunction in schizophrenia
- ☐ Identify issues and controversies regarding the safety, efficacy, and necessity of long-term pharmacotherapy with antipsychotic medications

The neurotic has problems. The psychotic has solutions.

– Thomas Szasz

Psychiatrist Thomas Szasz's appraisal of the fundamental nature of psychosis underscores the magnitude of belief-conviction and cognitive rigidity with which false fixed beliefs and perceptions are espoused. Goals of pharmacological treatment for psychosis can target a number of domains: medications may *loosen cognitive rigidity* and *dampen the intensity* of false beliefs and perceptions (without necessarily rendering perceptions as conforming more accurately to objective reality); they may reduce the *level of distress or agitation* associated with psychosis (again without necessarily altering the inaccuracy that somehow sustains fixed false ideas and perceptions); they may improve *social judgment* (such that someone may acquire sufficient awareness, if not true insight, to recognize where and with whom psychotic phenomena should and should not be discussed); they may *impose order on the form of thinking* to allow a more linear (if not logical) process by which they reach conclusions; or, sometimes, medications may actually *alter misperceptions* and allow for greater concordance between external reality and one's internal perception of it.

Taking a mainly neurocognitive approach to understanding these collective treatment goals, let us jump in by expanding on Figure 14.1, the "top-down/bottom-up" view of cognition described in the preceding chapter. If prefrontal/executive and limbic/emotional structures strive to maintain balance and homeostasis between "cold" and "hot" cognition, respectively (i.e., a functioning corticolimbic loop), we can envision this circuitry gone further awry when it frankly distorts perception and reality testing.

We all suspend reality testing, at least momentarily, when first viewing an optical illusion, or when bamboozled by a magic trick whose effect contradicts our internalized rules of physical reality. Something eventually jogs our internal capacity to realign our subjective perception with objective external reality, and then we usually are bemused (unless we are unable to find that internal affirmation). When we doubt our perceptions or our brains misperceive ideas or sensations we usually rely on others as a cross-check ("Did you hear that?" "Do you smell something burning?"). "Gaslighting" occurs when someone we trust as an external validator of our internal perception of reality deliberately (and usually malevolently) contradicts our internal experience of objective reality. At that point, the idealized equilibrium between "hot" and "cold" cognition becomes shaky and one or the other system tends to take charge.

> **Trivia**
>
> "Gaslight" was a 1938 play and later film in which sinister Charles Boyer diabolically tried to drive his on-screen wife Ingrid Bergman insane by invalidating and undermining the reality of her day-to-day perceptions and experiences – all in an effort to gain legal control over her finances. So much for routinely assuming benevolent intentions on the part of family members as collateral historians.

"Cold" cognition allows logical reasoning to prevail by allowing us to vet evidence that can support or refute a hypothesis. This largely forms the basis of cognitive therapy. ("It's certainly possible you didn't get the job because they were biased against you, but are there other possible explanations?") The same process comes into play when reality-testing frankly psychotic phenomena ("Is there a reason why the television would be talking about you?"). Or, for that matter, judging pharmacological cause-and-effect (see Chapter 1) – as when, say, deciding whether a physical sensation is a likely adverse drug effect. ("It's certainly possible that acetaminophen could worsen a fever, but consider the perhaps more likely explanation that it may simply be ineffective against the ailment causing it.")

By contrast, "hot" cognition hijacks the process by over-riding logic and plausibility. A threat to someone's basic welfare and sense of fundamental well-being unavoidably engages hot cognitive circuitry, if only for evolutionary reasons and the sake of preserving both the self and the species. Whether through autonomic hyperarousal (activating the limbic fight-or-flight response, and a self-protective harm-avoidant stance) or simply through bottom-up emotional overdrive of a prefrontal executive process (loudly shouting "Stop! Thief!" in a crowd, or "Fire!" in a movie theater, typically bypasses "cold" cognitive deliberation), factual accuracy gives way to urgency when survival stakes are sufficiently high. This is evolutionarily adaptive; there is not enough time to thoroughly gauge the validity of a possible threat and still maintain survival of the species.

Fight-or-flight "hot" cognition is thought to derive from hyperdopaminergic activation of mesolimbic circuitry. In particular, the amygdala and hippocampus together are thought to play a key role in detecting novelty in the environment and forming memories with high emotional valence (Blackford et al., 2010). Overactivity of this circuitry, depicted in Figure 15.1 as an expanded view from Figure 14.1 in Chapter 14, can drive autonomic hyperarousal and be a proximal contributor to agitation, psychosis, mania, and related states of hypervigilance.

> **Factoid**
>
> Paul Broca coined the term *le grand lobe limbique* ("limbus" meaning "border," denoting the curved rim of the cortex). Its exact structural subcomponents have been debated over time. Its role in emotional processing was described by James Papez (sometimes called "the Papez circuit").

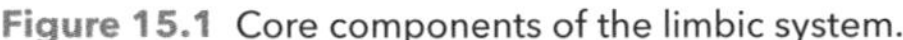

Figure 15.1 Core components of the limbic system.

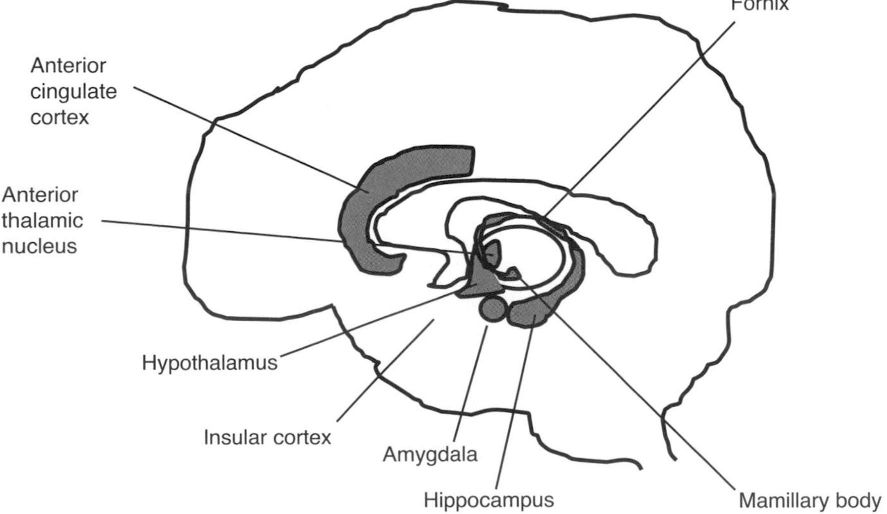

Pharmacotherapies that aim mainly to reduce anxiety and agitation, such as sedative-hypnotics (e.g., benzodiazepines), might literally dampen down the autonomic output from hyperactive mesolimbic activity, but that may not be synonymous with reducing the sense of perceived threat. Box 15.1 addresses the distinction between "fear" and "anxiety" with regards to presumed underlying neural circuitry and pharmacotherapy.

Box 15.1

Fear versus Anxiety

Some authorities point out that *fear* (a primal, visceral response to immediate threat) operates on limbic dopaminergic circuitry, while *anxiety* (a less immediate state of threat to fundamental safety and well-being, and in some ways an *over*deliberative process of weighing risks and implications) may reflect more serotonergic circuitry. Dopamine modulation may be more immediately relevant to fear circuitry than is the case for "just" anxiety and worry. DSM 5 also describes fear as "the emotional response to real or perceived imminent threat" while anxiety is "anticipation of future threat." Fear is considered a basic, discrete cognitive reaction that involves visual processing, whereas worry tends to be a more complex cognitive phenomenon based on learned experiences and more verbal than visual processing.

Antipsychotic drugs may be particularly useful when antifear rather than antianxiety circuitry has gone awry. Pure D_2 antagonists may offer a more direct method than benzodiazepines to down-regulate high dopamine tone emanating from hot cognitive circuitry, but pose the risk of also down-regulating other dopaminergic tracts that can sustain collateral damage (i.e., tuberoinfundibular or nigrostriatal) or may in themselves be hypotonic and in need of up-regulation (e.g., mesocortical DA circuitry in the setting of negative symptoms). D_2/D_3 partial agonists (i.e., aripiprazole, cariprazine, and brexpiprazole) represent a refinement over traditional pure D_2 antagonists by functioning more as a rheostat that modulates dopaminergic tone based on ambient DA functional activity. The theory of DA partial agonism posits that D_2/D_3 partial agonists would selectively increase dopaminergic tone where is it low (i.e., mesocortical pathways) and decrease it where it is too high (i.e., mesolimbic pathways). Put another way, imagine administering a tight D_2 antagonist (say, haloperidol) with a D_2 full agonist (say, methylphenidate) and hoping that the D_2 blocker will somehow show regional selectivity by binding to hyperactive mesolimbic brain circuitry (and not impede arousal and attention by blocking mesocortical DA tracts) while at the same time, hoping the DA agonist (methylphenidate) will selectively agonize mesocortical but not mesolimbic circuits. Partial agonism regulates this balance based on regionally ambient DA tone.

Figure 15.2 depicts the four main dopaminergic tracts in the brain: *mesocortical* and *mesolimbic circuits*, respectively, regulate attentional processing/executive function and emotional processing. Dopamine-blocking drugs can cause collateral damage to the *tuberoinfundibular* (prolactin-regulating) and *nigrostriatal* (extrapyramidal-regulating) tracts inasmuch

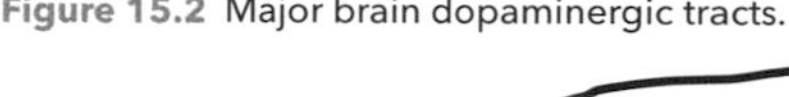

Figure 15.2 Major brain dopaminergic tracts.

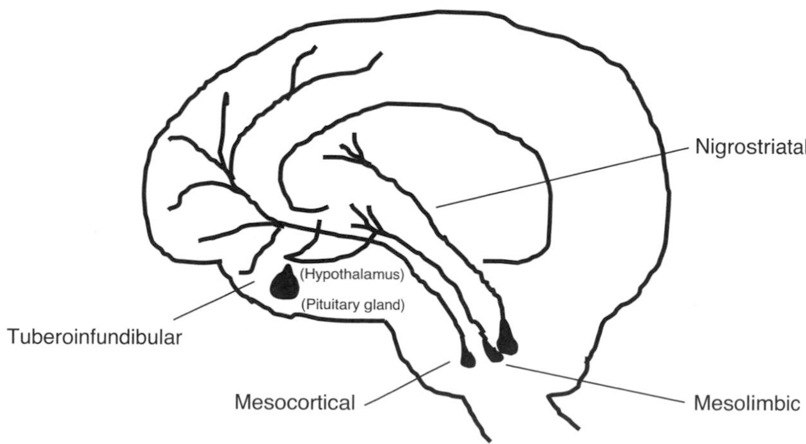

as: (a) DA released from the hypothalamus tonically inhibits prolactin release from the anterior pituitary (hence, DA blockers often cause hyperprolactinemia) and (b) DA projections from the substantia nigra to the extrapyramidal system tonically inhibit the release of acetylcholine; pharmacological blockade of nigrostriatal DA projections mimics parkinsonism by allowing release of excess extrapyramidal acetylcholine (which we then treat rather crudely with anticholinergic drugs – which in turn pose problems of their own for arousal and attentional processing). D_2 antagonists that (desirably) suppress mesolimbic DA hyperactivity in mania or psychosis unfortunately also (undesirably) suppress mesocortical DA activity, which in turn may exacerbate negative symptoms or otherwise lead to diminished arousal and attention, avolition, and apathy.

Recall from Chapter 1 Table 1.2 the varied functions of D_1, D_2, and D_3 receptor subtypes in the CNS. While all traditional antipsychotics (cf., pimavanserin) antagonize mesolimbic D_2 receptors, there is increasing interest in the role of D_3 receptors (involved in reward-based behavior) and D_1 receptor antagonism (relevant to antipsychotic and possible antidepressant effects). As an example of the latter, consider the novel antipsychotic drugs amisulpride and sulpiride (neither available orally in the USA), known for their potential value in depression at low doses (e.g., amisulpiride or sulpiride 50–300 mg/day), putatively attributed to blockade of presynaptic D_2/D_3 autoreceptors, in turn increasing dopamine release with increased postsynaptic binding at D_1 receptors that richly populate the striatum. Higher doses (e.g., amisulpride 400–1200 mg/day; sulpiride 600–1600 mg/day) are associated with postsynaptic D_2/D_3 antagonism in limbic regions, and presumably consequent antipsychotic efficacy. Amisulpride has a tighter D_2 receptor binding affinity (K_i ~ 3.0 nM) than does sulpiride (K_i ~ 9.8 nM).

A IS ATYPICALITY DEFINED BY $5HT_{2A}$ ANTAGONISM, D_2 FAST-OFFSET, OR OTHER PROPERTIES?

One oft-cited definition of "atypicality" of antipsychotics involves a molecule exerting a $5HT_{2A}$:D_2 receptor binding ratio >1 (Meltzer et al., 1989). $5HT_{2A}$ receptors have a reciprocal relationship with DA binding in that antagonizing $5HT_{2A}$ receptors increases DA release while $5HT_{2A}$ agonism decreases DA release. You might ask, what's so good about an antipsychotic increasing DA release? The answer lies in location. $5HT_{2A}$ receptors are densely distributed in the PFC, where increased DA tone is a desirable phenomenon with respect to attentional processing. and perhaps the treatment of negative symptoms. (There is also substantial $5HT_{2A}$ density in the nigrostriatal pathway. $5HT_{2A}$ blockade there can reduce D_2 antagonism in the dorsal striatum (caudate and putamen), effectively reducing, at least to some degree, the adverse iatrogenic motor effects caused by D_2 antagonists.)

Atypical-ish Typical Antipsychotics

PET imaging studies reveal at least some degree of postsynaptic $5HT_{2A}$ binding with some FGAs, including loxapine (Kapur et al., 1997a) and chlorpromazine (Trichard et al., 1998). The perphenazine metabolite *N*-dealkylperphenazine also has high $5HT_{2A}$ binding affinity (Sweet et al., 2000). $5HT_{2A}$:D_2 binding ratios of these FGAs do not exceed 1, technically making these antipsychotics (whose $5HT_{2A}$ occupancy is <80%) novel but not "atypical."

Another theory about atypicality arose when Kapur and Seeman (2001) proposed a hypothesis about the MOA of SGAs that became known as the "fast-on/fast-off" hypothesis. Briefly, it espoused that "atypicality" of an antipsychotic depended mainly on how rapidly a drug dissociated from the D_2 receptor after initially binding to it. These authors suggested that $5HT_{2A}$ blockade was less relevant (if at all relevant) to antipsychotic response than D_2 binding and dissociation. Later work then challenged this hypothesis by suggesting that drug accumulation in the lipophilic environment of the cell interior may underestimate the speed of dissociation from the D_2 receptor, showing wider variation in dissociation (Sahlholm et al., 2016).

The above notwithstanding, a key point of clinical relevance is the prospect that postsynaptic $5HT_{2A}$ antagonism could directly produce an antipsychotic effect. This is the basis for the antipsychotic efficacy of pimavanserin, presently FDA-approved only for the treatment of psychosis in patients with Parkinson's disease. Recall also from Chapter 13 Box 13.4 that the $5HT_{2A}$ binding properties of pimavanserin make it a compelling candidate treatment not only for psychosis

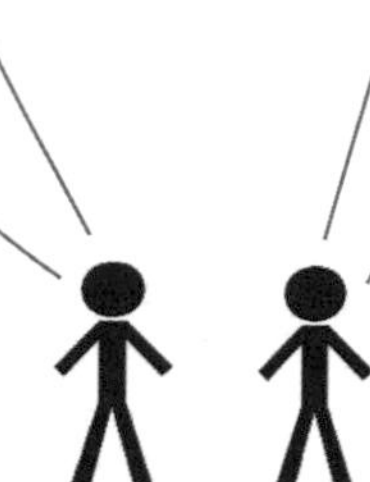
So if $5HT_{2A}$ and D_2 binding have reciprocal effects, why wouldn't a $5HT_{2A}$ *agonist*, rather than an *antagonist*, have an antipsychotic effect?
It might if $5HT_{2A}$ receptors were densely distributed in mesolimbic regions – where we'd like to down-regulate DA tone in psychosis. But it turns out there's not much $5HT_{2A}$ binding to be had in limbic regions.
Well if that's the case then how do $5HT_{2A}$ agonists like psilocybin cause psychosis? Don't they need somehow to increase mesolimbic DA?
$5HT_{2A}$ agonists are believed to act directly on pyramidal neurons in the cortex, ultimately driving mesolimbic dopamine release and thus causing psychosis. $5HT_{2A}$ antagonists can block hallucinogen-induced psychosis and to a degree may also improve positive symptoms in schizophrenia.

but also for depression – at least, based on its mechanistic rationale and initial proof-of-concept data. Similarly, the MOA of lumateperone – involving an approximate 60-fold greater binding affinity at $5HT_{2A}$ than D_2 receptors – should pique the interest of any psychopharmacologist wishing to minimize regionally undesired dopalytic effects (say, in the basal ganglia) when treating psychosis, and possible mood disorders as well.

Yet another consideration regarding antipsychotic pharmacodynamics involves nondopaminergic mechanisms altogether. The investigational drug ulotaront has no binding affinity at D_2 (or any other DA) receptor but is instead believed to exert a possible antipsychotic effect (and spare dopaminergic motor tracts altogether) via agonizing the trace amine-associated receptor 1 (TAAR1), as well as $5HT_{1A}$ receptors. An initial 4-week randomized comparison of ulotaront (50 or 75 mg/day) for relapsing schizophrenia was superior to placebo in positive and negative symptom total scores, with somnolence and gastrointenstinal complaints emerging as the most common adverse effects (Koblan et al., 2020).

B FGAs VERSUS SGAs: NEUROTOXICITY VERSUS NEUROPROTECTION?

SGAs differ from FGAs in their overall *somewhat* lesser propensity to cause adverse motor effects (EPS, acute dystonia, tardive dyskinesia). *They have not been shown to be more efficacious than FGAs to treat psychosis* (Crossley and Constante, 2010). Besides the role of $5HT_{2A}$ antagonism and the potential for fast offset of D_2 receptor binding, another point of distinction involves the potential neuroprotective effects of at least some SGAs relative to the possible nonprotective or even neurotoxic effects of some FGAs. The literature here involves a complex storyline.

Here goes: In 2007, it was reported that progressive gray-matter volume loss in schizophrenia patients was governed by a variant in the BDNF gene (Met allele carriers) as well as higher doses of antipsychotics (either FGAs or SGAs) – particularly in those who were antipsychotic-naïve (Ho et al., 2007). A later and larger neuroimaging study by that group found that among mostly first-episode schizophrenia patients, chronic exposure to both FGAs and SGAs was associated with age-inappropriate gray matter volume loss in all brain regions except the cerebellum (Ho et al., 2011). White matter volume also was diminished in higher-dose antipsychotic recipients, but modestly increased in low-dose recipients. A later naturalistic study of older adults with bipolar disorder also found that longer duration of antipsychotic exposure was related to lower gray-matter volumes (Gildengers et al., 2014).

Do these studies mean that antipsychotics *cause* loss of brain tissue, or that they merely fail to stave off inevitable, inexorable neuroprogression in schizophrenia? Unclear! Duration of psychosis has been shown to have a more detrimental effect than duration of antipsychotic therapy on brain volume (Andreason et al., 2013). Animal studies around this time also reported loss of total brain volume in macaque monkeys given haloperidol or olanzapine for up to 27 months (Dorph-Peterson et al., 2005).

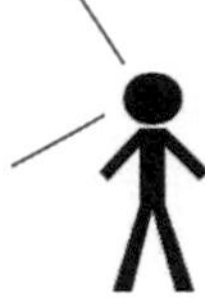

OK so if haloperidol is a neurotoxin tell me why we still use it in delirium?
Skip the mini-lecture. Just answer my question please.

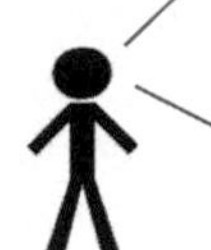

Delirium is a potentially lethal condition that reflects underlying gross brain dysfunction due to an acute process such as a toxic-metabolic syndrome, infection, neoplasm, head trauma, cardiac or renal failure, electrolyte imbalances…
Because there is a large database showing that it is safe, effective, and well-tolerated. Delirium is thought to reflect a hyperdopaminergic, low cholinergic state. Haloperidol has little anticholinergic or antihistaminergic activity and can be given IV or IM. There are data with a few SGAs in delirium – risperidone or olanzapine mainly – but mostly that's case reports or small open trials.

C IS THERE STILL A PLACE FOR FGAs?

Clinicians nowadays tend to beat up on FGAs because of their relatively higher liability than SGAs to cause tardive dyskinesia (~30% versus 20% prevalence, as noted in Chapter 10) and other movement disorders, hyperprolactinemia, as well as their comparatively lesser value for treating negative symptoms and mood symptoms. (In fact, in bipolar disorder, several studies show higher risks for inducing depression after a manic episode when using an FGA (e.g., haloperidol) than an SGA (e.g., olanzapine) (Tohen et al., 2003a) or even placebo (e.g., versus perphenazine; Zarate and Tohen, 2004)). So do FGAs still have a meaningful place in modern psychopharmacology?

FGA utility in the SGA era received something of a boost when the NIMH CATIE study (discussed further later in this chapter) reported the controversial finding that outcome (all-cause discontinuation) with perphenazine was comparable to that of quetiapine, risperidone, or ziprasidone, but was more cost-effective (Lieberman et al., 2005). Even more surprisingly, perphenazine was associated with greater improvement than olanzapine or risperidone in measures of cognitive function at 18 months (Keefe et al., 2007). The latter finding contrasts with prior meta-analyses that had suggested advantages in neurocognitive function with SGAs over FGAs. Consider the following:

- FGAs (particularly, haloperidol) are better-studied than SGAs in delirium
- Peak onset of action may be faster with FGAs than SGAs
- SGAs are unavailable in IV formulation (in contrast to haloperidol)
- Droperidol is a well-established postsurgical/ postanesthesia antinausea remedy
- Haloperidol and pimozide are well-established treatments for tics associated with Tourette's syndrome, and do so more effectively than α_2 agonists when comorbid ADHD is absent (Weissman and Qureshi, 2013)
- Chlorpromazine is the only medication FDA-approved to treat hiccups (dosed 25–50 mg PO QID PRN (as needed)); case reports also support the use of low-dose (0.5–1.5 mg) haloperidol
- In patients with existing diabetes or clinically significant metabolic syndrome for whom certain higher-liability SGAs (e.g., olanzapine, risperidone, quetiapine, among others) may be undesirable, and particularly if other SGAs with lower metabolic liability are ineffective, FGAs remain a viable option to treat psychosis or mania
- Low-dose low-potency FGAs such as chlorpromazine (e.g., 10–25 mg at a time) or loxapine (10 mg) can be useful as an anxiolytic, particularly when benzodiazepines may be undesirable (e.g., in the setting of substance use disorders; although beware the risk for lowering seizure threshold in patients with alcohol use disorders or those withdrawing from sedative-hypnotics, for whom benzodiazepines remain the treatment of choice for detoxification). Here, "ego glue" is the altogether nontechnical but conceptually fitting term commonly used to describe low-dose antipsychotics when used on an as-needed basis as a strategy to bind together anxiety or distress

that arises in the setting of internal crisis and turmoil.

High-potency FGAs possess minimal to no anticholinergic properties, consequently leading to their higher likelihood for causing EPS and the need to coprescribe an anticholinergic drug such as benztropine or trihexyphenidyl. Low-potency FGAs, in contrast, tend to possess stronger anticholinergic properties, resulting in less EPS (but more consequent sedation and adverse cognitive effects). Dosing with high-, medium-, and low-potency FGAs, respectively, is summarized in Tables 15.1–15.3 at the end of this chapter. The high potency FGA pimozide has historically received attention as possibly having unique value (or at least, an evidence base) in patients with delusional disorder. This is discussed in Box 15.2.

D ABERRANT DOPAMINE CIRCUITRY MAY JUST BE THE MESSENGER

While older theories about psychosis pointed to limbic hyperdopaminergic tone as being *the* putative site of dysfunction (and target of pharmacotherapy), latter-day theories have pointed to higher cortical processes that regulate downstream dopaminergic (and other) circuits – perhaps making mesolimbic dopamine more the fall guy than the perpetrator of psychosis.

This is really important

Enter glutamate, an abundant excitatory neurotransmitter. Intracellularly, it turns on other circuits; extracellularly,

If 80% saturation of D_2 receptors is optimal for psychosis, and achieved with haloperidol dosed just from 2-5 mg/day (Kapur et al., 1996; 1997b), why would we ever need to give a higher dose?

There are some reports that even higher (90%) D_2 occupancy may sometimes be more efficacious than the oft-cited 60-80% you mention (Kapur et al., 1997b). For severe psychotic agitation, the sedative effects of haloperidol or other antipsychotics may depend on other mechanisms besides D_2 blockade.

In which case, I'd be better off adding an adjunctive benzodiazepine for sedation?

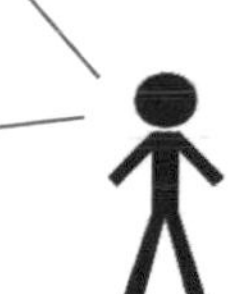
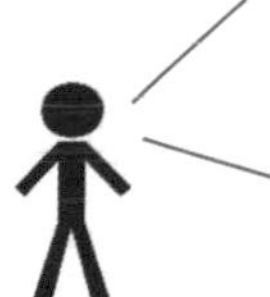

Very likely. IM haloperidol plus lorazepam has been shown to be noninferior to IM olanzapine for acute agitation in schizophrenia (Huang et al., 2015).

Box 15.2

Pimozide and Delusional Parasitosis

A single case report of delusional parasitosis improved by pimozide was reported in a dermatology journal in 1978 (Reilly et al., 1978), followed by a handful of additional case reports over ensuing years using this particular FGA for this unusual phenomenon. Further case reports then appeared using pimozide for other variants of delusional disorder, including litigious paranoia (Ungvari and Hollokoi, 1993), Capgras syndrome (Tueth and Cheong, 1992), and delusional jealousy (Soyka, 1995), among others. Review papers then created an "echo chamber" effect linking pimozide as an evidence-based treatment of choice for monosymptomatic hypochondriacal psychosis and all forms of delusional disorder. Its augmentation of fluoxetine for body dysmorphic disorder was no better than fluoxetine alone (Phillips, 2005). There has otherwise never been a randomized trial of pimozide for any form of delusional disorder. A Cochrane Review identified its efficacy for schizophrenia but noted a higher risk for parkinsonism than other FGAs, alongside the statement "There are no data to support or refute its use for... delusional disorder" (Sultana and McMonagle, 2000). Later case reports or retrospective case series have also described successful treatment of delusional parasitosis with risperidone, aripiprazole, quetiapine, paliperidone, ziprasidone, or olanzapine. No particular FGA or SGA stands out as being a more evidence-based treatment option than another either for delusional parasitosis or delusional disorder in its broader and more varied presentations.

it is excitotoxic. A key loop implicated in primary psychotic disorders such as schizophrenia involves the excitatory role of cortical glutamate in regulating downstream limbic dopamine circuitry. A central modern hypothesis in explaining schizophrenia posits that NMDA receptors (the same receptor discussed in regard to ketamine and depression in Chapter 13) hypofunction in the cortex, consequently failing to stimulate downstream corticolimbic circuitry. Inhibitory GABA interneurons represents the missing link in this circuit, as depicted in Figure 15.3.

What does this have to do with modern pharmacotherapy for psychosis? Unfortunately, not nearly as much as we would hope, since the pharmacological technology with which we attempt to treat psychosis remains confined to the downstream effects of excessive mesolimbic dopamine (in the case of positive symptoms – modulated by dopamine antagonism) and mesocortical dopamine (in the case of negative/deficit symptoms). This model postulates that restoring normal function of corticolimbic glutamate circuitry might ultimately depend on correcting faulty NMDA receptor function. Such technology, as yet, does not exist, although efforts toward advancing the field have sought to target *ionotropic* as well as *metabotropic glutamate receptors* in the hope of altering both psychosis

Box 15.3

More on NMDA Receptor Dysfunction and Potential Therapeutic Drug Targets in Schizophrenia

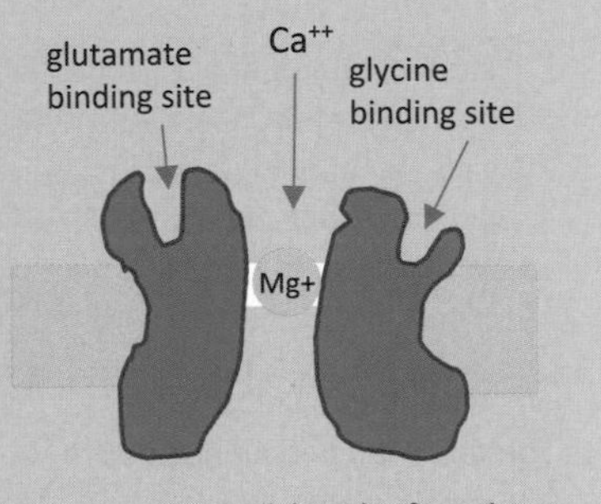

The NMDA receptor has a binding site for glutamate and another for glycine, as illustrated. The glycine binding (transporter) site (aka GlyT-1) also can become activated if D-serine or D-cycloserine binds there, and it is inhibited by sarcosine (aka *N*-methylglycine). For the NMDA receptor to become activated, binding at the glutamate and glycine sites must occur in order to dislodge a Mg^{+} plug in the ion channel which in turn then allows for Ca^{++} entry, depolarization, and activation of the receptor. Contemporary thinking is that in schizophrenia, faulty functioning of the NMDA receptor prevents downstream excitatory signaling of mesocortical pathways (contributing to negative symptoms) and corticolimbic glutamate pathways (which, in turn, regulate mesolimbic dopamine circuitry and result in positive symptoms), as depicted in Figure 15.3. In principle, pharmacotherapies that enhance binding of the glutamate or glycine regulatory sites of the NMDA receptor could (or, should) help to overcome dysfunctional circuitry. Evidence here has thus far been discouraging (albeit preliminary), with mostly negative RCTs of adjunctive D-sarcosine (e.g., Lane et al., 2006; Weiser et al., 2012), the GlyT1 inhibitor bitopertin (Bugarski-Kirola et al., 2016), or high dietary glycine (e.g., 30 g/day) (Potkin et al., 1999).

Figure 15.3 Corticoglutamatergic regulation of mesolimbic and mesocortical dopamine function.

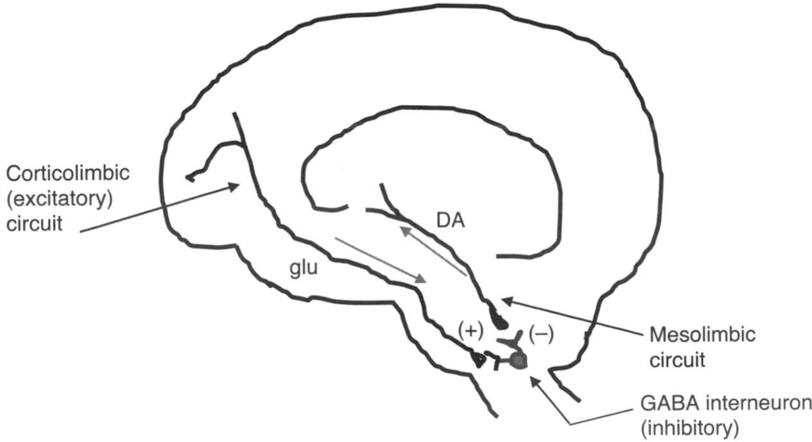

Ok, so, explain this to me. Phencyclidine (PCP) is a noncompetitive NMDA receptor antagonist (like ketamine) that causes psychosis (unlike ketamine). Why doesn't ketamine cause psychosis (not just dissociation), and why isn't PCP an antidepressant?

Remember from Chapter 13 that a host of NMDA receptor antagonists other than ketamine have failed to show value to treat depression, so we don't know for sure that NMDA receptor blockade per se is the key to its antidepressant properties, from among ketamine's many MOAs. PCP, another NMDA receptor antagonist as you point out, was studied for its possible antidepressant effects in animal models and found to be fairly weak. Oh, and ketamine can most definitely cause or exacerbate psychosis in schizophrenia patients. Think about patient-specific diatheses. And see, for instance, Malhotra et al., 1997.

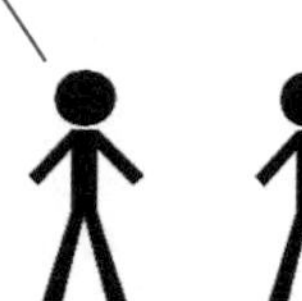

OK, so now…if schizophrenia patients already have hypofunctioning of their NMDA receptors, why doesn't that *protect* them from depression? It's like they have built-in ketamine, right?

Uh, not exactly. Remember, again, we can't really say that it's NMDA receptor antagonism that's producing an antidepressant effect. The fact that depression is so common in schizophrenia may even argue further against the hypothesis that NMDA receptor blockade produces an antidepressant effect in any sort of reliable way. Besides, even though ketamine does block NMDA receptors, it's probably the burst of synaptic glutamate and GABA in cortical pyramidal cells that's having the antidepressant effect – or at least, the neurotrophic effect.

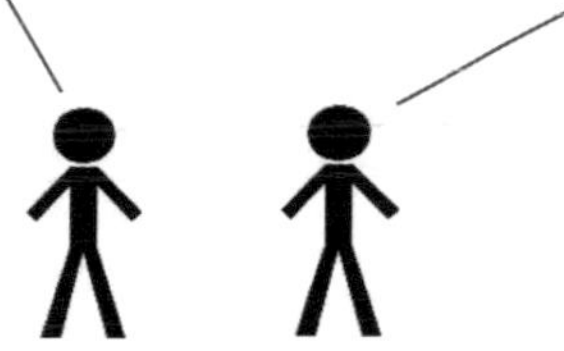

and depression. See Box 15.3 for further discussion about presumed NMDA receptor dysfunction in schizophrenia and its implications for targeted pharmacotherapy.

Recall from our ketamine discussion in Chapter 13 (see Box 13.12) that there are two types of glutamate receptors, ionotropic (of which there are three: NMDA, AMPA, and kainate) and metabotropic. Metabotropic glutamate receptors (mGlu) are thought to regulate presynaptic glutamate release. In particular the mGlu2 and 3 receptors (mGluR2/3) are autoreceptors believed to reduce hyperactive cortical pyramidal glutamate neurons. They also reduce glutamate release in reward circuitry (nucleus accumbens). Some day, we hope we might develop a way to overcome the faulty NMDA receptor function of corticolimbic glutamate circuitry in schizophrenia, as a more pathophysiologically sophisticated strategy to correct the downstream dysfunction it otherwise is believed to cause in mesolimbic dopamine signaling.

Efforts to treat psychosis via nondopalytic drugs have proven to be frustratingly limited. See Box 15.4 for the story behind one such endeavor meant to target the mGluR3 metabotropic glutamate receptor.

Our efforts to modulate psychosis, at least for the time being, remain focused primarily on altering mesolimbic and mesocortical DA function – preferably, by downregulating mesolimbic DA circuitry and sparing (or better yet, upregulating) mesocortical DA function. As mentioned at the beginning of this chapter, the three existing D_2/D_3 partial agonists (aripiprazole, brexpiprazole, and cariprazine) raise at least the prospect of better efficacy against negative symptoms, depression, and perhaps elements of cognitive dysfunction because of their potential for regional selectivity of DA modulation. While

Box 15.4

What Was Pomaglumetad and Why Should We Care?

Pomaglumetad was a prodrug for LY404039, a potent and selective agonist for Group II metabotropic glutamate mGluR2 and mGluR3 receptors that was studied as an antipsychotic in schizophrenia patients. Because it exerted no direct effects on dopamine, it represented a breakthrough dopamine-sparing drug mechanism to treat psychosis. An initial four-week proof-of-concept trial dosed at 40 mg PO BID (with olanzapine 15 mg/day as an active comparator for assay sensitivity) in 196 schizophrenia inpatients was favorable, improving both positive and negative symptoms significantly better than placebo (Patil et al., 2007). Then, in a subsequent RCT, neither pomaglumetad (dosed at 5, 20, 40, or 80 mg PO BID) nor olanzapine (as active comparator) separated from placebo, suggesting a failed rather than negative trial (Kinon et al., 2011). (An exploratory analysis looking for possible response predictors in a study subgroup found that patients who were early in their illness and previous D_2 antagonist recipients were more likely to respond to pomaglumetad than placebo (Kinon et al., 2015); although, searching for moderators of treatment response when an overall study finding is nonsignificant is methodologically not so kosher.) Finally, a later RCT using risperidone as an active comparator then also failed to separate from placebo (while risperidone did) (Downing et al., 2014). Other more exploratory RCTs (examining, for example, time until discontinuation versus TAU, or possible efficacy in negative-symptom-prone schizophrenia) also failed to show an advantage over placebo.

So does agonizing the mGluR2/3 autoreceptor increase or decrease presynaptic glutamate release? If the problem in schizophrenia is hypofunctioning of the NMDA receptor, wouldn't you want to increase, rather than decrease, intracellular glutamate transmission in, say, the corticolimbic glutamate tract?

The mGluR2/3 receptor is itself understudied. When pomaglumetad bit the dust it left open the question of whether it was just that particular drug that failed to treat psychosis or whether the Group II metabotropic glutamate system it was targeting was itself not as important as we had thought in the pathophysiology of schizophrenia. But, to your specific question, go back to that corticolimbic glutamate loop in Figure 15.3. Hypofunction of NMDA receptors means less stimulation of GABA inhibitory interneurons, in turn failing to *downregulate* pyramidal neuron glutamate release...causing excessive stimulation of AMPA and kainic acid glutamate receptors, leading to excitotoxic damage. mGluR2/3 agonists should decrease presynaptic glutamate release on excitatory neurons, alleviating the hyperglutamatergic excitotoxicity. Got all that?

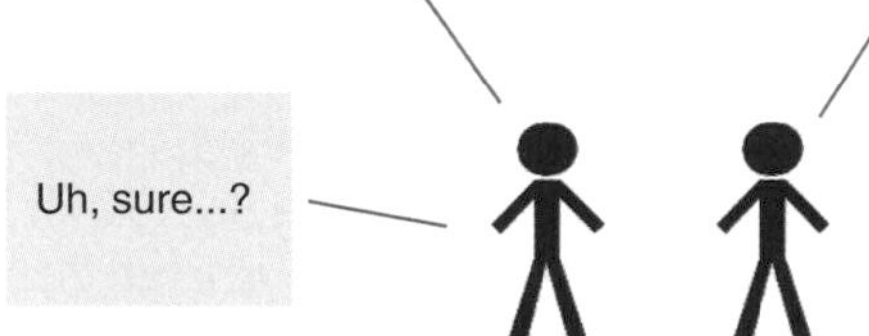

D_2 agonism appears to exert mainly a pro-attentional effect, D_3 circuitry receptor targeting has garnered increasing attention for its potential role in reward circuitry as well as possible antidepressant effects. (D_3 antagonists or partial agonists have been suggested to exert reward-based pro-cognitive effects in both animal and human studies, while the cognitive effects of drugs with D_3 pure agonism such as pramipexole, ropinirole, rotigotine, or bromocriptine are less clear.) Relative dissociation constants for D_2 and D_3 receptor binding across SGAs are summarized in Boxes 15.5 and 15.6, respectively.

E WHAT ABOUT D_1 RECEPTOR BINDING AND ANTIPSYCHOTIC ACTION?

D_1 receptors, which are exclusively postsynaptic, are found mainly in the striatum and prefrontal cortex. D_1 agonism influences monoaminergic function as well as phosphorylation of intracellular signaling proteins. This in turn may modulate cognition (e.g., working memory) favorably at low levels but adversely at high levels, following a so-called inverted U dose–response

Box 15.5

Relative D_2 Receptor Binding Affinities Across SGAs

SGA	Ki (nM)	Function	
Brexpiprazole	0.3	Partial agonist	
Cariprazine	0.49	Partial agonist	} Comparable to haloperidol (Ki = 0.74 nM)
Lurasidone	0.66	Antagonist	
Paliperidone	1.4	Antagonist	
Asenapine	1.7	Antagonist	
Aripiprazole	2.3	Partial agonist	
Risperidone	3.7	Antagonist	
Ziprasidone	4.75	Antagonist	
Iloperidone	8.3	Antagonist	
Olanzapine	30.8	Antagonist	
Lumateperone	32	Presynaptic partial agonist, postsynaptic antagonist	
Clozapine	147	Antagonist	
Quietapine	437	Antagonist	
Endogenous dopamine	540	–	

Source: Stahl, 2017
Pimavanserin has no appreciable binding to D_2 receptors

Box 15.6

Relative D_3 Receptor Binding Affinities Across SGAs

SGA	Ki (nM)	Function
Cariprazine	0.09	Partial agonist
Brexpiprazole	1.1	Partial agonist
Asenapine	1.8	Antagonist
Paliperidone	2.6	Antagonist
Aripiprazole	4.6	Partial agonist
Risperidone	7.3	Antagonist
Ziprasidone	7.3	Antagonist
Iloperidone	10.5	Antagonist
Lurasidone	15.7	Antagonist
Olanzapine	38.1	Antagonist
ENDOGENOUS DOPAMINE	60	-
Clozepine	310	Antagonist
Quietapine	394	Antagonist

Source: Stahl, 2017

curve (in other words, strong D_1 antagonists could worsen cognition). D_1 partial agonists (e.g., clozapine) in principle may aid cognition in schizophrenia. The novel antipsychotic lumateperone, FDA-approved for schizophrenia in late 2019, has a somewhat more complex MOA than existing SGAs. In addition to $5HT_{2A}$ antagonism (it has a 60-fold higher binding affinity at $5HT_{2A}$ than D_2 receptors), it also functions as a:

- presynaptic D_2 partial agonist/postsynaptic D_2 antagonist,
- D_1-regulated NMDA and AMPA receptor agonist,
- serotonin transporter reuptake inhibitor.

Preliminary studies in schizophrenia have shown greater improvement in positive and negative symptoms as compared either to placebo or risperidone, as well as cognitive and depressive symptoms (Lieberman et al., 2016). It also appears to have a relatively benign profile with respect to metabolic parameters (i.e., changes in weight, lipids, and glycemic markers).

Relative D_1 receptor binding affinities across SGAs are summaraized in Box 15.7

Another core aspect of psychosis involves executive functioning and the capacity for set-

Tip

Lumateperone requires only modest D_2 antagonism (see Table 15.9) because of its potent $5HT_{2A}$ antagonism.

shifting (especially with regard to reality-testing). Box 15.8 describes the concept of cognitive rigidity and the potential impact of antipsychotic drugs to facilitate cognitive flexibility.

Tip

Lumateperone is metabolized by both CYP450 3A4 and uridine 5′-diphosphaoglucutonosyl transferase (UGT). Because divalproex potently inhibits UGT, its coadministration with lumateperone is not recommended.

Box 15.7

Relative D_1 Receptor Binding Affinities Across SGAs[a]

SGA	Ki (nM)
Asenapine	2.9
Paliperidone	41
Lumateperone	41
Olanzapine	56.6
Ziprasidone	80
Iloperidone	129
Clozapine	240
Lurasidone	262
Riperidone	327
Brexpiprazole	164
Cariprazine	1000
Quietapine	1096
Aripiprazole	1173
ENDOGENOUS DOPAMINE	1766

Source: Stahl, 2017

F ARE THERE REALLY DIFFERENCES IN EFFICACY AMONG ANTIPSYCHOTICS?

When thinking through medication options among antipsychotics, one must once again appreciate factors such as efficacy (outcome under optimal conditions) versus effectiveness/tolerability, adherence, comorbidities, severity, chronicity, degree of treatment resistance, and acceptability (and the role of long half-life compounds or long-acting injectables). Effectiveness across antipsychotics was perhaps most extensively studied in the 18-month NIMH-sponsored CATIE trial, whose main finding was that 74% of schizophrenia patients prematurely discontinued their study participation. Reasons for premature study discontinuation from CATIE are depicted in Figure 15.4. Olanzapine had a significantly longer time until all-cause discontinuation as compared to quetiapine or risperidone, although criticisms of this observation include: (a) higher mean dosing of olanzapine; all antipsychotics were dosed within the parameters of their manufacturers' product labels (i.e., quetiapine 200–800 mg/day, mean dose 543.4 mg/day; risperidone 1.5–6 mg/day, mean dose 3.9 mg/day; ziprasidone 40–160 mg/day, mean dose 112.8 mg/day; perphenazine 8–32 mg/day, mean dose 20.8 mg/day) except olanzapine, which was dosed from 7.5 mg/day to a maximum of 30 mg/day (manufacturer's maximum 20 mg/day), mean dose 20.1 mg/day; and (b) significantly higher metabolic dysregulation (weight gain, hemoglobin A1c levels, cholesterol, and triglycerides) with olanzapine than other agents.

In first-episode psychosis, olanzapine has shown greater reduction in PANSS scores and negative symptom scores as compared to haloperidol, with fewer extrapyramidal side effects but more weight gain, and longer clinical trial retention (Lieberman et al., 2003).

Clozapine is regarded by many psychopharmacologists as *the* most efficacious antipsychotic, remaining relatively unrivalled

Box 15.8

Cognitive Rigidity and Antipsychotics

Set-shifting is the executive function task of redirecting one's sustainable attention one stimulus to another, or one core set of concepts to another. Cognitive therapy is largely an effort to enhance someone's capacity and flexibility for disengaging their focused attention from thinking patterns that are erroneous, maladaptive, or otherwise disturbing or disruptive to normal functioning. Cognitive rigidity or inflexibility is a term sometimes used to describe situations in which this task is unduly effortful, and is thought to reflect dysfunction in circuitry involving the medial PFC and subcortical (e.g., thalamo-cortical or cortical-ventral striatal) circuitry. Perseverative thinking, with an inability to disengage and redirect one's thinking patterns, may reflect similar underlying phenomena. Can antipsychotics act as a mental "lubricant" to lessen cognitive rigidity and improve set shifting? Studies in schizophrenia suggest that the COMT polymorphism may moderate this relationship (specifically, Met rather than Val carriers in the Val158Met SNP) make fewer perseverative and regressive errors during antipsychotic treatment (Nelson et al., 2018). Animal studies also suggest that clozapine (Li et al., 2007) and some antipsychotic drugs with $5HT_7$ antagonism such as asenapine (Tait et al., 2009) may also promote cognitive flexibility (Nikiforuk and Popik, 2013).

among medication options for treatment-resistant psychosis. Once viewed as a drug of last resort, or at least only after an inadequate response to at least two antipsychotics, contemporary data support the utility of pursuing a clozapine trial in early-stage schizophrenia after even one failed trial of another antipsychotic, with better outcomes seen than when olanzapine was chosen as an alternative second-line agent in the so-called OPTiMiSE trial (Optimization of Treatment and Management of Schizophrenia in Europe; Kahn et al., 2018).

Tip

All antipsychotics likely can have pro-arrhythmic effects and may prolong the QTc on ECG when dosed high enough; clinicians who elect to pursue ultra-high doses of any antipsychotics would be wise to follow serial ECGs and probably should avoid high dosing of any antipsychotic in patients with high baseline QTc intervals or other clinical risk factors for QTc prolongation (as described in Chapter 10, Box 10.2).

G HIGH-DOSE ANTIPSYCHOTICS

Instinct, if not evidence, often leads clinicians to raise medication doses in the context of an inadequate response to usual optimized dosages. In the case of antipsychotics, very limited data actually support this practice and mostly involve reports involving only several of the available agents. A meta-analysis of five trials (n = 348 schizophrenia patients) comparing high-dose versus standard dosing of haloperidol, fluphenazine, quetiapine, and ziprasidone after initial nonresponse to standard dosing found no significant differences between high versus standard dosing strategies relative to changes either in positive or negative symptoms (Dold et al., 2015b). On the other hand, among olanzapine recipients, one industry trial found that dosages up to 40 mg/day were more efficacious than lower doses only when baseline symptom severity was high (Kinon et al., 2008). Naturalistic studies suggest that high-dose antipsychotics are more often prescribed as part of antipsychotic polypharmacy than as monotherapy (Roh et al., 2014).

Findings from ultra-high-dose SGA studies in schizophrenia are summarized in Table 15.4.

What about *rapid antipsychotic dosing* titration schedules? So-called "rapid neuroleptization" is shunned with FGAs due to a substantial likelihood of causing dystonic reactions. In contrast, in the case of SGAs, data support the potential usefulness of rapid initial dosing

Figure 15.4 Reasons for premature study discontinuation in the CATIE Trial. Based on findings from Lieberman et al., 2005.

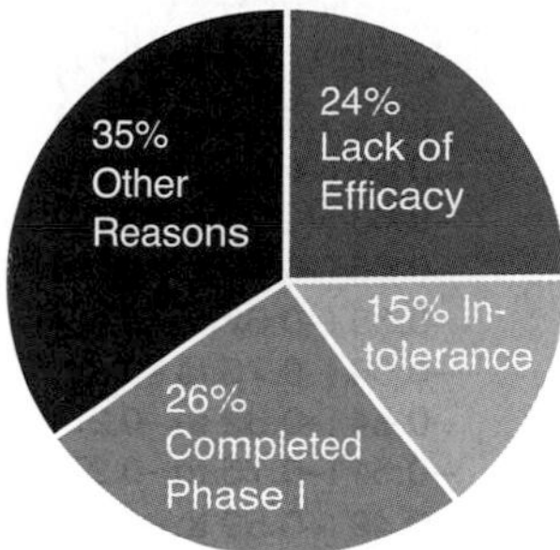

with several agents. In acute schizophrenia, quetiapine-IR dosed as 200 mg on Day 1, 400 mg on Day 2, 600 mg on Day 3, and 800 mg on Day 4 was compared to conventional dosing (50 mg on Day 1, 100 mg on Day 2, and increased in 100 mg/day increments to reach 400 mg on Day 5) in a group of 70 inpatients; no significant differences were seen between the two groups in frequency of adverse effects or dropout due to intolerance, but faster improvement in psychotic symptoms (by Day 4) was noted in subjects receiving rapid initial dosing (Pae et al., 2007). In studies of olanzapine for acute agitation in patients with schizophrenia or bipolar disorder, a decremental "reverse-loading" rapid initial dose escalation ("RIDE" strategy; up to 40 mg of oral olanzapine was allowed on Days 1 and 2, up to 30 mg on Days 3 and 4, and 5–20 mg/day thereafter) was compared to usual clinical practice (up to 10 mg/day on Days 1–4 then 5–10 mg/day thereafter); RIDE patients had greater reductions on PANSS "excited" subscale ratings at 24 hours and this group was superior to usual clinical practice on all measures of agitation by Day 4, with no observed significant difference from usual-care recipients in the incidence or severity of adverse effects (Baker et al., 2003).

H WHAT ARE EFFICACIOUS ANTIPSYCHOTICS IN SCHIZOPHRENIA?

Differences in the magnitude of clinical efficacy across most SGAs are fairly modest. In a important and comprehensive meta-analysis by Huhn et al. (2019) CrIs largely overlapped in standardized mean differences in symptom change scores (depicted in Figure 15.5), meaning there were no major differences across agents with respect to overall response – with the very notable exception of higher efficacy rates observed with clozapine as compared to other SGAs available in the United States. Table 15.5 describes antipsychotic dosing and receptor characteristics for the three available

Figure 15.5 Magnitude of overall change in symptoms: antipsychotic versus placebo. Adapted from Huhn et al., 2019.

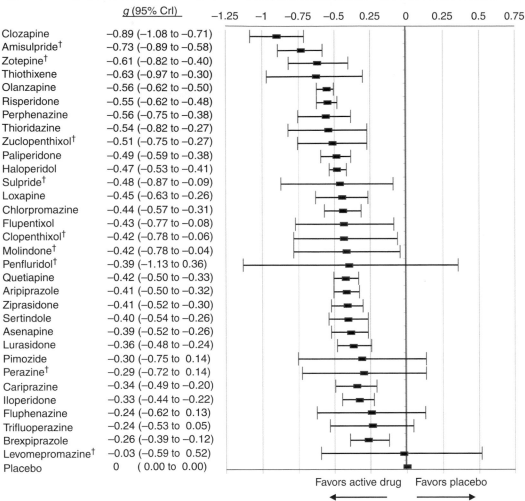

	g (95% Crl)
Clozapine	−0.89 (−1.08 to −0.71)
Amisulpride†	−0.73 (−0.89 to −0.58)
Zotepine†	−0.61 (−0.82 to −0.40)
Thiothixene	−0.63 (−0.97 to −0.30)
Olanzapine	−0.56 (−0.62 to −0.50)
Risperidone	−0.55 (−0.62 to −0.48)
Perphenazine	−0.56 (−0.75 to −0.38)
Thioridazine	−0.54 (−0.82 to −0.27)
Zuclopenthixol†	−0.51 (−0.75 to −0.27)
Paliperidone	−0.49 (−0.59 to −0.38)
Haloperidol	−0.47 (−0.53 to −0.41)
Sulpride†	−0.48 (−0.87 to −0.09)
Loxapine	−0.45 (−0.63 to −0.26)
Chlorpromazine	−0.44 (−0.57 to −0.31)
Flupentixol	−0.43 (−0.77 to −0.08)
Clopenthixol†	−0.42 (−0.78 to −0.06)
Molindone†	−0.42 (−0.78 to −0.04)
Penfluridol†	−0.39 (−1.13 to 0.36)
Quetiapine	−0.42 (−0.50 to −0.33)
Aripiprazole	−0.41 (−0.50 to −0.32)
Ziprasidone	−0.41 (−0.52 to −0.30)
Sertindole	−0.40 (−0.54 to −0.26)
Asenapine	−0.39 (−0.52 to −0.26)
Lurasidone	−0.36 (−0.48 to −0.24)
Pimozide	−0.30 (−0.75 to 0.14)
Perazine†	−0.29 (−0.72 to 0.14)
Cariprazine	−0.34 (−0.49 to −0.20)
Iloperidone	−0.33 (−0.44 to −0.22)
Fluphenazine	−0.24 (−0.62 to 0.13)
Trifluoperazine	−0.24 (−0.53 to 0.05)
Brexpiprazole	−0.26 (−0.39 to −0.12)
Levomepromazine†	−0.03 (−0.59 to 0.52)
Placebo	0 (0.00 to 0.00)

−1.25 −1 −0.75 −0.5 0.25 0 0.25 0.5 0.75

Favors active drug ← → Favors placebo

† Not available in the United States

I prefer to dose risperidone twice daily. Is that a problem?

Not a problem, but not really necessary. Once- or twice-daily risperidone dosing produced comparable response rates, time till response, and side-effect profiles – although plasma trough levels and median plasma concentrations in the first eight hours were somewhat higher with once- than twice-daily dosing, though that had no obvious clinical consequence (Nair, 1998).

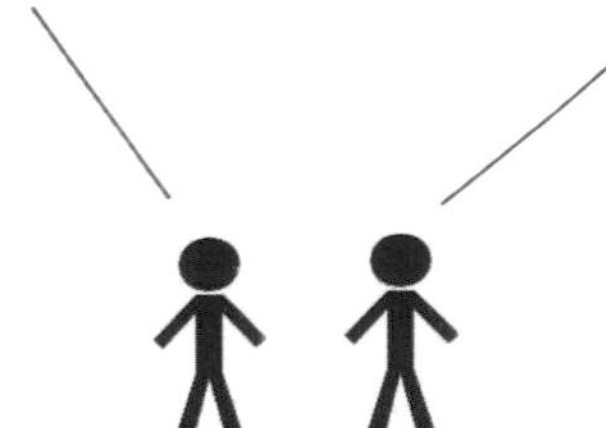

D_2/D_3 partial agonist SGAs. Tables 15.6–15.16 each individually discuss antipsychotic dosing and receptor features for currently available D_2 antagonist SGAs.

Linear dose–response relationships are often presumed with regard to antipsychotic efficacy. When patients do not improve at a particular dose, it is almost instinctive behavior on the part of many prescribers simply to raise the dose with expectations of a greater likelihood for efficacy. This is not always an evidence-based proposition, as illustrated by the example of lurasidone in Box 15.9.

That's all swell but the half-life of risperidone is only three hours. So why wouldn't you dose it more often than once a day?

Because the half-life of its active metabolite, 9-hydroxyrisperidone, is about 20-30 hours. Once a day is plenty frequent enough.

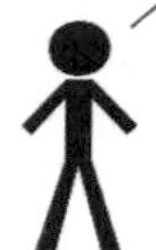

Box 15.9

Is There a Dose-Response Relationship with Lurasidone?

Five pivotal fixed-dose FDA registration trials of lurasidone in schizophrenia collectively failed to elucidate a clear signal regarding dose-response relationships with overall psychopathology outcome, and the observed findings can appear somewhat confusing. Fixed-dose comparisons versus placebo of either 40 mg/day or 120 mg/day were significant across three RCTs (Ogasa et al., 2013; Meltzer et al., 2011; Nasrallah et al., 2013), but (a) without a clear linear dose-response relationship or (b) showing significant separation from placebo at 80 mg/day but not 40 mg/day or 120 mg/day (Nasrallah et al., 2013). One can conclude that 80 mg/day was efficacious in every study at that dose but higher or lower doses were less reliable and dose escalation did not suggest progressive or commensurate increases in the magnitude of symptom reduction:

Notably, however, in patients who did not show at least a 20% symptom improvement after two weeks of lurasidone 80 mg/day, those whose dosages were then increased to 160 mg/day had a significantly greater reduction in positive and negative symptoms by six weeks (with a medium effect size) as compared to those who remained on 80 mg/day (Loebel et al., 2016).

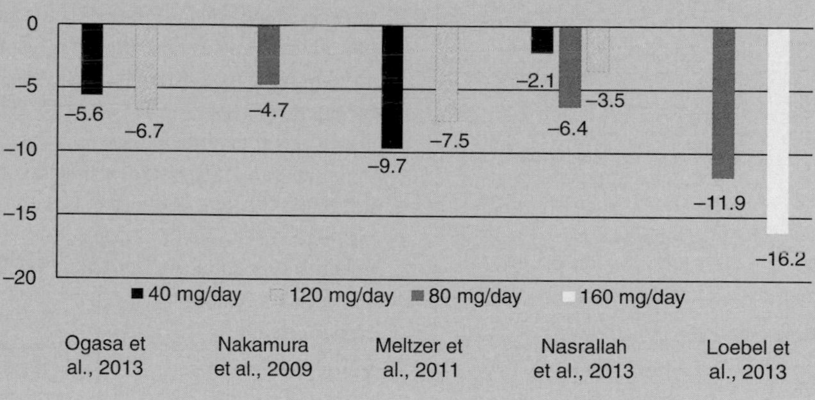

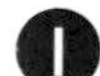

I SHORT-ACTING IM SGAs

Aripiprazole. Dosed at 9.75 mg up to three times/day, found to be superior to placebo and noninferior to IM haloperidol 6.5 mg IM at two hours postinjection (Andrezina et al., 2006). Direct subsequent transition to oral aripiprazole has been shown to ensue without an increased incidence of EPS, sedation, or other adverse effects.[1]

Olanzapine. Olanzapine for acute IM administration is dosed at 10 mg (may reduce to 5 or 7.5 mg if necessary) with a maximum of three doses at least two hours apart in 24 hours. Monitoring should occur for orthostatic hypotension. In a comparative RCT, greater reduction in agitation/excitation (and somnolence) was seen with olanzapine IM than aripiprazole IM at two hours but not 24 hours (Kittipeerachon and Chaichan, 2016). In 2005 a label warning cautioned against combining IM olanzapine with benzodiazepines following reports of

[1] In 2015 the short-acting IM formulation of aripiprazole was removed by its manufacturer from the US market for reasons unrelated to safety or efficacy.

fatalities, although subsequent observational studies have questioned the likelihood of significant adverse cardiovascular or cardiopulmonary outcomes (Williams, 2018).

Ziprasidone. IM ziprasidone to treat acute agitation is dosed at 10–20 mg/injection either as 10 mg IM every two hours or 20 mg IM every four hours (maximum daily dose 40 mg).

J LONG-ACTING INJECTABLE ANTIPSYCHOTICS

Long-acting injectable (LAI) antipsychotics have obvious value in patients with chronic psychotic disorders for whom adherence to oral medications is poor. Aripiprazole LAI has also been studied in relapse prevention for bipolar I disorder after an index manic episode. (Notably, in FDA registration trials of both aripiprazole monohydrate LAI and risperidone microspheres, efficacy was better than placebo for prevention of manic but not depressive episode relapses – however, a more fair appraisal of relapse prevention for depressive episodes would require a study design that initiated treatment following an index depressive episode, because existing trial designs were enriched for manic rather than depressive episodes (i.e., given that the polarity of the most recent episode is the more likely polarity of relapse.))

Tip

In addition to considering LAIs as a countermeasure for poor adherence, keep in mind that cariprazine has two active metabolites (desmethyl-cariprazine and didesmethyl-cariprazine) whose half-lives are one to three weeks – meaning that shaky adherence may be more pharmacologically forgiving. The long half-lives also may permit dosing less often than every day, should tolerability issues require especially low dosing.

On an overall basis, LAI antipsychotic pharmacotherapy in schizophrenia demonstrates strikingly higher rates of treatment adherence and lower rates of rehospitalization as compared to oral antipsychotics, as measured by claims-based data (e.g., Marcus et al., 2015). However, comparative studies of FGA versus SGA LAI preparations in schizophrenia have not demonstrated differences in rates of psychiatric rehospitalization, all-cause discontinuation, or hospital duration (Nielsen et al., 2015; Stone et al., 2018), making distinctions among treatment options more subject to patient preference/acceptability, adverse effect profiles, and cost than to differential efficacy.

Conversion of dosing from oral to long-acting injectable antipsychotics is summarized in Chapter 9, Table 9.6. Information to guide procedures after missed doses is summarized in Table 15.17.

Aripiprazole LAI achieves its steady-state pharmacokinetics by the fourth injection (as depicted in Figure 15.6); however, a clinically meaningful serum level (>100 ng/mL) is achieved after about one to two weeks. Note also that with no further injections after the 16th week, a clinically meaningful serum level is sustained for approximately another eight weeks.

K AUGMENTATION STRATEGIES FOR ANTIPSYCHOTIC DRUGS

A 2017 meta-analysis of 42 antipsychotic cotherapy combinations in schizophrenia revealed statistically significant advantages for a number of studied augmentations, depending on the outcome of interest (Correll et al., 2017). For treatment of *total psychopathology*, effect sizes for adjunctive pharmacotherapies that were significantly better than antipsychotic monotherapy are presented in Figure 15.7. *No significant effects* were seen with TCAs, testosterone, NMDA receptor antagonists, oxytocin, antipsychotics, pregnenolone, SSRIs, serotonin antagonist and reuptake inhibitors (SARIs), cholinesterase inhibitors, NERIs, H_2 blockers, divalproex, polyunsaturated fatty acids, MAO-B inhibitors, carbamazepine, DHEA, varenicline, or davunetide. Effect sizes observed for *positive symptoms* are presented in Figure 15.8.

Tip

Davunetide is a novel neuropeptide and antitau protein that is thought to confer neuroprotection via stabilizing microtubules.

For treatment of *positive symptoms*, notable common augmentation strategies that *failed* to reach statistical significance included lithium, additional antipsychotic(s), carbamazepine, NMDA receptor antagonists (e.g., memantine), acetylcholinesterase inhibitors, DHEA, and use of any antidepressant other than an NaSSA. In the case of schizophrenic negative symptoms inadequately responsive to an antipsychotic, common adjuncts

Figure 15.6 Mean serum plasma concentrations of aripiprazole after first injection. Adapted from Mallikaarjun et al., 2013.

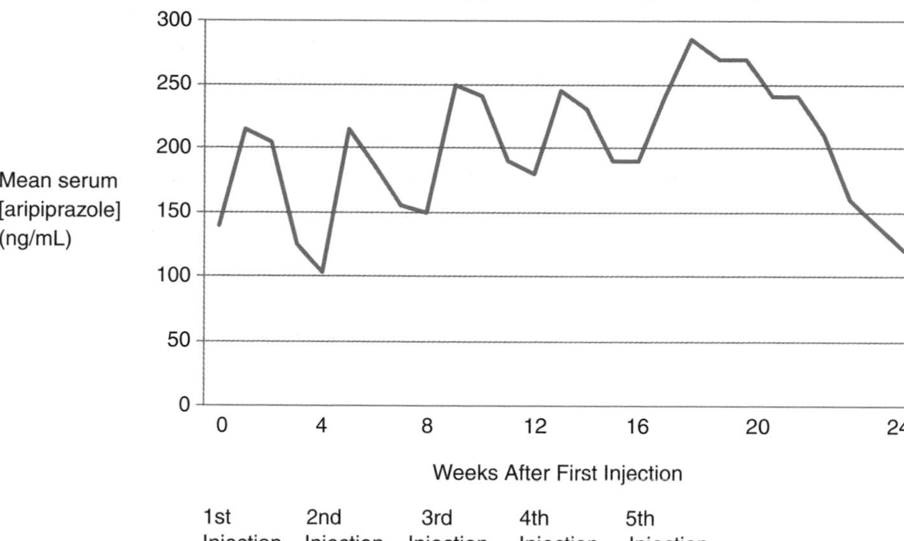

Figure 15.7 Effect sizes (g) for antipsychotic augmentation strategies: total psychopathology. Based on findings from meta-analysis by Correll et al. (2017).

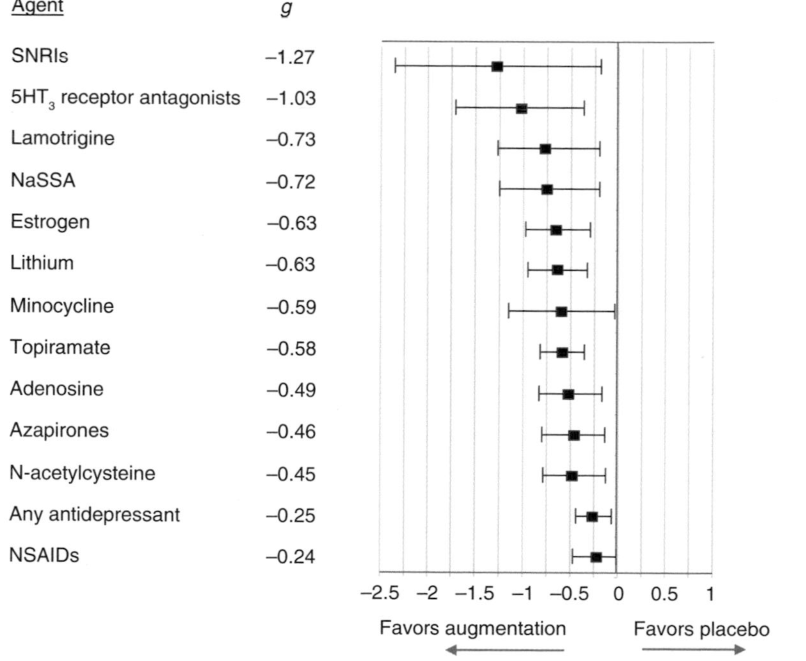

Figure 15.8 Effect sizes (*g*) for antipsychotic augmentation strategies: positive symptoms. Based on findings from meta-analysis by Correll et al. (2017).

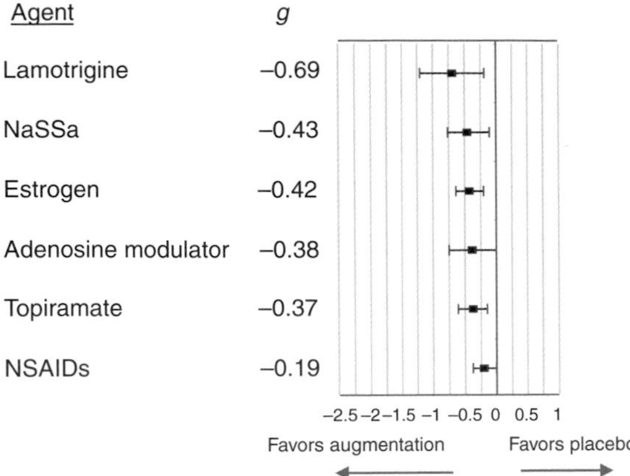

that failed to reach statistical significance included carbamazepine, lithium, pregnenolone, DHEA, adenosine modulators, NMDA receptor antagonists, and NSAIDs.

L POLY-ANTIPSYCHOTICS

Despite a dearth of evidence to support safety and efficacy, clinicians often combine two (or more) antipsychotics for a variety of reasons. These often include the hope for a faster onset, treatment of residual psychotic symptoms, targeted treatment of specific symptoms (e.g., agitation, anxiety, insomnia), hesitation to optimize the dose of a first antipsychotic (e.g., due to fears of adverse effects), or intended cross-tapers that never fully completed due either to fear of clinical worsening or the discovery of improvement mid-way through an intended cross-taper with an impression that synergy may have occurred and further tampering might be counterproductive. There is also at least some theoretical basis for using SGA polypharmacy to increase D_2 receptor occupancy while sparing some of the adverse effects that might otherwise arise from high-dose SGA monotherapy (Morrissette and Stahl, 2014).

The clinical trials literature regarding poly-antipsychotic use has been hampered by methodological inconsistencies (e.g., combining controlled and open trials, underpowered studies, variable trial durations, pooling of patients with varying levels of baseline severity, and variable optimization of a first antipsychotic before initiating the second). Few studies have also examined optimized dosing of both antipsychotics when the decision has been made to use multiple antipsychotics. (Sometimes, dosing optimization is presumed to be unnecessary, as in the example of purposefully using a low-dose antihistaminergic SGA such as quetiapine mainly for its sedative and pro-hypnotic rather than potential antipsychotic or antimanic/antidepressant properties, or using adjunctive ziprasidone as a possible cotherapy strategy mainly to counteract psychotropic weight loss (Wang et al., 2011).)

The largest meta-analysis to date examining poly-antipsychotic use identified 31 trials (n = 2073) (Galling et al., 2017). While an overall significant and clinically meaningful advantage for combination versus monotherapy was observed ($g = 0.53$), the effect was no longer significant when considering only double-blind studies or those otherwise considered high quality. However, adding a D_2 partial agonist (aripiprazole) to a full D_2 antagonist was found to further improve negative symptoms, as well as lower prolactin levels and decrease body weight. Contrary to expectations, no greater overall burden of adverse effects was seen when combining D_2 antagonists, except for higher prolactin levels than seen with D_2 antagonist monotherapy. A Cochrane Database review also found no advantage for combined versus monotherapy antipsychotics in schizophrenia for reducing relapse risk, rehospitalization rates, early treatment termination, or serious adverse events (Ortiz-Orendain et al., 2017).

M USING MOOD STABILIZERS AS ANTIPSYCHOTIC ADJUNCTS FOR PRIMARY PSYCHOTIC DISORDERS

A pharmacological conundrum in treating primary psychotic disorders is the relative lack of complementary MOAs from which combination drug regimens can thoughtfully be designed. Until viable antipsychotic MOAs involving circuitry other than direct modulation of dopamine pathways become feasible, clinicians are left essentially with the very limited options of combining antipsychotics (with prayers to the gods of pharmacodynamic synergy) or adding mood-stabilizing drugs (with prayers to the gods of extrapolation from nonaffective pharmacodynamics). Let us separately consider the existing database on "antimanic" mood stabilizers and other related compounds (perhaps best termed "antiglutamatergic anticonvulsants" for the present purposes).

In practice, adding antimanic mood stabilizers to *most* antipsychotics (with the possible exception of clozapine, as discussed separately in a later section) mainly seems to produce modest reductions in agitation/hostility or impulsivity in the context of treating nonaffective acute psychotic episodes. Adjunctive divalproex typically is begun at 15 mg/kg and may be increased as high as 35 mg/kg. Randomized data with divalproex-DR (see Table 15.18) reveal significantly greater initial improvement in delusions, excitation, poor judgment, impaired abstract thinking, and unusual thought content – however, advantages over a therapeutically dosed antipsychotic alone may be transient and serve mainly to accelerate overall improvement rather than produce a more enduring additive or synergistic effect on global mental state. A later, larger RCT with adjunctive extended-release divalproex found no advantage over olanzapine or risperidone alone – in fact, antipsychotic *monotherapy* was *better* than combined therapy with divalproex in reducing negative symptoms (Casey et al., 2009).

Tip

Antimanic mood stabilizers added to most antipsychotics (with the possible exception of clozapine; see later) may only transiently improve hostility/agitation, and not meaningfully diminish psychosis.

Perhaps divalproex simply provides an inadequate "antidote" to overcome the understimulation of mesolimbic GABA interneurons in schizophrenia (e.g., see Figure 15.3). What about other GABA analogues as adjuncts to antipsychotics in treating schizophrenia? Small, mostly open-label pilot studies and a handful of small randomized proof-of-concept studies have been conducted over the years with GABAergic agents such as gabapentin, pregabalin, and baclofen, among others. While such approaches are intriguing from a mechanistic standpoint, and some GABAergic compounds may help to reduce anxiety symptoms in schizophrenia patients, there is inadequate empirical data to draw conclusions about the utility of such approaches to treat psychosis after an incomplete response to dopamine antagonism. Moreover, some $GABA_A$-receptor-positive allosteric modulators such as barbiturates or benzodiazepines (e.g., lorazepam) *worsen* cognitive function (e.g., working memory) in schizophrenia. Lamotrigine stands apart from other "mood stabilizers" in that it is relatively devoid of GABAergic effects, and in fact is thought instead mainly to exert *antiglutamatergic* effects, which may account for its apparent greater value for depressive/internalizing rather than manic/externalizing symptoms (see also Chapter 13).

N LAMOTRIGINE

While lamotrigine does not directly affect glutamate receptors, it does diminish presynaptic glutamate release and as such represents a potentially attractive candidate for antipsychotic augmentation in psychotic disorders. The literature regarding lamotrigine augmentation of antipsychotics has been varied. Initial enthusiasm came from a positive RCT of lamotrigine or placebo augmentation of clozapine, followed by four subsequent RCTs lasting from 10–24 weeks; collectively, those five RCTs yielded an effect size (*g*) of 0.57 with an NNT of 4 (Tiihonen et al., 2009). A separate 10-week trial of adjunctive lamotrigine or placebo added to FGAs or SGAs then found no significant differences in the intent-to-treat study group but significant improvement was noted among the completer sample subgroup (Kremer et al., 2004). Two other placebo-controlled RCTs of adjunctive lamotrigine in schizophrenia patients resistant to SGAs then failed to replicate those initial findings (Goff et al., 2007). A more definitive meta-analysis of adjunctive pharmacotherapies after an inadequate response to clozapine, discussed separately below, failed to detect a significant signal with lamotrigine after removal of outliers from initial analyses.

Bottom Line

Adding lamotrigine to clozapine in treatment-resistant schizophrenia has an appealing theoretical rationale and may have some value based on the heterogeneity of study findings… but results have not been consistent or robust.

O OTHER ANTIGLUTAMATERGIC ANTICONVULSANTS: TOPIRAMATE

The anticonvulsant topiramate is, among other things, a glutamate-modulating drug (it exerts antiglutamatergic effects by binding to AMPA/kainate ionotropic glutamate receptors; it also binds to $GABA_A$ receptors) and, as such, holds at least theoretical relevance in the treatment of psychosis. A meta-analysis of 16 RCTs using topiramate as adjunctive therapy in schizophrenia (mean dose = 164.5 ± 70.4 mg/day) found a significant advantage over placebo for reducing PANSS or BPRS total scores with a medium effect size (*d* = 0.58), as well as PANSS positive symptoms (*d* = 0.37), negative symptoms (*d* = 0.58), and general psychopathology (*d* = 0.68) (Zheng et al., 2016b). Moderator analyses suggested that its effects were diminished in studies of short duration (<12 weeks) and when doses exceeded 150 mg/day. Dropout due to drug intolerance was no different than with comparator arms.

P ADJUNCTIVE ANTIDEPRESSANTS FOR PSYCHOSIS IN SCHIZOPHRENIA

A meta-analysis of 82 RCTs in which antidepressants were added to antipsychotics in schizophrenia revealed a significantly increased likelihood of response (RR = 1.52, 95% CI = 1.29–1.78; NNT = 5), though only fairly modest effects on positive symptoms (*d* = 0.17), negative symptoms (*d* = 0.30), or depressive symptoms (*d* = 0.25); risk for exacerbation of psychosis also appeared no higher than with comparator arms, suggesting that antidepressants overall represent a safe (if not robustly effective) adjunctive treatment option (Helfer et al., 2016). Unfortunately, subgroup analyses in that study failed to identify any particular patient types *most* helped by antidepressants – other than noting that effect sizes were generally somewhat higher when a pertinent target symptom domain (e.g., depression, or negative symptoms) was especially prominent at baseline (perhaps simply because greater variance existed from which to show changes over time). In meta-regressions, older age was associated with larger antidepressant–placebo differences for depression while higher baseline negative symptom scores showed larger antidepressant–placebo differences for reducing negative symptoms.

Studies of antidepressants specifically intended to target cognitive symptoms in schizophrenia have found statistically significant but clinically negligible differences in cognitive outcomes as compared to placebo (effect sizes ranging from 0.095 to 0.17) (Vernon et al., 2014).

Q OTHER ADJUNCTIVE STRATEGIES

Serotonin $5HT_3$ Antagonists. Postsynaptic $5HT_3$ receptors, usually thought of in relation to nausea, have garnered interest as a potential target for add-on pharmacotherapy in schizophrenia. A meta-analysis of six RCTs involving granisetron, ondansetron, or tropisetron found a significant and clinically meaningful advantage for PANSS total scores (*d* = 1.03) and PANSS negative symptom subscores (*d* = 1.10) but not PANSS positive symptom scores (*d* = 0.12) (Kishi et al., 2014).

Schizophrenia and $5HT_3$

$5HT_3$ receptor function is of theoretical interest in the pathogenesis of schizophrenia. Five RCTs of the $5HT_3$ antagonist ondansetron, dosed from 4-8 mg/day, showed a benefit in total psychopathology and negative symptoms, and may help EPS (Zheng et al., 2019). It was not so clearly of direct benefit to positive symptoms though.

NaSSAs. So-called noradrenergic and specific serotonergic antidepressants, as per NbN (NaSSAs), include mirtazapine and mianserin.[2] A meta-analysis of 12 RCTs as adjunctive pharmacotherapy in schizophrenia found a significant advantage with a large effect size for overall symptoms (*d* = 0.75), response rate (NNT = 4) and negative symptoms (*d* = 0.88) but not positive symptoms, depressive symptoms, or discontinuation rates versus placebo (Kishi and Iwata, 2014). NaSSAs also were associated with significantly lower rates of akathisia and EPS.

Anti-inflammatory Drugs. Interest in the association between serious forms of mental illness and inflammation has prompted studies of drugs with anti-inflammatory properties in the treatment of schizophrenia. NSAIDs are perhaps the best studied of agents in this overall class. An initial meta-analysis of five RCTs (n = 264) in schizophrenia, mainly examining celecoxib or acetylsalicylic acid, reported a significant effect on total symptoms (SMD = 0.43), positive symptoms (SMD = 0.34), and negative symptoms (SMD = 0.26) (Sommer et al., 2012). A later and larger meta-analysis (eight RCTs, n = 774) then found a statistically significant but clinically modest effect on positive symptoms (SMD = 0.19), with no significant change in negative symptoms (Andrade, 2014). A still later and broader meta-analysis of NSAIDs as well as other anti-inflammatory drugs involving 62 RCTs (including aspirin, celecoxib, omega-3 fatty acids, estrogen, selective estrogen receptor modulators, pregnenolone, *N*-acetylcysteine, minocycline, davunetide, and erythropoietin) found significant overall effects for

[2] Not available in the United States

reducing total (Hedge's $g = 0.41$), positive (Hedge's $g = 0.31$) and negative (Hedge's $g = 0.38$) symptoms, as well as cognitive improvements in particular with minocycline and pregnenolone (Cho et al., 2019). Within specific types of anti-inflammatory agents, adjunctive aspirin overall had the largest clinical impact. Effect sizes across specific anti-inflammatory drug classes from this latter study are depicted in Figure 15.9.

Statins. Statins are mainly thought to have at least theoretical relevance for treating positive and negative symptoms by virtue of their anti-inflammatory properties. A review of six RCTs (mostly small sample sizes and involving only 6–12 weeks of treatment) with simvastatin (40 mg/day), lovastatin (20 mg/day), atorvastatin (20 mg/day) or pravastatin (40 mg/day) found significant improvement in PANSS negative symptom ratings with simvastatin but no differences from placebo in the remaining studies (Kim et al., 2019).

Augmentation of Clozapine

Clozapine-resistant psychosis poses one of the most difficult pharmacological challenges in psychiatry, inasmuch as it is widely considered one of the most efficacious of all psychotropic drugs (see Figure 15.5), with no known better alternative pharmacotherapy for treatment-resistant psychotic disorders. (Though, as noted in Table 15.4, high-dose olanzapine may show comparable efficacy to clozapine in treatment-resistant schizophrenia.) Adding a second FGA or SGA to clozapine after an incomplete response is modestly supported by literature: in the previously mentioned meta-analysis by Galling et al. (2017) an overall significant ($p = 0.007$) medium effect ($g = 0.52$) was observed when either an FGA or SGA was added to clozapine, but findings were no longer significant when considering only studies deemed to be of high quality. Before embarking on augmentation strategies for clozapine, clinicians should first assure that fundamental aspects of clozapine therapy have occurred, including the features described in Box 15.10.

Tip

Adding aripiprazole to an SGA *other* than clozapine may worsen symptoms of psychosis due to the high D_2 binding affinity of aripiprazole (Freudenreich and Goff, 2002)

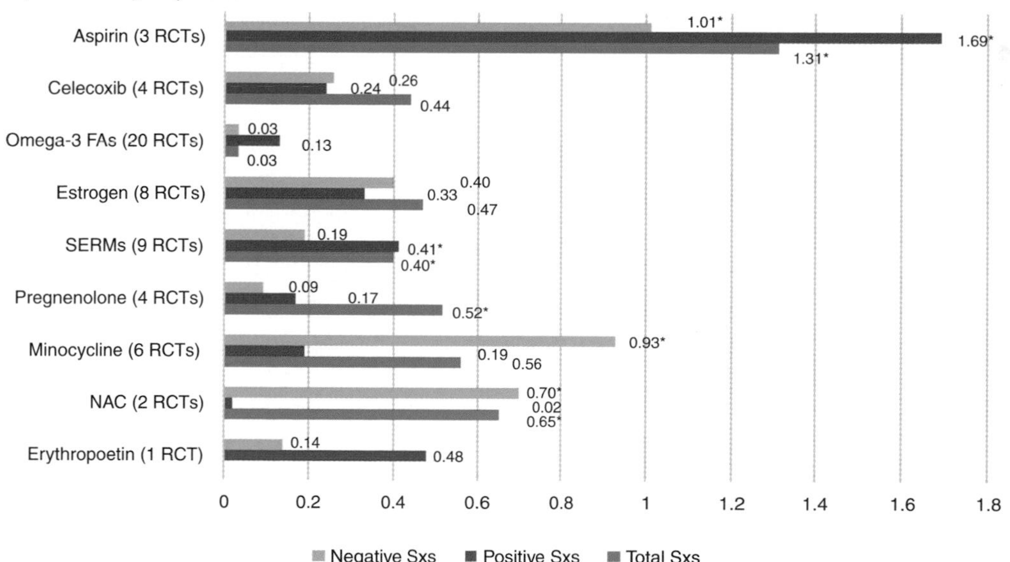

Figure 15.9 Effect sizes (Hedge's g) across anti-inflammatory RCTs in schizophrenia. Based on findings reported by Cho et al., 2019. Presented findings are statistically significant only where denoted (*) as such. "Total symptoms" not reported for erythropoietin.

Abbreviations: NAC = N-acetylcysteine; SERM = selective estrogen receptor modulator (i.e., raloxifene)

Box 15.10

Fundamental Aspects of Clozapine Therapy

- Assure clozapine has been optimally dosed in order to achieve a serum [clozapine] >350 ng/mL (see Chapter 7, Table 7.13). Note that clozapine efficacy has never been established via supratherapeutic dosing (i.e., dosages >900 mg/day and/or serum [clozapine] >1000 ng/mL)
- Assure reasonably good medication adherence
- Assure adequate duration of a clozapine trial - which in multidrug-resistant psychotic disorders may require several months or longer to form an accurate assessment
- Consider factors that can mediate (and attenuate) clozapine efficacy, such as cigarette smoking, alcohol or substance use disorders, or cotherapy with possible psychotomimetic agents such as amphetamine or methylphenidate
- Assess for presence of a comorbid and un(der)-treated mood disorder
- (Re)consider medical or neurological explanations for treatment-resistant psychosis, as illustrated by the case example in Clinical Vignette 15.1.

CLINICAL VIGNETTE 15.1

Persistent Psychosis Due to Another Medical Condition

Anthony was a 24-year-old man who dropped out of college following a severe acute psychotic episode, despite good premorbid functioning. Sequential adequate trials of several SGAs led to persistent adverse motor effects (akathisia, tremor, pseudoparkinsonism) but minimal antipsychotic efficacy. A clozapine trial was proposed. Over several months Anthony's dosage was increased to 500 mg/day with serum clozapine levels falling in the range 700–800 ng/mL. Sedation, cognitive dulling, and significant weight gain occurred, while tremor and EPS persisted with still minimal improvement in his complex delusional system: Anthony believed he was at the center of a government conspiracy and those around him were "operatives" sent to perform various psychological experiments and tests on him. His psychiatrist was struck by the persistence of Anthony's adverse motor effects, which displayed little change from one antipsychotic to another, including the time when clozapine was begun at low doses. A comprehensive metabolic panel was drawn and showed a mild transaminitis that Anthony's psychiatrist presumed reflected fatty liver due to his weight gain. Serology for hepatitis A, B, and C markers was negative, as was an abdominal ultrasound. Consultation with a gastroenterologist led to measurement of serum ceruloplasmin (found to be low) and 24-hour urine copper levels (found to be high). After a slit-lamp ophthalmology evaluation revealed the presence of Kayser–Fleischer rings, the diagnosis of Wilson's disease was made and chelation therapy with trietine was begun. The frequency and intensity of Anthony's delusional symptoms lessened as urinary copper levels eventually began to normalize.

Barring unusual clinical circumstances such as those present in Anthony's case, one might consider a number of pharmacological approaches when an incomplete response to clozapine occurs in severe/refractory psychosis. A meta-analysis focusing on augmentation strategies for clozapine identified 46 studies involving 25 intervention strategies (Siskind et al., 2018). Figure 15.10 depicts findings from studies adding FGAs or SGAs to clozapine. As is evident from the forest plot, aripiprazole and penfluridol[3] are the sole agents whose confidence intervals do not encompass zero, respectively exerting a medium or large effect size.

Figure 15.10 Effect sizes (g) for total psychotic symptoms with antipsychotics added to clozapine. Based on findings presented by Siskind et al., 2018.

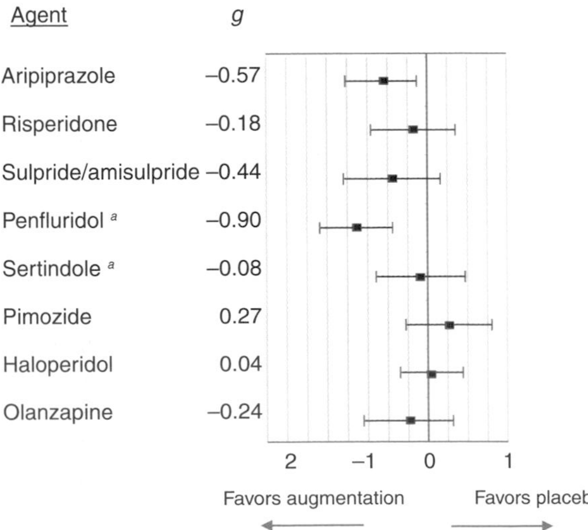

[a] Not available in the United States

[3] Not available in the USA

Other adjunctive agents that were found to significantly improve total psychotic symptoms when added to clozapine were fluoxetine ($g = 0.73$, 95% = −0.97 to −0.50) and divalproex ($g = 2.36$, 95% CI = −3.96 to −0.75), while adjunctive memantine improved negative symptoms ($g = -0.56$, 95% = −0.93 to −0.20); however, the authors note that many of the included studies were of poor quality, rendering their conclusions, at best, provisional.

The above findings dovetail with those of a separate meta-analysis focusing on anticonvulsant drugs added to clozapine in treatment-resistant schizophrenia, involving 22 RCTs (n = 1227) (Zheng et al., 2017b). That study found a significant benefit in positive symptoms and total psychopathology ratings for adjunctive divalproex (six RCTs, n = 430) as well as for topiramate (five RCTs, n = 270) (although topiramate had higher rates of all-cause discontinuation as compared to clozapine monotherapy (NNH = 7). Initial significant favorable effects of adjunctive lamotrigine became nonsignificant after outliers were removed from the meta-analysis.

In addition to the foregoing meta-analyses, significant improvement in both positive and negative symptoms was reported in a preliminary RCT of sodium benzoate 1–2 g PO qDay versus placebo added to clozapine in 60 poor clozapine responders (Lin et al., 2018).

Adjunctive ECT in Treatment-Resistant Schizophrenia

While our main focus throughout this text is on pharmacotherapies rather than devices or other biological interventions, we would note that ECT is sometimes considered a worthwhile intervention for refractory psychosis even in the absence of catatonia (where it represents the treatment of choice apart from benzodiazepines) or affective symptoms. A Cochrane Database review of 15 studies involving 1285 participants showed an advantage for clinical response (RR = 2.06, 95% CI = 1.75–2.42), though no advantage was observed when ECT was added to clozapine as compared to clozapine alone (Sinclair et al., 2019). Another meta-analysis of 11 RCTs (n = 818) reported a significant advantage and medium effect size ($g = 0.67$) for adding ECT to antipsychotics (other than clozapine) with NNT = 6 for response and NNT = 8 for remission (Zheng et al., 2016a).

Do Benzodiazepines Have Value in the Treatment of Schizophrenia?

Clinicians often use adjunctive benzodiazepines mainly to target agitation, insomnia, or anxiety in schizophrenia patients. The evidence base here again is unfortunately slim, perhaps reflecting more an absence of evidence than evidence of absence. A Cochrane Database review of 34 RCTs suggested only that benzodiazepine monotherapy provides short-term sedative benefit (measured in minutes to hours after administration) that was no different from antipsychotics, but confers no advantage over placebo with respect to more comprehensively assessed "response" rates (Dold et al., 2012).

Cannabidiol in Schizophrenia

A double-blind six-week exploratory RCT that examined CBD 1000 mg/day added to existing antipsychotics showed a significantly greater improvement in PANSS positive symptoms scale than with adjunctive placebo (p = 0.019) (McGuire et al., 2018). In reviewing the author's published data, we made use of a simple online effect size calculator to determine a Cohen's $d = 0.56$.

R COGNITION AS A PRIMARY TARGET OF TREATMENT IN SCHIZOPHRENIA

Global cognitive dysfunction that may worsen over time harkens to the original Kraepelinian construct of dementia praecox. Efforts to identify psychotropic interventions that can potentially leverage symptoms related to attentional processing, executive function, and memory have long been a holy grail of treatment studies, particularly because SGAs have generally not proven themselves to be effective remedies for cognitive dysfunction. Other strategies have thus far made only modest inroads in this endeavor, and both the quality and extent of data are limited:

- A meta-analysis of psychostimulants and atomoxetine in schizophrenia found consistent worsening of positive symptoms and relapse with methylphenidate; atomoxetine conferred some benefit for problem-solving skills while amphetamine showed a trend toward significance in improving executive function (Solmi et al., 2019). Balancing such observations are the potential psychotomimetic effects of both amphetamine and methylphenidate in individuals with a diathesis for psychosis (the so-called "dopamine supersensitivity" hypothesis in the pathophysiology of schizophrenia; Seeman, 2011).

- Limited data support the use of adjunctive modafinil to enhance pro-mnemonic, emotional processing, and problem-solving cognitive functions (Scoriels et al, 2013).
- Pro-cholinergics/acetylcholinesterase inhibitors (e.g., rivastigmine, donepezil, galantamine) have been shown to improve processing speed but not attention or working memory as compared to placebo in adults with schizophrenia (Santos et al., 2018).
- Adjunctive memantine, a weak NMDA receptor antagonist, has been shown to improve verbal recognition memory with medium effect size as well as both positive and negative symptoms (Veerman et al., 2016; de Lucena et al., 2009), but not executive functioning, with sustained effects over one year (Veerman et al., 2017). Dosed at 10 mg PO BID, its addition to risperidone also has been shown to improve attention, problem-solving, verbal learning, and cognitive flexibility better than placebo (Schaefer et al., 2019).
- α_7-Nicotinic acetylcholine receptor (α_7 nAChR) agonists have for many years been of theoretical interest in studies of cognitive dysfunction in schizophrenia and other conditions. While studies of animal models of psychosis have been encouraging, the existing database in human trials has been hampered by conflicting findings as well as potential cardiotoxicity and other (e.g., gastrointestinal) adverse effects (Beinat et al., 2015).
- A meta-analysis of intranasal oxytocin in schizophrenia found no overall benefit to improve social cognition but did suggest possible value in so-called "high-level" social cognition (e.g., mentalizing and theory of mind) (Bürkner et al., 2017).
- Novel strategies aimed at enhancing NMDA receptor function (recall Box 15.3) may hold promise for improving cognitive symptoms in schizophrenia, although studies remain preliminary. One such compound, sodium benzoate (an inhibitor of D-amino acid oxidase (DAAO), dosed at 1 g/day in combination with antipsychotics, has been shown to improve varied cognitive domains better than antipsychotics alone (Lane et al., 2013). Elsewhere, its addition to sarcosine resulted in better cognitive performance than seen with antipsychotics alone (unseen using adjunctive sarcosine *without* sodium benzoate) (Lin et al., 2017).

S LONG-TERM ANTIPSYCHOTICS IN SCHIZOPHRENIA

Finally, there remains debate about whether patients with chronic psychotic disorders such as schizophrenia or schizoaffective disorder routinely and expectably should remain on antipsychotic medications indefinitely (possibly permanently) after stabilization of an acute episode, or whether some subgroups actually fare better *not* taking long-term antipsychotic medications with respect to disease progression. The debate for versus against long-term/indefinite antipsychotic use is summarized in Table 15.19.

> *Nothing is known about the effects of antipsychotic drugs compared to placebo after three years.*
>
> - Leucht et al., 2012

"Good-prognosis" schizophrenia is often characterized by abrupt symptom onset, older age at onset, female sex, higher premorbid levels of psychosocial functioning (e.g., partnered, working), and an absence of comorbid substance use disorders (Correll et al., 2018). The presence of these characteristics, along with a marked remission of both positive and negative symptoms, would seem to be bare-minimum necessities for gauging the likelihood of successful candidacy for possible antipsychotic discontinuation in most patients with schizophrenia.

TAKE-HOME POINTS:

- Recognize that "treatment-resistant" psychosis can sometimes be confounded by poor adherence or suboptimal dosing/trial durations, comorbid substance abuse, a medical mimic, missed depression, or other unaddressed clinical idiosyncrasies.
- After two (and possibly even one) nonresponses to an adequate trial of an appropriate antipsychotic in schizophrenia or other conditions with prominent and persistent psychosis, consideration should be given to clozapine; dosed to a serum level >350 ng/mL but <1000 ng/mL. If necessary, counteract sedation, weight gain, or other side effects with strategies discussed in Chapter 10.
- It is reasonable to augment a partial response to clozapine with aripiprazole. Other SGAs or FGAs are less well-established in that role. Adjunctive lamotrigine could also be worth considering but data are mixed.
- Adjunctive divalproex (to clozapine) or topiramate (to any SGAs) are the best-studied mood stabilizer augmenters of SGAs. Not so much lithium.
- The literature does not strongly support efficacy from combining antipsychotics other than clozapine with aripiprazole (or possibly another SGA) in treatment-resistant psychosis, but there is little formal empirical study of poly-SGAs in treatment-resistant psychosis.
- Adding antidepressants to antipsychotics has not shown substantial value for treating positive symptoms in schizophrenia.
- Adjunctive ondansetron has preliminarily been shown to improve overall psychopathology, but not so clearly by exerting a specific effect on positive symptoms.
- Consider a role for ECT in treatment-resistant psychosis.

Table 15.1 FGA dosing: high-potency agents

Class	Specific agents	Dosing	Comments
Diphenylbutyl-piperidines	Pimozide	Begun at 1–2 mg/day, max 10 mg/day	Limited data suggesting utility in delusional parasitosis (see Box 15.2)
Butyrophenones	Droperidol	1.25–2.5 mg IM or slow IV	Used mainly for postoperative nausea/ vomiting; potential dose-related QTc prolongation
	Haloperidol	0.5–5 mg PO up to three times a day in schizophrenia. 2–5 mg IM in acute agitation	In severe agitation, doses may reach 40–100 mg/day. Dose-related risk for EPS/dystonia usually requires anticholinergic cotherapy. When given IV requires cardiac monitoring for QTc (ECG if not telemetry)

Abbreviations: IM = intramuscular; IV = intravenous; PO = by mouth; QTc = corrected QT interval; ECG = electrocardiogram

Tip

Remember pimozide has an increased risk for QTc prolongation, especially with CYP 2D6 inhibitors.

Tip

In severely ill inpatients with psychosis, capitalize on windows of opportunity by not skimping on adequate dosing when medications are willingly accepted.

Table 15.2 FGA dosing: medium-potency agents

Class	Specific agents	Dosing	Comments
Thioxanthenes	Thiothixene	Initially 5 mg PO BID, maintained at 20–30 mg/day, maximum 60 mg/day	A small, older literature also supports use at low doses in schizotypal and borderline personality disorders (see Chapter 20).
Dibenzepines	Loxapine	Initially dosed 10 mg PO BID, may titrate over 7–10 days to maximum of 50 mg/day	Comparable efficacy to risperidone or quetiapine; may cause more EPS than seen with SGAs (Chakrabarti et al., 2007). Inhaled formulation available (Adasuve®) to treat agitation associated with mania or psychosis (10 mg single-use inhaler given once q24 hours), carries risk for bronchospasm monitored through REMS program
	Trifluoperazine (piperazine side chain)	For psychosis, initially dosed 2–5 mg PO BID, maintenance dose 15–20 mg/day, maximum dose 40 mg/day; for anxiolysis, 1–2 mg PO BID (up to 6 mg/day)	Comparable efficacy to low-potency FGAs for treating psychosis (Tardy et al., 2014c). Superior to placebo for treating generalized anxiety disorder when dosed from 2–6 mg PO qDay (Mendels et al., 1986).
	Perphenazine (piperazine side chain)	For psychosis of moderate severity, usual dosing begins at 4–8 mg PO TID (maximum 24 mg/day; in severe psychosis, may dose as 8–16 mg PO BID–QID (maximum 64 mg/day)	Comparable efficacy to low-potency FGAs though with higher risk for akathisia (Tardy et al., 2014a).
	Fluphenazine (piperazine side chain)	For psychosis, usually begun as 2.5–10 mg PO every 4–6 hours (maximum 40 mg PO qDay) or 2.5–10 mg IM every 6–8 hours (maximum 10 mg/day); see Table 15.2 for long-acting injectable dosing	Comparable efficacy to low-potency FGAs for treating psychosis (Tardy et al., 2014b).

Abbreviations: BID = twice a day; EPS = extrapyramidal side effects; FGA = first-generation antipsychotic; IM = intramuscular; PO = by mouth; REMS = risk evaluation mitigation strategy; SGA = second-generation antipsychotic; TID = three times a day; qDay = once a day; QID = four times a day

Table 15.3 FGA dosing: low-potency agents

Class	Specific agents	Dosing	Comments
Phenothiazines	Chlorpromazine (aliphatic side chain)	10–25 mg PO TID as needed and tolerated for agitation associated with psychosis; as a primary antipsychotic in mania or schizophrenia, dosing may reach 1000 mg/day	May be more useful to treat agitation associated with psychosis than core elements of delusions or hallucinations, due to marked sedation and orthostatic hypotension at higher doses
	Thioridazine (piperadine side chain)	Usual initial dosing 50–100 mg PO TID, maintenance dose of 200–800 mg in divided dosing; low dosing (10–25 mg) used for anxiety, tension, and agitation	Boxed warning for dose-related QTc prolongation makes thioridazine appropriate only after failure to respond to other antipsychotics; contraindicated in combination with other drugs that cause QTc prolongation (see Chapter 10, Box 10.2); use also consequently not recommended in CYP450 2D6 PMs

Abbreviations: FGA = first-generation antipsychotic; PM = poor metabolizer; PO = by mouth; QTc = corrected QT interval; TID = three times a day

Table 15.4 Use of ultra-high-dose SGAs

Agent	Studies and outcomes
Aripiprazole	Safety data exist with dosing up to 90 mg/day. In general, doses >20 mg/day have not been shown to provide greater benefit as a group effect (Mace and Taylor, 2009). D_2 and D_3 receptor occupancy is ~95% with dosing at 30 mg/day (Yokoi et al., 2002). Case reports exist of therapeutic efficacy and safety up to 75 mg/day in treatment-resistant schizophrenia (Duggal and Mendhekar, 2006), but also of agitation and worsening psychosis with dosing of 60 mg/day (Thone, 2007)
Brexpiprazole	No data
Cariprazine	No data
Clozapine	No data >900 mg/day or with serum clozapine levels >1000 ng/mL. Risk for significant neurotoxicity and cardiotoxicity at supratherapeutic levels or when combined with potent CYP1A2 inhibitors such as ciprofloxacin. Use of adjunctive anticonvulsants to reduce risk for seizures is advisable with dosing >550 mg/day (Morrissette and Stahl, 2014) *This is really important!* ←
Iloperidone	No data. Concerns with supratherapeutic dosing (>24 mg/day) would involve the potential for significant orthostatic hypotension and sedation
Lumateperone	No data above 42 mg/day
Lurasidone	No data regarding efficacy. Doses of 240 mg/day in schizophrenia patients were associated with slowed attentional processing, impaired executive function, and reduced spatial working memory (Karpouzian-Rogers et al., 2020).
Olanzapine	- In a six-month RCT of clozapine (mean dose = 564 mg/day) versus high-dose olanzapine (mean dose = 34 mg/day, range 25–45 mg/day) in 40 treatment-resistant schizophrenia patients, both groups showed significant improvement from baseline with no significant between-group differences (although the study was not powered to demonstrate noninferiority) (Meltzer et al., 2008) - In contrast, another randomized double-blind crossover trial in 13 schizophrenia patients compared olanzapine 50 mg/day versus clozapine 450 mg/day, in which 6/13 olanzapine trials (46%) ended prematurely versus none of 10 clozapine trials; no olanzapine trials and 2/10 clozapine trials met "response" criteria, and effect sizes on BPRS subfactors were medium-to-large with clozapine but uniformly low with olanzapine (Conley et al., 2003) - Lastly, an open trial of olanzapine dosed up to 100 mg/day (mean dose = 31.3 mg/day) in 50 French schizophrenia inpatients or outpatients (mostly male smokers, ages 19–60) found a 68% response rate with generally good tolerability (adverse effects mostly involving involuntary movements (EPS, dystonia)) (Batail et al., 2014)
Paliperidone	No data
Quetiapine	Pierre et al. (2005) reported seven open cases of quetiapine dosed from 1200–2400 mg/day in treatment-refractory schizophrenia manifested mostly by positive symptoms and aggressive behaviors. Response times averaged 11 months, 4 of the 7 worsened after initially improving, and sedation, orthostatic hypotension, dysphagia and nocturnal startle reactions were common adverse effects. Another 12-week open case series (n = 12) targeting doses of 1200–1400 mg/day showed improvement in 4/12, but with poor tolerability (most subjects developed significant EPS, sedation, and weight gain and one developed diabetes mellitus) (Boggs et al., 2008).
Ziprasidone	An eight-week RCT compared dosing of 160 mg/day versus 360 mg/day in 75 schizophrenia patients who remained symptomatic despite treatment with 160 mg/day for three weeks; no significant differences were observed in symptom improvement but high-dose patients had lower diastolic blood pressures, more negative symptoms, and more QTc prolongation (Goff et al., 2013)

Abbreviations: BPRS = Brief Psychiatric Rating Scale; EPS = extrapyramidal side effects; QTc = corrected QT interval; RCT = randomized controlled trial; SGA = second-generation antipsychotic

Table 15.5 Dosing and use of SGAs: D_2/D_3 partial agonists

Agent	Notable receptor characteristics (apart from $5HT_{2A}$ antagonism)	Usual dosing in psychosis	Notable attributes
Aripiprazole	D_2/D_3 partial agonist, $5HT_{1A}$ partial agonist	Initial dosing in schizophrenia is 10–15 mg/day and 15 mg/day as monotherapy in mania. In our experience, particularly when other medications are present in a regimen, lower starting doses (i.e., 5 mg/day) are often appropriate and better tolerated. Titration to a maximum of 30 mg/day should occur based on response and tolerability	Long half-life (>75 hours) means the drug should auto-taper when stopped without the need for dosage reductions and that cross-tapers may require at least two weeks to reach either a steady state or terminal elimination half-life
Brexpiprazole	D_2/D_3 partial agonist, $5HT_{1A}$ partial agonist	Usually begun at 1 mg/day, may increase after four days to a target dose of 2 mg/day (days 5-7), then maximum of 4 mg/day by Day 8 and beyond	Long half-life (91 hours) holds similar pharmacokinetic implications as described above for aripiprazole
Cariprazine	D_2/D_3 partial agonist (*preferential D_3 > D_2 binding*), $5HT_{1A}$ partial agonist, $5HT_{1B}$ antagonist, modest H_1 antagonism	Usually begun at 1.5 mg/day, may increase to 3 mg on Day 2, usual range 3-6 mg/day; in schizophrenia dosing may go as high as 12 mg/day though unclear whether greater efficacy occurs at >6 mg/day	- Strong D_3 partial agonism may confer benefits in reward-based behavior - 72-week double-blind relapse prevention data in schizophrenia showed favorable metabolic profile (Durgam et al., 2016b) - Long half-life of two active metabolites

Abbreviations: SGA = second-generation antipsychotic

Table 15.6 Dosing and use of SGAs: asenapine

Receptor characteristics	Usual dosing in psychosis	Notable attributes
D_2 antagonist, $5HT_{1A}$ partial agonist	In schizophrenia, optimal dosing is 5 mg SL BID with no observed greater benefit at higher doses (10 mg SL BID) in FDA registration trials. In bipolar mania, recommended dosing is 5–10 mg SL BID.	Optimal bioavailability occurs via sublingual absorption (~35%) rather than oral administration (~2%) due to extensive first pass metabolism - Potent $5HT_7$ antagonism (Ki = 0.13 nM) prompts speculation about possible pro-cognitive effects, though little human data exists

Abbreviations: BID = twice a day; FDA = US Food and Drug Administration; SGA = second-generation antipsychotic; SL = sublingual

Table 15.7 Dosing and use of SGAs: clozapine

Receptor characteristics	Usual dosing in psychosis	Notable attributes
Loose D_2 antagonist; strong α_1 and H_1 antagonism	Usually begun at 12.5–25 mg/day, then increased by 25–50 mg/day every day, as tolerated, to a usual target range of 300–450 mg/day by two weeks. Subsequent increases should occur once or twice a week by ≤100 mg to a maximum of 600–900 mg/day, aiming for a serum clozapine level ≥350 ng/mL (see Chapter 7, Table 7.13). Dosing may be divided (BID or TID) to optimize tolerability, although in our experience most if not all of a therapeutic dose can be given at night. The manufacturer advises restarting from 25 mg/day in patients who have missed two or more days of medication with a potentially faster retitration to a previous effective dose if well-tolerated	No longer considered as strictly a drug of "last resort," clozapine has increasingly been acknowledged as warranting consideration after only one or two failed antipsychotic trials (Kahn et al., 2018)

Abbreviations: BID = twice a day; TID = three times a day; SGA = second-generation antipsychotic

Table 15.8 Dosing and use of SGAs: iloperidone

Receptor characteristics	Usual dosing in psychosis	Notable attributes
D_2 antagonist, strong α_1 and H_1 antagonism	Slow titration necessary to allow accommodation to significant α_1 antagonism: initiate at 1 mg PO BID on Day 1, 2 mg PO BID on Day 2, 4 mg PO BID on Day 3, 6 mg PO BID on Day 4, 8 mg PO BID on Day 5, 10 mg PO BID on Day 6, 10 mg PO BID on Day 7, then may increase to maximum of 12 mg PO BID on Day 8. In our experience, lower doses are often adequately effective	- Among the least likely of SGAs to cause EPS/akathisia - Beware potential for QTc prolongation with CYP2D6 inhibitors or genotypic PMs

Abbreviations: BID = twice a day; EPS = extrapyramidal side effects; PM = poor metabolizer; PO = by mouth; QTc = corrected QT interval; SGA = second-generation antipsychotic

Table 15.9 Dosing and use of SGAs: lumateperone

Receptor characteristics	Usual dosing in psychosis	Notable attributes
D_2 presynaptic partial agonist and postsynaptic antagonist	Dosing is 42 mg/day	May indirectly modulate glutamatergic neurotransmission, augmenting both NMDA and AMPA activity

Abbreviations: AMPA = α-amino-3-hydroxy-5-methyl-4-isoxazolepropionic acid; NMDA = *N*-methyl-D-aspartate; SGA = second-generation antipsychotic

Table 15.10 Dosing and use of SGAs: lurasidone

Receptor characteristics	Usual dosing in psychosis	Notable attributes
Minimal $5HT_{2C}$ and H_1 binding affinity; potent $5HT_7$ antagonism (K_i = 0.495 nM) and D_3 agonism (see Box 15.6) may contribute to potential cognitive benefits	Dosing in schizophrenia usually begins at 40 mg/day and may be increased up to 160 mg/day as per clinical judgment. Importantly, in fixed-dose FDA registration trials, there was no clear evidence of a linear dose–response relationship (Loebel et al., 2013)	- Relatively favorable metabolic profile (NNH for weight gain = 67 (Citrome, 2015)) - Possible cognitive benefit via $5HT_7$ antagonism

Abbreviations: FDA = US Food and Drug Administration; NNH = number needed to harm; SGA = second-generation antipsychotic

Table 15.11 Dosing and use of SGAs: olanzapine

Receptor characteristics	Usual dosing in psychosis	Notable attributes
Weak $5HT_{1A}$ antagonism	In schizophrenia, dosing is usually begun at 5–10 mg/day, aiming for a target dose of 10 mg/day. The manufacturer advises further dosage increases in increments of ≤5 mg/day no faster than once weekly to a maximum of 20 mg/day. (Maximal dosing in the CATIE trial was 30 mg/day.) Maintenance dosing of 10–20 mg/day is advised. In acute mania, initial dosing is 10–15 mg/day	- Considered among the more potent SGAs, set against a formidable metabolic adverse effect profile - Short-acting IM formulation available - Option of LAI for relapse prevention (see Chapter 9, Table 9.6)

Abbreviations: LAI = long-acting injectable; SGA = second-generation antipsychotic

Table 15.12 Dosing and use of SGAs: paliperidone

Receptor characteristics	Usual dosing in psychosis	Notable attributes
Tight D_2 antagonism, moderate $5HT_7$ blockade	In adults with schizophrenia or schizoaffective disorder, initial dosing is 6 mg PO qDay, titrated as per clinical judgment to a maximum of 12 mg/day or a minimum of 3 mg/day. The manufacturer advises upward dosing adjustments by increments of 3 mg/day no faster than every five days	- Uniquely carries FDA indication to treat schizoaffective disorder - Option of LAI for relapse prevention (see Chapter 9, Table 9.6)

Abbreviations: FDA = US Food and Drug Administration; LAI = long-acting injectable; PO = by mouth; qDay = every day; SGA = second-generation antipsychotic

Table 15.13 Dosing and use of SGAs: pimavanserin

Receptor characteristics	Usual dosing in psychosis	Notable attributes
Highly bound $5HT_{2A}$ inverse agonist and antagonist, less potent $5HT_{2C}$ inverse agonist/antagonist	For psychosis associated with Parkinson's disease, dosing is 34 mg PO qDay. In an initial Phase III trial as adjunctive therapy in schizophrenia, flexible dosing began at 20 mg/day and could vary from 10–34 mg/day; however, that trial failed to achieve statistical significance on its primary endpoint	Generally well tolerated; most common adverse effects include nausea, peripheral edema, confusion (all <10%)

Abbreviations: PO = by mouth; qDay = every day; SGA = second-generation antipsychotic

Table 15.14 Dosing and use of SGAs: quetiapine

Receptor characteristics	Usual dosing in psychosis	Notable attributes
Loose D_2 antagonist; strong α_1 and H_1 antagonism	Initial dosing in schizophrenia 25 mg PO BID titrated to target range of 150–750 mg/day (XR formulation initial dosing 300 mg PO qDay, titrated to 400–800 mg/day); bipolar mania initial dosing 50 mg PO BID titrated to target range of 400–800 mg/day (XR formulation initial dosing 300 mg PO qDay on Day 1 then 600 mg PO qDay on Day 2, titrated to target range of 400–800 mg PO qDay); bipolar depression initial dosing 50 mg PO qHS titrated to target dose of 300 mg/day (XR formulation dosed as 50 mg PO qDay on day 1, 100 mg PO qDay on Day 2, 200 mg PO qDay on Day 3, 300 mg PO qDay on Day 4)	Compelling anxiolytic profile, countered by formidable liability for weight gain and sedation acutely across indications **Tip** Quetiapine XR and IR both have ~7° half-lives; the IR formulation has a faster Tmax and higher Cmax; XR provides less variation from Cmax to Cmin.

Abbreviations: BID = twice a day; PO = by mouth; qDay = every day; qHS = every night; SGA = second-generation antipsychotic; XR = extended release

Table 15.15 Dosing and use of SGAs: risperidone

Receptor characteristics	Usual dosing in psychosis	Notable attributes
Highly bound $5HT_{2A}$ inverse agonist, potent antihistamine	Initial dosing in schizophrenia 2 mg/day (target dose ~4–8 mg/day), bipolar mania 2–3 mg/day (target dose ~1–6 mg/day)	Among the more high-liability SGAs for hyperprolactinemia; option for LAI for relapse prevention (see Chapter 9, Table 9.6).

Abbreviations: LAI = long-acting injectable; PO = by mouth; SGA = second-generation antipsychotic

Table 15.16 Dosing and use of SGAs: ziprasidone

Receptor characteristics	Usual dosing in psychosis	Notable attributes
$5HT_{1A}$ partial agonism, potent $5HT_{2C}$ partial agonism, modest H_1 antagonism	In schizophrenia, dosing begins at 20 mg PO BID titrated upward every two days up to 80 mg PO BID (usual target) or maximum of 100 mg PO BID. For acute agitation, dosing of 10–20 mg IM every two hours (maximum 40 mg/day) is appropriate. Dosing in acute mania begins at 40 mg PO BID, titrating upward to usual target range of 40–80 mg PO BID	- Greater bioavailability when administered with food - Among the more weight-neutral of SGAs - Short-acting IM formulation available - History of QTc prolongation is a relative contraindication

Abbreviations: BID = twice a day; PO = by mouth; QTc = corrected QT interval; SGA = second-generation antipsychotic

Table 15.17 How to address missed doses of SGA LAIs

SGA	Length of time since last injection		
Aripiprazole monohydrate			
If 2nd or 3rd scheduled dose is missed:	4–5 weeks: administer next dose as soon as possible		
if >4th scheduled dose is missed:	4–6 weeks: administer next dose as soon as possible >6 weeks: restart oral aripiprazole × 14 days with next injection		
Aripiprazole lauroxil			
Dose at last injection:			
441 mg	≤6 weeks	>6 but ≤7 weeks	>7 weeks
662 mg	≤8 weeks	>8 but ≤12 weeks	>12 weeks
882 mg	≤8 weeks	>8 but ≤12 weeks	>12 weeks
1064 mg	≤10 weeks	>10 but ≤12 weeks	>12 weeks
Dosage at readministration	No supplementation required	Supplement with single IM dose	Single IM dose or single 30 mg PO dose or 21 days PO
Olanzapine pamoate	No specific recommendations		
Paliperidone palmitate (Invega Sustenna®)			
If missed dose follows 1st injection:			
If less than four weeks since 1st injection:	156 mg IM (deltoid) as soon as possible, then 117 mg IM (deltoid or gluteal) five weeks later, then resume usual monthly schedule (deltoid or gluteal)		
If four to seven weeks since 1st injection:	156 mg IM (deltoid) as soon as possible, then repeat (same dose) one week later, then resume usual monthly schedule (deltoid or gluteal)		
If more than seven weeks since 1st injection:	234 mg IM (deltoid) as soon as possible, then 156 mg IM one week later (± four days), then resume usual monthly schedule (deltoid or gluteal)		
If missed dose follows a monthly injection:			
If four to six weeks since last monthly injection:	Resume usual monthly dosing as soon as possible		
If six weeks to six months since last monthly injection:	Usual IM dose (deltoid) as soon as possible, then repeat (same dose) after one week, then resume usual monthly schedule (deltoid or gluteal)		
If more than six months since last monthly injection:	234 mg IM (deltoid) initially then 156 mg IM (deltoid) one week later, then resume usual monthly schedule (deltoid or gluteal)		
Paliperidone palmitate (Invega Trinza®)			
If 14 weeks to four months since last dose:	Administer previous dose as soon as possible, then resume usual three-month dosing		

Table 15.17 (Cont.)

SGA	Length of time since last injection
If four to nine months since last dose:	Reinitiate as follows: If *last dose* was *273 mg*, give 78 mg IM on Day 1 and Day 8 (deltoid), then 273 mg IM one month later (deltoid or gluteal) If *last dose* was *410 mg*, give 117 mg IM on Day 1 and Day 8 (deltoid), then 410 mg IM one month later (deltoid or gluteal) If *last dose* was *546 mg*, give 156 mg IM on Day 1 and Day 8 (deltoid), then 546 mg IM one month later (deltoid or gluteal) If *last dose* was *819 mg*, give 156 mg IM on Day 1 and Day 8 (deltoid), then 819 mg IM one month later (deltoid or gluteal)
If more than nine months:	Reinitiate with Invega Sustenna® as per guidelines for its administration
Risperidone microspheres	No specific recommendations

Abbreviations: IM = intramuscular; LAI = long-acting injectable; PO = by mouth; SGA = second-generation antipsychotic

Table 15.18 Adding antimanic mood stabilizers to antipsychotics

Mood stabilizer	Study	Outcomes	Implications
Divalproex			
Casey et al., 2003	N = 249; 28-day RCT; divalproex-DR mean dose (BID) ~2300 mg/day (mean [VPA]~100 μg/mL) or placebo added to olanzapine (mean dose = 15 mg/day) or risperidone (mean dose = 6 mg/day)	Significantly better and faster reductions in PANSS scores for first three weeks but no significant difference by four weeks. Greater somnolence (29%), headache (20%), stomach upset (18%), and weight gain (12%)	Adjunctive divalproex may speed global improvement and facilitate hospital discharge but may not show a continued advantage beyond the first few weeks
Casey et al., 2009	N = 402; 12-week RCT; divalproex-ER mean dose (qDay) (mean [VPA] ~ 98 μg/mL) or placebo	No differences in PANSS total or positive symptom scores over the study period	No clear benefit
Lithium			
Leucht et al., 2015	Meta-analysis of 22 RCTs (N = 763)	1.8 × better response with lithium augmentation of antipsychotics but only when including schizoaffective disorder patients; little information on tolerability	Possible adjunctive value when affective symptoms are present; no direct effect on improving psychosis
Carbamazepine			
Leucht et al., 2014	Meta-analysis of 10 trials (N = 283 subjects)	No observed differences from placebo as adjunct to antipsychotics, or on reducing relapse rates	Existing studies are small and of variable quality. Concern that hepatic enzyme induction may cause reduced serum levels of concomitant antipsychotic drugs

Abbreviations: BID = twice a day; DR = delayed release; ER = extended release; PANSS = Positive and Negative Syndrome Scale; qDay = every day; RCT = randomized controlled trial; VPA = valproic acid

Table 15.19 Pros and cons of long-term/indefinite antipsychotic use in schizophrenia

Argument favoring indefinite antipsychotic use	Arguments opposing indefinite antipsychotic use
Most (~75%) schizophrenia patients who stop antipsychotic medications relapse within 12–18 months (Correll et al., 2018)	There is little to no systematic, randomized data supporting the safety and efficacy of continued antipsychotic therapy beyond three years' duration
Studies that purport good outcomes for schizophrenia patients not taking long-term medications are confounded by indication (i.e., good-prognosis patients are more likely to remain well off medications, while those who are prescribed long-term medications are likely to be more severely ill)	A definable subgroup of good-prognosis patients remain well without long-term antipsychotic treatment
Long-term (e.g., two-year) studies of antipsychotic dose reductions after acute stabilization have found higher relapse rates as compared to patients who continue without dosage reductions (Wunderink et al., 2013)	About 20% of patients from dose-reduction studies remain relapse-free at two-year follow-up, and by five-year follow-up relapse rates were comparable between those who had stopped versus continued antipsychotics (Wunderink et al., 2013)
	Eight very long-term naturalistic outcome studies (e.g., up to 20 years' duration) do not show routinely better global outcomes for patients who have taken versus not taken antipsychotic medications for more than two years (reviewed by Harrow and Jobe, 2018)

16 Deficit States and Negative Symptoms

LEARNING OBJECTIVES

- ☐ Differentiate negative symptoms from depressive states
- ☐ Describe the strengths and limitations of existing pharmacotherapies, including antidepressants, stimulants and other pro-dopaminergic drugs, antiglutamatergic agents, and hormonal therapies to treat negative symptoms
- ☐ Identify emerging and experimental pharmacotherapies to treat negative symptoms

Schizophrenia cannot be understood without understanding despair.

- R.D. Laing

A THE FOUR "A"s

Swiss psychiatrist Eugen Bleuler, who coined the term schizophrenia, identified **a**ffect, **a**ssociation, **a**mbivalence and **a**utism as the so-called "Four As" of negative symptom schizophrenia. Latter-day observers have sometimes added **a**logia, **a**nergia, **a**nhedonia, and **a**pathy/**a**motivation to the original list.

Negative symptoms, as classically associated with schizophrenia, refer to the absence of normal function (hence, they are "deficit" states), as contrasted with positive symptoms (that is, the *excess* presentations of otherwise normal brain functions). In that sense, negative symptoms also differ fundamentally from depression insofar as the latter represents a kind of positive symptom, one characterized by the "feelingful" presence of emotions (anguish, despair) – quite different from the emotional vacancy of flat (rather than sad) affect. The schizophrenia literature often refers explicitly to "the deficit syndrome." True negative symptoms can be among the hardest of symptoms to leverage pharmacologically. (Indeed, for the conventional operational definition of "response" for negative symptoms, the bar has generally been lowered so as to achieve only a 20% (or more) improvement from baseline symptom severity.) Clinicians sometimes cross their fingers with the hope that deficit states may just represent depression, and prescribe antidepressants vigorously and often sequentially (possibly even convincing themselves that nonresponse to antidepressants affirms the presence of TRD, rather than a different condition for which antidepressants may not be so helpful). Yet, the likely pathophysiology of negative symptoms is different from that seen with depression, making effective management a different kind of undertaking than that used in TRD.

A prevailing view is that negative symptoms arise from hypofunctioning of mesocortical DA circuitry, as touched upon earlier in Chapter 15 (e.g., see Figure 15.2). Once again, the notion of relative balance of dopaminergic functioning in different brain pathways bears on our understanding of positive versus negative symptoms. In the same vein, one might differentiate *primary* negative symptoms (arising from inherent hypodopaminergic tone in mesocortical pathways) from *secondary* negative symptoms as being more iatrogenic phenomena that result from the collateral damage to D_2 mesocortical circuitry caused by D_2 blockade from most if not all FGAs and some SGAs.

But what leads to the hypodopaminergic tone of mesocortical circuitry that is thought to account for negative symptoms? Recall from Chapter 15 (Figure 15.3) that in the case of positive symptoms, prevailing thinking is that *hyper*dopaminergic function in mesolimbic pathways is a downstream consequence of diminished corticolimbic glutamatergic excitation (believed to result from faulty cortical pyramidal neuron NMDA receptor functioning); GABA interneurons that would ordinarily inhibit mesolimbic DA tracts are understimulated and therefore fail to do so, giving mesolimbic DA free rein to run amok. In the case of mesocortical DA, it is thought that once again, faulty glutamatergic stimulation

Figure 16.1 Mesocortical dysfunction and negative symptoms.

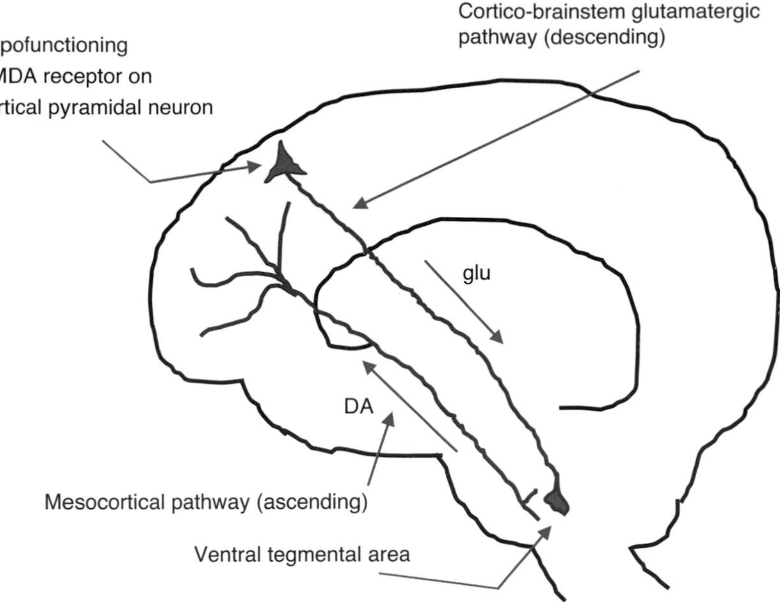

descending from the VMPFC to the ventral tegmental area (VTA) fails to "turn on" mesocortical DA, resulting in direct understimulation. No GABAergic middle-men this time.

Clinicians should have a clear concept of the phenomenology of negative symptoms and understand how to categorize and quantify their features and severity. Examples of relevant elements to note when interviewing a patient would include features such as an unchanging facial expression, decreased spontaneous movements, a paucity of expressive gestures, poor eye contact, lack of vocal inflections, poverty of content of speech, thought blocking, and an increased latency of response to questions. In most modern clinical trials, negative symptoms are quantified using either the negative symptoms factor subscale of the Positive and Negative Syndrome Scale (PANSS; Kay et al., 1987) or else the Schedule for the Assessment of Negative Symptoms (SANS; Andreason, 1982). Component items of these scales are summarized in Box 16.1.

Box 16.1

Measurement Scales and Subcomponents for Negative Symptoms

PANSS negative symptom factors	Schedule for the Assessment of Negative Symptoms (SANS)
• Blunted affect	• Affective flattening
• Emotional withdrawal	• Alogia
• Poor rapport	• Avolition–apathy
• Apathetic withdrawal	• Anhedonia–asociality
• Difficulty thinking	• Attentional impairment
• Lack of spontaneity	
• Stereotyped thinking	

B PHARMACOTHERAPY: ANTIPSYCHOTICS

The emergence of SGAs brought renewed optimism about the potential to impact negative symptoms, possibly via $5HT_{2A}$ antagonism (with consequent increases in prefrontal DA release). A reciprocal relationship exists between $5HT_{2A}$ and D_2 receptors such that, at least in principle, $5HT_{2A}$ antagonism should increase DA release. And, because of the relatively high density of $5HT_{2A}$ receptors in the prefrontal cortex, it would seem like a win–win proposition for most SGAs to capitalize on the potential for thus indirectly raising prefrontal DA tone while blocking mesolimbic DA (see Figure 16.2). Indeed, early favorable studies adding the $5HT_2/_{1C}$ antagonist ritanserin to FGAs to treat negative symptoms (Duinkerke et al., 1993) lent support to the hypothesis that SGAs might confer greater value than FGAs to improve deficit states.

Figure 16.2 Reciprocal relationship between $5HT_{2A}$ and mesocortical dopamine.

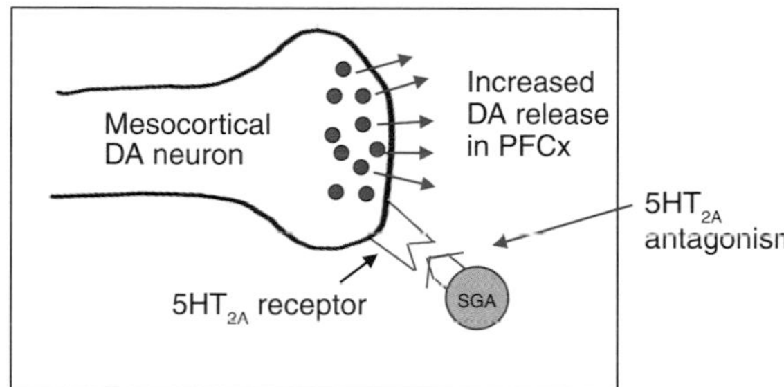

However, reality has not spectacularly borne out this expectation; while SGAs can treat negative symptoms, their impact is not that dramatic. A possible exception may be an as-yet unpublished favorable Phase II 26-week RCT with pimavanserin for negative symptoms, yielding a statistically significant advantage over placebo but with a small effect ($d = 0.21$).

One network meta-analysis of 11 studies involving eight antipsychotics (including FGAs (haloperidol, molidone) and SGAs (aripiprazole, olanzapine, risperidone, paliperidone, quetiapine, and ziprasidone)) found *no* significant effect of any agent on negative symptoms (Harvey et al., 2016) though another larger meta-analysis of 38 SGAs produced a moderate overall effect size for negative symptoms of $g = -0.579$ (95% CI = −0.755 to −0.404) (Fusar-Poli et al., 2015). FGAs in that meta-analysis, in contrast, had only a slightly smaller effect size ($g = -0.531$) but their difference from placebo was not significant (based on overlapping confidence intervals; 95% CI= −1.104 to 0.041). Another meta-analysis involving 21 RCTs of antipsychotics for negative symptoms concluded that olanzapine was superior to haloperidol, while cariprazine, olanzapine, and quetiapine were all more effective than risperidone (Krause et al., 2018b). Figure 16.3 depicts relative effect sizes reported in a meta-analysis of findings from 10

Figure 16.3 Impact of specific antipsychotics on negative symptoms. Based on findings reported by Leucht et al., 2009.

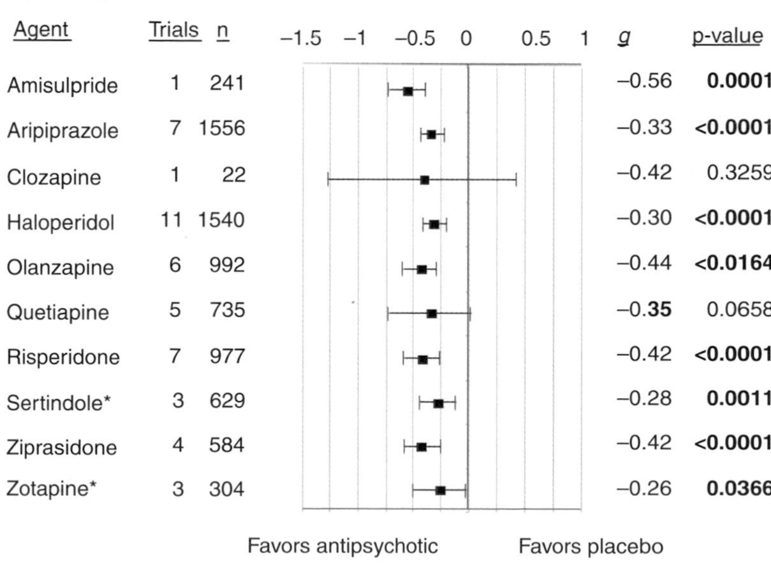

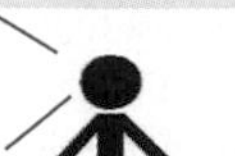

Um...I thought clozapine was supposed to be really good for negative symptoms. Why is its effect so piddly in that meta-analysis?
Where'd you hear that?
Uh, residency? Supervisor? Not sure...
Clozapine has not proven itself to be very effective for negative symptoms. A small early comparison to haloperidol showed a minor advantage for negative symptoms (Breier et al., 1994) that was not seen in later larger randomized comparisons (Buchanan et al., 1998; Kane et al., 2001); or, if there was an impact on negative symptoms, it was lost after controlling for its effect on positive symptoms (Rosenheck et al.,1999).

I read in Chapter 15 that adding aripiprazole to clozapine was effective in clozapine nonresponders. But if you add a D_2 partial agonist to a full antagonist, what's the net effect at the D_2 receptor, and couldn't that just make negative symptoms worse?
You're speculating that the D_2 antagonist and the partial agonist will inevitably wind up playing musical chairs in the mesolimbic and mesocortical pathways – which drug kicks the other off the D_2 receptor? But it's hard to predict the actual pharmacodynamic effects. Remember that in the tuberinfundibular pathway we get less prolactin elevation by adding aripiprazole to a D_2 full antagonist. So, read on.

antipsychotic RCTs reported by Leucht et al. (2009). Table 16.1 at the end of this chapter summarizes findings from RCTs across SGAs targeting negative symptoms.

In a meta-analysis of 18 trials (n = 931 subjects) of poly-antipsychotic therapy, negative symptoms showed greater improvement with poly-antipsychotic therapy than monotherapy ($g = -0.38$, 95% CI = −0.63 to −0.13, $p < 0.003$), but this occurred only in studies augmenting with aripiprazole (eight studies, N = 532, $g = -0.41$, 95% CI = −0.79 to −0.03, p = 0.036), and was just barely nonsignificant when two D_2 antagonists were combined (n = 10 trials involving 399 subjects; $g = -0.36$, 95% CI = −0.72 to 0.01, p = 0.056) (Galling et al., 2017). It is presently unknown whether the addition of other D_2/D_3 partial agonists (i.e., cariprazine, brexpiprazole) or lumateperone (a D_2 presynaptic partial agonist and postsynaptic antagonist) to a D_2 antagonist might similarly confer an advantage specifically for treatment of negative symptoms.

C ANTIDEPRESSANTS

In the pre-SGA literature, tricyclic antidepressants (imipramine, maprotiline) and MAOIs (tranylcypromine) represented the usual pharmacological approach to negative symptoms, and phenomenological parallels (rather than distinctions) were drawn between negative symptoms and postpsychotic depression. Early RCTs that reported benefit with tricyclics for negative symptoms also used relatively coarse outcome measures (e.g., clinical global impression (CGI) scores) (e.g., Siris et al., 1988). After SSRIs were introduced in the late 1980s and early 1990s, preliminary RCTs began to report improvement in negative symptoms with the addition of fluoxetine to FGAs (e.g., Spina et al., 1994).

A meta-analysis of 26 antidepressants for treatment of negative symptoms yielded a somewhat more modest pooled effect size than seen collectively with SGAs ($g = -0.349$, 95% CI = −0.551 to −0.146) (Fusar-Poli et al., 2015). Another meta-analysis of 42 studies (n = 1934 subjects) found that antidepressants in general more effectively treated negative symptoms when added to FGAs than SGAs (Galling et al., 2018). Changes in overall symptom burden were driven more by improvement in negative symptoms ($g = -0.25$, 96% CI = −0.44 to 0.06; p = 0.01).

Figure 16.4 summarizes findings from a meta-analysis involving 83 trials (n = 3251 subjects) prescribed antidepressants for negative symptoms.

Figure 16.4 Impact of specific antidepressants on negative symptoms. Based on findings from meta-analysis reported by Helfer et al., 2016.

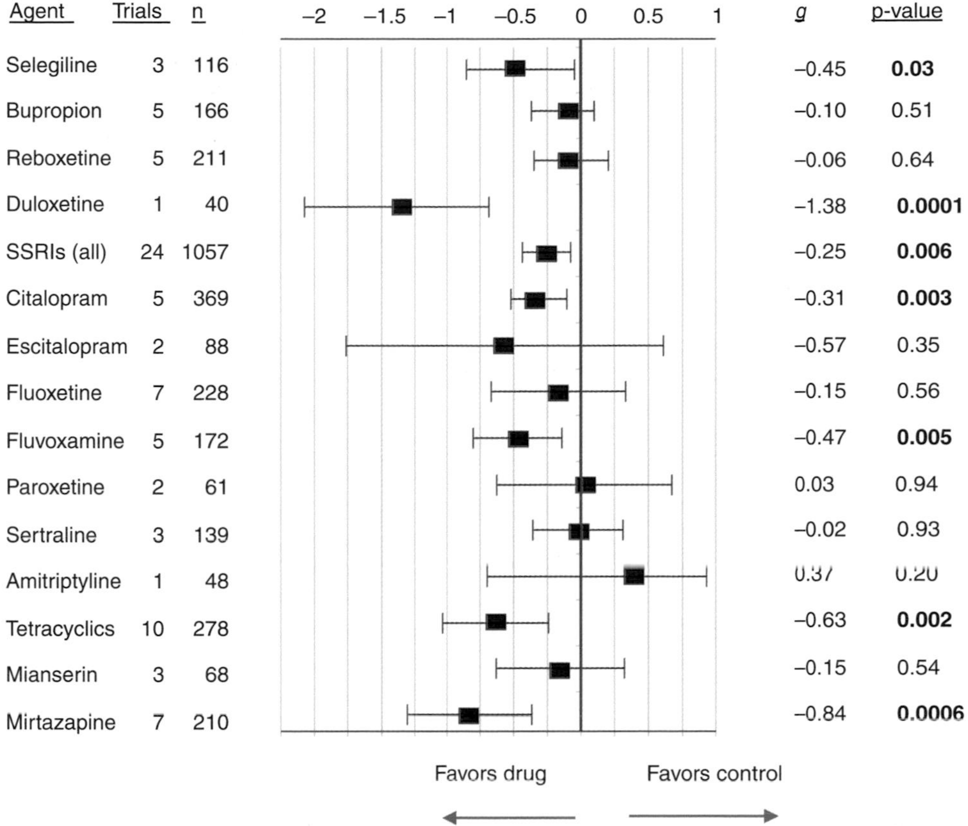

Agent Trials n
−2 −1.5 −1 −0.5 0 0.5 1
g p-value
Selegiline 3 116 −0.45 0.03
Bupropion 5 166 −0.10 0.51
Reboxetine 5 211 −0.06 0.64
Duloxetine 1 40 −1.38 0.0001
SSRIs (all) 24 1057 −0.25 0.006
Citalopram 5 369 −0.31 0.003
Escitalopram 2 88 −0.57 0.35
Fluoxetine 7 228 −0.15 0.56
Fluvoxamine 5 172 −0.47 0.005
Paroxetine 2 61 0.03 0.94
Sertraline 3 139 −0.02 0.93
Amitriptyline 1 48 0.37 0.20
Tetracyclics 10 278 −0.63 0.002
Mianserin 3 68 −0.15 0.54
Mirtazapine 7 210 −0.84 0.0006
Favors drug
Favors control

Looks like duloxetine and mirtazapine are both pretty impactful for schizophrenic negative symptoms. Hey, you think I could maybe combine both for their complementary MOAs and get like a rocket fuel type thing going?

You could certainly try combining them. That would be blending an evidence-based and rationale-based approach to a difficult clinical problem.

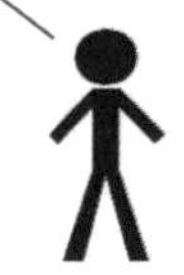

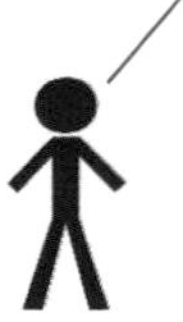

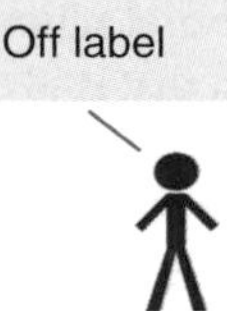

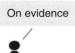

D PRO-DOPAMINERGIC AGENTS

Pro-dopaminergic drugs, including psychostimulants, represent among the more mechanistically obvious strategies to treat negative symptoms, presumably by countering hypodopaminergic mesocortical tone. The physiological challenge with such medications involves their unfortunate regional nonspecificity; the practical task is to increase mesocortical DA tone while sparing undesired pro-dopaminergic effects in mesolimbic pathways. An early effort in this regard involved adding pramipexole to haloperidol in 15 schizophrenia patients (Kasper et al., 1997), noting "response" (i.e., >20% improvement from baseline PANSS scores) in 9/15 but worsening in 3/15. A later small (n = 24) 12-week pilot RCT found adjunctive pramipexole (mean dose = 4.25 mg/day) better than placebo for improving both negative and positive symptoms in schizophrenia with good overall tolerability (Kelleher et al., 2012). Single case reports also describe success when adding ropinirole (up to 4 mg/day) or bromocriptine (10–20 mg/day) to antipsychotics in efforts to target negative symptoms.

What about (ar)modafinil, given its function as a DA receptor agonist? A meta-analysis of eight RCTs (n = 872) involving adjunctive (ar)modafinil for negative symptoms found a small but significant impact (g = −0.26, 95% CI = −0.48 to −0.04), improving PANSS negative subscale scores by a mean of only 0.27 points (Andrade et al., 2015). Surprisingly, that meta-analysis also found no significant effect for (ar)modafinil versus placebo on fatigue or daytime drowsiness, although may clinicians (us included) often regard this drug as having potential utility to counter iatrogenic sedation from antipsychotic drugs. We would also note the potential value of the novel antinarcoleptic drug solriamfetol (available as 75 or 150 mg/day); as a DA and NE reuptake inhibitor it offers conceptual appeal for negative symptoms, although studies have not, as yet, emerged involving its use for that purpose.

E AMPHETAMINES

Schizophrenia patients who misuse psychostimulants at least in some instances may genuinely be "self-medicating" insofar as they may be trying to use a potent D_2 agonist to compensate for mesocortical hypodopaminergic tone. In early literature, open trials reported significant improvement in negative symptoms from baseline following intravenous dextroamphetamine (van Kammen and Boronow, 1988). A later preliminary RCT (n = 37) reported only modest improvement in negative symptoms with oral adjunctive amphetamine versus placebo; however, that study involved only a single oral dose over one day (Sanfilipo et al., 1996). In a later and more traditional RCT, lisdexamfetamine (20–70 mg/day; median dose = 50 mg/day) plus existing antipsychotics was studied in a multicenter trial involving an initial 10-week open period followed by a four-week randomized discontinuation (Lasser et al., 2013).

After open treatment, 53% of subjects met responder criteria (>20% improvement from baseline SANS score) but at the conclusion of the double-blind withdrawal phase there was no significant difference between lisdexamfetamine and placebo.

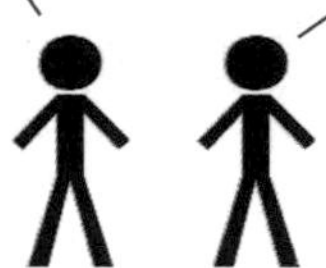

So net–net "negative" on stimulants for negative symptoms?
Not necessarily. Findings thus far truly are mixed and further studies are warranted.

In their overall literature review of psychostimulants in schizophrenia, Lindenmayer and colleagues (2013) found variable outcomes: some randomized trials of dextroamphetamine dosed up to 60 mg/day found no differences in negative symptoms relative to placebo, while others noted increased paranoia, belligerence, and hostility, as well as adverse cardiovascular effects in up to 8%. Data with methylphenidate are comparatively less extensive and involve relatively small numbers of subjects. With no definitive, adequately powered RCTs of adjunctive amphetamine for negative symptoms in schizophrenia, the available evidence base limits our ability to draw firm conclusions about their relative safety (are there identifiable moderators to gauge their patient-specific risk for inducing psychosis or agitation?) and efficacy.

F NMDA RECEPTOR MODULATORS

Given that presumptive hypoactive NMDA receptor function is thought to contribute significantly to the pathogenesis of both positive and negative symptoms in schizophrenia, innovative research efforts have increasingly looked for strategies that could potentially enhance NMDA receptor functioning either directly or through the glycine or other modulatory sites on the receptor. All are of interest with respect to both positive and negative symptoms. Several molecules have been studied, and all presently remain more of interest to clinical investigators than everyday practitioners. These include several amino acids that can potentially coactivate the NMDA receptor by agonizing or partially agonizing the glycine regulatory site (see Chapter 15, Figure 15.3) – specifically, D-serine, D-cycloserine, sarcosine, and glycine. Mixed findings exist with most agents. For example, in RCTs of D-cycloserine for negative symptoms, once-weekly dosing of 50 mg over eight weeks improved SANS scores better than did placebo (Goff et al., 2008), but elsewhere, 22 male schizophrenia patients randomized to D-cycloserine 50 mg PO qDay did not differ in SANS scores from placebo recipients after four weeks (Duncan et al., 2004). Oral glycine itself (dosed at 0.4 mg/kg/day, or about 30 mg/day) has been shown to improve negative symptoms significantly, albeit modestly (by ~15%) (Javitt et al., 1994), though possibly with greater effect at higher doses (i.e., 60 mg PO qDay) (Heresco-Levy et al., 1996). Similarly, some data with sarcosine have been favorable – for example, a six-week RCT in 65 Taiwanese schizophrenia patients receiving 2 g PO qDay (versus placebo) added to risperidone found significant reductions in SANS total and subscale scores, particularly for improving alogia and blunted affect (Lane et al., 2005) – but a meta-analysis of four RCTs produced a nonsignificant overall finding for negative symptoms relative to placebo, as discussed further below.

A meta-analysis of 32 NMDA receptor modulators (n = 1413 subjects with chronic schizophrenia) found an overall modest effect on negative symptoms ($g = -0.27$; p = 0.01) (Singh and Singh, 2011). Notably, in that study no NMDA receptor modulators were found to improve negative symptoms when added to clozapine. A summary of findings from this meta-analysis is presented in Figure 16.5. (Additionally, a later and larger meta-analysis of studies involving only *N*-acetylcysteine in schizophrenia (n = 7 trials including 220 subjects randomized to NAC and 220 to placebo) found a significant overall effect ($g = -0.72$, 95% CI = −1.20 to −0.25, p = 0.003) (Yolland et al., 2019).)

The amino acid antioxidant carnosine may also exert some effect on NMDA receptor modulation, although it has been less extensively studied than other such molecules. An initial eight-week study as augmentation to risperidone in 60 schizophrenia patients treated in Iran found greater improvement in PANSS negative syndrome subscores than with adjunctive placebo ($d = 0.79$, p = 0.004) (Ghajar et al., 2018b).

Figure 16.5 Effect sizes of NMDA receptor modulators for negative symptoms in schizophrenia

Agent	Usual Dosing Range	Trials	n	g	p-value
CX516	2700 mg/day	2	123	0.09	0.63
D-alanine	7000 mg/day	1	31	−0.81	**0.03**
D-cycloserine	50–200 mg/day	10	360	0.12	0.55
D-serine	2000 mg/day	5	203	−0.53	**<0.001**
Glycine	2000–60000 mg/day	7	268	−0.39	0.13
Memantine	20 mg/day	2	156	−1.51	0.32
N-acetylcysteine	2000 mg/day	1	140	−0.45	**0.01**
Sarcosine	2000 mg/day	4	132	−0.32	0.07

−4 −3 −2 −1 0 1

Favors drug ← → Favors control

So when it comes to NMDA receptor modulators for negative symptoms in schizophrenia, go with D-serine, *N*-acetylcysteine or D-alanine and bag the rest?

Whoa, slow down there partner. These are all highly experimental agents that pertain to one presumed underlying mechanism relevant to schizophrenia…but all are far from established and ready for mainstream use in the clinic.

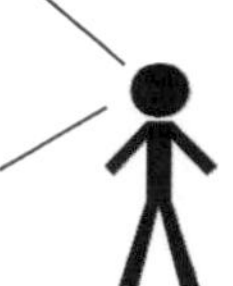

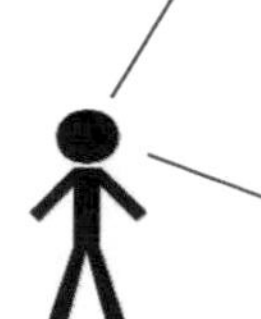

Then why are you even showing this information?

Because negative symptoms are very hard to treat and there is no established best treatment. These are all options to be aware of and possibly consider, recognizing the very preliminary nature of the data.

G OTHER ANTIGLUTAMATERGIC AGENTS

Minocycline. The antibiotic minocycline has been reported to exert both anti-inflammatory and antiglutamatergic properties. A meta-analysis of six RCTs (n = 215 subjects taking minocycline, n = 198 taking placebo), usually at a target dose of 200 mg PO qDay, found superiority over placebo on the PANSS negative symptom subscale ($g = -0.76$, 95% CI = −1.22 to −0.31; p = 0.001) and executive functioning ($g = 0.22$, 95% CI = 0.01–0.44; p = 0.04) (but not attention or memory) (Solmi et al., 2017). Tolerability was comparable to placebo.

Bitopertin. The glycine reuptake inhibitor bitopertin, though found to be unhelpful for positive symptoms in schizophrenia (see Chapter 15, Box 15.3), was shown at 10 mg or 30 mg PO qDay in a randomized proof-of-concept study to improve negative symptoms significantly better than placebo over eight weeks (about a 25% improvement from baseline with either dose) (Umbricht et al., 2014a).

Pregnenolone with *L*-Theanine

Pregnenolone is a neurosteroid with diverse actions related to cognition and neuronal growth and development. It also is a precursor to other neurosteroids such as allopregnanolone (known to affect mood and stress response via modulation of $GABA_A$ receptors) and pregnenolone sulfate (a positive allosteric modulator of NMDA receptors) (Marx et al., 2011). An initial RCT adding pregnenolone 50 mg PO qDay or placebo to existing antipsychotics over eight weeks in symptomatic nonchronic schizophrenia patients suggested *significant improvement in negative symptoms* with a large effect size ($d = 0.79$) (Ritsner et al., 2014). A later controlled adjunctive trial with risperidone in women with schizophrenia preliminarily found a significant reduction in negative symptoms that was not sustained after Bonferroni correction (Kashani et al., 2017). Negative studies have also been reported, with a meta-analysis concluding no significant overall effect on negative symptoms for pregnenolone (Heringa et al., 2015).

l-Theanine, an amino acid found in green tea (see Chapter 11), has a chemical structure similar to that of glutamate and has been shown to increase glutamate and glutamine density in frontal and inferior parietal regions among schizophrenia patients (Ota et al., 2015). The rationale for its pairing with pregnenolone involves its potential complementary neuroprotective function in either an additive or synergistic fashion. In an 8-week RCT comparison of placebo versus pregnenolone 50 mg PO qDay plus *l*-theanine (400 mg PO qDay) in 40 chronic schizophrenia or schizoaffective disorder patients, the combination produced a significantly greater reduction in negative symptoms than with placebo, yielding moderate effect sizes (Kardashev et al., 2018). These initial favorable findings await replication.

Dehydroepiandosterone (DHEA)

DHEA is a precursor to both testosterone and estrogen, and is thought to have neuroprotective properties. In schizophrenia, high DHEA levels have in some studies been associated with lower symptom severity (Harris et al., 2001). However, an 8-week RCT in 58 patients with chronic schizophrenia or schizoaffective disorder *failed to show a difference* from placebo (Ritsner et al., 2010).

Oxytocin

The pituitary hormone oxytocin has garnered increasing interest for its role in aspects of social "salience" (e.g., empathy, trust, awareness of social cues) as well as a potential direct effect on psychosis (the latter potentially mediated via its direct effects on DA regulation). However, a review of six RCTs (with intranasal dosing ranging from 24–80 IU/day) found *no significant effect* on negative symptoms (g = 0.33, p = 0.159) (Heringa et al., 2015).

Estrogen

A meta-analysis of seven RCTs using estrogen involving 479 patients (one study enrolling men only) found a modest effect on negative symptoms ($g = 0.23$, p = 0.027) (though a somewhat greater effect on positive symptoms ($g = 0.41$, p = 0.002)) and total symptom severity (g = 0.71, p = 0.003); findings were negligibly different when focus was confined only to female subjects (Heringa et al., 2015). Estradiol, the more potent agonist of estrogen receptors, may produce larger effects than other estrogen formulations for negative symptoms (Begemann et al., 2012). Raloxifene, a selective estrogen receptor modulator (mixed estrogen agonist/antagonist), dosed at 120 mg/day for 12 weeks in postmenopausal women, has been shown to improve total and general symptoms on PANSS ratings better than placebo, but no significant effect on negative symptoms has been demonstrated (Kulkarni et al., 2016).

Testosterone

A single RCT of 1% testosterone gel 5 g nightly versus placebo added to existing antipsychotic (and other) medications in 30 schizophrenic men (ages 20–49) found a significant effect on negative symptoms ($g = 0.82$, $p = 0.027$) though no significant effect on positive symptoms or total symptom severity (Ko et al., 2008).

Ondansetron

As noted in Chapter 15, the $5HT_3$ antagonist ondansetron has been shown to exert a greater benefit than placebo as an adjunct to antipsychotics in improving PANSS total scores, based on meta-analysis of three RCTs (n = 171, SMD = −1.06, 95% CI = −2.10 to −0.02). More specifically, it appears better than placebo in improving negative symptoms (meta-analysis including four RCTs, n = 209, SMD = −0.96 (95% CI = −1.71 to −0.22) but had only a marginally significant effect on positive symptoms (p = 0.05) (Zheng et al., 2019). RCTs (mostly involving augmentation to haloperidol or risperidone) studying oral dosing of 8 mg/day for up to 12 weeks also have reported improvement in EPS and gastrointestinal adverse effects from antipsychotics (e.g., Zhang et al., 2006).

Citicoline

Citicoline is a nutritional supplement with possible neuroprotective properties (see Chapter 11, Table 11.10). A preliminary RCT from Iran found that citicoline 2500 mg/day led to greater improvement in PANSS negative syndrome subscores as compared to placebo (Ghajar et al., 2018a).

Cannabidiol

In contrast to an encouraging preliminary finding for positive symptoms (see Chapter 14), RCT data have shown no significant impact of CBD (dosed at 1000 mg/day) for PANSS negative symptoms when added to existing antipsychotics in schizophrenia patients (McGuire et al., 2018).

TAKE-HOME POINTS

- Negative symptoms are hard to treat and have no "gold standard" remedy nor any specific agents that exert a large effect size.
- Negative symptoms differ fundamentally from depression; monoaminergic antidepressants tend not to be very effective - with the possible exceptions of mirtazapine and/or duloxetine.
- SGAs as a class have only modest value and there are no dramatic differences among them in efficacy for negative symptoms. Adding aripiprazole to a full D_2 antagonist may be somewhat helpful.
- Data are mixed, but at least somewhat encouraging, with the addition of lisdexamfetamine. Augmentation with pregnenolone (50 mg PO qDay) or with *l*-theanine (400 mg PO qDay) appears safe and has some preliminary supportive evidence, as does ondansetron 8 mg PO qDay.
- Premenopausal women who are gynecologically eligible for estradiol may notice a benefit for negative symptoms.
- D-serine and *N*-acetylcysteine also appear to be safe nutraceuticals that may have some value in a treatment regimen targeting negative symptoms.

Table 16.1 Effects of SGAs on negative symptom scale scores across FDA registration trials in schizophrenia

SGA	Change from baseline in negative symptoms
Aripiprazole	Across five pooled 4–6-week acute trials in schizophrenia, mean change from baseline = -0.35 (versus -0.9 with placebo) (p <0.001); significantly greater reductions than with placebo in all PANSS negative symptom domains except for blunted affect (Kane et al., 2008)
Asenapine	Dosing at 5 mg PO BID (but not 10 mg PO BID) was superior to placebo on the PANSS negative subscale at Weeks 5 and 6 (Kane et al., 2010)
Brexpiprazole	A pooled analysis of two Phase III studies found a mean PANSS negative subscale score drug-placebo difference of −1.2 points at 2 mg/day (p = 0.0015; *d* = 0.24) and −1.28 points at 4 mg/day (p = 0.0007; *d* = 0.25), with no significant changes observed at dosages of 0.25 or 1 mg/day; a Phase II placebo-controlled study (with aripiprazole as an active comparator) found no significant changes from baseline in PANSS negative subscale scores with any dose studied (0.25, 1 mg, 2.5 mg, 5 mg) (but also no change was observed with aripiprazole 15 mg/day) (Correll et al., 2016)
Cariprazine	With dosing of 1.5–3 mg/day: LSMD = -2.0, ES = 0.41; slightly over half met "responder" criteria; with dosing of 4.5–6 mg/day: LSMD = -3.4, *g* = 0.71; about 70% met "responder" criteria (Earley et al., 2019b)
Clozapine	A meta-analysis of seven short-term randomized comparisons to other SGAs found a small-to-medium effect (*g* = –0.25, 95% CI = –0.40 to –0.10) favoring clozapine (led mainly by one comparative study with risperidone) and eight long-term randomized comparisons to other SGAs found no significant difference (*g* = –0.11, 95% CI = –0.39 to 0.16) (Siskind et al., 2016)
Iloperidone	Based on pooled data from seven acute clinical trials (four placebo- and active-controlled and three noninferiority active-comparator trials), significantly greater reduction in PANSS negative symptom subscale for dosing at 10–16 mg/day (but not 20–24 mg/day) relative to placebo (Citrome et al., 2011)
Lurasidone	A pooled analysis of patient-level data from five 6-week fixed-dose (40–160 mg/day) RCTs revealed a significant reduction in PANSS negative symptoms (p < 0.001) with an effect size (Cohen's *d*) - 0.33 (Loebel et al., 3015)
Lumateperone	In a randomized comparison of lumateperone versus placebo, PANSS negative subscale scores were not significantly different from placebo either at a dosage of 28 mg/day (p = 0.03, ES = 0.11) or 42 mg/day (p = 0.09, ES = 0.20) (Correll et al., 2020)
Olanzapine	Across a range of dosages, significantly greater reductions in SANS scores than with placebo (by about 26–27%) (Beasley et al., 1996); in an internationally conducted randomized comparison of olanzapine (5–20 mg/day) with haloperidol (5–20 mg/day), significantly greater reductions in PANSS negative syndrome subscale scores with olanzapine (mean change = –4.5) than haloperidol (mean change = -3.2) (p = 0.03; *d* = -0.21) (Tollefson et al., 1997)
Paliperidone	- In a six-week comparison of 6, 9, or 12 mg/day of oral paliperidone, PANSS negative factor scores were significantly improved from baseline at all doses (-4.2, -3.5, and -5.0 points, respectively (we calculate Cohen's *d* (relative to placebo) = 0.53, 0.44, and 0.67, respectively) (Kane et al., 2007) - Another six-week RCT compared 6, 9 or 15 mg/day with placebo (and olanzapine 10 mg/day as an active comparator) and again found significant reductions from baseline PANSS negative factor scores at all doses (-3.9, -3.9, and -4.2 points, respectively, corresponding to (our calculated) *d* (relative to placebo) = 0.52, 0.53, and 0.59, respectively) (Davidson et al., 2007) - A third six-week RCT, comparing 6 or 12 mg/day of paliperidone to placebo or olanzapine 10 mg/day, found significant reductions in negative factor scores with both paliperidone doses (means and SDs not reported, making effect sizes not calculable) (Marder et al., 2007)

SGA	Change from baseline in negative symptoms
Quetiapine	- A six-week Phase II flexibly dosed RCT (mean dose = 307 mg/day) found significantly greater improvement in SANS scores than with placebo (Borison et al., 1996) - In a six-week Phase II trial, change in PANSS negative syndrome subscale scores with quetiapine (mean dose = 407 mg/day) was no different from chlorpromazine (mean dose = 384 mg/day) (Peuskens and Link, 1997) - In another Phase II study, quetiapine dosed up to 750 mg/day did *not* differ from placebo on PANSS negative syndrome subscale scores but did separate on the SANS (Small et al., 1997) - In a six-week Phase III RCT, SANS scores significantly improved with quetiapine 300 mg/day but not 75 mg/day, 150 mg/day, 600 mg/day, or 750 mg/day (Gunasekara and Spencer, 1998) - A six-week Phase III RCT found significantly greater improvement in SANS scores with dosing at 225 mg PO BID (but not 25 mg PO BID or 150 mg PO BID) than placebo (King et al., 1998)
Risperidone	A meta-analysis of six RCTs with dosing from 4–8 mg/day found a 1.43-fold greater likelihood of achieving "response" on negative symptoms (>20% improvement from baseline) as compared to FGAs (Carman et al., 1995)
Ziprasidone	Doses of either 80 mg/day or 160 mg/day reduced PANSS negative syndrome subscale scores significantly better than placebo over six weeks (Daniel et al., 1999), but no significant difference from placebo in a four-week RCT dosed at 40 or 120 mg/day in schizophrenia or schizoaffective disorder patients (Keck et al., 1998). During a one-year placebo-controlled relapse prevention study, greater reductions in PANSS negative syndrome subscale scores were observed versus placebo at highest doses (i.e., 160 mg/day = –4.2 point difference (p <0.001); 80 mg/day = –1.0 point difference (p = 0.011); 40 mg/day = –1.9 point difference (p <0.001) (Arato et al., 2002)

Abbreviations: BID = twice a day; ES = effect size; FDA = US Food and Drug Administration; FGA = first-generation antipsychotic; LSMD = least square mean differences; PANSS = Positive and Negative Syndrome Scale; PO = by mouth; RCT = randomized controlled trial; SANS = Schedule for the Assessment of Negative Symptoms; SGA = second-generation antipsychotic

17 Anxiety

LEARNING OBJECTIVES

- ☐ Appreciate that anxiety symptoms and disorders are often less benign and more insidious than one might initially think
- ☐ Distinguish preventative from abortive pharmacotherapy strategies for management of anxiety and their relative appropriateness for a given patient
- ☐ Understand the demonstrated anxiolytic properties of specific antidepressants, benzodiazepines, anticonvulsants, and antipsychotics, as well as antihistamines, β-blockers, α agonists, and cannabidiol

Present fears are less than horrible imaginings.

- Shakespeare (Macbeth)

Ostensibly innocuous, yet deceptively so, like Monty Python's fabled Killer Rabbit of Caerbannog (but with no Holy Hand Grenade of Antioch to lob as a countermeasure), anxiety often stands underappreciated for its pernicious and often devastating ill effects. Less profound and baffling than the perceptual and ideational anomalies of psychosis, less emotionally wrenching or blatantly lethal than suicidal melancholy, and less relentlessly haunting than the psychic sequelae of trauma, anxiety may be the prime example of a normal human emotion gone awry. While "normal" anxiety cues vigilance to environmental threats, demands, and rewards, *aberrant* anxiety paralyzes cognitive function, overrides judgment, subverts harm appraisal, drives impulsive action, and generally worsens the prognosis and treatment responsiveness of any coexisting psychiatric problem. It is also easily mistaken for other forms of psychopathology that involve autonomic hyperarousal and psychomotor activation, potentially driving wrong pharmacotherapy decisions.

Tip

Anxiety follows an inverted U-shaped curve, sometimes known as the Yerkes-Dodson law; a minimum threshold of anxiety is necessary for arousal, vigilance and motivation, but beyond an *optimum point* leads to disorganization and impaired performance.

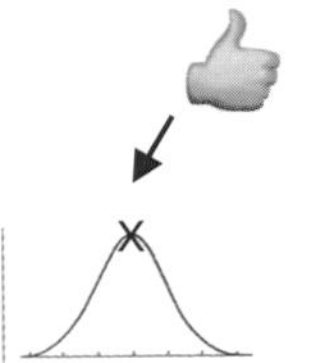

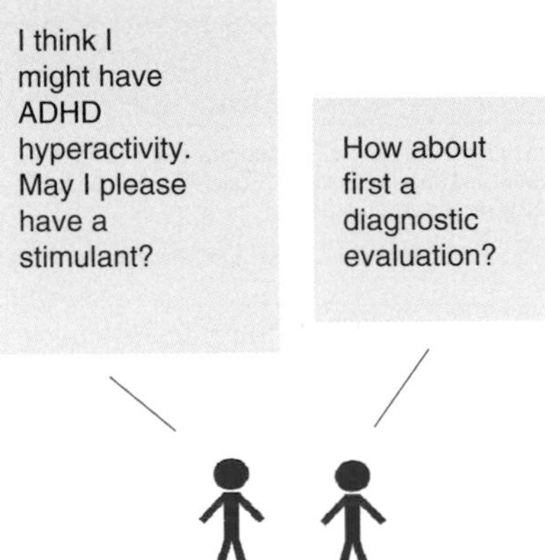

I think I might have ADHD hyperactivity. May I please have a stimulant?
How about first a diagnostic evaluation?

Collectively, anxiety disorders are the most common psychiatric condition in the United States, annually afflicting about 18% of adults. They are also among the most heterogeneous of disorders, cutting across virtually all forms of psychopathology, with implications for likely shared underlying neural circuitry. Their diverse phenomenology can involve psychomotor hyperactivity, somatization, disruption to the sleep–wake cycle and sleep architecture, eating dysregulation (restriction; comfort/binge eating), relief-based addiction behaviors, cognitive/executive dysfunction ("Can you consider the possibility that there may be alternative explanations for how you are interpreting events?"), rumination, and harm appraisal.

It is useful to differentiate anxiety *symptoms* from formal *disorders*, and the extent to which they may be comorbidities versus artifacts of other free-standing conditions. Anxiety is often (but not always) linked with affective disorders. Asking patients if they perceive a chronology (does anxiety precede depression or vice-versa? Or are they entirely coincidental?) may help gauge whether one of the two represents the more driving force, with possible pharmacological implications. Subthreshold anxiety symptoms often color the presentation of virtually all other psychiatric disorders. It is also, therefore, especially useful to clarify what exact problems patients are actually referring to when they invoke language involving the concept of "anxiety."

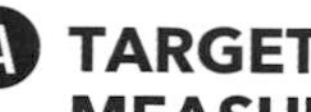

TARGET SYMPTOMS AND THEIR MEASUREMENT

Because the term "anxiety" can encompass many diverse emotional states, and in the spirit of defining the goals of treatment, clinicians should aim to delineate specific target signs and symptoms of anxiety before embarking on its pharmacotherapy. Box 17.1 provides a kind of informal glossary that may help to "translate" patients' subjective complaints about anxiety into more definable and tangible symptoms that become targets of treatment.

Box 17.1

Defining The Signs and Symptoms of "Anxiety"

The Term ...	... Really Means ...
"Activation"	Medications that can induce a state of psychomotor acceleration or hyperarousal (such as stimulants or some antidepressants) may cause patients to complain of "anxiety"
"Agitation"	A state of feeling keyed-up and restless; motor hyperactivity tends not to be goal-directed
"Akathisia"	Subjective and/or objective restlessness caused by dopamine antagonists
"Delirium"	Delirious patients, with an acutely altered sensorium with waxing and waning consciousness, may identify themselves as feeling "anxious" when they actually mean "grossly cognitively disorganized" and "unable to process basic information due to unalertness"
"Dementia"	Dementia patients may use the term "anxiety" to capture subjective feelings of distress associated with confusion, disorientation, memory loss, or other aspects of cognitive disorganization
"Depression"	Clinically depressed patients may misidentify anxiety as a predominant emotional state when sadness or despair may be more accurate descriptors of their internal experience
"Hyperactivity"	In ADHD, hyperactivity is a hyperkinetic phenomenon involving fidgetiness or squirminess, impatience, difficulty taking turns, and a sense of urgency
"Mania"	The psychomotor activation of (hypo)mania is purposeful and goal-directed, in contrast to the more diffuse sense of tension and distress associated with agitation
"Obsession"	The repetition of a(n often senseless) thought that intrudes into one's awareness, from which it is difficult to redirect sustained attention elsewhere
"Panic"	A brief, time-limited autonomic hyperarousal state that involves tachypnea, tachycardia, and feelings of dread; "anxiety" may pertain to an anticipatory state of recurrences
"Paranoia"	Someone who expects harm or mistreatment by others may identify their apprehension as "anxiety" without necessarily registering the nefarious intent they attribute to others
"Racing thoughts"	The phenomenon in which one thought follows another at an accelerated rate, often making it difficult to discern their specific content, usually associated with the psychomotor acceleration of mania/hypomania
"Ruminations"	Excessive and repeated focusing on thoughts and feelings related to distress

Anxiety features can be captured and quantified based on their frequency and intensity using formal rating scales such as those used in RCTs (see Table 17.1 at the end of this chapter) – or by simply having patients self-rate symptoms using a 0 to 10 Likert-type scale. Formal anxiety rating scales used in clinical trials vary in the phenomena they measure (e.g., psychic worry, somatic symptoms, panic attacks). It is helpful for clinicians to choose some metric that patients will find user-friendly enough to objectify and track anxiety symptoms over time – particularly in the case of a symptom that, by definition, can be prone to embellishment or overdramatization by its inherent nature.

B ABORTIVE VERSUS PREVENTATIVE THERAPY

Pharmacotherapy is sometimes geared toward immediate/"abortive" relief, either on a usually short-term basis (e.g., short-acting benzodiazepines) or long-term (e.g., low- or medium-potency FGAs), or explicitly long-term prevention of occurrences (e.g., SSRIs, SNRIs, GABAergic agents, some SGAs). Here, analogies to migraine headaches or asthma may be useful to frame the focus of treatment as being mainly a preventative endeavor for most anxiety disorders (which, by definition, usually must persist for at least six months), where medication is taken daily rather than viewed as mainly an as-needed, on-the-spot remedy for "breakthrough" anxiety.

A wide range of psychotropic drug classes has been studied, carrying varying degrees of evidence to treat different components of anxiety, as summarized in brief in Box 17.2.

From an overall pharmacotherapy perspective, consider findings from one comparative study of relative effect sizes across 24 agents studied in GAD from 1987 to 2003 which found that all medications studied had a collective effect size (Cohen's *d*) of 0.39 (Hidalgo et al., 2007). Individual values from that analysis are summarized in Box 17.3.

As depicted in Figure 17.1, the $GABA_A$ receptor has five subunits with distinct binding sites for these ligands (the exact binding site of ethanol at the $GABA_A$ receptor is controversial). Configurations involving α, β, and γ subunits vary across brain regions, and may also include δ and ρ subunits. Activation of the receptor

Box 17.2

Pharmacotherapy Options For Anxiolysis

Agent	Rationale
α_2-Agonists	Clonidine, guanfacine dexmedetomidine diminish sympathetic outflow and can blunt autonomic hyperarousal
Anticonvulsants	Anxiolytic anticonvulsants (e.g., gabapentin, pregabalin) can increase GABAergic tone, dampening neuronal excitation via increased inhibitory signaling
Antidepressants	SSRIs, SNRIs, NaSSAs, MAOIs, and TCAs all have varying degrees of evidence to reduce anxiety symptoms either in free-standing anxiety disorders or when anxiety arises in the context of treating major depression
Antihistamines	H_1 antagonists (e.g., diphenhydramine, hydroxyzine, and promethazine) can diminish anxiety symptoms in the context of reducing arousal and wakefulness
Antipsychotics	Anti-dopaminergic effects can down-regulate fear circuitry
Benzodiazepines	GABAergic effects are sedating and directly anxiolytic
Beta-blockers	Cardioselective beta-blockers (propranolol, atenolol) can diminish central sympathetic outflow that would otherwise amplify autonomic hyperarousal. Beta-blockers tend to be most useful for social or performance-based anxiety by blunting its somatic manifestations and consequent feedback mechanisms to the central nervous system. The evidence base does not strongly support their value for generalized anxiety or panic attacks
Buspirone	The prototype $5HT_{1A}$ partial agonist; $5HT_{1A}$ knockout mice display anxiety-like phenotypes (Garcia-Garcia et al., 2014)

Abbreviations: GABA = gamma aminobutyric acid; MAOI = monoamine oxidase inhibitor; SNRI = serotonin norepinephrine reuptake inhibitor; SSRI = selective serotonin reuptake inhibitor; TCA = tricyclic antidepressant

Box 17.3

Relative Effect Sizes Across Anxiolytic Drugs and Drug Classes for GAD

Agent	*d*
Pregabalin	0.50
Hydroxyzine	0.45
Venlafaxine XR	0.42
Benzodiazepines	0.38
SSRIs	0.36
Buspirone	0.17
Complementary/alternative medicine (= kava and homeopathy)	-0.31

Figure 17.1 The $GABA_A$ receptor.

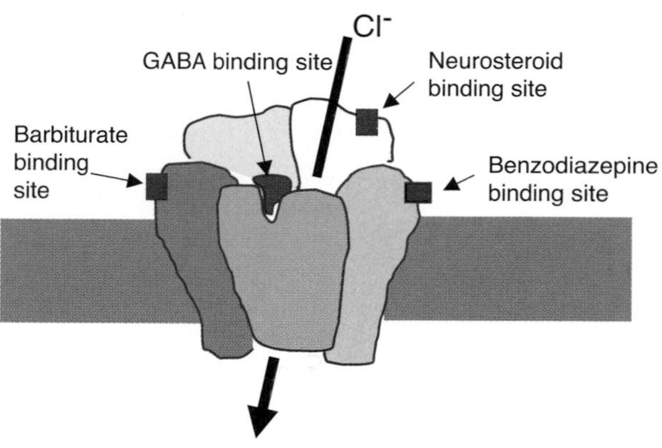

causes influx of Cl^- from the extracellular to the intracellular compartment and hyperpolarization (reduced excitability) of the nerve cell membrane.

Tip

$GABA_A$ and $GABA_C$ receptors are ligand-gated while $GABA_B$ receptors are G-protein coupled.

Benzodiazepines bind to *some* $GABA_A$ receptors – namely, those having a γ subunit. These benzodiazepine-sensitive $GABA_A$ receptors mediate phasic inhibitory neurotransmission and are postsynaptic. So-called "Z-drug" hypnotics (i.e., zolpidem, eszopiclone, and zaleplon), neuroactive steroids (e.g., allopregnanolone), some anesthetics, alcohol, and perhaps barbiturates also bind somewhere to these same benzodiazepine-sensitive $GABA_A$ receptors. However, there is another class of $GABA_A$ receptors that do not bind benzodiazepines or Z-drug hypnotics, but do bind naturally occurring neuroactive steroids, including those with antidepressant properties, anesthetics, alcohol, and barbiturates. These benzodiazepine-insensitive $GABA_A$ receptors contain a δ subunit, mediate tonic inhibitory neurotransmission, and are extrasynaptic.

$GABA_A$ modulators are cross-tolerant, which is why benzodiazepines can be used to detoxify someone from alcohol or barbiturates. Gabapentinoids have no binding affinities at $GABA_A$ or $GABA_B$ receptors; they antagonize voltage-sensitive calcium channels by binding to $\alpha_2\delta$ subunits, effectively inhibiting the release of glutamate. Other GABAergic anticonvulsants, such as divalproex, are thought to increase brain GABA levels by blocking GABA's catabolic enzyme, GABA transaminase.

Z-drugs are benzodiazepine analogues that function as $GABA_A$ agonists and are most often used as sedative-hypnotics (sleep aids). As compared to benzodiazepines, they tend to have a lower abuse potential, are less prone to cause tolerance during long-term use, have less risk for respiratory suppression, and incur less retrograde memory impairment (Wagner and Wagner, 2000).

So, can I use allopregnanolone to detox a patient from alcohol or benzodiazepines, if they're all cross-tolerant at the $GABA_A$ receptor? Or, use it to facilitate a benzo or alcohol detox? Or... can you withdraw from allopregnanolone?

Not sure! Tolerance can develop to allopregnanolone (long-term exposure leads to down-regulation of $GABA_A$ receptors), the same way as with any other $GABA_A$ positive allosteric modulator – at least in preclinical studies (Turkmen et al., 2011). What that might mean in humans though is more speculative.

Why aren't Z-drugs used to treat anxiety?

They haven't really been formally studied for their possible anxiolytic, as opposed to hypnotic, effects.The anxiolytic effects of traditional benzodiazepines are thought to relate to their agonism at the $GABA_A$ α_2, α_3, and α_5 subunits. Z-drugs more selectively bind to the α_1 subunit, which corresponds to hypnotic but not anxiolytic effects.

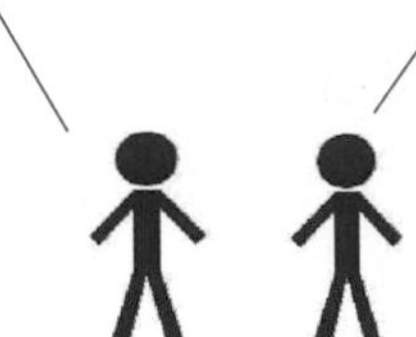

Benzodiazepines are used by about 3–13% of adults in the general population (Airagnes et al., 2019; Maust et al., 2019). Among clinical groups, they are commonly used on a regular basis in about one-quarter of MDD patients (Rivzi et al., 2015) or bipolar patients after remission from an acute episode (Perlis et al., 2010). Collectively, they are formally indicated for the short-term relief of anxiety symptoms (package insert information advises no longer than *two to four weeks' duration*), and FDA registration trials of safety and efficacy do not exist beyond four months' duration. Despite concerns in all patients for the potential for both physical and psychological dependence, as well as tolerance and withdrawal, long-term prescriptions (more than six to eight months' duration) reportedly occur in up to 10–15% of adults (Takeshima et al., 2016; Takano et al., 2019), with 5% continuing uninterrupted for up to eight years (Takeshima et al., 2016). Clinical subpopulations vary in prevalence rates, as might be expected. For example, a Swedish database registry of 21 833 individuals with bipolar disorder found that 29% began a benzodiazepine or benzodiazepine agonist, with 20% of that subgroup becoming long-term users (Wingård et al., 2018).

Clonazepam has its FDA approval in panic disorder based on pivotal trials lasting from six to nine weeks. It also has been shown to be superior

Tip

Adding clonazepam to an SSRI in MDD patients with comorbid panic disorder, but not comorbid social anxiety disorder, may yield faster improvement of anxiety symptoms (Seedat and Stein, 2004).

Tip

In patients receiving long-term/preventative pharmacotherapies for anxiety disorders (e.g., SSRIs, GABAergic anticonvulsants), advise them to track the necessity of as-needed "abortive" benzodiazepine use as its own outcome measure for the success of the primary preventative medication (analogous to the need for triptan rescues when using anticonvulsant drugs for migraine prevention).

That's kinda subjective, don't ya think? What if my day-to-day life is more stressful than yours, just suppose?

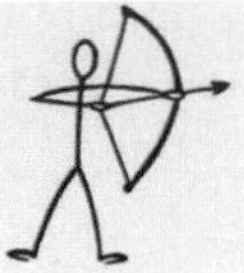

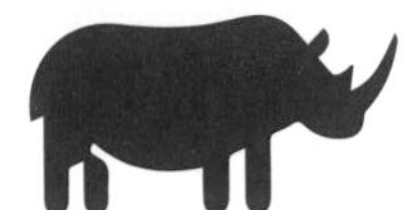

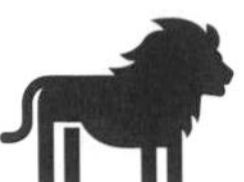

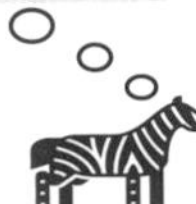

Quotable:

"Anxiety or tension associated with the stress of everyday life usually does not require treatment with an anxiolytic"
- Package insert information for all benzodiazepines

to placebo for treatment of social anxiety disorder "off label" (Davidson et al., 1993). The FDA psychotropic indication for lorazepam is "for the management of anxiety disorders or for the short-term relief of the symptoms of anxiety or anxiety associated with depressive symptoms."

See Table 9.7 in Chapter 9 for information about approximate dosing equivalents among benzodiazepines.

Physical dependence can occur within a few weeks to months of regular use – nearly one in three individuals who takes a benzodiazepine for at least four weeks will develop physical dependence (Marriott and Tyrer, 2012). Naturalistic studies of benzodiazepine use for up to nine years' duration have been associated with the development of diverse neurocognitive deficits that may be substantial (Barker et al., 2004).

Benzodiazepine dosing often becomes a point of contention between clinicians and patients when concerns are not equally shared about the potential for tolerance and dependence as well as adverse cognitive and motor effects, or factors such as diversion. As a rule of thumb, less is more with respect to both dosing and duration.

In some clinical populations, naturalistic studies have identified chronic benzodiazepine use as a correlate of poorer outcomes or particular symptom patterns – although causality is difficult to infer from nonrandomized studies, inasmuch as poorer-prognosis patients or those with more severe overall psychopathology may be those who are more likely to be prescribed benzodiazepines. For example, in adults with bipolar disorder, long-term benzodiazepine use was associated with an increased risk for affective relapse while controlling for confounding variables (HR = 1.21, 95% CI = 1.01–1.45; Perlis et al., 2010). In MDD, benzodiazepine use has been shown to be more likely when anhedonic features are present (Rivzi et al., 2015). In schizophrenia, a Cochrane Database review found no clinical benefit from benzodiazepines (added to antipsychotics, in comparison to antipsychotics alone) other than desired sedation following acute administration (Dold et al., 2012).

Characteristics that have been found to describe patients who tend to receive benzodiazepines on a long-term basis, within naturalistic/observational studies, are summarized in Table 17.2 at the end of this chapter.

At the same time, there are undeniable patient subgroups who clearly benefit from long-term use of benzodiazepines for anxiety disorders whose conditions worsen without benzodiazepines and for whom alternative anxiolytic pharmacotherapies have unequivocally suboptimal efficacy. In MDD, combined treatment using an antidepressant plus a benzodiazepine appears more effective than an antidepressant alone in reducing overall depressive symptom severity during the first few weeks of treatment ($g = -0.25$, 95% CI = −0.46 to −0.03), but not thereafter ($g = -0.18$, 95% CI= −0.40 to 0.03); curiously, adjunctive benzodiazepines have not been shown to significantly improve concomitant anxiety symptoms when added to antidepressants for treatment of MDD (Ogawa et al., 2019). Combined pharmacotherapy patients also tend to have less premature dropout in MDD clinical trials as compared to antidepressant monotherapy recipients.

TRIVIA
The brand name ATIVAN came about from the marketing concept of "anxiety and tension vanish."

Patient preference for long-term benzodiazepines over other pharmacotherapies, in the context of chronic anxiety, can pose delicate challenges and potentially lead to nonproductive struggles, as illustrated in Clinical Vignette 17.1.

CLINICAL VIGNETTE 17.1

Annie is a 57-year-old divorced woman chronically maintained (>20 years) on alprazolam 1 mg three to four times daily for "constant worry," mostly about what will happen to her in life. She has a strongly external locus of control, dependent personality traits, and perseverates about "not feeling whole or complete" without being in a relationship. She has never had a major depressive episode or (hypo)manic episode, and has never been psychotic. Though she has never made a suicide attempt she chronically feels life is not worth living if it means being alone, and finds negative emotional states intolerable. Her condition has been conceptualized as generalized anxiety disorder, persistent depressive disorder (formerly dysthymic disorder), and dependent personality disorder, but it historically has not improved despite adequate trials of SSRIs, SNRIs, gabapentin, or adjunctive aripiprazole or quetiapine. She has been in cognitive behavioral therapy, dialectical behavior therapy, and insight-oriented psychotherapy and says therapy has "never done anything for [her]." She calls alprazolam "the only thing that keeps [her] going" but feels she has become tolerant to it and is now requesting a higher dosage.

The appropriateness of chronic benzodiazepine use is problematic and suffers as much from there being a dearth of controlled long-term trials as from the biases of clinicians from whom benzodiazepines are often sought. Annie's case exemplifies several pertinent issues. First and foremost involves diagnostic clarification – hers being an instance where the presence (or, as importantly, the ambiguity) of a categorical diagnosis *does matter*: does Annie have an ailment (GAD or some variant thereof?) for which benzodiazepines are indicated and appropriate, especially if other options such as serotonergic antidepressants fail to render relief? Part of the challenge in her case involves discriminating "generalized anxiety" from sheer distress intolerance. Past nonresponse to multiple appropriate pharmacotherapies for GAD is certainly not diagnostic of anything, but points us toward either: (a) the presence of a highly treatment-resistant form of GAD or (b) a diagnosis other than GAD for which GAD-appropriate treatments may fail because Annie has either a different or more complex condition than the type for which medications for GAD are both evidence-based and relevant. As noted in Box 17.1, "anxiety" can be a problematic term because its colloquial use often denotes an array of dysphoric emotional states that correspond only superficially to "anxiety" when defined as a clinical entity – in this instance, potentially relating more to low frustration tolerance, distress intolerance, feeling empty or incomplete, a poor capacity to self-soothe, and difficulty with self-regulating normal negative emotions. Such "*pseudo*"-anxious patients who find benzodiazepines "likeable" may be at especially high risk for seeking insatiably high doses and using them more as a coping strategy to self-regulate negative emotions than to target specific symptoms of abnormal anxiety.

Tip

The term "likeability" is often used in relation to controlled substances to describe the positive psychoactive component of a drug that increases its likelihood for recreational misappropriation.

Across specific anxiety disorders, the magnitude of benefit from benzodiazepines varies. For example, a Cochrane Database review of benzodiazepine use for panic disorder found an RR for response (relative to placebo) of 1.65 (95% CI = 1.39–1.96) with an NNT = 4 (95% CI = 3–7); for remission, the RR = 1.61 (95% CI =1.38–1.88) (Breilmann et al., 2019).

Risk factors for benzodiazepine dependence or misuse that have been identified in the literature (as summarized by Kan et al., 2004) include the following:

- Longer duration of benzodiazepine use
- Higher benzodiazepine dose
- Younger age

In the case of GAD per se, a network meta-analysis of 91 RCTs involving 14 812 participants, and encompassing both pharmacological as well as psychosocial/psychotherapeutic interventions, found that all pharmacotherapies except for serotonin modulators and SGAs had greater effects than did placebo; most pharmacological interventions also had larger effects than psychological interventions (Chen et al., 2019c).

So do you just tell Annie you're going to taper off her alprazolam because you think it's inappropriate for her to continue it now that she's become tolerant? What if there isn't a better pharmacological alternative? What if it's harm reduction to continue it? If you cut her off she might resort to other more hazardous things to make herself feel better.

In Annie's case we don't have a history suggesting that she is prone to abuse other drugs. Hers is a complicated situation because you can't really just declare a moratorium on the chronic use of alprazolam without having some alternative treatment strategy in mind. Pharmacologically, there's really just two options, short of maintaining the status quo: (a) review all her past med trials and suggest something from Box 17.2 that she hasn't taken (or, optimally taken), or (b) relegate pharmacotherapy to a more minor role in her overall treatment and refocus her toward more concentrated skills-based psychosocial treatment approaches. It's tempting to think of an addiction treatment program, even though she hasn't "abused" benzodiazepines – in no small part for the support and coping skills that, say, 12-step groups might offer her.

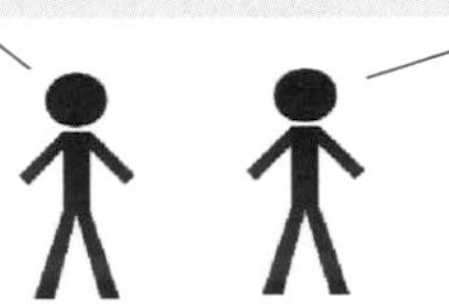

Another network meta-analysis of 89 RCTs involving 25 411 subjects, examining mean score changes in HAM-A ratings in GAD trials, determined that duloxetine had the largest mean difference (MD = −3.13, 95% CrI = −4.13 to −2.13), followed by pregabalin (MD = −2.79, 95% CrI = −3.69 to −1.91), then venlafaxine (MD = −2.69, 95% CrI = −3.50 to −1.89), and then escitalopram (MD = −2.45, 95% CrI = −3.27 to −1.63) (Slee et al., 2019).

What happens when patients who take benzodiazepines on a long-term basis for anxiety disorders stop taking them? See the discussion in Box 17.4.

Box 17.4

Stopping Chronic Benzodiazepines

The empirical literature on discontinuing long-term benzodiazepines in patients with anxiety disorders is limited. A Cochrane review found the greatest benefit for successfully tapering off chronic benzodiazepines with divalproex (RR = 2.55, 95% CI = 1.08-6.03) or tricyclic antidepressants (RR = 2.20, 95% CI = 1.27-3.82) (Baandrup et al., 2018). The lowest anxiety symptoms at the end of detoxification were associated with use of carbamazepine, pregabalin, captodiame,[1] paroxetine, and flumazenil (however, use of the latter agent was associated with increased panic attacks, as well as junctional or ventricular tachyarrhythmias and seizures, while eventual relapse of benzodiazepine use was lowest with divalproex or cyamemazine.[2]

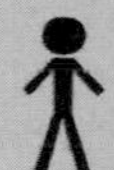
A study of 107 GAD patients who had been taking benzos for over eight years found that imipramine was better than either buspirone or placebo in facilitating a successful taper-off (over 80% of patients) (Rickels et al., 2000).
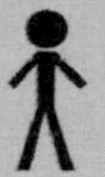
Impressive.

1 Captodiame is an antihistamine and $5HT_{2C}$ antagonist and α_1 agonist available outside of the USA.
2 Cyamemazine is a phenothiazine FGA available outside of the USA.

Ⓒ BUSPIRONE AND REVISITING YET AGAIN THE ROLE OF $5HT_{1A}$ AGONISM IN ANXIETY

Buspirone is a wonderful example of a drug that *should* work better in reality than it actually seems to, based on its mechanism of action, alongside its particularly benign side-effect profile. It belongs to a drug class called azapirones, a group of relatively short half-life compounds with pharmacodynamic effects primarily via partial agonism at the $5HT_{1A}$ receptor. Others azapirones include gepirone, ipsapirone, and tandospirone (used mostly in China and Japan).

Recall from previous chapters the dense distribution of presynaptic $5HT_{1A}$ autoreceptors in the dorsal raphe nuclei, along with postsynaptic $5HT_{1A}$ heteroreceptors located mainly on pyramidal neurons and GABAergic interneurons within the prefrontal cortex and limbic structures such as the amygdala and hippocampus.

Why isn't buspirone by itself an effective antidepressant?
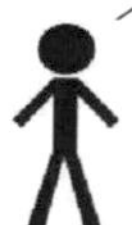
Probably because it doesn't exert very potent partial agonist effects on postsynaptic 5HT1A heteroreceptors.

A Cochrane Database review of azapirones (mainly buspirone) for *GAD* found an NNT = 4 (based on CGI scores) and lesser efficacy than seen with benzodiazepines (Chessick et al., 2006). RCT data with buspirone in *social anxiety disorder* have been negative (van Vliet et al., 1997). In *panic disorder*, an eight-week RCT comparing buspirone to placebo found no significant difference from placebo (though better tolerability than imipramine, which was an active comparator) (Sheehan et al., 1988; 1990). Another study of high-dose buspirone in *panic disorder* (5–100 mg/day; mean dose = 61 mg/day) again found no difference from placebo (in contrast to alprazolam; mean dose = 5.2 mg/day) (Sheehan et al., 1993). However, that study has inspired some practitioners to advocate (anecdotally) higher-than-usual dosing of buspirone (e.g., as much as 90–120 mg/day) for possibly greater anxiolytic efficacy in GAD.

$5HT_{1A}$ partial agonism also has potential bearing on improvement of sexual dysfunction of hypoactive sexual desire, as in the case of flibanserin and possibly also relevant to the mechanism of action of the α_2 antagonist yohimbine. Gepirone is another $5HT_{1A}$ partial agonist for which FDA regulatory approval for any indication has been fruitless. See Box 17.5.

Box 17.5

What is Gepirone and Why Has It Repeatedly Failed to Gain FDA Approval?

Gepirone is an azapirone with stronger binding affinity than buspirone as a $5HT_{1A}$ presynaptic partial agonist; at higher doses it functions predominantly as a pure agonist. It has a storied history, having been developed in 1986 but then rejected by the FDA multiple times as an anxiolytic and novel antidepressant based on impressions that its efficacy was not sufficiently demonstrated. In 2016 the FDA granted an appeal to overturn prior denials of approvals in MDD for its extended-release formulation, based on two positive Phase II RCTs in MDD. It continues to remain an investigational compound in MDD, as well as in GAD and possibly as a treatment for hypoactive sexual desire.

Notably, vilazodone also has a strong binding affinity at the $5HT_{1A}$ receptor where it too functions as a partial agonist; however, preclinical data are presently unavailable on its Ki. The manufacturer reports an IC_{50} of 2.1 nM at the $5HT_{1A}$ receptor (i.e., the half-maximal inhibitory concentration, another means of expressing receptor binding affinity).

Box 17.6

$5HT_{1A}$ Receptor Binding Affinities Across SGAs and Serotonergic Antidepressants/Related Compounds

Agent	Ki (nM)	Function
Brexpiprazole	0.12	Partial agonist
Aripiprazole	1.7–5.6	Partial agonist
Ziprasidone	2.5–76	Partial agonist
Cariprazine	2.6	Partial agonist
Lurasidone	6.75	Partial agonist
Asenapine	8.6	Partial agonist
Vortioxetine	15	Full agonist
Pindolol	15–81	Presynaptic antagonist
Buspirone	28.6	Presynaptic full agonist, postsynaptic partial agonist
Cyproheptadine	59	Antagonist
Nefazodone	80	Partial agonist
Clozapine	123.7	Partial agonist
Iloperidone	168	Uncertain
Quetiapine	320-432	Partial agonist
Yohimbine	346	Partial agonist
Escitalopram	>1000	Uncertain
Olanzapine	2063-2,720	Partial agonist
Mirtazapine	3300-5010	(Little to no affinity)
Paroxetine	21,200	(Little to no affinity)
Sertraline	>35,000	(Little to no affinity)

Vilazodone, Vortioxetine, and $5HT_{1A}$

Vortioxetine and vilazodone stand out among serotonergic antidepressants as uniquely exerting not only potent reuptake inhibition at the serotonin transporter but also partial agonism at $5HT_{1A}$ receptors. Intuitively, one would think this mechanistic pairing could make for: (a) a more potent antidepressant strategy (say, as compared to SSRIs with little to no $5HT_{1A}$ binding affinity) and (b) particular value in the setting of anxiety (with or without depression). The former of these hypotheses has not been formally tested in RCTs

Why are SSRIs anxiolytic, if their Kis for $5HT_{1A}$ are so awful? And, obviously they're not at all GABAergic. Is anxiolysis just mediated via their serotonin reuptake inhibition?

SSRIs, TCAs, and MAOIs all increase postsynaptic $5HT_{1A}$ signaling but their effects are not necessarily via direct ligand binding.

for TRD, nor have post hoc analyses in MDD with either of these two compounds examined the potential impact on concurrent anxiety symptoms as a possible moderator of antidepressant response. There are some post hoc data regarding the latter hypothesis. Let us then consider what data do exist for each of these novel serotonergic agents with respect to anxiolysis.

One small (n = 40) RCT of *vortioxetine* for MDD with comorbid social anxiety disorder found no significant difference in CGI scores (the primary outcome), but secondary analyses showed a significant and clinically meaningful advantage for vortioxetine over placebo on MADRS depression scores ($d = 0.672$) and on LSAS anxiety scores ($d = 0.714$) (Liebowitz et al., 2017).

In FDA registration trials for *vortioxetine* in MDD, secondary analyses examining the impact of concurrent anxiety symptoms have yielded only modest findings. The individual studies found the results shown in Box 17.7.

Box 17.7

Is Vortioxetine Anxiolytic?

- In a Phase III trial comparing vortioxetine 15 or 20 mg/day with placebo, a nominally significant difference in HAM-A scores was observed (Boulenger et al., 2014).
- In a Phase III comparison of vortioxetine 10 or 20 mg/day versus placebo, no significant reduction in HAM-A scores at eight weeks was observed (Jacobson et al., 2015).
- Another early RCT found that in MDD patients with baseline HAM-A scores >20, greater reductions were seen in 24-item HAM-D scores with vortioxetine (1 mg/day ($p = 0.004$, $d = 0.40$), 5 mg/day ($p = 0.002$, $d = 0.48$), or 10 mg/day ($p = 0.001$, $d = 0.49$) than placebo (Henigsberg et al., 2012).
- A randomized comparison of vortioxetine 2.5 mg/day, 5 mg/day, and 10 mg/day (then known as Lu AA21004) versus placebo (with duloxetine 60 mg/day as an active comparator) in MDD found significant improvement with vortioxetine 5 mg/day or 10 mg/day, as compared to placebo, in reducing HAM-A scores from baseline when using a mixed model repeated measures analysis or an observed cases analysis (but not with LOCF analysis) (Baldwin et al., 2012).
- A randomized comparison of vortioxetine 5 mg/day or 10 mg/day versus placebo (with venlafaxine up to 225 mg/day as an active comparator) in MDD found significant reductions from baseline HAM-A with all doses of both active treatments (Alvarez et al., 2012).

What do you make of the better anxiolytic efficacy of vilazodone at low rather than high doses?

You can't conclude anything. These were post hoc analyses, not powered either to assess anxiety or compare specific doses. I wouldn't make any inferences about dosing for anxiety.

But...if you were going to design an a priori study, might you favor low doses based on these data?

Maybe.

In the case of *vilazodone* for MDD, a pooled post hoc analysis of two Phase III FDA registration trials found a surprisingly greater magnitude of improvement in depressive symptoms among anxious rather than nonanxious depressed subjects (note that 82% of the study population had anxious depression) (Thase et al., 2014). (We say "surprisingly" because, to our knowledge, this is one of the very few studies within the literature showing a *greater* antidepressant effect when MDD co-occurs with prominent anxiety.) Significantly greater improvement also was noted with vilazodone than placebo on the HAM-A psychic anxiety subscale ($p < 0.001$; $d = 0.31$) but not the somatic anxiety subscale ($p = 0.069$, $d = 0.13$), as well as on both the psychic anxiety ($p < 0.003$, $d = 0.21$) and somatic anxiety ($p = 0.019$, $d = 0.17$) subscales of the 17-item HAM-D.

In a separate clinical trials initiative with vilazodone for GAD, three acute large studies (mean dose = 31.4 mg/day; n = 844 randomized to vilazodone versus n = 618 to placebo) collectively showed significant reduction in HAM-A scores over eight weeks but with only a modest effect for response (NNT = 10) (Zareifopoulos and Dylja, 2017). Poor tolerability, mainly due to high incident rates of nausea and diarrhea (NNH = 14; likelihood to be helped or harmed (LHH) = 1.14), ultimately led to abandonment of commercial interest in exploring vilazodone as a stand-alone anxiolytic pharmacotherapy.

Recap

As noted in Chapter 10, drugs with potent $5HT_{1A}$ binding affinities tend to incur significant upper GI adverse effects.

Does that mean I wouldn't need to coprescribe so much benzos for my anxiously depressed patients?

Maybe!

D OTHER MONOAMINERGIC ANTIDEPRESSANTS AS ANXIOLYTICS

Collectively, monoaminergic antidepressants have an NNT = 7 for panic disorder according to a Cochrane Review meta-analysis (Bighelli et al., 2018). For GAD, antidepressants in a 2003 Cochrane Database review identified an NNT = 5 (Kapciski et al., 2003). If we collectively consider and compare the specific anxiolytic properties of monoaminergic antidepressants other than vortioxetine and vilazodone, we can summarize the major findings in Tables 17.3–17.10.

What would happen if you paired pindolol, a $5HT_{1A}$ full antagonist, with, say, buspirone or vilazodone – both partial agonists? Would their anxiolytic or other pharmacodynamic effects synergize?

Pindolol, as we learned in Chapters 6 and 13, blocks $5HT_{1A}$ presynaptic autoreceptors and thus could, at least in principle, jump-start an SSRI response by tricking the autoreceptor into thinking it needs to spit out more presynaptic serotonin. You're basically asking what might happen if you paired that with partial agonism at the *postsynaptic* $5HT_{1A}$ heteroreceptor (via buspirone or vilazodone). Nobody has done that experiment yet, but it's conceivable it might have a beneficial additive or synergistic pharmacodynamic effect for mood or anxiety.

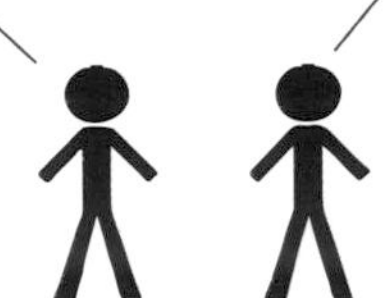

E ANTICONVULSANTS AS ANXIOLYTICS

GABAergic anticonvulsants, as least in principle, should represent viable pharmacotherapy options for anxiolysis by virtue of increasing inhibitory neurotransmission in limbic and prefrontal cortical structures related to anxiety and fear circuitry. Mechanisms vary across agents; for example, divalproex increases the activity of glutamic acid decarboxylase (which converts glutamate to GABA) and at high doses also down-regulates GABA transaminase (responsible for degradation of GABA). Gabapentinoids (see also Box 17.8), as noted earlier, bind to the $\alpha_2\delta$ subunit of voltage-gated calcium channels, thereby inhibiting presynaptic release of excitatory neurotransmitters. Lamotrigine, as a purely antiglutamatergic (and non-GABAergic) compound, shows little anxiolytic efficacy. Tables 17.11–17.17 at the end of this chapter summarize information on anxiolytic efficacy observed across anticonvulsant drugs.

Anxiolytic properties have been assessed both as a concurrent symptom in the context of treating another disorder (e.g., depression) or as an intervention for a specific anxiety disorder.

Box 17.8

A Word on Gabapentinoid Dosing

Gabapentin is popularly used "off label" as an anxiolytic in part because of its polite pharmacokinetic profile (no P-K interactions, renally excreted) and good tolerability (mainly, sedation). It is absorbed via low-capacity solute transporters in the small intestines which become saturated at doses much above 900–1200 mg/day (bioavailability drops to ≤40% at doses above 1600 mg/day), which, together with its short half-life (five to seven hours) necessitates multiple daily dosings. Gabapentin enacarbil is a pro-drug that is rapidly hydrolyzed by esterases to gabapentin and absorbed via high-capacity nutrient transporters (monocarboxylase transporter type 1 (MCT-1) and sodium-dependent multivitamin transporter (SMVT) distributed throughout the GI tract. As such, once-daily dosing is feasible and doses as high as 6000 mg/day are well absorbed. **Dosing conversion from gabapentin enacarbil to gabapentin is approximately 1:2 (i.e., gabapentin enacarbil dosing from 2400–6000 mg is approximately proportional to 1250–3125 mg/day gabapentin) (Lal et al., 2009)**.

Pregabalin has also been used to facilitate tapering-off long-term benzodiazepine use in GAD patients. Hadley et al. (2012) gave 106 GAD patients who had been taking a benzodiazepine for up to one year pregabalin 300–600 mg/day for up to 12 weeks while reducing their benzodiazepine dose by 25% per week. Anxiety symptoms and withdrawal symptoms were significantly better in subjects taking pregabalin than placebo, and although more pregabalin than placebo recipients were numerically benzodiazepine-free by study completion, that difference was nonsignificant (although a high dropout in the placebo group – over 60% – with consequent loss of power may have caused the failure to detect a true difference in the primary outcome).

F ANTIPSYCHOTICS AS ANXIOLYTICS

Apart from their sedative effects (keep in mind that FGAs have been termed "major tranquilizers," in contrast to benzodiazepines as "minor tranquilizers"), antidopaminergic drugs are relevant to the modulation of fear circuitry (recall our discussion of fear versus anxiety in Chapter 15). Comparative studies of antipsychotics for anxiolysis have not clearly parsed the relative contributions of D_2 blockade from other pertinent mechanisms, such as H_1 antagonism or serotonergic effects (in the case of SGAs) – leaving open the question of whether putative anxiolytic efficacy reflects a specific impact on, say, fear circuitry, or simply a more general kind of sedating effect. Antidopaminergic drugs may have some advantage in the setting of ill-defined or free-floating "raw" feelings of anxiety, as opposed to apprehension with more substantive content base (recall the notion of "ego glue" from Chapter 15). Clinically, antipsychotic medication can seem especially compelling in contexts where there is ambiguity between fear versus anxiety (back again to Box 15.1!), or the often gray line between an obsession and a delusion, particularly when the sufferer does not perceive the implausibility of the content of their worry. Consider Clinical Vignette 17.2.

Two FGAs carry formal FDA indications for the short-term treatment of nonpsychotic anxiety: trifluoperazine (dosed from 2–6 mg/day for GAD (Mendels et al., 1986)) and perphenazine (the latter in combination with amitriptyline for treatment of "moderate to severe anxiety and/or agitation and depressed mood," as the proprietary combination agent Triavil®). Among SGAs, quetiapine is popularly used at low doses for its putative

CLINICAL VIGNETTE 17.2

Emma was a 47-year-old stay-at-home mother, diagnosed with GAD (germ phobias, constant health fears, and preoccupations with imagined catastrophes) and OCD (the latter mainly involving contamination fears and preoccupations with orderliness). Her longstanding pharmacotherapy regimen consisted of *fluoxetine 80 mg/day with gabapentin 600 mg/day*[3] and lorazepam 1 mg at night. After receiving a summons to serve on jury duty she became intensely preoccupied with the idea that if she were to serve on a jury and "said the wrong thing" or "convicted an innocent person" then "they" would come after her. She had an uncharacteristically difficult time reality-testing the likelihood of this proposition, which she said seemed plausible to her though she did not know why – and, yet, she acknowledged that if a friend came and told her the same thing, she would find the idea absurd. Unable to accurately appraise this perceived threat and see the implausibility of its content, the idea of delusional disorder was entertained, although the treating psychiatrist found that diagnosis not entirely satisfying conceptually because her complaints seemed to be an extreme elaboration of her baseline thematic worry, embellished by histrionic overtones. Nevertheless, a decision was made to target her symptoms with adjunctive aripiprazole (initially 5 mg/day, eventually increased to 10 mg/day) based on its evidence-based value as an adjunct to SSRIs in OCD (recall from Chapter 14 its effect size of $d = 1.11$) as well as its inherent antipsychotic properties.

[3] This combination was first described for refractory OCD in a case series of intramural patients at NIMH by Corá-Locatelli et al. (1998).

anxiolytic properties (though, as shown in Table 17.19, it has extensive RCT data in GAD). Quetiapine is a highly potent H_1 antagonist, with binding affinity (Ki = 7 nM) comparable to that of chlorpromazine (Ki = 2 nM), promethazine (Ki = 1 nM), and doxepin (Ki = 0.2 nM). There are unfortunately no published randomized comparisons with any FGAs or SGAs relative to antihistaminergic drugs that have no antidopaminergic properties (e.g., diphenhydramine, hydroxyzine); such a study would be quite useful in helping clarify the extent to which low-dose antipsychotics deliver anxiolytic effects for mechanistic reasons other than antihistaminergic sedation. Tables 17.18 and 17.19, respectively, summarize information about the specific anxiolytic effects of D_2/D_3 partial agonists and D_2 antagonists.

G ANTIHISTAMINES

H_1 antagonists have long been used for both abortive and preventative anxiolytic purposes, particularly in clinical groups for whom controlled substances are considered inappropriate (e.g., patients detoxifying from substances or who are in recovery from chemical addictions). As noted earlier, there remains debate about how much the anxiolytic effects of quetiapine, mirtazapine, and low-potency FGAs such as chlorpromazine arise from mechanisms beyond their H_1 antagonism.

A Cochrane Database review of hydroxyzine for GAD found an OR = 0.30 (95% CI = 0.15–0.58) as compared to placebo with comparable efficacy, acceptability, and tolerability as compared to chlordiazepoxide (OR = 0.75, 95% CI = 0.35–1.62) or buspirone (OR = 0.76, 95% CI = 0.40–1.42) (Guaiana, 2010).

H BETA-BLOCKERS

Cardioselective beta-blockers that do not cross the blood–brain barrier can help to mitigate anxiety, mainly by blocking or blunting anxiety-based peripheral autonomic somatic effects – such as tachycardia/palpitations, tremor, and sweating. Despite early reports suggesting their potential value in GAD (Peet, 1988), the anxiolytic properties of beta-blockers today are generally considered to be mainly limited to social anxiety, particularly stage fright. Propranolol

Tip

Beta-blockers are not very effective for panic attacks.

Tip

Lipophilic beta-blockers (propranolol, metoprolol, pindolol) cross the blood–brain barrier while hydrophilic ones (e.g., atenolol, nadolol, labetolol, nebivolol) do not.

and atenolol remain the best-studied agents within the class. The former is typically dosed from 10–20 mg about 30–90 minutes before a performance event; when used in an ongoing fashion for social anxiety, daily dosing from 40–120 mg/day has shown efficacy relative to placebo (reviewed by Bourgeois, 1991). Atenolol for anxiolysis is typically dosed at 50 mg daily for one week, then (if no response) increased to 50 mg twice daily.

Tip

Parsimony especially favors beta-blockers for social anxiety when comorbid migraine headaches or tremor may also be present (extra points if also akathetic), and asthma or sick sinus syndrome are absent.

In the case of specific phobias other than performance anxiety, a modest literature supports the potential value of atenolol 50–100 mg preflight in reducing somatic anxiety symptoms associated with flight phobias (Ekeberg et al., 1990).

Tip

Contrary to urban legend, beta-blockers have not compellingly been shown to cause depression (Ko et al., 2002) or cognitive dysfunction (Palac et al., 1990)

I ALPHA AGONISTS AND AUTONOMIC HYPERAROUSAL

Noradrenergic α_2 agonists such as clonidine and guanfacine have considerable, often underappreciated, psychotropic versatility. In addition to their potential utility in ADD/ADHD (see Chapter 21), value in opiate detoxification (see Chapter 18) and potential role in trauma and nightmares (see Chapter 19), they can have anxiolytic value in dampening "fight-or-flight" responses. Use of long-acting clonidine can help to minimize the potential for occasional rebound daytime hypertension that might otherwise occur from solely night-time dosing of immediate-release clonidine.

Tip

Guanfacine binds more selectively to α2a subreceptors as compared to clonidine (which binds to α2a, -2b, and -2c receptors); α2b and -2c activation is thought to contribute more directly (than -2a agonism) to sedation.

J WHAT ABOUT CBD OIL FOR ANXIETY?

Basic information about cannabidiol (CBD) and its differentiation from THC was summarized in Chapter 11 (Box 11.4). The evidence base for its potential value

So tell me something. If beta-blockers in general aren't all that great for anxiety other than social phobia, what about using pindolol for anxiety? Does its $5HT_{1A}$ antagonism that you keep harping on about make it kind of a super beta-blocker plus?

What a great question! One small RCT in panic disorder found that adding pindolol 2.5 mg TID to fluoxetine was better than fluoxetine plus placebo (Hirschmann et al., 2000), while another RCT in social phobia found 5 mg TID was no better than placebo added to paroxetine (Stein et al., 2001). And that is the world's literature on pindolol as an anxiolytic. Maybe you want to go do a study…?

Why does clonidine cause sedation?

Clonidine suppresses noradrenergic output from the locus coeruleus, which in turn is necessary to maintain arousal and wakefulness.

as an anxiolytic likely involves the pharmacodynamic inhibitory effects of the cannabinoid type 1 receptor (CB_1 R), expressed on GABAergic and glutamatergic neurons; CBD also acts as a $5HT_{1A}$ agonist (Russo et al., 2005) or allosteric modulator (Rock et al., 2012). A review of clinical trials examining CBD as an anxiolytic identified six RCTs and several case reports and case series, mostly involving treatment of social-phobia-like symptoms in healthy adults (Skelley et al., 2019). If we confine our focus to clinically anxious populations, where CBD dosages have varied from 25–600 mg/day, only two RCTs are available: one study by Bergamaschi et al. (2011) compared effects of a single dose of oral CBD 600 mg/day in 24 social anxiety disorder patients and 12 healthy controls administered 90 minutes before a simulated public speaking task; subjective anxiety ratings (using a visual analog scale) were significantly lower among CBD than placebo recipients. Crippa et al. (2011) treated 10 treatment-naïve men with social anxiety disorder with a single dose of CBD 400 mg using a placebo-crossover design; as compared to placebo, CBD treatment was associated with significantly lower subjective anxiety ratings alongside a number of single photon emission computed tomography (SPECT) imaging uptake patterns in various limbic structures. Ongoing studies of CBD in PTSD use doses as high as 600 mg/day.

A meta-analysis of seven RCTs involving pharmaceutical-grade cannabinoids (i.e., THC with or without CBD) for anxiety symptoms in a medically ill population (mostly chronic noncancer pain or multiple sclerosis patients) found a modest though significant reduction in anxiety symptoms relative to placebo ($g = -0.25$, 95% CI = −0.49 to −0.01) (Black et al., 2019). These latter authors conclude, "There is scarce evidence to suggest that cannabinoids improve depressive disorders and symptoms, anxiety disorders, attention-deficit hyperactivity disorder, Tourette syndrome, post-traumatic stress disorder, or psychosis." While CBD remains an over-the-counter product with no federal agency oversight for quality assurance, and in the absence of a meaningful controlled-trials database, it is presently difficult to advise patients from an evidence-based standpoint on either its safety or efficacy for treating anxiety symptoms or disorders, relative to more established compounds.

TAKE-HOME POINTS

- Anxiety syndromes and symptom profiles vary qualitatively (e.g., psychic, somatic) in the specific target symptoms they present for pharmacotherapy.
- Strive to reserve benzodiazepines for short-term anxiolysis and favor other agents for long-term preventative use in persistent anxiety disorders; track the need for "rescue" dosing with benzodiazepines as a potential measure of success for the primary preventative treatment.
- Depression with concurrent anxiety symptoms is a common presentation that tends to diminish antidepressant responsivity, though initial data with vilazodone suggest a possibly more robust effect.
- Serotonergic antidepressants are generally the first-line approach for most anxiety disorders.
- Among anticonvulsants, gabapentin and pregabalin have a strongly emerging database, particularly for GAD, social anxiety disorder, and panic disorder.
- FGAs and SGAs vary in their demonstrated anxiolytic properties, and in their relative efficacies when treating formal anxiety disorders versus anxiety symptoms that co-occur in other major psychiatric disorders. Parsing the relative antihistaminergic versus other (e.g., antidopaminergic) mechanisms of possible relevance specific to treating anxiety remains an understudied challenge.
- Consider α-agonists (notably, clonidine) in the context of autonomic hyperarousal, particularly when there may be parsimonious value as a hypnotic for sleep, pro-attentional effects, and a desire to avoid controlled substances (e.g., in the setting of recovery from substance use disorders).
- CBD is a popular and potentially promising compound for anxiolysis but there does not presently exist an empirical database from which to offer evidence-based recommendations regarding its safety and efficacy.

Table 17.1 Anxiety rating scales

Measure	Description with strengths and weaknesses
General symptoms	
HAM-A (Hamilton, 1959)	The HAM-A is a 14-item clinician-administered scale, with each item scored individually from 0 ("absence") to 4 ("very severe"). Total scores <17 are considered to reflect mild anxiety, 18–24 equate to moderate anxiety, and scores >25 are considered severe. Subscales capture *psychic anxiety* (e.g., anxious mood, tensions, fears) and *somatic anxiety* (e.g., musculoskeletal, cardiovascular, respiratory, gastrointestinal, and genitourinary complaints). Some experts feel the overall scale may be unduly weighted toward somatic components
Beck Anxiety Inventory (Beck et al., 1988)	21-item self-report tool thought to have less "contamination" from content related to depression. Scores of 0-7 reflect minimal anxiety, 8–15 = mild anxiety, 16-25 = moderate anxiety, and 26-63 = severe anxiety
STAI (State-Trait Anxiety Inventory)	40 self-report questions (20 capturing state- ("S-anxiety") and 20 identifying trait- ("T-anxiety") features), each on a four-point Likert scale. Total scores for each scale range from 20 to 80 with higher scores reflecting greater severity
Zung Anxiety Scale (Zung, 1971)	20-item self-report measure that taps cognitive, autonomic, motor and central nervous system aspects of anxiety, with each item scored from 1 ("a little of the time") to 4 ("most of the time"). Total raw scores can range from 20 to 80; ≤44 is considered normal, 45–59 reflects mild to moderate anxiety, 60–74 indicates marked to severe anxiety, and ≥75 reflects extreme anxiety
Specific symptoms	
Liebowitz Social Anxiety Scale (LSAS) (Liebowitz, 1987)	24-item self-report or clinician-rated index; contains 13 questions regarding performance anxiety and 11 related to concerns involving social interactions. Each item is rated from 0 to 3, higher scores reflect greater severity. Total scores <30 reflect an absence of clinically significant symptoms, scores from 31-60 are considered "probable," scores from 61-90 are considered "very probable," and scores ≥90 are "highly probable" of SAD
Brief Social Phobia Scale (BSPS) (Davidson et al., 1991; Wilson, 1993)	11-item checklist designed to capture changes in the frequency and severity of symptoms (each rated from 0 to 4) over time. A total score as well as subscores reflecting fear, avoidance, and physiology can be calculated
Marks Fear Questionnaire (Marks and Mathews, 1979)	17-item self-rated measure; each item scored from "0" ("would not avoid it") to "8" ("always avoid it"). The sum of items 2–6 gives a range from 0 to 120. Scores ≥30 are clinically significant
Penn State Worry Questionnaire (Meyer et al., 1990)	16-item self-report questionnaire capturing trait worry. Questions rated from "1" ("not at all typical of me") to "5" ("very typical of me"). Total scores range from 16 to 80. Scores of 26-39 reflect "low worry," 50-59 indicates "moderate worry," and 60-80 reflect "high worry"
Social Phobia and Anxiety Inventory (SPAI) (Turner et al., 1989)	45-item self-report form that captures social-situational anxiety, somatic symptoms, and phobic cognitions. Individual items are rated on seven-point scales. Scores ≥60 = clinically significant social phobia
Social Phobia Inventory (SPIN) (Connor et al., 2000)	17-item self-rated form capturing fear, avoidance, and physiological/somatic dimensions of social anxiety. Each item is rated from "0" ("not at all") to "4" ("extremely"), range from 0 to 68; scores ≥19 taken as a cut-off for casehood
Panic and Agoraphobia Scale (PAS) (Bandelow, 1995)	13-item inventory measuring panic attacks, agoraphobic avoidance, anticipatory anxiety, disability, and health-related worries, clinician- or self-rated

Abbreviations: HAM-A = Hamilton Ratings Scale for Anxiety; SAD = social anxiety disorder

Table 17.2 Factors associated with long-term benzodiazepine use

Factor	Findings
Older age	Age ≥60 years: OR = 1.93, 95% CI = 1.46–2.53 (Wingård et al., 2018); age >50 years: HR = 0.82, 95% CI = 0.89–0.94 (Takeshima et al., 2016); age ≥65: HR = 0.77, 95% CI = 0.65–0.91 (Hata et al., 2018)
Male sex	61.5% (versus 50.3% with only short-term use) (Takano et al., 2019)
Concomitant stimulant therapy	OR = 1.78, 95% CI = 1.33–2.39 (Wingård et al., 2018)
Presence of a mood disorder diagnosis	34.4% (versus 14.1% with only short-term use) (Takano et al., 2019)
Simultaneous prescription of two or more benzodiazepines/Z-drugs	25.7% (versus 9.6% with only short-term use) (Takano et al., 2019); OR = 2.46, 95% CI = 1.79–3.38 (Wingård et al., 2018)
High benzodiazepine dosages	Dosing equivalent ≥5 mg diazepam: HR = 0.69, 95% CI = 0.55–0.87 (Hata et al., 2018)

Abbreviations: CI = confidence interval; HR = hazard ratio; OR = odds ratio

Table 17.3 Antidepressants as anxiolytics: SSRIs

Drug class	Findings
SSRIs	**Generalized anxiety disorder:** For SSRIs collectively in GAD, overall *g* = –0.67 (95% CI = –0.90 to –0.43) (Chen et al., 2019c) Escitalopram: four acute RCTs demonstrated efficacy (dosed from 10–20 mg/day) relative to placebo, while a 76-week placebo-controlled relapse prevention RCT found a fourfold higher chance of relapse with placebo than escitalopram (Pelissolo, 2008) **Panic disorder:** Escitalopram: a 10-week RCT (dosing from 5–10 mg/day) reduced panic attack frequency more than did placebo and was faster in onset than citalopram (Pelissolo, 2008) Paroxetine: in three 10-week RCTs, paroxetine CR (n = 444, dosing from 25–75 mg/day) was superior to placebo in achieving panic-free status (73% with paroxetine, 60% with placebo) (Sheehan et al., 2005) Fluvoxamine: a 12-week RCT compared fluvoxamine 150 mg/day with the MAOI brofaromine; 33% of fluvoxamine recipients were judged responders (as were 47% of subjects prescribed brofaromine), with both agents viewed as having comparable efficacy (Van Vliet et al., 1994) **Social anxiety disorder:** Sertraline: a 10-week placebo-controlled crossover trial of sertraline in 12 outpatients demonstrated significant reductions in LSAS scores (Katzelnick et al., 1995). A 20-week RCT in 204 outpatients found significantly better global improvements scores and MFQ scores with sertraline than with placebo (Van Ameringen et al., 2001) Escitalopram: two RCTs (12 and 24 weeks) with dosing from 10–20 mg/day found escitalopram better than placebo and comparable to paroxetine in reducing LSAS scores, as well as longer time to relapse than with placebo (Pelissolo, 2008) Fluvoxamine: a small (n = 30) 12-week RCT of fluvoxamine (150 mg/day) found a greater proportion of active drug recipients with "substantial improvement" (i.e., "response") (46%) than placebo (7%) on the LSAS (Van Vliet et al., 1994) Paroxetine: a large, multicenter 12-week RCT with dosing up to 50 mg/day found significantly greater reductions in LSAS scores, and global improvement in 55% of paroxetine recipients versus 24% of placebo recipients (Stein et al., 1998); elsewhere, a 12-week placebo-controlled randomized discontinuation trial following 11 weeks of open-label treatment found fewer relapses with continued paroxetine than placebo (Stein et al., 1996)

Abbreviations: CI = confidence interval; CR = controlled release; GAD = generalized anxiety disorder; LSAS = Liebowitz Social Anxiety Scale; MAOI = monoamine oxidase inhibitor; MFQ = Mood and Feelings Questionnaire; SSRI = selective serotonin reuptake inhibitor; RCT = randomized controlled trial

Table 17.4 Antidepressants as anxiolytics: SNRIs

Drug class	Findings
SNRIs	Overall $g = -0.54$ (95% CI = -0.79 to -0.30 (Chen et al., 2019c) **Panic disorder:** - In 664 nondepressed outpatients with panic disorder, a 12-week comparison of venlafaxine ER (75 mg/day or 150 mg/day) or paroxetine (40 mg/day) found greater improvement in achieving freedom from full-symptom panic attacks with either active drug relative to placebo (Pollack et al., 2007) **Social anxiety disorder:** - A 12-week RCT of venlafaxine ER (mean dose = 201.7 mg/day) found comparable efficacy to paroxetine (mean dose = 46.0 mg/day) and superiority to placebo (both active drugs) in reducing LSAS and SPIN scores (Liebowitz et al., 2005) - Another 12-week RCT of venlafaxine ER (192.4 mg/day) or paroxetine (mean dose 44.2 mg/day) found significantly greater improvements in LSAS scores with both active treatments relative to placebo, with response rates of 69% (venlafaxine), 66% (paroxetine), and 36% (placebo) (Allgulander et al., 2004) - A 12-week RCT of paroxetine CR (12.5–37.5 mg/day) or placebo found significantly greater improvement in LSAS scores with a 57% overall response rate with active drug (Lepola et al., 2004) - In a 24-week relapse prevention trial, 78% of paroxetine recipients (n = 136) had sustained global improvement as compared to 51% of placebo recipients (n = 121) (Stein et al., 2002a) **GAD:** - A meta-analysis of eight RCTs with duloxetine found significant difference from placebo in total HAM-A and HAM-A psychic anxiety scores, but not somatic anxiety ratings (Li et al., 2018) - A meta-analysis of 10 RCTs with venlafaxine XR found a significant advantage over placebo in reducing total HAM-A scores or achieving response or remission (Li et al., 2017)

Abbreviations: CI = confidence interval; CR = controlled release; ER = extended release; GAD = generalized anxiety disorder; HAM-A = Hamilton Ratings Scale for Anxiety; LSAS = Liebowitz Social Anxiety Scale; SPIN = Social Phobia Inventory; SNRI = serotonin-norepinephrine reuptake inhibitor; RCT = randomized controlled trial; XR = extended release

Table 17.5 Antidepressants as anxiolytics: TCAs

Drug class	Overall findings
TCAs	Tertiary amine tricyclics (particularly imipramine) have long been a gold standard treatment for panic disorder, as well as treatment of depression with concurrent anxiety. There have been surprisingly few contemporary reviews of meta-analyses of antidepressants (including tricyclics) for the specific treatment of anxiety disorders. For GAD, imipramine, paroxetine, and venlafaxine all demonstrate efficacy over placebo with a collective NNT of 5.15 (Schmitt et al., 2005). RCT data support the use of nortriptyline over placebo for poststroke depression with comorbid GAD (Kimura et al., 2003), but empirical trials using secondary amine TCAs specifically for anxiety disorders are otherwise limited. Imipramine has long been an established treatment for panic disorder; optimal response has been associated with a serum [imipramine] of 110–140 ng/mL (Mavissakalian and Perel, 1995). A 16-week crossover comparison of clomipramine or desipramine in panic disorder found efficacy with either drug but a greater effect with clomipramine than desipramine (Sasson et al., 1999). Another 12-week comparison of clomipramine versus paroxetine in panic disorder found comparable efficacy but better tolerability (less dropout) with paroxetine than clomipramine (Lecrubier and Judge, 1997)

Abbreviations: CI = confidence interval; GAD = generalized anxiety disorder; NNT = number needed to treat; RCT = randomized controlled trial; TCA = tricyclic antidepressant

Table 17.6 Antidepressants as anxiolytics: MAOIs

Drug class	Findings
MAOIs	**Social anxiety disorder:** - An eight-week RCT revealed a higher response rate with phenelzine (64%) than atenolol (30%) or placebo (23%) (Liebowitz et al., 1992) - An eight-week comparison of phenelzine and the RIMA moclobemide found superiority of both drugs to placebo but better tolerability with moclobemide than phenelzine (Versiani et al., 1992); in contrast, a later 12-week placebo-controlled RCT of moclobemide found no advantages at any studied doses (75 mg/day, 150 mg/day, 300 mg/day, 600 mg/day, 900 mg/day) (Noyes et al., 1997) **Panic disorder:** - A double-blind RCT of tranylcypromine (30 or 60 mg/day) for panic disorder with concurrent social anxiety disorder found that 68–70% of subjects became free of panic attacks over 12 weeks, with greater efficacy at 60 mg/day (Nardi et el., 2010)

Abbreviations: MAOI = monoamine oxidase inhibitor; RCT = randomized controlled trial; RIMA = reversible inhibitor of MAO-A

Table 17.7 Antidepressants as anxiolytics: bupropion

Agent	Overall findings
Bupropion	As noted in Chapter 5 (Box 5.3), bupropion and SSRIs appear to exert comparable degrees of efficacy in anxious depression. In GAD, a pilot RCT of 24 subjects achieved similar improvement in HAM-A scores with bupropion XL 150–300 mg/day as with escitalopram 10–20 mg/day (Bystritsky et al., 2008)

Abbreviations: GAD = generalized anxiety disorder; HAM-A = Hamilton Ratings Scale for Anxiety; SSRI = selective serotonin reuptake inhibitor; RCT = randomized controlled trial; XL = extended release

Table 17.8 Antidepressants as anxiolytics: nefazodone and trazodone

Agent	Overall findings
Nefazodone	A small (n = 14) eight-week open trial for panic disorder, dosed from 200–600 mg/day, found 10/14 subjects "much" or "very much" improved (DeMartinis et al., 1996). A meta-analysis of six RCTs in MDD showed improvement in depression symptoms regardless of baseline HAM-A scores; overall HAM-A scores improved significantly more with mirtazapine than placebo, as did HAM-D somatic anxiety scores (Fawcett et al., 1995)
Trazodone	An eight-week trial of trazodone (300 mg/day) was superior to placebo for panic disorder in a small (n = 11) RCT (Mavissakalian et al., 1987)

Abbreviations: HAM-A = Hamilton Ratings Scale for Anxiety; HAM-D = Hamilton Ratings Scale for Depression; MDD = major depressive disorder; RCT = randomized controlled trial

Table 17.9 Antidepressants as anxiolytics: mirtazapine

Agent	Overall findings
Mirtazapine	- An eight-week open randomized comparison of mirtazapine (15–30 mg/day) or paroxetine (10–20 mg/day) for MDD patients with prominent anxiety (baseline HAM-A scores >18) showed comparable overall efficacy in HAM-A scores but faster improvement in the first two weeks with mirtazapine (Kim et al., 2011). An earlier meta-analysis of eight RCTs in MDD with prominent anxiety found significant overall improvement as compared to placebo and significant improvement in HAM-D items related to anxiety and agitation (Fawcett and Barkin, 1998) **Social anxiety disorder:** - A 12-week RCT of mirtazapine (n = 30, dosing = 30–45 mg/day) versus placebo (n = 30) found no between-group differences (Schutters et al., 2010) - Another 10-week RCT of mirtazapine (n = 30, dosing = 30 mg/day) versus placebo (n = 33) in women found significantly greater improvement in LSAS and social phobia inventory scores with mirtazapine than placebo (Muehlbacher et al., 2005) **Generalized anxiety disorder:** A 12-week open trial (30 mg/day) in 44 outpatients reported response in 80% and remission in 36% based on changes in HAM-A scores from baseline (Gambi et al., 2005)

Abbreviations: HAM-A = Hamilton Ratings Scale for Anxiety; LSAS = Liebowitz Social Anxiety Scale; MDD = major depressive disorder; RCT = randomized controlled trial

Table 17.10 SSRI and SNRI dosing for anxiety disorders based on FDA registration trials

Agent	Dosing
SSRIs	
Escitalopram	Generalized anxiety disorder: initial dose = 10 mg/day; manufacturer's package insert information advises that dosage increases may occur after one week. FDA clinical trials have not extended beyond eight weeks but extended use if left to the discretion of the prescriber
Fluoxetine	Panic disorder: 10 mg/day
Paroxetine	Generalized anxiety disorder: target dose = 20 mg/day; higher doses (up to 50 mg/day) have shown no greater benefit compared to placebo Panic disorder: target dose = 40 mg/day (studied for up to three months in FDA registration trials) Social anxiety disorder: target dose = 20 mg/day; higher doses, up to 60 mg/day, have shown no greater benefit compared to placebo
Sertraline	Generalized anxiety disorder: initiate at 25 mg/day, maximum 200 mg/day Social anxiety disorder: initiate at 25 mg/day, maximum 200 mg/day
SNRIs	
Duloxetine	Generalized anxiety disorder: 60 mg/day (initial dose = target dose)
Venlafaxine	Generalized anxiety disorder: initially 37.5–75 mg/day, target dose = 75 mg/day, maximum dose = 225 mg/day Panic disorder: initially 37.5 mg/day, target dose = 75 mg/day, maximum dose = 225 mg/day Social anxiety disorder: initially 75 mg/day, target dose = maximum dose = 75 mg/day

Abbreviations: FDA = US Food and Drug Administration; SNRI = serotonin-norepinephrine reuptake inhibitor; SSRI = selective serotonin reuptake inhibitor

Table 17.11 Anxiolytic properties of anticonvulsants: carbamazepine

Anticonvulsant	Empirical findings
Carbamazepine	**Panic disorder:** - Tondo and colleagues (1989) reported outcomes for 34 patients receiving open-label carbamazepine (mean dose = 419 mg/day) for 2–12 months; "good response" (no formal rating scales used) was judged in 58.8% of subjects - Lack of efficacy was reported in a small (n = 14) NIMH intramural trial using a mean dose of 679 mg/day over a mean of 66 days (Uhde et al., 1988)

Abbreviations: NIMH = National Institute of Mental Health

Table 17.12 Anxiolytic properties of anticonvulsants: divalproex

Anticonvulsant	Empirical findings
Divalproex	**Panic disorder:** A small (n = 12) six-week low-dose (500 mg/day) open trial found moderate to marked improvement (by CGI scores) in all subjects (Woodman et al., 1994) **Social anxiety disorder**: - A small (n=17) 12-week open-label trial found a 41.1% response rate in LSAS scores (Kinrys et al., 2003) In two small placebo-controlled studies of acute bipolar depression, reductions in baseline HAM-A scores were significantly greater with divalproex than placebo (Davis et al., 2005; Ghaemi et al., 2007)

Abbreviations: CGI = Clinical Global Impressions; HAM-A = Hamilton Ratings Scale for Anxiety; LSAS = Liebowitz Social Anxiety Scale

Table 17.13 Anxiolytic properties of anticonvulsants: lamotrigine

Anticonvulsant	Empirical findings
Lamotrigine	There is very little empirical support for the use of lamotrigine for treatment of anxiety, either syndromally or as a concurrent feature in mood-disorder patients. Small case reports suggest potential value as an adjunct when dosed up to 200 mg/day in panic disorder (Masdrakis et al., 2010) but no large-scale trials. Some authors view baseline anxiety as a negative predictor for lamotrigine response in trials for mood disorders.

Table 17.14 Anxiolytic properties of anticonvulsants: topiramate

Anticonvulsant	Empirical findings
Topiramate	Topiramate has received little formal study of its potential anxiolytic properties, despite its potential GABAergic effects via modulation at the GABA-A nonbenzodiazepine recognition site. One small (n = 23) open trial in social anxiety disorder (completed only by slightly more than half of enrollees), with dosing up to 400 mg/day (by Week 9), found nearly a 30% (significant) reduction from baseline in LSAS scale scores, with 9 of 12 completers judged to be "responders" after 16 weeks, and 6 of 23 ITT subjects (26.1%) deemed remitters (Van Ameringen et al., 2004).

Abbreviations: GABA = gamma aminobutyric acid; ITT = intent-to-treat; LSAS = Liebowitz Social Anxiety Scale

Table 17.15 Anxiolytic properties of anticonvulsants: tiagabine

Anticonvulsant	Empirical findings
Tiagabine	- A small randomized comparison of the GABA reuptake inhibitor tiagabine (n = 20; begun at 4 mg/day and increased by 2 mg/day increments; mean dose = 10 mg/day) or paroxetine (n = 20; mean dose = 27 mg/day) found significant reductions from baseline HAM-A scores in both groups with good tolerability (Rosenthal, 2003) - Three 10-week RCTs in GAD compared 4, 8, or 12 mg/day fixed dosing or 4–16 mg/day flexible dosing arms. All failed to show a difference from placebo in HAM-A scores (primary outcome) (Pollack et al., 2008)

Abbreviations: GABA = gamma aminobutyric acid; GAD = generalized anxiety disorder; HAM-A = Hamilton Ratings Scale for Anxiety; RCT = randomized controlled trial

Table 17.16 Anxiolytic properties of anticonvulsants: levetiracetam

Anticonvulsant	Empirical findings
Levetiracetam	**Social anxiety disorder:** - One small (n = 20) open trial (dosed up to 1500 mg PO BID) found significant improvement from baseline in LSAS and HAM-A scores (Simon et al., 2004) - A small (n = 16) seven-week RCT (dosing from 500–3000 mg/day) found no difference from placebo (Zhang et al., 2005) **Panic disorder**: - A small (n = 18) 12-week open trial found significant reductions from baseline in frequency of panic attacks as well as HAM-A scores and global improvement (mean dose = 1138 mg/day) (Papp, 2006)

Abbreviations: BID = twice a day; HAM-A = Hamilton Ratings Scale for Anxiety; LSAS = Liebowitz Social Anxiety Scale; PO = by mouth; RCT = randomized controlled trial

Table 17.17 Anxiolytic properties of anticonvulsants: gabapentinoids

Anticonvulsant	Empirical findings
Gabapentin	**Social anxiety disorder:** - A 14-week RCT found significantly greater improvement in LSAS scores with gabapentin (n = 34; most subjects received ≥2100 mg/day; maximum 3600 mg/day) than with placebo (n = 35) (Pande et al., 1999) **Panic disorder:** - Eight-week RCT versus placebo yielded no significant difference on PAS scores but secondary analyses showed separation from placebo when controlling for baseline severity as a moderating factor (Pande et al., 2000b)
Pregabalin	**Generalized anxiety disorder:** A meta-analysis of eight RCTs (n = 2299) calculated a small-to-medium effect size (g = 0.37, 95% CI = 0.30–0.44) (Generoso et al., 2017) (cf. somewhat higher effect size identified in studies up until 2003, as noted in Table 17.4). Acute (e.g., six-week) studies have found superiority to placebo in both psychic and somatic anxiety HAM-A subscores at doses of 200 mg/day, 400 mg/day, or 450 mg/day with generally good tolerability (Pohl et al., 2005), as well as comparable anxiolytic efficacy (at doses of 300 mg/day, 450 mg/day, or 600 mg/day) to alprazolam 1.5 mg/day over four weeks (Rickels et al., 2005), or at 400 mg/day to low-dose venlafaxine (75 mg/day) over six weeks (Montgomery et al., 2006); 200 mg PO TID pregabalin also showed comparable efficacy to lorazepam 2 mg PO TID (n = 68) in a trial for which the magnitude of symptom improvement from placebo was numerically greater with pregabalin than with lorazepam, and separation from placebo was evident by one week (Feltner et al., 2003) **Social anxiety disorder**: - A 10-week open trial (450 mg/day), then 26-week randomized comparison versus placebo found better LSAS scores and MFQ total phobia and social phobia scores with active drug (Greist et al., 2011) - An 11-week RCT found significantly greater improvements in LSAS scores with 600 mg/day (but not 300 or 450 mg/day) than with placebo (Feltner et al., 2011) - A 10-week RCT found significantly greater improvements in LSAS scores with 600 mg/day (but not 150 mg/day) than with placebo (Pande et al., 2004)

Abbreviations: CI = confidence interval; HAM-A = Hamilton Ratings Scale for Anxiety; LSAS = Liebowitz Social Anxiety Scale; PAS = Panic and Agoraphobia Scale; MFQ = Marks Fear Questionnaire; PO = by mouth; RCT = randomized controlled trial; TID = three times a day

Table 17.18 SGA trials for treatment of specific anxiety disorders: D_2/D_3 partial agonists

Agent	Findings
Aripiprazole	**Generalized anxiety disorder:** - A small (n = 9) six-week open trial (mean dose = 13.9 mg/day) added to existing antidepressants yielded "much" or "very much" improved global impressions (Menza et al., 2007).
Brexpiprazole	- A six-week open-label trial of brexpiprazole 1–3 mg/day added to antidepressants in 37 MDD patients with prominent anxiety found significant improvement from baseline in both MADRS depression scores and HAM-A scores (Davis et al., 2016) - In FDA registration trials for adjunctive use with an antidepressant in MDD, HAM-A scores showed significantly greater reductions with brexpiprazole 2 mg/day (Thase et al., 2015a) or 1 or 3 mg/day (Thase et al., 2015b) than placebo
Cariprazine	Post hoc analyses of two FDA registration trials for acute bipolar depression each found significantly greater reductions in HAM-A scores with cariprazine than placebo dosed at 1.5 mg/day but not 3 mg/day (Earley et al., 2019a; 2020)

Abbreviations: FDA = US Food and Drug Administration; HAM-A = Hamilton Ratings Scale for Anxiety; MADRS = Montgomery–Åsberg Depression Rating Scale; MDD = major depressive disorder; SGA = second-generation antipsychotic

Table 17.19 SGA trials for treatment of specific anxiety disorders: D_2 antagonists[a]

Agent	Findings
Lurasidone	In secondary analyses of FDA registration trials for bipolar depression, HAM-A scores improved significantly more, and comparably, with either low-dose (20–60 mg/day) or high-dose (80–120 mg/day) lurasidone than placebo (Loebel et al., 2014a)
Olanzapine	In secondary analyses of RCTs for bipolar depression, olanzapine (both alone and with fluoxetine) improved HAM-A symptoms better than placebo (Tohen et al., 2003b) **Generalized anxiety disorder**: a small six-week RCT of olanzapine (n = 9; mean dose = 8.7 mg/day) or placebo (n = 12) added to SSRIs found greater reductions in HAM-A with active drug (*d* = 0.58) (Pollack et al., 2006) **Social anxiety disorder**: a small RCT of olanzapine (n = 7, mean dose = 9 mg/day) versus placebo found significantly greater improvement in BSPS and SPIN scores with active drug (Barnett et al., 2002)
Quetiapine	In FDA registration trials for bipolar depression, HAM-A scores improved significantly more with quetiapine (300 or 600 mg/day) in bipolar I but not bipolar II depressed subjects (Hirschfeld et al., 2006) **Generalized anxiety disorder**: three RCTs in GAD (n = 2248 subjects) found response and remission rates greater than placebo with quetiapine doses of 50 or 150 (but not 300) mg/day (NNT = 8.4) (Maneeton et al., 2016). Notably, in a network meta-analysis of 89 RCTs for GAD, quetiapine had the largest effect on HAM-A of all studied agents but poor tolerability as compared to placebo (Slee et al., 2019) **Social anxiety disorder**: one small (n = 15; likely underpowered) negative RCT versus placebo in social anxiety disorder (Vaishnavi et al., 2007) In bipolar disorder patients with comorbid GAD or panic disorder, quetiapine XR (mean dose = 186.4 mg/day) showed greater improvement than placebo or divalproex on HAM-A and CGI anxiety scores (Sheehan et al., 2013)
Risperidone	**Generalized anxiety disorder**: a five-week randomized comparison of risperidone (n = 19; dosing 0.5–1.5 mg/day) or placebo (n = 20) added to existing anxiolytics for GAD found greater reductions with risperidone in HAM-A total and psychic anxiety subscores, though overall response rates were not significantly higher (Brawman-Mintzer et al., 2005). Another four-week comparison of risperidone (n = 196) or placebo (n = 194) added to SSRIs for GAD found no significant improvement in a global measure of anxiety symptoms taken as the primary outcome (Pandina et al., 2007) **Panic disorder:** a single-blind RCT found comparable efficacy, though faster improvement, with low-dose risperidone (mean dose = 0.53 mg/day) than paroxetine on panic attack frequency and severity as well as HAM-A scores (Prosser et al., 2009) In bipolar disorder patients with co-occurring GAD or panic disorder, risperidone (mean dose = 2.5 mg/day) was no different from placebo in reducing anxiety symptoms (Sheehan et al., 2009) An open trial of risperidone (mean dose = 1.12 mg/day) in 30 patients with refractory panic disorder, social anxiety disorder or GAD was shown to improve HAM-A and global impression scores significantly from baseline (Simon et al., 2006b)
Ziprasidone	**Generalized anxiety disorder**: an eight-week RCT of ziprasidone (n = 41, mean dose = 50.2 mg/day) found no significant difference from placebo (n = 21) in HAM-A scores (Lohoff et al., 2010), while an earlier small (n = 13) seven-week open-label trial suggested potential benefit (Snyderman et al., 2005) In bipolar disorder patients with comorbid panic disorder or GAD, ziprasidone (mean dose = 146.7 mg/day) was no better than placebo in improving anxiety symptoms (Suppes et al., 2014)

[a] No data available, as of yet, with asenapine, clozapine, iloperidone, lumateperone, paliperidone, or pimavanserin

Abbreviations: BSPS = Brief Social Phobia Scale; CGI = Clinical Global Impressions; FDA = US Food and Drug Administration; GAD = generalized anxiety disorder; HAM-A = Hamilton Ratings Scale for Anxiety; NNT = number needed to treat; RCT = randomized controlled trial; SGA = second-generation antipsychotic; SPIN = Social Phobia Inventory; SSRI = selective serotonin reuptake inhibitor; XR = extended release

18 Addiction and the Reward Pathway

LEARNING OBJECTIVES

- ☐ Understand the mechanics of the mesolimbic reward pathway, its dysregulation in addiction, and the rationale for pharmacotherapies targeting its circuitry
- ☐ Describe evidence-based pharmacotherapies and strategies for managing acute withdrawal from alcohol and controlled substances
- ☐ Discuss the efficacy of antidepressants, anticonvulsants, opiate antagonists, antipsychotics, and antiglutamatergic drugs for relapse prevention in chemical addictions
- ☐ Describe controversies and pharmacological management strategies for the phenomenon of postacute withdrawal syndromes
- ☐ Describe the strengths and limitations of currently available pharmacotherapies to treat behavioral addictions, including compulsive gambling

> I have absolutely no pleasure in the stimulants in which I sometimes so madly indulge. It has not been in the pursuit of pleasure that I have periled life and reputation and reason. It has been the desperate attempt to escape from torturing memories, from a sense of insupportable loneliness and a dread of some strange impending doom.
>
> *- Edgar Allan Poe*

Addictions are, fundamentally, disorders of the reward pathway. Clinicians, patients or family members are sometimes dissatisfied with the pronouncement that an addiction is its own diagnosis, preferring instead to search for additional psychiatric conditions (such as mood or anxiety disorders) from which addiction behaviors might be secondary offshoots – perhaps in part because of the more extensive range of pharmacotherapy options available to treat mood and anxiety disorders than addictions. True dual diagnoses certainly exist, in which mood or thinking problems occur as free-standing entities, but unless they chronologically antecede an addiction it becomes difficult if not impossible to discriminate them from the symptoms caused by repeated intoxication and withdrawal states. Still, intrinsic disorders of the reward pathway can be complex and often inherently involve problems with mood, thinking, perception, impulse control, self-regulation, compulsivity, and a host of psychopathology dimensions described in earlier chapters. In this chapter we will focus on the pharmacotherapy of primary addictions – that is, the pathological pursuit of chemical or behavioral experiences that activate the reward pathway despite disrupting adaptation and functioning.

Tip

Some observers point out that social isolation may be a mediating factor in the pathogenesis of addiction. Preclinical studies suggest that social deprivation in early life alters synaptic plasticity in the reward pathway and may predispose to addiction (Whitaker et al., 2013).

At the risk of oversimplification, and for purposes of anticipating pharmacotherapy targets and their likely outcomes, let us grossly divide addiction behaviors into those driven by *relief-seeking* and *reward-seeking*. The former implies an internal emotional discomfort or negative affective state for which certain kinds of high-intensity chemical or behavioral stimuli are pursued mainly to alleviate distress. The latter, in contrast, bears less on seeking relief from internal distress than on procuring high-intensity positive affective states. Neuroscientists who conceptualize addictions as disorders of the

Figure 18.1. The reward pathway.

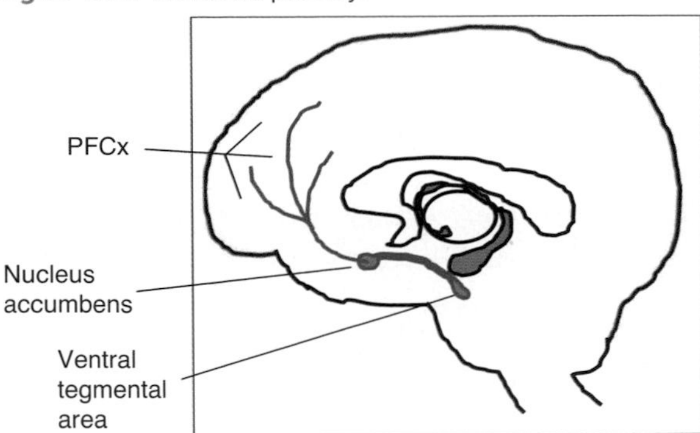

reward pathway (see Figure 18.1) posit that an inordinately high threshold of dopaminergic stimulation is needed to overcome dysregulation of motivational circuitry.

Tip

Alcohol cues (e.g., pictures) activate the ventral striatum, a phenomenon blocked by naltrexone ± ondansetron (Myrick et al., 2008).

Taking this model a step further, some authors (perhaps including Edgar Allan Poe, as noted above) describe dysfunction in three domains as underlying the compulsive behavior associated with addiction behavior: (1) *binge-intoxication* (involving DA and opioid-based circuitry in the basal ganglia (called "exaggerated incentive salience," driving craving and the pursuit of reward)), (2) *withdrawal and negative affect* (involving negative emotional states and distress intolerance related to amygdala and habenula circuitry), and (3) *preoccupation and anticipation* (involving craving, impulsivity, and executive dysfunction, reflecting dysregulation of the PFCx and insula) (Koob and Volkow, 2016). An appeal of this model for clinicians is that it accommodates various psychiatric symptoms (anxiety, dysphoria, compulsivity, and impulsivity, among others) as it falls squarely within the addiction framework without the need necessarily to invoke additional disorders when identifying pharmacotherapy rationales and goals.

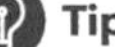

Tip

The term "dry drunk," originating from Alcoholics Anonymous (AA), is meant to describe individuals with the disease of alcoholism who abstain from drinking but continue to encounter problems with *unmanageability* (put in the language of AA) – that is, craving, emotional dysregulation, preoccupation, and interpersonal or other psychosocial consequences of past use.

Medication strategies to manage addictions are often underused, perhaps because they are limited in number and breadth of spectrum. The few that carry FDA indications for chemical addictions (none do for behavioral addictions) are limited to alcohol (e.g., naltrexone, disulfiram, acamprosate) or opiates (e.g., methadone, buprenorphine) and tend to have modest effect sizes. The evidence base for pharmacotherapies useful for other abusable substances (e.g., sedative-hypnotics, stimulants/cocaine, cannabis, hallucinogens, organic solvents) is modest, confined mostly to small proof-of-concept trials, and largely nonreplicated. Ancillary pharmacotherapies (e.g., targeting anxiety, impulse control, dysphoria, or executive dysfunction) are largely more rationale- than evidence-based. The evidence base is also unfortunately scant for treating addictions in patients with established comorbid major psychiatric disorders (e.g., alcoholism in schizophrenia or bipolar disorder; stimulant use disorders in adults with ADHD). Ancillary to pharmacotherapies and support groups such as 12-step programs for managing addictions, clinical trials also sometimes involve adjunctive behavioral interventions such as contingency management, described in Box 18.1.

Box 18.1

What is Contingency Management?

Substance-abuse treatment studies often include comparisons with contingency management (CM), an evidence-based behavioral therapy involving motivational incentives (e.g., rewards such as monetary vouchers or prizes) shown to enhance retention in treatment studies of stimulant-, opiate-, cannabis-, alcohol-, and benzodiazepine-use disorders; CM also appears efficacious in nicotine dependence and weight loss/exercise programs.

We will consider each of the above issues as practical challenges, organizing our discussion around the pharmacotherapy base for specific addictions rather than overviewing every potentially relevant agent with respect to every conceivable form of addiction (but recognizing that many individuals with addictions nevertheless incur problems with more than one substance of abuse). Lastly, while DSM-5 has replaced the nosological categories of substance abuse and dependence with the overarching term "substance use disorders," we will maintain our focus on the construct of addiction per se in keeping with the types of target symptoms described above.

A OUTCOME MEASURES

Objective clinical measures are useful for tracking outcomes when targeting substance misuse as a focus of pharmacotherapy. In addition to performing random urine toxicology screens, clinical intervention studies often track variables related to the frequency and quantity of use. For example, in the case of alcohol use, common outcome measures involving consumption include:

- the number of drinks per drinking day,
- the proportion of heavy drinking days, and
- number of drinks per heavy drinking day.

The urge to drink is often measured using the Obsessive-Compulsive Drinking Scale (Anton et al., 1996), a 14-item self-administered scale adapted from the YBOCS. It was developed based on conceptual similarities between OCD and the compulsivity and persistent urges associated with alcoholism, alongside observations that the term "craving" can be ambiguous and fails to capture the strong driving elements of urgency associated with addictions.

During acute detoxifications, objective measures (mostly reflecting autonomic parameters) include the Clinical Institute Withdrawal Assessment for Alcohol Revised (CIWA-Ar), a 10-item scale which tracks nausea/vomiting, tremor, sweating, anxiety, agitation, tactile sensations, auditory or visual disturbances, headache, and orientation, with each item scored from 0 to 7 (except for orientation, scored from 0 to 4) and a maximum score of 67 (Sullivan et al., 1989); scores of 0–8 indicate minimal withdrawal, 9–15 indicate moderate withdrawal, and >16 indicate severe withdrawal. The CIWA-Ar counterpart measure in opiate withdrawal, the Clinical Opiate Withdrawal Scale (COWS), is an 11-item scale that captures autonomic phenomena (e.g., heart rate, pupillary dilatation, tremor, piloerection) and related somatic features (e.g., yawning, bone aches, rhinorrhea) (Wesson and Ling, 2003). Scores of 5–12 are considered to reflect "mild" withdrawal, 13–24 = "moderate," 25–36 = "moderately severe," and >36 = "severe" withdrawal.

Laboratory markers relevant for tracking actual substance use include urine toxicology screens (summarized in Table 18.1) as well as breathalyzer tests for alcohol, which can detect alcohol for up to 24 hours. Alcohol has a half-life of about four to five hours and is metabolized at a rate of about 0.15% per hour. This means that a blood alcohol level of 0.08 (equivalent to two drinks in a 120 pound woman or four drinks in a 180 pound man) will require about five hours to clear to 0. Table 18.2 at the end of this chapter provides a summary of drugs that are commonly known to cause false-positive findings for illicit or controlled substances on commercial drug toxicology screens.

Detectable biological consequences of heavy use are available mostly in the case of alcohol. Relevant laboratory measures include serum *carbohydrate-deficient transferrin* (CDT), a biomarker for heavy alcohol use over the preceding two weeks (typically reflected by a %CDT >2.6). Heavy alcohol use (more than five drinks/day) interferes with the ability of hepatocytes to manufacture transferrin (an iron transport glycoprotein) with its normal complement of carbohydrate side chains (hence the name). Once a baseline CDT value is established, clinicians sometimes gauge abstinence or resumption of heavy drinking over time based on an observed CDT decrease or increase, respectively, of at least 30%. Other hepatic enzymes relevant to heavy drinking include serum *aspartate aminotransferase* (AST) and *alanine aminotransferase* (ALT). Both are often elevated in the context of recent acute alcohol intoxication, with an AST:ALT ratio >2 often seen in the setting of alcoholic liver disease, particularly when accompanied by elevated *gamma-glutamyl transferase* (GGT; sometimes also referred to as gamma-glutamyl-transpeptidase). Additional biological stigmata of heavy alcohol use include high mean corpuscular volume (MCV) anemia.

B ALCOHOL AND ALCOHOLISM

The term "alcoholism" is medically nontechnical and, along with the constructs of "abuse" and "dependence," has been replaced in modern nosology with the term alcohol (or other substance) "use disorder." Historically, however, it hearkens to a basic tenet from Alcoholics Anonymous (AA) that emphasizes the loss of control over drinking (or other substances) resulting in unmanageable psychosocial consequences. Descriptors of alcohol misuse vary based on patterns of periodic binge drinking versus more continual maintenance drinking. Quantitative definitions, such as those by the National Institute on Alcohol Abuse and Alcoholism (NIAAA), identify an increased risk for alcohol-related problems in men who consume more than 14 drinks per week or four drinks per day or women who consume more than seven drinks per week or three drinks per day. Definitions of alcohol dependence in DSM-IV and its earlier editions emphasized the concepts of physiological tolerance, dependence, and withdrawal. In 2018, the National Survey on Drug Use and Health (NSDUH) identified 7.9% of American adults as having alcohol use disorder.

Diagnostically, the DSM-5 definition of alcohol use disorder and DSM-IVTR alcohol abuse or dependence differ mainly in that DSM-5 added craving and removed legal consequences from alcohol as part of its descriptive criteria. Box 18.2 provides some basic definitions relevant to alcohol use and misuse.

Box 18.2

Definitions

One *drink* = 12 oz beer or 8 oz malt liquor or 5 oz wine or 1.5 oz distilled spirits or liquor

Intoxication is legally defined as a blood alcohol concentration (BAC) >0.08

Binge drinking is defined by the Substance Abuse and Mental Health Services Administration (SAMSHA) as five or more drinks for men or four or more drinks for women per drinking occasion

Heavy alcohol use is defined by SAMSHA as binge drinking on five or more days in the past month

Alcohol withdrawal syndrome is defined by a cluster of physical symptoms arising after stopping a period of heavy alcohol use, manifested usually by headache, agitation, nausea, vomiting, tachycardia, sweating, and insomnia

Delirium tremens (DTs) involve tremor, autonomic instability, fever, disorientation, and visual hallucinations

The term "maintenance moderation" (see Box 18.3) arose to describe the sometimes controversial treatment goal of moderate or "controlled" drinking as a possible viable alternative to abstinence.

Descriptors of patterns of problem drinking behavior, in addition to "maintenance" and "binge" drinking, include the so-called Apollonian/Dionysian distinction between clustered characteristics that may have implications for differential therapeutic approaches, described in Box 18.4.

Box 18.3

Moderation Management

Abstinence from alcohol has long been a traditional optimal component of successful treatment for alcohol use disorders. The alternative concept of "moderation" or "controlled drinking" considers the possibility that some patients who use alcohol excessively may be able to reduce rather than entirely eliminate alcohol use. An eight-year follow-up study found that only about 14% of subjects at follow-up were able to maintain "controlled but asymptomatic" drinking; successful moderation management was strongly inversely related to the extent and severity of alcohol use and alcohol-related problems at baseline (Miller et al., 1992).

Box 18.4

Type A versus Type B (Apollonian/Dionysian) Alcoholism

One conceptual framework for classifying subtypes of alcoholism, and possible treatment approaches, used cluster analyses to identify two groups: Type "A" or "I" (also called "Apollonian" drinkers) had a *later* age at onset, fewer childhood risk factors, less severe dependence, fewer alcohol-related problems, and less overall psychopathology; Type "B" or "II" (also called "Dionysian" drinkers) had an *earlier* age at onset, higher familiality of alcoholism, more poly-drug abuse, greater severity of dependence, more prominent antisocial features (Babor et al., 1992), and were usually men (Carpenter and Hasin, 2001). Type B alcoholics benefit more than Type A alcoholics from coping-skills-based psychosocial interventions (Litt et al., 1992). Type B alcoholism may reflect greater serotonergic dysfunction and has been hypothesized to benefit more from serotonergic pharmacotherapies (though, see Table 18.4).

A Drinking Dichotomy

Apollo and Dionysus were both sons of Zeus in Greek mythology - the former embodying rational thinking and order, the latter emotionality and chaos. Their contradistinction is often invoked in both literature and science to characterize the "cerebral" versus the "emotional" dichotomies.

C TREATMENT OF ACUTE ALCOHOL WITHDRAWAL

Benzodiazepines are generally the preferred treatment for acute alcohol withdrawal because of their cross-tolerance with alcohol at the $GABA_A$ receptor (see Chapter 17,

Figure 17.1). The overarching goal of detoxification is to prevent withdrawal seizures (typical onset = 24–48 hours after stopping heavy alcohol use) and a consequent risk for delirium tremens (DTs; typical onset = 48–72 hours after stopping heavy alcohol use), which in turn carry a mortality rate (even with ICU support) of 5–15% due to respiratory collapse and cardiac arrhythmias. While all benzodiazepines are comparably effective for treating alcohol withdrawal syndrome (Mayo-Smith, 1997), lorazepam or oxazepam (both relatively short-acting) or chlordiazepoxide and diazepam (both longer-acting) are typically favored agents. Longer half-life agents have the advantage of a lesser risk for rebound symptoms to occur later in the course of recovery, although their metabolic requirements can sometimes pose a risk for patients with liver disease. Dosing generally occurs either based on a *symptom-triggered regimen* (STR) according to CIWA-Ar ratings (usually ≥8) or a similar monitoring system, or a *fixed-tapering-dose regimen* (FTDR), where dosing occurs regardless of objective symptom ratings (as might occur in an outpatient detoxification setting without regular frequent intervals of objective assessment).

D DO ANTICONVULSANTS AID ACUTE ALCOHOL WITHDRAWAL?

Anticonvulsant drugs, though generally safe, are less well-established than benzodiazepines for managing both the psychological/physiological distress and risk for seizures and DTs associated with alcohol withdrawal syndromes. Among those best studied, the following may be noted:

Carbamazepine: Limitations of using carbamazepine in the setting of alcohol detoxification mainly involve its pharmacokinetic interactions and potential for hepatotoxicity. A review of seven RCTs found that carbamazepine (typically dosed initially at 800 mg/day) was superior to placebo (and comparable to oxazepam) in reducing acute withdrawal symptoms; however, it failed to show efficacy in reducing alcohol withdrawal seizures or DTs (Barrons and Roberts, 2010). Nevertheless, it has been shown elsewhere to decrease cravings after withdrawal, reduce alcohol use after acute detoxification, and prevent rebound withdrawal symptoms.

Oxcarbazepine: A six-day RCT during inpatient alcohol detoxification found no significant differences from placebo in withdrawal symptom ratings or the need for benzodiazepine rescue medications (Koethe et al., 2007).

Divalproex: Adding divalproex-DR 500 mg PO TID to oxazepam over four to seven days during acute alcohol detoxification has shown superiority over adding placebo to reduce CIWA-Ar scores, overall benzodiazepine requirements, and seizure risk (Reoux et al., 2001).

Gabapentin: During outpatient alcohol detoxification, gabapentin (typically begun at 1200 mg/day in divided doses with reductions by 300 mg/day every few days subsequently) has been shown to reduce CIWA-Ar scores in comparable fashion to lorazepam (Myrick et al., 2009) or chlordiazepoxide (Stock et al., 2013), reduce the probability of drinking (Myrick et al., 2009), and improve sedation and craving (Stock et al., 2013). In addition to good tolerability, it has the unique advantage among anticonvulsants of undergoing no hepatic metabolism and having no pharmacokinetic interactions either with alcohol or other drugs.

Pregabalin: Though well-tolerated, no differences from placebo were found (dosing of 300 mg/day for six days) in reducing the need for diazepam to counter withdrawal symptoms by CIWA-Ar (Förg et al., 2012). Other studies using higher doses have suggested pregabalin may nevertheless be of value in reducing craving and general psychiatric symptoms when used during and after acute alcohol detoxification.

E ANTICRAVING DRUGS

Naltrexone, acamprosate, and disulfiran are perhaps the best formally studied pharmacotherapies for alcohol addiction, with topiramate often under-recognized for its "off-label" efficacy in reducing alcohol craving and drinking behavior. A comparative meta-analysis of 61 RCTs with either naltrexone or acamprosate concluded that naltrexone overall appeared to be more efficacious for reducing heavy drinking and craving, while acamprosate was more efficacious in promoting abstinence overall (findings summarized in Table 18.3) (Maisel et al., 2013). Note the uniformly and discouragingly low magnitude of effect across the agents studied.

Naltrexone. Naltrexone is a relatively pure μ and δ opioid receptor antagonist. It is often regarded as having utility in binge drinking, more so than for continual or "maintenance" drinking. A meta-analysis involving 53 RCTs (n = 9140 subjects) with oral naltrexone (50 mg/day) reported an NNT (to prevent "return to heavy drinking") of 12 (95% CI = 8–26) (Jonas et al., 2014). Injectable naltrexone showed a significant advantage in that review for "reduction in *heavy* drinking days" as compared to placebo, which was not evident with oral naltrexone. Another meta-analysis of 30 studies involving naltrexone plus a structured psychotherapy found that naltrexone significantly reduced alcohol use and GGT levels, but not cravings, and that adjunctive psychotherapy was not more efficacious than naltrexone alone (Ahmed et al., 2018b). Theoretical concerns that naltrexone could potentially induce dysphoria via blockade of endorphins are discussed in Box 18.5.

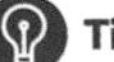

Tip

There is some pharmacogenetic evidence to suggest that naltrexone may be associated with lower relapse rates in subjects possessing the Asp40 (rather than Asn40) allelic variant of the μ opioid receptor (OPRM1) (Oslin et al., 2003).

Chapter 8 said not to do pharmacogenetic testing. Now you're saying I should get OPRM1 genotyping before giving naltrexone?

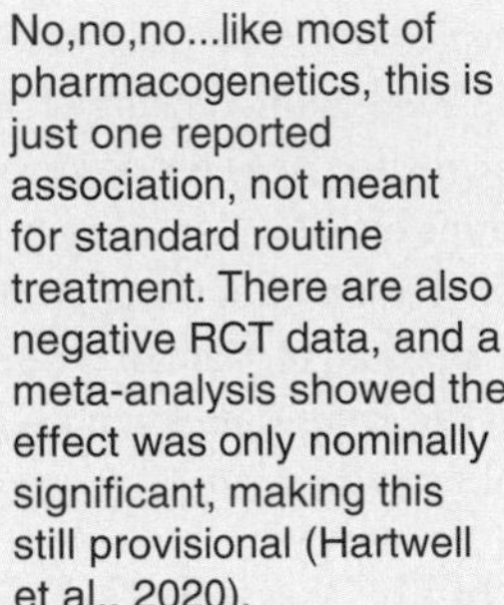

No,no,no...like most of pharmacogenetics, this is just one reported association, not meant for standard routine treatment. There are also negative RCT data, and a meta-analysis showed the effect was only nominally significant, making this still provisional (Hartwell et al., 2020).

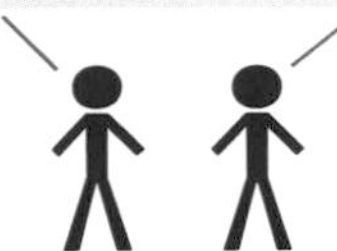

Acamprosate. Acamprosate is a novel compound believed to modulate NMDA and $GABA_A$ transmission, and to down-regulate glutamate during periods of alcohol withdrawal. Its effects on alcohol use are considered to be modest, as noted in one of the historically largest multisite pharmacotherapy RCTs in alcohol dependence, comparing 16 weeks of naltrexone (100 mg/day) or acamprosate (3 g/day), their combination, or placebo, all administered with or without a behavioral intervention (the so-called COMBINE study (Anton et al., 2006)). Using either the percentage of days abstinent or the time until relapse to heavy drinking as primary outcome measures, acamprosate had no significant effect (either alone or in combination with naltrexone), in contrast to naltrexone, which was efficacious either alone or in combination with medical management and/or a behavioral intervention (naltrexone significantly reduced the risk of a heavy drinking day: HR = 0.72 (95% CI = 0.53–0.98, p = 0.02)). Remarkably, in the COMBINE trial, *none* of the effect sizes for the primary outcome variables (percentage of days abstinent or the hazard ratio for a return to heavy drinking) were statistically significant except for naltrexone alone (i.e., minus acamprosate or CBI (a combined behavioral intervention)). Even then, the effect size was small ($d = 0.22$, 95% CI = 0.03–0.40) and the reduction of risk for return to heavy drinking was a somewhat modest 0.28.

Box 18.5

Can Naltrexone Induce Dysphoria?

At least on theoretical grounds, it is reasonable to ask whether naltrexone can induce dysphoria in some patients by blocking endorphins. Some authors have suggested that such a phenomenon, if it truly exists, is rare (Miotto et al., 2002 note that the incidence of depression as an adverse effect in naltrexone RCTs is 1.4%) but might be confounded by *comorbid* depression. A history of depression has not formally been identified in clinical trials as a moderator of adverse outcomes in any naltrexone RCTs. Some authors have suggested that dysphoria arising after naltrexone initiation could reflect a protracted abstinence syndrome (discussed further at the end of this chapter), anecdotally noting the potential value of adding bupropion (Williams and Ziedonis, 2003). That strategy would be especially intriguing and parsimonious should overweight/obesity or nicotine dependence also be present.

Why on earth would naltrexone *work less well* when paired with acamprosate? Or with a behavioral therapy augmentation?
Was that just a typo?

It was indeed a surprise and contrary to the authors' hypotheses based on their preliminary data. All subjects received intensive medical management, and it's possible that the effect of that aspect of the intervention may have been so substantial as to overshadow any further effects from an additional treatment besides high-dose naltrexone.

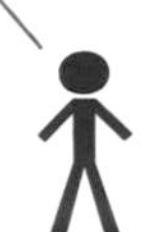

A meta-analysis of 27 RCTs using acamprosate (n = 7519) reported an NNT for "return to *any* drinking" of 12 (95% CI = 8–26) (Jonas et al., 2014). That meta-analysis found no statistically significant difference between acamprosate and oral naltrexone in "return to any drinking" (RR = 0.02, 95% CI = −0.03 to 0.08) or "return to heavy drinking" (RR = 0.01, 95% CI = −0.05 to 0.06). A post hoc analysis of seven European RCTs found that relapse prevention was predicted by severity of baseline craving and anxiety, but not a negative family history of alcoholism, late age at drinking onset, or degree of physiological dependence on alcohol at baseline (Verheul et al., 2005). Dosing is 666 mg by mouth three times daily.

Disulfiram. Disulfiram blocks aldehyde dehydrogenase, preventing the degradation of acetaldehyde (the immediate breakdown product of alcohol; see Chapter 12, Box 12.3), leading to intense nausea and a flushing reaction if someone consumes alcohol (including through mouthwashes or perfumes). It essentially creates a behavioral operant conditioning paradigm that serves to counter the reinforcing effects associated with alcohol. A meta-analysis of 22 RCTs in adult alcoholism found a medium effect size (g = 0.58, 95% CI = 0.35–0.82), although interestingly, superiority to control conditions was found only in open-label (and not blinded) randomized trials, suggesting an important (and useful) role for expectancy bias (Skinner et al., 2014).

Nalmefene. Nalmefene is a κ opioid receptor partial agonist. It was approved as an IV formulation in 1995 by the FDA to treat opioid overdose, and was later approved as an oral formulation by the European Medicines Agency for alcohol dependence. It has been the subject of considerable debate in the literature because of its apparent modest effect and high attrition rates in clinical trials (Palpacuer et al., 2015). The oral form (available in 18 mg tablets) is manufactured in Europe but not the United States. A meta-analysis by Palpacuer et al. (2018) reported a small effect size (g = −0.19, 95% CI = −0.29 to −0.10). Some studies advocate using either naltrexone or nalmefene only prior to consuming alcohol as a strategy to mitigate heavy drinking; see Box 18.6.

Box 18.6

The Sinclair Method

The "Sinclair Method" is a popular, patented method developed by American psychologist David Sinclair that is intended to treat alcoholism by having patients take a single dose of naltrexone or nalmefene shortly before consuming alcohol as a strategy to block the positive reinforcing effects of drinking, leading to behavioral extinction via classical conditioning. Limited empirical data suggest that targeted use of naltrexone (i.e., only when craving alcohol) plus coping-skills therapy was significantly better than coping skills plus placebo for reducing heavy drinking over a several-month period (Heinälä et al., 2001).

Topiramate. The anticonvulsant topiramate, often viewed as an anti-impulsivity/anticraving drug (e.g., in binge eating), has one of the largest and most underappreciated databases for efficacy to treat alcohol use disorders; based mainly on the studies by Johnson and colleagues (2003; 2007), topiramate at a target dose of 300 mg/day significantly robustly reduces the percentage of heavy drinking days, percentage of days abstinent, and drinks per drinking day. A meta-analysis of four placebo-controlled trials demonstrated a large effect size for reducing total alcohol consumption (g = −0.77, 95% CI = −1.12 to −0.42) (Palpacuer et al., 2018); indirect comparisons in that meta-analysis also showed topiramate to be superior to naltrexone, acamprosate, or nalmefene.

Tip

A preliminary pharmacogenetics study found that a GRIK1 polymorphism moderated the effects of topiramate on heavy drinking (Kranzler et al., 2014)

Gabapentin. Dosed at 1200 mg/day, it has been shown to be no different from placebo in reducing alcohol

Can combining naltrexone plus disulfiram be synergistic to reduce alcohol craving or heavy use?

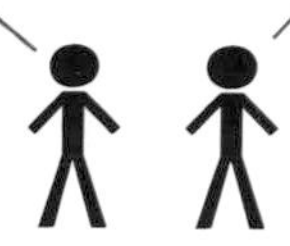

Not especially, but it may vary by subgroups. Among depressed alcoholics, that combination didn't outperform either monotherapy (Petrakis et al., 2007), but in patients with both alcohol- and cocaine-use disorders, the pairing was most likely to produce at least three consecutive weeks of abstinence (Pettinati et al., 2008).

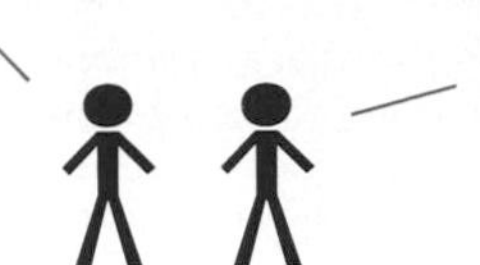

Why would topiramate reduce heavy drinking behavior? Is it because its memory and related cognitive side effects make you forget about drinking? Nyuk-nyuk-nyuk...
Or maybe you just can't find the booze! Heh, heh, heh.

Uh, no, I think the more likely explanation has to do with topiramate's modulation of glutamate signaling and pro-GABAergic effects to decrease midbrain extracelluar DA release, with consequent effects on the reward pathway...

craving or drinking behavior in a laboratory setting (Myrick et al., 2007), but at 1800 mg/day was superior to placebo in promoting abstinence (NNT = 8) or reducing the likelihood to resume heavy drinking (NNT = 5), while also significantly improving mood, sleep, and craving better than placebo (Mason et al., 2014). Also, adding gabapentin (1200 mg/day) to naltrexone has been shown to significantly improve drinking outcomes shortly after cessation of drinking as compared to naltrexone alone (Anton et al., 2011). Even with dosing as low as 300 mg twice daily, following an initial seven-day detoxification with diazepam, gabapentin was significantly better than placebo in reducing drinking behavior (number of drinks per day, mean percentage of heavy drinking days, percentage of days abstinent) in a 90-day study of 60 Brazilian men with chronic heavy alcohol dependence (mean = 17 drinks/day for the 90 days preceding detoxification) (Furieri and Nakamura-Palacios, 2007).

Baclofen. A Cochrane Database review of 12 RCTs (dosing range from 10 to 150 mg/day) found no significant difference from placebo in return to any drinking, percentage of days abstinent, or percentage of heavy drinking days, craving, or anxiety; surprisingly, baclofen *increased* the number of drinks per drinking day (mean difference = 1.55, 95% CI = 1.32–1.77) and also appeared to increase depressive symptoms as compared to placebo ($g = 0.27$, 95% CI = 0.05–0.48) (Minozzi et al., 2018).

Ondanasetron. The dense mesolimbic distribution of 5HT$_3$ receptors is thought to regulate DA release, making the 5HT$_3$ antagonist ondansetron a reasonable candidate drug to affect reward-based alcohol use. Johnson et al. (2000) compared oral ondansetron (dosed at 1 μg/kg, 4 μg/kg, or 16 μg/kg twice daily) with placebo over 11 weeks, stratifying for early- versus late-onset alcoholism subtypes. Early-onset drinkers randomized to ondansetron at all doses had significantly fewer drinks per day and drinks per drinking day, while dosing at 4 μg/kg was associated with significantly more days abstinent than placebo. However, effect sizes even at maximal dosing were relatively small across outcome measures (d ranging from 0.17–0.22).

F ANTICONVULSANTS BEYOND THE DETOXIFICATION PERIOD

A Cochrane Database review of anticonvulsants, collectively, for alcohol dependence (25 trials, 2641 participants) found no significant differences from placebo in continuous abstinence, although

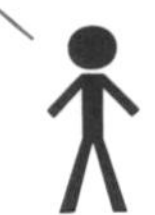

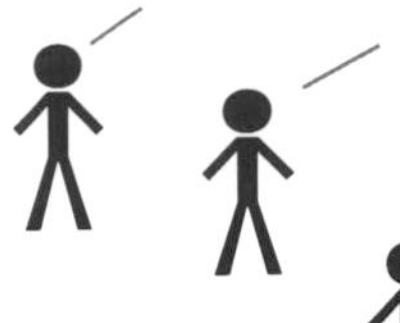

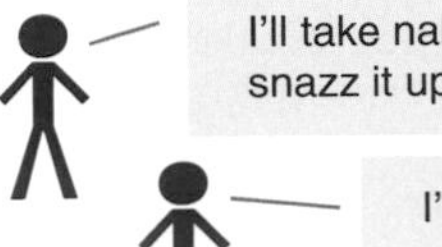

So what's the best drug for alcoholism?

I'll take naltrexone for binge drinking, and you can snazz it up with bupropion to lose weight
I'm partial to placebo, but I read ahead

anticonvulsants as a class did reduce number of drinks per drinking day (mean difference = −1.49 drinks/drinking day) and heavy drinking (g = −0.35, 95% CI = −0.51 to −0.19) (Pani et al., 2014). Significant findings were driven mainly by topiramate and to a lesser extent by gabapentin or divalproex. In comparison to naltrexone, no significant differences were found in that meta-analysis for anticonvulsants with respect to severe relapse or days until severe relapse.

G ANTIDEPRESSANTS AND ALCOHOL USE DISORDER

Tip

The use of antidepressants to treat alcohol use disorder has a weaker evidence base unless comorbid depression also exists.

A Cochrane Database review of antidepressant trials for co-occurring MDD and alcohol use disorders (33 studies, 2242 participants) found an overall small effect of antidepressants versus placebo in reducing depressive symptoms (g = −0.27, 95% CI = −0.49 to −0.04), which became nonsignificant after eliminating trials with a high risk of bias (Agabio et al., 2018). Antidepressants were found to increase abstinence from alcohol during trials (RR = 1.71, 95% CI = 1.22–2.39) and decreased the number of drinks per drinking day (mean difference = −1.13 drinks per drinking day). Head-to-head comparative trials of specific antidepressants were too preliminary and few in number to draw meaningful inferences.

Tip

Beware of the possible pro-convulsant effects of bupropion, psychostimulants or low potency FGAs in the setting of acute alcohol (or benzodiazepine) detoxification, and be mindful of their subsequent potential contribution to seizure risk should alcohol relapse recur.

Tip

Sustained abstinence from alcohol or other substance of abuse (e.g., more than one month) may be a practical necessity in order for any pharmacotherapy for depression to be efficacious; even then, the cumulative neurotoxic effects of previous substance misuse can still exert a negative moderating effect on treatment outcome.

Part of the complexity in judging the effects of antidepressants (based both on the empirical literature as well as clinical practice) involves the high comorbidity of alcohol use disorder with other addictions among those who are clinically depressed. For example, one early study of fluoxetine or placebo in cocaine-dependent versus non-cocaine-dependent heavy alcohol users found that cocaine abuse markedly worsened the prognosis for treating depressive symptoms (Cornelius et al., 1998).

Findings from RCTs of antidepressants in the treatment of alcohol use disorders are presented in Table 18.4.

H ANXIETY AND ALCOHOL USE DISORDER

A Cochrane Database review identified five placebo-controlled RCTs that examined sertraline, paroxetine, or buspirone for trials each ranging from 8–24 weeks (Ipser et al., 2015).

Paroxetine had about a twofold greater and significant likelihood of "global response" than did placebo; interestingly, a significant reduction specifically in anxiety symptom severity was observed with buspirone but not paroxetine, and slightly over 40% of paroxetine recipients dropped out of treatment prematurely due to adverse effects. Separately, a dedicated RCT comparing paroxetine or placebo for social anxiety disorder patients with alcohol dependence found that while paroxetine was better than placebo for reducing anxiety symptoms, it was not different from placebo in reducing drinking behavior (Thomas et al., 2008).

So much for the popular self-medication hypothesis that alcohol misuse would vanish if only anxiety was treated successfully...?

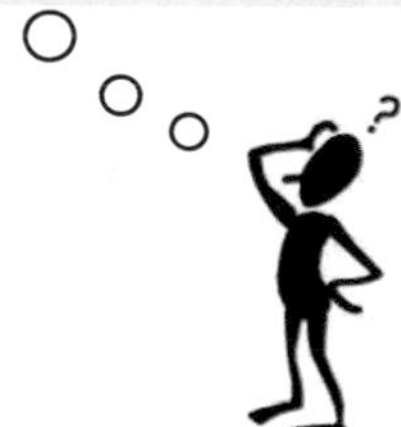

Wait, why are you assuming that anxiety is necessarily the object of self-medication? Why can't it be depression? Or trauma? Or simply feeling emotionally overwhelmed by everyday life stresses?

I ANTIPSYCHOTICS FOR ALCOHOL USE DISORDER

A meta-analysis of 13 RCTs focusing on FGAs or SGAs (including amisulpride, aripiprazole, olanzapine, quetiapine, tiapride, or flupenthixol decanoate) for primary alcohol dependence found no advantages as compared to placebo for alcohol relapse prevention, craving, or time until first alcohol consumption or resumed heavy drinking, and in fact, placebo was better than antipsychotics in the number of days abstinent or time until all-cause discontinuation (Kishi et al., 2013).

Think topiramate plus placebo might outperform topiramate alone?

Only if your patient thought they were taking an antipsychotic

J NOVEL PHARMACOTHERAPIES IN ALCOHOL USE DISORDERS

The NMDA receptor antagonist memantine was preliminarily studied in open-label fashion at a low dose (5 mg/day) in conjunction with divalproex in 45 bipolar II outpatients with comorbid alcohol dependence (Lee et al., 2018). Significant reductions from baseline were observed in depression, mania, and alcohol-use parameters, although the lack of a placebo or other comparator group limits interpretability of the findings.

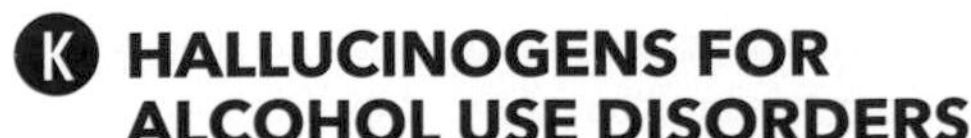

K HALLUCINOGENS FOR ALCOHOL USE DISORDERS

A pooled meta-analysis of six RCTs of single-dose lysergic acid diethylmide (LSD) for alcohol use disorders (n = 536 participants, median dose = 500 μg [i.e. micrograms] found early a highly significant, twofold increased likelihood for benefit (NNT = 6) (Krebs and Johansen, 2012). The likelihood of sustained treatment response remained significant after six months post treatment (OR = 1.66, 95% CI = 1.11–2.47, p = 0.01) but not at 12-month follow-up (OR = 1.19, 95% CI = 0.74–1.90, p = 0.47). Alcohol abstinence was significantly greater than for controls at one to three months, but not at six months. Adverse effects included agitation, confusion and GI upset.

L STIMULANT AND COCAINE USE DISORDERS

According to the SAMHSA, 1.9% of US adults have misused prescription stimulants at least once, and 0.2% would meet diagnostic criteria for stimulant use disorder – often in pursuit of cognitive enhancement (Compton et al., 2018). Cocaine addiction afflicts about 0.6% of the US population, with 1.4% of young adults reporting any use in the past month (Center for Behavioral Health Statistics and Quality, 2015).

Pharmacological RCTs for treatment of psychostimulant misuse unfortunately are not extensive. A Cochrane Database review of 11 trials found that prescribed stimulants (dextroamphetamine or methylphenidate, as well as modafinil or bupropion) had no significant impact on reducing amphetamine use or craving and did not increase sustained abstinence (Pérez-Mañá et al., 2013). The use of long- versus slow-release stimulants for individuals who abuse stimulants is discussed in Box 18.7.

In studies of psychostimulants for cocaine dependence, various pharmacological strategies have been studied, but none has shown consistent or dramatic

My adult ADHD patient has substance abuse, as do a quarter of ADHD patients (Levin et al., 1998). Does that mean I must avoid stimulant therapy, and just stick with atomoxetine or alpha agonists?

Treatment of ADHD with stimulants in patients with amphetamine-use disorder is controversial. However, stimulant treatment of pediatric ADHD actually *lowers* the risk for later substance abuse about twofold (Wilens et al., 2003a), and delayed initiation of stimulants in youth with ADHD may *protect* against later conduct disorder (Mannuzza et al., 2008)

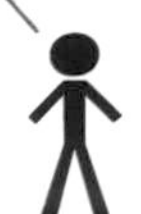

Box 18.7

Long-acting Slow-release Stimulants in Individuals with Stimulant Abuse?

Does lisdexamfetamine have a lower potential for abuse than short-acting formulations of amphetamine? Because lisdexamfetamine is a pro-drug that gradually liberates free dextroamphetamine via hydrolysis of its *l*-lysine moieties, it is often considered to have lower likelihood for inducing euphoria or prompting abuse. However, this remains a point of speculation. In children and adolescents with ADHD, Tmax for the pro-drug is 1 hour while for its dextroamphetamine metabolite it is 5 hours (range: 4.5–6 hours); for mixed amphetamine salts XR, Tmax is 6.6 hours (range: 3–12 hours). However, IV infusion of lisdexamfetamine 50 mg/day had no greater subjective "likeability" than placebo, in contrast to IV dextroamphetamine 20 mg, in one study of adults with histories of stimulant abuse (Jasinski and Krishnan, 2009a). Those authors later found that oral lisdexamfetamine 50 or 100 mg in adults with stimulant abuse produced less "likeability" as compared to 40 mg of oral dextroamphetamine IR (though, lisdexamfetamine 150 mg showed higher likeability than placebo (Jasinski and Krishnan, 2009b).

The bottom line? Lisdexamfetamine has a rationale and at least some database to favor its use over mixed amphetamine salts among individuals considered to be at risk for stimulant abuse.

efficacy to promote abstinence. One initially compelling line of investigation involved the use of modafinil, beginning with a much-publicized (at the time) eight-week RCT showing greater efficacy (dosed at 400 mg/day) than placebo to reduce cocaine use (Dackis et al., 2005), followed by a larger negative replication trial by the same investigators (Dackis et al., 2012). A subsequent Cochrane Database review examined dextroamphetamine, lisdexamfetamine, methylphenidate, modafinil, mazindol, methamphetamine, and mixed amphetamine salts, as well as bupropion and selegiline, finding an overall improved likelihood for sustained cocaine abstinence (RR = 1.36, 95% CI = 1.05–1.77, p = 0.02), but none was found to significantly reduce cocaine use (g = 0.16, 95% CI = −0.02 to 0.33); overall efficacy was greatest for bupropion and dextroamphetamine (Castells et al., 2016).

Part of the clinical challenge and treatment complexity may reflect a high incidence of polysubstance misuse (for example, 60% or more of patients seen in methadone maintenance programs have both opiate and cocaine dependence (Kosten et al., 2003)). Among patients with dual-substance misuse of cocaine and opioids who were receiving buprenorphine (mean dose = 16 mg/day) and CM, 12 weeks of adjunctive desipramine (150 mg/day) was superior to adjunctive placebo in leading to fewer cocaine-positive urine toxicology screens (Kosten et al., 2003). Interestingly, a post-hoc analysis of this latter study found that desipramine was more effective than placebo in leading to drug-free urine toxicology screens when a history of major depression was absent rather than present – suggesting a possible intrinsic anticraving effect for desipramine unrelated to its antidepressant properties (or restricting the use of desipramine only to depressed cocaine-abusing opiate-dependent patients) (Gonzalez et al., 2003).

Among methamphetamine abusers, topiramate was found to be no better than placebo in promoting abstinence (Elkashef et al., 2012). In cocaine-dependent patients, findings with topiramate are mixed, as summarized in Table 18.5 at the end of this chapter. In a meta-analysis of five studies, topiramate use was more likely associated with continued abstinence (RR = 2.43, 95% CI = 1.31–4.53, p = 0.005) and craving reduction was observed in one of five studies, but no significant differences from placebo were seen in treatment retention (Singh et al., 2016).

Among anticonvulsants other than topiramate:

- An RCT of gabapentin found no difference from placebo (Bisaga et al., 2006)
- A 12-week placebo-controlled RCT of tiagabine (20 mg/day; n = 141) found no differences from placebo (Winhusen et al., 2007)

Traditional antidepressants have received moderate attention in the RCT literature focusing on cocaine misuse, as summarized in Table 18.6 at the end of this chapter.

Ⓜ ANTIPSYCHOTICS AND COCAINE USE DISORDER

It makes intuitive sense to think that because cocaine misuse so potently influences the reward pathway, modulation of DA circuitry (particularly, perhaps, via DA partial agonism) would offer a logical treatment strategy. In reality, available evidence may actually suggest a surprisingly opposite and undesired effect: aripiprazole has been shown to increase rather than decrease cocaine self-administration (Haney et al., 2011). A Cochrane Database review of 14 RCTs found no significant advantage over placebo or an active comparator for the use of any antipsychotic with respect to cocaine craving, abstinence, or money spent on use (Indave et al., 2016). We could identify no other RCTs involving aripiprazole or other D_2/D_3 partial agonists (brexpiprazole or cariprazine) for treatment of cocaine use disorder, leaving open the question of the effects of such agents (particularly in light of the association between D_3 receptor function and reward/reinforcement) in the context of cocaine use.

N CITICOLINE AND COCAINE OR METHAMPHETAMINE USE DISORDER

Cytidine-5′-diphosphate choline (CDP-choline, or citicoline) is a neuroprotective agent involved in intracellular signaling (see Chapter 11, Table 11.10) for which several preliminary RCTs suggest potential value for reducing cocaine use in patients with bipolar disorder. (It is available as an over-the-counter nutritional supplement in the USA and by prescription in Japan and Europe.) Dosing in RCTs typically has begun at 500 mg/day, increasing to 1000 mg/day after one week, then 1500 mg/day by Week 4 and finally 2000 mg/day by Week 6. It may improve memory in the course of treating addiction symptoms (Brown et al., 2007). In some trials, initial benefits were shown to diminish over the course of several weeks (Brown et al., 2015). Citicoline also has provisionally shown greater improvement than placebo in reducing both depressive symptoms and methamphetamine use in unipolar or bipolar patients (Brown and Gabrielson, 2012).

O CANNABIS

Cannabinoids activate endogenous cannabinoid receptors in the brain which in turn cause release of mesolimbic dopamine. Δ-9-tetrahydrocannabinol (THC) causes hippocampal neurotoxicity (Chan et al., 1998), persistent and pervasive neurocognitive deficits with chronic heavy use starting in adolescence (Mejer et al., 2012), leads to amotivational states and impaired reward learning (Lawn et al., 2016), induces paranoia in individuals at risk for psychosis (Freeman et al., 2015), worsens treatment response and long-term remission rates in bipolar disorder (Kim et al., 2015), and is associated with higher psychiatric symptom severity among individuals with mood and anxiety disorders (Mammen et al., 2018). THC is considered to be more psychologically than physiologically addictive, although "withdrawal" phenomena have been described that mainly involve craving, restlessness, nervousness, insomnia, and negative affect states; the latter have been shown to attenuate (among tobacco nonusers or nonheavy users) via placement of a 7 mg nicotine patch over 15 days (Gilbert et al., 2020). Insomnia associated with cannabis withdrawal has (mostly anecdotally) been treated with gabapentin, lofexidine, mirtazapine, quetiapine, or zolpidem, although adequate RCTs are lacking. Overall "withdrawal" symptoms have been reported to remit spontaneously and without need for pharmacological intervention within about 16 days of cannabis cessation.

There are no well-established pharmacotherapies with demonstrated efficacy to promote abstinence from cannabis. Antidepressant RCTs have generally produced disappointing results (e.g., a large 12-week comparison of venlafaxine or placebo in depressed cannabis-dependent patients found significantly *lower* abstinence rates with venlafaxine than placebo, and little to no effect on mood improvement (Levin et al., 2013)). However, an intriguing preclinical study found that pregnenolone inhibits the CB1 receptor, creating a negative feedback loop that reduces the effects of THC (Vallée et al., 2014); however, some authors have cautioned that these preclinical data should not be construed as the basis necessarily for recommending pregnenolone in the treatment of cannabis addiction, citing the failure of the CB1 receptor antagonist rimonabant (SR141718) because of possible induction of suicidal ideation and depression or other signs of mood dysregulation. Another promising but preliminary treatment approach involves *N*-acetylcysteine: when dosed at 1200 mg PO BID, a significant reduction in cannabis use was observed (with a 2.4-fold reduction in positive urine toxicology screens over eight weeks) in adolescents (Gray et al., 2012), but that finding was not replicated in a similar 12-week trial with adults (Gray et al., 2017).

Studies of the synthetic THC analogue dronabinol have largely failed to show benefit in treatment of cannabis dependence (Levin et al., 2011). Preliminary findings with the synthetic cannabinoid agonist nabilone (begun at 0.5 mg/day for seven days, then 1 mg/day for seven days, then 1.5 mg/day for seven days, then 2 mg/day thereafter) also failed to demonstrate efficacy for reducing cannabis use, but did show a reduction in some self-reported craving measures, with good tolerability (Hill at al., 2017).

P OPIATE USE DISORDERS

According to the 2015 National Survey on Drug Use and Health (NSDUH), 4.7% of US adults prescribed an opiate misused them, and 0.8% would meet diagnostic criteria for opiate use disorder (Han et al., 2017). A reminder of opiate metabolic breakdown products is summarized in Figure 18.2.

Pharmacodynamic goals in managing opiate dependence involve efforts to provide safe blockade of opiate receptors. While pure agonism via methadone maintenance represents a well-established strategy, buprenorphine has emerged in recent years as a simpler office-based alternative that provides at least comparable (if not in some respects greater) efficacy. Buprenorphine is a partial agonist at the μ opiate receptor, as well as an antagonist at κ and δ receptors. Controlled trials also suggest that at low doses it may also have pharmacodynamic value in treating depression and reducing suicidal ideation (Serafini et al., 2018).

Tip

Beware if and when opiate-dependent patients on methadone maintenance request dosage reductions; it may signal relapse intentions.

Tip

Buprenorphine manages opiate withdrawal, symptom severity, and likelihood of completing opiate detox more effectively than clonidine; however, studies are lacking of their possible combined synergy

Buprenorphine has a ceiling (maximum) effect on respiratory depression, meaning that increasing doses do not pose a greater cardiopulmonary hazard, unlike pure opioid agonists. On an overall basis among opioid-dependent patients, buprenorphine and methadone show comparable rates of retention in treatment and reduced opioid misuse (as measured by urine toxicology screens) (Strain et al., 1994). When opioid and cocaine use disorders co-occur, methadone maintenance has been shown to be superior to buprenorphine for promoting abstinence from both substances (Schottenfeld et al., 2005).

Table 18.7 at the end of this chapter summarizes evidence-based pharmacotherapies relevant to opiate withdrawal and relapse prevention.

Q POST-ACUTE WITHDRAWAL SYNDROME

"Post-acute withdrawal syndrome" (PAWS) is a popularly described though medically controversial phenomenon meant to refer to "late"-occurring physical complaints and symptoms following acute withdrawal from alcohol, opiates, or sedative-hypnotics. The construct validity of PAWS has been a subject of debate in the medical literature because no clear physiological explanation or anatomical model for its occurrence has been identified. Nor do randomized intervention trials exist from which inferences can be drawn about optimal management strategies.

Pitfalls involving purported protracted withdrawal states, as well as the potential for misuse of noncontrolled substances, are illustrated in Clinical Vignettes 18.1 and 18.2.

Figure 18.2 Metabolism of opiates.

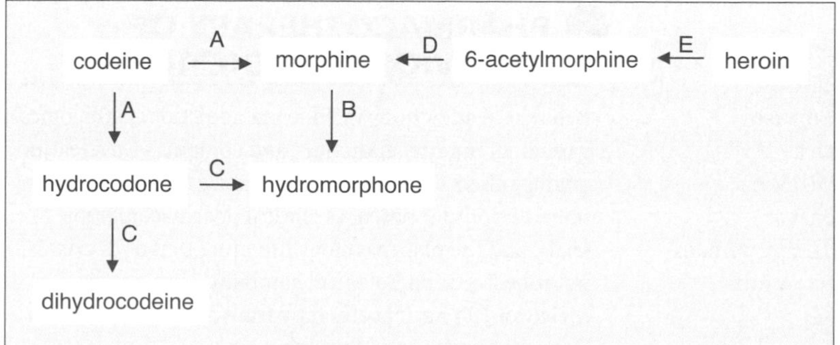

Enzymatic pathways: A = *O*-demethylation via CYP2D6 and glucuronidation via UGT2B7; B = glucuronidation via UGT2B7 and UGT1A3; C = Demethylation via CYP2D6, *N*-demethylation via CYP34; D = carboxylesterase; E = pseudocholinesterase (Kamendulis et al., 1996; Holmquist, 2009; Anderson et al., 2015)

CLINICAL VIGNETTE 18.1

Protracted Benzodiazepine Withdrawal, or Craving and Distress Intolerance

Lou was a 42-year-old divorced man with a history of intermittent, near-daily cannabis use since his early teenage years, as well as chronic depression and anxiety. He claimed to be taking alprazolam up to 18 mg/day (partly prescribed by his previous psychiatrist and supplemented by borrowing from friends) for the past four years, and said he occasionally required an extra 1–2 mg/day for "breakthrough anxiety." In an outpatient detoxification program his alprazolam was converted to clonazepam (though dosing equivalency is generally considered 1:1, he was autonomically stable taking clonazepam 8 mg/day after 10 days, and the treatment program was skeptical of the amount of alprazolam he claimed to have actually been taking). Over the next two months his dosage was gradually further decreased to 6 mg/day by 0.5 mg/week increments, then by 0.25 mg/week and then by 0.125 mg/week increments as he increasingly complained of feeling "edgy, cold, and numb." He reported being unable to tolerate further reductions from 5.125 mg/day due to a wide range of diffuse physical complaints. His CIWA-Ar score remained persistently at 9, due mainly to ratings of anxiety and agitation. His psychiatrist expressed skepticism that his physical complaints reflected physiological withdrawal in the absence of observable autonomic signs, coupled with the very gradual timeframe and seemingly miniscule magnitude of dosage reductions. Successive trials of adjunctive gabapentin, hydroxyzine, quetiapine, aripiprazole, and low-dose chlorpromazine (10 mg) all failed to alleviate his discomfort. He pleaded to resume a higher dose because he "could no longer humanly tolerate the intensity of his withdrawal symptoms."

CLINICAL VIGNETTE 18.2

Misuse of Noncontrolled Substances

Conrad was a 26-year-old man living with his parents and working part-time as a messenger, struggling with off-and-on recovery from benzodiazepine, alcohol, and opiate use disorders. He had found clonidine to be useful in managing internal feelings of distress after having initially taken it as part of an opiate detoxification program. After his psychiatrist read a clinical trial showing that buprenorphine plus clonidine (up to 0.3 mg/day) was better than buprenorphine alone in maintaining abstinence from opiates (Kowalczyk et al., 2015), she was happy to continue prescribing it for him to possibly help prevent relapse. Conrad struggled greatly with managing impulses and negative feelings and maintaining emotional self-regulation in the face of daily stresses, and began to self-increase his clonidine use from 0.3 mg nightly to as much as 1.2 mg three to four times daily. He ultimately was brought by paramedics to the emergency department (ED) when his parents found him unresponsive. In the ED he was bradycardic, markedly hypotensive and hypothermic (the latter helping to differentiate initial erroneous suspicions that he had relapsed on opiates) but recovered with fluid resuscitation and monitoring. Subsequently, in his recovery program he added clonidine to the list of substances over which he was powerless and experienced unmanageability.

R HALLUCINOGEN MISUSE

As serotonergic psychedelics such as psilocybin gain increasing interest and attention for their possible therapeutic value for treating depression, there is strikingly little to no formal literature on pharmacological strategies to treat their misuse. Nor is there a well-defined literature on the pharmacological management of the misuse of so-called empathogen-entactogens such as 3,4-methylenedioxymethamphetamine (MDMA). Behavioral approaches, such as motivational enhancement and cognitive-behavioral therapy, remain more the cornerstones of psychiatric interventions.

In patients with for phencyclidine (PCP) intoxication, antipsychotics should be avoided because of their potential to increase the risk for PCP-induced hyperthermia, seizures, dystonia, or anticholinergic reactions. Benzodiazepines remain the preferred method for pharmacological management.

S PHARMACOTHERAPY OF BEHAVIORAL ADDICTIONS

Behavioral addictions include sex addiction, pathological gambling, internet addiction, and compulsive overeating, among others. The empirical literature on behavioral interventions far outpaces clinical pharmacotherapy trials, and the pharmacology literature that does exist is not robust. For pathological gambling, findings from a review of 19 pharmacotherapy trials are summarized in Table 18.8 at the end of this chapter.

Among other behavioral addictions, internet use disorder (though unacknowledged in DSM-5 or the International Classification of Diseases (ICD-10)) has been a focus of increasing attention, with treatment structured mainly around cognitive or similar behavioral therapy approaches; pharmacotherapy tends to be reserved mainly for associated conditions (e.g., antidepressants for depression, psychostimulants for ADHD) rather than for primarily targeting addiction behavior. Compulsive sexual disorders often represent an interface between obsessive-compulsive and impulse-control disorders, and addictions as defined in this chapter based on dysfunction of the reward pathway. RCTs of any pharmacotherapy are scarce, and the literature mostly contains open trials or retrospective reports focusing on serotonergic antidepressants (e.g., SSRIs, nefazodone), with some suggestion that sexual obsessions may respond better than paraphilias (Stein et al., 1992), as well as single case reports suggesting potential value for naltrexone or topiramate for compulsive sexual behavior.

TAKE-HOME POINTS

- Addictions are complicated disorders unto themselves that likely have their own neurobiology, even though they are often comorbid with other psychiatric conditions. They tend to require their own treatment.
- Naltrexone or topiramate seem to have the biggest effects to reduce heavy drinking.
- Gabapentin can help reduce emotional distress symptoms during alcohol detox and afterwards during relapse prevention.
- Don't use imipramine, fluvoxamine, paroxetine, or mirtazapine in depressed alcoholics and hope for much benefit in drinking behavior – better off with desipramine, sertraline, or fluoxetine from an evidence-based standpoint.
- Cocaine addiction is particularly hard to treat pharmacologically. There is a modest evidence base favoring topiramate and desipramine. Citicoline up to 2000 mg/day may help reduce cocaine use, especially in people with bipolar disorder.
- In ADHD patients at risk for stimulant abuse, don't withhold stimulant therapy but favor long-acting formulations to minimize abuse potential.
- For cannabis use disorder, consider *N*-acetylcysteine in younger patients and pregnenolone in adults.
- Think about buprenorphine in the context of depression when considering options for opioid relapse prevention.

Table 18.1 Substances of abuse and their usual detection windows

Drug	Analyte tested	Approximate detection window in urine
Amphetamine	Amphetamine	48 hours
Barbiturates	Amobarbital, pentobarbital, secobarbital (short-acting); phenobarbital (long-acting)	2–4 days for short-acting, up to 30 days for long-acting
Benzodiazepines	Alprazolam, temazepam, clonazepam, lorazepam; chlordiazepoxide, diazepam	1–10 days 10–14 days
Buprenorphine	Buprenorphine, norbuprenorphine	1–7 days
Cocaine	Benzoylecgonine	1–3 days
Codeine	Codeine, morphine	1–2 days
Ecstasy (3,4-methylenedioxy-methamphetamine; MDMA)	3,4-Methylenedioxy-methamphetamine; 4-hydroxy-3-methoxy-amphetamine (HMA)	2–4 days
Ethanol	Ethanol; ethyl gluconoride (EtG) or ethyl sulfate (EtS)	10–12 hours 40–130 hours
Heroin	Morphine; 6-acetylmorphine	1–3 days
Hydrocodone	Hydrocodone; hydromorphone	1–2 days
Hydromorphone	Hydromorphone	30–60 hours
Ketamine	Ketamine, norketamine	1–4 days
Lysergic acid diethylamide (LSD)	Lysergic acid diethylamide	8–96 hours
Marijuana	Tetrahydrocannabinol	1–3 days for casual use; up to 30 days for chronic use
Methadone	Methadone	2–4 days
Morphine, oxycodone	Morphine	1–3 days
Oxycodone	Oxymorphone	1–4 days
Phencyclidine	Phencyclidine	Up to 8 days in chronic users

Table 18.2 False positive findings on drug toxicology screens [a]

False-positive findings of ...	... May be caused by ...
Amphetamines	Amantadine, atomoxetine, brompheniramine, bupropion, chlorpromazine, desipramine, desoxyephedrine, doxepin, ephedrine, isometheptene, isoxsuprime, labetolol, metformin, phentermine, phenylephrine, phenylpropanolamine, promethazine, pseudoephedrine, ranitidine, selegiline, thioridazine, trazodone, trimethobenzamide, trimipramine
Benzodiazepines	Efavirenz, oxaprozin, sertraline
Barbiturates	Ibuprofen, naproxen
Cannabinoids	Dronabinol, efavirenz, ibuprofen, naproxen, piroxicam, promethazine, proton pump inhibitors, sulindac, tolmetin
Lysergic acid diethylamide (LSD)	Amitriptyline, dicyclomine, sumatriptan
Methadone	Chlorpromazine, clomipramine, diphenhydramine, doxylamine, ibuprofen, quetiapine, thioridazine, verapamil
Opiates	Dextromethorphan, diphenhydramine, fluoroquinolones, naltrexone, poppy seeds, rifampin
Phencyclidine	Dextroamphetamine, dextromethorphan, diphenhydramine, ibuprofen, imipramine, ketamine, lamotrigine, meperidine, thioridazine, tramadol, venlafaxine, zolpidem

[a] Findings as reported by Li et al., 2019

Table 18.3 Effects of naltrexone or acamprosate on alcohol-use behavior [a]

Outcome	Medications	*g*	95% CI	p-value	Number of studies
Abstinence	Naltrexone	0.116	0.049–0.183	0.001	36
	Acamprosate	0.359	0.246–0.472	<0.001	15
Heavy drinking	Naltrexone	0.189	0.123–0.255	<0.001	39
	Acamprosate	0.072	-0.078–0.221	0.346	5
Craving	Naltrexone	0.144	0.045–0.244	0.005	26
	Acamprosate	0.034	-0.0036–0.104	0.347	9
Heavy drinking and craving	Naltrexone	0.180	0.118–0.243	<0.001	42
	Acamprosate	0.041	-0.029–0.112	0.246	9

a Based on meta-analysis of 61 placebo-controlled RCTs reported by Maisel et al. (2013)
Abbreviations: CI = confidence interval

Table 18.4 Antidepressants in alcohol use disorders

Antidepressant	Positive trials	Negative trials
Citalopram	An early four-month placebo-controlled trial in 62 nondepressed alcohol-dependent patients showed significantly greater reductions in drinking behavior than with placebo (Tiihonen et al., 1996)	(-) 12-week RCT found citalopram (20–40 mg/day) recipients had *more* heavy drinking days and smaller changes in alcohol frequency and consumption than seen with placebo (Charney et al., 2015) Citalopram + naltrexone did not produce better mood or drinking outcomes than did naltrexone alone in 138 depressed alcoholics (Adamson et al., 2015)
Desipramine	Among alcohol-dependent patients, desipramine improved depression symptoms and maintained abstinence better than did placebo in depressed (but not nondepressed) alcoholics (Mason et al., 1996) In PTSD combat veterans with an alcohol use disorder, desipramine was superior to paroxetine or naltrexone in reducing alcohol use (Petrakis et al., 2012)	None
Imipramine	None	A 12-week RCT of imipramine in 69 actively drinking depressed patients showed improvement in mood but not drinking behavior (McGrath et al., 1996)
Fluoxetine	A 12-week RCT of fluoxetine (n = 25; mean maximal dose = 25 mg/day) found significantly less total alcohol use and a greater reduction in depression versus placebo (n = 26) (Cornelius et el., 1997)	A 12-week RCT of fluoxetine (n = 46, dosed up to 60 mg/day) in 101 depressed alcoholics improved depression symptoms but not drinking behavior better than placebo (n = 49) (Kranzler et al., 1995)
Fluvoxamine	None	A one-year RCT of fluvoxamine (up to 300 mg/day) or placebo in 493 nondepressed alcoholics found a trend for poorer abstinence and relapse rates with fluvoxamine (Chick et al., 2004)
Paroxetine	None	1 (-) 16-week RCT in alcohol-dependent outpatients with social anxiety disorder (Thomas et al., 2008)
Mirtazapine	None	An eight-week RCT of mirtazapine 30 mg/day was no better than placebo in reducing drinking (de Bejczy and Söderpalm, 2015)
Sertraline	Sertraline (200 mg/day) + naltrexone (100 mg/day) was superior to either monotherapy or placebo in 170 depressed alcoholics to promote abstinence and longer time until heavy drinking relapse (Pettinati et al., 2010)	No significant differences in alcohol-use parameters were observed when comparing lower-dose naltrexone monotherapy (60 mg/day) with sertraline 100 mg/day over 10 weeks (Farren et al., 2009)

Abbreviations: PTSD = post-traumatic stress disorder; RCT = randomized controlled trial

Table 18.5 RCTs of topiramate for cocaine abuse or dependence

Positive findings	Negative findings
A 13-week double-blind pilot trial (n = 40) found higher rates of cocaine abstinence with topiramate (target dose = 200 mg/day) than placebo (Kampman et al., 2004)	In 170 newly abstinent cocaine- and alcohol-dependent subjects, topiramate 300 mg/day for 13 weeks was no better than placebo in sustaining reductions in cocaine use or craving, or alcohol use (Kampman et al., 2013)
A 12-week RCT found that a target dose of 300 mg/day was better than placebo in increasing the proportion of nonuse days, craving, and urinary cocaine-free weeks (Johnson et al., 2013)	A 12-week open randomized comparison of cognitive behavior therapy ± topiramate 200 mg/day in 74 crack-cocaine-dependent outpatients found no reduction in cocaine use, possibly mediated by low adherence (Nuijten et al., 2014)
A 12-week RCT among 60 crack-cocaine-dependent subjects, using a target dose of 200 mg/day, found more frequent negative urine toxicology screens for benzoylecgonine and less quantity and frequency of cocaine use, but results were significant only for the first four weeks (Baldaçara et al., 2016)	In 170 methadone-maintained patients with cocaine dependence randomized to topiramate (induction over seven weeks, maintenance over eight weeks; target dose = 300 mg/day) or placebo, no differences in abstinence were observed (Umbricht et al., 2014b)

Abbreviations: RCT = randomized controlled trial

Table 18.6. RCTs of antidepressants for cocaine dependence

Positive findings	Negative findings
In a six-month RCT among 106 methadone-maintained veterans, cocaine-free urine drug screens were significantly more frequent when CM was paired with bupropion (300 mg/day) than placebo (Poling et al., 2006)	A 12-week placebo-controlled RCT of bupropion (dosing = 300 mg/day) showed no differences in cocaine-use frequency, depressive symptoms, or psychosocial functioning (Margolin et al., 1995)
Adjunctive desipramine was superior to placebo in reducing cocaine use among cocaine- and opioid-dependent outpatients also receiving buprenorphine (Kosten et al., 2003)	In a 33-week RCT, 145 methadone-maintained dual diagnosis (opiate and cocaine) nondepressed outpatients fared better with voucher incentives than fluoxetine in reducing cocaine use (Winstanley et al., 2011)
A 13-week RCT of desipramine (150 mg/day) showed superiority to placebo for reducing both cocaine and opioid use among 180 opioid-dependent cocaine abusers maintained on methadone or buprenorphine (Oliveto et al., 1999)	A 12-week RCT of mirtazapine 45 mg/day (n = 11) or placebo (n = 13) in depressed cocaine-dependent outpatients found no differences in reducing cocaine use, but mirtazapine was better for reducing depression and improving sleep (Afshar et al., 2012)
A 12-week RCT of desipramine (up to 300 mg/day) or placebo in 111 cocaine-dependent outpatients with comorbid MDD found significantly greater improvement in both mood and cocaine use with desipramine than placebo; no *direct* effect of desipramine on cocaine use was observed (McDowell et al., 2005)	A 12-week RCT of venlafaxine (up to 300 mg/day) in 130 depressed cocaine-dependent patients found no differences from placebo in any mood or cocaine-use outcomes (Raby et al., 2014)
In a 12-week trial of recently abstinent cocaine-dependent patients with depression, sertraline (up to 200 mg/day) was superior to placebo in delaying time until relapse and also led to a reduction in depressive symptoms (Oliveto et al., 2012)	
In a 12-week trial of recently abstinent cocaine-dependent patients with depression, sertraline (up to 200 mg/day) (but not sertraline plus gabapentin (1200 mg/day)) was superior to placebo for reduced cocaine use (Mancino et al., 2014)	

Abbreviations: CM = contingency management; RCT = randomized controlled trial

Table 18.7 Pharmacotherapies for opiate withdrawal and relapse prevention

Agent	Rationale/comment
Clonidine	Decreases noradrenergic presynaptic release to diminish autonomic hyperarousal symptoms associated with opiate withdrawal; additionally, has been shown to decouple stress from craving in everyday life as an ongoing pharmacotherapy after completion of acute detoxification (Kowalczyk et al., 2015)
Opiate antagonists: naltrexone	A Cochrane Database review found no significant differences between oral naltrexone and placebo across varied measures of opioid relapse (Minozzi et al., 2011)
Opiate agonists: methadone	Cochrane Database reviews report no significant differences between methadone and buprenorphine in opioid detoxification duration or intensity of withdrawal symptoms (Gowing et al., 2017) or self-reported opioid use, opioid-positive urine drug screens, retention in maintenance treatment, or adverse events (Nielsen et al., 2016)
Opiate partial agonists: buprenorphine	A Cochrane Database review found no difference between buprenorphine and methadone in opiate withdrawal treatment duration, less severe withdrawal symptoms than with clonidine or lofexidine; as compared to clonidine or lofexidine, buprenorphine produced better withdrawal scores with a low-to-medium effect size (g = –0.43, 95% CI = –0.58 to –0.28) and a higher rate of completion (NNT = 4) (Gowing et al., 2017). Insurance registry studies show that about one-quarter of opiate-dependent patients who begin oral buprenorphine discontinue within the first month, as predicted by low initial dose (≤4 mg/day), male sex, younger age, minority race/ethnicity, comorbid substance use disorders, presence of hepatitis C, and having a history of opioid overdose (Samples et al., 2018)
Cannabidiol	Oral administration of 400 or 800 mg once a day for three days reduced both craving and anxiety induced by salient drug cues (Hurd et al., 2019)

Abbreviations: CI = confidence interval; NNT = number needed to treat

Table 18.8 Summary of pharmacotherapy RCTs for pathological gambling [a]

Agent	Positive findings	Negative findings
Bupropion	No data	One (-) 12-week RCT (mean dose = 324 mg/day) using PG-YBOCS
Fluvoxamine	One (+) 16-week RCT (mean dose = 195 mg/day) using PG-CGI and PG-YBOCS	One (-) six-month RCT (mean dose = 200 mg/day) on money spent on gambling per week
Lithium carbonate	No data	One (-) 10-week RCT (mean dose = 1150 mg/day) on PG-YBOCS and PG-CGI-I
N-acetylcysteine	Two (+) RCTs (one 12-week, dosing range from 1200–3000 mg/day; the second eight-week open-label then 16 weeks randomized discontinuation) on PG-YBOCS	No data
Nalmefene	One (+) 16-week RCT; dosing of 50 or 100 mg/day superior to placebo using PG-YBOCS	One (-) 16-week RCT (dosing = 20–40 mg/day) using PG-YBOCS
Naltrexone	Two (+) 12–18 week RCTs using dosages from 50–200 mg/day	Two (-) 11–20 week RCTs with dosages up to 250 mg/day
Olanzapine	No data	Two (-) RCTs (one seven-week (dosing 2.5–10 mg/day) and one 12-week RCT (mean dose = 8.9 mg/day)) on PG-YBOCS
Paroxetine	1 (+) 8-week RCT (mean dose = 51.7 mg/day) using GSAS, PG-CGI	One (-) 16-week RCT (mean dose = 50 mg/day) using PG-CGI
Sertraline	No data	One (-) RCT, mean dose = 95 mg/day using CCPGQ
Topiramate	One (+) RCT (mean dose = 180.7 mg/day) with significantly greater reduction in gambling craving than placebo	One (-) 14-week RCT (mean dose = 222.5 mg/day) using PG-YBOCS

[a] Based on findings by Kraus et al., 2020

Abbreviations: CCPGQ = Criteria for Control of Pathological Gambling Questionnaire; GSAS = Gambling Symptom Assessment Scale; PG-CGI = pathological gambling Clinical Global Impressions scale; PG-YBOCS = pathological gambling modification of the Yale–Brown Obsessive-Compulsive Scale; RCT = randomized controlled trial

19 Trauma and Post-traumatic Stress Disorder

LEARNING OBJECTIVES

- [ ] Recognize the impact of trauma, particularly during early development, as a moderator of poor outcome across many psychiatric disorders
- [ ] Describe the importance of resilience and its enhancement as a treatment goal across psychiatric disorders
- [ ] Recognize the varied symptom targets of treatment in PTSD
- [ ] Describe the strengths and limitations of existing evidence-based pharmacotherapies for acute stress disorders
- [ ] Identify controversies regarding the use of benzodiazepines in patients with PTSD
- [ ] Discuss the evidence base for antidepressants, anticonvulsants, antipsychotics, α agonists, ketamine, and novel/emerging pharmacotherapies for PTSD

> That which does not kill us makes us stronger.
>
> *- Friedrich Nietzsche*

Trauma and dissociation are together often thought of as falling more within the treatment realm of cognitive-behavioral psychotherapy than psychopharmacology. Indeed, in the case of PTSD, trauma-focused psychotherapies collectively exert larger effect sizes than seen with pharmacotherapies (Watts et al., 2013; Lee et al., 2016), which in the aggregate yield response rates only of about 20–30%. Yet, in order to understand the potential relevance of pharmacotherapy to psychological trauma, one must first appreciate the interplay between trauma's psychological and neurobiological corollaries. Traumatic events form durable, emotionally based memories consolidated through limbic circuitry – in turn affecting emotional regulation and broad cognitive domains (attentional processing and vigilance, executive function, and impulse control). Environmental cues that become associated with threats to one's physical and/or emotional well-being become aversive and can elicit fear responses, involving autonomic hyperarousal and vigilance, and can prompt intrusive, repetitive thought patterns laced with negative affect states. PTSD itself is viewed by some as fundamentally a behavioral disorder involving abnormal fear extinction. Furthermore, trauma and abuse occurring in childhood may influence neuronal development, perhaps thereby imposing one of the more devastating moderators of treatment outcome across a range of psychiatric disorders.

Whether or not formal diagnoses of PTSD ensue after traumatic exposures, survivors of significant trauma in both childhood and adulthood can incur brain volumetric (e.g., hippocampal) changes (Woon et al., 2010); some studies suggest that small hippocampal volume may result from, rather than predispose to, the development of PTSD in adult trauma victims (Winter and Irle, 2004). Trauma challenges resilience (see Box 19.1) yet at the same time can shape and strengthen it. Developmentally, it disrupts the formation of normal attachment styles and patterns, and at any stage in life can impart punitive expectations in response to life stresses through operant conditioning, and the fostering of learned helplessness.

Box 19.1

What is Resilience?

The term "resilience" is often used to describe an intact capacity for effective coping in response to stress. Resilience also implies an ability to withstand adversity without developing consequent psychopathology. It likely contributes to overall risk for developing depression, anxiety, and PTSD (among other conditions), as well as being a moderator of treatment outcomes. Charney (2004) links resilience with intact reward and motivation, fear responsiveness, and adaptive social behaviors (such as altruism and social bonding); it is also thought to involve a cognitive style characterized by accurate (rather than excessively positive or negative) threat appraisal (Southwick et al., 2015).

So, we need a resilience pill?

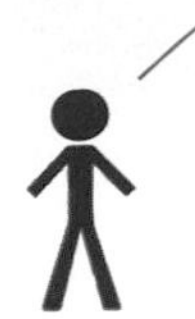

Not sure about that as a categorical thing but when any patient seems to show poor resilience maybe think about pharmacology approaches that can enhance cognitive flexibility and capacity for set-shifting, help them to frame accurate threat appraisals by modulating fear circuitry, and foster optimism by treating depression or anxiety if and when those exist.

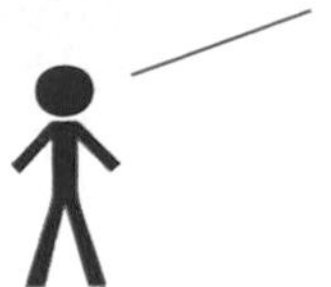

Sounds like a benzo.

From the above, one could envision an array of potential pharmacotherapy targets.

It is not difficult to envision trauma and abnormal or exaggerated stress responses as widely impacting the trajectory of psychopathology across virtually all domains of emotional, perceptual, cognitive, and behavioral functioning. Our approach in this chapter will therefore be no less dimensional than in previous chapters. Beyond the DSM-5/ICD-10 categories of PTSD (for which only two medications carry FDA indications (sertraline and paroxetine and acute stress disorders (where no drugs carry regulatory agency approval), we will consider the rationales and evidence base for varied drug classes and putative mechanisms, focusing as always on having clearly defined goals of treatment.

A STRESS, DISTRESS, AND TRAUMA

Stress involves any environmental stimulus that demands a response from the individual. In some conceptualizations, stresses may be beneficial or fortuitous (so-called "eustress," e.g., job promotions, marriages, having a child) or detrimental ("distress," encompassing reversals of fortune, illness, unreasonable work or social demands, loss of social supports). Stresses can become traumatic when they overwhelm someone's ability to cope and threaten one's basic sense of physical and emotional safety and well-being. Abuse is a type of trauma that involves deliberate and purposefully inflicted harm that violates someone's personal boundaries, jeopardizing one's physical or emotional safety and well-being. It may be overtly physical, emotional, verbal, or sexual, and may involve acts of commission or omission (e.g., assault versus physical or emotional neglect).

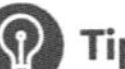

Tip

It can be useful to ask patients to compare themselves to themselves at their prior personal best. Do they think the magnitude of their anxiety or distress in response to a given stress is commensurate with the situation, and on par with their usual reaction in relative rather than absolute terms?

It becomes difficult and subjective to quantify the magnitude of psychological distress resulting from any stressor – particularly since people can easily differ in how they experience or interpret the same objective stressor. Nevertheless, Holmes and Rahe (1967) devised a 43-item measure of stressful life events (referred to in the literature as the Holmes–Rahe Scale, or the Social Readjustment Rating Scale; see Box 19.2) that has become widely adopted in studies attempting to quantify

Box 19.2

Ten Leading Stressful Life Events and their Quantification [a]

Life event	Mean value
Death of spouse [b]	100
Divorce	73
Marital separation	65
Imprisonment	63
Death of close family member	63
Personal injury or loss	53
Marriage	50
Fired from work	47
Marital reconciliation	45
Retirement	45

[a] Adapted from Holmes and Rahe, 1967

[b] Some authors have modified the original Holmes-Rahe scale also to include death of a child, alongside death of spouse, as the most devastating of stressful life events

stress and trauma. Particular life stresses are accorded a numerical score (identified as "life-changing units"); in their original studies, total scores above 300 were associated with the highest probability of developing a significant medical illness, while scores <150 carried the least risk, and those 150–299 held moderate risk. Critics have noted that the scale does not differentiate events that involve eustress versus distress, are sudden versus planned, or acute from chronic.

An example of emotional trauma related to persistent depression is presented in Clinical Vignette 19.1.

That knocks out most of the Holmes–Rahe top 10 stresses...

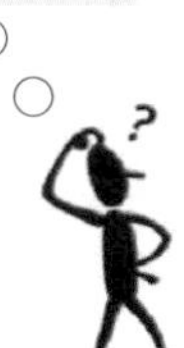

Tip

DSM-5 requires that a violent or life-threatening trauma occur either first-hand or be witnessed *in person* to constitute a trauma that might lead to PTSD.

CLINICAL VIGNETTE 19.1

Manny was a 19-year-old undergraduate with significant social anxiety, risk aversion, and avoidant behavior. He took an academic medical leave of absence after failing two classes during a major depressive episode. Within three months of starting duloxetine his mood and vegetative symptoms improved, but he had persistent low motivation and minimal structured daily activity. Low motivation was construed as a residual depressive symptom but did not improve with optimized dosing, adjunctive bupropion, stimulants, or aripiprazole. In psychotherapy he described his "low motivation" as a paralysis driven by fears of being "criticized and ridiculed" and feeling mortified about past failures. Rather than pursue "amotivation and apathy" as signs of anhedonia, his therapist suggested that he felt paralyzed by fear and a sense of trauma over the consequences of his depression and pre-existing social anxiety. She advised augmenting his pharmacotherapy with a structured psychotherapy approach that challenged his phobic avoidance and distorted beliefs about himself, and his expectations of repeated failure, as emotional consequences from the trauma associated with his depression.

B PTSD AS A CATEGORICAL CONSTRUCT

Prior to DSM-5, PTSD was conceptualized as an anxiety-disorder subtype; the comparative literature on treatment outcomes therefore often incorporates PTSD RCTs alongside those of other anxiety disorders, both past and present (e.g., OCD). The decision to remove PTSD from the broader nosological category of anxiety disorders came partly from observations that trauma-related psychopathology often involves prominent features that are separate from anxiety, such as shame, guilt, and anger. The term "trauma" itself was operationally redefined from DSM-IV (a threat to physical integrity) to "actual or threatened death, serious injury, or sexual violence" (American Psychiatric Association, 2013, p. 271). Intense fear, horror, or helplessness, included in the DSM-IV conceptualization of PTSD, were removed in DSM-5.

Tip

According to the World Health Organization, PTSD occurs in about 4% of individuals who experience a traumatic event.

As a nosological entity, PTSD was originally viewed in DSM-III and DSM-IV as having three core domains: *intrusive thoughts* that involve re-experiencing/reliving the trauma, *avoidance/numbing*, and *hyperarousal* (e.g., an exaggerated startle response). DSM-5 added to these features the construct of *negative alterations in cognition or mood*. DSM-5 also eliminated "acute" and "chronic" specifiers for characterizing PTSD.

Tip

Factors thought to protect against developing PTSD among trauma survivors include social support, perceptions of belongingness, high resilience, nonavoidant coping strategies, and positive expectancies (hope, optimism, and coping-specific self-efficacy).

Complex PTSD (often abbreviated c-PTSD), not included either in DSM-IV or DSM-5, was a construct initially proposed by Herman (1988) that describes psychiatric problems in the aftermath of prolonged or repeated interpersonal trauma. In addition to core PTSD elements of intrusive thoughts, avoidance and hyperarousal, other symptoms may include impulsivity, aggression, mood dysregulation or affective lability, dissociation, somatic complaints, and chaotic interpersonal relationships. Traumas that may predispose to c-PTSD may include prolonged childhood sexual abuse or adult experiences involving prolonged captivity, domestic violence, or physical or sexual exploitation (e.g., human trafficking). Similar to noncomplex PTSD, the cornerstone of treatment mainly involves psychotherapy based on trauma recovery, such as prolonged exposure. Pharmacotherapy usually assumes secondary importance for associated or comorbid symptoms (e.g., substance use disorders, insomnia, depressive syndromes) rather than for psychopathology dimensions (such as emotional dysregulation) that are intrinsic to c-PTSD itself.

Tip

PTSD is more common in women than men, although risk may stratify by type of traumatic event.

Tip

About one-third of PTSD patients have a chronic course (i.e., a symptomatic duration more than three months).

In patients with MDD, a history of childhood trauma is a substantial moderator of poor outcome. No particular pharmacotherapy regimen has demonstrated better antidepressant efficacy than any other in the setting of childhood trauma.

 MEASURES

Clinicians, knowingly or unknowingly, often choose pharmacotherapies in PTSD patients directed toward one or more of the traditional symptom clusters (avoidance, intrusive thoughts and re-experiencing and reliving, and sleep disturbances (notably, nightmares)). In RCTs, PTSD symptoms are often globally rated using the 17-item Clinician-Administered PTSD Scale (CAPS), for which baseline scores >50 are generally considered to reflect significant levels of symptom severity (0–19 is generally considered "minimally symptomatic" or asymptomatic; 20–39 reflects "subthreshold" or mild symptoms, 40–59 reflects "threshold" to moderate severity, 60–79 is considered "severe," and scores >80 are considered "extreme" (Weathers et al., 2001). The CAPS scale includes measures of core PTSD subcomponents including re-experiencing (Cluster "B"), avoidance/numbing (Cluster

Can I have PTSD without having had a distinct traumatic event happen to me? My life is just generally stressful in ways that feel traumatic.
I hear ya, bro'. This has been a longstanding debate in psychiatry. Some authors call it the "Criterion 'A' problem" since the way we define trauma is subjective and its impact can vary greatly from person to person. For better or worse, though, the concept now bears solely on catastrophically violent or otherwise life-threatening events.
I see. So if I'm just really stressed out by life and it's not PTSD…can I have a benzo then?
Better you should go reread Chapter 17

DSM-5 also includes "reckless or self-destructive behaviors" in its definition of PTSD. Does that mean it becomes a kind of variant of bipolar disorder, or borderline personality disorder, and I should treat it with drugs for those conditions?
No, not necessarily. This is another good example of a conceptually overlapping symptom that has no diagnostic specificity. Like Chapter 1 said, diagnosis matters most if there is a coherent constellation of signs and symptoms. Otherwise, we're looking at dimensions of psychopathology. Track its course alongside the other symptoms you're treating with whatever treatment you choose.

"C"), and hyperarousal (Cluster "D"). The threshold for gauging "response" in PTSD is conventionally taken to be a CAPS improvement from baseline of ≥20–30%. Some studies (e.g., Feder et al., 2014) identify a CAPS score of ≤50 as an indicator of "significant improvement" in RCTs. Also of note, acute clinical trial durations in PTSD often extend up to 12 weeks to gauge response.

The Impact of Events Scale (IES) is also often used to track symptoms involving the three core PTSD domains of intrusive thoughts, avoidance symptoms, and hyperarousal.

The Davidson Trauma Scale is a 17-item self-rated measure yielding a frequency score of 0–68, severity score of 0–68, and total score of 0–136 (Davidson et al., 1997a).

The PTSD Checklist-Civilian Version (PCL-C) and -Military Version (PCL-M) are each a 17-item self-report measure with scores ranging from 17–85 (Blanchard et al., 1996).

The State–Trait Anxiety Inventory (STAI; see Chapter 17, Table 17.2) is sometimes incorporated in PTSD clinical trials as an index of overall anxiety symptoms.

So then, does treatment of acute stress disorder forestall or prevent the onset of PTSD?

A meta-analysis of 19 RCTs (Astill Wright et al., 2019) found no value for propranolol, oxytocin, gabapentin, fish oil, dexamethasone, escitalopram, imipramine, or chloral hydrate. Hydrocortisone (see later in the chapter), after a severe physical injury, was better than placebo, except its side effects and limited database make it impractical and premature to recommend for general use to prevent PTSD after a traumatic event. (Plus, remember, not all trauma survivors inevitably develop PTSD. Go back to assessing risk factors.)

Excuse me. The psychotherapy literature shows that prolonged exposure or cognitive therapy in symptomatic trauma survivors with acute stress disorder leads to a significantly reduced risk for developing PTSD after five months (Shalev et al., 2012).

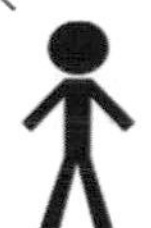

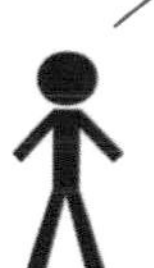

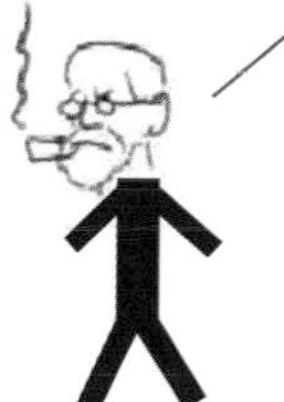

So hold on. In adjustment disorders we often use benzodiazepines or drugs like trazodone or Z-drugs for insomnia. Is that so different in an acute stress disorder? Or in crisis work? Say…helping an otherwise nonpsychiatrically ill person manage intense fears during a pandemic?

Not so different – that's essentially exactly the same concept, and keep in mind DSM-5 has reconceptualized adjustment disorders as "trauma- and stressor-related conditions." But here's an area where evidence-based studies are greatly lacking to inform best practices. As noted in a review by Stein (2018), formal studies are small, underpowered, and exist mostly for alprazolam and for a handful of not-so-mainstream options – such as *Gingko biloba*, *S*-adenosylmethionine, kava-kava, an extract called euphytose, and several putative anxiolytic/antidepressant agents that are not available in the USA, such as etifoxine, mianserin, and tianeptine. So, in the absence of much evidence, taking an empirical, symptom-targeted pharmacotherapy approach such as the kind you describe for this phenomenon is entirely reasonable.

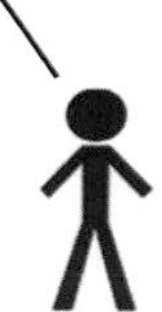

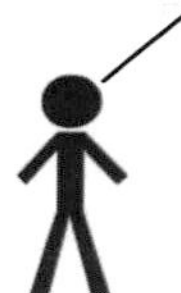

The emotional, cognitive and physiological/autonomic sequelae of a traumatic or stressful event that arises during only the first month after exposure to the event is termed an "acute stress disorder" in DSM-5. Persistence of symptoms beyond this time period may in turn lead to the development of PTSD. The question of whether and when pharmacotherapy is relevant to acute stress disorders is discussed in Box 19.3.

Tip

Cognitive therapy is often a preferred psychotherapy modality over exposure-based therapies in the setting of extreme emotional dysregulation or dissociation because exposure exercises may be less feasible and exacerbate such extreme stress response symptoms.

Box 19.3

Acute Stress Disorders and their Treatment

The phenomenon of an "acute stress disorder" is meant to describe a range of psychopathology symptoms that arise in the immediate aftermath (within one month) of a catastrophic traumatic event. Phenomenology is similar to that of PTSD but is more proximal in time to the trauma (whereas PTSD symptoms are defined by their emergence at least one month afterward). Psychotherapy-based treatments, such as CBT, are the preferred first-line intervention. Short-term (less than one month) use of a benzodiazepine may be appropriate for anxiety, agitation, or insomnia, based on anecdotal impressions. RCTs of SSRIs (notably, escitalopram across several studies (Shalev et al., 2012; Suliman et al., 2015; Zohar et al., 2018)) for acute stress disorder have shown no advantage over placebo, although secondary analyses from one study (Zohar et al., 2018) found a possible preventative effect against PTSD following deliberate or intentional traumatic events (physical assaults, rape, missile attacks).

 D COVID-19

The COVID-19 pandemic warrants special discussion in the context of traumatic stress. It stands as a unique, once-in-a-lifetime form of massive and chronic disruption and threat to life as we have known it in virtually every sphere of importance starting from the most basic platform of Maslow's (1943) hierarchy of needs, shown in Figure 19.1. The prolonged nature of its associated multifaceted stresses and uncertainties about basic physical safety and emotional well-being strongly resembles the kind of stresses associated with chronic PTSD as seen among prisoners of war or victims of chronic emotional, physical, sexual, or sociopolitical abuse.

Figure 19.1 Maslow's hierarchy of needs.

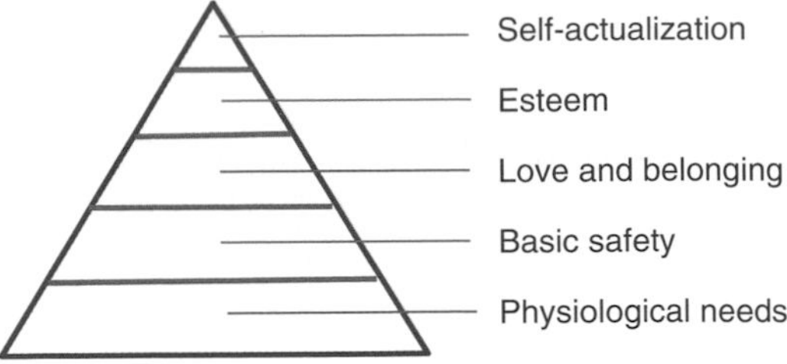

The concept of resilience presumes that people who endure even extraordinary levels of stress, but possess the elements described in Box 19.1 that can help people to bounce back from adversity, may derive some measure of protection against developing subsequent PTSD. That said, the unique and extraordinary world-wide ramifications of the COVID-19 pandemic pose challenges that are unprecedented in modern times. Basic pharmacological considerations may involve symptom-based approaches (e.g., managing insomnia or anxiety regardless of the presence of a formal psychiatric syndrome). "Anxiety" that rises to the level of more fulminant or abject distress may justify intervention with dopalytic anxiolytic drugs in the sense of antipsychotics sometimes being referred to as "major tranquilizers." Monoaminergic antidepressants remain clinically indicated for the treatment of depressive episodes and anxiety disorders, with a lesser evidence base for the treatment of subthreshold depressive symptoms in the context of adjustment disorders.

We offer in Box 19.4 a pharmacological toolbox for key management issues in assessing stress-related psychopathology in the context of COVID-19.

E CORE PHARMACOTHERAPY OF PTSD

Sertraline (mean dose in registration trials of about 150 mg/day) and paroxetine are the sole two medications carrying FDA indications for PTSD. RCTs with sertraline have shown more robust efficacy for PTSD clusters of avoidance/numbing and arousal, but not re-experiencing/

Box 19.4

COVID-19 Stress-related Psychopathology: Assessment and Management

- Differentiate circumstances, even those that are dire, from disease. The presence of a depressive episode, an anxiety disorder, a substance use disorder, or a trauma-related condition warrants its own treatment no differently than when we treat angina or hay fever regardless of whether those problems only manifest themselves "situationally." In other words, assess for historical pre-existing conditions as psychiatric vulnerability markers when assessing survivorship of COVID-19 associated stresses.
- Be cognizant of the risk for increased alcohol- or substance-use problems, and their neurotoxic/psychotoxic effects, even among highly stressed individuals without a clear or declared history of alcohol or substance use disorders. Intervene when appropriate in ways discussed in Chapter 18.
- Resist the temptation simply to prescribe or increase existing dosages of benzodiazepines or other sedative-hypnotics in response to complaints of "stress" without first assessing patients.
- In patients being treated for COVID-19, recognize potential end-organ risks for QTc prolongation from experimental drugs such as hydroxychloroquine; be mindful of the potential risks for benzodiazepines to depress respiratory drive, particularly when anxiety is linked with hypoxia and air-hunger; assure proper hematological monitoring of drugs that carry risks for blood dyscrasias, recognizing that COVID-19 tends to suppress lymphocyte more than neutrophil counts.
- Mobilize and optimize nonpharmacological supports, particularly when issues related to social isolation pose especially prominent hazards to emotional equilibrium.

intrusion (Brady et al., 2000). In registration trials with sertraline, acute response was demonstrated over 10 weeks, with relapse prevention studied for up to 28 weeks in acute responders to an open-label 24-week trial. Efficacy of paroxetine in PTSD was shown in two 12-week FDA registration trials (about 40% of enrolled subjects also had comorbid MDD or anxiety disorders). A first, fixed-dose study showed efficacy at either 20 or 40 mg/day, but no additional benefit with 40 versus 20 mg/day. Two additional dose studies (20–50 mg/day) showed significantly greater CAPS score reductions than with placebo.

Tip

Some authorities advocate that it may take up to 12 weeks to judge response from an adequate pharmacotherapy trial in PTSD.

Tip

Optimal treatment duration to prevent relapse after an acute response is likely *at least 24 months* (based on randomized discontinuation findings with sertraline (Davidson et al., 2001a).

Among other SSRIs, citalopram has shown no difference from placebo, although escitalopram dosed up to 20 mg/day (Robert et al., 2006) or 40 mg/day (achieved by four-week titration; Qi et al., 2017) has shown significant improvements in CAPS scores as well as global impressions in 12-week open trials.

Tip

SSRIs are less effective in chronic than acute PTSD.

A meta-analysis of pharmacotherapies for PTSD by Watts et al. (2013) (results depicted in Figure 19.2) identified the largest effect sizes for topiramate, paroxetine, risperidone, and venlafaxine (nonsignificant findings are boxed in gray). An overall medium effect size was observed for pharmacotherapies, collectively (g = 0.42, 95% CI = 0.31–0.53; 56 studies involving 5357 subjects) – as contrasted with a larger effect size observed across most forms of psychotherapy (g = 1.14, 95% CI = 0.97–1.30, 76 studies involving 3771 subjects), particularly cognitive-behavioral therapy (g = 1.26), eye movement desensitization and reprocessing (EMDR; g = 1.01), psychodynamic psychotherapy (g = 0.78), and hypnotherapy (g = 0.72). On the other hand, a large 24-week multisite US Department of Veterans Affairs (VA) study of combat-related PTSD among war veterans found no outcome differences among those randomized to receive sertraline, prolonged exposure therapy, or their combination (Rauch et al., 2019). In the meta-analysis by Watts et al. (2013), a moderator analysis showed significantly larger effects in women than men and in nonveterans than veterans.

Tip

In the meta-analysis by Watts et al. (2013), antidepressants had an overall medium effect size (g = 0.43).

Figure 19.2 Meta-analysis of pharmacotherapies for PTSD (g (95% CI)).

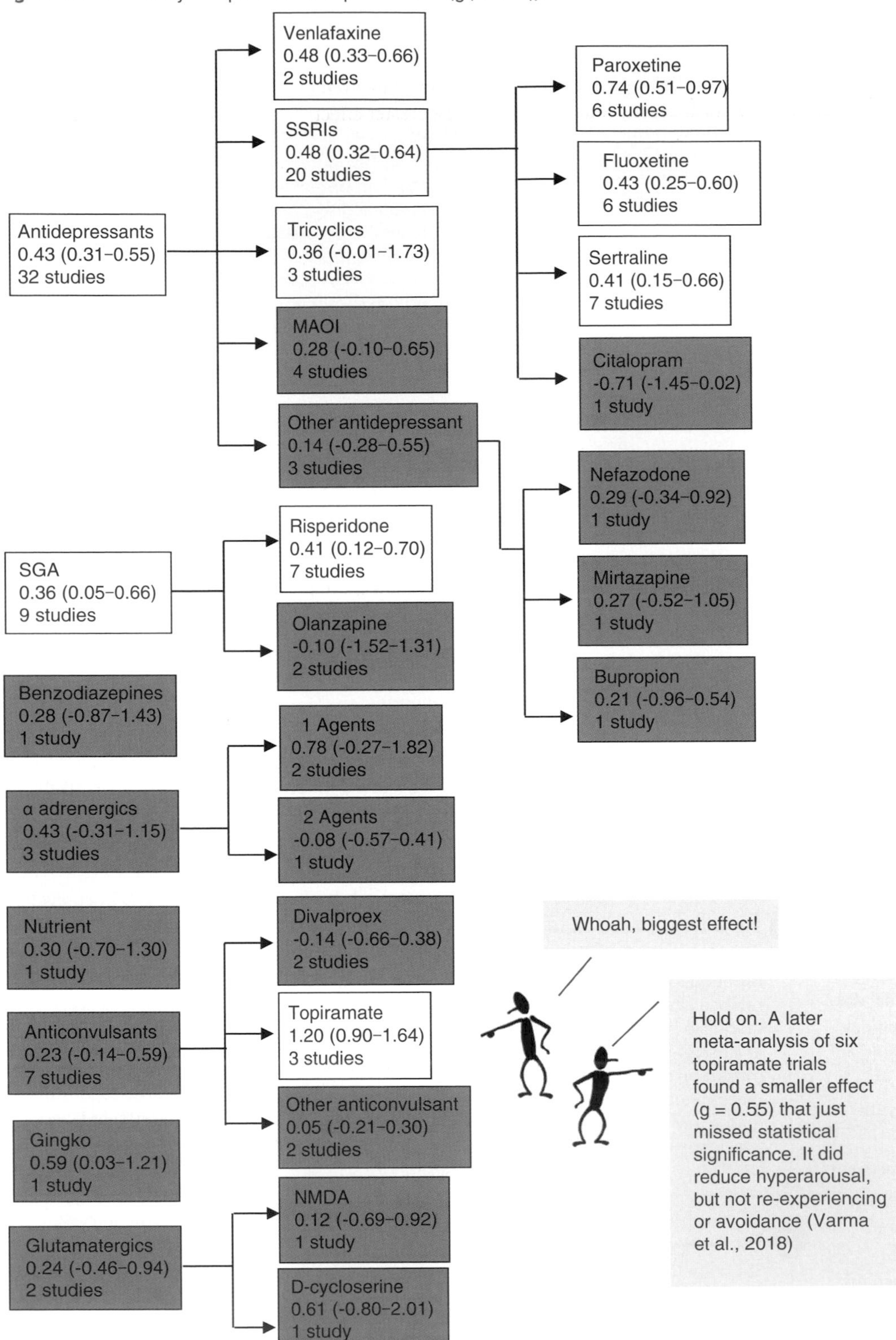

A separate retrospective comparative effectiveness study among 2931 US veterans found no significant outcome differences among those who had been prescribed fluoxetine, paroxetine, sertraline, topiramate, or venlafaxine (that is, all appeared equally effective, producing about the same magnitude of improvement on PTSD rating scales), while the criteria for meeting the diagnosis of PTSD itself persisted in over 80% of patients after six months of treatment (Shiner et al., 2018).

When considering subcomponents of PTSD as a syndrome, RCTs have shown efficacy with venlafaxine for re-experiencing and avoidance/numbing but not autonomic hyperarousal (Davidson et al., 2006). Open-label escitalopram trials report greater reductions from baseline severity of avoidance/numbing and hyperarousal than in re-experiencing (Robert et al., 2006). Tricyclics have been observed to exert a greater effect on intrusive thoughts, as well as depressive and anxiety symptoms, with less impact on avoidance symptoms (Sutherland and Davidson, 1994).

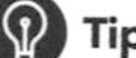

Tip

PTSD RCTs show no advantage for augmenting exposure therapy with an SSRI as compared to exposure therapy alone (Simon et al., 2008; Popiel et al., 2015; Rauch et al., 2019).

Table 19.1 at the end of the chapter summarizes findings from randomized trials of combination pharmacotherapy approaches for PTSD.

The use of benzodoazepines in PTSD patients is often controversial. Reasons for this are discussed in detail in Box 19.5.

Tip

Among benzodiazepines, temapezam (15–30 mg PO qHS for seven days) was studied in a small (n = 22) RCT versus placebo in non-combat-related PTSD and found to improve sleep duration with a trend for fewer wakenings after sleep onset (Mellman et al., 2002). Temazepam did not directly improve core PTSD symptoms, but reduced awakenings correlated with improved PTSD symptoms.

My PTSD patient has neuropathic pain. Can I get a two-fer by using an SNRI or TCA?

Maybe. Venlafaxine has positive data in PTSD, TCAs less so. By the way, as you'll see in Table 19.2, there's very little PTSD data with gabapentin or pregabablin.

Doesn't the type of trauma matter in gauging response to one medicine over another? Combat versus civilian PTSD? Motor vehicle accident versus hurricane? Sexual versus physical versus emotional abuse?

Among depressed or anxious patients with a history of childhood trauma or abuse, outcomes are poorer than when such a history is absent, regardless of the specific type of abuse. In PTSD trials, generally speaking, medications tend to be less effective for military veterans with chronic PTSD than civilian populations (Friedman et al., 2007). Military veterans with chronic PTSD who enroll in RCTs also tend to have higher CAPS scores as compared to civilian PTSD (Zohar et al., 2002).

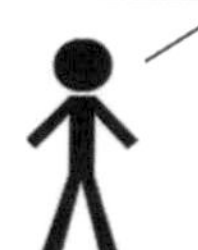

Box 19.5

Are Benzodiazepines Detrimental in PTSD?

Benzodiazepine use in PTSD is condemned by many authors because of a purported lack of demonstrated efficacy against core PTSD symptoms, as well as an increased risk for complications involving substance use disorders. Like so many areas in psychiatry, controversy abounds and is driven more by absence of evidence than true evidence of absence, coupled with opinion-based admonitions. As elegantly discussed by Roth (2010), most of the literature claiming that benzodiazepines fail to lessen PTSD symptoms, may *worsen* PTSD risk, or aggravate concerns about substance misuse are based mainly on older anecdotal observations, small open trials, comparative studies that failed to control for baseline symptom severity, or the use of short-acting benzodiazepines which were discontinued without tapers of adequate duration. Roth points out that most practice guidelines that caution against using benzodiazepines for PTSD tend repeatedly to cite one single small (n = 10) crossover trial of alprazolam in which improvement actually *did* occur in anxiety and avoidance/intrusion (but no other PTSD core symptoms) (Braun et al., 1990), and misinterpret another study of adverse outcomes in eight alprazolam recipients that explicitly advocated for long- versus short-acting benzodiazepines to minimize withdrawal effects (e.g., Risse et al., 1990).

Concerns that benzodiazepines would expectably worsen comorbid substance use disorder actually were not borne out in a one-year naturalistic outcome study of 370 veterans with PTSD in which prescribed benzodiazepine use was in fact associated with significant *reductions* in alcohol-related problems, violence, and healthcare service utilization (Kosten et al., 2000).

Thus, it becomes difficult to interpret meta-analyses that conclude benzodiazepines "should be considered relatively contraindicated for patients with PTSD or recent trauma" – while acknowledging benzodiazepines improve sleep and anxiety but not core PTSD symptoms (e.g., Guina et al., 2015) – because of the extensive design limitations, unexplored interaction effects (e.g., sleep improvement vis-à-vis PTSD symptom domains) and confounding factors in the small existing literature. We would offer our anecdotal observation that a moderator for poor outcomes with benzodiazepines in PTSD patients may be comorbidity with borderline personality disorder or other conditions involving impaired capacity for emotional self-regulation and impulse control (see also Chapter 20).

Clinical decisions, once again, must be made on a case-by-case basis depending on the particular characteristics of any given patient.

F ADRENERGIC MODULATION AND PTSD

Beta-Blockers

A conceptually compelling theory regarding the pathogenesis of PTSD as a disorder of fear extinction circuitry involves the idea that a traumatic event becomes "learned" and its memory traces become encoded as aversive emotional reactions because of high and prolonged adrenergic tone associated with the fight-or-flight response. Therefore, interest has coalesced around the possible utility of beta-blockers that cross the blood–brain barrier (notably, propranolol) as a way to mitigate memory "over"-consolidation and perhaps prevent PTSD after trauma exposure via blunting the adrenergic "learning" context. Prompt introduction of propranolol relative to the traumatic event is considered fundamental to the paradigm. (Some authors believe that the window of opportunity may be as short as six hours following trauma exposure.) In clinical reports, propranolol dosing has been 40 mg PO TID or QID for 7–10 days, usually begun within one day of the traumatic event. Initial optimism was spurred by early pilot observations of reduced physiological activation relative to placebo (Pitman et al., 2002) and a reduced incidence of PTSD in comparison to trauma victims refusing propranolol (Vaiva et al., 2003). However, a meta-analysis of five trials (three randomized, one open, one retrospective) involving 214 physical trauma victims presenting to emergency departments found no difference between propranolol and placebo in the relative risk for eventual emergence of PTSD (RR = 0.92, 95% CI = 0.55–1.55) (Argolo et al., 2015). The small number of studies in that meta-analysis, along with its focus on physical-injury patients presenting to an emergency department, limits the ability to form more generalizable conclusions about the possible utility (and timing) of propranolol as a strategy to mitigate the consolidation of traumatic memories or the development of PTSD.

A notable placebo-controlled randomized trial of propranolol as a "memory reconsolidation blocker" was undertaken in the context of a 90-minute pretreatment during a six-week course of psychotherapy sessions involving once-weekly memory reactivation; propranolol use was associated with significantly lower CAPS scores than with placebo, though with a large within-group effect size both for propranolol ($d = 1.76$) and for placebo ($d = 1.25$) (Brunet et al., 2018). In chronic PTSD patients, a single dose of propranolol has been shown to improve processing speed on neuropsychological performance tasks better than placebo (Mahabir et al., 2016).

Alpha-1 Antagonists

Initial studies lasting up to 20 weeks examined the α_1 antagonist prazosin specifically to address nightmares and related sleep disturbances in military veterans with combat-related PTSD. Dosing typically begins at 1 mg PO HS for at least three nights followed by upward titration to a range of 3–15 mg nightly (mean doses usually have been about 10 mg/day). A meta-analysis (George et al., 2016) found an improvement in the incidence of nightmares ($g = 1.022$, $p = 0.001$) and overall sleep quality ($g = 1.14$, $p < 0.01$). Sleep latency and duration were numerically better with prazosin than placebo ($g = 0.93$) but only at a marginal level of statistical significance ($p = 0.05$). No significant effects on systolic or diastolic blood pressure were noted.

Tip

α_1-receptors are densely distributed throughout the limbic system.

Trazodone is an α_1 antagonist – why can't we just use that for PTSD nightmares?
You sure can.There's even open-trial data to support that specific use, dosed from 50-200 mg nightly (Warner et al., 2001).

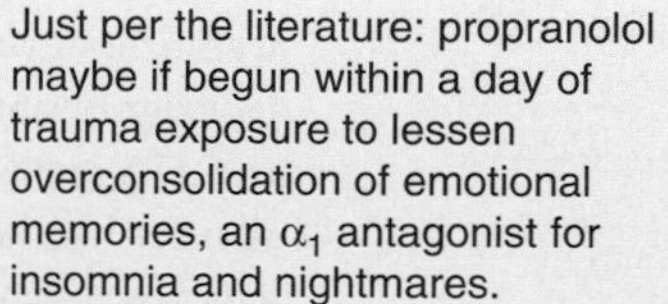

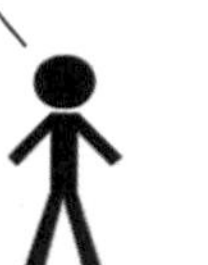

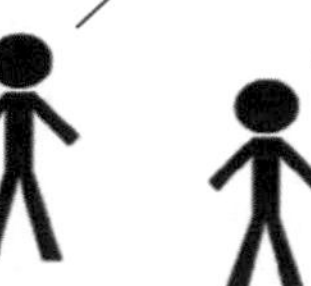

Could you do both?
That's unstudied, may be riskier cardiovascularly, and not sure there's a rationale for synergy.

Tip

Abrupt cessation of centrally acting α_2 agonists can cause rebound hypertension. This is a concern with clonidine or guanfacine, but not with α_1 antagonists such as prazosin.

A subsequent large ($n = 304$) multisite VA collaborative RCT in chronic combat-related PTSD failed to replicate findings from smaller previous RCTs, finding no differences from placebo in nightmares or sleep quality; supine systolic blood pressure after 10 weeks decreased by a mean of 6.7 mmHg with prazosin (Raskind et al., 2018).

The authors of this latter report suggested that their study population, though chronic, may have been "too stable" for antiadrenergic therapy to exert a benefit. In post-hoc analyses, systolic hypertension was suggested as a possible moderator of a favorable prazosin response.

What about α_2 agonists, such as clonidine or guanfacine, to reduce sympathetic tone in the context of presumed hyperadrenergic states following significant traumatic events? Recall that CNS α_2 receptors are postsynaptic autoreceptors that functionally down-regulate central norepinephrine outflow. Of these two agents, guanfacine has the more extensive clinical trials database and the findings are mostly negative: an eight-week

Tip

Clonidine binds to α_{2a} as well as α_{2b} and α_{2c} subreceptors, which are thought to drive its comparatively greater sedating effects as compared to guanfacine, which has greater affinity just for the α_{2a} subreceptor.

RCT in combat veterans given guanfacine dosed from 0.5–3 mg nightly found no advantage over placebo in improving CAPS or IES scores (Neylan et al., 2006). A similarly designed RCT in 36 combat veterans (most of whom were already taking an SSRI) also showed no benefit in PTSD symptoms as compared to placebo (Davis et al., 2008b). Studies with clonidine involve mostly a handful of successful single case reports using from 0.5 to 1 mg up to three times daily. Its sedating properties may offer a sometimes incidental advantage with respect to both sleep problems and possible anxiolytic effects secondary to its sedative properties.

G ANTICONVULSANTS

Theoretical interest in the potential role for anticonvulsants in trauma partly involves the concept of kindling of limbic nuclei as a neurophysiological consequence of re-experiencing and reliving in the pathogenesis and perpetuation of PTSD symptoms. Generally speaking, anticonvulsants as a class have failed to gain much favor in the pharmacotherapy of trauma or PTSD. Divalproex and topiramate are among the more extensively studied compounds. Findings from RCTs are summarized in Table 19.2 at the end of this chapter.

H ANTIPSYCHOTICS

A meta-analysis of eight SGA RCTs in PTSD found an overall weighted mean difference in CAPS scores of −5.89 (95% CI = −9.21 to −2.56, p = 0.0005) with significant improvement noted in CAPS intrusion and hyperarousal subscores (Liu et al., 2014). The meta-analysis by Watts et al. (2013) summarized in Figure 19.2 found a pooled effect size (nine studies) of $g = 0.36$ – lower than that seen with serotonergic antidepressants. Another meta-analysis of nine RCTs (n = 497) involving mainly olanzapine, risperidone, or quetiapine (as well as one trial with ziprasidone) found only a small pooled effect size for total CAPS score improvements relative to placebo ($g = -0.29$, 95% CI = −0.471 to −0.106, p = 0.002), with a somewhat greater magnitude of change seen in CAPS intrusion subscores ($g = -0.373$, 95% CI = −0.568 to −0.178, p <0.0001) (Han et al., 2014).

Olanzapine, risperidone, and quetiapine represent the SGAs with the most extensive formal database in PTSD (partly perhaps as an artifact of their having been available for study longer than most other agents). A summary of existing trial findings across SGAs is presented in Table 19.3 at the end of this chapter.

I KETAMINE

One initial proof-of-concept study found that a single IV ketamine infusion produced rapid improvement in global PTSD symptoms (IES symptoms were significantly better at 24 hours as compared to midazolam (an active control)), as well as depressive features, in 41 patients with chronic PTSD (Feder et al., 2014). A later small (n = 15) study of six open-label IV ketamine infusions in a group of MDD patients with PTSD found that 80% achieved remission from PTSD and the mean time until relapse was 41 days (Albott et al., 2018).

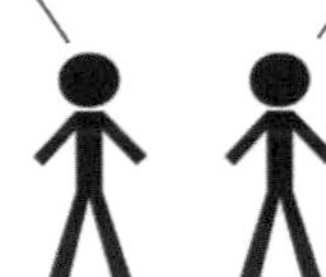

So then what do you do for acute ketamine responders to maintain improvement after the initial infusion?
You could try giving repeated ketamine infusions. In the single-infusion PTSD study, CAPS scores were no longer different from midazolam at Day 7.

J NOVEL THERAPEUTICS

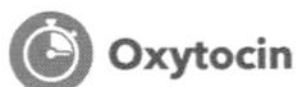

Oxytocin

The neuropeptide oxytocin modulates glucocorticoid and autonomic stress responses to perceived threat, and promotes anxiolytic and pro-social effects that may contribute to how individuals process traumatic events. One multicenter RCT with 120 mostly accident victims compared placebo with intranasal oxytocin dosed at 40 IU twice daily for eight days, begun within 12 days of a traumatic accident (van Zuiden et al., 2017). No overall difference between treatment groups was observed at six weeks; however, high baseline severity was a moderator that significantly differentiated magnitude of change in CAPS scores with drug versus placebo. IN oxytocin also has been shown to reduce the intensity of provoked avoidance symptoms in known female PTSD patients (Sack et al., 2017).

Hydrocortisone

Glucocorticoids facilitate extinction learning, decrease retrieval of fear memories, and enhance memory consolidation and reconsolidation. Based on such observations, preliminary studies have examined the impact of the synthetic glucocorticoid hydrocortisone as an augmentation of prolonged exposure therapy in treatment of PTSD. In one RCT, hydrocortisone 30 mg was compared to placebo orally dosed 20 minutes prior to each of seven sessions of prolonged exposure therapy in 24 military veterans (Yehuda et al., 2015). Hydrocortisone reduced CAPS scores significantly more than placebo, with a between-group effect size of $d = 0.43$.

N-Acetylcysteine

N-acetylcysteine dosed at 2400 mg/day for eight weeks was found to be superior to placebo in a group of 25 veterans with PTSD and a substance use disorder (Back et al., 2016). Significant improvements occurred in overall PTSD symptoms as well as craving measures. All subjects also received CBT.

D-Serine

A six-week pilot RCT of *D*-serine 30 mg/kg/day versus placebo in 22 chronic PTSD subjects found improvement in CAPS scores at a trend level of significance, with significant improvement in anxiety and other secondary outcome measures (Heresco-Levy et al., 2009).

Creatine

Creatine, thought to improve brain energy metabolism, was studied in a preliminary four-week open trial in 10 chronic PTSD patients who continued to take existing medications; formulated as creatine monohydrate and dosed at 3 mg PO qDay for one week then 4 mg PO qDay, a modest but significant improvement was observed from baseline in CAPS and depressive symptom scores (Amital et al., 2006).

3,4-Methylenedioxymethamphetamine (MDMA)

Novel pharmacotherapy approaches to PTSD include psychotherapy augmentation with MDMA, with a rationale based on its potential to catalyze emotional engagement, feelings of trust and empathy, and an enhanced capacity to revisit traumatic experiences and promote fear extinction while avoiding emotional detachment or dissociation. Empirical studies of MDMA as an adjunct to psychotherapy for PTSD were essentially prohibited until the early twenty-first century because of its Schedule I federal drug classification. Based on limited data, a meta-analysis of five RCTs showed a roughly 3.5-fold increased likelihood of response and 2.5-fold probability of remission, with a large effect size ($g = 1.30$), with good tolerability (Bahji et al., 2020). Magnitude of the potential improvement from baseline seems impressive, with one RCT in chronic military PTSD reporting an effect size (after 75 mg dosing) of $d = 2.8$ (Mithoefer et al., 2018).

Cannabidiol

Cannabidiol is thought to mitigate fear memory by disrupting memory consolidation. The existing database relevant to PTSD mostly involves preclinical studies (e.g., using fear extinction paradigms) or preliminary studies in anxiety states (broadly defined) in healthy control subjects. Studies in PTSD subjects using oral dosages ranging from 300–600 mg/day remain ongoing.

Stellate Ganglion Block

The stellate (cervicothoracic) ganglion plays a key role in modulating sympathetic outflow. Its interruption either by surgical ablation or anesthetic injection has historically been used to manage certain regional pain syndromes and forms of autonomic dysfunction such as hyperhidrosis or Raynaud's phenomenon. Initial case reports suggested potential value for this procedure to counter autonomic hyperarousal symptoms in PTSD. Early small RCTs yielded mixed results (both positive and negative (e.g., Hanling et al., 2016) studies), with greatest effects from positive trials in irritability or angry outbursts, difficulty concentrating, and sleep disturbance (Lynch et al., 2016). A subsequent large, multisite RCT of right-sided stellate ganglion block at zero and two weeks in 113 military PTSD subjects led to greater magnitude of improvement in CAPS scores as compared to sham injections, with a medium effect size ($d = 0.56$) (Rae Olmsted et al., 2020).

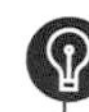

Tip

Risks of stellate ganglion blockade include Horner's syndrome, difficulty swallowing, and vocal cord paralysis.

K DISSOCIATION

Dissociative phenomena are considered to be a psychological phenomenon related to defense mechanisms in managing anxiety related to psychological trauma. The mainstays of treatment involve psychosocial/psychotherapeutic interventions such as prolonged exposure therapy, EMDR, narrative exposure therapy, cognitive processing therapy, and trauma memory processing, among other modalities. State dissociation has been recognized as a moderator of poor outcome in PTSD behavioral therapy trials, although the so-called "dissociative subtype" of PTSD is nevertheless felt to be responsive to exposure-based behavioral therapies (Wolf et al., 2016). An RCT of paroxetine (dosed up to 60 mg/day) in 70 mostly ethnic minority adults with chronic PTSD found a greater improvement in dissociative symptoms than seen with placebo (Marshall et al., 2007).

Tip

"Dissociative features" were identified in DSM-5 as a specifier term relevant for PTSD. The phenomenon is also seen across other conditions, including borderline personality disorder, schizophrenia, epilepsy, and autism spectrum disorders, among others.

There is sometimes a clinical temptation to use antipsychotic medications for symptoms related to dissociative phenomena simply on the grounds that dissociation reflects a kind of breakdown in reality testing, or perhaps signals a role for "ego glue" noted in earlier chapters. However, we are aware of no formal studies examining the potential efficacy of antipsychotic drugs for dissociative symptoms (or, for that matter, derealization or depersonalization). One small (n = 14) open trial of single-dose clonidine (0.75–1.5 mg) in women with borderline personality disorder noted brief postdose reductions in aversive inner tension, self-injurious urges, and dissociative symptoms (Philipsen et al., 2004a), suggesting a possible adrenergic component to dissociative content (at least in the context of broader symptoms related to borderline personality disorder). Another proof-of-concept small open trial suggested potential reductions in dissociative symptoms that arise alongside flashbacks using high-dose naltrexone (25–100 mg PO QID) in women with borderline personality disorder (Bohus et al., 1999), although such findings have not been affirmed in randomized placebo-controlled trials (Schmahl et al., 2012). A single dose of IV naloxone also was no better than placebo in reducing dissociative states in another small crossover trial in nine patients with borderline personality disorder (Philipsen et al., 2004b).

L DISSOCIATIVE IDENTITY DISORDER

Dissociative identity disorder (DID) remains a controversial diagnostic entity based on its phenomenological overlap with borderline personality disorder and other conditions for which traumatic events are thought to be catalytic if not etiological (e.g., PTSD, dissociative amnesia). Its psychological dimensions, particularly with respect to defense mechanisms, have been a main focus of interventional studies, which have mainly been psychotherapy-based. Apart from treatment of possible co-occurring conditions or symptoms such as depression, anxiety, or insomnia, is there a distinct role for pharmacotherapy? Once again, we encounter a psychopathological phenomenon for which there is not an extensive evidence base. Some textbooks proffer that benzodiazepines might exacerbate dissociation, although such observations are largely more impressionistic than systematic. One contemporary review of pharmacotherapy for DID cites a litany of pharmacotherapy options (e.g., antidepressants, beta-blockers, clonidine, anticonvulsants, SGAs, naltrexone) based mainly on conjecture and conceptual appeal rather than empirical observations (which derive, at best, from single case reports) (Gentile et al., 2013).

TAKE-HOME POINTS

- Trauma histories in general – but especially in childhood – worsen the prognosis of most if not all psychiatric disorders.
- Don't expect SSRIs to do all that much for acute stress reactions; cognitively oriented psychotherapies remain the most evidence-based intervention.
- In PTSD, SSRIs are the first-line and best-studied pharmacotherapy class. Sertraline and paroxetine carry FDA indications, but chances are other agents within-class probably work just as well.
- SGAs, particularly olanzapine and quetiapine, show modest benefit for core PTSD symptoms – they may be selectively useful for avoidance – but the data are not extensive or robust and tolerability can be problematic.
- Benzodiazepines, contrary to urban legend, are not categorically evil in the world of trauma, although they are largely understudied; they may help sleep and anxiety – at least in the short run which – could, in turn, possibly secondarily help lessen some core PTSD symptoms.
- α-Agonists such as prazosin have gained great popularity for PTSD-related nightmares and possibly other aspects of autonomic hyperarousal, but the evidence base remains mixed.
- Magnitude of improvement in PTSD remains modest. There is optimism from preliminary studies involving novel compounds, including enactogens such as MDMA, cannabidiol, hydrocortisone, and oxytocin.

Table 19.1 Combination pharmacotherapy RCTs in PTSD

Regimen	Outcome
Positive trials	
SSRI (fluoxetine, sertraline or paroxetine) + olanzapine (n = 10, mean dose = 15 mg/day) or placebo (n = 9)	Significantly greater improvement with olanzapine in CAPS, depression scores, sleep problems over eight weeks (Stein et al., 2002)
Citalopram + baclofen	Greater reductions in overall PTSD symptoms, and hyperarousal and avoidance measures in particular, as compared to citalopram alone (Manteghi et al., 2014)
Negative trials	
Sertraline + mirtazapine	No difference between groups in CAPS scores (primary outcome) but significantly higher remission rates by 24 weeks with combination (39%) versus sertraline alone (11%), with NNT of 3.5 (Schneier et al., 2015).
Sertraline + risperidone	Among 45 civilian PTSD patients, nonresponders (≥30% improvement in CAPS) to eight weeks of open-label sertraline, further improvement was no different for those randomized to adjunctive risperidone or placebo, although nominally significant improvement was seen on a secondary outcome measure (the Davidson Trauma Scale) (Rothbaum et al., 2008)
SSRI + risperidone	In 247 military-related PTSD patients unresponsive to more than two SSRI trials, six months of adjunctive risperidone (mean dose = 2.74 mg/day) was no better than placebo in improving CAPS or MADRS (depression) symptoms (Krystal et al., 2011)
SSRI (paroxetine or sertraline) + ziprasidone	No significant differences in CAPS scores after eight weeks in SSRI nonresponders randomized to adjunctive ziprasidone (n = 9) or placebo (n = 15) (Hamner et al., 2019)

Abbreviations: CAPS = Clinician-Administered PTSD Scale; PTSD = post-traumatic stress disorder; SSRI = selective serotonin reuptake inhibitor; MADRS = Montgomery–Åsberg Depression Rating Scale; NNT = number needed to treat; RCT = randomized controlled trial

Table 19.2 Anticonvulsants in the treatment of PTSD

Agent	Findings
Carbamazepine	Early open trials reported subjective improvement without formal assessment measures. One five-week open trial (carbamazepine mean dose = 780 mg/day) found "moderate" or "very much" improved status in 7/10 subjects (Lipper et al., 1986)
Divalproex	- An eight-week RCT in 85 combat veterans with PTSD (mean dose = 2309 mg/day, mean serum [valproate] = 82 mg/L) found no significant differences from placebo in CAPS scores (Davis et al., 2008a) - 16 combat veterans treated openly with low-dose divalproex (mean dose = 109.3 mg/day) had significant improvement in hyperarousal and avoidance, although standardized rating scales were not utilized (Fesler, 1991) - An eight-week open trial in 16 patients (mean dose = 365 mg/day) significantly reduced hyperarousal, intrusive thoughts, and HAM-D and HAM-A scores (Clark et al., 1999) - 14 military veterans with PTSD received open-label divalproex for up to eight weeks (mean dose = 1840 mg/day, mean serum [valproate] = 69 μg/mL) with significant improvement from baseline in CAPS total and subscores and HAM-D and HAM-A scores (Petty et al., 2002)
Gabapentin	Apart from single case reports, one retrospective review of 30 PTSD patients reported improved sleep parameters including nightmares (Hamner et al., 2001)
Lamotrigine	A small, preliminary RCT (n = 15, dosing up to 500 mg/day) reported "response" in 5/10 lamotrigine recipients versus 1/4 placebo recipients, significant reductions in re-experiencing and avoidance/numbing symptom clusters (Hertzberg et al., 1999)
Levetiracetam	Over a mean of 9.7 weeks, 23 civilian PTSD patients unresponsive to antidepressants received (mostly adjunctive) open-label levetiracetam (mean dose = 1967 mg/day), with 13 (56%) deemed responders by PCL-C scores (Kinrys et al., 2006)
Oxcarbazepine	Data limited to single case reports
Pregabalin	One small (n = 37) six-week RCT from Iran found a just-significant benefit with pregabalin (dose = 300 mg/day) over placebo on PCL-M scores in combat-related PTSD (Baniasadi et al., 2014)
Tiagabine	A 12-week open trial (mean dose = 10.8 mg/day) in 29 PTSD patients followed by a 24-week double-blind randomized discontinuation showed greater sustained improvement across varied PTSD measures than those crossed over to placebo (Connor et al., 2006)
Topiramate	- A retrospective chart review involving 35 patients with civilian PTSD found significant reductions from baseline in the frequency of nightmares (79%) and flashbacks (86%); most subjects judged to be responders were receiving dosages ≤100 mg/day (Berlant and Van Kammen, 2002). A second four-week study by the same investigators, evaluating 33 civilian PTSD outpatients, found a mean 49% decline in total PTSD symptoms, with significant reductions in subscales related to re-experiencing, avoidance/numbing, and hyperarousal, with an overall response rate of 77% (median time to response = nine days, mean dose = 50 mg/day) (Berlant, 2004). - A 12-week RCT in 35 Brazilian patients with combat-related PTSD found significant improvement in CAPS scores related to flashbacks, intrusive memories, nightmares, avoidance/numbing, social isolation, with overall good tolerability (mean dose = 103 mg/day) (Yeh et al., 2011) - A 12-week RCT in 38 civilian-related PTSD patients found no significant difference from placebo in total CAPS scores but did significantly improve re-experiencing symptoms (Tucker et al., 2007) - A seven-week RCT in combat-related PTSD in 40 male veterans found no significant difference from placebo, although high dropout due to adverse effects (55% of topiramate recipients) likely resulted in a failed rather than negative trial (Lindley et al., 2007)

Abbreviations: CAPS = Clinician-Administered PTSD Scale; HAM-A = Hamilton Ratings Scale for Anxiety; HAM-D = Hamilton Ratings Scale for Depression; PCL-C = PTSD Checklist-Civilian Version; PCL-M = PTSD Checklist-Military Version; PTSD = post-traumatic stress disorder; RCT = randomized controlled trial

Table 19.3 SGAs RCTs in PTSD [a]

SGA	Outcomes
Aripiprazole	A meta-analysis of six (mostly military veteran) trials (three monotherapy (all open label), three adjunct (one open label, one retrospective review, one RCT) found significant improvements in primary outcomes (CAPS or similar global measures) from baseline scores (Britnell et al., 2017); however, the sole RCT (Naylor et al., 2015) found no significant difference from placebo in subjects who completed either four weeks (n = 14) or eight weeks (n = 12)
Asenapine	One small (n = 15) open pilot study (mean dose = 13.6 mg/day) reported significant improvements from baseline CAPS total scores and all three subclusters; 10/18 (56% were deemed responders (CAPS score improvements ≥30%) (Pilkinton et al., 2016)
Olanzapine	Following an array of small open acute trials with favorable findings (within-group improvement from baseline symptom severity), three RCTs have been reported: - An eight-week trial in 28 civilian PTSD patients found significantly greater improvement than with placebo (mean dose = 9.3 mg/day) in CAPS total (*d* = 0.43) and avoidance (but not hyperarousal or intrusion) scores, though 6/14 olanzapine subjects had significant weight gain (Carey et al., 2012) - An adjunctive 12-week RCT (mean dose = 15 mg/day) in 19 SSRI-nonresponders found significantly greater improvement than with placebo on CAPS total scores and secondary outcome measures involving depression and sleep, alongside a mean weight change of 13 lbs (Stein et al., 2002b) - A 10-week trial with 15 subjects found no significant differences in any outcome measures (Butterfield et al., 2001)
Quetiapine	A 12-week RCT found significantly greater improvement with quetiapine (n = 42, mean dose = 258 mg/day; maximum = 800 mg/day) than with placebo (n = 38) in CAPS total, re-experiencing, and hyperarousal subscores, as well as anxiety, depression, and BPRS scores; substantial premature dropout (Villarreal et al., 2016)
Risperidone	Initial controlled trials showed significant improvement among chronic PTSD veterans, particularly with respect to intrusive thoughts, psychotic symptoms, and aggressive features (reviewed by Pae et al., 2008). However, two subsequent large multisite RCTs showed no advantage for risperidone versus placebo, as already noted briefly in Table 19.1 - In 25 civilian PTSD nonremitters after eight weeks of sertraline who were then randomized to eight weeks of adjunctive risperidone or placebo, no significant treatment group differences were observed in the primary outcome (CAPS total scores) (Rothbaum et al., 2008) - In a six-month RCT with 367 veterans with PTSD, *no significant differences from placebo* were observed in CPS total scores, nor were there between-group differences in depression or anxiety symptoms or other secondary outcome measures (Krystal et al., 2011)
Ziprasidone	Alongside several favorable small, open case reports, there exists one small negative adjunctive trial with an SSRI, as noted in Table 19.1.

[a] No clinical trials with cariprazine, iloperidone, lumateperone, lurasidone, or pimavanserin; an RCT of paliperidone was withdrawn (ClinicalTrials.gov Identifier: NCT00766064); and a favorable and promising, as-yet unpublished Phase II RCT of brexpiprazole plus sertraline (ClinicalTrials.gov Identifier: NCT04174170) has shown preliminary efficacy (not evident with either monotherapy) with a large effect size.

Abbreviations: BPRS = Brief Psychiatric Rating Scale; CAPS = Clinician-Administered PTSD Scale; PTSD = post-traumatic stress disorder; RCT = randomized controlled trial; SGA = second-generation antipsychotic

20 Personality Disorders and Traits

LEARNING OBJECTIVES

- ☐ Describe the overall symptom-targeted role, alongside general strengths and limitations, of pharmacotherapy in the treatment of personality disorders
- ☐ Discuss efficacy findings from studies of antipsychotic pharmacotherapy for Cluster A personality disorders intended to mitigate their possible evolution to schizophrenia
- ☐ Describe the symptom domains most effectively treated by psychotropic medication in borderline personality disorder
- ☐ Describe the emerging database with hormonal therapies, antiglutamatergic drugs and other novel compounds in the treatment of personality disorders

> People with borderline personality disorder are like people with third degree burns over 90% of their bodies. Lacking emotional skin, they feel agony at the slightest touch or movement.
>
> *- Marsha Linehan*

No psychotropic drug has ever been developed specifically to treat any personality disorder, and the extent to which personality in all its developmental and biopsychosocial complexity even lends itself to the "disease" model – for which pharmacotherapy can be "reparative" – remains an open and debated issue. Personality represents the confluence of temperament, genetic predispositions, cohesion of identity, moral compass, interpersonal responsivity, and coping patterns that are shaped and developed over the course of early life experiences. Personality traits often reflect the interpersonally driven behavioral characteristics described in earlier chapters such as introversion/ extroversion, internalizing/ externalizing, aggression, harm avoidance/novelty-seeking, empathy and social cognition, antisocial behavior and interpersonal exploitativeness, and the use of developmentally primitive versus mature defense mechanisms. To the extent that personality traits may be maladaptive (e.g., impairing interpersonal effectiveness, leading to self-sabotage or self-harm) and are ego-dystonic, they represent targets for modification and change.

Tip

MDD patients responsive to paroxetine significantly improve in neuroticism and extraversion. In fact, after statistically controlling for the effects of paroxetine on those personality features, changes in symptoms of major depression no longer differ from those seen with placebo (Tang et al., 2009)

Tip

In patients with body dysmorphic disorder (BDD), more than half have been shown to have comorbid personality disorders, most often avoidant > dependent > obsessive-compulsive > paranoid; fluvoxamine-responsive BDD significantly decreases the diagnosability of these comorbid personality disorders (Phillips and McElroy, 2000)

If medication does have a distinct role in the treatment of personality disorders, it is likely not as the antidote to a discrete syndrome but more targeted to facets of aberrant mood, thinking, cognitive processing, behavior, perception, and impulse control. In the world of personality disorders, traditional thinking has long been to search for diagnosable comorbid psychiatric conditions responsive to pharmacotherapy, then attribute residual psychopathology as more likely reflective of personality and potentially more amenable to psychotherapeutic interventions. Some clinicians outright ignore psychopathology features of personality disorders and convince themselves that symptom etiologies arise from other comorbid psychiatric conditions that may not necessarily be present (such as major depression, bipolar disorder, or anxiety disorders). While it is certainly true that an untreated major psychiatric syndrome can color anyone's personality – and neglecting to treat a major depression or psychotic episode could lead to erroneous diagnoses of a personality (or cognitive, or other) disorder – the opposite extreme of misattributing personality psychopathology to other explanations brings its own hazards. Such an approach runs the risk of being scientifically disingenuous on several counts:

- It presumes with all-or-none thinking that medications only treat diseases and have no role for targeted dimensions of psychopathology seen in personality disorders
- It invites overdiagnosis of nonpersonality disorders with the hope and expectation that such nosologic reclassifications will somehow magically improve outcomes or make diagnostic formulations more palatable to patients, insurers, or other stakeholders in the patient's functioning
- It presumes that findings from RCTs of conditions such as major depression, bipolar disorder, schizophrenia, or syndromal anxiety disorders should neatly extrapolate to other conditions with superficial overlapping features – and then runs the risk of classifying cases as "treatment-resistant" when the actual ailment may be a personality disorder as an altogether different entity.

Tip

Successful treatment of PTSD has been shown to "eliminate" personality disorder diagnoses in about half of PTSD patients initially assessed as having paranoid, obsessive-compulsive, or avoidant personality disorders (Markowitz et al., 2015).

The RCT evidence base for mood, anxiety or psychotic disorders extrapolates better to the symptom-targeted treatment of personality disorders when one first considers overlapping versus divergent characteristics across study populations. This is why in Chapter 3 we emphasized the importance of gleaning carefully from the Method section of a clinical trial the description of the study sample. Only then can one formulate hypotheses about plausible symptom targets. Consider, for example, the use of antipsychotics in borderline personality disorder: as discussed further below, the evidence base most strongly favors targeting anger, hostility, and paranoia, rather than, say, depression (in fact, haloperidol

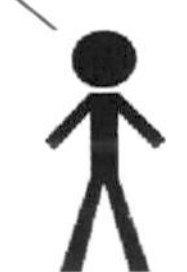
My patient has emotional lability and anger outbursts provoked by interpersonal conflicts. Which bipolar meds would be most evidence-based for those symptoms?

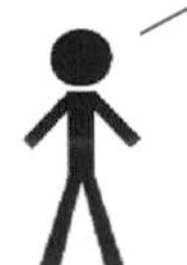
You're assuming that medicines for bipolar disorder would necessarily be helpful for her condition if she doesn't have other psychomotor symptoms of mania?

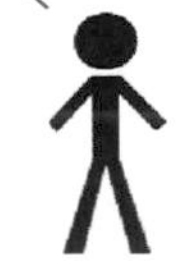
My patient's dyspnea hasn't improved with azithromycin or clarithromycin. Which broader-spectrum pneumonia drugs should I try?

You're assuming that she has an infectious disease just because she coughs and her lungs rattle?

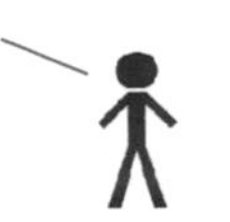
I pretty much use SGAs for everything, that way I don't have to think about what's really wrong with the patient

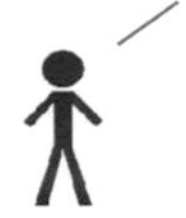
I use macrolide antibiotics for everything that rattles. Maybe try them for anger outbursts?

has shown a meaningful benefit for anger but may *worsen* depressive symptoms in borderline personality disorder (Mercer et al., 2009)).

When considering overlapping versus nonoverlapping features between bipolar and borderline personality disorders as a Venn diagram (Figure 20.1), we cannot assume from RCTs in bipolar disorder that an antimanic mood stabilizer such as lithium or divalproex will necessarily exert the same overall effect on emotional lability or aggression in the absence of nonoverlapping features such as high energy or rapid speech. Does this mean it would be a waste of time to consider mood stabilizers for overlapping symptoms when nonoverlapping symptoms are absent? Certainly not – so long as the prescriber recognizes and appreciates that such an empirical trial may be more experimental than would be the case if the clear syndrome for which the drug was originally studied was also present.

The bulk of this chapter will therefore consider the strength of evidence that does (and does not) exist for pharmacotherapy trials directed at personality disorder symptoms, alongside the database for extrapolating to personality disorders from pharmacotherapy trials of non-personality-disorder conditions. A caveat in this venture is that most clinical pharmacotherapy trials for personality disorders are comprised either of case reports or open-label studies, with relatively few RCTs (much less adequately powered or replicated RCTs).

An unfortunate reality for afficionados of evidence-based medicine is that there appears to be little incentive for the pharmaceutical industry to devote its resources to conducting regulatory trials in pursuit of a labeling indication for a condition such as borderline personality disorder – either because of the lack of historical precedent for such an undertaking or, perhaps, skepticism on the part of pharmaceutical manufacturers that such an effort would be feasible and acceptable to stakeholders. Indeed, because the presence of a significant personality disorder tends to confer a poorer prognosis when it occurs comorbidly with many other psychiatric disorders, one must recognize that large-scale industry-sponsored FDA registration pharmacotherapy trials in mood, psychotic, anxiety, and other disorders often exclude enrollment of subjects with significant personality disorders – making extrapolations to the care of such patients all the more difficult for the practitioner.

Ⓐ THINKING ABOUT PERSONALITY DISORDERS

Since DSM-III, modern psychiatric nosology has broadly divided personality disorders into three overarching domains or clusters, commonly referred to as "A" (paranoid, schizoid, and schizotypal), "B" (borderline, histrionic, narcissistic, and antisocial), and "C" (avoidant, dependent, and obsessive-compulsive). While imperfect (e.g., avoidant personality disorders bear conceptual overlap with social anxiety disorder; schizoid versus avoidant features can sometimes be hard to differentiate; borderline and narcissistic pathology both can involve lack of empathy and aggression, but probably for

Figure 20.1 Phenomenological overlaps between bipolar and borderline personality disorders.

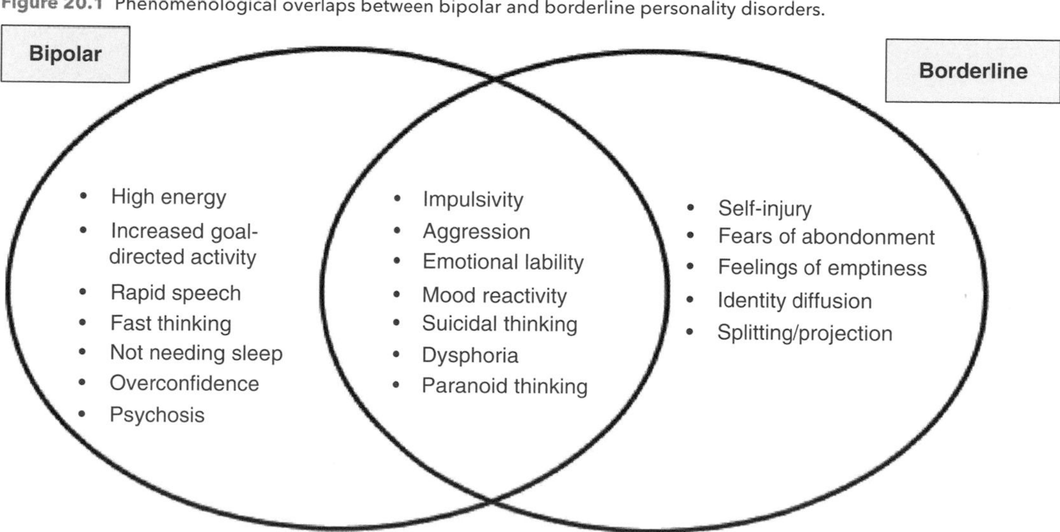

different reasons), we find it can be a useful organizing framework for understanding the core psychopathology of personality disorders, particularly with respect to dimensions that represent viable targets for treatment.

B CLUSTER A: PARANOID, SCHIZOID, SCHIZOTYPAL

Cluster A personality disorders are viewed by some (including Kraepelin) as attenuated variants of schizophrenia, with greater or lesser degrees of positive symptoms (e.g., the oddness and peculiarity of schizotypal features) or negative symptoms (e.g., the isolation and seeming indifference to social contact (rather than avoidance of expected rejection) associated with schizoid personality disorders). There has been considerable focus on the idea of early intervention for patients with "subthreshold symptoms" of schizophrenia, including paranoid or odd/schizotypal features, in the hopes that doing so might lessen the risk for developing presentations of more frank psychosis such as schizophrenia, schizoaffective disorder, or psychotic mood disorders. Empirical studies have shown that the risk for transition from subthreshold "psychosis-like" symptoms to schizophrenia is higher in men and may be reducible through integrated (pharmacological plus psychosocial) interventions (Nordentoft et al., 2006). While prospective follow-up trials are not extensive, a limited database has yielded mixed findings on whether cognitive therapy plus low-dose antipsychotics (risperidone being among the more extensively studied agents) effectively delays the transition to first-episode psychosis, with both positive (McGorry et al., 2002) and negative (Yung et al., 2011) findings. There is some evidence that the severity and manifestations of Cluster A personality disorders may become more pronounced over time in comparison to Cluster B or C disorders (Sievewright et al., 2002).

Fun Fact

It is estimated that 5–10% of the general population at some point has transient ideas of reference, odd beliefs, and excessive suspiciousness (van Os, 2003)

With respect to pharmacotherapy trials aimed to reduce symptoms of Cluster A personality disorders per se, as illustrated in Clinical Vignette 20.1, the empirical literature is remarkably sparse. What modest empirical information does exist has not shown especially robust efficacy for treating longstanding paranoia or trait-like odd thinking patterns that technically fall short of delusional intensity.

A search of the peer-reviewed literature revealed *no* treatment studies specifically focusing on schizoid personality disorder and only a handful of small case series reports (with n <10) involving FGAs (mostly flupentixol) over a period of several weeks or months

Which antipsychotic should I use to best forestall the transition from schizotypal personality disorder to schizophrenia?

I wish I could give you an empirically informed answer to that question. There are no direct comparative pharmacotherapy trials. The literature on interventions for youth at risk for schizophrenia amalgamates those with attenuated psychotic or negative symptoms plus a family history of psychosis. Up to 70% of such people go on to meet the definition of schizophrenia by 10-year follow-up (Hambrecht et al., 2002).

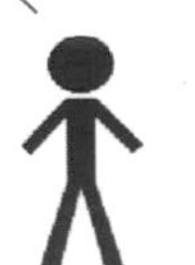

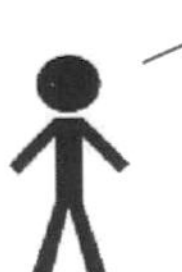

OK, but as far as treatment goes, rates of developing frank psychosis after one year in at-risk youth were numerically lower with olanzapine (16%) than placebo (38%) in one major study *but the difference wasn't significant* – although the mean weight gain with olanzapine was about 20 pounds (McGlashan et al., 2006). And in the above-mentioned McGorry et al. study of risperidone, 10% of at-risk subjects getting risperidone plus CBT developed frank psychosis after six months as compared to 36% getting no specific treatment, which was a significant difference.

CLINICAL VIGNETTE 20.1

In her psychopharmacology supervision, Dr. Edirplusima discussed the case of a very socially isolated 23-year-old man with odd, paranoid beliefs and a predilection for heavy use of hallucinogens and cannabis, the latter condition purportedly in "relative" remission. His family appeared invested in the diagnosis of schizotypal personality disorder rather than the more probable "label" of schizophrenia with hallucinogen use disorder. A prior trial of aripiprazole was stopped after causing a dystonic reaction at 10 mg/day within a few weeks of initiation, and the patient refused to continue a subsequent trial of quetiapine 250 mg/day due to sedation. Dr. Edirplusima felt compelled to offer clozapine, having read the OPTiMiSE trial (see Chapter 15), which advised initiating clozapine after a single failed antipsychotic trial – though she envisioned that the patient, whose insight was poor and sobriety probably equivocal, might not follow through with hematological monitoring.

In addition to obtaining regular urine toxicology screens, the supervisor suggested that an alternative pharmacological tactic might be to "side" with the family's investment in the Cluster "A" diagnosis and offer next a trial of olanzapine on the grounds of its evidence-based potential to forestall the emergence of frank schizophrenia – noting also, to Dr. Edirplusima, that her patient's two prior SGA trials allow one to conclude less about failed efficacy than tolerability, alongside the potential confounding psychotomimetic effects of unquantified substance misuse. Said differently, the patient may ultimately be a better *future* candidate for accepting clozapine if he and his family were the ones to declare that prior antipsychotics were ineffective, and *they* were the ones to then ask if a more potent and viable remedy existed.

with improvement assessed only on the basis of global impression scale scores (Birkeland, 2013).

Tip

Best-studied pharmacotherapies for schizotypal personality disorder are thiothixene, haloperidol, olanzapine, risperidone, or fluoxetine – but all existing trials are limited by small sample sizes, heterogeneous patient enrollment, and few randomized study designs.

In schizotypal personality disorder, a comprehensive review by Jakobsen et al. (2017) identified only four RCTs, from among a larger total of 16 evaluable case series and formal open or randomized controlled studies from 1972–2012. Strongest findings from that review, focusing on the RCT data, included:

Thiothixene – a 12-week trial in 50 patients with either schizotypal or borderline personality disorder found that thiothixene (mean dose = 8.7 mg/day) was superior to placebo in improving illusions, ideas of reference, psychoticism, obsessive-compulsiveness, and anxiety (Goldberg et al., 1986)

Risperidone – dosed at 2 mg/day for nine weeks was superior to placebo in reducing PANSS general symptoms as well as positive and negative symptoms (Koenigsberg et al., 2003). Another RCT focusing solely on neurocognitive functioning with risperidone found no differences from placebo (McClure et al., 2009)

Amisulpride – dosed at 400 mg/day was superior to placebo on measures of neurocognitive performance (Koychev et al., 2012)

I understand there are minimal data using antipsychotics to treat paranoid personality disorder, but there's certainly a rationale to try them, right?

You certainly can try, if the patient will allow you…but beware the dynamics at play when the patient is mistrustful and suspicious of others' intentions…and there you come offering to put a technically experimental substance into them. Good luck with that.

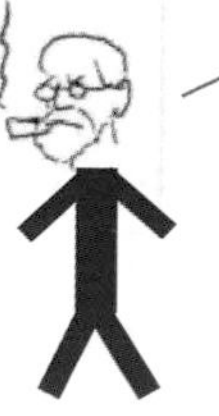

You'd need a pretty strong therapeutic alliance first, and even then, it's no easy proposition.

Other open trials (excluding single case reports) involving antipsychotics focusing on schizotypal personality disorder have suggested greater benefit with thiothixene (mean 9.4 mg/day) than haloperidol (mean 3 mg/day) based on a study of 52 patients with either schizotypal or borderline personality disorder (Serban and Siegel, 1984). An open trial of haloperidol (mean dose = 3.6 mg/day) in 17 schizotypal personality disorder patients led to mild to moderate overall symptom improvement but high dropout (Hymowitz et al., 1986). An open 26-week trial with olanzapine (mean dose = 9.3 mg/day, n=11) showed significant improvements from baseline in global symptoms and functioning, but early dropout in 8/11 subjects, and concomitant medications (usually mood stabilizers or SSRIs) limited the interpretation of study findings (Keshavan et al., 2004). Finally, one 12-week open trial of fluoxetine in 22 schizotypal or borderline personality disorder patients had reduced self-injury and improvement in global symptoms from baseline (Markovitz et al., 1991).

The α_2 agonist guanfacine holds interest for addressing cognitive processing deficits in schizotypal personality disorder by virtue of its postsynaptic binding in PFC circuitry relevant to working memory and context processing. An eight-week RCT comparing guanfacine (n = 15, dosed at 2 mg/day) or placebo (n = 13) augmentation of cognitive remediation and social-skills training revealed greater improvement in reasoning and problem-solving (i.e., solving mazes) among active drug recipients (McClure et al., 2019). Guanfacine previously has been shown to improve context processing on cognitive performance-based laboratory tasks in people with schizotypal personality disorder (McClure et al., 2007).

Tip

Context processing allows people to disambiguate cues and recognize situation-specific meanings (e.g., grasping "inside" jokes, sarcasm, double entendres). It bears on both attention processing and social cognition (see also Chapter 21, Table 21.1).

C CLUSTER B: BORDERLINE, HISTRIONIC, ANTISOCIAL

Borderline personality disorder is perhaps the most phenomenologically complex of all personality disorders because it entails elements of virtually all domains of psychopathology.

In its original conceptualization, "borderline" referred to the ambiguous boundary between psychosis and neurosis, thought breachable by stress. At one time it was also described as "pseudo-neurotic schizophrenia" or "ambulatory schizophrenia," with greater emphasis placed on disturbances of thinking and perception than on mood. In later years, attention shifted from this original distinction between borderline personality disorder and schizophrenia to the overlap between borderline personality disorder and bipolar disorder, focusing instead on the phenomenon of affective instability in both conditions. Studies of affective lability differentiate its presentation in borderline personality disorder from bipolar disorder in several key areas:

- Mood lability or emotion dysregulation appears driven more by situations involving interpersonal conflicts
- The timeframe for mood "swings" in borderline personality disorder is typically on the order of minutes to hours, in contrast to days to weeks in bipolar disorder
- Mood "swings" or manifestations of impulsivity in borderline personality disorder may not be linked to changes in energy and the sleep–wake cycle as occurs in mania/hypomania

So does that mean that if my schizotypal personality disorder patient takes guanfacine before going on a job interview they'll catch on faster to the interviewer's questions?

No, I wouldn't make that assumption. Possibly they might pay better attention, but don't necessarily expect them to become more nimble at picking up on social cues.

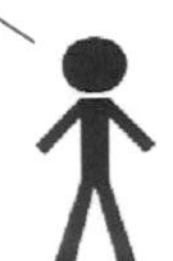

- Qualitatively, affective instability in borderline personality disorder involves substantially more emotional excursions from euthymia, depression, or anxiety to *fulminant anger* (and seldom elation) than occurs in bipolar disorder (Henry et al., 2001)

For identifying therapeutic targets, as well as anticipating potential interpersonal conflicts in treatment, we find pragmatic value in Millon's (Millon and Davis, 1996) phenomenological subtyping of borderline personality disorder (i.e., "discouraged" (appearing quiet, dependent, somber and clingy, with more inward- than outward-directed anger), "impulsive" (appearing energetic and charismatic alternating with cold and hostile), "petulant," (characterized by feelings of unworthiness, irritability, explosive anger, jealous or controlling behavior and resentment), and "self-destructive" (manifested by high-strung, moody or reckless behaviors and self-destructive acts)).

The varied domains of borderline personality disorder differ in their accessibility to pharmacological intervention. Studies that report outcomes based only on global impression scale scores yield less informative data than do measures that capture key components of borderline psychopathology. For example, composite measures such as the Zanarini Rating Scale for Borderline Personality Disorder (ZAN-BPD; Zanarini et al., 2003) encompass four major symptom domains: disturbances in affect, cognition, impulsivity, and interpersonal relationships. The Borderline Personality Disorder Severity Index (BPDSI) captures feelings of abandonment, relationships, impulsivity, suicidal behavior, affective instability, feelings of emptiness, anger outbursts, dissociation and paranoid thinking, and identity diffusion (Arntz et al., 2003). Other pertinent outcome measures in studies of borderline pathology include self-harm (e.g., the Self-Harm Inventory (SHI; Sansone et al., 1998) and the State–Trait Anger Expression Inventory (STAXI), a 57-item inventory developed by Spielberger et al. (1983).

A 2010 Cochrane Database review noted that, while "some beneficial effects" were evident with SGAs, mood stabilizers, and omega-3 fatty acids, no drug exerted a significant effect on total symptom severity, and no pharmacotherapy has been shown to alleviate core symptoms such as feelings of emptiness, identity disturbances, and fears of abandonment (Stoffers et al., 2010).

D ANGER

Outbursts of anger and primitive rage, mainly in the context of frustration intolerance, occur prominently across Cluster B personality disorders. The phenomenon

I have a binge-eating Millon-petulant and self-destructive borderline who's an SLC6A4 s/s homozygote with the Asn40 SNP on OPRM1. Would that lessen your enthusiasm for using naltrexone either for self-mutilation behavior or binge-eating and weight loss?

Interesting. You're positing that there may be less of an endorphin effect from cutting than if she had the Asp40 OPRM1 SNP, as has been suggested from preliminary studies for naltrexone response in alcohol-use disorders? Interesting idea, but I don't know. You didn't ask if her s/s homozygosity would make an SSRI trial less compelling. You might be slightly more keen on that idea if she were *l/l genotype*, based on MDD studies, but you'll note from Table 20.1 below that the database with SSRIs is rather weak for depression in borderline personality disorder.

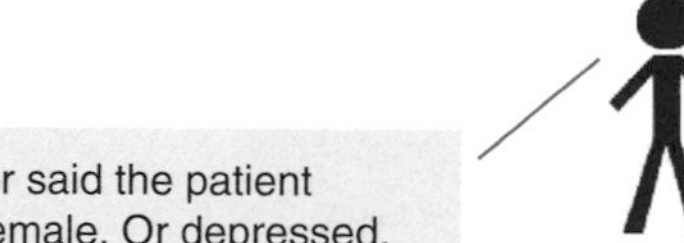

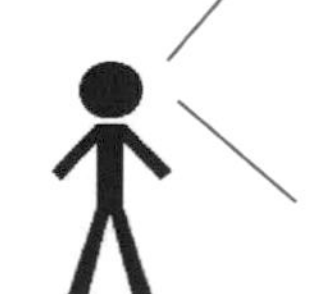

I never said the patient was female. Or depressed.

Ahh....well...uhh, the pharmacogenetics database with SLC6A4 is stronger in women than men, and pertains more to depression than other outcomes.

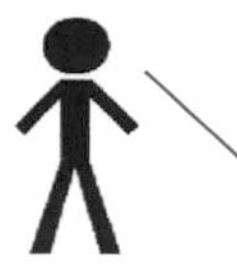

Um, you know, the "literature" on naltrexone for cutting behavior is a whopping six open cases. Go look back at Table 14.5 in Chapter 14, why don't you.

is especially well-recognized in borderline personality disorder, where overt and often sudden anger and rage attacks, typically in response to interpersonal conflicts, are regarded by some as *sine qua non* features. The concept of inwardly versus outwardly directed anger is captured by measures such as the STAXI and often immediately palpable without the need for formal quantification during clinical assessments. A 2009 meta-analysis observed that mood stabilizers, as a broad class, exerted the largest effect size against anger as a target symptom, followed by antidepressants and then antipsychotics (see Box 20.1).

Box 20.1

Effect Sizes Across Broad Drug Classes Targeting Anger in Borderline Personality Disorder

Drug class	*d* (95% CI)
Mood stabilizers	-1.75 (-2.77 to -0.74)
Antidepressants	-0.74 (-1.27 to -0.21)
Antipsychotics	-0.59 (-1.04 to -0.15)

Based on meta-analysis by Mercer et al. (2009)

The meta-analysis by Mercer et al. (2009) found that among SGAs, aripiprazole demonstrated the largest effect against anger symptoms. Studies of divalproex (see Table 20.2) suggest antiaggression efficacy in short-term studies, but those of longer duration had smaller effects. The prominent antianger effect of antidepressants as a class in that meta-analysis was driven largely by one study of fluoxetine (Coccaro and Kavoussi, 1997) having an especially large impact, although drug effects on depressive symptoms per se were not necessarily covaried for examining effects on anger outcomes.

E DISTRESS INTOLERANCE

Distress tolerance is the ability to withstand negative affective states while in pursuit of a goal. Disrupted functioning is believed to reflect corticolimbic dysregulation. The capacity to tolerate distress or frustration is linked with both resilience and anxiety, and can be problematic not only for patients with borderline personality disorder but also those with addictions, PTSD, and anxiety disorders, among other relevant conditions. Low distress tolerance also has been linked with obsessional thinking, but not frank OCD. It remains a cornerstone focus of DBT skills training. A Medline search of the terms "distress intolerance" and "trial" yielded multiple studies of DBT, mindfulness training, exercise, and other psychosocial interventions but no pharmacotherapy trials. In our view distress intolerance represents an understudied yet fundamental target for pharmacotherapy outcome studies across all relevant agents.

F NONSUICIDAL SELF-INJURY

Recall from Chapter 14 the available database using SSRIs, SGAs, anticonvulsants, and opioid antagonists to target self-injurious behavior. Problematic with much of the available empirical information is that it is largely based on anecdotal case reports, and also blends together populations with borderline personality disorder, substance use disorders, developmental disabilities, and other forms of psychopathology that may reflect diverse underlying neurobiological processes.

G CHRONIC SUICIDAL IDEATION

It is worth noting that, with the exception of intranasal esketamine, no drug has ever shown a specific pharmacodynamic effect to reduce suicidal ideation. Lithium and clozapine, both regarded as having antisuicide properties in mood disorders and schizophrenia, respectively, have been shown in controlled trials to lower the risk of suicide attempts, but not ideation (presumably via indirect effects on impulse control). There is remarkably little empirical study of the

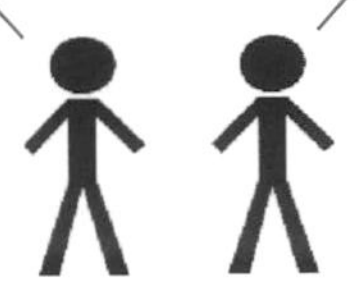

So then what is the best drug to use for self-mutilation behavior?
There isn't a "best" drug. There are no no large RCTs, only open trials and case reports. Maybe fluoxetine or sertraline have "more" data because there exist more than 10 cases with each.

phenomenon of *chronic* suicidal ideation (as occurs often in borderline personality disorder), or clinical scenarios in which patients ruminate in prolonged deliberative (i.e., nonimpulsive) fashion about situations under which suicidal behavior holds conceptual appeal. There is also the related issue of *contingent* suicidal thinking – for example, advanced declarations that suicidal intent will arise if some event should occur or fail or occur, rather like making a hostage threat. Such phenomena are not clearly tied either to depression or poor impulse control (in fact, the executive planning involved in such circumstances by definition requires intense "top-down" cold cognitive processing). One could speculate about more obsessional or ruminative than depressive or impulsive neural circuitry at play, but at present no specific pharmacotherapy has shown robust efficacy for chronic suicidal thinking. Notably, while initial open trials of repeatedly dosed IV ketamine have shown efficacy for chronic suicidal thinking in MDD (Ionescu et al., 2016b), a subsequent placebo-controlled RCT failed to affirm an effect (Ionescu et al., 2019).

H DEPRESSION, ANTIDEPRESSANTS, AND BORDERLINE PERSONALITY DISORDER

Generally speaking, antidepressants exert a more modest effect on depressive or most features of borderline personality disorder than was once thought. The Cochrane Database analysis by Mercer et al. (2009; see Box 20.2) found that antidepressants as a class exerted a greater effect on anger than on depression – consistent with findings on the use of SSRIs for impulsive aggression as described in Chapter 14. Antipsychotics, collectively, exerted a lesser (and statistically nonsignificant) antidepressant effect, relative to mood stabilizers or antidepressants.

Box 20.2

Effect Sizes Across Broad Drug Classes Targeting Depression in Borderline Personality Disorder

Drug class	*d* (95% CI)
Mood stabilizers	-0.63 (-0.99 to -0.27)
Antidepressants	-0.37 (-0.69 to -0.05)
Antipsychotics	-0.46 (-0.94 to 0.03)

Based on meta-analysis by Mercer et al. (2009)

Among traditional antidepressants, serotonergic antidepressants have garnered the most interest (say, as compared to secondary amine tricyclics, or bupropion) based on hypothesized links between serotonergic regulation of limbic arousal and function. As shown in the summary in Table 20.1, however, RCTs of SSRIs have yielded mixed findings. Notably, though, most have been of short duration and are likely underpowered.

I MAOIs

A small RCT in 16 women with borderline personality disorder found that tranylcypromine (mean dose = 40 mg/day) was superior to placebo in improving depression and rejection sensitivity, but not behavioral dyscontrol (Cowdry and Gardner, 1988).

Leibowitz and Klein (1981) postulated that a particular constellation of symptoms – histrionic personality, rejection sensitivity, brief periods of depressed mood, and atypical depressive features (notably, hypersomnia and hyperphagia) – which they termed "hysteroid dysphoria," could be a subtype of atypical depression common in borderline personality disorder that may be particularly responsive to MAOIs

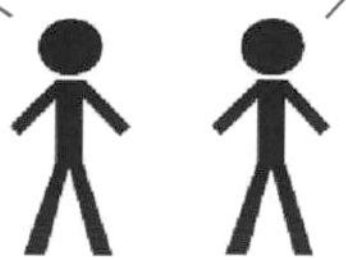
You know, at least in MDD, the Met/Met variant of the BDNF Val66Met SNP may moderate the antisuicide effect of ketamine (Chen et al., 2019b)
You've really got a thing going about pharmacogenetics, don't you. Bit of a fetish maybe?

(phenelzine) over TCAs (amitriptyline) (Kayser et al., 1985). Subsequent investigations focusing on hysteroid dysphoria also found phenelzine to be superior to placebo or to haloperidol after acute treatment on measures of global symptoms, anxiety, anger, and hostility, but no distinct benefit for depressive symptoms (Soloff et al., 1993). A 16-week continuation trial found haloperidol to have sustained advantage over placebo for reducing irritability but high premature dropout (64%), with phenelzine demonstrating only modest benefits for depression coupled with observations of "excitement and reactivity" (Cornelius et al., 1993).

Separately, a randomized comparison of phenelzine, imipramine, or placebo for atypical depression, including 40 subjects with borderline personality disorder, found significantly higher response rates (by CGI) for depression with the MAOI (89%) than the tricyclic (31%) or placebo (20%) (Parsons et al., 1989).

J MOOD STABILIZERS

One must appreciate that the term "mood stabilizer" connotes something of a semantic misnomer, inasmuch as no drug commonly referred to in that category has formally been studied specifically to treat moment-to-moment changes in emotional state, or the extent to which intense mood reactivity or affective lability is reduced using a day-to-day or even hour-by-hour timescale. From the literature on bipolar disorder (see Chapter 13), we also know that some agents are known to exert more antimanic than antidepressant properties (e.g., lithium, divalproex, carbamazepine), while fewer are predominantly antidepressant (i.e., lamotrigine). Table 20.2 summarizes information from open and controlled trials in borderline personality disorder using anticonvulsants with established "mood-stabilizing" properties in bipolar disorder.

Of note, some clinicians have a penchant for favoring lamotrigine as a presumptive antidote for moment-to-moment affective instability in mood-unstable patients with ambiguous "bipolar spectrum" diagnoses. Is that because they read and were enamored by the study by Reich et al. (2009) where 15 borderline personality disorder patients taking lamotrigine showed less affective lability than those taking placebo? Despite a much larger one-year negative RCT by Crawford et al (2018)? Or rather, if prescribing instead reflects a subjective perception that lamotrigine is simply a more user-friendly, relatively low-risk medication option if a bipolar diagnosis is "soft"? Here may be an instance where the evidence base collides with clinical experience, leaving "the truth" buried in a morass of empirical uncertainty.

K FGAs AND SGAs

An early literature described efficacy using low doses of FGAs in borderline personality disorder. For example, an open trial of thioridazine (mean dose = 92 mg/day)

Can SSRIs function like mood stabilizers to help regulate moment-to-moment mood shifts?

The study of fluoxetine by Rinne et al. (2002) found improvement on the "rapid mood shifts" items of the BPDSI – so that technically makes it more of a "mood" stabilizer than even a "mood stabilizer."

Um, what about lithium in borderline personality disorder, y'know, for impulsivity and what-not? Assuming risk for toxicity in overdose was, say, not a major concern?

Not a ton of data. A somewhat complicated small (n = 17) crossover study compared lithium (mean dose = 985.7 mg/day) with desipramine (mean dose = 162.5 mg/day) or placebo (Links et al., 1990). Rating scale outcomes were no different among groups.

in 11 DSM-IIIR outpatients with borderline personality disorder reported significant improvements from baseline in BPRS scores (Teicher et al., 1989). Another early RCT found that haloperidol (mean dose = 7.2 mg/day) was superior to both placebo and amitriptyline (mean dose = 147.62 mg/day) on a composite outcome measure encompassing depression, anxiety, hostility, paranoid ideation, and psychoticism (Soloff et al., 1986); post hoc analyses found that a better response to haloperidol was associated with "hostile depression," suspiciousness, and severity of schizotypal symptoms (Soloff et al., 1989).

SGAs as a class, as noted by Mercer et al. (2009), have not been shown to exert a significant effect on depressive symptoms in borderline personality disorder (Box 20.2), but may be more efficacious for managing *anger* (Box 20.1). Individual findings from specific open or randomized trials of SGAs are presented in Table 20.3. Of note, more RCTs exist with olanzapine or quetiapine than other agents, although study designs are mixed (e.g., olanzapine trials include mono- as well as combination pharmacotherapies, or adjuncts to DBT). We would offer here our completely anecdotal impression that low-dose clozapine for diverse symptoms in borderline personality disorder may be among the better-kept secret weapons in psychopharmacology with regard to therapeutic efficacy – as limited, obviously, by its potential pitfalls of sedation, weight gain, and other metabolic dysregulation, along with the "hassle" factor of hematological monitoring. Newer agents such as cariprazine, brexpiprazole, or lumateperone, which may be conceptually appealing and spare the metabolic adverse burden of some older SGAs, remain too new to have accrued empirical data.

My patient with borderline personality disorder feels that her medications need to be "tweaked" every few days. Are those the "necessary clinical adjustments" (NCAs) that were referred to in Chapter 1?

Probably not. Steady-state pharmacokinetic changes in most psychotropic medications generally don't occur on the scale of hours, or from one day to the next. I'd wonder if she's construing medicines as a way to self-soothe when she experiences negative affects, and if she continues to feel unsoothed she may perceive that as a reason to tweak medications. Oh, and she may get belligerent if you fail to appease her wishes.

So then what should I do for that?

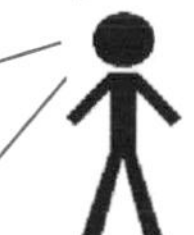

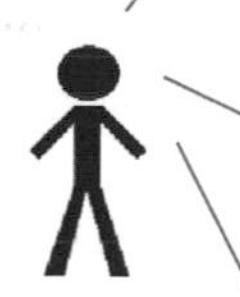

Psychotherapy, to provide emotional reassurance and to help her learn better skills for coping and self-regulating unpleasant emotional states....and not automatically equating unpleasant emotional states with the need for medication tweaks.

What's psychotherapy?

Another book.

My patient with borderline personality disorder got so much better after starting lamotrigine in the hospital for two weeks and then her mood swings relapsed the day after she left. Why did the lamotrigine suddenly stop working so fast?

My hunch would be that her "relapse" had less to do with the pharmacodynamic properties of lamotrigine over two weeks than with the nonpharmacodynamic properties of being in the hospital. Borderline personality disorder is highly influenced by interpersonal and psychosocial factors. That's why some borderline personality disorder patients seem better almost instantly when hospitalized, and also sometimes regress in their coping skills and ability to adapt to stress when hospitalizations are prolonged.

L BENZODIAZEPINES VERSUS USE OF COPING SKILLS: EITHER/OR? BOTH/AND?

Poor resilience, and having a limited repertoire of adaptive coping skills, sets the stage for patients to seek potentially maladaptive strategies, with varying degrees of desperation, to self-soothe when stressed. Desperation to relieve emotional distress heightens the allure of hazardous high-reward behaviors that can serve to alleviate distress (at least momentarily) and replace it with pleasure. Having a reliable "mental toolbox" of adaptive strategies to cope with distress becomes a key element of psychotherapies such as DBT. Pharmacotherapies such as benzodiazepines or other scheduled drugs (e.g., psychostimulants, opiates) run a particular risk for abuse in borderline personality disorder particularly because the quest to avoid negative affect states may feel constant and unsatisfiable. For these reasons, coupled with the lack of an evidence base to support their long-term use in this population, benzodiazepines remain especially controversial. As one notable example, Cowdry and Gardner (1988) found that alprazolam (mean dose = 4.7 mg/day) was associated with worsening of suicidality and behavioral dyscontrol, and no improvement in any outcome measures. Patients with borderline personality disorder often convey an insatiable hunger to avoid distress or negative affect states, linked with poor internal self-regulation. Such factors collectively place highly vulnerable patients at increased risk for consuming excessive medication doses, incurring more adverse events, and having trouble following parameter limits when using controlled substances. Borderline personality disorder patients who find themselves exceeding the prescribed quantity of a medication or who relentlessly seek ever-increasing amounts or types of drug remedies for distress intolerance tend to be poor candidates for controlled substances.

M MEMANTINE

Bearing on theories that glutamatergic dysfunction in depression extends to patients with borderline personality disorder, memantine dosed at 20 mg/day (n = 17) was superior to placebo + treatment as usual (n = 16) in improving ZAN-BPD scores with good tolerability over an eight-week study period (Kulkarni et al., 2018).

N OMEGA-3 FATTY ACIDS

A 12-week RCT of omega-3 fatty acids (n = 23; dosed as eicosopentanoic acid (EPA) 1.2 g/day plus docosahexanoic acid (DHA) 0.8 g/day) or placebo (n = 20) in conjunction with divalproex (dosed from 800–1300 mg/day) found no significant between-group differences in BPDSI total scores or subscales assessing abandonment, interpersonal relationships, identity disturbance, parasuicidal thoughts, affective instability or feelings of emptiness or dissociation – however, significant differences occurred favoring EPA/DHA on BPDSI subscales for impulsivity and anger outbursts (Bellino et al., 2014).

O YI-GAN

An open trial of the Chinese herbal medicine yi-gan san (mean daily dose = 6.4 g; range = 2.5–7.5 g/day) found significant improvements from baseline in BPRS total scores and subitems related to anxiety, depressed mood, hostility, suspiciousness, motor retardation, uncooperativeness, and excitement over 12 weeks in 20 female outpatients with borderline personality disorder. (Miyaoka et al., 2008).

My emotionally dysregulated patient with poor coping skills has begun compulsively shopping and started drinking heavily. I guess that makes her bipolar, huh?

No, those could just be maladaptive coping strategies that are motivated and driven by inner tension or her intolerance of negative or aversive emotions. Do address the alcohol use and ways to expand her repertoire of alternative coping skills, but don't go down the "bipolar path" unless there is a clear signal of high energy and psychomotor activation (like not needing sleep, without next-day fatigue) that's a departure from her norm.

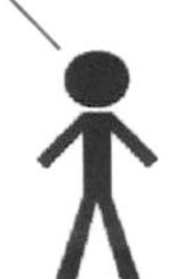

P OXYTOCIN

Oxytocin has been suggested as a pharmacological strategy to counter deficits in affective empathy in people with borderline personality disorder. In one RCT, a single dose of 24 IU oxytocin IN in 51 mid-luteal phase women was superior to placebo in improving affective empathy and approach motivation (Domes et al., 2019). A review of 11 RCTs in borderline personality disorder found that IN oxytocin improved social cognition (e.g., laboratory-based recognition and discrimination of emotions and hypervigilance to social threats (Servan et al., 2018)).

Q PSYCHOSTIMULANTS

Impaired decision-making represents another known symptom domain, and potential treatment target, in borderline personality disorder. A single dose of methylphenidate has been shown to be superior to placebo on decision-making using a laboratory paradigm (The Iowa Gambling Task) (Gvirts et al., 2018). Earlier open-label trials of methylphenidate also have shown improvement in attentional processing as well as aggressive behaviors.

Clinical Vignette 20.2 illustrates the common pitfalls when controlled substances become a focal point for patients with mood dysregulation, identity diffusion, and poor capacity to self-regulate negative affect states.

CLINICAL VIGNETTE 20.2

Amy is a 23-year-old unemployed single woman living alone with what both her parents and therapist called "failure to launch." Moody, sulky, disgruntled, quietly angry, and lacking in a daily structured routine, she self-soothes by vaping cannabis nightly, occasionally using IN cocaine, and cutting her arms with scissor points when she feels "too stressed out." She has varied and disconnected somatic complaints for which no unifying established medical diagnosis could be made. Her relationships are tumultuous and when she feels rejected she talks about wanting to kill herself. She says she feels lonely and isolated but is "afraid of getting close" to anyone. From among a large number of past pharmacotherapy trials involving antidepressants, mood stabilizers, SGAs, and α agonists, among others, the only medications she has ever really found to be helpful are benzodiazepines and amphetamine – both of which she has taken at higher-than prescribed dosages. She thinks she must be an ultra-rapid drug metabolizer and now requests pharmacogenetic testing because she hopes that the results will convince her psychiatrist to prescribe higher doses of "the only drugs that help."

Amy's is a difficult case. Apart from likely diagnoses of multiple substance use (cannabis, cocaine, and possibly benzodiazepine and amphetamine) disorders, she conveys features of "discouraged" and "self-destructive" borderline traits in Millon's conceptualization. What are reasonable goals for a psychopharmacologist, given the absence of other clear diagnostic entities with plausible targets for pharmacotherapy? We would offer the following thoughts as the blueprint for a meaningful consultation:

- Prioritize abstinence from substance use as a necessary step for discerning comorbid from artifactual signs of psychopathology. This likely would require environmental changes (such as sober living and regular drug toxicology screens). Consider the possibility that Amy may be taking other psychoactive substances than the ones she self-reports. Tapering of benzodiazepines is probably advisable (given that she takes more than prescribed and is not clearly reaping benefits over risks) and will likely be a gradual process depending on her actual dose and duration of use. Little can occur for her until we can control for this "confounding" factor.
- Systematically assess the current and lifetime presence or absence of any major psychiatric syndromes, including major depressive or manic/hypomanic episodes, psychotic episodes, and anxiety syndromes. Recognize that this becomes all the more difficult because of the critical confounding effects of substance use. Collateral history as well as family history data may help.
- Review past medication trials to gauge dosing, duration, and adherence relative to pertinent symptom targets.
- Amy's creative hypothesis that she is an ultra-rapid metabolizer likely has little bearing on her desire to take higher doses of benzodiazepines and amphetamine. (Arguably, if she were taking lisdexamfetamine, she may be unable to metabolize the pro-drug to active amphetamine – except, pharmacokinetic conversion of lisdexamfetamine to free amphetamine occurs via gut hydrolysis, rather than hepatic enzymes.) Her escalating use of benzodiazepines probably more likely reflects tolerance and physiological dependence than "ultra-rapid metabolism" but either way, further dosage increases of a benzodiazepine are unlikely to be wise or beneficial.
- Formulate specific symptom targets of treatment – potentially including expression of anger-in and

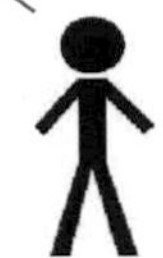
Identity diffusion...got a pill?

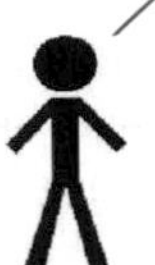
Not so much the stuff of pharmacotherapy

There are no established medications for histrionic personality disorder per se. If someone with a histrionic personality develops atypical depressive features then it's entirely reasonably to favor phenelzine as having the most data, but probably only after an SSRI or two proves to not help, since that'd be much easier to try first.

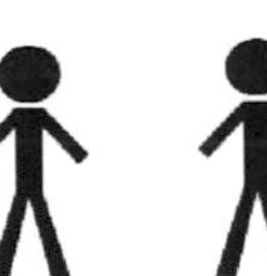
Antisocial personality traits. Got a pill?
For *impulsive aggression*, there are a number of options, as discussed in Chapter 14. However, for *premeditated* or willful and purposeful aggression, or interpersonal manipulativeness, or lack of empathy...not so much.

anger-out, self-injurious behavior, and anxiety. Position the role of pharmacotherapy as being a possible adjunct to supplement, rather than replace, the core psychosocially based treatments she more immediately needs to regain a sense of control over her life.

R CLUSTER C: AVOIDANT, DEPENDENT, AND OBSESSIVE-COMPULSIVE

Formal studies of pharmacotherapy for Cluster C personality disorders are neither extensive nor encouraging. In avoidant personality disorder, most intervention studies have largely focused on patients with anxiety disorders (e.g., social anxiety disorder) with or without avoidant personality disorder as a comorbidity. For example, a 26-week RCT with assessments at 6 and 12 months in 102 such subjects found that cognitive therapy was superior to paroxetine or placebo but not to the combination (Nordahl et al., 2016). A post hoc analysis of nefazodone, psychotherapy, or their combination for chronic depression patients found that the presence of a comorbid Cluster C personality disorder did not negatively moderate treatment outcome (Maddux et al., 2009).

TAKE-HOME POINTS

- Personality disorders involve heterogeneous psychopathology that weaves together neurobiological and psychological factors. Much of the pharmacotherapy literature is based on case reports, open trials, or small underpowered studies in mixed samples, limiting the ability to make broad recommendations. Decision-making often must be driven more by plausible rationales than evidence-based data. Pharmacology is mostly an ancillary treatment to psychotherapy for most significant personality disorders.
- In Cluster A disorders, risperidone, olanzapine, and some FGAs (thiothixene, haloperidol) have modest data targeting attenuated psychotic symptoms. Monitor younger patients for progression to schizophrenia or other frank psychotic disorders – as well as risks for metabolic dysregulation or tardive dyskinesia during long-term treatment.
- In Cluster B disorders, aripiprazole and divalproex both seem to have slightly more robust data for impulsive aggression; SSRIs are commonly still used first line for depression but their evidence base specifically for depression is modest and limited by small sample sizes. An older literature supports value for MAOIs, especially phenelzine, in atypical depressive presentations in borderline personality disorder.
- In Cluster C disorders, pharmacotherapy data mostly involve targeting comorbid social anxiety disorder. There are promising initial findings with oxytocin to target elements of social cognition, and omega-3 fatty acids as novel therapeutics.

Table 20.1 RCTs of serotonergic antidepressants in borderline personality disorder

Antidepressant	Outcome
Fluoxetine	A 13-week RCT found greater improvement in anger and depression with fluoxetine (n = 13, dosing 20–60 mg/day) than placebo (n = 9) (Salzman et al., 1994)
	A 12-week RCT in 40 MDD, bipolar, or schizophrenia subjects (including 13 with borderline personality disorder) found significantly greater improvement with fluoxetine than placebo in irritability and aggression but not depression (Coccaro and Kavoussi, 1997)
	A 12-week RCT of DBT + fluoxetine (n = 9) or placebo (n = 11) found no advantage for active drug to reduce depressive symptoms (Simpson et al., 2005)
Fluvoxamine	A 12-week RCT in 38 female borderline patients found that fluvoxamine (dosed from 150-250 mg/day) was superior to placebo in reducing "rapid mood shifts" but not impulsivity or aggression (Rinne et al., 2002)

Abbreviations: DBT = dialectical behavior therapy; MDD = major depressive disorder; RCT = randomized controlled trial

Table 20.2 Anticonvulsants in borderline personality disorder

Anticonvulsant	Outcome
Carbamazepine	**Positive trials:** - A double-blind crossover trial in 11 female patients found greater improvement in behavioral dyscontrol than with placebo (Gardner and Cowdry, 1986) **Negative trials:** - A one-month RCT in 20 patients found no significant outcome differences from placebo (de la Fuente and Lotstra, 1994)
Divalproex	**Positive trials:** - Open eight-week trial with 11 patients (8 completers), in whom half showed significant reductions from baseline on symptom measures of anxiety, anger, rejection sensitivity, and impulsivity (Stein et al., 1995a) - An eight-week open trial in 10 SSRI-nonresponsive patients (having "at least one personality disorder") reported significant decreases from baseline in irritability and overt aggression (Kavoussi and Coccaro, 1998) - A small RCT of divalproex (n = 12) or placebo (n = 4) in borderline personality disorder reported superiority of active drug based on global impression scores (Hollander et al., 2001) - In 52 outpatients, divalproex (mean modal dose = 1325 mg/day) was better than placebo in reducing impulsive aggression, irrespective of baseline affective instability (Hollander et al., 2005). Similar findings favoring divalproex's effects on impulsive aggression and irritability were then affirmed in a larger multisite RCT in borderline personality disorder (n = 96) as well as intermittent explosive disorder (n = 116) and post-traumatic stress disorder (n = 34) (Hollander et al., 2003b) - A six-month double-blind comparison in 30 female subjects with borderline personality disorder and comorbid bipolar II disorder randomized to divalproex (mean dose = 850 ± 249 mg/day), and 10 to placebo, found significantly greater improvement with divalproex in reducing interpersonal sensitivity and anger/hostility, with minimal adverse effects (Frankenburg and Zanarini, 2002)
Gabapentin	- No formal clinical trials
Lamotrigine	**Positive trials:** - A 12-week preliminary randomized comparison of adjunctive lamotrigine (n = 15, mean final dose = 106.7 mg/day) vs. placebo (n = 12) found significantly greater reductions in affective lability and impulsivity among those taking active drug, but no notable improvements in feelings of emptiness, identity disturbance, or self-mutilation/suicidality (Reich et al., 2009). - An eight-week randomized comparison of lamotrigine (brought to a target dose of 200 mg/day via standard titration) or placebo found greater reductions in all anger (STAXI) measures except anger-in (Tritt et al., 2005); benefits remained observable for the group as a whole on STAXI measures across six-month follow-ups over 18 months (Leiberich et al., 2008) **Negative trials:** - A 52-week RCT of lamotrigine (up to 200 mg/day) in 276 patients with borderline personality disorder found no significant differences from placebo using the Zanarini Rating Scale for Borderline Personality Disorder (ZAN-BPD) or in secondary outcome measures (e.g., depressive symptoms, deliberate self-harm, quality of life) (Crawford et al., 2018)
Oxcarbazepine	- Open trial in 17 outpatients (dosing = 1200–1500 mg/day); CGI and BPRS scores significantly improved from baseline, as did BPDSI items related to interpersonal relationships, impulsivity, affective instability, anger outbursts; adverse effects included headache, dizziness, nausea (Bellino et al., 2005)

Table 20.2 (Cont.)

Anticonvulsant	Outcome
Topiramate	**Positive trials:** - An eight-week double-blind comparison of topiramate (n = 21; titration was to a target dose of 250 mg/day by six weeks) or placebo (n = 10) found significantly greater reductions with active drug on STAXI measures (state-anger, trait-anger, anger-out, anger-control), with good tolerability (Nickel et al., 2004) - A 10-week randomized comparison of topiramate (n = 28; 25–200 mg/day) or placebo (n = 28) found significantly greater improvements than with placebo on measures of somatization, interpersonal sensitivity, anxiety, hostility, phobic anxiety and global severity (Loew et al., 2006) - An eight-week randomized comparison of topiramate (n = 22; target dose = 250 mg/day) or placebo (n = 20) found greater improvements in aggression (measured by STAXI subscales) with topiramate than placebo (Nickel et al., 2005)

Abbreviations: BPDSI = Borderline Personality Disorder Severity Index; BPRS = Brief Psychiatric Rating Scale; CGI = Clinical Global Impressions; RCT = randomized controlled trial; SSRI = selective serotonin reuptake inhibitor; STAXI = State–Trait Anger Expression Inventory

Table 20.3 SGAs in borderline personality disorder

SGA	Outcome
Aripiprazole	- A 12-week trial of adjunctive therapy (dosing from 10–15 mg/day) in 21 nonresponders to sertraline (dosing from 100–200 mg/day): 9/16 completers (56%) responded, 24% dropped out due to adverse effects (Bellino et al., 2008)
Asenapine	- A 12-week randomized comparison of asenapine (n = 21; dosing = 5–10 mg/day) found superiority to olanzapine (n = 19; 5–10 mg/day) in reducing affective instability; inferior to olanzapine in reducing paranoid ideation and dissociation (Bozzatello et al., 2017)
Clozapine	- No RCTs are available. A meta-analysis of 12 studies (limited to case reports and small open trials, generally all in highly refractory cases) found substantial benefit for psychotic symptoms, impulsivity, aggression, self-injury, need for adjunctive anxiolytic medications, and overall functioning (Beri and Boydell, 2014)
Olanzapine	**Positive RCTs:** - A six-month RCT of olanzapine in 28 female patients showed greater improvement than placebo in improving all domains studied (anxiety, paranoia, anger-hostility, and interpersonal sensitivity) except depression (Zanarini and Frankenburg, 2001) - A 12-week RCT in 40 male and female patients found greater clinical global improvement with olanzapine (2.5–20 mg/day) than placebo (Bogenschutz and Nurnberg, 2004) - A 12-week RCT of fixed dose/ranges of olanzapine (2.5 or 5–10 mg/day) versus placebo in 451 outpatients found modestly greater reductions on ZAN-BPD total scores with only the 5–10 mg/day dose (*d* = 0.29); significantly higher response rates occurred with 5–10 mg/day dosing (73.6%) than 2.5 mg/day (60.1%) or placebo (57.8%); and significantly greater weight gain with either dose than placebo (Zanarini et al., 2011); a subsequent 12-week open-label extension/continuation phase of that study showed further improvements in ZAN-BPD symptoms (Zanarini et al., 2012) - Dialectical behavior therapy (DBT) augmented with olanzapine or placebo was studied in two RCTs: a first 12-week trial (mean dose = 8.8 mg/day) in 60 patients found greater improvement in depression, anxiety, and impulsivity/aggression than seen with placebo (Soler et al., 2005); another six-month study found that DBT + olanzapine (mean dose = 4.46 mg/day) yielded less irritability, aggression, depression, and self-injury (Linehan et al., 2008) - An eight-week RCT comparing olanzapine (n = 16), fluoxetine (n = 14) or both (OFC; n = 15) found greater improvement in depression and overt aggression with OFC or olanzapine than fluoxetine alone (Zanarini et al., 2004) **Negative RCTs:** - A 12-week RCT of flexibly dosed olanzapine (n = 155) found *no* significant differences from placebo (n = 159) in ZAN-BPD total scores (Schulz et al., 2008)
Paliperidone	- A 12-week open trial in 18 outpatients (dosing = 3-6 mg/day) found significant improvement from baseline in global symptoms, impulse control, anger, and cognitive-perceptual disturbances (Bellino et al., 2011)
Quetiapine	- A 14-week open trial (mean dose = 309 mg/day) in 14 outpatients; significant improvements from baseline in BPDSI "impulsivity" and "outbursts of anger" items; 21% dropout due to somnolence or nonadherence (Bellino et al., 2006) - A 12-week open trial (mean dose = 540 mg/day) in 29 outpatients; significant improvement from baseline in BPRS hostility and suspiciousness scales as well as HAM-D and CGI scales (Perrella et al., 2007)

Table 20.3 (Cont.)

SGA	Outcome
	- A 12-week open trial in 23 outpatients (mean dose = 251 mg/day); significant improvement from baseline in impulsivity as well as measures of hostility, depression, anxiety, and global functioning (Villeneuve and Lemelin, 2005) - A 12-week open trial in 41 outpatients (dosing range =100–800 mg/day); significant improvements from baseline were observed in impulsivity, hostility, affective lability, depression, and anxiety (Van den Eynde et al., 2008)
Ziprasidone	- A 12-week RCT in 60 patients found no significant differences from placebo (mean dose = 84.1 mg/day) on global impressions (Pascual et al., 2008)

No studies with brexpiprazole, cariprazine, iloperidone, lumateperone, or pimavanserin

Abbreviations: BPDSI = Borderline Personality Disorder Severity Index; BPRS = Brief Psychiatric Rating Scale; CGI = Clinical Global Impressions; HAM-D = Hamilton Ratings Scale for Depression; OFC = olanzapine/fluoxetine combination; RCT = randomized controlled trial; SGA = second-generation antipsychotic; ZAN-BPD = Zanarini Rating Scale for Borderline Personality Disorder

21 Cognition

LEARNING OBJECTIVES

- ☐ Recognize and differentiate the major cognitive domains of attention, memory, and executive function; appreciate how deficits in one or more of these areas can manifest across a range of psychiatric disorders
- ☐ Understand basic methods for objectively evaluating subjective cognitive complaints
- ☐ Recognize the relative impact of antidepressants, antipsychotics, and anticonvulsants on cognitive functioning
- ☐ Describe the relative effect of agents studied in RCTs to treat adult ADHD
- ☐ Describe management strategies for pharmacological tolerance to stimulants in adult ADHD
- ☐ Describe the evidence base to support the use of currently available pharmacotherapies targeting major cognitive impairment, including pro-cholinergics and NMDA receptor modulators

The chief function of the body is to carry the brain around.

- Thomas Edison

Attentional problems are among the most ubiquitous and nonpathognomonic of psychiatric complaints. Nearly all psychiatric disorders impact cognitive functioning in one form or another, and it can be a challenge for clinicians to differentiate free-standing disorders of cognition (e.g., adult ADHD or dementia) from those that are iatrogenic (due to psychotropic or nonpsychotropic medications) or the epiphenomena of other conditions (such as depression, mania, anxiety, or schizophrenia). Cognitive problems involve distinct domains that can form unique constellations and present differently from one psychiatric disorder to another (e.g., skip ahead to Table 21.2). Sometimes they may be just one facet of a more complex, heterogeneous phenotype. Consequently, pharmacotherapies for cognitive problems in one disorder (say, dementia) may not so neatly extrapolate to those of another (say, ADHD). Cognitive problems may be profound and all-encompassing (as in dementia, some developmental disorders, or schizophrenia), artifactual (as in depression-related cognitive dysfunction (formerly called pseudodementia)), or subtle (as might occur in anxiety disorders or high-functioning patients with mood disorders).

Let us begin with some practical definitions regarding key components of cognition, as reviewed in Table 21.1 at the end of this chapter. Hierarchical models of cognitive functioning in general are often described as a pyramid (depicted in Figure 21.1) in which arousal and attention stand as prerequisite functions for target detection, comprehension, and sustained attention (vigilance); attention also depends on processing speed. Learning and memory are subservient to attentional processes, and all of these functions must precede planning, organizing, and logical reasoning.

The concept of executive function involves higher-level processing and manipulation of complex information. Its elements are described in more detail in Box 21.1.

Memory involves the encoding and retrieval of information; it entails short- and long-term components, verbal and nonverbal elements, and emotional and nonemotional content. Like attention, it may be influenced by numerous psychiatric (e.g., anxiety/fear, distress, depression) and somatic (e.g., pain, fatigue, hunger) factors. Long-term memory is traditionally subdivided into the domains summarized in Figure 21.1.

Figure 21.1. Subtypes of long-term memory.

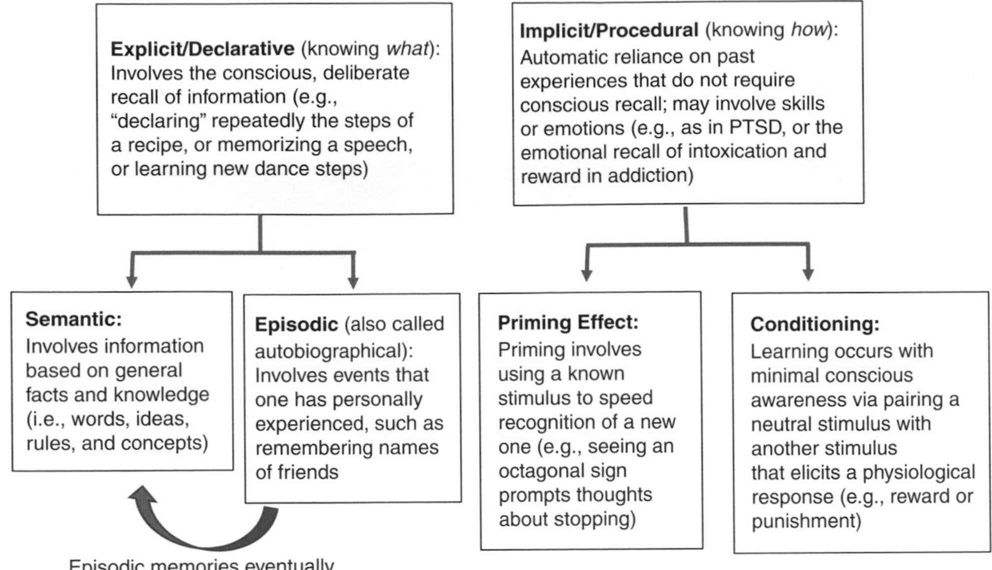

Box 21.1

The Components of Executive Function

The term "executive function" broadly encompasses an array of "top-down" higher cognitive processes that includes attentional control, planning and logical reasoning, decision-making, impulse control and cognitive inhibition, working memory, verbal fluency, organizational skills, and cognitive flexibility/set-shifting. It is fundamental to problem-solving, creativity, self-regulation, and coping and resilience. Cognitive neuroscientists often conceptualize executive function as involving three core components: inhibition and interference control, working memory, and cognitive flexibility. As discussed in Chapter 1, the DLPFC is the primary seat of executive functioning which, along with the VMPFC (the prefrontal seat of emotional processing), is balanced by "bottom-up" or "hot" cognitive functions driven by limbic and paralimbic structures.

A FORMAL MEASURES

For initial bedside assessments, the Montreal Cognitive Assessment (MoCA) is a quick (10–12 minute), easily administered brief neuropsychological performance test developed for assessment of dementia and mild cognitive impairment, capturing orientation, short-term/delayed recall, executive functioning/visuospatial processing, language, abstraction, and verbal fluency (Nasreddine et al., 2005). Scored from 0 to 30, scores >26 are considered normal; mild cognitive impairment subjects during field-testing had a mean score of 22.1, while those with Alzheimer's dementia had a mean score of 16.2. The Screen for Cognitive Impairment for Psychiatry (SCIP) is another relatively brief (approximately 15 minute) tool to assess working memory, immediate and delayed verbal recall, verbal fluency, and psychomotor speed (Purdon et al., 2005). The Folstein Mini-Mental Status Exam (MMSE) is a commonly used tool that is better-suited to capturing gross cognitive deficits (as in dementia) but is nonstandardized, poorly captures mild cognitive impairment, may overestimate cognitive deficits in older adults without dementia, and may be influenced by education and IQ (Naugle et al., 1989). Formal neuropsychological testing may be useful to follow up abnormalities on initial screens or to tease out more complex diagnostic issues.

Even within a given psychiatric disorder, cognitive variations may be evident that define clinical subgroups. For example, in bipolar disorder, some subgroups can demonstrate social cognition that is superior to healthy controls, while other groups may show select deficits in processing speed, attention, verbal learning and social cognition, while still others manifest global cognitive impairment nearly as profound and extensive as seen in schizophrenia (Burdick et al., 2014). In major depression, only about one-fifth of patients manifest

Figure 21.2 The pyramid of cognitive function.

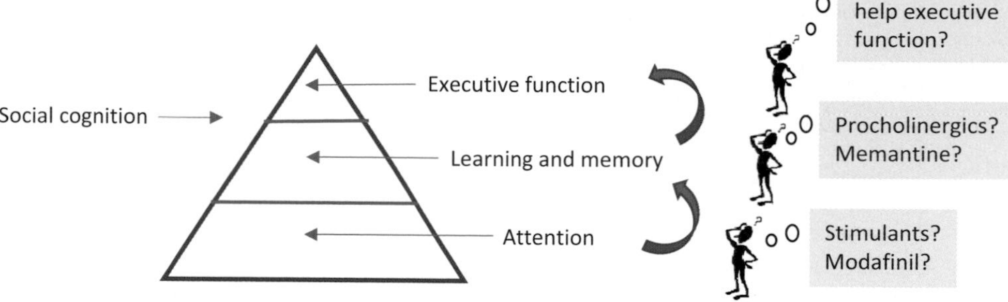

global impairment across most cognitive domains (Mohn and Rund, 2016). Table 21.2 at the end of this chapter provides a comparison of impairment across cognitive domains in schizophrenia and affective disorders.

Hierarchical models of cognitive functioning in general are often described as a pyramid (depicted in Figure 21.2) in which arousal and attention stand as prerequisite functions for target detection, comprehension, and sustained attention (vigilance); attention also depends on processing speed. Learning and memory are subservient to attentional processes, and all of these functions must precede planning, organizing, and logical reasoning.

In the parlance of cognitive neuroscience, general cognitive ability, often termed "g" or "g factor" broadly connotes general mental ability and is thought to account for about 40–50% of interindividual variability across diverse cognitive tasks that are thought to be inter-related. For clinicians, there are a number of implications for accurately defining cognitive domains:

- Patients who complain of problems in a particular domain (such as "memory" or "attention") may be identifying an altogether different kind of problem than they are perceiving (such as, performance anxiety or problems with set-shifting)
- Patients with cognitive complaints such as executive dysfunction may seek treatment for "ADD" when in fact medications that can improve attentional processing may not necessarily help deficits in executive function, memory or other domains subservient to attention
- Studies that assess "cognitive effects" of psychotropic drugs (either beneficial or adverse) may actually assess only narrow cognitive functions (such as processing speed) or broad constructs (such as "g") without using validated measures. The digit symbol substitution test (DSST), a subcomponent of the Wechsler Adult Intelligence Scale, is among the more widely used measures of overall cognitive functioning inasmuch as it taps attention, processing speed, visuospatial motor skills, and correlates with everyday functional capabilities. For better or worse, it is considered more sensitive than specific in its ability to discern deficits in specific cognitive domains.

Self-reported cognitive function also may not reliably capture true functioning as accurately as can performance-based tasks (which may be more time-consuming or require more resources as a secondary outcome measure in a clinical trial than may be feasible). In other words, just because a patient reports that they are having subjective problems with attention or memory does not necessarily mean that they are having objective cognitive deficits.

B CLINICAL ASSESSMENT OF COGNITIVE COMPLAINTS

The following general concepts may be useful in assessing cognitive complaints:

- Recognize that subjective cognitive complaints may not necessarily accurately reflect objective cognitive deficits
- Clarify subjective complaints with respect to timing, onset, and persistent versus episodic presentations
- Identify psychiatric or medical problems that can directly cause cognitive complaints (depression, anxiety, psychosis, dementia). Pay particular attention to parsing the timing of symptoms (e.g., ADD is a childhood disorder that persists into adulthood in about half of cases; de novo adult-onset ADD as a valid construct is controversial)
- Determine whether cognitive deficits may be resulting from any current medications (antihistamines, anticholinergics, topiramate), alcohol, or other substances (e.g., opiates, cannabis)

- Particularly if and when cognitive complaints (such as subjective memory deficits) track poorly alongside symptoms of an established or suspected psychiatric disorder, attempt to document and quantify objective (performance-based) cognitive deficits using a bedside assessment tool
- Choose pharmacotherapies for mood, anxiety or psychotic disorders that minimize adverse cognitive effects, as feasible
- Consider the role for targeted pharmacotherapy interventions intended to diminish or ameliorate cognitive symptoms, as appropriate

Tip

Topiramate is associated with reversible, dose-related memory and language processing deficits in 10% or more of treated patients across diagnoses (i.e., migraine, epilepsy, binge eating). Case reports suggest that adjunctive donepezil may help mitigate the extent of cognitive problems (Wheeler, 2006).

Tip

Amantadine often can counteract extrapyramidal adverse effects from antipsychotics as effectively as benztropine or trihexyphenidyl but without incurring anticholinergic effects, in turn potentially sparing adverse cognitive consequences.

C COGNITIVE DYSFUNCTION IN MOOD DISORDERS

At least half of adults with bipolar disorder complain of attentional or other cognitive problems, although interestingly there tends to be a poor correlation between patients' subjective cognitive complaints and objectively measured cognitive deficits (Burdick et al., 2005). Depression slows cognitive processing and disrupts executive functioning (hence the challenge for cognitive therapists who attempt to guide depressed patients to see things from alternative points of view when examining cognitive distortions). Patients even with low-grade depression or anxiety who sometimes self-diagnose ADD, perceiving a sense of inefficient attention, disengagement, or being easily distracted, may be recognizing the cognitive stigmata of depression, and at the very least warrant a careful assessment for coincident depressive or other affective features before one can attribute attentional complaints in the context of depression to anything other than the mood disorder itself.

A minority of psychotropic drugs relevant to treating depression can cause or exacerbate cognitive complaints – mainly, antihistaminergic (e.g., some SGAs, mirtazapine, trazodone, hydroxyzine) or anticholinergic drugs (e.g., tricyclics, paroxetine) or benzodiazepines, so-called "Z"-drugs, or other hypnotics. SSRIs, SNRIs, MAOIs and bupropion are largely (at worst) neutral with respect to adverse cognitive effects and if anything, may be expected to improve cognitive function by virtue of improving depression. In particular, the novel serotonergic agent vortioxetine was studied for its potential pro-cognitive effect using a statistical design that controlled for the effects of vortioxetine on depressive symptoms while showing an independent effect on processing speed, as measured using the DSST (McIntyre et al., 2016). Recall from Chapter 3, Box 3.9, the concept of pseudospecificity, and concerns about drawing possible misleading conclusions that a drug uniquely improves a nonspecific symptom within a broader symptom constellation (e.g., sertraline can improve insomnia in the context of treating depression – but there is no evidence of its broader sedative-hypnotic effects for other conditions). In the case of vortioxetine in MDD, McIntyre et al. (2016) elegantly averted the hazards of an otherwise pseudospecific observation by using path analysis (an extension of multiple regression) to demonstrate that changes in DSST were not simply mediated by changes in depression symptom score – i.e., cognitive improvement was not merely an artifact of treating depression.

We might ask, "Can some psychotropic medications directly enhance cognitive function, or is improvement in cognitive function more often a pseudospecific artifact of treating a broader clinical syndrome?" This issue is discussed in Box 21.2.

Baune and colleagues (2018) performed a meta-analysis of

Tip

Practice effects refer to the neuropsychological phenomenon in which repeated learning efforts result in greater fluency - limiting the confidence with which one can attribute an observed alleged cognitive benefit of a drug as opposed to the sheer repetition of a testing procedure.

Box 21.2

Pseudospecificity Revisited: Cognitive Dysfunction and Nootropic Drug Effects

"Nootropic" effects refer to the ability of a drug to enhance cognitive function. Psychostimulants are sometimes suggested to possess nootropic effects: for example, in healthy volunteers, methylphenidate has been shown to enhance implicit/procedural memory (Klinge et al., 2018), while modafinil demonstrably improves planning and working memory (Müller et al., 2013) and reaction time (Turner et al., 2003). However, in schizophrenia, methylphenidate increases perseverative errors and worsens overall cognitive disorganization (Szeszko et al., 1999), and findings regarding the possible pro-cognitive effects of modafinil in schizophrenia are mixed (Turner et al., 2004b). In patients with alcohol-related cognitive deficits, modafinil may improve short-term memory but not planning and selective attention (Joos et al., 2013). Vortioxetine appears to improve attentional processing in MDD but not in adult ADHD (Biederman et al., 2019).

Psychopharmacologists must therefore ask, when is it reasonable to consider attentional complaints as free-standing phenomena potentially amenable to any possibly nootropic drug that could, say, enhance processing speed, or, when is their contextual boundary (such as ADHD versus schizophrenia versus alcohol use disorders) critical for anticipating pharmacotherapy outcomes? The answers are likely complex, patient-specific, and probably ones for which broad class effects cannot be taken for granted.

Box 21.3

Cognitive Function and the $5HT_7$ Receptor

Serotonergic $5HT_7$ receptors in the CNS are located throughout the cortex, as well as the hypothalamus and thalamus. Preclinical studies suggest that $5HT_7$ antagonism may influence learning and memory, as well as modulate circadian rhythms and regulate inhibitory neurons that in turn regulate serotonergic activity in the dorsal raphe nucleus.

DSST changes during antidepressant RCTs for MDD across 72 published studies. As shown in Figure 21.3, most robust, and significant, differences were observed with vortioxetine versus placebo and sertraline versus nortriptyline.

Psychotropic drugs with $5HT_7$ antagonism are regarded as viable candidates for improving cognitive function. Vortioxetine and lurasidone are two prominent such examples from among many others. Relative binding affinities at the $5HT_7$ receptor across varied psychotropic medications are presented in Box 21.4.

Procholinergics. Studies of acetylcholinesterase inhibitors (AChIs) in mood disorders have focused mainly on adjunctive use in older adult mood disorder populations. Among those with MDD, a review of four RCTs found that adjunctive donepezil improved global cognition at one year but not two years, while RCTs of adjunctive galantamine found no discernible benefit either for cognitive or depressive symptoms (McDermott and

Figure 21.3 Meta-analysis of changes in DSST (effect sizes) with antidepressants across MDD RCTs. Based on meta-analysis by Baune et al., 2018.

Agent/comparator	g (95% CI)
Vortioxetine vs. placebo	0.34 (0.18, 0.49)
Duloxetine vs. placebo	0.13 (−0.03, 0.28)
Sertraline vs. placebo	−0.17 (−0.57, 0.22)
Citalopram vs. placebo	−0.04 (−0.33, 0.26)
Escitalopram vs. placebo	−0.25 (−0.57, 0.06)
Phenelzine vs. placebo	−0.02 (−0.52, 0.48)
Nortriptyline vs. placebo	0.01 (−0.56, 0.58)
Vortioxetine vs. duloxetine	0.13 (−0.03, 0.28)
Fluoxetine vs. sertraline	−0.27 (−0.53, −0.01)
Sertraline vs. nortriptyline	0.52 (0.20, 0.85)
Fluoxetine vs. desipramine	−0.26 (−1.24, 0.72)
Phenelzine vs. nortriptyline	−0.03 (−0.53, 0.47)

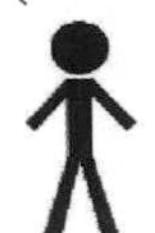
Isn't bupropion good for attention? Putative dopamine agonist, and all that?

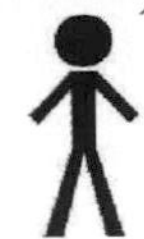
As a matter of fact, there are RCT data showing efficacy for bupropion to improve ADHD symptoms in adult ADHD patients (Wilens et al., 2001, 2005a), and even open trial data in those with histories of comorbid bipolar disorder (and with no reactivation or worsening of mania symptoms!) (Wilens et al., 2003b). A Cochrane Database review of four RCTs determined an overall medium effect size (g = –0.50) for improving ADHD symptom severity (Verbeeck et al., 2017).

Except nobody's looked much at attentional processing as a secondary outcome measure with bupropion in MDD RCTs.

Box 21.4

$5HT_7$ Receptor Binding Affinities Across Antipsychotics, Antidepressants, and Anxiolytics

Agent	Ki (nM)
Lurasidone	0.495
Pimozide	0.5
Brexpiprazole	3.7
Ziprasidone	6–9.3
Risperidone	6.60
Aripiprazole	9.3–39
Asenapine	9.9
Amisulpride	11.5
Clozapine	17.95
Vortioxetine	19
Amoxapine	41
Maprotiline	50

Agent	Ki (nM)
Loxapine	88
Amitriptyline	92.8-123
Olanzapine	105-365
Paliperidone	105-365
Cariprazine	111
Clomipramine	127
Mirtazapine	265
Quetiapine	307
Buspirone	375-381
Haloperidol	377.2
Imipramine	>1000

Gray, 2012). Galantamine is a relatively weak AChI but a potent modulator of nicotinic receptors (Woodruff-Pak et al., 2002). Adjunctive donepezil appears inferior to placebo for averting progression from mild cognitive impairment to dementia in MDD patients (Reynolds et al., 2011).

D COGNITIVE DYSFUNCTION IN BIPOLAR DISORDER

Data exist regarding possible pro-cognitive effects of psychotropic medications mainly from secondary analysis of RCTs designed with primary outcomes focusing on noncognitive aspects of psychopathology (e.g., improvement in depression or anxiety). Findings may be summarized as follows:

Lamotrigine – Post hoc analyses from two pooled RCTs of lamotrigine for relapse prevention in bipolar I disorder examined changes from baseline subjective cognitive complaints during the initial 8–16 week open-label stabilization phase; significant improvements were noted from baseline (Khan et al., 2004). Notably, although cognitive improvements correlated with improvements in depression symptoms, subjective cognitive improvements remained significant while controlling for changes in MADRS depression scores, suggesting a possible inherent pro-cognitive effect.

Lurasidone – One of the few RCTs devoted to examining cognitive function was a six-week randomized comparison of open lurasidone (n = 17) versus

ECT is believed to cause mainly retrograde amnesia, but can some patients develop anterograde amnesia?

Meta-analyses show that retrograde amnesia from ECT usually diminishes shortly after the last treatment. Anterograde amnesia is rare but may be related to age or underlying disease as well as ECT technical parameters (e.g., bilateral lead placement). There are small preliminary RCTs suggesting a possible lowered risk for delayed memory deficits after ECT when patients receive galantamine (8 mg/day) (Matthews et al., 2013) or donepezil (Prakash et al., 2006), and case reports of benefit with rivastigmine.

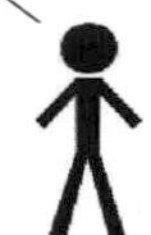

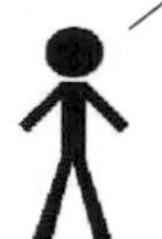

treatment as usual (n = 17) in euthymic bipolar patients; those randomized to lurasidone (mean dose = 48 mg/day) had significantly greater improvement in global cognitive functioning ($d = 0.46$) – although no specific individual subcomponent domains of cognitive function differed from placebo, perhaps due to underpowering of the study to detect more than a global effect (Yatham et al., 2017).

Withania somnifera – Also known as ashwaganda, or Indian ginseng. An eight-week double-blind RCT in 53 patients found that 500 mg/day was well-tolerated and superior to placebo on digit span ($d = 0.51$) (i.e., auditory working memory), an executive function test of stimulus discrimination ($d = 0.62$), and had a somewhat lesser but significant impact on social cognition ($d = 0.26$) (Chengappa et al., 2013).

Pramipexole – As discussed in Chapter 13, this D_2/D_3 agonist useful in TRD and bipolar depression has also been a focus of investigation in efforts to treat cognitive complaints in bipolar disorder. An eight-week double-blind RCT in 50 affectively stable bipolar outpatients found no overall benefit for cognitive function except in a small subgroup of "strictly euthymic" patients (free from even low-grade affective symptoms) in whom attentional processing (digit span) and executive function (Stroop color–word interference) were better than placebo (Burdick et al., 2012).

Creatine monohydrate. As mentioned in Chapter 11, the role of creatine in energy metabolism has prompted interest in its potential effects on neuronal plasticity and enhanced cognitive function. As a post hoc analysis to a negative RCT of creatine monohydrate in bipolar depression (fixed dose = 6 g/day), pre- and post-treatment cognitive testing in a subgroup (n = 18) noted significant improvement in verbal fluency, but no other neuropsychological domains (Toniolo et al., 2017).

E COGNITIVE DYSFUNCTION IN SCHIZOPHRENIA

Schizophrenia involves diffuse cognitive deficits in multiple domains, as summarized in Table 21.2. It was at one time thought that SGAs might exert benefit for the cognitive symptoms of schizophrenia, but by and large this has not proven to be the case. In fact, in the CATIE schizophrenia trial, only clinically small (though statistically significant) neurocognitive improvements were noted after two and six months with olanzapine, quetiapine, risperidone, and perphenazine (no differences among groups), but by 18 months improvement in cognitive function was unexpectedly greatest in subjects taking the FGA perphenazine (Keefe et al., 2007).

Emotion perception was unimproved by any antipsychotics used in CATIE (Penn et al., 2009). Notably, SGAs have been shown in several meta-analyses to cause fewer adverse cognitive effects than do FGAs (e.g., Keefe et al., 2004, Bilder et al., 2002, Good et al., 2005), but not to improve any dimensions of cognition from baseline in adult schizophrenia patients. From their perspective, patients with schizophrenia or other psychosis-spectrum disorders may misconstrue cognitive dysfunction as necessarily equating to ADD, and reflexively request stimulants, as described in Clinical Vignette 21.1.

CLINICAL VIGNETTE 21.1

Donny was a 25-year-old man with schizotypal personality disorder involving extensive preoccupations with the occult and instances of thought blocking and impoverished thinking. He complained of trouble focusing his attention and an inability to remember names and details, which he attributed to a suspected ill-defined underlying neurological problem. He sought consultation requesting stimulants in the hope that would improve his concentration and memory.

If Donny had hallucinations or discrete delusions, a formal diagnosis of schizophrenia would likely be more compelling, as would a conceptualization of his cognitive problems as being inherent to a schizophrenia spectrum disorder. Though he may self-identify his problems as fundamentally involving attention, and believe that a stimulant would be appropriate, a more detailed assessment would likely point to his psychotic-like experiences as accounting more directly for his cognitive problems than either a diagnosis of ADHD or an occult/underlying neurological problem.

When considering the potential impact on cognition in schizophrenia of psychotropic medications other than antipsychotics, the clinical trials literature indicates the following:

Modafinil. One RCT in 20 chronic schizophrenia patients found that modafinil dosed at 200 mg/day improved attentional set-shifting and short-term verbal memory span, and slowed response latency on spatial planning tasks, though no effect was observed on stop-signal performance (Turner et al., 2004b).

Procholinergics. Studies of procholinergic drugs ((i.e., AChIs), including donepezil, galantamine, and rivastigmine) added to antipsychotics suggest weak effects, if any, for treating cognitive symptoms in schizophrenia. In a review of nine RCTs, an overall significant benefit was seen on processing speed (g = −0.52, 95% CI = −0.79 to −0.25, p = 0.0002); however placebo significantly outperformed AChIs in attention and no significant drug–placebo differences were observed in working memory (Santos et al., 2018). A later review of 11 studies in schizophrenia (Hsu et al., 2018) more specifically found no effect on any cognitive function domains with galantamine (five RCTs), rivastigmine (one RCT), or donepezil (three RCTs), although one small (n = 13) open trial with donepezil found significant improvements from baseline in set-shifting, learning ability, and attention (Chung et el., 2009).

Putative NMDA receptor modulators. Studied drugs in this category include memantine, *D*-cycloserine, glycine, *D*-serine, sodium benzoate, and *l*-carnosine. As collectively reviewed in a meta-analysis by Hsu et al. (2018), the following observations can be made:

- Seven trials involving memantine (including both open and randomized blinded designs) found modest but significant positive findings on composite memory measures in clozapine-refractory schizophrenia patients (d = 0.30) as well as several short-term (six-week) studies reporting improvements on MMSE performance scores.
- Two RCTs (from 8–16 weeks) with *D*-cycloserine or glycine found no differences from placebo in cognitive performance, though an open trial of *D*-serine dosed at 60 mg/kg was associated with improvement across multiple cognitive domains, except for working memory.
- A six-week RCT of sodium benzoate (which inhibits *D*-amino acid oxidase (DAAO)) in 52 schizophrenia patients found that dosing at 1 g PO qday was superior to placebo in improving processing speed and visual learning and memory.
- The antioxidant *l*-carnosine, dosed at 2 mg PO qDay over three months in 75 symptomatically stable schizophrenia patients, found several indicators of better executive functioning than with placebo (namely, nonreversal set-shifting, strategic efficiency, and fewer perseverative errors).

Dehydroepiandrosterone (DHEA). One 12-week RCT found no impact of DHEA on any cognitive domains (reviewed by Hsu et al., 2018).

Raloxifene. The selective estrogen receptor modulator raloxifene dosed at 60 mg/day has been shown preliminarily to improve attention, processing speed, and memory in postmenopausal female schizophrenia patients (Huerta-Ramos et al., 2014).

Pregnenolone. The neurosteroid pregnenolone was studied (dose = 50 mg/day) targeting cognition in recent-onset schizophrenia (n = 60) during an eight-week RCT versus placebo (Kreinin et al., 2017). Significantly greater improvements in visual attention were found with pregnenolone than placebo (d = 0.42), as well as significant improvements in sustained attention and spatial working memory.

N-Acetylcysteine. A review of seven RCTs found significant effects for *N*-acetylcysteine over placebo by 24 weeks in improving working memory in schizophrenia (g = 0.56, p = 0.005), while an effect on processing speed was nonsignificant (Yolland et al., 2019).

α7 Nicotinic receptor agonists. Agonists and positive allosteric modulators of α_7 nicotinic acetylcholine receptors are conceptually appealing targets for the possible treatment of cognitive problems in both schizophrenia and dementia, among other conditions. Nicotine is itself a nonselective agonist at the nicotinic ACh receptor, and is known to improve sensory deficits in schizophrenia. A number of α_7 nicotinic ACh receptor partial agonists have been the focus of investigation but most efforts have been confined to

Figure 21.4 Meta-analysis comparing relative effect sizes across pharmacotherapies for adult ADHD. Based on meta-analysis by Cortese et al. (2018).

Agent	g (95% CI)
Amphetamines	−0.79 (−0.99 to −0.58)
Atomoxetine	−0.45 (−0.58 to −0.32)
Bupropion	−0.46 (−0.85 to −0.07)
Methylphenidate	−0.49 (−0.64 to −0.35)
Modafinil	0.16 (−0.28 to 0.59)

−1 −0.5 0 0.5 1

Favors drug ← → Favors placebo

preclinical studies. Most clinical trials in humans have failed to demonstrate a benefit for cognitive function, either due to unexpectedly high placebo response rates, cross-reactivity and nonselectivity over $5HT_3$ receptor targets, or toxicity from positive allosteric modulators. The antismoking drug varenicline is a nicotinic receptor partial agonist (binding to the $\alpha_4\beta_2$ receptor) and a potent α_7 receptor full agonist; a meta-analysis of four RCTs focusing on cognitive dysfunction in schizophrenia found no significant differences from placebo in overall cognitive functioning, attention, executive function, or processing speed (nor were differences evident in effects on psychosis, and smoking status was not a moderator of outcomes in studies of cognition) (Tanzer et al., 2020).

F ADULT ADHD

Remember old-fashioned analog radios? You had to dial in a station that was set against the backdrop of staticky background noise. High quality target detection requires a strong signal-to-noise (S:N) ratio, as illustrated in Figure 21.5. The DLPFC is like an analog radio searching for a salient signal. In ADD, the DLPFC picks up too much background noise (distraction) that overshadows the intensity of the signal (that is, the stimulus we want to focus on). Psychostimulants boost the DLPFC's ability to detect the signal, improving the S:N ratio and voilà: patients report an almost immediate "organizing" effect as background noise no longer competes so vividly with signal detection.

Figure 21.5 Analog radio and signal-to-noise ratio

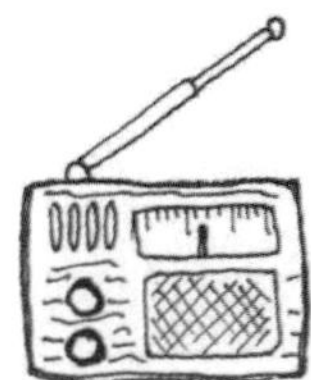

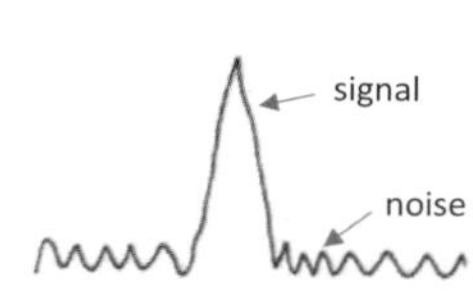

When considering attentional problems in adults to be their own disorder, one must assure that cognitive complaints are not better accounted for by a different condition, as noted above. Consensus among nosologists remains that ADHD is, by definition, a childhood disorder that may persist into adulthood in up to half of individuals – although there are birth cohort and other prospective studies to suggest, with some controversy, that adult-onset ADHD may be a valid and distinct diagnostic construct (Caye et al., 2016).

A network meta-analysis of pharmacotherapies for adult ADHD found medium effects with most agents and a large effect with amphetamine, though mostly with overlapping confidence internals across different studied compounds (Cortese et al., 2018), as illustrated in Figure 21.4. Data were unavailable in adult ADHD for guanfacine or clonidine.

Psychostimulants remain the usual core treatment for ADHD and can broadly be divided into amphetamine-based and methylphenidate-based. There are more pharmacodynamic similarities than differences between these two major subclasses – although with respect to dosing, as noted in Chapter 9, amphetamine is about twice as potent as methylphenidate (i.e., 1 mg of methylphenidate is equivalent to about 0.5 mg of amphetamine). We are aware of no direct comparative studies showing superiority of one compound over the other. Studies in *adult* ADHD in general are more extensive with amphetamine than methylphenidate. A Cochrane Database review found a large effect size for amphetamine in reducing ADHD symptom severity across 13 RCTs ($g = -0.90$) (Castells et al., 2018), while another meta-analysis found a lower effect size with methylphenidate in adult ADHD ($g = -0.49$) (Cortese et al., 2018). Across 185 RCTs in child or adolescent ADHD, a larger effect size was noted for methylphenidate ($g = -0.77$) in a Cochrane Database review (Storebø et al., 2015). A comparative analysis by Arnold (2000), focusing mostly on a child and adolescent ADHD literature, noted the following possible differences, of at-most subtle magnitude:

- In the setting of comorbid Tourette's disorder, overall efficacy may be somewhat greater with methylphenidate (as well as a lesser exacerbation of tics)
- Amphetamine may have a somewhat greater effect on oppositional/conduct-disordered symptoms such as aggression, irritability, and explosiveness
- Amphetamine may show more day-to-day consistency of response

- Some studies report more anorexia and more sleep disruption with amphetamine than methylphenidate
- Methylphenidate has been associated with more depression/apathy than seen with amphetamine in some reports.

Importantly, crossover trials have shown that a nonresponse to either agent does not meaningfully diminish the likelihood of response to the other; indeed, an overall response rate of >87% has been noted if both agents are successively tried following nonresponse to an initial one (Arnold, 2000). Differences among psychostimulants with respect to long-acting delivery systems are discussed in Box 21.5.

Stimulants and Executive Function

In the context of treating ADHD, there are compelling data that psychostimulants, particularly lisdexamfetamine, can improve symptoms of executive dysfunction. Notably, in adult AHDH, a 10-week multisite fixed-dose comparison of lisdexamfetamine 30 mg/day, 50 mg/day, 70 mg/day, or placebo found a significantly greater improvement across all active drug doses than with placebo using a composite measure of executive function with an effect size of 0.74 (Adler et al., 2013). Executive function improvements were evidenced by both clinician- and self-rated assessments (Weisler et al., 2017). Adolescents and young adults receiving amphetamine or methylphenidate have demonstrated significantly better sustained attention and verbal learning as compared to untreated ADHD subjects, but less robust effects on organization and planning, working memory and set-shifting (Biederman et al., 2008b). Elsewhere in the child ADHD literature, methylphenidate use has been shown to improve spatial working memory (Barnett et al., 2001).

Modafinil. Modafinil was shown to treat ADHD symptoms in youths across three RCTs (Wigal et al.,

Box 21.5

Long-Acting Stimulant Delivery Systems

There are several long-acting formulations of psychostimulants:

- Lisdexamfetamine is a molecule composed of dextroamphetamine bound to lysine moieties that render the active drug into an inactive pro-drug; free dextroamphetamine is then liberated after its lysine moieties are hydrolyzed in the GI tract. Dosing ranges from 10–70 mg/day.
- An osmotic-release oral delivery system (OROS) formulation of methylphenidate (Concerta®) uses a rigid tablet within a semi-permeable outer membrane through which water is absorbed, extruding the active drug into the GI tract, providing approximately 12 hours' bioavailability. Dosing is 18-54 mg once daily, with a maximum of 54 mg/day in children and adolescents and 72 mg/day in adults. 18 mg of OROS methylphenidate is approximately equivalent to 15 mg of methylphenidate.
- A time-released formulation of high-dose methylphenidate (Adhansia XR®), dosed from 25 to 85 mg, exerts an effect for up to 16 hours. Another time-released methylphenidate product, (Jornay PM®), dosed at 20, 40, 60, 80, or 100 mg, is administered in the early evening and exerts its effects via a delayed and extended release beginning the next morning.
- Methylphenidate transdermal system (Daytrana®) is a once-daily patch that can be worn for up nine hours, usually applied on the hip. It delivers an hourly methylphenidate dose of either 1.1 mg (10 mg patch, containing 27.5 mg/patch), 1.6 mg (15 mg patch, containing 41.3 mg/patch), 2.2 mg (20 mg patch, containing 55 mg/patch), or 3.3 mg (30 mg patch, containing 82.5 mg/patch). Dosing usually begins with one 10 mg patch/day that can be increased weekly as needed. Dosing is based on pediatric study groups and is considered an "off-label use in adults," although there are a small number of published open trials in adult ADHD.

Impulse control is an executive function. Would impulsive borderline patients benefit from amphetamine or methylphenidate if they do not also have ADHD?

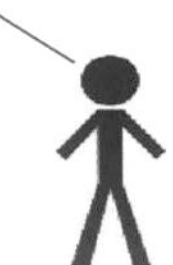

Good question and hard to know in the absence of formal studies. Remember from Chapter 20 that the literature on stimulants for executive function in borderline personality disorder is very limited. They may exacerbate vulnerability to psychosis and carry addiction risk. On the other hand, provisional data do suggest possible benefit at least from a single-dose laboratory study of methylphenidate in decision-making (Gvirts et al., 2018).

2006) but in 2006 failed to achieve FDA approval for that indication due to several observed cases of serious cutaneous reactions, including Stevens–Johnson syndrome. In adult ADHD patients, modafinil has been shown in RCTs to improve inhibitory control, in turn leading to improved memory (memory span, visual memory) and spatial planning, slowed response latency, and decreased impulsive responding (Turner et al., 2004a) – however, as noted in Figure 21.4, its observed effect size in adult ADHD is small.

G STIMULANTS AND EMOTIONAL LABILITY

ADHD may inherently involve emotional dysregulation (Shaw et al., 2014) – making it fair to ask whether stimulants are more likely to improve or worsen emotional dysregulation. A review of five RCTs in both child and adult ADHD by Posner et al. (2014) uniformly found improvement in measures of emotion regulation in studies lasting up to 24 weeks, with effect sizes ranging from d = 0.28–0.40. (The largest observed effect size on emotional dysregulation was with OROS methylphenidate (0.75 mg/kg dosing) in adult ADHD (d = 0.70); Reimherr et al., 2007.) Irritability exacerbated by stimulants was noted to occur in "a small minority" of subjects across trials. A later meta-analysis focusing on the relationship between stimulant or atomoxetine use and emotional lability solely in adult ADHD (nine RCTs) found an overall effect size of g = –0.41 (95% CI = –0.57 to –0.25) (Moukhtarian et al., 2017).

The issue of physiological tolerance or tachyphylaxis to stimulants is discussed in Box 21.6.

Atomoxetine. Comparable to the findings reported in Figure 21.4 by Cortese et al. (2018), a separate meta-analysis of 13 RCTs with atomoxetine in adult ADHD found an overall significant difference and medium effect size (g = –0.45) as compared to placebo, as well as relative to measures of inattention specifically (g = –0.42), and a significant but somewhat lesser magnitude of impact on impulsivity/hyperactivity (g = –0.36) (Ravishankar et al., 2016). A review of five head-to-head comparative trials of atomoxetine versus stimulants for ADHD found greater improvement and higher response rates with OROS methylphenidate than atomoxetine, and comparability in ADHD symptom ratings between atomoxetine versus methylphenidate immediate release or versus extended-release mixed amphetamine salts (Gibson et al., 2006). While the manufacturer advises initial atomoxetine dosing at 40 mg/day for three days, then escalation to a target dose of 80 mg/day and a possible maximum dose of 100 mg/day after an additional two to four weeks, naturalistic studies suggest that a little over one-third of adult ADHD patients are underdosed when treated under ordinary

Box 21.6

What to Do When Tolerance to Stimulants Occurs

Both amphetamine and methylphenidate can lead to pharmacological tolerance, hypothesized to result at least in part from increased density of striatal DA transporter receptors (Wang et al., 2009), correlated with duration of drug exposure. Long-term studies in pediatric ADHD suggest that the need for an approximate 25% increase in stimulant dosing over one year is common (e.g., Wilens et al., 2005b). There has been surprisingly little empirical study of specific strategies to manage tolerance to stimulants in ADHD patients, leaving most recommendations as based more on opinion than systematic empirical evidence. Such strategies include: (a) optimizing/maximizing doses, (b) supratherapeutic stimulant dosing, (c) drug holidays with eventual reintroductions after one month or more, (d) replacement of one stimulant with another, and (e) augmentation of an existing stimulant with a nonstimulant agent such as atomoxetine, bupropion, or an α agonist. Anecdotal and/or retrospective observations in the child/adolescent ADHD literature suggest that after either substitution of a different medication or time off from the current stimulant, efficacy of the original drug is often evident upon subsequent retrial (Ross et al., 2002).

So what do stimulants do in people without ADHD, besides increase energy?

A review by Bagot and Kaminer (2014) found that modafinil can improve reaction time, logical reasoning, and problem-solving. Methylphenidate can improve performance of attention-based tasks and reduce planning latency. Amphetamine improves consolidation of information and recall.

conditions (mean observed dose was 68.5 mg/day), most often occurring in women and those who had undergone fewer treatments with other ADHD medications prior to starting atomoxetine (Kabul et al., 2015).

Antidepressants. Among traditional monoaminergic antidepressants, tricyclics have been studied extensively in child and adolescent ADHD. In particular, as noted in a Cochrane Database review, desipramine (for which more RCTs exist than for other TCAs) has been shown to exert a large effect based on assessments by parents ($g = -1.42$) or teachers ($g = -0.97$) (Otasowie et al., 2014). As noted in Figure 21.4, bupropion was shown to have a medium effect size for targeting overall symptoms in adult ADHD. And, as noted in Box 21.2, while vortioxetine has demonstrated benefits for attentional processing in MDD, RCTs in ADHD have been negative.

Dasotraline. Dasotraline is a triple reuptake inhibitor of monoamines (serotonin, norepinephrine, and dopamine) that was originally submitted by its manufacturer for FDA consideration as a treatment for ADHD, based on acute (four-week) RCT positive findings in both child and adult ADHD. In adults, dosing at 8 mg/day (but not 4 mg/day) separated significantly from placebo on the primary endpoint measure of a standardized ADHD rating scale (Koblan et al., 2015). In children, an RCT found that 4 mg/day but not 2 mg/day improved ADHD symptoms. Based on the existing data the FDA declined to approve an indication for ADHD and requested further studies from the manufacturer to better clarify both efficacy and safety. Appetite suppression was noted as an adverse effect across ADHD clinical trials, prompting a separate effort by the manufacturer to pursue a possible indication in binge-eating disorder.

α Agonists. α_2 Agonists such as clonidine or guanfacine can improve cognitive functioning in ADD/ADHD by increasing noradrenergic outflow from the locus coeruleus to the PFCx. Clonidine and guanfacine are the α agonists that have been best studied in ADHD, and the literature is again more extensive in children/adolescents than adults. Also, as noted in Chapter 19, agents that bind more selectively to α_{2A} than α_{2B} or α_{2C} subreceptors e.g., guanfacine) may be less prone to cause sedation. A meta-analysis of 11 trials using clonidine in pediatric ADHD found a medium overall effect size ($d = 0.58$) (Connor et al., 1999), making it less impactful than the magnitude of effect for improving attentional symptoms seen with stimulants.

Tip

While stimulants can precipitate or exacerbate motor tics, α agonists can suppress them.

Amantadine. A limited RCT database, solely in pediatric ADHD, suggests possible value of the dopamine agonist amantadine (100–150 mg/day); a small (n = 40) six-week trial found comparable improvement to methylphenidate in parent and teacher ADHD symptom rating scales, although that study was not statistically powered for noninferiority (Mohammadi et al., 2010), and the absence of placebo-controlled trials or adult ADHD RCTs limits the evidence base for using amantadine in ADHD on a broader basis.

Memantine. A small database suggests value for memantine in adult ADHD. One RCT in 40 subjects found greater improvement than seen with placebo over six weeks on measures of inattention/memory, hyperactivity/restlessness, and impulsivity/emotional lability (Mohammadzadeh et al., 2019). Another small (n = 26) 12-week RCT found that adjunctive memantine was no better than placebo for improving executive function in adult ADHD when added to methylphenidate (Biederman et al., 2017).

So how is it that α_2 agonists can both increase attention yet cause sedation? And hypotension?

Seemingly counterintuitive, eh? Different regional targets and receptor subtypes. Agonism of presynaptic α_{2a} receptors increases sympathetic tone from the locus coeruleus to the cortex (specifically, the DLPFC), thereby increasing attention, while α_{2b} and α_{2c} agonism in the locus coeruleus causes sedation. And in the brainstem, α_{2a} agonism of presynaptic autoreceptors dampens sympathetic outflow, decreasing peripheral vascular resistance, and thus lowering blood pressure.

Gingko biloba. Touted for its possible pro-cognitive/memory-enhancing effects mostly from anecdotal reports, *Gingko biloba* (dosed from 80–120 mg/day) was found in one six-week RCT (n = 50) to be less effective than methylphenidate in improving child/adolescent ADHD symptoms (Salehi et al., 2010). Another adjunctive trial in pediatric ADHD found that *Gingko biloba* (n = 31) was better than placebo (n = 29) when added to methylphenidate (20–30 mg/day) for improving parent and teacher ADHD ratings of inattention (Shakibaei et al., 2015).

H DEMENTIA AND MAJOR COGNITIVE IMPAIRMENT

Pharmacotherapies for dementia aim to address not only cognitive deficits but also domains such as agitation, psychosis, and dysregulation of circadian rhythms. With respect to cognitive targets of treatment, the mainstays of therapy remain pro-cholinergic drugs and memantine. A meta-analysis and meta-regression involving 80 trials found approximately two fold greater efficacy in Parkinson's dementia or dementia with Lewy bodies than in Alzheimer's dementia or vascular dementia (Knight et al., 2018). Table 21.3 presents a summary of effect sizes reported across agents at successive time intervals based on that meta-analysis.

In patients with mild cognitive impairment, donepezil was shown in one multisite RCT to exert a small but significant improvement in cognitive function ratings as compared to placebo (Doody et al., 2009). A Cochrane Database review of 13 studies in Alzheimer's disease of mild, moderate, or severe intensity found better outcomes for cognitive function than with placebo at 26 weeks, but no difference in behavioral symptoms (Birks and Harvey, 2018).

When considering the utility of SGAs for cognitive symptoms of dementia, findings are largely unfavorable despite modest evidence for the utility of low-dose AGAs such as respiridone to manage psychosis or control agitation (Katz et al., 1999). A meta-analysis of 16 RCTs (involving aripiprazole, olanzapine, quetiapine, and risperidone versus placebo) found small effects (g <0.20) deemed not clinically meaningful on varied cognitive measures (Schneider et al., 2006). In the Clinical Antipsychotic Trials of Intervention Effectiveness-Alzheimer's Disease Study (CATIE-AD), subjects had deterioration in cognitive functioning over 36 months regardless of treatment intervention, and SGA use was associated with worse cognitive functioning than seen with placebo (Vigen et al., 2011). Randomized study drugs consisted of olanzapine (mean dose = 5.5 mg/day), risperidone (mean dose = 1.0 mg/day) or quetiapine (mean dose = 56.5 mg/day).

Elsewhere, although SSRIs have not shown much benefit for cognitive problems in dementia, one large RCT found significantly more improvement with citalopram than placebo to diminish agitation – however, citalopram recipients had more worsening than seen with placebo on measures of cognitive function (Porsteinsson et al., 2014). Yet, on the other hand, SSRI treatment of existing depression in patients with dementia has also been shown to lessen the negative effects of depression on cognitive function (Rozzini et al., 2010).

TAKE-HOME POINTS

- Cognitive dysfunction encompasses diverse phenomenology and unique contexts across psychiatric disorders.
- Assure proper assessment of subjective cognitive complaints relative to other forms of psychopathology that patients may sometimes misconstrue as synonymous with objective cognitive deficits.
- Attempt to minimize the impact of psychotropic agents that can cause or aggravate cognitive problems (notably, anticholinergics, antihistamines, sedative-hypnotics, topiramate).
- Recognize differences in attentional processing versus components of memory or executive dysfunction when characterizing the nature and extent of suspected cognitive problems.
- Consider the rationale for, and potential evidence base to support, pro-cognitive effects of certain psychotropic agents (e.g., vortioxetine, lurasidone) alongside the use of novel compounds and stimulant drugs for targeting suspected deficits in attentional processing and executive dysfunction.

Table 21.1 Major cognitive domains

Cognitive domain	Practical definition	Bedside tests
Processing speed	The time it takes to perform a mental task and process information	Trail-making, digit symbol substitution (DSST)
Attention	The ability to concentrate on a discrete stimulus and ignore other perceivable stimuli; often divided into *selective attention* (focusing on one stimulus from among several), *divided attention* (processing responses to two or more stimuli), *sustained attention* (focusing on one stimulus for an extended period of time), and *executive attention* (e.g., choosing from among varied responses in a conflict situation)	Digit span; continuous performance tasks (e.g., detecting a specific letter or number when presented with a series); trail-making (captures visual attention and task-switching)
Working memory	A component of short-term memory that involves temporarily holding multiple pieces of information in mind at the same time. Examples would include keeping score while rolling the dice during a board game, or remembering a shopping list while scanning for items when walking down a supermarket aisle	Memory span (e.g., reciting up to seven random numbers forward and backward)
Verbal fluency	Measures vocabulary size, lexical access speed, and inhibition ability; abnormalities may be relevant to numerous brain disorders, including dementia, schizophrenia, traumatic brain injury, Parkinson's disease, and developmental disorders, among others	Controlled oral word association tests (COWATs) are timed tests of category (semantic) fluency (e.g., "name as many animals as you can that are found in a zoo"), or letter (phonemic) fluency ("name as many things as you can that begin with the letter "f")
Social cognition	A psychological function involving people's capacity to encode, store, retrieve, and process information related to social interactions (e.g., emotion recognition, understanding etiquette, gestures, and inferences); may be impaired in schizophrenia, autism, and traumatic brain injury, among other disorders	Facial-affect recognition tasks, other normed tests of social inference (e.g., the Penn Emotional Acuity Test)

Table 21.2 Impaired cognitive domains across major psychiatric conditions

Disorder	Processing speed	Attention	Working memory	Verbal learning	Visual learning	Reasoning and problem-solving	Social cognition
Schizophrenia	Impaired	Impaired	Impaired	Impaired	Impaired	Impaired	Impaired
Bipolar disorder	+/- Impaired	Impaired	Moderately impaired	Impaired	Intact	Intact	+/- Impaired
Major depressive disorder	Impaired	Impaired	Intact	+/- Impaired [a]	+/- Impaired	+/- Impaired [b]	+/- Impaired [c]

[a] May be linked with slow processing speed (Zaremba et al., 2019)

[b] May be linked with slow processing speed (Mohn and Rund, 2016)

[c] May be linked with poor cognitive flexibility (Förster et al., 2018)

Table 21.3 Effect sizes for acetylcholinesterase inhibitors or memantine in dementia (g, 95% CI)

Agent	3 months	6 months	12 months
Donepezil 3–5 mg/day	1.15 (0.69–1.61)	1.52 (0.74–2.30)	–
Donepezil 10 mg/day	1.07 (0.91–1.23)	1.13 (0.94–1.33)	1.52 (0.38–2.66)
Galantamine	1.10 (0.83–1.36)	1.39 (0.79–2.00)	0.58 (0.27–0.90)
Rivastigmine	0.98 (0.32–1.63)	0.69 (0.43–0.95)	1.40 (1.12–1.68)
Memantine	0.65 (0.37–0.94)	0.40 (0.05–0.75)	0.41 (–0.44 to 1.26)

22 Putting It All Together

The perfect is the enemy of the good.

- Voltaire

We have, we hope, covered a large but not unwieldy swath of territory of practical relevance for the everyday clinician trying to make pharmacological decisions informed by evidence. As illustrated throughout the preceding pages, the availability of empirical data to guide treatment decisions varies greatly within and across disorders. It probably matters more that clinicians know *how to think empirically* – that is, knowing when, where, and how to look up information pertinent to a given case – rather than try to tackle the impossible task of comprehensively knowing the ever-changing clinical trials database for all disorders. Wisdom equally involves recognizing when evidence is lacking, prompting reliance on opinion, extrapolation, and plausible rationales – but not conflating those guideposts with an empirical database.

It is time now to cull the principles we have tried to illustrate and summarize what we would consider to be basic maxims for practical psychopharmacology.

A CHANGE ONLY ONE VARIABLE AT A TIME

Apart from making good general sense, this axiom also serves as an excellent starting point in any complex clinical case. Among its virtues, such a strategy imposes an element of reflective delay and deliberation, requiring both clinician and patient to resist their own limbically driven urges and temptations to make critical decisions with undue haste, or unwittingly inflict iatrogenic sources of confusion by making messy situations even messier. Changing one variable at a time also means allowing enough time to elapse in order to judge the effect of what one has just done before causing additional changes to the system. In any multivariate equation, holding all but one variable constant also can be one of the most powerful ways to leverage clarity out of complexity, letting ambiguities unfold and resolve without the added confusion of desperate and possibly capricious meddling.

However, there are times when changing only one variable at a time may not be feasible. In real-world practice, patients are seldom if ever treated under tightly controlled environments where all key moderators and mediators of outcome can be held constant so as to allow for more certain inferences about probable cause-and-effect relationships. Sometimes clinical urgency demands altering more than one pharmacological parameter at a time – as in the case of stopping a drug that has become inappropriate (such as an antidepressant during mania) or deleterious (such as a stimulant or MAOI in the setting of a hypertensive crisis). From a purely scientific perspective, it would be informative to stop an antidepressant in the setting of emerging suspected mania and simply observe whether signs of psychomotor activation spontaneously attenuate (suggesting a direct adverse drug effect, as opposed to a catalytic effect that should persist despite removal of the triggering agent); but, on a practical level, disaster could result from withholding an appropriate remedy for here-and-now severe symptoms. Therein lies the trade-off between gathering evidence and providing sensible and compassionate care. The pragmatic compromise often involves simply acknowledging to oneself and one's patient that cause-and-effect relationships may be hard to know with confidence, yet one must persevere nevertheless.

B IDENTIFY AND TRACK THE SPECIFIC TARGETS OF TREATMENT

Formal "measurement-based care" involves using standardized rating instruments to track symptom severity and changes over time, akin to the manner done in a clinical research trial. Without having some metric for tracking symptoms, it becomes nearly impossible to glean anything more than a gestalt or subjective impression about clinical status. However, on the downside of such an approach, everyday practitioners may not have received formal training in how to properly administer and score observer-based rating scales, and some measures can be time-consuming to rate. For practitioners, validated *self-rated* measures can become a true time-saver, fostering expedience and efficiency when reviewed during appointments, and flagging attention to the most critical and compelling facets of a complex problem.

Good care almost always should involve some objective measure by which one can track the recognized targets of treatment, whether those are full syndromes (e.g., major depression) or individual symptoms (e.g., insomnia, suicidal thinking, self-injury events, or episodes of alcohol or substance use). Even having patients track global symptoms (say, "anxiety") using a simple 10-point Likert or visual analogue scale provides useful information over time, especially when performed at regular intervals, when seeking to judge treatment effects. Such scales also can yield clues about timing and context (e.g., diurnal variation? relation to sleep or menstrual cycle?). Even more rudimentary, one could simply ask patients at each visit if they perceive a target symptom or condition to be "better," "the same," or "worse" than when previously seen, giving some longitudinal sense of the trajectory of improvement, or lack thereof. Tangible events such as panic attacks, days of substance use, or binge-eating episodes also lend themselves to simple quantification and tracking (e.g., number of events per week), in ways analogous to tracking number of headaches or seizures per unit time. If a medication is helping with a clinically meaningful effect (i.e., a presumably medium or large effect size), a reduction in events, or Likert scale scores, should give a reliable indication over a designated time period.

When reading the clinical trials literature, "global improvement" is often a secondary outcome in RCTs across many disorders. While it is a supportive construct, it imparts little information about what actually has or has not changed following a treatment intervention. Near the end of Chapter 1 we discussed identifying the intended goals and symptom targets of treatment before embarking on any pharmacotherapy regimen. The counterpoint to that approach involves surveying what symptoms actually have or have not been leveraged once an adequate treatment trial has become established. One might presume that an antihistaminergic SGA is serving mainly as a hypnotic, when in fact it might also prove itself to be an effective anxiolytic. Residual symptoms sometimes beg the question of comorbidities, as was illustrated by the phobic avoidance and trauma that emerged after treatment of a severe depression in Clinical Vignette 19.1 (Chapter 19).

C APPRECIATE THE CHALLENGE OF DIFFERENTIATING DRUG EFFECTS FROM THE NATURAL COURSE OF ILLNESS

Chapter 1 began with a discussion of how to form attributions and recognize causality and plausibility in the world of treatment interventions. These concepts hold equally true for suspected benefits as well as suspected adverse effects. Keep in working memory the dilemma of "post hoc ergo propter hoc," especially when pharmacotherapy can serve as the ready scapegoat for misconstruing unresolved or worsening symptoms as drug side effects. When depressed patients report suicidal thoughts after starting an antidepressant, clarify if they were truly absent before the medication was started, and gauge whether or not other associated symptoms within a broader constellation also may have worsened (suggesting progression of the underlying problem, and lack of efficacy thus far for the intended remedy, rather than an iatrogenic effect). Consider plausibility; diverse and unrelated symptom complaints that are diffuse and lack a unifying pathophysiology may have a more psychological than pharmacodynamic origin. In particular, patients with somatic symptom disorder (or otherwise, high levels of somatization, as noted in Chapter 12) or paranoid patients may be especially prone to attribute negative affect states or unacceptable bodily sensations to perceived harm from medications given to them.

Accounting for changing variables includes not only pharmacotherapies but also relevant environmental factors. Imagine a patient with severe asthma who begins taking a daily inhaled steroid and simultaneously moves to a dry climate. It would be hard to know to which of those two relevant interventions deserves credit, or for that matter, whether the net result reflected an additive or even synergistic effect rather than a single-cause effect (where one intervention was potent and the other irrelevant). From the patient's perspective, who cares? If they are better, does the cause behind their improvement matter on a practical level? It might not if they were indifferent about both their geographic relocation and their ongoing use of a potentially unnecessary drug. It matters more if maintaining a potentially unnecessary intervention poses a hazard or hardship. It matters especially if we expect the ailment to recur and want to plan for how best to manage it again in the future.

D WHATEVER YOU DO, HAVE A CLEAR RATIONALE

We like telling patients that the one thing we can promise them is a *rationale* for any recommendations made. Discern purposeful from random treatment suggestions. If one opts to raise or lower a dose, or add or subtract a medication, or otherwise make "necessary clinical adjustments," let there be no ambiguity or uncertainty as to the reasoning and purpose behind the recommendation. Know what can reasonably be expected from making "large-scale" versus incremental changes to a regimen. For example, increasing a sertraline dose from 150 to 200 mg/day in the setting of ongoing depression or anxiety is more likely to fine-tune an established incomplete response rather than convert an outright nonresponse to a response.

The existing evidence base for many conditions is limited by availability – remember to distinguish absence of evidence from evidence of absence. As an example, consider that in the case of borderline personality disorder the only published RCT data with SSRIs are with fluoxetine or fluvoxamine (Chapter 20, Table 20.1); what, then, is the likelihood that sertraline or paroxetine might be efficacious for depressive symptoms, or mood instability, especially given other data supporting the use of those agents in PTSD (Chapter 19). While the answer is technically an unknown, it is not much of a stretch to devise a plausible rationale.

Beware of random versus rationale-based treatment suggestions. While it is usually true that "there is always something else one could consider trying," it becomes disingenuous and unrealistic beyond a certain point to offer iterative treatment options that have no basis or likelihood for working when other established interventions that have larger effect sizes, or have already been studied in treatment-resistant settings, have failed to yield a benefit.

E THINK ABOUT BACKUP SYSTEMS AND THE VIRTUES OF REDUNDANCY

The only thing better than having a good plan is having a good backup plan, and then a backup to the backup plan. Good engineering anticipates glitches and includes contingent strategies if a first approach fails. Good psychopharmacology should operate no differently. In fact, when one considers that first-round interventions often

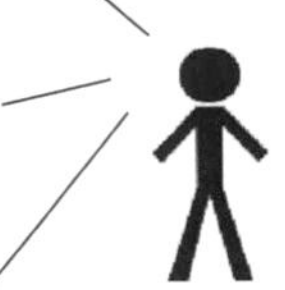
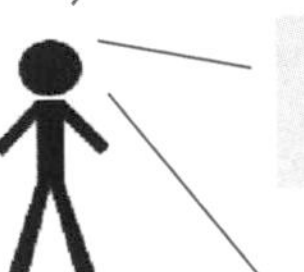
My multi-drug-resistant depressed patient hasn't improved after adequate trials of sertraline, desvenlafaxine plus brexpiprazole, fluoxetine plus olanzapine, nortriptyline plus lithium, and tranylcypromine plus modafinil, as well as 18 bilateral ECT treatments and nine ketamine infusions.
Hmm. Have you considered trying fluvoxamine?
Uh, no, not especially. Why? Are there particular data for its efficacy after multiple prior nonresponses?
No. But if you haven't tried it, it's something else to try.
Well, I guess that's technically true. But after multiple nonresponses the chances of success with anything keep declining. You could always pick *something* to try simply because it hasn't previously been tried, but with no a priori reason to think it will work better than anything else it becomes more and more random. And then if the patient starts to improve it'd be hard to know if that's just the natural course of illness.
So? If the patient improves who cares why he's better?

fully succeed in fewer than half of patients with significant mood, anxiety, or psychotic disorders, it becomes rather disingenuous for clinicians *not* to think ahead about logical next steps and fall-back operations. In this regard there also often arises a delicate balance between persevering with an adequate trial on the one hand (especially in more severe, chronic, or otherwise refractory presentations) versus recognizing when the time has come to halt an ineffective treatment and move on.

Iterative or sequential treatment strategies are like blueprints that should be mapped out from Day 1, and when the operation is planned wisely and with foresight it should reflect more elegance than randomness. Consider, for instance, a TRD patient already taking fluoxetine for whom the decision is made to add olanzapine (creating synergy from OFC, i.e. DIY Symbyax® rather than a random SGA, or switching to another) antidepressant. Should that plan fail, it would be handy to build in a failsafe contingency bridge that will accommodate the long terminal elimination half-life of fluoxetine before then starting an MAOI. Such a bridge plan might include pramipexole, an SGA, high-dose thyroid hormone, or lithium. In persistent psychotic disorders, recall the rationale in Clinical Vignette 20.1 from Chapter 20, in which clozapine was viewed as a likely inevitable treatment, but the route by which one arrived there (including the patient's own acceptability of the option) was at the heart of decisions about *which* SGAs to try first. Nobody likes the idea of random medical decision-making. Even if there is no way to guarantee an end result, one can try to assure a clear and non-capricious pathway leading to whatever end result arises.

F AIN'T BROKE, DON'T FIX

There is simple wisdom in the idea that little is to be gained from tampering with a stable system in equilibrium. Recall our discussion of Newtonian psychopharmacology in earlier chapters; a stable condition ought to remain on an unchanging trajectory unless acted upon by some force. In the psychopathological universe, such forces are many and may include medication nonadherence, resurgence of residual symptoms or comorbidities, life stresses such as those found in Box 19.2, drug interactions, seasonal and circadian disruptions, and inherent unpredictability of the natural course of illness. In many ways, prescribers stand guard over such forces, recognizing their potential disruptions to homeostasis.

As one example, consider the perennial question of when to stop antidepressants after successful treatment for bipolar depression. Newtonian psychopharmacology would argue not to tamper with success by disrupting homeostasis, and make no alterations unless forces acting on the system change (e.g., mania symptoms emerge). Of course, Bayesian psychopharmacology would invite broader consideration of past treatment outcomes and risk for mood destabilization based on an individual-specific previous illness course – meaning that the best strategy for someone with past-year rapid cycling or recent mania might be different from someone with no recent mania. The very act of *considering* such moderating factors would, at least, provide a more empirical than arbitrary foundation for decision-making.

G IF A STABLE CONDITION DESTABILIZES, RETRACE MOST RECENT STEPS

When clinical equilibrium goes awry, it is often helpful to retrace one's psychopharmacological footsteps. What was the last change made? If a drug was stopped because it was presumed to be ineffective, subsequent deterioration may be just the very empirical data one needed in order to know that it was in fact helping, even if only partially. If a drug was stopped or a dosage was lowered in an effort to address an undesirable but nonhazardous side effect (such as weight gain), restoring the previous dose usually makes sense if for no other reason than to establish whether the drug was unequivocally helpful. Furthermore, restoring a regimen to re-establish homeostasis places the patient in a more advantageous position from which to later decide whether to continue to retain a helpful drug and try to manage its side effects or to switch to something else. In the latter instance, though, it is far easier to change medications for the sake of tolerability when clinical symptoms are well-controlled rather than poorly controlled.

H THOSE WHO DO NOT LEARN FROM HISTORY ARE DOOMED TO REPEAT IT

While past performance is certainly no guarantee of what the future may bring, it is not a bad place to start. George Santayana's admonition applies no less to psychopharmacology than to any other human endeavor. If a treatment was helpful in the past, it makes little sense to discard that information and embark on other untried remedies without a clear and compelling reason (such as an insurmountable side effect or reason to think

That drug gave me awful tinnitus which went away when I stopped it, but since then I'm back to feeling depressed and actively suicidal.

How about if we undertake a two-step operation: first, resume the drug that helped in order to most reliably get you feeling better, and from there we could then try changing it to something more tolerable that might help prevent relapse – rather than gamble on a complete unknown, if you're now suicidal.

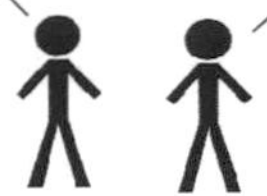
Why not just give him ketamine for suicidal depression?
You sure could, except there's no guarantee that would work better, and you already have something that you know has worked *for him*.

that an alternative proposed treatment option is likely to work better). This problem often surfaces in the context of treatment nonadherence, when patients discontinue an otherwise efficacious treatment and the dilemma arises as to whether simply to resume it and address nonadherence through psychosocial means, or to seize upon the occasion and knowingly opt not to resume a known efficacious option in favor of an unknown but perhaps compelling alternative (e.g., a long-acting injectable SGA? A longer half-life antidepressant? A next-best agent that spares the side effect identified as the driving force behind nonadherence?). Once again, whatever ultimate treatment decision emerges, having an established rationale remains paramount.

I PRACTICE PHARMACO-ARCHAEOLOGY

An anthropological cousin to CSI psychopharmacology (see Chapter 1), we define pharmaco-archaeology as the forensic task of reconstructing how an existing pharmacotherapy regimen came into being. Extensive combination pharmacotherapy regimens sometimes arise by random accrual from the collective efforts of two or more previous prescribers, without necessarily taking into account the ongoing relevance, possible pharmacokinetic interactions, or risk–benefit ratios of all drugs that are continued. When reviewing a past or current pharmacotherapy regimen, one can often make reasonable inferences and speculations about past treaters' clinical impressions based on the pharmacology trail they leave behind. For example, patients with a purported diagnosis of bipolar disorder who mainly have had subtherapeutic doses of mood stabilizing/antimanic drugs, or use of drugs with more ill-established mood-stabilizing efficacy (such as gabapentin or oxcarbazepine) to the exclusion of more well-established medications (such as lithium, divalproex, or olanzapine) suggest at least the possibility of diagnostic uncertainty on the part of previous prescribers. Were past prescriptions for fluvoxamine suggestive of impressions about OCD? Were past low doses of antipsychotics signs of concern about benzodiazapine misuse, or indicators of a previous clinician's uncertainty about the boundary between psychotic versus nonpsychotic agitation or anxiety? Did someone previously knowingly choose fluoxetine because of its long half-life, tipping off their concerns about nonadherence? You get the idea.

J REMEMBER TO DISTINGUISH DRUG INTOLERANCES FROM LACK OF EFFICACY WHEN ASSESSING A TREATMENT HISTORY

As basic and fundamental as this concept may be, even the best of clinicians may be susceptible to labeling a complex case as "treatment resistant" when the reality of circumstances may instead suggest that adverse effects have led to aborted rather than failed trials.

K APPRECIATE PLACEBO AND NOCEBO EFFECTS, AND CAPITALIZE ON THE NONPHARMACODYNAMIC EFFECTS OF PRESCRIBING

It never hurts to underpromise and overdeliver. While paradoxical injunctions tend to work better in the context of an established therapeutic relationship, the basic principle involves recognizing that the effect sizes of most psychotropic drugs relative to placebo are much more modest than one might think (look back at Chapter 3, Box 3.6). This probably has more to do with the efficacy of placebo than the inherent pharmacodynamic shortcomings of drugs for a placebo-responsive ailment. Go ahead and endorse your patient's preference for paroxetine over other SSRIs just because her friend had a positive experience with it. Argue why?

L CONSIDER THE "SLIDING SCALE" APPROACH

We often treat insulin-dependent diabetes mellitus by using a standing daily dose of insulin in conjunction with a "sliding scale" supplemental dose, if and when needed, based on day-to-day observed hyperglycemia. Such an approach is sometimes analogized for treating anxiety, as when advising patients about parameters for taking an as-needed benzodiazepine or similar on-the-spot anxiolytic. "PRN" antidepressant dosing on a day-to-day basis is unlikely to have utility based on the time scale with which we think most monoaminergic antidepressants work. However, a "sliding scale" approach to dosing supplemental antipsychotic medications might be viable when used to treat psychotic or other target symptoms that may wax and wane without sufficient persistence to justify outright daily dose increases. Consider Clinical Vignette 22.1.

CLINICAL VIGNETTE 22.1

George was a 24-year-old single man living with his parents who had transdiagnostic symptoms involving features of OCD and psychosis, including germ phobias and preoccupations about past environmental exposures that he felt may have caused him irreparable brain damage. His belief-conviction around his concerns varied over time. After several SSRI and/or SGA trials his condition improved markedly with olanzapine 5 mg/day except for occasional "breakthrough" lapses in reality testing. He was comfortable for the most part on his standing olanzapine 5 mg daily dose, and was reluctant to increase it further due to side-effect concerns, as well as a sense that his breakthrough symptoms occurred only a minority of the time. A plan was made in which George would each day track on a 0–10 Likert scale the intensity, frequency, and distress he felt regarding his concerns, and his ability to use cognitive skills to "quarantine" and compartmentalize his concerns about environmental toxicities. For days scoring ≥7/10 he would supplement his standing olanzapine with a "sliding scale" additional dose of 2.5 mg; for weeks in which sliding scale supplementation was needed on three or more days, the sliding scale supplement would be "folded in" to his standing dose. George appreciated the way in which this plan helped him recognize and quantify his distress and afforded him more of a sense of control and empowerment over his medication dosing.

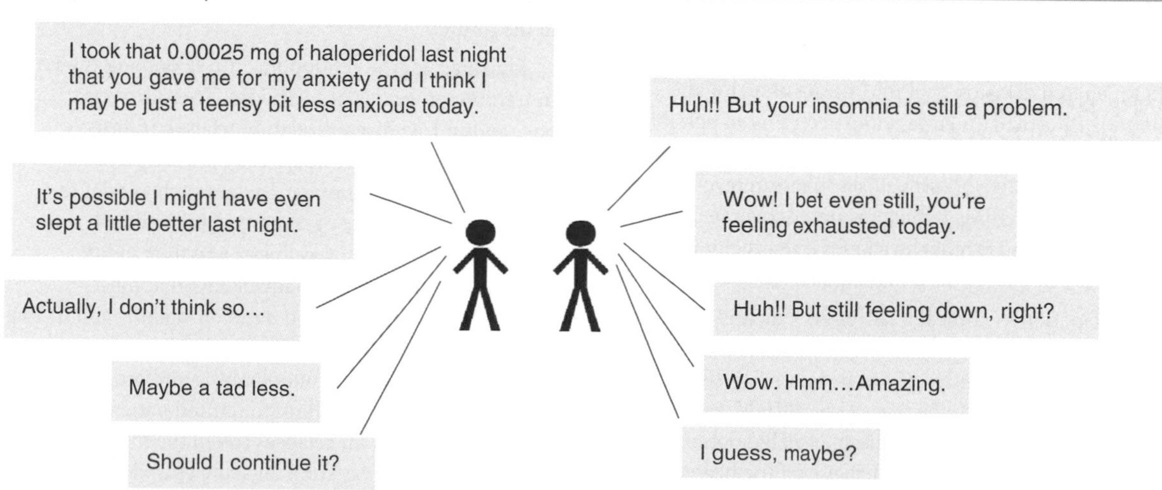
I took that 0.00025 mg of haloperidol last night that you gave me for my anxiety and I think I may be just a teensy bit less anxious today.
Huh!! But your insomnia is still a problem.
It's possible I might have even slept a little better last night.
Wow! I bet even still, you're feeling exhausted today.
Actually, I don't think so…
Huh!! But still feeling down, right?
Maybe a tad less.
Wow. Hmm…Amazing.
Should I continue it?
I guess, maybe?

M USE TECHNOLOGY WISELY AND PURPOSEFULLY

Order laboratory tests, including pharmacogenetics, serum drug levels, or neuroimaging, because you think they will help to answer a specific question (such as, respectively, to affirm suspicions that someone may be an ultra-rapid metabolizer, or is nonadherent, or harboring a pituitary origin to biochemical hypothyroidism with a normal TSH). Do not forget to consider the potential value of neuropsychological testing – but frame the specific question for which an answer is sought (e.g., "I suspect a cortical dementia, but was wondering about psychosis in the differential diagnosis"). Avoid "shotgun" diagnostic approaches unless they seem justifiable and necessary. Do not let laboratory assays become the psychiatric equivalent of an exploratory laparotomy; have a hypothesis and use technology, when appropriate, to test it.

N UNDERTAKE "HEROIC" PHARMACOTHERAPIES WITH CAUTION, WISDOM, DELIBERATION, AND SHARED DECISION-MAKING

Much the way an oncologist might tell a seriously ill patient that certain chemotherapy strategies can be riskier than others, but could yield better results, so too can a psychopharmacologist lay out for patients with treatment-resistant psychiatric conditions options that may be considered heroic. Examples include high-dose MAOIs in TRD (and, even higher risk, augmenting high-dose MAOIs with psychostimulants – a bold and potentially hazardous maneuver supported only by case reports in a handful of highly treatment-resistant cases, where "shared decision-making" means assuring the patient is informed and aware and accepting of possible cardiovascular, cerebrovascular, or related risks) or cautiously pushing clozapine doses to serum levels near the therapeutic ceiling, with appropriate coverage for seizure risk, because other strategies (even including poly-SGA use) have proven inadequate.

Participation in clinical trials offers a means of access to investigational compounds when multiple "standard" approaches are ineffective. It can be informative, and even empowering, to peruse the www.clinicaltrials.gov website side-by-side with patients in search of viable options that may be nonconventional or otherwise off the beaten path.

O STRIVE FOR REMISSION BUT RECOGNIZE WHEN MORE AGGRESSIVE PHARMACOLOGY BECOMES HAZARDOUS

Everything is a risk–benefit analysis. Voltaire's admonition that perfection is the enemy of the good holds wisdom and value when navigating the world of complex pharmacotherapy. Remember the tale of overzealous Icarus pharmacology from Chapter 6 – nobody wants to risk melting their polypharmacological wings by flying too close to the sun. De-prescribe treatments whose value seems dubious, and capitalize wisely on pharmacological parsimony when two (or more) therapeutic objectives can be accomplished in one fell swoop. Advocate to retain more "cumbersome" treatments (such as clozapine or lithium) when the alternatives are unequivocally inferior, relative benefits are unrivaled, and the stakes are high because the nature of the ailment could be potentially life-threatening. Recognize instances in which "further tinkering" with a regimen may lead to diminishing returns (e.g., more adverse effects without greater benefit) or set unrealistic expectations about likely magnitude of response. We are humbled by disease states for which the field defines "response" as a mere 20% or 30% improvement from baseline (e.g., PTSD and schizophrenia, respectively). We must simultaneously recognize present limitations while looking to the future with the hope of continued technological advances. "Cautious optimism," even in the face of limited successes, sometimes gets a boost from reminding patients that many drugs used in the present did not exist a generation ago, and it can be hard to forecast where technology (and the evidence base) will be in the future.

Pharmacological "endpoints" are seldom discussed in training programs or textbooks. There are very few randomized discontinuation trials to inform decisions about when one should optimally stop a potential long-term therapy. Factors such as relapse proneness, magnitude of response (and residual symptoms), duration of wellness, and tolerability problems are among the many factors that must configure for individualized decision-making about drug discontinuations. All too often, medication cessations occur at random or without planning and proper monitoring. It can be helpful to remind patients about high-risk windows for relapses (often the first four to six months after recovery from an acute episode), warning signs to watch for, and the distinction between stopping a pharmacotherapy and stopping ongoing monitoring in order to prevent relapse.

P DO NOT MISCONSTRUE PSYCHOPHARMACOLOGY AS THE SUBSTITUTE FOR NEEDING A HIGHER LEVEL OF CARE

There are times when crises and out-of-control distress seep into many facets of someone's life such that they warrant not only potential changes to a pharmacotherapy but also environmental changes, relief from obligations, modification of lifestyle habits, psychotherapeutic tactics, or other situations for which pharmacotherapy may play more of a secondary or supportive rather than primary and fundamental role. Recognize the appropriate treatment setting. Heart attack patients need an emergency room more than an outpatient cardiologist. So too, it often takes a village to manage complex, difficult psychiatric conditions. In patients with severe, overwhelming, far-reaching interpersonal or psychosocial problems the idea that a medication alone will provide a definitive remedy is often simply unrealistic. Patients with chronic, unrelenting problems sometimes mainly need compassionate long-term management more than stoked hopes for miraculous remedies that may not exist.

Pharmacotherapy changes are not synonymous with training patients in strategies that enhance coping skills, any more than changes to an eyeglass prescription do not alone make someone a better driver – but, the right technology can help to surmount biological imperfections, allowing someone to make the most of their skillsets and survival know-how.

The Last Word

Our final word is one of humility. The brain is complex and we can barely understand, much less predict, how it functions from one person to the next in response to a given biological or psychosocial stimulus. We encourage every psychopharmacologist to adopt the mindset of a clinical investigator, who, together with the patient, comprises an "n-of-1" trial. Investigators can and should masterfully describe everything they see and then process the data, consult sources of expertise (think: PubMed), look to the patient's own personal history for clues about what may be helpful, deliberate, and think aloud alongside the patient to assure they understand the thought process behind any recommendations. Our treatments continue to evolve. The future depends on favoring scientific methods over guesswork, and empiricism over impressionism. This works best when we do not simply interpret the literature but, moreover, fit it to the clinical profile, personal preferences, and distinct presentation of every unique patient encounter.

References

Adamson SJ, Sellman JD, Foulds JA, et al. A randomized trial of combined citalopram and naltrexone for nonabstinent outpatients with co-occurring alcohol dependence and major depression. *J Clin Psychopharmacol* 2015; 35: 143–149

Adan-Manes J, Novalbos J, López-Rodríguez R, et al. Lithium and venlafaxine interaction: a case of serotonin syndrome. *J Clin Pharm Ther* 2006; 31: 397–400

Adler LA, Dirks B, Deas PF, et al. Lisdexamfetamine dimesylate in adults with attention-deficit/hyperactivity disorder who report clinically significant impairment in executive function: results from a randomized, double-blind, placebo-controlled study. *J Clin Psychiatry* 2013; 74: 694–702

Afshar M, Knapp CM, Sarid-Segal O, et al. The efficacy of mirtazapine in the treatment of cocaine dependence with comorbid depression. *Am J Drug Alcohol Abuse* 2012; 38: 181–186

Agabio R, Trogu E, Pani PP. Antidepressants for the treatment of people with co-occurring depression and alcohol dependence. *Cochrane Database Syst Rev* 2018; 4: CD008581

Agarwal LJ, Berger CE, Gill L. Naltrexone for severe self-harm: a case report. *Am J Psychiatry* 2011; 168: 437–438

Agid O, Siu CO, Potkin SG, et al. Meta-regression analysis of placebo response in antipsychotic trials, 1970–2010. *Am J Psychiatry* 2013; 170: 1335–1344

Aguglia A, Mineo L, Rodolico A, et al. Asenapine in the management of impulsivity and aggressiveness in bipolar disorder and comorbid borderline personality disorder: an open-label uncontrolled study. Int Clin Psychopharmacol 2018; 33: 121–130

Ahmed AO, Richardson J, Buckner A, et al. Do cognitive deficits predict negative emotionality and aggression in schizophrenia? *Psychiatry Res* 2018a; 259: 350–357

Ahmed R, Kotapati VP, Khan AM, et al. Adding psychotherapy to the naltrexone treatment of alcohol use disorder: a meta-analytic review. *Cureus* 2018b; 10: e3107

Aiken CB, Orr C. Rechallenge with lamotrigine after a rash. *Psychiatry (Edgmont)* 2010; 7: 27–32

Airagnes G, Lemogne C, Renuy A, et al. Prevalence of prescribed benzodiazepine long-term use in the French general population according to sociodemographic and clinical factors: findings from the CONSTANCS cohort. *BMC Public Health* 2019; 19: 566

Albers LJ, Ozdemir V, Marder SR. Low-dose fluvoxamine as an adjunct to reduce olanzapine therapeutic dose requirements: a prospective dose adjusted drug interaction strategy. *J Clin Psychopharmacol* 2005; 25: 170–174

Albertini E, Ernst CL, Tamaroff RS. Psychopharmacological decision making in bipolar disorder during pregnancy and lactation: a case-by-case approach to using current evidence. *Focus* 2019; 17: 249–258

Albott CS, Lim KO, Forbes MK, et al. Efficacy, safety, and durability of repeated ketamine infusions for comorbid posttraumatic stress disorder and treatment-resistant depression. *J Clin Psychiatry* 2018; 79: 17m11684

Alexopoulos GS, Canuso CM, Gharabawi GM, et al. Placebo-controlled study of relapse prevention with risperidone augmentation in older patients with resistant depression. *Am J Geriatr Psychiatry* 2008; 16: 21–30

Alexopoulos GS, Katz IR, Reynolds CF 3rd, et al. The expert consensus guideline series. Pharmacotherapy of depressive disorders in older patients. *Postgrad Med* 2001; Spec No Pharmacotherapy: 1–86

Allan ER, Alpert M, Sison CE, et al. Adjunctive nadolol in the treatment of acutely aggressive schizophrenic patients. *J Clin Psychiatry* 1996; 57: 455–459

Allen MH, Hirschfeld RM, Wozniak PJ, et al. Linear relationship of valproate serum concentration to response and optimal serum levels for acute mania. *Am J Psychiatry* 2006; 163: 272–275

Allgulander C, Mangano R, Zhang J, et al. Efficacy of Venlafaxine ER in patients with social anxiety disorder: a double-blind, placebo-controlled, parallel-group comparison with paroxetine. *Hum Psychopharmacol* 2004; 19: 387–396

Alpert M, Allan ER, Citrome L, et al. A double-blind, placebo-controlled study of adjunctive nadolol in the management of violent psychiatric patients. *Psychopharmacol Bull* 1990; 26: 367–371

Alphs L, Davis JM. Noncatecholaminergic treatments of tardive dyskinesia. *J Clin Psychopharmachol* 1982; 2: 380–385

Altemus M, Neeb CC, Davis A, et al. Phenotypic differences between pregnancy-onset and postpartum-onset major depressive disorder. *J Clin Psychiatry* 2012; 73: e1485–e1491

Altshuler LL, Bauer M, Frye MA, et al. Does thyroid supplementation accelerate tricyclic antidepressant response?: a review and meta-analysis of the literature. *Am J Psychiatry* 2001; 158: 1617–1622

Altshuler LL, Post RM, Hellemann G, et al. Impact of antidepressant continuation after acute positive or partial treatment response for bipolar depression: a blinded, randomized study. *J Clin Psychiatry* 2009; 70: 450–457

Altshuler L, Suppes T, Black D, et al. Impact of antidepressant discontinuation after acute bipolar depression remission on rates of depressive relapse at 1-year follow-up. *Am J Psychiatry* 2003; 160: 1252–1262

Altshuler LL, Suppes T, Black DO, et al. Lower switch rate in depressed patients with bipolar II than bipolar I disorder treated adjunctively with second-generation antidepressants. *Am J Psychiatry* 2006; 163: 313–315

Alvarez E, Perez V, Dragheim M, et al. A double-blind, randomized, placebo-controlled, active reference study of Lu AA21004 in patients with major depressive disorder. *Int J Neuropsychopharmacol* 2012; 15: 589–600

American Psychiatric Association. *Practice Guideline for the Treatment of Major Depressive Disorder*, 3rd Edn. Arlington, VA: American Psychiatric Association; 2010

American Psychiatric Association. *Diagnostic and Statistical Manual of Mental Disorders*, 5th Edn. Arlington, VA: American Psychiatric Association; 2013

American Society of Hospital Pharmacists. ASHP statement on pharmaceutical care. *Am J Hosp Pharm.* 1993; 50: 1720-1723

Amerio A, Ossola P, Scagnelli F, et al. Safety and efficacy of lithium in children and adolescents: a systematic review in bipolar illness. *Eur Psychiatry* 2018; 54: 85–97

Amerio A, Stubbs B, Odone A, et al. The prevalence and predictors of comorbid bipolar disorder and obsessive-compulsive disorder: a systematic review and meta-analysis. *J Affect Disord* 2015; 186: 99–109

Amieva H, LeGoff M, Millet X, et al. Prodromal Alzheimer's disease: successive emergence of the clinical symptoms. *Ann Neurol* 2008; 64: 492–498

Amital D, Vishne T, Roitman S, et al. Open study of creatine monohydrate in treatment-resistant posttraumatic stress disorder. *J Clin Psychiatry* 2006; 67: 836–837

Amsterdam JD, Berwish NJ. High dose tranylcypromine therapy for refractory depression. *Pharmacopsychiatry* 1989; 22: 21–25

Amsterdam JD, Fawcett J, Quitkin FM, et al. Fluoxetine and norfluoxetine plasma concentrations in major depression: a multicenter study. *Am J Psychiatry* 1997; 154: 963–969

Amsterdam JD, Li Y, Soeller I, et al. A randomized, double-blind, placebo-controlled trial of oral Matricaria recutita (chamomile) extract therapy for generalized anxiety disorder. *J Clin Psychopharmacol* 2009; 29: 378–382

Anand A, Charney DS, Oren DA, et al. Attenuation of the neuropsychiatric effects of ketamine with lamotrigine: support for hyperglutamatergic effects of N-methyl-D-aspartate receptor antagonists. *Arch Gen Psychiatry* 2000; 57: 170–176

Anderson M, Björkhem-Bergman L, Beck O. Possible mechanism for inhibition of morphine formation from 6-acetylmorphine after intake of street heroin. *Forensic Sci Int* 2015; 252: 150–156

Andrade C. Nonsteroidal anti-inflammatory drugs and 5-HT3 serotonin receptor antagonists as innovative antipsychotic augmentation treatments for schizophrenia. *J Clin Psychiatry* 2014; 75: e707–e709

Andrade C. Antidepressant exposure during pregnancy and risk of autism in the offspring: 1: meta-review of meta-analyses. *J Clin Psychiatry* 2017; 78: e1047–e1051

Andrade C, Kisely S, Monteiro I, et al. Antipsychotic augmentation with modafinil or armodafinil for negative symptoms of schizophrenia: systematic review and meta-analysis of randomized controlled trials. *J Psychiatry Res* 2015; 60: 14–21

Andrade C, Sandarsh S, Chetan KB, et al. Serotonin reuptake inhibitor antidepressants and abnormal bleeding: a review for clinicians and a reconsideration of mechanisms. *J Clin Psychiatry* 2010; 71: 1565–1575

Andreason NC. Negative symptoms in schizophrenia: definition and reliability. *Arch Gen Psychiatry* 1982; 39: 784–788

Andreason NC, Liu D, Ziebell S, et al. Relapse duration, treatment intensity, and brain tissue loss in schizophrenia: a prospective longitudinal MRI study. *Am J Psychiatry* 2013; 170: 609–615

Andreason NC, Pressler M, Nopoulos P, et al. Antipsychotic dose equivalents and dose-years: a standardized method for comparing exposure to different drugs. *Biol Psychiatry* 2010; 67: 255–262

Andrezina R, Josiassen RC, Marcus RN, et al. Intramuscular aripiprazole for the treatment of acute agitation in patients with schizophrenia or schizoaffective disorder: a double-blind, placebo-controlled comparison of intramuscular haloperidol. *Psychopharmacology (Berl)* 2006; 188: 281–292

Anglin RES, Samaan Z, Walter SD, et al. Vitamin D deficiency and depression in adults: systematic review and meta-analysis. *Br J Psychiatry* 2013; 202: 100–107

Anton RF, Moak DH, Latham PK. The obsessive compulsive drinking scale: a new method of assessing outcome in alcoholism treatment studies. *Arch Gen Psychiatry* 1996; 53: 225–231. Erratum in: *Arch Gen Psychiatry* 1996; 53: 576

Anton RF, Myrick H, Wright TM, et al. Gabapentin combined with naltrexone for the treatment of alcohol dependence. *Am J Psychiatry* 2011; 168: 709–717

Anton RF, O'Malley SS, Ciraulo DA, et al. Combined pharmacotherapies and behavioral interventions for alcohol dependence: the COMBINE study. A randomized controlled trial. *J Am Med Assoc* 2006; 295: 2003–2017

Anttila S, Viikki M, Huuhka K, et al. TPH2 polymorphisms may modify clinical picture in treatment-resistant depression. *Neurosci Lett* 2009; 464: 43–46

Appelberg BG, Syvälahti EK, Koskinen TE, et al. Patients with severe depression may benefit from buspirone augmentation of selective serotonin reuptake inhibitors: results from a placebo-controlled, randomized, double-blind, placebo wash-in study. *J Clin Psychiatry* 2001; 62: 448–452

Appelhof BC, Fliers E, Wekking EM, et al. Combined therapy with levothyroxine and liothyronine in two ratios, compared with levothyroxine monotherapy in primary hypothyroidism: a double-blind, randomized, controlled clinical trial. *J Clin Endocrinol Metab* 2005; 90: 2666–2674

Arato M, O'Connor R, Meltzer HY, et al. A 1-year, double-blind, placebo-controlled trial of ziprasidone 40, 80 and 160 mg/day in chronic schizophrenia: the Ziprasidone Extended Use in Schizophrenia (ZEUS) study. *Int Clin Psychopharmacol* 2002; 17: 207–215

Argolo FC, Cavalcanti-Ribeiro P, Netto LR, et al. Prevention of posttraumatic stress disorder with propranolol: a meta-analytic review. *J Psychosom Res* 2015; 79: 89–93

Argyropoulou P, Patakas D, Koukou A, et al. Buspirone effect on breathlessness and exercise performance in patients with chronic obstructive pulmonary disease. *Respiration* 1993; 60: 214–220

Arnold LE. Methylphenidate vs. amphetamine: comparative review. *J Attention Disord* 2000; 4: 200–211

Arnold LM, Mutasim DF, Dwight MM, et al. An open clinical trial of fluvoxamine treatment of psychogenic excoriation. *J Clin Psychopharmacol* 1999; 19: 15–18

Arnow BA, Blasey C, Williams LM, et al. Depression subtypes in predicting antidepressant response: a report from the iSPOT-D trial. *Am J Psychiatry* 2015; 172: 743–750

Arns M, Bruder G, Hegerl U, et al. EEG alpha asymmetry as a gender-specific predictor of outcome to acute treatment with different antidepressant medications in the randomized iSPOT-D study. *Clin Neurophysiol* 2016; 17: 509–519

Arntz A, Van den Hoorn M, Cornelis J. Reliability and validity of the borderline personality disorder severity index. *J Pers Disord* 2003; 17: 45–59

Aronson R, Offman HJ, Joffe RT, et al. Triiodothyronine augmentation in the treatment of refractory depression: a meta-analysis. *Arch Gen Psychiatry* 1996; 53: 842–848

Askari N, Moin M, Sanati M, et al. Granisetron adjunct to fluvoxamine for moderate to severe obsessive-compulsive disorder: a randomized, double-blind, placebo-controlled trial. *CNS Drugs* 2012; 26: 883–892

Astill Wright L, Sijbrandij M, Sinnerton R, et al. Pharmacological prevention and early treatment of post-traumatic stress disorder and acute stress disorder: a systematic review and meta-analysis. *Transl Psychiatry* 2019; 9: 334

AstraZeneca. A multi-center, double-blind, randomized-withdrawal, parallel-group, placebo-controlled Phase III study of the efficacy and safety of quetiapine fumarate extended release (Seroquel XR™) as monotherapy in the maintenance treatment of patients with major depressive disorder following an open-label stabilization period (AMETHYST study). www.astrazenecaclinicaltrials.com/_mshost800325/content/clinical-trials/resources/pdf/8579609 ClinicalTrials.gov ID NCT00278941. Study code: D1448C00005. 2008

Astrup A, Caterson I, Zelissen P, et al. Topiramate: long-term maintenance of weight loss induced by a low-calorie diet in obese subjects. *Obes Res* 2004; 12: 1658–1669

Avgerinos KI, Spyrou N, Bougioukas KI, et al. Effects of creatine supplementation on cognitive function of healthy individuals: a systematic review of randomized controlled trials. *Exp Gerontol* 2018; 108: 166–173

Awortwe C, Makiwane M, Reuter H, et l. Critical evaluation of causality assessment of herb-drug interactions in patients. *Br J Clin Pharmacol* 2018; 84: 679–693

Azuma K, Takaesu Y, Soeda H, et al. Ability of suvorexant to prevent delirium in patients in the intensive care unit: a randomized controlled trial. *Acute Med Surg* 2018; 5: 362–368

Baandrup L, Ebdrup BH, Rasmussen JØ, et al. Pharmacological interventions for benzodiazepine discontinuation in chronic benzodiazepine users. *Cochrane Database Syst Rev* 2018; 3: CD011481

Babor TF, Hofmann M, DelBoca FK, et al. Types of alcoholics, I: evidence for an empirically derived typology based on indicators of vulnerability and severity. *Arch Gen Psychiatry* 1992; 49: 599–608

Bacaltchuk J, Hay P, Mari JJ. Antidepressants versus placebo for the treatment of bulimia nervosa: a systematic review. *Aust N Z J Psychiatry* 2000; 34: 310–317

Back SE, McCauley JL, Korte KJ, et al. A double-blind, randomized, controlled pilot study of N-acetylcysteine in veterans with posttraumatic stress disorder and substance use disorders. *J Clin Psychiatry* 2016; 77: e1439–e1446

Bagby RM, Ryder AG, Cristi C. Psychosocial and clinical predictors of response to pharmacotherapy for depression. *J Psychiatry Neurosci* 2002; 27: 250–257

Bahji A, Forsyth A, Groll D, et al. Efficacy of 3,4-methylenedioxymethamphetamine (MDMA)-assisted psychotherapy for posttraumatic stress disorder: a systematic review and meta-analysis. *Prog Neuropsychopharmacol Biol Psychiatry* 2020; 96: 109735

Baillon SF, Narayana U, Luxenberg JS, et al. Valproate preparations for agitation in dementia. *Cochrane Database Syst Rev* 2018; 10: CD003945

Bak M, Weltens I, Bervoets C, et al. The pharmacological management of agitated and aggressive behaviour: a systematic review and meta-analysis. *Eur Psychiatry* 2019; 57: 78–100

Baker RW, Kinon BJ, Maguire GA, et al. Effectiveness of rapid initial dose escalation of up to forty milligrams per day of oral olanzapine in acute agitation. *J Clin Psychopharmacol* 2003; 23: 342–348

BALANCE Investigators and Collaborators; Geddes JR, Goodwin GM, Rendell J, et al. Lithium plus valproate combination therapy versus monotherapy for relapse prevention in bipolar I disorder (BALANCE): a randomised open-label trial. *Lancet* 2010; 375: 385–395

Baldaçara L, Cogo-Moreira H, Parreira BL, et al. Efficacy of topiramate in the treatment of crack cocaine dependence: a double-blind, randomized, placebo-controlled trial. *J Clin Psychiatry* 2016; 77: 398–406

Baldessarini RJ, Vázques G, Tondo L. Treatment of cyclothymic disorder: commentary. *Psychother Psychosom* 2011; 80: 131–135

Baldwin DS, Loft H, Dragheim M. A randomised, double-blind, placebo controlled, duloxetine-referenced, fixed-dose study of three dosages of Lu AA21004 in acute treatment of major depressive disorder (MDD). *Eur Neuropsychopharmacol* 2012; 22: 482–491

Bali V, Chatterjee S, Carnahan RM, et al. Risk of dementia among elderly nursing home patients using paroxetine and other selective serotonin reuptake inhibitors. *Psychiatr Serv* 2015; 66: 1333–1340

Ballenger JC, Davidson JR, Lecrubier Y, et al. Consensus statement on panic disorder from the International Consensus Group on Depression and Anxiety. *J Clin Psychiatry* 1998; 59(Suppl 8): 47–54

Bandelow B. Assessing the efficacy of treatments for panic disorder and agoraphobia. II. The Panic and Agoraphobia Scale. *Int Clin Psychopharmacol* 1995; 2: 73–81

Baniasadi M, Hosseini G, Bordbar MRF, et al. Effect of pregabalin augmentation in treatment of patients with combat-related chronic posttraumatic stress disorder: a randomized controlled trial. *J Psychiatr Pract* 2014; 20: 419–427

Banzi R, Cusi C, Randazzo C, et al. Selective serotonin reuptake inhibitors (SSRIs) and serotonin-norepinephrine reuptake inhibitors (SNRIs) for the prevention of migraine in adults. *Cochrane Database Syst Rev* 2015; 4: CD002919

Barbee JG, Thompson TR, Jamhour NJ, et al. A double-blind placebo-controlled trial of lamotrigine as an antidepressant augmentation agent in treatment-refractory unipolar depression. *J Clin Psychiatry* 2011; 72: 1405–1412

Bareggi SR, Bianchi L, Cavallaro R, et al. Citalopram concentrations and response in obsessive-compulsive disorder. Preliminary results. *CNS Drugs* 2004; 18: 329–335

Barker MJ, Greenwood KM, Jackson M, et al. Cognitive effects of long-term benzodiazepine use: a meta-analysis. *CNS Drugs* 2004; 18: 37–48

Barnett R, Maruff P, Vance A, et al. Abnormal executive function in attention deficit hyperactivity disorder: the effect of stimulant medication and age on spatial working memory. *Psychol Med* 2001; 31: 1107–1115

Barnett SD, Kramer ML, Casat CD, et al. Efficacy of olanzapine in social anxiety disorder: a pilot study. *J Psychopharmacol* 2002; 16: 365–368

Barrons R, Roberts N. The role of carbamazepine and oxcarbazepine in alcohol withdrawal syndrome. *J Clin Pharm Ther* 2010; 35: 153–167

Barsky AJ, Saintfort R, Rogers MP, et al. Nonspecific medication side effects and the nocebo phenomenon. *J Am Med Assoc* 2002; 287: 622–627

Batail JM, Langrée B, Robert G, et al. Use of very-high dose olanzapine in treatment-resistant schizophrenia. *Schizophr Res* 2014; 159: 411–414

Batelaan NM, Bosman RC, Muntingh A, et al. Risk of relapse after antidepressant discontinuation in anxiety disorders, obsessive-compulsive disorder, and post-traumatic stress disorder: systematic review and meta-analysis of relapse prevention trials. *Br Med J* 2017; 358: j3927

Bauer M, Dell'Osso L, Kasper S, et al. Extended-release quetiapine fumarate (quetiapine XR) monotherapy and quetiapine XR or lithium as add-on to antidepressants in patients with treatment-resistant major depressive disorder. *J Affect Disord* 2013; 151: 209–219

Bauer MS, Whybrow PC. Rapid cycling bipolar affective disorder. II. Treatment of refractory rapid cycling with high-dose levothyroxine: a preliminary study. *Arch Gen Psychiatry* 1990; 47: 435–440

Baune BT, Brignone M, Larsen KG. A network meta-analysis comparing effects of various antidepressant classes on the digit symbol substitution test (DSST) as a measure of cognitive dysfunction in patients with major depressive disorder. *Int J Neuropsychopharmacol* 2018; 21: 97–107

Bazire SR. Sudden death associated with switching monoamine oxidase inhibitors. *Drug Intell Clin Pharm* 1986; 20: 954–956

Beasley CM Jr, Tollefson G, Tran P, et al. Olanzapine versus placebo and haloperidol: acute phase results of the North American double-blind olanzapine trial. *Neuropsychopharmacology* 1996; 14: 111–123

Beck AT, Epstein N, Brown G, et al. An inventory for measuring clinical anxiety: psychometric properties. *J Consult Clin Psychol* 1988; 56: 893–897

Begemann MJ, Dekker CF, van Lunenburg M, et al. Estrogen augmentation in schizophrenia: a quantitative review of current evidence. *Schizophr Res* 2012; 141: 179–184

Beinat C, Banister SD, Herrera M, et al. The therapeutic potential of α7 nicotinic acetylcholine receptor (α7 nAChR) agonists for the treatment of the cognitive deficits associated with schizophrenia. *CNS Drugs* 2015; 29: 529–542

Bellatuono C, Tofani S, Di Sciascio G, et al. Benzodiazepine exposure in pregnancy and risk of major malformations: a critical overview. *Gen Hosp Psychiatry* 2013; 35: 3–8

Bellino S, Paradiso E, Bogetto F. Oxcarbazepine in the treatment of borderline personality disorder: a pilot study. *J Clin Psychiatry* 2005; 66: 1111–1115

Bellino S, Paradiso E, Bogetto F. Efficacy and tolerability of quetiapine in the treatment of borderline personality disorder: a pilot study. *J Clin Psychiatry* 2006; 67: 1042–1046

Bellino S, Paradiso E, Bogetto F. Efficacy and tolerability of aripiprazole augmentation in sertraline-resistant patients with borderline personality disorder. *Psychiatry Res* 2008; 161: 206–212

Bellino S, Bozzatello P, Rinaldi C, et al. Paliperidone ER in the treatment of borderline personality disorder: a pilot study of efficacy and tolerability. *Depress Res Treat* 2011; 2011: 680194

Bellino S, Bozzatello P, Rocca G, et al. Efficacy of omega-3 fatty acids in the treatment of borderline personality disorder: a study of the association with valproic acid. *J Psychopharmacol* 2014; 28: 125–132

Bellino S, Paradiso E, Bozzatello P, et al. Efficacy and tolerability of duloxetine in the treatment of patients with borderline personality disorder: a pilot study. *J Psychopharmacol* 2010; 24: 333–339

Benazzi F. Characteristics of bipolar II patients with interpersonal rejection sensitivity. *Psychiatr Clin Neurosci* 2001; 54: 499–501

Bergamaschi MM, Queiroz RH, Chagas MH, et al. Cannabidiol reduces the anxiety induced by simulated public speaking in treatment-naïve social phobia patients. *Neuropsychopharmacology* 2011; 36: 1219–1226

Bergero-Miguel T, García-Encinas MA, Villena-Jimena A, et al. Gender dysphoria and social anxiety: an exploratory study in Spain. *J Sex Med* 2016; 13: 1270–1278

Beri A, Boydell J. Clozapine in borderline personality disorder: a review of the evidence. *Ann Clin Psychiatry* 2014; 26: 139–144

Berk M, Dean OM, Cotton SM, et al. The efficacy of adjunctive N-acetylcysteine in major depressive disorder: a double-blind, randomized, placebo-controlled trial. *J Clin Psychiatry* 2014; 75: 628–636

Berlant J. Prospective open-label study of add-on and monotherapy topiramate in civilians with chronic nonhallucinatory posttraumatic stress disorder. *BMC Psychiatry* 2004; 4: 24

Berlant J, van Kammen DP. Open-label topiramate as primary or adjunctive therapy in chronic civilian posttraumatic stress disorder: a preliminary report. *J Clin Psychiatry* 2002; 63: 15–20

Berlin HA, Koran LM, Jenike MA, et al. Double-blind, placebo-controlled trial of topiramate augmentation in treatment-resistant obsessive-compulsive disorder. *J Clin Psychiatry* 2011; 72: 716–721

Berman M, Marcus RN, Swanink R, et al. The efficacy and safety of aripiprazole as adjunctive therapy in major depressive disorder: a multicenter, randomized, double-blind, placebo-controlled study. *J Clin Psychiatry* 2007; 68: 843–853

Berman RM, Fava M, Thase ME, et al. Aripiprazole augmentation in major depressive disorder: a double-blind, placebo-controlled study in patients with inadequate response to antidepressants. *CNS Spectr* 2009; 14: 197–206

Bersudsky Y. Phenytoin: an anti-bipolar anticonvulsant? *Int J Neuropsychopharmacol* 2006; 9: 479–484

Berwaerts J, Lane R, Nuamah IF, et al. Paliperidone extended-release as adjunctive therapy to lithium or valproate in the treatment of acute mania: a randomized, placebo-controlled study. *J Affect Disord* 2011; 129: 252–260

Berwaerts J, Melkote R, Nuamah I, et al. A randomized, placebo- and active-controlled study of paliperidone extended-release as maintenance treatment in patients with bipolar I disorder after an acute manic or mixed episode. *J Affect Disord* 2012b; 138: 247–258

Berwaerts J, Xu H, Nuamah I, et al. Evaluation of the efficacy and safety of paliperidone extended-release in the treatment of acute mania: a randomized, double-blind, dose-response study. *J Affect Disord* 2012a; 136: e51–e60

Beucke JC, Sepulcre J, Talukdar T, et al. Abnormally high degree connectivity of the orbitofrontal cortex in obsessive-compulsive disorder. *JAMA Psychiatry* 2013; 70: 619–629

Bhatara VS, Magnus RD, Paul KL, et al. Serotonin syndrome induced by venlafaxine and fluoxetine: a case study in polypharmacy and potential pharmacodynamic and pharmacokinetic mechanisms. *Ann Pharmacother* 1998; 32: 432–436

Biederman J, Faraone SV, Keenan K, et al. Evidence of familial association between attention deficit disorder and major affective disorders. *Arch Gen Psychiatry* 1991a; 48: 633–642

Biederman J, Faraone SV, Keenan K, et al. Familial association between attention deficit disorder and anxiety disorders. *Am J Psychiatry* 1991b; 148: 251–256

Biederman J, Fried R, Tarko L, et al. Memantine in the treatment of executive function deficits in adults with ADHD. *J Atten Disord* 2017; 21: 343–352

Biederman J, Joshi G, Mick E, et al. A prospective open-label trial of lamotrigine monotherapy in children and adolescents with bipolar disorder. *CNS Neurosci Ther* 2010; 16: 91–102

Biederman J, Krishnan S, Zhang Y, et al. Efficacy and safety of lisdexamfetamine (NRP-104) in children with attention-deficit/hyperactivity disorder: a phase 3, randomized, multicenter, double-blind, parallel-group study. *Clin Ther* 2007; 29: 450–463

Biederman J, Lindsten A, Sluth LB, et al. Vortioxetine for attention deficit hyperactivity disorder in adults: a randomized, double-blind, placebo-controlled, proof-of-concept study. *J Psychopharmacol* 2019; 33: 511–521

Biederman J, Petty CR, Wilens TE, et al. Familial risk analyses of attention deficit hyperactivity disorder and substance use disorders. *Am J Psychiatry* 2008a; 165: 107–115

Biederman J, Seidman LJ, Petty CR, et al. Effects of stimulant medication on neuropsychological functioning in young adults with attention-deficit/hyperactivity disorder. *J Clin Psychiatry* 2008b; 69: 1150–1156

Biel MG, Peselow E, Mulcare L, et al. Continuation versus discontinuation of lithium in recurrent bipolar illness: a naturalistic study. *Bipolar Disord* 2007; 9: 435–442

Bighelli I, Castellazzi M, Cipriani A, et al. Antidepressants versus placebo for panic disorder in adults. *Cochrane Database Syst Rev* 2018; 4: CD010676

Bilder RM, Goldman RS, Volavka J, et al. Neurocognitive effects of clozapine, olanzapine, risperidone, and haloperidol in patients with chronic schizophrenia or schizoaffective disorder. *Am J Psychiatry* 2002; 159: 1018–1028

Binder RL, Levy R. Extrapyramidal reactions in Asians. *Am J Psychiatry* 1981; 138: 1243–1244

Birkeland SF. Psychopharmacological treatment and course in paranoid personality disorder: a case series. *Int Clin Psychopharmacol* 2013; 28: 283–285

Birks JS, Harvey RJ. Donepezil for dementia due to Alzheimer's disease. *Cochrane Database Syst Rev* 2018; (6): CD001190

Birmingham CL, Goldner EM, Bakan R, et al. Controlled trial of zinc supplementation in anorexia nervosa. *Int J Eat Disord* 1994; 15: 231–235

Bisaga A, Aharonovich E, Garawi F, et al. A randomized placebo-controlled trial of gabapentin for cocaine dependence. *Drug Alcohol Depend* 2006; 81: 267–274

Bishara D, Olofinjana O, Sparshatt A, et al: Olanzapine: a systematic review and meta-regression of the relationships between dose, plasma concentration, receptor occupancy, and response. *J Clin Psychopharmacol* 2013; 33: 329–335

Bishop JR, Moline J, Ellingrod VL, et al. Serotonin 2A-1438 G/A and G-protein Beta3 subunit C825T polymorphisms in patients with depression and SSRI-associated sexual side-effects. *Neuropsychopharmacology* 2006; 31: 2281–2288

Bisol LW, Lara DR. Low-dose quetiapine for patients with dysregulation of hyperthymic and cyclothymic temperaments. *J Psychopharmacol* 2001; 24: 421–424

Bivard A, Lillicrap T, Krishnamurthy V, et al. MIDAS (Modafinil in Debilitating Fatigue After Stroke): a randomized, double-blind, placebo-controlled, cross-over trial. *Stroke* 2017; 48: 1293–1298

Bixby AL, VandenBerg A, Bostwick JR. Clinical management of bleeding risk with antidepressants. *Ann Pharmacother* 2019; 53: 186–194

Black DW, Gabel J, Hansen J, et al. A double-blind comparison of fluvoxamine versus placebo in the treatment of compulsive buying disorder. *Ann Clin Psychiatry* 2000; 12: 205–211

Black N, Stockings E, Campbell G, et al. Cannabinoids for the treatment of mental disorders and symptoms of mental disorders: a systematic review and meta-analysis. *Lancet Psychiatry* 2019; 6: 995–1010

Blackford JU, Buckholtz JW, Avery SN, et al. A unique role for the human amygdala in novelty detection. *Neuroimage* 2010; 50: 1188–1193

Blanchard EB, Jones-Alexander J, Buckley TC, et al. Psychometric properties of the PTSD checklist (PCL). *Behav Res Ther* 1996; 34: 699–673

Blessing EM, Steenkamp MM, Manzanares J, et al. Cannabidiol as a potential treatment for anxiety disorders. *Neurotherapeutics* 2015; 12: 825–836

Blier P, Bergeron R, de Montigny C. Selective activation of postsynaptic 5-HT1A receptors induces rapid antidepressant response. *Neuropsychopharmacology* 1997; 16: 333–338

Blier P, Ward HE, Tremblay P, et al. Combination of antidepressant medications from treatment initiation for major depressive disorder: a double-blind randomized study. *Am J Psychiatry* 2010; 167: 281–288

Bloch M, Schmidt PJ, Danaceau MA, et al. Dehydroandrosterone treatment of mid-life dysthymia. *Biol Psychiatry* 1999; 45: 1533–1541

Bloch MH, Landeros-Weisenberger A, Dombrowski P, et al. Systematic review: pharmacological and behavioral treatment for trichotillomania. *Biol Psychiatry* 2007; 62: 839–846

Bloch MR, Elliott M, Thompson H, et al. Fluoxetine in pathological skin-picking: open-label and double-blind results. *Psychosomatics* 2001; 42: 314–319

Blodgett JC, Del Re AC, Maisel NC, et al. A meta-analysis of topiramate's effects for individuals with alcohol use disorders. *Alcohol Clin Exp Res* 2014; 38: 1481–1488

Blom TJ, Mingione CJ, Guerdjikova AI, et al. Placebo response in binge eating disorder: a pooled analysis of 10 clinical trials from one research group. *Eur Eat Disord Rev* 2014; 22: 140–146

Bocchetta A, Ardau R, Fanni T, et al. Renal function during long-term lithium treatment: a cross-sectional and longitudinal study. *BMC Med* 2015; 13: 12

Boeker T. Ziprasidone and migraine headache. *Am J Psychiatry* 2002; 159: 1435–1436

Bogenschutz MP, Nurnberg GH. Olanzapine versus placebo in the treatment of borderline personality disorder. *J Clin Psychiatry* 2004; 65: 104–109

Boggs DL, Kelly DL, Feldman S, et al. Quetiapine at high doses for the treatment of refractory schizophrenia. *Schizophr Res* 2008; 101: 347–348

Bohus MJ, Landwehrmeyer GB, Stiglmayr CE, et al. Naltrexone in the treatment of dissociative symptoms in patients with borderline personality disorder: an open label trial. *J Clin Psychiatry* 1999; 60: 598–603

Bonari L, Pinto N, Ahn E, et al. Perinatal risks of untreated depression during pregnancy. *Can J Psychiatry* 2004; 49: 726–735

Bondolfi G, Chautems C, Rochat B, et al. Non-response to citalopram in depressive patients: pharmacokinetic and clinical consequences of a fluvoxamine augmentation. *Psychopharmacology (Berl)* 1996; 128: 421–425

Bondolfi G, Lissner C, Kosel M, et al. Fluoxetine augmentation in citalopram non-responders: pharmacokinetic and clinical consequences. *Int J Neuropsychopharmacol* 2000; 3: 55–60

Bonn-Miller MO, Loflin MJE, Thomas BF, et al. Labeling accuracy of cannabidiol extracts sold online. *J Am Med Assoc* 2017; 218: 1708–1709

Boonstra E, de Kleijn R, Colzato LS, et al. Neurotransmitters as food supplements: the effects of GABA on brain and behavior. *Front Psychol* 2015; 6: 1520

Borison RL, Arvanitis LA, Miller BG. ICI 204,636, an atypical antipsychotic: efficacy and safety in a multicenter, placebo-controlled trial in patients with schizophrenia. U.S. SEROQUEL Study Group. *J Clin Psychopharmacol* 1996; 16: 158–169

Borras L, Huguelet P, Eytan A. Delusional "pseudotranssexualism" in schizophrenia. *Psychiatry* 2007; 70: 175–179

Bortnick B, El-Khalili N, Banov M, et al. Efficacy and tolerability of extended release quetiapine fumarate (quetiapine XR) monotherapy in major depressive disorder: a placebo-controlled, randomized study. *J Affect Disord* 2011; 128: 83–94

Bose A, Li D, Gandhi C. Escitalopram in the acute treatment of depressed patients aged 60 years or older. *Am J Geriatr Psychiatry* 2008; 16: 14–20

Bottlender R, Rudolf D, Strauß A, et al. Mood-stabilisers reduce the risk of developing antidepressant-induced maniform states in acute treatment of bipolar I depressed patients. *J Affect Disord* 2001; 63: 79–83

Boulenger J-P, Loft H, Florea I. A randomized clinical study of LuAA21004 in the prevention of relapse in patients with major depressive disorder. *J Psychopharmacol* 2012; 26: 1408–1416

Boulenger J-P, Loft H, Olsen CK. Efficacy and safety of vortioxetine (Lu AA21004), 15 and 20 mg/day: a randomized, double-blind, placebo-controlled, duloxetine-referenced study in the acute treatment of adult patients with major depressive disorder. *Int Clin Psychopharmacol* 2014; 29: 138–149

Bourgeois JA. The management of performance anxiety with beta adrenergic-blocking agents. *Jefferson J Psychiatry* 1991; 9: 13–28

Bourgeois BF, D'Souza J. Long-term safety and tolerability of oxcarbazepine in children: a review of clinical experience. *Epilepsy Behav* 2005; 7: 375–382

Bowden CL, Calabrese JR, Sachs G, et al. A placebo-controlled 18-month trial of lamotrigine and lithium maintenance treatment in recently manic or hypomanic patients with bipolar I disorder. *Arch Gen Psychiatry* 2003; 60: 392–400

Bowden CL, Janicak PG, Orsulak P, et al. Relation of serum valproate concentration to response in mania. *Am J Psychiatry* 1996; 153: 765–770

Bowden CL, Keck PE Jr., McElroy SL, et al. A randomized, placebo-controlled 12 month trial of divalproex and lithium in treatment of outpatients with bipolar I disorder. Divalproex Maintenance Study Group. *Arch Gen Psychiatry* 2000; 57: 481–489

Bowden CL, Singh R, Weisler P, et al. Lamotrigine vs. lamotrigine plus divalproex in randomized, placebo-controlled maintenance treatment for bipolar depression. *Acta Psychiatr Scand* 2012; 126: 342–350

Bowden CL, Vieta E, Ice KS, et al. Ziprasidone plus a mood stabilizer in subjects with bipolar I disorder: a 6-month, randomized, placebo-controlled, double-blind trial. *J Clin Psychiatry* 2010; 71: 130–137

Bowtell M, Eaton S, Thien K, et al. Rates and predictors of relapse following discontinuation of antipsychotic medication after a first episode of psychosis. *Schizophr Res* 2018; 195: 231–236

Bozzatello P, Rocca P, Uscinska M, et al. Efficacy and tolerability of asenapine compared with olanzapine in borderline personality disorder: an open-label randomized controlled trial. *CNS Drugs* 2017; 31: 809–819

Brady K, Pearlstein T, Asnis G, et al. Efficacy and safety of sertraline treatment of posttraumatic stress disorder: a randomized controlled trial. *J Am Med Assoc* 2000; 283: 1837–1844

Braun P, Greenberg S, Dasberg H, et al. Core symptoms of posttraumatic stress disorder unimproved by alprazolam treatment. *J Clin Psychiatry* 1990; 51: 236–238

Brawman-Mintzer O, Knapp RG, Nietert PJ. Adjunctive risperidone in generalized anxiety disorder: a double-blind, placebo-controlled study. *J Clin Psychiatry* 2005; 66: 1321–1325

Breier A, Buchanan RW, Kirkpatrick B, et al. Effects of clozapine on positive and negative symptoms in outpatients with schizophrenia. *Am J Psychiatry* 1994; 151: 20–60

Breilmann J, Girlanda F, Guaiana G, et al. Benzodiazepines versus placebo for panic disorder in adults. *Cochrane Database Syst Rev* 2019; (3): CD010677

Breitbart W, Rosenfeld B, Kaim M, et al. A randomized, double-blind, placebo-controlled trial of psychostimulants for the treatment of fatigue in ambulatory patients with human immunodeficiency virus disease. *Arch Intern Med* 2001; 161: 411–420

Brekhman II, Dardymov IV. New substances of plant origin which increase nonspecific resistance. *Ann Rev Pharmacol* 1969; 9: 419–430

Bremner JD, Shearer K, McCaffery P. Retinoic acid and affective disorders: the evidence for an association. *J Clin Psychiatry* 2012; 73: 37–50

Briggs-Gowan MJ, Carter S, Bosson-Heenan J, et al. Are infant-toddler social-emotional and behavioral problems transient? *J Am Acad Child Adolesc Psychiatry* 2006; 45: 849–858

Britnell SR, Jackson AD, Brown JN., et al. Aripiprazole for post-traumatic stress disorder: a systematic review. *Clin Neuropharmacol* 2017; 40: 273–278

Bro SP, Kjaersgard MI, Parner ET, et al. Adverse pregnancy outcomes after exposure to methylphenidate or atomoxetine during pregnancy. *Clin Epidemiol* 2015; 7: 139–147

Brown WA. Placebo as a treatment for depression. *Neuropsychopharmacology* 1994; 10: 265–269

Brown ES, Gabrielson B. A randomized double-blind, placebo-controlled trial of citicoline for bipolar and unipolar depression and methamphetamine dependence. *J Affect Disord* 2012; 143: 257–260

Brown ES, Gorman AR, Hynan LS. A randomized, placebo-controlled trial of citicoline add-on therapy in outpatients with bipolar disorder and cocaine dependence. *J Clin Psychopharmacol* 2007; 27: 498–502

Brown ES, Todd JP, Hu T, et al. A randomized, double-blind, placebo-controlled trial of citicoline for cocaine dependence in bipolar I disorder. *Am J Psychiatry* 2015; 172: 1014–1021

Bruder GE, Sedoruk JP, Stewart JW, et al. Electroencephalographic alpha measures predict therapeutic response to a selective serotonin reuptake inhibitor antidepressant: pre- and post-treatment findings. *Biol Psychiatry* 2008; 63: 1171–1177

Brunet A, Saumier D, Liu A, et al. Reduction of PTSD symptoms with pre-reactivation propranolol therapy: randomized controlled trial. *Am J Psychiatry* 2018; 175: 427–433

Brunner E, Tohen M, Osuntokun O, et al. Efficacy and safety of olanzapine/fluoxetine combination vs fluoxetine monotherapy following successful combination therapy of treatment-resistant major depressive disorder. *Neuropsychopharmacology* 2014; 39: 2549–2559

Bruno A, Micò U, Pandolfo G, et al. Lamotrigine augmentation of serotonin reuptake inhibitors in treatment-resistant obsessive-compulsive disorder: a double-blind, placebo-controlled study. *J Psychopharmacol* 2012; 26: 1456–1462

Buchanan RW, Breier A, Kirkpatrick B, et al. Positive and negative symptoms response to clozapine with and without the deficit syndrome. *Am J Psychiatry* 1998; 155: 751–760

Bugarski-Kirola D, Iwata N, Sameliak S, et al. Efficacy and safety of adjunctive bitopertin versus placebo in patients with suboptimally controlled symptoms of schizophrenia treated with antipsychotics: results from three phase 3, randomised, double-blind, parallel-group, placebo-controlled, multicentre studies in the SearchLyte clinical trial programme. *Lancet Psychiatry* 2016; 3: 1115–1128

Buitelaar JK, Sobanski E, Stieglitz RD, et al. Predictors of placebo response in adults with attention-deficit/hyperactivity disorder: data from 2 randomized trials of osmotic-release oral system methylphenidate. *J Clin Psychiatry* 2012; 73: 1097–1102

Burdick KE, Endick CJ, Goldberg JF. Assessing cognitive deficits in bipolar disorder: are self-reports valid? *Psychiatry Res* 2005; 136: 43–50

Burdick KE, Braga RJ, Nnadi CU, et al. Placebo-controlled adjunctive trial of pramipexole in patients with bipolar disorder: targeting cognitive dysfunction. *J Clin Psychiatry* 2012; 73: 103–112

Burdick KE, Russo M, Frangou S, et al. Empirical evidence for discrete neurocognitive subgroups in bipolar disorder: clinical implications. *Psychol Med* 2014; 44: 3083–3096

Bürkner PC, Williams DR, Simmons TC, et al. Intranasal oxytocin may improve high-level social cognition in schizophrenia, but not social cognition or neurocognition in general: a multilevel Bayesian meta-analysis. *Schizophr Bull* 2017; 43: 1291–1303

Butterfield MI, Becker ME, Connor KM, et al. Olanzapine in the treatment of post-traumatic stress disorder: a pilot study. *Int Clin Psychopharmacol* 2001; 16: 197–203

Bystritsky A, Kerwin L, Feusner JD, et al. A pilot controlled trial of bupropion XL versus escitalopram in generalized anxiety disorder. *Psychopharmacol Bull* 2008; 41: 46–51

Cain JW. Poor response to fluoxetine: underlying depression, serotonergic overstimulation, or a "therapeutic window"? *J Clin Psychiatry* 1992; 53: 272–277

Cakir S, Kulakisizoglu IB. The efficacy of mirtazapine in agitated patients with Alzheimer's disease: a 12-week open-label pilot study. *Neuropsychiatr Dis Treat* 2008; 4: 963–966

Calabrese JR, Bowden CL, Sachs G, et al. A placebo-controlled 18-month trial of lamotrigine and lithium maintenance treatment in recently depressed patients with bipolar I disorder. *J Clin Psychiatry* 2003; 64: 1013–1024

Calabrese JR, Bowden CL, Sachs GS, et al. A double-blind placebo-controlled study of lamotrigine monotherapy in outpatients with bipolar I depression. *J Clin Psychiatry* 1999; 60: 79–88

Calabrese JR, Keck PE Jr, Starace A, et al. Efficacy and safety of low- and high-dose cariprazine in acute and mixed mania associated with bipolar I disorder: a double-blind, placebo-controlled study. *J Clin Psychiatry* 2015; 76: 284–292

Calabrese JR, Pikalov A, Streicher C, et al. Lurasidone in combination with lithium or valproate for the maintenance treatment of bipolar I disorder. *Eur Neuropsychopharmacol* 2017a; 27: 865–876

Calabrese JR, Sanchez R, Jin N, et al. Efficacy and safety of aripiprazole once-monthly in the maintenance treatment of bipolar I disorder: a double-blind, placebo-controlled, 52-week randomized withdrawal study. *J Clin Psychiatry* 2017b; 78: 324–331

Calabrese JR, Shelton MD, Rapport DJ, et al. A 20-month, double-blind, maintenance trial of lithium versus divalproex in rapid-cycling bipolar disorder. *Am J Psychiatry* 2005; 162: 2152–2161

Calabrese JR, Suppes T, Bowden CL, et al. A double-blind, placebo-controlled, prophylaxis study of lamotrigine in rapid-cycling bipolar disorder: Lamictal 614 Study Group. *J Clin Psychiatry* 2000; 61: 841–850

Campbell M, Adams PB, Small AM, et al. Lithium in hospitalized aggressive children with conduct disorder: a double-blind and placebo-controlled study. *J Am Acad Child Adolesc Psychiatry* 1995; 34: 445–453

Campbell M, Small AM, Green WH, et al. Behavioral efficacy of haloperidol and lithium carbonate: a comparison in hospitalized aggressive children with conduct disorder. *Arch Gen Psychiatry* 1984; 41: 650–656

Canuso CM, Singh JB, Fedgchin M, et al. Efficacy and safety of intranasal esketamine for the rapid reduction of symptoms of depression and suicidality in patients at imminent risk for suicide: results of a double-blind, randomized, placebo-controlled study. *Am J Psychiatry* 2018; 175: 620–630

Carbon H, Hsieh CH, Kane JM, et al. Tardive dyskinesia prevalence in the period of second-generation antipsychotic use: a meta-analysis. *J Clin Psychiatry* 2017; 78: e264–e278

Cardenas D. Let not thy food be confused with thy medicine: the Hippocratic misquotation. *E-SPEN* 2013; 8: e260–e262

Careri JM, Draine AE, Hanover R, et al. A 12-week double-blind, placebo-controlled, flexible-dose trial of vilazodone in generalized social anxiety disorder. *Prim Care Companion CNS Disord* 2015; 17: 10.4088/PCC.15m01831

Carey P, Suliman S, Ganesan K, et al. Olanzapine monotherapy in posttraumatic stress disorder: efficacy in a randomized, double-blind, placebo-controlled study. *Hum Psychopharmacol* 2012; 27: 386–391

Carhart-Harris RL, Bolstridge M, Dy CMJ, et al. Psilocybin with psychological support for treatment-resistant depression: six-month follow-up. *Psychopharmacology (Berl)* 2018; 235: 399–408

Carman J, Peuskens S, Vangeneugden A. Risperidone in the treatment of negative symptoms of schizophrenia: a meta-analysis. *Int Clin Psychopharmacol* 1995; 10: 207–213

Caroff SN, Mann SC. Neuroleptic malignant syndrome. *Med Clin North Amer* 1993; 77: 185–202

Carpenter KM, Hasin DS. Reliability and discriminant validity of the Type I/II and Type A/B alcoholic subtype classifications in untreated problem drinkers: a test of the Apollonian–Dionysian hypothesis. *Drug Alcohol Depend* 2001; 63: 51–67

Casamassima F, Huang J, Fava M, et al. Phenotypic effects of bipolar liability gene among individuals with major depressive disorder. *Am J Med Genet B Neuropsychiatr Genet* 2010; 153B: 303–309

Casey DE, Daniel DG, Tamminga C, et al. Divalproex ER combined with olanzapine or risperidone for treatment of acute exacerbations of schizophrenia. *Neuropsychopharmacology* 2009; 34: 1330–1338

Casey DE, Daniel DG, Wassef AA, et al. Effect of divalproex combined with olanzapine or risperidone in patients with an acute exacerbation of schizophrenia. *Neuropsychopharmacology* 2003; 28: 182–192

Castells X, Blanco-Silvente L, Cunill R. Amphetamines for attention deficit hyperactivity disorder (ADHD) in adults. *Cochrane Database Syst Rev* 2018; 8: CD007813

Castells X, Cunill R, Pérez-Mañá C, et al. Psychostimulant drugs for cocaine dependence. *Cochrane Database Syst Rev* 2016; 9: CD007380

Castro VM, Roberson AM, McCoy TH, et al. Stratifying risk for renal insufficiency among lithium-treated patients: an electronic health record study. *Neuropsychopharmacology* 2016; 41: 1138–1143

Catalá-López F, Hutton B, Núñez-Beltrán A, et al. The pharmacological and non-pharmacological treatment of attention deficit hyperactivity disorder in children and adolescents: a systematic review with network meta-analyses of randomised trials. *PLoS One* 2017; 12: e0180355

Caye A, Rocha TB, Anselmi L, et al. Attention-deficit/hyperactivity disorder trajectories from childhood to young adulthood: evidence from a birth cohort supporting a late-onset syndrome. *JAMA Psychiatry* 2016; 73: 705–712

Center for Behavioral Health Statistics and Quality (CBHSQ). *Behavioral Health Trends in the United States: Results from the 2014 National Survey on Drug Use and Health. HHS Publication No. SMA 15-4927, NSDUH Series H-50.* Rockville, MD: Substance Abuse and Mental Health Services Administration; 2015

Chakrabarti A, Bagnall A, Chue P, et al. Loxapine for schizophrenia. *Cochrane Database Syst Rev* 2007; (4): CD001943

Chambers CD, Hernandez-Diaz S, Van Marter LJ, et al. Selective serotonin-reuptake inhibitors and risk of persistent pulmonary hypertension of the newborn. *New Engl J Med* 2006; 354: 579–587

Chan GC, Hinds TR, Impey S, et al. Hippocampal neurotoxicity of Delta9-tetrahydrocannabinol. *J Neurosci* 1998; 18: 5322–5332

Chang K, Saxena K, Howe M. An open-label study of lamotrigine adjunct or monotherapy for the treatment of adolescents with bipolar depression. *J Am Acad Child Adolesc Psychiatry* 2006; 45: 298–304

Chang HY, Tseng PT, Stubbs B, et al. The efficacy and tolerability of paliperidone in mania of bipolar disorder: a preliminary meta-analysis. *Exp Clin Psychopharmacol* 2017; 25: 422–433

Chang SS, Liu CM, Lin SH, et al. Impaired flush response to niacin skin patch among schizophrenia patients and their nonpsychotic relatives: the effect of genetic loading. *Schizophr Bull* 2009; 35: 213–221

Charney DS. Psychobiological mechanisms of resilience and vulnerability: implications for successful adaptation to extreme stress. *Am J Psychiatry* 2004; 161: 195–216

Charney DA, Heath LM, Zikos E, et al. Poorer drinking outcomes with citalopram treatment for alcohol dependence: a randomized, double-blind, placebo-controlled trial. *Alcohol Clin Exp Res* 2015; 39: 1756–1765

Chaudhry IB, Neelam K, Duddu V, et al. Ethnicity and Psychopharmacology. *J Psychopharmachol* 2008; 22: 673–680

Chekroud AM, Gueorguieva R, Krumholz HM, et al. Reevaluating the efficacy and predictability of antidepressant treatments: a symptom clustering approach. *JAMA Psychiatry* 2017; 74: 370-378

Chen JJ, Hua H, Massihi L, et al. Systematic literature review of quetiapine for the treatment of psychosis in patients with parkinsonism. *J Psychiatry Clin Neurosci* 2019a; 31: 188–195

Chen JX, Su YA, Bian QT, et al. Adjunctive aripiprazole in the treatment of risperidone-induced hyperprolactinemia: a randomized, double-blind, placebo-controlled, dose-response study. *Psychoneuroendocrinology* 2015; 58: 130–140

Chen MH, Lin WC, Wu HJ, et al. Antisuicidal effect, BDNF Val66Met polymorphism, and low-dose ketamine infusion: reanalysis of adjunctive ketamine study of Taiwanese patients with treatment-resistant depression (AKSTP-TRD). *J Affect Disord* 2019b; 251: 162–169

Chen TR, Huang HC, Hsu JH, et al. Pharmacological and psychological interventions for generalized anxiety disorder in adults: a network meta-analysis. *J Psychiatr Res* 2019c; 118: 73–83

Chen YF, Wang SJ, Khin NA, et al. Trial design issues and treatment effect modeling in multi-regional schizophrenia trials. *Pharm Stat* 2010; 9: 217–229

Chengappa KNR, Brar JS, Gannon JM, Schlicht PJ. Adjunctive use of a standardized extract of *Withania somnifera* (ashwaganda) to treat symptom exacerbation in schizophrenia: a randomized, double-blind, placebo-controlled study. *J Clin Psychiatry* 2018; 79: 17m11826

Chengappa KN, Bowie CR, Schlicht PJ, et al. Randomized placebo-controlled adjunctive study of an extract of *Withania somnifera* for cognitive dysfunction in bipolar disorder. *J Clin Psychiatry* 2013; 74: 1076–1083

Chessick CA, Allen MH, Thase M, et al. Azapirones for generalized anxiety disorder. *Cochrane Database Syst Rev* 2006; (3) :CD006115

Chiappini S, Schifano F. A decade of gabapentinoid misuse: an analysis of the European Medicines Agency's "Suspected Adverse Drug Reactions" database. *CNS Drugs* 2016; 30: 647–654

Chick J, Aschauer H, Hornik K, et al. Efficacy of fluvoxamine in preventing relapse in alcohol dependence: a one-year, double-blind, placebo-controlled multicentre study with analysis by typology. *Drug Alcohol Depend* 2004; 74: 61–70

Cho M, Lee TY, Kwak YB, et al. Adjunctive use of anti-inflammatory drugs for schizophrenia: a meta-analytic investigation of randomized controlled trials. *Aust N Z J Psychiatry* 2019; 53: 742–759

Chollet F, Tardy J, Albucher JF. Fluoxetine for motor recovery after stroke (FLAME): a randomised placebo-controlled trial. *Lancet Neurol* 2011; 10: 123–130

Choy Y, Peselow ED, Case BG, et al. Three-year medication prophylaxis in panic disorder: to continue or discontinue? A naturalistic study. *Compr Psychiatry* 2007; 48: 419–425

Christensen J, Grønborg TK, Sørensen MJ. Prenatal valproate exposure and risk of autism spectrum disorders and childhood autism. *J Am Med Assoc* 2013; 309: 1696–1703

Christenson GA, MacKenzie TB, Mitchell JE, et al. A placebo-controlled, double-blind crossover study of fluoxetine in trichotillomania. *Am J Psychiatry* 1991; 148: 1566–1571

Chung YC, Lee CR, Park TW, et al. Effect of donepezil added to atypical antipsychotics on cognition in patients with schizophrenia: an open-label trial. *World J Biol Psychiatry* 2009; 10: 156–162

Cipriani A, Furukawa TA, Salanti G, et al. Comparative efficacy and acceptability of 21 antidepressant drugs for the acute treatment of adults with major depressive disorder: a systematic review and network meta-analysis. *Lancet* 2018; 391: 1357–1366

Citrome L. The ABCs of dopamine receptor partial agonists – aripiprazole, brexpiprazole, and cariprazine: the 15-min challenge to sort these agents out. *Int J Clin Pract.* 2015; 69: 1211–1220

Citrome L. Activating and sedating adverse effects of second-generation antipsychotics in the treatment of schizophrenia and major depressive disorder: absolute risk increase and number needed to harm. *J Clin Psychopharmacol* 2017a; 37: 138–147

Citrome L, Meng X, Hochfeld M. Efficacy of iloperidone in schizophrenia: a PANSS five-factor analysis. *Schizophr Research* 2011; 131(1–3): 75–81

Citrome L, Durgam S, Lu K, et al. The effect of cariprazine on hostility associated with schizophrenia: post hoc analyses from 3 randomized controlled trials. *J Clin Psychiatry* 2016a; 77: 109–115

Citrome L, Ota A, Nagamizu K, et al. The effect of brexpiprazole (OPC-34712) and aripiprazole in adult patients with acute schizophrenia: results from a randomized, exploratory study. *Int Clin Psychopharmacol* 2016b; 31: 192–201

Citrome L, Landbloom R, Chang CT, et al. Effects of asenapine on agitation and hostility in adults with acute manic or mixed episodes associated with bipolar I disorder. *Neuropsychiatr Dis Res* 2017b; 13: 2955–2963

Citrome L, Volavka J, Czobor P, et al. Effects of clozapine, olanzapine, risperidone, and haloperidol on hostility among patients with schizophrenia. *Psychiatr Serv* 2001; 52: 1510–1514

Ciudad A, Alvarez E, Roca M, et al. Early response and remission as predictors of a good outcome of a major depressive episode at 12-month follow-up: a prospective, longitudinal, observational study. *J Clin Psychiatry* 2012; 73: 185–191

Claes L, Bouman WP, Witcomb G, et al. Non-suicidal self-injury in trans people: associations with psychological symptoms, victimization, interpersonal functioning, and perceived social support. *J Sex Med* 2015; 12: 168–179

Clark CT, Klein AM, Perel JM, et al. Lamotrigine dosing for pregnant patients with bipolar disorder. *Am J Psychiatry* 2013; 170: 1240–1247

Clark RD, Canive JM, Calais LA, et al. Divalproex in posttraumatic stress disorder: an open-label clinical trial. *J Trauma Stress* 1999; 12: 395–401

Clayton AH, Stewart RS, Fayyad R, et al. Sex differences in clinical presentation and response in panic disorder: pooled data from sertraline treatment studies. *Arch Womens Ment Health* 2006; 9: 151–157

Clemons WE, Makela E, Young J. Concomitant use of modafinil and tranylcypromine in a patient with narcolepsy: a case report. *Sleep Med* 2004; 5: 509–511

Cloninger CR. *The Temperament and Character Inventory (TCI): A Guide to its Development and Use*. St. Louis, MO: Washington University; Center for Psychobiology of Personality; 1994

Cloninger CR, Przybeck TR, Svrakic DM. The Tridimensional Personality Questionnaire: US normative data. *Psychol Rep* 1991; 69: 1047–1057

Cloninger CR, Zohar AH, Hirschmann S, et al. The psychological costs and benefits of being highly persistent: personality profiles distinguish mood disorders from anxiety disorders. *J Affect Disord* 2012; 136: 758–766

Clyde PW, Harari AE, Getka EJ, et al. Combined levothyroxine plus liothyronine compared with levothyroxine alone in primary hypothyroidism: a randomized controlled trial. *J Am Med Assoc* 2003; 290: 2952–2958

Coccaro EF, Kavoussi RJ. Fluoxetine and impulsive aggressive behavior in personality disordered subjects. *Arch Gen Psychiatry* 1997; 54: 1081–1088

Coccaro EF, Lee RJ, Kavoussi JR. A double blind, randomized, placebo-controlled trial of fluoxetine in patients with intermittent explosive disorder. *J Clin Psychiatry* 2009; 70: 653–662

Coccaro EF, Adan F, Allen D, et al. Plasma-serum differences in the assessment of tricyclic antidepressant blood levels. *Int Clin Psychopharmacol* 1987; 2: 217–224

Cohen JM, Hernández-Díaz S, Bateman BT, et al. Placental complications associated with psychostimulant use in pregnancy. *Obstet Gynecol* 2017; 130: 1192–1201

Cohen JM, Huybrechts KF, Patorno E, et al. Anticonvulsant mood stabilizer and lithium use and risk of adverse pregnancy outcomes. *J Clin Psychiatry* 2019; 80: 18m12572

Cohen LG, Chesly S, Eugenio S, et al. Erythromycin-induced clozapine toxic reaction. *Arch Intern Med* 1996; 156: 675–677

Cohen LS, Soares CN, Poitras JR, et al. Short-term use of estradiol for depression in perimenopausal and postmenopausal women: a preliminary report. *Am J Psychiatry* 2003; 160: 1519–1522

Cohen LS, Viguera AC, McInerney KA, et al. Reproductive safety of second-generation antipsychotics: current data from the Massachusetts General Hospital National Pregnancy Registry for Atypical Antipsychotics. *Am J Psychiatry* 2016; 173: 263–270

Cohen NL, Ross EC, Bagby RM, et al. The 5-factor model of personality and antidepressant medication compliance. *Can J Psychiatry* 2004; 49: 106–113

Cole JD, Kazarian SS. The Level of Expressed Emotion Scale: a new measure of expressed emotion. *J Clin Psychol* 1988; 44: 392-397

Comer JS, Olfson M, Mojtabai R. National trends in child and adolescent psychotropic polypharmacy in office-based practice, 1996–2007. *J Am Acad Child Adolesc Psychiatry* 2010; 49: 1001–1010

Compton WM, Han B, Blanco C, et al. Prevalence and correlates of prescription stimulant use, misuse, use disorders, and motivations for misuse among adults in the United States. *Am J Psychiatry* 2018; 175: 741–755

Conley RR, Kelly DL, Richardson CM, et al. The efficacy of high-dose olanzapine versus clozapine in treatment-resistant schizophrenia: a double-blind crossover study. *J Clin Psychopharmacol* 2003; 23: 668–671

Connor DF, Fletcher KE, Swanson JM, et al. A meta-analysis of clonidine for symptoms of attention-deficit hyperactivity disorder. *J Am Acad Child Adolesc Psychiatry* 1999; 38: 1551–1559

Connor KM, Davidson JRT, Churchill LE, et al. Psychometric properties of the Social Phobia Inventory. *Br J Psychiatry* 2000; 176: 379-386

Connor KM, Davidson JR, Weisler RH, et al. Tiagabine for posttraumatic stress disorder: effects of open-label and double-blind discontinuation treatment. *Psychopharmacology* 2006; 184: 21–25

Connor KM, Hidalgo RB, Crockett B, et al. Predictors of treatment response in patients with posttraumatic stress disorder. *Prog Neuropsychopharmacol Biol Psychiatry* 2001; 25: 337–345

Conus P, Cotton SM, Francey SM, et al. Predictors of favourable outcome in young people with a first episode psychosis without antipsychotic medication. *Schizophr Res* 2017; 185: 130–136

Cook IA, Hunter AM, Gilmer WS, et al. Quantitative electroencephalogram biomarkers for predicting likelihood and speed of achieving sustained remission in major depression: a report from the Biomarkers for Rapid Identification of Treatment Effectiveness in Major Depression (BRITE-MD) trial. *J Clin Psychiatry* 2013; 74: 51–56

Cools R, Robbins TW. Chemistry of the adaptive mind. *Philos Trans A Math Phys Eng Sci* 2004; 362: 2871–2888

Cooper TB, Bergner PE, Simpson GM. The 24-hour serum lithium level as a prognosticator of dosage requirements. *Am J Psychiatry* 1973; 130: 601–603

Cooper-Karaz R, Apter JT, Cohen R, et al. Combined treatment with sertraline and liothyronine in major depression: a randomized, double-blind, placebo-controlled trial. *Arch Gen Psychiatry* 2007; 64: 679–688

Corá-Locatelli G, Greenberg BD, Martin J, et al. Gabapentin augmentation for fluoxetine-treated patients with obsessive-compulsive disorder. *J Clin Psychiatry* 1998; 59: 480–481

Cordás TA, Tavares H, Calderoni DM, et al. Oxcarbazepine for self-mutilating bulimic patients. *Int J Neuropsychopharmacol* 2006; 9: 769–771

Cornelius JR, Salloum IM, Ehler JG, et al. Fluoxetine in depressed alcoholics: a double-blind, placebo-controlled trial. *Arch Gen Psychiatry* 1997; 54: 700–705

Cornelius JR, Salloum IM, Thase ME, et al. Fluoxetine versus placebo in depressed alcoholic cocaine abusers. *Psychopharmacol Bull* 1998; 34: 117–121

Cornelius JR, Soloff PH, George A, et al. Haloperidol vs. phenelzine in continuation therapy of borderline disorder. *Psychopharmacol Bull* 1993; 29: 333–337

Correll CU, Kane JM. One-year incidence rates of tardive dyskinesia in children and adolescents treated with second-generation antipsychotics: a systematic review. *J Child Adolesc Psychopharmacol* 2007; 17: 647–656

Correll CU, Davis RE, Weingart M, et al. Efficacy and safety of lumateperone for treatment of schizophrenia: a randomized trial. *JAMA Psychiatry* 2020; 77: 349–358

Correll CU, Leucht S, Kane JM. Lower risk for tardive dyskinesia associated with second-generation antipsychotics: systematic review of 1-year studies. *Am J Psychiatry* 2004; 161: 414–425

Correll CU, Rubio JM, Kane JM. What is the risk-benefit ratio of long-term antipsychotic treatment in patients with schizophrenia? *World Psychiatry* 2018; 17: 149–160

Correll CU, Manu P, Olshanskiy V, et al. Cardiometabolic risk of second-generation antipsychotic medications during first-time use in children and adolescents. *J Am Med Assoc* 2009; 302: 1765–1773

Correll CU, Rubio JM, Inczedy-Farkas G, et al. Efficacy of 42 pharmacologic cotreatment strategies added to antipsychotic monotherapy in schizophrenia: systematic overview and quality appraisal of the meta-analytic evidence. *JAMA Psychiatry* 2017; 74: 675–684

Correll CU, Skuban A, Hobart M, et al. Efficacy of brexpiprazole in patients with acute schizophrenia: review of three randomized, double-blind, placebo-controlled studies. *Schizophr Res* 2016; 174: 82–92

Cortese S, Adamo N, Del Giovane C, et al. Comparative efficacy and tolerability of medications for attention-deficit hyperactivity disorder in children, adolescents, and adults: a systematic review and network meta-analysis. *Lancet Psychiatry* 2018; 5: 727–738

Corya SA, Williamson D, Sanger TM, et al. A randomized, double-blind comparison of olanzapine/fluoxetine combination, olanzapine, fluoxetine, and venlafaxine in treatment-resistant depression. *Depress Anxiety* 2006; 23: 364–372

Coryell W, Winokur G, Solomon D, et al. Lithium and recurrence in a long-term follow-up of bipolar affective disorder. *Psychol Med* 1997; 27: 281–289

Costi S, Soleimani L, Glasgow A, et al. Lithium continuation therapy following ketamine in patients with treatment resistant unipolar depression: a randomized controlled trial. *Neuropsychopharmacol* 2019; 44: 1812–1819

Coupland CAC, Hill T, Dening T, et al. Anticholinergic drug exposure and the risk of dementia: a nested case-control study. *JAMA Intern Med* 2019; 179: 1084–1093

Cowdry RW, Gardner DL. Pharmacotherapy of borderline personality disorder: alprazolam, carbamazepine, trifluoperazine, and tranylcypromine. *Arch Gen Psychiatry* 1988; 45: 111–119

Crawford MJ, Sanatinia R, Barrett B, et al. The clinical effectiveness and cost-effectiveness of lamotrigine in borderline personality disorder: a randomized placebo-controlled trial. *Am J Psychiatry* 2018; 175: 756–764

Crippa JA, Derenusson GN, Ferrari TB, et al. Neural basis of anxiolytic effects of cannabidiol (CBD) in generalized social anxiety disorder: a preliminary report. *J Psychopharmacol* 2011; 25: 121–130

Cristancho P, Lenze EJ, Dixon D, et al. Executive function predicts antidepressant treatment noncompletion in late-life depression. *J Clin Psychiatry* 2018; 79: 16m11371

Cross-Disorder Group of the Psychiatric Genomics Consortium. Genetic relationship between five psychiatric disorders estimated from genome-wide SNPs. *Nat Genet* 2013; 45: 984–994

Crossley NA, Constante M. Efficacy of atypical v typical antipsychotics in the treatment of early psychosis: meta-analysis. *Br J Psychiatry* 2010; 196: 434–439

Crossley NA, Marques TR, Taylor H, et al. Connectomic correlates of response to treatment in first-episode psychosis. *Brain* 2017; 140: 487–496

Cummings JL, Lyketsos CG, Peskind ER, et al. Effect of dextromethorphan-quinidine on agitation in patients with Alzheimer disease dementia: a randomized clinical trial. *J Am Med Assoc* 2015; 314: 1242–1254

Cutler AJ, Montgomery SA, Feifel D, et al. Extended release quetiapine fumarate monotherapy in major depressive disorder: a placebo- and duloxetine-controlled study. *J Clin Psychiatry* 2009; 70: 526–539

Czerwensky F, Leucht S, Steimer W. MC4R rs489693: a clinical risk factor for second generation antipsychotic-related weight gain? *Int J Neuropsychopharmacol* 2013; 16: 2103–2109

Czobor P, Volavka J, Meibach RC. Effect of risperidone on hostility in schizophrenia. *J Clin Psychopharmacol* 1995; 15: 243–249

D'Abreu A, Friedman JH. Tardive dyskinesia-like syndrome due to drugs that do not block dopamine receptors: rare or non-existent. Literature review. *Tremor Other Hyperkinet Mov (NY)* 2018; 8: 570

Dackis CA, Kampman KM, Lynch KG, et al. A double-blind, placebo-controlled trial of modafinil for cocaine dependence. *Neuropsychopharmacol* 2005; 30: 205–211

Dackis CA, Kampman KM, Lynch KG, et al. A double-blind, placebo-controlled trial of modafinil for cocaine dependence. *J Subst Abuse Treat* 2012; 43: 303–312

Dager SR, Khan A, Cowley DS, et al. Characteristics of placebo response during long-term treatment of panic disorder. *Psychopharmacol Bull* 1990; 26: 273–278.

Daly C, Griffin E, Ashcroft DM, et al. Intentional drug overdose involving pregabalin and gabapentin: findings from the National Self-Harm Registry Ireland, 2007–2015. *Clin Drug Investig* 2018a; 38: 373–380

Daly J, Singh JB, Fedgchin M, et al. Efficacy and safety of intranasal esketamine adjunctive to oral antidepressant therapy in treatment-resistant depression: a randomized clinical trial. *JAMA Psychiatry* 2018b; 75: 139–148

Daly J, Trivedi MH, Janik A, et al. Efficacy of esketamine nasal spray plus oral antidepressant treatment for relapse prevention of patients with treatment-resistant depression: a randomized clinical trial. *JAMA Psychiatry* 2019; 76: 893–903

Daniel DG, Zimbroff DL, Potkin SG, et al. Ziprasidone 80 mg/day and 160 mg/day in the acute exacerbation of schizophrenia and schizoaffective disorder: a 6-week placebo-controlled trial. Ziprasidone Study Group. *Neuropsychopharmacology* 1999; 20: 491–505

Dannlowski U, Baune BT, Böckemann I, et al. Adjunctive antidepressant treatment with quetiapine in agitated depression: positive effects on symptom reduction, psychopathology and remission rates. *Hum Psychopharmacol* 2008; 23: 587–593

Daray FM, Thommi SB, Ghaemi SN. The pharmacogenetics of antidepressant-induced mania: a systemic review and meta-analysis. *Bipolar Disord* 2010; 12: 702–706

Darbinyan V, Aslanyan G, Amroyan E, et al. Clinical trial of Rhodiola rosea L. extract SHR-5 in the treatment of mild to moderate depression. *Nord J Psychiatry* 2007; 61: 343–348

Davanzano R, Dal Bo S, Bua J, et al. Antiepileptic drug and breastfeeding. *Ital J Pediatr* 2013; 39: 50

Davidson J, Baldwin D, Stein DJ, et al. Treatment of posttraumatic stress disorder with venlafaxine extended release: a 6-month randomized controlled trial. *Arch Gen Psychiatry* 2006; 63: 1158–1165

Davidson J, Pearlstein T, Londborg P, et al. Efficacy of sertraline in preventing relapse of posttraumatic stress disorder: results of a 28-week double-blind, placebo-controlled study. *Am J Psychiatry* 2001a; 158: 1974–1981

Davidson J, Stein DJ, Rothbaum BO, et al. Resilience as a predictor of treatment response in patients with posttraumatic stress disorder treated with venlafaxine extended release or placebo. *J Psychopharmacol* 2012; 26: 778–783

Davidson JR, Book SW, Colket JT, et al. Assessment of a new self-rating scale for post-traumatic stress disorder. *Psychol Med* 1997a; 27: 153–160

Davidson JR, Malik ML, Sutherland SN. Response characteristics to antidepressants and placebo in post-traumatic stress disorder. *Int Clin Psychopharmacol* 1997b; 12: 291–296

Davidson JR, Potts N, Richichi E, et al. Treatment of social phobia with clonazepam and placebo. *J Clin Psychopharmacol* 1993; 13: 423–428

Davidson JR, Potts NL, Richichi EA, et al. The Brief Social Phobia Scale. *J Clin Psychiatry* 1991; (52 Suppl): 48S–51S

Davidson JR, Rothbaum BO, van der Kolk BA et al. Multicenter, double-blind comparison of sertraline and placebo in the treatment of posttraumatic stress disorder. *Arch Gen Psychiatry* 2001b; 58: 485–492

Davidson M, Emsley R, Kramer M, et al. Efficacy, safety and early response of paliperidone extended-release tablets (paliperidone ER): results of a 6-week, randomized, placebo-controlled study. *Schizophr Res* 2007; 93: 117–130

Davis JM. Dose equivalence of the antipsychotic drugs. *J Psychiatr Res* 1974; 11: 65–69

Davis LL, Barotlucci A, Petty F. Divalproex in the treatment of bipolar depression: a placebo-controlled study. *J Affect Disord* 2005; 85: 259–266

Davis LL, Davidson JR, Ward LC, et al. Divalproex in the treatment of posttraumatic stress disorder: a randomized, double-blind, placebo-controlled trial in a veteran population. *J Clin Psychopharmacol* 2008a; 28: 84–88

Davis LL, Ota A, Perry P, et al. Adjunctive brexpiprazole in patients with major depressive disorder and anxiety symptoms: an exploratory study. *Brain Behav* 2016; 6: e00520

Davis LL, Ward C, Rasmussen C, et al. A placebo-controlled trial of guanfacine for the treatment of posttraumatic stress disorder in veterans. *Psychopharmacol Bull* 2008b; 41: 8–18

Davison JM, Dunlop W. Renal hemodynamics and tubular function in normal human pregnancy. *Kidney Int* 1980; 18: 152–161

de Bejczy A, Söderpalm B. The effects of mirtazapine versus placebo on alcohol consumption in male high consumers of alcohol: a randomized, controlled trial. *J Clin Psychopharmacol* 2015; 35: 43–50

Debonnel G, Saint-André E, Hébert C, et al. Differential physiological effects of a low dose and high doses of venlafaxine in major depression. *Int J Neuropsychopharmacol* 2007; 10: 51–61

De Hert M, Sermon J, Geerts P, et al. The use of continuous treatment versus placebo or intermittent treatment strategies in stabilized patients with schizophrenia: a systematic review and meta-analysis of randomized controlled trials with first- and second-generation antipsychotics. *CNS Drugs* 2015; 29: 637–658

DeKosky ST, Williamson JD, Fitzpatrick AL, et al. Ginkgo biloba for prevention of dementia: a randomized controlled trial. *J Am Med Assoc* 2008; 300: 2253–2262

de la Fuente JM, Lotstra F. A trial of carbamazepine in borderline personality disorder. *Eur Neuropsychopharmacol* 1994; 4: 479–486

de Leon J, Wynn G, Sandson NB. The pharmacokinetics of risperidone versus paliperidone. *Psychosomatics* 2010; 51: 80–88

de Lucena D, Fernandes BS, Berk M, et al. Improvement of negative and positive symptoms in treatment-refractory schizophrenia: a double-blind, randomized, placebo-controlled trial with memantine as add-on therapy to clozapine. *J Clin Psychiatry* 2009; 70: 1416–1423

DeMartinis A, Schweizer E, Rickels K. An open-label trial of nefazodone in high comorbidity panic disorder. *J Clin Psychiatry* 1996; 57: 245–248

Deng L, Sun X, Qiu S, et al. Interventions for management of post-stroke depression: a Bayesian network meta-analysis of 23 randomized controlled trials. *Sci Rep* 2017; 7: 16466

Dennis CL, Ross LE, Herxheimer A. Oestrogens and progestins for preventing and treating postpartum depression. *Cochrane Database Syst Rev* 2008;(4):CD001690

de Oliveira IR, de Sena EP, Pereira EL, et al. Haloperidol blood levels and clinical outcome: a meta-analysis of studies relevant to testing the therapeutic window hypothesis. *J Clin Pharm Ther* 1996; 21: 229–236

DePetris AE, Cook BL. Differences in diffusion of FDA antidepressant risk warnings across racial-ethnic groups. *Psychiatr Serv* 2013; 64: 466–471

De Picker L, Van Den Eede F, Dumont G, et al. Antidepressants and the risk of hyponatremia: a class-by-class review of literature. *Psychosomatics* 2014; 55: 536–537

Depping AM, Komossa K, Kissling W, Leucht S. Second generation antipsychotics for anxiety disorders. *Cochrane Database Syst Rev* 2010; (12): CD008120

de Silva VA, Suraweera C, Ratnatuga SS, et al. Metformin in prevention and treatment of antipsychotic induced weight gain: a systematic review and meta-analysis. *BMC Psychiatry* 2016; 16: 341

de Vries C, van Bergen A, Regeer EJ, et al. The effectiveness of restarted lithium treatment after discontinuation: reviewing the evidence for discontinuation-induced refractoriness. *Bipolar Disord* 2013; 15: 645–649

Devulapalli KK, Nasrallah HA. An analysis of the high psychotropic off-label use in psychiatric disorders. The majority of psychiatric diagnoses have no approved drug. *Asian J Psychiatry* 2009; 2: 29–36

DeYoung CG, Hirsh JB, Shane MS, et al. Testing predictions from personality neuroscience: brain structure and the big five. *Psychol Sci* 2010; 21: 820–828

Di Florio A, Forty L, Gordon-Smith K, et al. Perinatal episodes across the mood disorder spectrum. *JAMA Psychiatry* 2013; 70: 168–175

DiMascio A, Bernardo DL, Greenblatt DJ, et al. A controlled trial of amantadine in drug-induced extrapyramidal disorders. *Arch Gen Psychiatry* 1976; 33: 599–602

Dinz JB, Shavitt RG, Fossaluza V, et al. A double-blind, randomized, controlled trial of fluoxetine plus quetiapine or clomipramine versus fluoxetine plus placebo for obsessive-compulsive disorder. *J Clin Psychopharmacol* 2011; 31: 763–768

Docherty JP, Sack DA, Roffman M, et al. A double-blind, placebo-controlled, exploratory trial of chromium picolinate in atypical depression: effect on carbohydrate craving. *J Psychiatr Pract* 2005; 11: 302–314

Dodd S, Dean OM, Berk M. A review of the theoretical and biological understanding of the nocebo and placebo phenomena. *Clin Ther* 2017; 39: 469–476

Dodd S, Berk M, Kelin K, et al. Treatment response for acute depression is not associated with number of previous episodes: lack of evidence for a clinical staging model for major depressive disorder. *J Affect Disord* 2013; 150: 344–349

Dodd S, Schacht A, Kelin K, et al. Nocebo effects in the treatment of major depression: results from an individual study participant-level meta-analysis of the placebo arm of duloxetine clinical trials. *J Clin Psychiatry* 2015; 76: 702–711

Dodd S, Walker AJ, Brnabic JM, et al. Incidence and characteristics of the nocebo response from meta-analyses of the placebo arms of clinical trials of olanzapine for bipolar disorder. *Bipolar Disord* 2019; 21: 142–150

Dold M, Aigner M, Lanzenberger R, Kasper S. Antipsychotic augmentation of serotonin reuptake inhibitors in treatment-resistant obsessive-compulsive disorder: an update meta-analysis of double-blind, randomized, placebo-controlled trials. *Int J Neurpharmacol* 2015a; 18: pyv047

Dold M, Bartova L, Rupprecht R, et al. Dose escalation of antidepressants in unipolar depression: a meta-analysis of double-blind, randomized controlled trials. *Psychother Psychosom* 2017; 86: 283–291

Dold M, Fugger G, Aigner M, et al. Dose escalation of antipsychotic drugs in schizophrenia: a meta-analysis of randomized controlled trials. *Schizophr Res* 2015b; 166: 187–193

Dold M, Li C, Tardy M, et al. Benzodiazepines for schizophrenia. *Cochrane Database Syst Rev* 2012; (11): CD006391

Domes G, Ower N, von Dawans B, et al. Effects of intranasal oxytocin administration on empathy and approach motivation in women with borderline personality disorder: a randomized controlled trial. *Transl Psychiatry* 2019; 9: 328

Doody RS, Ferris SH, Salloway S, et al. Donepezil treatment of patients with MCI: a 48-week randomized, placebo-controlled trial. *Neurology* 2009; 72: 1555–1561

Dorph-Petersen KA, Pierri JN, Perel JM, et al. The influence of chronic exposure to antipsychotic medications on brain size before and after tissue fixation: a comparison of haloperidol and olanzapine in macaque monkeys. *Neuropsychopharmacol* 2005; 30: 1649–1661

Downing AM, Kinon BJ, Millen BA, et al. A double-blind, placebo-controlled comparator study of LY2140023 monohydrate in patients with schizophrenia. *BMC Psychiatry* 2014; 14: 351

Drevets WC, Zarate CA Jr., Furey ML. Antidepressant effects of the muscarinic cholinergic receptor antagonist scopolamine: a review. *Biol Psychiatry* 2013; 73: 1156–1163

Duffy A, Heffer N, Goodday SM, et al. Efficacy and tolerability of lithium for the treatment of acute mania in children with bipolar disorder: a systematic review: a report from the ISBD-IGSLi joint task force on lithium treatment. *Bipolar Disord* 2018; 20: 583–593

Duggal HS, Mendhekar DN. High-dose aripiprazole in treatment-resistant schizophrenia. *J Clin Psychiatry* 2006; 67: 674–675

Duinkerke SJ, Botter PA, Jansen AA, et al. Ritanserin, a selective 5-HT2/1C antagonist, and negative symptoms in schizophrenia. A placebo-controlled double-blind trial. *Br J Psychiatry* 1993; 163: 451–455

Dumon JP, Catteau J, Lanvin F, et al. Randomized, double-blind, crossover, placebo-controlled comparison of propranolol and betaxolol in the treatment of neuroleptic-induced akathisia. *Am J Psychiatry* 1992; 149: 647–650

Dumville JC, Miles JN, Porthouse J, et al. Can vitamin D supplementation prevent winter-time blues? A randomised trial among older women. *J Nutr Health Aging* 2006; 10: 151–153

Duncan EJ, Szilagyi S, Schwartz MP, et al. Effects of D-cycloserine on negative symptoms in schizophrenia. *Schizophr Res* 2004; 71: 239–248

Dunkley EJ, Isbister GK, Sibbritt D, et al. The Hunter Serotonin Toxicity Criteria: simple and accurate diagnostic decision rules for serotonin toxicity. *QJM* 2003; 96: 635–642

Dunlop BW, Kelley ME, Aponte-Rivera V, et al. Effects of patient preferences on outcomes in the Predictors of Remission in Depression to Individual and Combined Treatments (PReDICT) study. *Am J Psychiatry* 2017; 174: 546–556

Dunner DL, Fieve RR. Clinical factors in lithium carbonate prophylaxis failure. *Arch Gen Psychiatry* 1974; 30: 229–233

Dunner DL, Amsterdam JD, Shelton RC, et al. Efficacy and tolerability of adjunctive ziprasidone in treatment-resistant depression: a randomized, open-label, pilot study. *J Clin Psychiatry* 2007; 68: 1071–1077

Dupuis B, Catteau J, Dumon JP, et al. Comparison of propranolol, sotalol, and betaxolol in the treatment of neuroleptic-induced akathisia. *Am J Psychiatry* 1987; 144: 802–805

Durgam S, Earley W, Guo H, et al. Efficacy and safety of adjunctive cariprazine in inadequate responders to antidepressants: a randomized, double-blind, placebo-controlled study in adult patients with major depressive disorder. *J Clin Psychiatry* 2016a; 77: 371–378

Durgam S, Earley W, Li R, et al. Long-term cariprazine treatment for the prevention of relapse in patients with schizophrenia: a randomized, double-blind, placebo-controlled trial. *Schizophr Res* 2016b; 176: 264–271

Durgam S, Gommoll C, Forero G, et al. Efficacy and safety of vilazodone in patients with generalized anxiety disorder: a randomized, double-blind, placebo-controlled, flexible-dose trial. *J Clin Psychiatry* 2016c; 77: 1687–1694

Durgam S, Satlin A, Vanover K, et al. Lumateperone (ITI-007) in the treatment of bipolar depression: results from a randomized clinical trial. Poster presented at the Annual Meeting of the American College of Neuropsychopharmacology, Orlando, Florida, December 8–11, 2019

Durgam S, Starace A, Li D, et al. The efficacy and tolerability of cariprazine in acute mania associated with bipolar I disorder: a phase II trial. *Bipolar Disord* 2015; 17: 63–75

Earley W, Burgess MV, Rekeda L, et al. Cariprazine treatment of bipolar depression: a randomized double-blind placebo-controlled phase 3 study. *Am J Psychiatry* 2019a; 176: 439–448

Earley WR, Burgess MV, Khan B, et al. Efficacy and safety of cariprazine in bipolar I depression: a double-blind, placebo-controlled phase 3 study. *Bipolar Disord* 2020; 22: 372–384

Earley W, Guo H, Daniel D, et al. Efficacy of cariprazine on negative symptoms in patients with acute schizophrenia: a post hoc analysis of pooled data. *Schizophr Res* 2019b; 204; 282–288

Earley WR, Guo H, Németh G, et al. Cariprazine augmentation to antidepressant therapy in major depressive disorder: results of a randomized, double-blind, placebo-controlled trial. *Psychopharmacol Bull* 2018; 48: 62–80

Egbe A, Uppu S, Lee S, et al. Congenital malformations in the newborn population: a population study and analysis of the effect of sex and prematurity. *Pediatr Neonatol* 2015; 56: 25–30

Eison AS, Mullins UL. Regulation of central 5HT2A receptors: a review of in vivo studies. *Behav Brain Res* 1996; 73: 177–181

Ekeberg O, Kjeldsen SE, Greenwood DT, et al. Effects of selective beta-adrenoceptor blockade on anxiety associated with flight phobia. *J Psychopharmacol* 1990; 4: 35–41

el-Ganzouri AR, Ivankovich AD, Braverman B, et al. Monoamine oxidase inhibitors: should they be discontinued preoperatively? *Anesth Analg* 1985; 64: 592–596

Elkashef A, Kahn R, Yu E, et al. Topiramate for the treatment of methamphetamine addiction: a multi-center placebo-controlled trial. *Addiction* 2012; 107: 1297–1306

El-Khalili N, Joyce M, Atkinson S, et al. Extended-release quetiapine fumarate (quetiapine XR) as adjunctive therapy in major depressive disorder (MDD) in patients with an inadequate response to ongoing antidepressant treatment: a multicentre, randomized, double-blind, placebo-controlled study. *Int J Neuropsychopharmacol* 2010; 13: 917–932

El-Mallakh RS, Vöhringer PA, Ostacher MM, et al. Antidepressants worsen rapid-cycling course in bipolar depression: a STEP-BD randomized clinical trial. *J Affect Disord* 2015; 184: 318–321

Emamzadehfard S, Kamaloo A, Paydary K, et al. Riluzole in augmentation of fluvoxamine for moderate to severe obsessive-compulsive disorder: randomized, double-blind, placebo-controlled study. *Psychiatry Clin Neurosci* 2016; 70: 332–341

Erland LAE, Saxena PK. Melatonin natural health products and supplements: presence of serotonin and significant variability of melatonin content. *J Clin Sleep Med* 2017; 13: 275–281

Ernst CL, Goldberg JF. The reproductive safety profile of mood stabilizers, atypical antipsychotics, and broad-spectrum psychotropics. *J Clin Psychiatry* 2002; 63(Suppl 4): 42–55

Etkin A, Patenaude B, Song YJ, et al. A cognitive-emotional biomarker for predicting remission with antidepressant medications: a report from the iSPOT-D trial. *Neuropsychopharmacology* 2015; 40: 1332–1342

Etminan M, Sodhi M, Procyshyn RM, et al. Risk of hair loss with different antidepressants: a comparative retrospective cohort study. *Int Clin Psychopharmacol* 2018; 33: 44–48

Faedda GL, Tondo L, Baldessarini RJ, et al. Outcome after rapid vs gradual discontinuation of lithium treatment in bipolar disorders. *Arch Gen Psychiatry* 1993; 50: 448–455

Fallon BA. Pharmacotherapy of somatoform disorders. *J Psychosom Res* 2004; 56: 455–460

Fang H, Zhen YF, Liu XY, et al. Association of the BDNF Val66Met polymorphism with BMI in chronic schizophrenic patients and healthy controls. *Int Clin Psychopharmacol* 2016; 31: 353–357

Faridhossinie F, Sadeghi R, Farid L, et al. Celecoxib: a new augmentation strategy for depressive mood episodes: a systematic review and meta-analysis of randomized placebo-controlled trials. *Hum Psychopharmacol* 2014; 29: 216–223

Farnia V, Gharebaghi H, Alikhani M, et al. Efficacy and tolerability of adjunctive gabapentin and memantine in obsessive compulsive disorder: double-blind, randomized, placebo-controlled trial. *J Psychiatr Res* 2018; 104: 137–143

Farren CK, Scimeca M, Wu R, et al. Double-blind, placebo-controlled study of sertraline with naltrexone for alcohol dependence. *Drug Alcohol Depend* 2009; 99: 317–321

Fava M. Weight gain and antidepressants. *J Clin Psychiatry* 2000; 61(Suppl 11): 37–41

Fava M, Rosenbaum JF. Anger attacks in depression. *Depress Anxiety* 1998; 8(Suppl 1): 59–63

Fava GA, Benasi G, Lucente M, et al. Withdrawal symptoms after serotonin-noradrenaline reuptake inhibitor discontinuation: systematic review. *Psychother Psychosom* 2018a; 87: 195–203

Fava GA, Gatti A, Belaise C, et al. Withdrawal symptoms after selective serotonin reuptake inhibitor discontinuation: a systematic review. *Psychother Psychosom* 2015; 84: 72–81

Fava M, Durgam S, Earley W, et al. Efficacy of adjunctive low-dose cariprazine in major depressive disorder: a randomized, double-blind, placebo-controlled trial. *Int Clin Psychopharmacol* 2018b; 33: 312–321

Fava M, Evins AE, Dorer DJ, et al. The problem of the placebo response in clinical trials for psychiatric disorders: culprits, possible remedies, and a novel study design approach. *Psychother Psychosom* 2003; 72: 115–127

Fava M, Ménard F, Davidsen CK, et al. Adjunctive brexpiprazole in patients with major depressive disorder and irritability: an exploratory study. *J Clin Psychiatry* 2016; 77: 1695–1701

Fava M, Mischoulon D, Iosifescu D, et al. A double-blind, placebo-controlled study of aripiprazole adjunctive to antidepressant therapy among depressed outpatients with inadequate response to prior antidepressant therapy (ADAPT-A Study). *Psychother Psychosom* 2012; 81: 87–97

Fava M, Nierenberg AA, Quitkin FM, et al. A preliminary study on the efficacy of sertraline and imipramine on anger attacks in atypical depression and dysthymia. *Psychopharmacol Bull* 1997; 33: 101–103

Fava M, Rappe SM, Pava JA, et al. Relapse in patients on long-term fluoxetine treatment: response to increased fluoxetine dose. *J Clin Psychiatry* 1995; 56: 52–55

Fava M, Rush AJ, Alpert JE, et al. Difference in treatment outcome in outpatients with anxious versus nonanxious depression: a STAR*D report. *Am J Psychiatry* 2008; 165: 342–351

Fawcett J, Barkin RL. A meta-analysis of eight randomized, double-blind, controlled clinical trials of mirtazapine for the treatment of patients with major depression and symptoms of anxiety. *J Clin Psychiatry* 1998; 59: 123–127

Fawcett J, Marcus RN, Anton SF, et al. Response of anxiety and agitation symptoms during nefazodone treatment of major depression. *J Clin Psychiatry* 1995; 56 (Suppl 6): 37–42

Fawcett J, Rush AJ, Vukelich J, et al. Clinical experience with high-dose pramipexole in patients with treatment-resistant depressive episodes in unipolar and bipolar disorder. *Am J Psychiatry* 2016; 173: 107–111

Feder A, Parides MK, Murrough JW, et al. Efficacy of intravenous ketamine for treatment of chronic posttraumatic stress disorder: a randomized clinical trial. *JAMA Psychiatry* 2014; 71: 681–688

Fedgchin M, Trivedi M, Daly EJ, et al. Efficacy and safety of fixed-dose esketamine nasal spray combined with a new oral antidepressant in treatment-resistant depression: results of a randomized, double-blind, active-controlled study (TRANSFORM-1). *Int J Neuropsychopharmacol* 2019; 22: 616–630

Fein S, Paz V, Rao N, et al. The combination of lithium carbonate and an MAOI in refractory depressions. *Am J Psychiatry* 1988; 145: 249–250

Feinberg SS. Combining stimulants with monoamine oxidase inhibitors: a review of uses and one possible additional indication. *J Clin Psychiatry* 2004; 65: 1520–1524

Feltner DE, Crockatt JG, Dubovsky SJ, et al. A randomized, double blind, placebo-controlled, fixed-dose, multicenter study of pregabalin in patients with generalized anxiety disorder. *J Clin Psychopharmacol* 2003; 23: 240–249

Feltner DE, Liu-Dumaw M, Schweizer E, et al. Efficacy of pregabalin in generalized social anxiety disorder: results of a double-blind, placebo-controlled, fixed-dose study. *Int Clin Psychopharmacol* 2011; 26: 213–220

Ferreria-Garcia R, da Rocha Freire RC, Appolinário JC, et al. Tranylcypromine plus amitriptyline for electroconvulsive therapy-resistant depression: a long-term study. *J Clin Psychopharmacol* 2018; 38: 502–504

Ferrando SJ. Psychopharmacologic treatment of patients with HIV/AIDS. *Curr Psychiatry Rep* 2009; 11: 235–242

Ferrnadon SJ, Freyberg Z. Treatment of depression in HIV positive individuals: a critical review. *Int Rev Psychiatry* 2008; 20: 61–71

Fesler FA. Valproate in combat-related post-traumatic stress disorder. *J Clin Psychiatry* 1991; 52: 361–364

Fiedorowicz JG, Endicott J, Leon AC, et al. Subthreshold hypomanic symptoms in progression from unipolar major depression to bipolar disorder. *Am J Psychiatry* 2011; 168: 40–48

Figueroa Y, Rosenberg DR, Birmaher B, et al. Combination treatment with clomipramine and selective serotonin reuptake inhibitors for obsessive-compulsive disorder in children and adolescents. *J Child Adolesc Psychopharmacol* 1998; 8: 61–67

Findling RL, Ginsberg LD. The safety and effectiveness of open-label extended-release carbamazepine in the treatment of children and adolescents with bipolar I disorder suffering from a manic or mixed episode. *Neuropsychiatr Dis Treat* 2014; 10: 1589–1597

Findling RL, Chang K, Robb A, et al. Adjunctive maintenance lamotrigine for pediatric bipolar I disorder: a placebo-controlled, randomized withdrawal study. *J Am Acad Child Adolesc Psychiatry* 2015; 54: 1020–1031

Florio V, Porcelli S, Saria A, et al. Escitalopram plasma levels and antidepressant response. *Eur Neuropsychopharmacol* 2017; 27: 940–944

Focosi D, Azzarà A, Kast RE, et al. Lithium and hematology: established and proposed uses. *J Leukoc Biol* 2009; 85: 20–28

Foglia JP, Pollock BG, Kirschner MA, et al. Plasma levels of citalopram enantiomers and metabolites in elderly patients. *Psychopharmacol Bull* 1997; 33: 109–112

Ford AC, Lacy BE, Harris LA, et al. Antidepressants and psychological therapies in irritable bowel syndrome: an updated systematic review and meta-analysis. *Am J Gastroenterol* 2019; 114: 21–39

Forester BP, Harper DG, Georgakas J, et al. Antidepressant effects with open label treatment with coenzyme Q10 in geriatric bipolar depression. *J Clin Psychopharmacol* 2015; 35: 338–340

Förg A, Hein J, Volkmar K, et al. Efficacy and safety of pregabalin in the treatment of alcohol withdrawal syndrome: a randomized placebo-controlled trial. *Alcohol* 2012; 47: 149–155

Fornaro M, Anastasia A, Novello S, et al. Incidence, prevalence and clinical correlates of antidepressant-emergent mania in bipolar depression: a systematic review and meta-analysis. *Bipolar Disord* 2018; 20: 195–227

Förster K, Jörgens S, Air TM, et al. The relationship between social cognition and executive function in major depressive disorder in high-functioning adolescents and young adults. *Psychiatr Res* 2018; 263: 139–146

Fournier JC, DeRubeis RJ, Hollon SD, et al. Antidepressant drug effects and depression severity: a patient-level meta-analysis. *J Am Med Assoc* 2010; 303: 47–53

Franchini L, Serretti A, Gasperini M, et al. Familial concordance of fluvoxamine response as a tool for differentiating mood disorder pedigrees. *J Psychiatr Res* 1998; 32: 244–259

Frank C. Pharmacologic treatment of depression in the elderly. *Can Fam Physician* 2014; 60: 121–126

Frank J. Managing hypertension using combination therapy. *Am Fam Physician* 2008; 77: 1279–1286

Frank E, Prien RF, Jarrett RB, et al. Conceptualization and rationale for consensus definitions of terms in major depressive disorder. Remission, recovery, relapse, and recurrence. *Arch Gen Psychiatry* 1991; 48: 851–855

Frankenburg FR, Zanarini MC. Divalproex sodium treatment of women with borderline personality disorder and bipolar II disorder: a double-blind placebo-controlled pilot study. *J Clin Psychiatry* 2002; 63: 442–446

Freeman D, Dunn G, Murray RM, et al. How cannabis causes paranoia: using the intravenous administration of Δ9-tetrahydrocannabinol (THC) to identify key cognitive mechanisms leading to paranoia. *Schizophr Bull* 2015; 41: 391–399

Freeman EW, Rickels K, Arredondo R, et al. Full- or half-cycle treatment of severe premenstrual syndrome with a serotonergic antidepressant. *J Clin Psychopharmacol* 1999; 19: 3–8

Freudenreich O, Goff DC. Antipsychotic combination therapy in schizophrenia: a review of efficacy and risks of current combinations. *Acta Psychiatr Scand* 2002; 106: 323–330

Frieder A, Fersh M, Hainline R, et al. Pharmacotherapy of postpartum depression: current approaches and novel drug development. *CNS Drugs* 2019; 33: 265–282

Friedman RA, Mitchell J, Kocsis JH. Retreatment for relapse following desipramine discontinuation in dysthymia. *Am J Psychiatry* 1995; 152: 926–928

Friedman MJ, Marmar CR, Baker DG, et al. Randomized, double-blind comparison of sertraline and placebo for posttraumatic stress disorder in a Department of Veterans Affairs setting. *J Clin Psychiatry* 2007; 68: 711–720

Frye MA, Helleman G, McElroy SL, et al. Correlates of treatment-emergent mania associated with antidepressant treatment in bipolar depression. *Am J Psychiatry* 2009; 166: 164–172

Frye MA, Ketter TA, Kimbrell TA, et al. A placebo-controlled study of lamotrigine and gabapentin monotherapy in refractory mood disorders. *J Clin Psychopharmacol* 2000; 20: 607–614

Fujii H, Goel A, Bernard N, et al. Pregnancy outcomes following gabapentin use: results of a prospective comparative cohort study. *Neurology* 2013; 80: 1565–1570

Furieri FA, Nakamura-Palacios EM. Gabapentin reduces alcohol consumption and craving: a randomized, double-blind, placebo-controlled trial. *J Clin Psychiatry* 2007; 68: 1691–1700

Furmark T, Appel L, Henningssohn S, et al. A link between serotonin-related gene polymorphisms, amygdala activity, and placebo-induced relief from social anxiety. *J Neurosci* 2008; 28: 13066–13074

Furu K, Kieler H, Haglund B, et al. Selective serotonin reuptake inhibitors and venlafaxine in early pregnancy and risk of birth defects: population based cohort study and sibling design. *Br Med J* 2015; 350: h1798

Furukawa TA, Cipriani A, Atkinson LZ, et al. Placebo response rates in antidepressant trials: a systematic review of published and unpublished double-blind randomised controlled trials. *Lancet* 2016; 3: 1059–1066

Furukawa TA, Cipriani A, Leucht S, et al. Is placebo response in antidepressant trials rising or not? A reanalysis of datasets to conclude this long-lasting controversy. *Evid Based Ment Health* 2018a; 21: 1–3

Furukawa TA, Levine SZ, Tanaka S, et al. Initial severity of schizophrenia and efficacy of antipsychotics: participant-level meta-analysis of 6 placebo-controlled studies. *JAMA Psychiatry* 2015; 72: 14–21

Furukawa TA, Maruo K, Noma H, et al. Initial severity of major depression and efficacy of new generation antidepressants: individual participant data meta-analysis. *Acta Psychiatr Scand* 2018b; 137: 450–458

Fusar-Poli P, Cappucciati M, Rutigiano G, et al. Diagnostic stability of ICD/DSM first episode psychosis diagnoses: meta-analysis. *Schizophr Bull* 2016; 42: 1395–1406

Fusar-Poli P, Papanasatiou E, Stahl D, et al. Treatments of negative symptoms in schizophrenia: meta-analysis of 168 randomized placebo-controlled trials. *Schizophr Bull* 2015; 41: 892–899

Gadde KM, Kopping MF, Wagner HT 2nd, et al. Zonisamide for weight reduction in obese adults: a 1-year randomized controlled trial. *Arch Intern Med* 2012; 172: 1557–1564

Gallagher P, Young AH. Mifepristone (RU-486) treatment for depression and psychosis: a review of the therapeutic implications. *Neuropsychiatr Dis Treat* 2006; 2: 33–42

Galling B, Roldán A, Hagi K, et al. Antipsychotic augmentation vs. monotherapy in schizophrenia: systematic review, meta-analysis and meta-regression analysis. *World Psychiatry* 2017; 16: 77–89

Galling B, Vernon JA, Pagsberg AK, et al. Efficacy and safety of antidepressant augmentation of continued antipsychotic treatment in patients with schizophrenia. *Acta Psychiatr Scand* 2018; 137: 187–205

Gambi F, De Berardis D, Campanella D, et al. Mirtazapine treatment of generalized anxiety disorder: a fixed dose, open label study. *J Psychopharmacol* 2005; 19: 483–487

Garakani A, Martinez JM, Marcus S, et al. A randomized, double-blind, and placebo-controlled trial of quetiapine augmentation of fluoxetine in major depressive disorder. *Int Clin Psychopharmacol* 2008; 23: 269–275

Garcia-Garcia AL, Newman-Tancredi A, Leonardo ED. 5-HT(1A) [corrected] receptors in mood and anxiety: recent insights into autoreceptor versus heteroreceptor function. *Psychopharmacol (Berl)* 2014; 231: 623–636

Gardini S, Cloninger CR, Venneri A. Individual differences in personality traits reflect structural variance in specific brain regions. *Brain Res Bull* 2009; 79: 265–270

Gardner DL, Cowdry RW. Positive effects of carbamazepine on behavioral dyscontrol in borderline personality disorder. *Am J Psychiatry* 1986; 143: 519–522

Gardner DM, Shulman KI, Walker SE, et al. The making of a user friendly MAOI diet. *J Clin Psychiatry* 1996; 57: 99–104

Garlow SJ, Dunlop BW, Ninan PT, et al. The combination of triiodothyronine (T3) and sertraline is not superior to sertraline monotherapy in the treatment of major depressive disorder. *J Psychiatr Res* 2012; 46: 1406–1413

Gatti F, Bellini L, Gasperini M, et al. Fluvoxamine alone in the treatment of delusional depression. *Am J Psychiatry* 1996; 153: 414–416

Gaul C, Diener H-C, Danesch U, et al. Improvement of migraine symptoms with a proprietary supplement containing riboflavin, magnesium and Q10: a randomized, placebo-controlled, double-blind, multicenter trial. *J Headache Pain* 2015; 16: 516

Geddes JR, Calabrese JR, Goodwin GM. Lamotrigine for treatment of bipolar depression: independent meta-analysis and meta-regression of individual patient data from five randomised trials. *Br J Psychiatry* 2009; 194: 4–9

Geddes JR, Burgess S, Hawton K, et al. Long-term lithium therapy for bipolar disorder: systematic review and meta-analysis of randomized controlled trials. *Am J Psychiatry* 2004; 161: 217–222

Geddes JR, Gardiner A, Rendell J, et al. Comparative evaluation of quetiapine plus lamotrigine combination versus quetiapine monotherapy (and folic acid versus placebo) in bipolar depression (CEQUEL): a 2 x 2 factorial randomised trial. *Lancet Psychiatry* 2016; 3: 31–39

Geers AL, Helfer SG, Kosbab K, et al. Reconsidering the role of personality in placebo effects: dispositional optimism, situational expectations, and the placebo response. *J Psychosom Res* 2005; 58: 121–127

Gelaye B, Rondon M, Araya R, et al. Epidemiology of maternal depression, risk factors, and child outcomes in low-income and middle-income countries. *Lancet Psychiatry* 2016; 3: 973–982

Gelenberg AJ, Kane JM, Keller MB, et al. Comparison of standard and low serum levels of lithium for maintenance treatment of bipolar disorder. *N Engl J Med* 1989; 321: 1489–1493

Generoso MB, Trevizol AP, Kasper S, et al. Pregabalin for generalized anxiety disorder: an updated systematic review and meta-analysis. *Int Clin Psychopharmacol* 2017; 32: 49–55

Gengo F, Timko J, D'Antonio J, et al. Prediction of dosage of lithium carbonate: use of a standard predictive model. *J Clin Psychiatry* 1980; 41: 319–320

Gentile JP, Dillon KS, Gillig PM. Psychotherapy and pharmacotherapy for patients with dissociative identity disorder. *Innov Clin Neurosci* 2013; 10: 22–29

Genuis SJ, Schwalfenberg G, Siy A-K J, et al. Toxic element contamination of natural health products and pharmaceutical preparations. *PLoS One* 2012; 7: e49676

George KC, Kebejian L, Ruth LJ, et al. Meta-analysis of the efficacy and safety of prazosin versus placebo for the treatment of nightmares and sleep disturbances in adults with posttraumatic stress disorder. *J Trauma Dissociation* 2016; 17: 494–510

Georgotas A, McCue RE, Hapworth W, et al. Comparative efficacy and safety of MAOIs versus TCAs in treating depression in the elderly. *Biol Psychiatry* 1986; 21: 1155–1166

Gerner R, Estabrook W, Steur J, et al. Treatment of geriatric depression with trazodone, imipramine, and placebo: a double-blind study. *J Clin Psychiatry* 1980; 41: 216–220

Gex-Fabry M, Gervasoni N, Eap CB, et al. Time course of response to paroxetine: influence of plasma level. *Prog Neuropsychopharmacol Biol Psychiatry* 2007; 31: 892–900

Ghaemi SN, Gilmer WS, Goldberg JF, et al. Divalproex in the treatment of acute bipolar depression: a preliminary double-blind, randomized, placebo-controlled pilot study. *J Clin Psychiatry* 2007; 68: 1840–1844

Ghaemi SN, Ostacher MM, El-Mallakh RS, et al. Antidepressant discontinuation in bipolar depression: a Systematic Treatment Enhancement Program for Bipolar Disorder (STEP-BD) randomized clinical trial of long-term effectiveness and safety. *J Clin Psychiatry* 2010; 71: 372–380

Ghajar A, Gholamian F, Tabatabei-Motlagh M, et al. Citicoline (CDP-choline) add-on therapy to risperidone for treatment of negative symptoms in patients with stable schizophrenia: a double-blind, randomized placebo-controlled trial. *Hum Psychopharmacol* 2018a; 33: e2662

Ghajar A, Khoaie-Ardakani MR, Shahmoradi Z, et al. L-carnosine as an add-on to risperidone for treatment of negative symptoms in patients with stable schizophrenia: a double-blind, randomized placebo-controlled trial. *Psychiatry Res* 2018b; 262: 94–101

Ghanizadeh A, Nikseresht MS, Sahraian A. The effect of zonisamide on antipsychotic-associated weight gain in patients with schizophrenia: a randomized, double-blind, placebo-controlled clinical trial. *Schizophr Res* 2013; 147: 110–115

Ghio L, Gotelli S, Marcenaro M, et al. Duration of untreated illness and outcomes in unipolar depression: a systematic review and meta-analysis. *J Affect Disord* 2014; 152–154: 45–51

Giacobbe P, Rakita U, Lam R, et al. Efficacy and tolerability of lisdexamfetamine as an antidepressant augmentation strategy: a meta-analysis of randomized controlled trials. *J Affect Disord* 2018; 226: 294–300

Gibson AP, Bettinger TL, Patel NC, et al. Atomoxetine versus stimulants for treatment of attention deficit/hyperactivity disorder. *Ann Pharmacother* 2006; 40: 1134–1142

Gilaberte I, Montejo AL, de la Gandara J, et al. Fluoxetine in the prevention of depressive recurrences: a double-blind study. *J Clin Psychopharmacol* 2001; 21: 417–424

Gilbert DG, Rabinovich NE, McDaniel JT. Nicotine patch for cannabis withdrawal symptom relief: a randomized controlled trial. *Psychopharmacol (Berl)* 2020; 237: 1507–1519

Gildengers AG, Chung K-H, Huang S-H, et al. Neuroprogressive effects of lifetime illness duration in older adults with bipolar disorder. *Bipolar Disord* 2014; 16: 617–623

Gilles M, Deuschle M, Kellner S, et al. Paroxetine serum concentrations in depressed patients and response to treatment. *Pharmacopsychiatry* 2005; 38: 118–121

Gilmor ML, Owens MJ, Nemeroff CB. Inhibition of norepinephrine uptake in patients with major depression treated with paroxetine. *Am J Psychiatry* 2002; 159: 1701–1710

Ginde AA, Liu MC, Camargo CA Jr. Demographic differences and trends of vitamin D insufficiency in the US population, 1988–2004. *Arch Intern Med* 2009; 169: 626–632

Ginsberg LD. Carbamazepine extended-release capsules: a retrospective review of its use in children and adolescents. *Ann Clin Psychiatry* 2006; 18(Suppl 1): 3–7

Glantz MD, Anthony JC, Berglund PA, et al. Mental disorders as risk factors for later substance dependence: estimates of optimal prevention and treatment benefits. *Psychol Med* 2009; 39: 1365–1377

Glassman AH, O'Connor CM, Califf RM, et al. Sertraline treatment of major depression in patients with acute MI or unstable angina. *J Am Med Assoc* 2002; 288: 701–709

Gleeson M. Dosing and efficacy of glutamine supplementation in human exercise and sport training. *J Nutr* 2008; 138: 2045S–2049S

Goedhard LE, Stolker JJ, Heerdink ER, et al. Pharmacotherapy for the treatment of aggressive behavior in general adult psychiatry: a systematic review. *J Clin Psychiatry* 2006; 67: 1013–1024

Goff DC, Cather C, Gottlieb JD, et al. Once-weekly D-cycloserine effects on negative symptoms and cognition in schizophrenia: an exploratory study. *Schizophr Res* 2008; 106: 320–327

Goff DC, Keefe R, Citrome L, et al. Lamotrigine as add-on therapy in schizophrenia: results of 2 placebo-controlled trials. *J Clin Psychopharmacol* 2007; 27: 582–589

Goff DC, McEvoy JP, Citrome L, et al. High-dose oral ziprasidone versus conventional dosing in schizophrenia patients with residual symptoms: the ZEBRAS study. *J Clin Psychopharmacol* 2013; 33: 485–490

Goldberg JF. Complex combination pharmacotherapy for bipolar disorder: knowing when less is more or more is better. *Focus* 2019; 17: 218–231

Goldberg JF, Ernst CL. *Managing the Side Effects of Psychotropic Medications*, 2nd Edn. Washington, DC: American Psychiatric Association Publishing; 2019

Goldberg JF, Whiteside JE. The association between substance abuse and antidepressant-induced mania in bipolar disorder: a preliminary study. *J Clin Psychiatry* 2002; 63: 791–795

Goldberg JF, Bowden CL, Calabrese JR, et al. Six-month prospective life charting of mood symptoms with lamotrigine versus placebo in rapid cycling bipolar disorder. *Biol Psychiatry* 2008; 63: 125–130

Goldberg JF, Calabrese JR, Saville BR, et al. Mood stabilization and destabilization during acute and continuation phase treatment for bipolar I disorder with lamotrigine or placebo. *J Clin Psychiatry* 2009; 70: 1273–1280

Goldberg JF, Freeman MP, Balon R, et al. The American Society of Clinical Psychopharmacology survey of psychopharmacologists' practice patterns for the treatment of mood disorders. *Depress Anxiety* 2015; 32: 605–613

Goldberg SC, Schulz SC, Schulz PM, et al. Borderline and schizotypal personality disorders treated with low-dose thiothixene vs placebo. *Arch Gen Psychiatry* 1986; 43: 680–686

Golden JC, Goethe JW, Wooley SB. Complex psychotropic polypharmacy in bipolar disorder across varying mood polarities: a prospective cohort study of 2712 patients. *J Affect Disord* 2017; 221: 6–10

Goldlewska BR, Olajossy-Hilkesberger L, Ciwoniuk M, et al. Olanzapine-induced weight gain is associated with the -759C/T and -697G/C polymorphisms of the HTR2C gene. *Pharmacogenomics J* 2009; 9: 234–241

Goldstein TR, Frye MA, Denicoff KD, et al. Antidepressant discontinuation-related mania: critical prospective observation and theoretical implications in bipolar disorder. *J Clin Psychiatry* 1999; 60: 563–567

Gómez JM, Teixidó Perramón C. Combined treatment with venlafaxine and tricyclic antidepressants in depressed patients who had partial response to clomipramine or imipramine: initial findings. *J Clin Psychiatry* 2000; 61; 285–289

Gomez AF, Barthel AL, Hofmann SG. Comparing the efficacy of benzodiazepines and serotonergic antidepressants for adults with generalized anxiety disorder: a meta-analytic review. *Expert Opin Pharmacother* 2018; 19: 883–894

Gonul AS, Akdeniz F, Donat O, et al. Selective serotonin reuptake inhibitors combined with venlafaxine in depressed patients who had partial response to venlafaxine: four cases. *Prog Neuropsychopharmacol Biol Psychiatry* 2003; 27: 889–891

Gonzalez G, Feingold A, Oliveto A, et al. Comorbid major depressive disorder as a prognostic factor in cocaine-abusing buprenorphine-maintained patients treated with desipramine and contingency management. *Am J Drug Alcohol Abuse* 2003; 29: 497–514

Good KP, Kiss I, Buiteman C, et al. A meta-analysis of neuropsychological change to clozapine, olanzapine, quetiapine, and risperidone in schizophrenia. *Int J Neuropsychopharmacol* 2005; 8: 457–472

Goodnick PJ. Blood levels and acute response to bupropion. *Am J Psychiatry* 1992; 149: 399–400

Goodnick PJ, Puig A, DeVane CL, Freund BV. Mirtazapine in major depression with comorbid generalized anxiety disorder. *J Clin Psychiatry* 1999; 60: 446–468

Goodwin FK, Fireman B, Simon GE, et al. Suicide risk in bipolar disorder during treatment with lithium and divalproex. *J Am Med Assoc* 2003; 290: 1467–1473

Gorwood P, Demyttenare K, Vaiva G, et al. An increase in joy after two weeks is more specific of later antidepressant response than a decrease in sadness. *J Affect Disord* 2015; 185: 97–103

Gorwood P, Weiller E, Lemming O, et al. Escitalopram prevents relapse in older patients with major depressive disorder. *Am J Geriatr Psychiatr* 2007; 15: 581–593

Goss AJ, Kaser M, Costafreda SG, et al. Modafinil augmentation therapy in unipolar and bipolar depression: a systematic review and meta-analysis of randomized controlled trials. *J Clin Psychiatry* 2013; 74: 1101–1107

Gowing L, Ali R, White JM, Mbewe D. Buprenorphine for managing opioid withdrawal. *Cochrane Database Sys Rev* 2017; (2): CD002025

Grace AA. Phasic versus tonic dopamine release and the modulation of dopamine system responsivity: a hypothesis for the etiology of schizophrenia. *Neurosci* 1991; 41: 1–24

Grant JE, Kim SW, Odlaug BL. A double-blind, placebo-controlled study of the opiate antagonist, naltrexone, in the treatment of kleptomania. *Biol Psychiatry* 2009; 65: 600–606

Grant JE, Odlaug BL, Kim SW. Lamotrigine treatment of pathologic skin picking: an open-label study. *J Clin Psychiatry* 2007; 68: 1384–1391

Grant JE, Odlaug BL, Kim SW. N-acetylcysteine, a glutamate modulator, in the treatment of trichotillomania: a double-blind, placebo-controlled study. *Arch Gen Psychiatry* 2009a; 66: 756–763

Grant JE, Odlaug BL, Chamberlain SR, et al. A double-blind, placebo-controlled trial of lamotrigine for pathological skin picking: treatment efficacy and neurocognitive predictors of response. *J Clin Psychopharmacol* 2010; 30: 396–403

Grant JE, Chamberlain SR, Redden SA, et al. N-Acetylcysteine in the treatment of excoriation disorder: a randomized clinical trial. *JAMA Psychiatry* 2016; 73: 490–496

Grant JE, Odlaug BL, Chamberlain SR, et al. Dronabinol, a cannabinoid agonist, reduces hair pulling in trichotillomania: a pilot study. *Psychopharmacol (Berl)* 2011; 218: 493–502

Grant JE, Odlaug BL, Schreiber LR, et al. The opiate antagonist, naltrexone, in the treatment of trichotillomania: results of a double-blind, placebo-controlled study. *J Clin Psychopharmacol* 2014; 34: 134–138

Gray KM, Carpenter MJ, Baker NL, et al. A double-blind randomized controlled trial of N-acetylcysteine in cannabis-dependent adolescents. *Am J Psychiatry* 2012; 169: 805–812

Gray KM, Sonne SC, McClure EA, et al. A randomized placebo-controlled trial of N-acetylcysteine for cannabis use disorder in adults. *Drug Alcohol Depend* 2017; 177: 249–257

Greden JF, Parikh SV, Rothschild AJ, et al. Impact of pharmacogenomics on clinical outcomes in major depressive disorder in the GUIDED trial: a large, patient- and rater-blinded, randomized controlled study, *J Psychiatr Res* 2019; 111: 59–67

Greendyke RM, Kanter DR. Therapeutic effects of pindolol on behavioral disturbances associated with organic brain disease: a double-blind study. *J Clin Psychiatry* 1986; 47: 423–426

Greist JH, Liu-Dumaw M, Schweizer E, et al. Efficacy of pregabalin in preventing relapse in patients with generalized social anxiety disorder: results of a double-blind, placebo-controlled 26-week study. *Int Clin Psychopharmacol* 2011; 26: 243–251

Grieve SM, Korgaonkur MS, Gordon E, et al. Prediction of nonremission to antidepressant therapy using diffusion tensor imaging. *Clin Psychiatry* 2016; 77: e436–e443

Grigoriadis S, Graves L, Peer M, et al. Benzodiazepine use during pregnancy alone or in combination with an antidepressant and congenital malformations: systematic review and meta-analysis. *J Clin Psychiatry* 2019; 80: 18r12412

Grof P, Duffy A, Cavazzoni P, et al. Is response to prophylactic lithium a familial trait? *J Clin Psychiatry* 2002; 63: 942–947

Grossman E, Messerli FH, Grodzicki T, et al. Should a moratorium be placed on sublingual nifedipine capsules given for hypertensive emergencies and pseudoemergencies? *J Am Med Assoc* 1996; 276: 1328–1331

Grunze H, Kotlik E, Costa R, et al. Assessment of the efficacy and safety of eslicarbazepine acetate in acute mania and prevention of recurrence: experience from multicenter, double-blind, randomised phase II clinical studies in patients with bipolar disorder I. *J Affect Disord* 2015; 174: 70–82

Guaiana G, Barbui C, Cipriani A. Hydroxyzine for generalised anxiety disorder. *Cochrane Database Syst Rev* 2010; (12): CD006815

Guina J, Rossetter SR, DeRhodes BJ, et al. Benzodiazepines for PTSD: a systematic review and meta-analysis. *J Psychiatr Pract* 2015; 21: 281–303

Guitivano J, Sullivan PF, Stuebe AM, et al. Adverse life events, psychiatric history, and biological predictors of postpartum depression in an ethnically diverse sample of postpartum women. *Psychol Med* 2018; 48: 1190–1200

Gunasekara NS, Spencer CM. Quetiapine: a review of its use in schizophrenia. *CNS Drugs* 1998; 9: 325–340

Gunn RL, Finn PR. Impulsivity partially mediates the association between reduced working memory capacity and alcohol problems. *Alcohol* 2013; 47: 3–8

Gvirts HZ, Lewis YD, Dvora S, et al. The effect of methylphenidate on decision making in patients with borderline personality disorder and attention-deficit/hyperactivity disorder. *Int Clin Psychopharmacol* 2018; 33: 233–237

Gyurak A, Patenaude B, Korgaonkar MS, et al. Frontoparietal activation during response inhibition predicts remission to antidepressants in patients with major depression. *Biol Psychiatry* 2016; 79: 274–281

Hackam DG, Mrobrada M. Selective serotonin reuptake inhibitors and brain hemorrhage: a meta-analysis. *Neurology* 2012; 79: 1862–1865

Haddy TB, Rana SR, Castro O. Benign ethnic neutropenia: what is the normal absolute neutrophil count? *J Lab Clin Med* 1999; 133: 15–22

Hadley SJ, Mandel FS, Schweizer E. Switching from long-term benzodiazepine therapy to pregabalin in patients with generalized anxiety disorder: a double-blind, placebo-controlled trial. *J Clin Psychopharmacol* 2012; 26: 461–470

Hagos FT, Daood MJ, Ocque JA, et al. Probenecid, an organic anion transporter 1 and 3 inhibitor, increases plasma and brain exposure of N-acetylcysteine. *Xenobiotica* 2017; 47: 346–353

Haji EO, Tadić A, Wagner S, et al. Association between citalopram serum levels and clinical improvement of patients with major depression. *J Clin Psychopharmacol* 2011; 31: 281–286

Halikas JA. Org 3770 (mirtazapine) versus trazodone: a placebo controlled trial in depressed elderly patients. *Hum Psychopharmacol* 1995; 10(Suppl 2): S125–S133

Hall K, Lembo AJ, Kirsch I, et al. Catechol-o-methyltransferase val158met polymorphism predicts placebo effect in irritable bowel syndrome. *PLoS ONE* 2012; 7: e48135

Hall KT, Loscalzo J, Kaptchuk TJ. Genetics and the placebo effect. *Trends Mol Med* 2015; 2: 285–294

Hambrecht M, Lammertink M, Klosterktter J, et al. Subjective and objective neuropsychological abnormalities in a psychosis prodrome clinic. *Br J Psychiatry Suppl* 2002; 43: S30–S37

Hamilton MW. The assessment of anxiety states by rating. *Br J Med Psychol* 1959; 32: 10–16

Hamner MB, Brodrick PS, Labatte LA. Gabapentin in PTSD: a retrospective, clinical series of adjunctive therapy. *Ann Clin Psychiatry* 2001; 13: 141–146

Hamner MB, Hernandez-Tejada MA, Zuschlag ZD, et al. Ziprasidone augmentation of SSRI antidepressants in posttraumatic stress disorder: a randomized, placebo-controlled pilot study of augmentation therapy. *J Clin Psychopharmacol* 2019; 39: 153–157

Han B, Compton WM, Blanco C, et al. Prescription opioid use, misuse, and use disorders in U.S. adults: 2015 National Survey on Drug Use and Health. *Ann Int Med* 2017; 167: 293–301

Han C, Pae C-U, Wang S-M, et al. The potential role of atypical antipsychotics for the treatment of posttraumatic stress disorder. *J Psychiatr Res* 2014; 56: 72–81

Hanania NA, Singh S, El-Wali R, et al. The safety and effects of the beta blocker, nadolol, in mild asthma: an open-label pilot study. *Pulm Pharmacol Ther* 2008; 21: 134–141

Haney M, Rubin E, Foltin RW. Aripiprazole maintenance increases smoked cocaine self-administration in humans. *Psychopharmacol (Berl)* 2011; 216: 379–387

Hanling SR, Hickey A, Lesnik I, et al. Stellate ganglion block for the treatment of posttraumatic stress disorder: a randomized, double-blind, controlled trial. *Reg Anesth Pain Med* 2016; 41: 494–500

Hansen LB, Larsen NE, Vestergard P. Plasma levels of perphenazine (Trilafon) related to development of extrapyramidal side effects. *Psychopharmacol (Berl)* 1981; 74: 306–309

Haroon E, Daguanno AW, Woolwine BJ, et al. Antidepressant treatment resistance is associated with increased inflammatory markers in patients with major depressive disorder. *Psychoneuroendocrinology* 2018; 95: 43–49

Harris DS, Wolkowitz OM, Reus VI. Movement disorder, memory, psychiatric symptoms and serum DHEA levels in schizophrenic and schizoaffective patients. *World J Biol Psychiatry* 2001; 2: 99–102

Harrow M, Jobe TH. Does long-term treatment of schizophrenia with antipsychotic medications facilitate recovery? *Schizophr Bull* 2013; 39: 962–965

Harrow M, Jobe TH. Long-term antipsychotic treatment of schizophrenia: does it help or hurt over a 20-year period? *World Psychiatry* 2018; 17: 162–163

Härtter S, Wetzel H, Hammes E, et al. Serum concentrations of fluvoxamine and clinical effects: a prospective open clinical trial. *Pharmacopsychiatry* 1998; 31: 199–200

Hartwell EE, Feinn R, Morris PE, et al. Systematic review and meta-analysis of the moderating effect of rs1799971 in OPRM1, the mu-opioid receptor gene, on response to naltrexone treatment of alcohol use disorder. *Addiction* 2020; 115: 1426–1437

Harvey RC, James AC, Shields GE. A systematic review and network meta-analysis to assess the relative efficacy of antipsychotics for the treatment of positive and negative symptoms in early-onset schizophrenia. *CNS Drugs* 2016; 30: 27–39

Hata T, Kanazawa T, Hamada T, et al. What can predict and prevent the long-term use of benzodiazepines? *J Psychiatr Res* 2018; 97: 94–100

Hawkins RA. The blood-brain barrier and glutamate. *Am J Clin Nutr* 2009; 90: 867S–874S

Hayasaka Y, Purgato M, Magni LR, et al. Dose equivalents of antidepressant: evidence-based recommendations from randomized controlled trials. *J Affect Disord* 2015; 180: 179–184

Hedayati SS, Gregg LP, Carmody T, et al. Effect of sertraline on depressive symptoms in patients with chronic kidney disease without dialysis dependence: the CAST randomized clinical trial. *J Am Med Assoc* 2017; 318: 1876–1890

Hegerl U, Mergl R, Sanders C, et al. A multi-centre, randomised, double-blind, placebo-controlled clinical trial of methylphenidate in the initial treatment of acute mania (MEMAP study). *Eur Neuropsychopharmacol* 2018; 28: 185–194

Heidari M, Zarei M, Hosseini SM, et al. Ondansetron or placebo in the augmentation of fluvoxamine response over 8 weeks in obsessive-compulsive disorder. *Int Clin Psychopharmacol* 2014; 29: 344–350

Heinälä P, Alho H, Kiianmaa K, et al. Targeted use of naltrexone without prior detoxification in the treatment of alcohol dependence: a factorial double-blind, placebo-controlled trial. *J Clin Psychopharmacol* 2001; 21: 287–292

Hieronymous F, Nilsson S, Eriksson E. A mega-analysis of fixed-dose trials reveals dose-dependency and a rapid onset of action for the antidepressant effect of three selective serotonin reuptake inhibitors. *Transl Psychiatry* 2016; 6: e34

Helfer B, Samara MT, Huhn M, et al. Efficacy and safety of antidepressants added to antipsychotics for schizophrenia: a systematic review and meta-analysis. *Am J Psychiatry* 2016; 173: 876–886

Hendricks J, Greenway FL, Westman EC, et al. Blood pressure and heart rate effects, weight loss and maintenance during long-term phentermine pharmacotherapy for obesity. *Obesity* 2011; 19: 2351–2360

Henigsberg N, Mahableshwarkar A, Jacobsen P, et al. A randomized, double-blind, placebo-controlled 8-week trial of the efficacy and tolerability of multiple doses of Lu AA21004 in adults with major depressive disorder. *J Clin Psychiatry* 2012; 73: 953–959

Henry C, Mitropoulou V, New AS, et al. Affective instability and impulsivity in borderline personality and bipolar II disorders: similarities and differences. *J Psychiatr Res* 2001; 35: 307–312

Henssler J, Kurschus M, Franklin J, et al. Trajectories of acute antidepressant efficacy: how long to wait for response? *J Clin Psychiatry* 2018; 79: 17r11470

Heresco-Levy U, Javitt D, Ermilov M, et al. Double-blind, placebo-controlled, crossover trial of glycine adjuvant therapy for treatment-resistant schizophrenia. *Br J Psychiatry* 1996; 169: 610–617

Heresco-Levy U, Vass A, Bloch B, et al. Pilot controlled trial of D-serine for the treatment of post-traumatic stress disorder. *Int J Neuropsychopharmacol* 2009; 12: 1275–1282

Herman J. *Trauma and Recovery: the Aftermath of Violence from Domestic Abuse to Political Terror*. New York, NY: Basic Books; 1988

Heringa SM, Begemann MJH, Goverde AJ, et al. Sex hormones and oxytocin augmentation strategies in schizophrenia: a quantitative review. *Schizophr Res* 2015; 168: 603–613

Herring WJ, Connor KM, Snyder E, et al. Suvorexant in elderly patients with insomnia: pooled analyses of data from phase III randomized controlled clinical trials. *Am J Geriatr Psychiatry* 2017; 25: 791–802

Hertzberg MA, Butterfield MI, Feldman ME, et al. A preliminary study of lamotrigine for the treatment of posttraumatic stress disorder. *Biol Psychiatry* 1999; 45: 1226–1229

Hesdorffer DC, Berg AT, Kanner AM. An update on antiepileptic drugs and suicide: are there definitive answers yet? *Epilepsy Curr* 2010; 10: 137–145

Hewett K, Chrzanowski W, Jokinen R, et al. Double-blind, placebo-controlled evaluation of extended-release bupropion in elderly patients with major depressive disorder. *J Psychopharmacol* 2010; 24: 521–529

Heylens G, Elaut E, Kreukels BP, et al. Psychiatric characteristics in transsexual individuals: multicenter study in four European countries. *Br J Psychiatry* 2014; 204: 151–156

Hidaka T, Fujii K, Funahashi I, et al. Safety assessment of coenzyme Q10 (CoQ10). *Biofactors* 2008; 32: 199–208

Hidalgo RB, Tupler LA, Davidson JR. An effect-size analysis of pharmacological treatments for generalized anxiety disorder. *J Psychopharmacol* 2007; 21: 864–872

Hidese S, Ota M, Wakbayashi C, et al. Effects of chronic l-theanine administration in patients with major depressive disorder: an open-label study. *Acta Neuropsychiatr* 2017; 29: 72–79

Hieber R, Dellenbaugh T, Nelson LA. Role of mirtazapine in the treatment of antipsychotic-induced akathisia. *Ann Pharmacother* 2008; 42: 841–846

Hiemke C, Bergemann N, Clement HW, et al. Consensus guidelines for therapeutic drug monitoring in neuropsychopharmacology: update 2017. *Pharmacopsychiatry* 2018; 51: 9–62

Hiemke C, Peled A, Jabarin M, et al. Fluvoxamine augmentation of olanzapine in chronic schizophrenia: pharmacokinetic interactions and clinical effects. *J Clin Psychopharmacol* 2002; 22: 502–506

Hill AB. The environment and disease: association or causation? *Proc Royal Soc Med* 1965; 58: 295–300

Hill KP, Palastro MD, Gruber SA, et al. Nabilone pharmacotherapy for cannabis dependence: a randomized, controlled pilot study. *Am J Addict* 2017; 26: 795–801

Hinz M, Stein A, Uncini T. Relative nutritional deficiencies are associated with centrally acting monoamines. *Int J Gen Med* 2012; 5: 413–430

Hirsch LJ, Weintraub D, Du Y, et al. Correlating lamotrigine serum concentrations with tolerability in patients with epilepsy. *Neurology* 2004; 63: 1022–1026

Hirschmann S, Dannon P, Iancu I, et al. Pindolol augmentation in patients with treatment-resistant panic disorder: a double-blind, placebo-controlled trial. *J Clin Psychopharmacol* 2000; 20: 556–559

Hirschfeld RM, Russell JM, Delgado PL, et al. Predictors of response to acute treatment of chronic and double depression with sertraline or imipramine. *J Clin Psychiatry* 1998; 59: 669–675

Hirschfeld RM, Weisler RH, Raines SR, et al. Quetiapine in the treatment of anxiety in patients with bipolar I or II depression: a secondary analysis from a randomized, double-blind, placebo-controlled study. *J Clin Psychiatry* 2006; 67: 355–362

Ho BC, Andreasen NC, Dawson JD, et al. Association between brain-derived neurotrophic factor Val66Met gene polymorphism and progressive brain volume changes in schizophrenia. *Am J Psychiatry* 2007; 164: 1890–1899

Ho BC, Andreasen NC, Ziebell S, et al. Long-term antipsychotic treatment and brain volumes: a longitudinal study of first-episode schizophrenia. *Arch Gen Psychiatry* 2011; 68: 128–137

Hoes MJ, Zeijpveld JH. Mirtazapine as a treatment for serotonin syndrome. *Pharmacopsychiatry* 1996; 29: 81

Hoffer A. Schizophrenia: an evolutionary defence against severe stress. *J Orthomolec Med* 1994; 9: 205–221

Hollander E, Allen A, Lopez RP, et al. A preliminary double-blind, placebo-controlled trial of divalproex sodium in borderline personality disorder. *J Clin Psychiatry* 2001; 62: 199–203

Hollander E, Koran LM, Goodman WK, et al. A double-blind, placebo-controlled study of the efficacy and safety of controlled-release fluvoxamine in patients with obsessive-compulsive disorder. *J Clin Psychiatry* 2003a; 64: 640–647

Hollander E, Swann AC, Coccaro EF, et al. Impact of trait impulsivity and state aggression on divalproex versus placebo response in borderline personality disorder. *Am J Psychiatry* 2005; 162: 621–624

Hollander E, Tracey KA, Swann AC, et al. Divalproex in the treatment of impulsive aggression: efficacy in cluster B personality disorders. *Neuropsychopharmacology* 2003b; 28: 1186–1197

Holmes TH, Rahe RH. The social readjustment rating scale. *J Psychosom Res* 1967; 11: 213–218

Holmquist GL. Opioid metabolism and effects of cytochrome P450. *Pain Med* 2009; 10 (Suppl 1): S20–S29

Holst J, Bäckström T, Hammarbäck S, et al. Progestogen addition during oestrogen replacement therapy – effects on vasomotor symptoms and mood. *Maturitas* 1989; 11: 13–20

Hooley JM, Parker HA. Measuring expressed emotion: an evaluation of the shortcuts. *J Fam Psychol* 2006; 20: 386–396.

Horing B, Weimer K, Muth ER, et al. Prediction of placebo responses: a systematic review of the literature. *Front Psychol* 2014; 5: 1079

Horvath AO, Symonds BD. Relation between working alliance and outcome in psychotherapy: a meta-analysis. *J Counsel Psychol* 1991; 38: 139–149

Horvitz-Lennon M, Mattke S, Predmore Z. The role of antipsychotic plasma levels in the treatment of schizophrenia. *Am J Psychiatry* 2017; 174: 421–426

Howes OD, Kambeitz J, Kim E, et al. The nature of dopamine dysfunction in schizophrenia and what this means for treatment. *Arch Gen Psychiatry* 2012; 69: 776-786

Hrøbjartsson A, Gøtzsche PC. Is the placebo powerless? An analysis of clinical trials comparing placebo with no treatment. *N Engl J Med* 2001; 344: 1594–1602

Hsu W-Y, Lane H-Y, Li C-H. Medications used for cognitive enhancement in patients with schizophrenia, bipolar disorder, Alzheimer's disease, and Parkinson's disease. *Front Psychiatry* 2018; 9: 91

Huang CL, Hwang TJ, Chen YH, et al. Intramuscular olanzapine versus intramuscular haloperidol plus lorazepam for the treatment of acute schizophrenia with agitation: an open-label, randomized controlled trial. *J Formos Med Assoc* 2015; 114: 438–445

Huband N, Ferriter M, Nathan R, et al. Antiepileptics for aggression and associated impulsivity. *Cochrane Database Syst Rev* 2010; (2): CD003499

Hudson JI, Hiripi E, Pope HG Jr., et al. The prevalence and correlates of eating disorders in the National Comorbidity Survey Replication. *Biol Psychiatry* 2007; 61: 348–358

Huerta-Ramos E, Iniesta R, Ochoa S, et al. Effects of raloxifene on cognition in postmenopausal women with schizophrenia: a double-blind, randomized, placebo-controlled trial. *Eur Neuropsychopharmacol* 2014; 24: 223–231

Huhn M, Nikolakopoulou A, Schneider-Thoma J, et al. Comparative efficacy and tolerability of 32 oral antipsychotics for the acute treatment of adults with multi-episode schizophrenia: a systematic review and network meta-analysis. *Lancet* 2019; 394: 939–951

Hurd YL, Spriggs S, Alishayev J, et al. Cannabidiol for the reduction of cue-induced craving and anxiety in drug-abstinent individuals with heroin use disorder: a double-blind randomized placebo-controlled trial. *Am J Psychiatry* 2019; 176: 911–922

Hymowitz P, Frances A, Jacobsberg LB, et al. Neuroleptic treatment of schizotypal personality disorders. *Compr Psychiatry* 1986; 27: 267–271

Imaz ML, Torra M, Soy D, et al. Clinical lactation studies of lithium: a systematic review. *Front Pharmacol* 2019; 10: 1005

Indave BI, Minozzi S, Paolo Pani P, et al. Antipsychotic medications for cocaine dependence. *Cochrane Database Syst Rev* 2016; (3): CD006306

Insel TR, Hamilton JA, Guttmacher LB, et al. D-amphetamine in obsessive-compulsive disorder. *Psychopharmacol (Berl)* 1983; 80: 231–235

Ionescu DF, Bentley KH, Eikermann M, et al. Repeat-dose ketamine augmentation for treatment-resistant depression with chronic suicidal ideation: a randomized, double blind, placebo controlled trial. *J Affect Disord* 2019; 243: 516–524

Ionescu DF, Fava M, Kim DJ, et al. A placebo-controlled crossover study of iloperidone augmentation for residual anger and irritability in major depressive disorder. *Ther Adv Psychopharmacol* 2016a; 6: 4–12

Ionescu DF, Swee MB, Pavone KJ, et al. Rapid and sustained reductions in current suicidal ideation following repeated doses of intravenous ketamine: secondary analysis of an open-label study. *J Clin Psychiatry* 2016b; 77: e719–e725

Ipser JC, Wilson D, Akindipe TO, et al. Pharmacotherapy for anxiety and comorbid alcohol use disorders. *Cochrane Database Syst Rev* 2015; 1: CD007505

ISIS-2 Collaborative Group. Randomised trial of intravenous streptokinase, oral aspirin, both, or neither among 17,187 cases of suspected acute myocardial infarction: ISIS-2. ISIS-2 (Second International Study of Infarct Survival) Collaborative Group. *Lancet* 1988; 2: 349–360

Isojärvi JI, Laatikainen TJ, Pakarinen AJ, et al. Polycystic ovaries and hyperandrogenism in women taking valproate for epilepsy. *N Engl J Med* 1993; 329: 1383–1388

Jacobs-Pilipski MJ, Wilfley DE, Crow SJ, et al. Placebo response in binge eating disorder. *Int J Eat Disord* 2007; 40: 204–211

Jacobsen FM. Low-dose trazodone as a hypnotic in patients treated with MAOIs and other psychotropics: a pilot study. *J Clin Psychiatry* 1990; 51: 298–302

Jacobson PL, Mahableshwarkar AR, Serenko M, et al. A randomized, double-blind, placebo-controlled study of the efficacy and safety of vortioxetine 10 mg and 20 mg in adults with major depressive disorder. *J Clin Psychiatry* 2015; 76: 575–582

Jafferany M, Osuagwu FC. Use of topiramate in skin-picking disorder: a pilot study. *Prim Care Companion CNS Disord* 2017; 19(1)

Jahangard L, Akbarian S, Haghighi M, et al. Children with ADHD and symptoms of oppositional defiant disorder improved in behavior when treated with methylphenidate and adjuvant risperidone, though weight gain was also observed: results from a randomized, double-blind, placebo-controlled clinical trial. *Psychiatry Res* 2017; 251: 182–191

Jain FA, Hunter AM, Brooks III JO, et al. Predictive socioeconomic and clinical profiles of antidepressant response and remission. *Depress Anxiety* 2013; 30: 624–630

Jakobsen KD, Skyum E, Hashemi N, et al. Antipsychotic treatment of schizotypy and schizotypal personality disorder: a systematic review. *J Psychopharmacol* 2017; 31: 397–405

Jakubczyk A, Wrzosek M, Łukaszkiewicz J, et al. The CC genotype in HTR2A T102C polymorphism is associated with behavioral impulsivity in alcohol-dependent patients. *J Psychiatr Res* 2012; 46: 44–49

Jakubovski E, Varigonda AL, Freemantle N, et al. Systematic review and meta-analysis: dose-response relationship of selective serotonin reuptake inhibitors in major depressive disorder. *Am J Psychiatry* 2016; 173: 174–183

Jana U, Sur TK, Maity LN, et al. A clinical study on the management of generalized anxiety disorder with Centella asiatica. *Nepal Med Coll J* 2010; 12: 8–11

Janowsky DS, Davis JM, el-Yousef MK, et al. A cholinergic-adrenergic hypothesis of mania and depression. *Lancet* 1972; 300: 632–635

Jarivavilas A, Thavichachart N, Kongsakon R, et al. Effects of paliperidone extended release on hostility among Thai patients with schizophrenia. *Neuropsychiatr Dis Treat* 2017; 13: 141–146

Jasinski D, Krishnan S. Abuse liability and safety of oral lisdexamfetamine dimesylate in individuals with a history of stimulant abuse. *J Psychopharmacol* 2009b; 23: 419–427

Jasinski DR, Krishnan S. Human pharmacology of intravenous lisdexamfetamine dimesylate: abuse liability in adult stimulant abusers. *J Psychopharmacol* 2009a; 23: 410–418

Javitt DC, Zylberman I, Zukin SR, et al. Amelioration of negative symptoms in schizophrenia by glycine. *Am J Psychiatry* 1994; 151: 1234–1236

Jentink J, Loane, MA, Dolk H, et al. Valproic acid monotherapy in pregnancy and major congenital malformations. *N Engl J Med* 2010; 362: 2185–2193

Jiang H, Ling Z, Zhang Y, et al. Altered microbiota composition in patients with major depressive disorder. *Brain Behav Immun* 2015; 48: 186–194

Jin W, Zheng H, Shan B, et al. Changes of serum trace elements level in patients with alopecia areata: a meta-analysis. *J Derm* 2017; 44: 588–591

Joffe RT, Swinson RP, Levitt AJ. Acute psychostimulant challenge in primary obsessive-compulsive disorder. *J Clin Psychopharmacol* 1991; 11: 237–241

Joffe H, Cohen LS, Suppes T, et al. Valproate is associated with new-onset oligoamenorrhea with hyperandrogenism in women with bipolar disorder. *Biol Psychiatry* 2006; 59: 1078–1086

Joffe H, Petrillo LF, Viguera AC, et al. Treatment of premenstrual worsening of depression with adjunctive oral contraceptive pills: a preliminary report. *J Clin Psychiatry* 2007; 68: 1954–1962

Johnson BA, Ait-Daoud N, Bowden CL, et al. Oral topiramate for treatment of alcohol dependence: a randomised controlled trial. *Lancet* 2003; 361: 1677–1685

Johnson BA, Ait-Daoud N, Wang XQ, et al. Topiramate for the treatment of cocaine addiction: a randomized clinical trial. *JAMA Psychiatry* 2013; 70: 1338–1346

Johnson BA, Roache JD, Javors MA, et al. Ondansetron for reduction of drinking among biologically predisposed alcoholic patients: a randomized controlled trial. *Arch Gen Psychiatry* 2000; 284: 23–30

Johnson BA, Rosenthal N, Capece JA, et al. Topiramate for treating alcohol dependence: a randomized controlled trial. *J Am Med Assoc* 2007; 298: 1641–1651

Jonas DE, Amick HR, Feltner C, et al. Pharmacotherapy for adults with alcohol use disorders in outpatient settings: a systematic review and meta-analysis. *J Am Med Assoc* 2014; 311: 1889–1900

Jones JM, Aldrich J, Gillham R, et al. Efficacy of mood stabilisers in the treatment of impulsive or repetitive aggression: systematic review and meta-analysis. *Br J Psychiatry* 2011; 198: 93–98

Joos L, Goudriaan A, Schmaal L, et al. Effect of modafinil on cognitive functions in alcohol dependent patients: a randomized, placebo-controlled trial. *J Psychopharmacol* 2013; 27: 998–1006

Jorge RE, Acion L, Moser D, et al. Escitalopram and enhancement of cognitive recovery following stroke. *Arch Gen Psychiatry* 2010; 67: 187–196

Ju SY, Lee YJ, Jeong SN. Serum 25-hydroxyvitamin D levels and the risk of depression: a systematic review and meta-analysis. *J Nutr Health Aging* 2013; 17: 447–455

Kabul S, Altorre C, Motejano LB, et al. Real-world dosing patterns of atomoxetine in adults with attention-deficit/hyperactivity disorder. *CNS Neurosci Ther* 2015; 21: 936–942

Kagawa S, Mihara K, Nakamura A, et al. Relationship between plasma concentrations of lamotrigine and its early therapeutic effect of lamotrigine augmentation therapy in treatment-resistant depressive disorder. *Ther Drug Monit* 2014; 36: 730–733

Kahn RS, van Rossum IW, Leucht S, et al. Amisulpride and olanzapine followed by open-label treatment with clozapine in first-episode schizophrenia and schizophreniform disorder (OPTiMiSE): a three-phase switching study. *Lancet Psychiatry* 2018; 5: 797–807

Kalivas J, Kalivas L, Gilman D, et al. Sertraline in the treatment of neurotic excoriations and related disorders. *Arch Dermatol* 1996; 132: 589–590

Kamarck TW, Haskett RF, Muldoon M, et al. Citalopram intervention for hostility: results of a randomized clinical trial. *J Consult Clin Psychol* 2009; 77: 174–188

Kamendulis LM, Brzezinski MR, Pindel EV, et al. Metabolism of cocaine and heroin is catalyzed by the same human liver carboxylesterases. *J Pharmacol Exp Ther* 1996; 279: 713–717

Kamijima K, Higuchi T, Ishigooka J, et al. Aripiprazole augmentation to antidepressant therapy in Japanese patients with major depressive disorder: a randomized, double-blind, placebo-controlled study (ADMIRE study). *J Affect Disord* 2013; 151: 899–905

Kampman KM, Pettinati HM, Lynch KG, et al. A double-blind, placebo-controlled trial of topiramate for the treatment of comorbid cocaine and alcohol dependence. *Drug Alcohol Depend* 2013; 133: 94–99

Kampman KM, Pettinati H, Lynch KG, et al. A pilot trial of topiramate for the treatment of cocaine dependence. *Drug Alcohol Abuse* 2004; 75: 233–240

Kan CC, Hilberink SR, Breteler MH. Determination of the main risk factors for benzodiazepine dependence using a multivariate and multidimensional approach. *Compr Psychiatry* 2004; 45: 88–94

Kane JM, Assunção-Talbott S, Eudicone JM, et al. The efficacy of aripiprazole in the treatment of multiple symptom domains in patients with acute schizophrenia: a pooled analysis of data from the pivotal trials. *Schizophr Res* 2008; 105: 208–215

Kane JM, Canas F, Kramer M, et al. Treatment of schizophrenia with paliperidone extended-release tablets: a 6-week placebo-controlled trial. *Schizophr Res* 2007; 90: 147–161

Kane JM, Cohen M, Zhao J, et al. Efficacy and safety of asenapine in a placebo- and haloperidol-controlled trial in patients with an acute exacerbation of schizophrenia. *J Clin Psychopharmacol* 2010; 30: 106–115

Kane JM, Marder SR, Schooler NR, et al. Clozapine and haloperidol in moderately refractory schizophrenia: a 6-month randomized and double-blind comparison. *Arch Gen Psychiatry* 2001; 58: 965–972

Kaneriya SH, Robbins-Welty GA, Smaqula SF, et al. Predictors and moderators of remission with aripiprazole augmentation in treatment-resistant late-life depression: an analysis of the IRL-GRey randomized clinical trial. *JAMA Psychiatry* 2016; 73: 329–336

Kanes S, Colquhoun H, Gunduz-Bruce H, et al. Brexanolone (SAGE-547 injection) in post-partum depression: a randomised controlled trial. *Lancet* 2017; 390: 480–489

Kapciski F, Lima MS, Souza JS, Schmitt R. Antidepressants for generalized anxiety disorder. *Cochrane Database Syst Rev* 2003; (2): CD003592

Kapur S, Seeman P. Does fast dissociation from the dopamine D_2 receptor explain the action of atypical antipsychotics? A new hypothesis. *Am J Psychiatry* 2001; 158: 360–369

Kapur S, Remington G, Jones C, et al. High levels of dopamine D2 receptor occupancy with low-dose haloperidol treatment: a PET study. *Am J Psychiatry* 1996; 153: 948–950

Kapur S, Zipursky R, Remington G, et al. PET evidence that loxapine is an equipotent blocker of 5-HT_2 and D_2 receptors: implications for the therapeutics of schizophrenia. *Am J Psychiatry* 1997a; 154: 1525–1529

Kapur S, Zipursky R, Roy P, et al. The relationship between D2 receptor occupancy and plasma levels on low dose oral haloperidol: a PET study. *Psychopharmacol (Berl)* 1997b; 131: 148–152

Kardashev A, Ratner Y, Ritsner MS. Add-on pregnenolone with L-theanine to antipsychotic therapy relieves negative and anxiety symptoms of schizophrenia: an 8-week, randomized, double-blind, placebo-controlled trial. *Clin Schizophr Relat Psychoses Spring* 2018; 12: 31-41

Karpouzian-Rogers T, Stocks J, Meltzer HY, et al. The effect of high vs. low dose lurasidone on eye movement biomarkers of prefrontal abilities in treatment-resistant schizophrenia. *Schizophr Res* 2020; 215: 314–321

Kashani L, Shams N, Moazen-Zadeh E, et al. Pregnenolone as an adjunct to risperidone for treatment of women with schizophrenia: a randomized double-blind placebo-controlled clinical trial. *J Psychiatr Res* 2017; 94: 70–77

Kasper S, Dold M. Factors contributing to the increasing placebo response in antidepressant trials. *World Psychiatry* 2015; 14: 304-306

Kasper S, de Swart H, Friis-Andersen H. Escitalopram in the treatment of depressed elderly patients. *Am J Geriatr Psychiatry* 2005; 13: 884–891

Kasper S, Barnas C, Heiden A, et al. Pramipexole as adjunct to haloperidol in schizophrenia: safety and efficacy. *Eur Neuropsychopharmacol* 1997; 7: 65–70

Katila H, Mezhebovsky I, Mulroy A, et al. Randomized, double-blind study of the efficacy and tolerability of extended release quetiapine fumarate (quetiapine XR) monotherapy in elderly patients with major depressive disorder. *Am J Geriatr Psychiatry* 2013; 21: 769–784

Kato H, Fukatsu N, Noguchi T, et al. Lamotrigine improves aggression in patients with temporal lobe epilepsy. *Epilepsy Behav* 2011; 21: 173–176

Katona C, Hansen T, Olsen CK. A randomized, double-blind, placebo-controlled, duloxetine-referenced, fixed-dose study comparing the efficacy and safety of Lu AA21004 in elderly patients with major depressive disorder. *Int Clin Psychopharmacol* 2012; 27: 215–223

Katz IR, Jeste DV, Mintzer JE, et al. Comparison of risperidone and placebo for psychosis and behavioural disturbances associated with demetia: a randomized, double-blind trial. *J Clin Psychiatry* 1999; 60: 107–115

Katzelnick DJ, Kobak KA, Greist JH, et al. Sertraline for social phobia: a double-blind, placebo-controlled crossover study. *Am J Psychiatry* 1995; 152: 1368–1371

Kavoussi RJ, Coccaro EF. Divalproex sodium for impulsive aggressive behavior in patients with personality disorder. *J Clin Psychiatry* 1998; 59: 676–680

Kavoussi RJ, Liu J, Coccaro EF. An open trial of sertraline in personality disordered patients with impulsive aggression. *J Clin Psychiatry* 1994; 55: 137–141

Kawada K, Ohta T, Tanaka K, et al. Addition of suvorexant to ramelteon therapy for improved sleep quality with reduced delirium risk in acute stroke patients. *Stroke Cerebrovasc Dis* 2019; 28: 142–148

Kay SR, Fiszbein A, Opler LA. The positive and negative syndrome scale (PANSS) for schizophrenia. *Schizophr Bull* 1987; 13: 261–276

Kayser A, Robinson DS, Nies A, et al. Response to phenelzine among depressed patients with features of hysteroid dysphoria. *Am J Psychiatry* 1985; 142: 486–488

Kazemi A, Noorbala AA, Azam K, et al. Effect of probiotic and prebiotic vs. placebo on psychological outcomes in patients with major depressive disorder: a randomized clinical trial. *Clin Nutr* 2019; 38: 522–528

Keck P Jr., Buffenstein A, Ferguson J, et al. Ziprasidone 40 and 120 mg/day in the acute exacerbation of schizophrenia and schizoaffective disorder: a 4-week placebo-controlled trial. *Psychopharmacol (Berl)* 1998; 140: 173–184

Keck PE Jr., Bowden CL, Meinhold JM, et al. Relationship between serum valproate and lithium levels and efficacy and tolerability in bipolar maintenance therapy. *Intl J Psychiatry Clin Pract* 2005; 9: 271–277

Keck PE Jr., Calabrese JR, McIntyre RS, et al. Aripiprazole monotherapy for maintenance therapy in bipolar I disorder: a 100-week, double-blind study versus placebo. *J Clin Psychiatry* 2007; 68: 1480–1491

Keck PE Jr., McElroy SL, Tugrul KC, et al. Valproate oral loading in the treatment of acute mania. *J Clin Psychiatry* 1993; 54: 305–308

Keck PE Jr., Strakowski SM, Hawkins JM, et al. A pilot study of rapid lithium administration in the treatment of acute mania. *Bipolar Disord* 2001; 3: 68–72

Keck PE Jr., Versiani M, Potkin S, et al. Ziprasidone in the treatment of acute bipolar mania: a three-week, placebo-controlled, double-blind, randomized trial. *Am J Psychiatry* 2003; 160: 741–748

Keefe RS, Bilder RM, Davis SM, et al. Neurocognitive effects of antipsychotic medications in patients with chronic schizophrenia in the CATIE Trial. *Arch Gen Psychiatry* 2007; 64: 633–647

Keefe RSE, Seidman LJ, Christensen BK, et al. Comparative effect of atypical and conventional antipsychotic drugs on neurocognition in first-episode psychosis: a randomized, double-blind trial of olanzapine versus low doses of haloperidol. *Am J Psychiatry* 2004; 161: 985–995

Keitner GI, Garlow SJ, Ryan CE, et al. A randomized, placebo-controlled trial of risperidone augmentation for patients with difficult-to-treat unipolar, non-psychotic major depression. *J Psychiatr Res* 2009; 43: 205–214

Kelleher JP, Centorrino F, Huxley NA, et al. Pilot randomized, controlled trial of pramipexole to augment antipsychotic treatment. *Eur Neuropsychopharmacol* 2012; 22: 415–418

Kelley JM, Kaptchuk TJ, Cusin C, et al. Open-label placebo for major depressive disorder: a pilot randomized controlled trial. *Psychother Psychosom* 2012; 81: 312–314

Kellner CH, Knapp RG, Petrides G, et al. Continuation electroconvulsive therapy vs pharmacotherapy for relapse prevention in major depression: a multisite study from the Consortium for Research in Electroconvulsive Therapy (CORE). *Arch Gen Psychiatry* 2006; 63: 1337–1344

Kelly LE, Poon S, Madadi P, et al. Neonatal benzodiazepines exposure during breastfeeding. *J Pediatr* 2012; 161: 448–451

Kemp DE, Ganocy SJ, Brecher M, et al. Clinical value of early partial symptomatic improvement in the prediction of response and remission during short-term treatment trials in 3369 subjects with bipolar I or II depression. *J Affect Disord* 2011; 130: 171–179

Kemp DE, Gao K, Fein EB, et al. Lamotrigine as add-on treatment to lithium and divalproex: lessons learned from a double-blind, placebo-controlled trial in rapid-cycling bipolar disorder. *Bipolar Disord* 2012; 14: 780–789

Kendell RE, Cooper JE, Gourlay AJ. Diagnostic criteria of American and British psychiatrists. *Arch Gen Psychiatry* 1971; 25: 123–130

Kennedy SH, Lam RW, McIntyre RS, et al. Canadian Network for Mood and Anxiety Treatments (CANMAT) 2016: Clinical Guidelines for the Management of Adults with Major Depressive Disorder Section 3. Pharmacological Treatments. *Can J Psychiatry* 2016; 61: 540–560

Kennel KA, Drake MT, Hurley DL. Vitamin D deficiency in adults: when to test and how to treat. *Mayo Clin Proc* 2010; 85: 752–758

Keshavan M, Shad M, Soloff P, et al. Efficacy and tolerability of olanzapine in the treatment of schizotypal personality disorder. *Schizophr Res* 2004; 71: 97–101

Kessler DS, MacNeill SJ, Tallon D, et al. Mirtazapine added to SSRIs or SNRIs for treatment resistant depression in primary care: phase III randomised placebo controlled trial (MIR). *Br Med J* 2018; 363: k4218

Kessler RC, Adler LA, Barkley R, et al. Patterns and predictors of attention-deficit/hyperactivity disorder persistence into adulthood: results from the National Comorbidity Survey Replication. *Biol Psychiatry* 2005a; 57: 1442–1451

Kessler RC, Adler L, Barkley R, et al. The prevalence and correlates of adult ADHD in the United States: results from the National Comorbidity Survey Replication. *Am J Psychiatry* 2006; 163: 716–723

Kessler RC, Birnbaum H, Demler O, et al. The prevalence and correlates of nonaffective psychosis in the National Comorbidity Survey Replication (NCS-R). *Biol Psychiatry* 2005b; 58: 668–676

Kessler RC, Chiu WT, Demler O, et al. Prevalence, severity, and comorbidity of 12-month DSM-IV disorders in the National Comorbidity Survey Replication. *Arch Gen Psychiatry* 2005c; 62: 617–627

Ketter TA, Post RM, Theodore WH. Positive and negative psychiatric effects of antiepileptic drugs in patients with seizure disorders. *Neurology* 1999; 53 (5 Suppl 2): S53–S67

Ketter TA, Post RM, Parekh PI, et al. Addition of monoamine oxidase inhibitors to carbamazepine: preliminary evidence of safety and antidepressant efficacy in treatment-resistant depression. *J Clin Psychiatry* 1995; 56: 471–475

Keuthen N, Jameson M, Loh R, et al. Open-label escitalopram treatment for pathological skin picking. *Int Clin Psychopharmacol* 2007; 22: 268–274

Khan A, Redding N, Brown WA. The persistence of the placebo response in antidepressant clinical trials. *J Psychiatr Res* 2008; 42: 791–796

Khan A, Brodhead AE, Schwartz KA, et al. Sex differences in antidepressant response in recent antidepressant clinical trials. *J Clin Psychopharmacol* 2005; 25: 318–324

Khan A, Fahl Mar K, Faucett J, et al. Has the rising placebo response impacted antidepressant clinical trial outcome? Data from the US Food and Drug Administration 1987–2013. *World Psychiatry* 2017; 16: 181–192

Khan A, Ginsberg LD, Asnis GM, et al. Effect of lamotrigine on cognitive complaints in patients with bipolar I disorder. *J Clin Psychiatry* 2004; 65: 1483–1490

Khan SJ, Fersh ME, Ernst C, et al. Bipolar disorder in pregnancy and postpartum: principles of management. *Curr Psychiatry Rep* 2016; 18: 13

Khera R, Murad MH, Chandar AK, et al. Association of pharmacological treatments for obesity with weight loss and adverse events: a systematic review and meta-analysis. *J Am Med Assoc* 2016; 315: 2424–2434

Kim HJ, Kim JE, Cho G, et al. Associations between anterior cingulate cortex glutamate and gamma-aminobutyric acid concentrations and the harm avoidance temperament. *Neurosci Lett* 2009; 464: 103–107

Kim JE, Yoon SJ, Kim J, et al. Efficacy and tolerability of mirtazapine in treating major depressive disorder with anxiety symptoms: an 8-week open-label randomised paroxetine-controlled trial. *Int J Clin Pract* 2011; 65: 323329

Kim SW, Dodd S, Berk L, et al. Impact of cannabis use on long-term remission in bipolar I and schizoaffective disorder. *Psychiatry Investig* 2015; 12: 349–355

Kim S-W, Kang H-J, Jhon M, et al. Statins and inflammation: new therapeutic opportunities in psychiatry. *Front Psychiatry* 2019; 10: 103

Kimmel M, Hess E, Roy PS, et al. Family history, not lack of medication use, is associated with the development of postpartum depression in a high-risk sample. *Arch Womens Ment Health* 2015; 18: 113–121

Kimura M, Tateno A, Robinson RG. Treatment of poststroke generalized anxiety disorder comorbid with poststroke depression: merged analysis of nortriptyline trials. *Am J Geriatr Psychiatry* 2003; 11: 320–327

King DJ, Link CGG, Kowalcyk B. A comparison of bd and tid dose regimens of quetiapine (Seroquel) in the treatment of schizophrenia. *Psychopharmacology* 1998; 137: 139–146

Kinon BJ, Millen BA, Zhang L, et al. Exploratory analysis for a targeted patient population responsive to the metabotropic glutamate 2/3 receptor agonist pomaglumetad methionil in schizophrenia. *Biol Psychiatry* 2015; 78: 754–762

Kinon BJ, Volavka J, Stauffer V, et al. Standard and higher dose of olanzapine in patients with schizophrenia or schizoaffective disorder: a randomized, double-blind, fixed-dose study. *J Clin Psychopharmacol* 2008; 28: 392–400

Kinon BJ, Zhang L, Millen BA, et al. A multicenter, inpatient, phase 2, double-blind, placebo-controlled dose-ranging study of LY2140023 monohydrate in patients with DSM-IV schizophrenia. *J Clin Psychopharmacol* 2011; 31: 349–355

Kinrys G, Pollack MH, Simon NM, et al. Valproic acid for the treatment of social anxiety disorder. *Int Clin Psychopharmacol* 2003; 18: 169–172

Kinrys G, Wygant LE, Pardo TB, et al. Levetiracetam for treatment refractory posttraumatic stress disorder. *J Clin Psychiatry* 2006; 67: 211–214

Kirsch I, Deacon BJ, Huedo-Medina TB, et al. Initial severity and antidepressant benefits: a meta-analysis of data submitted to the Food and Drug Administration. *PLoS Med* 2008; 5: e45

Kishi T, Iwata N. Meta-analysis of noradrenergic and specific serotonergic antidepressant use in schizophrenia. *Int J Neuropsychopharmacol* 2014; 17: 343–354

Kishi T, Mukai T, Matsuda Y, et al. Selective serotonin 3 receptor antagonist treatment for schizophrenia: meta-analysis and systematic review. *Neuromolecular Med* 2014; 16: 61–69

Kishi T, Sevy S, Chekuri R, et al. Antipsychotics for primary alcohol dependence: a systematic review and meta-analysis of placebo-controlled trials. *J Clin Psychiatry* 2013; 74: e642–e654

Kittipeerachon M, Chaichan W. Intramuscular olanzapine versus intramuscular aripiprazole for the treatment of agitation in patients with schizophrenia: pragmatic double-blind randomized trial. *Schizophr Res* 2016; 176: 231–238

Kleinstäuber M, Witthöft M, Steffanowski A, et al. Pharmacological interventions for somatoform disorders in adults. *Cochrane Database Syst Rev* 2014; (11): CD010628

Klinge C, Shuttleworth C, Muglia P, et al. Methylphenidate enhances implicit learning in healthy adults. *J Psychopharmacol* 2018; 32: 70–80

Knegtering R, Baselmans P, Castelein S, et al. Predominant role of the 9-hydroxy metabolite of risperidone in elevating blood prolactin levels. *Am J Psychiatry* 2005; 162: 1010–1012

Knight R, Khondoker M, Magill N, et al. A systematic review and meta-analysis of the effectiveness of acetylcholinesterase inhibitors and memantine in treating the cognitive symptoms of dementia. *Dementia Geriatr Cogn Disord* 2018; 45: 131–151

Ko DT, Herbert PR, Coffey CS, et al. Beta-blocker therapy and symptoms of depression, fatigue, and sexual dysfunction. *J Am Med Assoc* 2002; 288: 351–357

Ko YH, Lew YM, Jung SW, et al. Short-term testosterone augmentation in male schizophrenics: a randomized, double-blind, placebo-controlled trial. *J Clin Psychopharmacol* 2008; 28: 375–383

Koblan KS, Hopkins SC, Sarma K, et al. Dasotraline for the treatment of attention-deficit/hyperactivity disorder: a randomized, double-blind, placebo-controlled, proof-of-concept trial in adults. *Neuropsychopharmacology* 2015; 40: 2745–2752

Koblan KS, Kent J, Hopkins SC, et al. A non-D2-receptor-binding drug for the treatment of schizophrenia. *N Engl J Med* 2020; 382: 1497–1606

Kocsis JH, Thase ME, Trivedi MH, et al. Prevention of recurrent episodes of depression with venlafaxine ER in a 1-year maintenance phase from the PREVENT study. *J Clin Psychiatry* 2007; 68: 1014–1023

Koenig AM, Butters MA, Begley A, et al. Response to antidepressant medications in late-life depression across the spectrum of cognitive functioning. *J Clin Psychiatry* 2014; 75: e100–e107

Koenigsberg HW, Reynolds D, Goodman M, et al. Risperidone in the treatment of schizotypal personality disorder. *J Clin Psychiatry* 2003; 64: 628–634

Koethe D, Juelicher A, Nolden BM, et al. Oxcarbazepine – efficacy and tolerability during treatment of alcohol withdrawal: a double-blind, randomized, placebo-controlled multicenter pilot study. *Alcohol Clin Exp Res* 2007; 31: 1188–1194

Köhler O, Benros ME, Nordentoft M, et al. Effect of anti-inflammatory treatment on depression, depressive symptoms, and adverse effects: a systematic review and meta-analysis of randomized clinical trials. *JAMA Psychiatry* 2014; 71: 1381–1391

Koob GF, Volkow ND. Neurobiology of addiction: a neurocircuitry analysis. *Lancet Psychiatry* 2016; 3: 760–773

Koran LM, Aboujaoude E, Gamel NN. Double-blind study of dextroamphetamine versus caffeine augmentation for treatment-resistant obsessive-compulsive disorder. *J Clin Psychiatry* 2009; 70: 1530–1535

Koran LM, Aboujaoude EN, Gamel NN. Escitalopram treatment of kleptomania: an open-label trial followed by double-blind discontinuation. *J Clin Psychiatry* 2007; 68: 422–427

Koran LM, Cain JW, Dominguez RA, et al. Are fluoxetine plasma levels related to outcome in obsessive-compulsive disorder? *Am J Psychiatry* 1996; 153: 1450–1454

Koran LM, Chuong HW, Bullock KD, et al. Citalopram for compulsive shopping disorder: an open-label study followed by double-blind discontinuation. *J Clin Psychiatry* 2003; 64: 793–798

Koran LM, Gamel NN, Choung HW, et al. Mirtazapine for obsessive-compulsive disorder: an open trial followed by double-blind discontinuation. *J Clin Psychiatry* 2005; 66: 515–520

Koran LM, Gelenberg AJ, Kornstein SG, et al. Sertraline versus imipramine to prevent relapse in chronic depression. *J Affect Disord* 2001; 65: 27–36

Korgaonkar MS, Williams LM, Song YJ, et al. Diffusion tensor imaging predictors of treatment outcomes in major depressive disorder. *Br J Psychiatry* 2014; 205: 321–328

Kornstein SG, Bose A, Li D, et al. Escitalopram maintenance treatment for prevention of recurrent depression: a randomized, placebo-controlled trial. *J Clin Psychiatry* 2006; 67: 1767–1775

Kornstein SG, Schatzberg AF, Thase ME, et al. Gender differences in treatment response to sertraline versus imipramine in chronic depression. *Am J Psychiatry* 2000; 157: 1445–1452

Kosten T, Oliveto A, Feingold A, et al. Desipramine and contingency management for cocaine and opiate dependence in buprenorphine maintained patients. *Drug Alcohol Depend* 2003; 70: 315–325

Kosten TR, Fontana A, Sernyak MJ, et al. Benzodiazepine use in posttraumatic stress disorder among veterans with substance abuse. *J Nerv Ment Dis* 2000; 188: 454–459

Kotov R, Gamez W, Schmidt F, et al. Linking "big" personality traits to anxiety, depressive, and substance use disorders: a meta-analysis. *Psychol Bull* 2010; 136: 768–821

Kowalczyk WJ, Phillips KA, Jobes ML, et al. Clonidine maintenance prolongs opioid abstinence and decouples stress from craving in daily life: a randomized controlled trial with ecological momentary assessment. *Am J Psychiatry* 2015; 172: 760–767

Kowatch RA, Suppes T, Carmody TJ, et al. Effect size of lithium, divalproex sodium, and carbamazepine in children and adolescents with bipolar disorder. *J Am Acad Child Adolesc Psychiatry* 2000; 39: 713–720

Koychev I, McMullen K, Lees J, et al. A validation of cognitive biomarkers for the early identification of cognitive enhancing agents in schizotypy: a three-center double-blind placebo-controlled study. *Eur Neuropsychopharmacol* 2012; 22: 469–481

Kozel FA, Trivedi MH, Wisniewski SR, et al. Treatment outcomes for older depressed patients with earlier versus late onset of first depressive episode: a Sequenced Treatment Alternatives to Relieve Depression (STAR*D) report. *Am J Geriatr Psychiatry* 2008; 16: 58–64

Kraemer HC. Messages for clinicians: moderators and mediators of treatment outcome in randomized clinical trials. *Am J Psychiatry* 2016; 173: 672–679

Kranz GS, Wadsak W, Kayfmann U, et al. High-dose testosterone treatment increases serotonin transporter binding in transgender people. *Biol Psychiatry* 2015; 78: 525–533

Kranzler HR, Armeli S, Tennen H, et al. A double-blind, randomized trial of sertraline for alcohol dependence: moderation by age of onset [corrected] and 5-hydroxytryptamine transporter linked promoter region genotype. *J Clin Psychopharmacol* 2011; 31: 22–30

Kranzler HR, Burleson JA, Korner P, et al. Placebo-controlled trial of fluoxetine as an adjunct to relapse prevention in alcoholics. *Am J Psychiatry* 1995; 152: 391–397

Kranzler HR, Covault J, Feinn R, et al. Topiramate treatment for heavy drinkers: moderation by a GRIK1 polymorphism. *Am J Psychiatry* 2014; 171: 445–452

Kraus RP. Pindolol augmentation of tranylcypromine in psychotic depression. *J Clin Psychopharmacol* 1997; 17: 225–226

Kraus SW, Etuk R, Potenza MN. Current pharmacotherapy for gambling disorder: a systematic review. *Expert Opin Pharmacother* 2020; 21: 287–296

Krause M, Huhn M, Schneider Thoma J, et al. Antipsychotic drugs for elderly patients with schizophrenia: a systematic review and meta-analysis. *Eur Neuropsychopharmacol* 2018a; 28: 1360–1370

Krause M, Zhu Y, Huhn M, et al. Antipsychotic drugs for patients with schizophrenia and predominant or prominent negative symptoms: a systematic review and meta-analysis. *Eur Arch Psychiatry* 2018b; 268: 625–639

Krebs TS, Johansen PØ. Lysergic acid diethylamide (LSD) for alcoholism: meta-analysis of randomized controlled trials. *J Psychopharmacol* 2012; 26: 994–1002

Kreinin A, Bawakny N, Ritsner MS. Adjunctive pregnenolone ameliorates the cognitive deficits in recent-onset schizophrenia: an 8-week, randomized, double-blind, placebo-controlled trial. *Clin Schizophr Relat Psychoses* 2017; 10: 201–210

Kremer I, Vass A, Gorlik I, et al. Placebo-controlled trial of lamotrigine added to conventional and atypical antipsychotics in schizophrenia. *Biol Psychiatry* 2004; 56: 441–446

Krivoy A, Balicer RD, Feldman B, et al. The impact of age and gender on adherence to antidepressants: a 4-year population-based cohort study. *Psychopharmacol (Berl)* 2015; 232: 3385–3390

Krivoy A, Onn R, Vilner Y, et al. Vitamin D supplementation in chronic schizophrenia patients treated with clozapine: a randomized, double-blind, placebo-controlled trial. *EBioMedicine* 2017; 26: 138–145

Krymchantowski AV, Jevoux C, Moreira PF. An open pilot study assessing the benefits of quetiapine for the prevention of migraine refractory to the combination of atenolol, nortriptyline, and flunarizine. *Pain Med* 2010; 11: 48–52

Krystal JH, Rosenheck RA, Cramer JA, et al. Adjunctive risperidone treatment for antidepressant-resistant symptoms of chronic military service-related PTSD: a randomized trial. *J Am Med Assoc* 2011; 306: 493–502

Kulkarni J, Gavrilidis E, Gwini S, et al. Effect of adjunctive raloxifene therapy on severity of refractory schizophrenia in women. A randomized clinical trial. *JAMA Psychiatry* 2016; 73: 947–954

Kulkarni J, Thomas N, Hudaib AB, et al. Effect of the glutamate NMDA receptor antagonist memantine as adjunctive treatment in borderline personality disorder: an exploratory, randomised, double-blind, placebo-controlled trial. *CNS Drugs* 2018; 32: 179–187

Kupfer DJ, Frank E, Perel JM, et al. Five-year outcome for maintenance therapies in recurrent depression. *Arch Gen Psychiatry* 1992; 49: 769–773

Kuruvilla K, Shaji KS. How reliable is 24 hour serum lithium level after a test dose of lithium in predicting optimal lithium dose? *Indian J Psychiatry* 1989; 31: 70–72

Kushner SF, Khan A, Lane R, et al. Topiramate monotherapy in the management of acute mania: results of four double-blind placebo-controlled trials. *Bipolar Disord* 2006; 8: 15–27

Laib AK, Brünen S, Pfeifer P, et al. Serum concentrations of hydroxybupropion for dose optimization of depressed patients with bupropion. *Ther Drug Monit* 2014; 36: 473–479

Laird KT, Lavretsky H, St Cyr N, et al. Resilience predicts remission in antidepressant treatment of geriatric depression. *Int J Geriatr Psychiatry* 2018; 33: 1596–1603

Lakhan SE, Vieira KF. Nutritional and herbal supplements for anxiety and anxiety-related disorders: systematic review. *Nutr J* 2010; 9: 42.

Lal R, Sukbuntherng J, Luo W, et al. Pharmacokinetics and tolerability of single escalating doses of gabapentin enacarbil: a randomized-sequence, double-blind, placebo-controlled crossover study in healthy volunteers. *Clin Ther* 2009; 31: 1776–1786

Lane HY, Chang YC, Liu YC, et al. Sarcosine or D-serine add-on treatment for acute exacerbation of schizophrenia: a randomized, double-blind, placebo-controlled study. *Arch Gen Psychiatry* 2005; 62: 1196–1204

Lane HY, Huang CL, Wu PL, et al. Glycine transporter I inhibitor, N-methylglycine (sarcosine), added to clozapine for the treatment of schizophrenia. *Biol Psychiatry* 2006; 60: 645–649

Lane HY, Lin CH, Green MF, et al. Add-on treatment of benzoate for schizophrenia: a randomized, double-blind, placebo-controlled trial of D-amino acid oxidase inhibitor. *JAMA Psychiatry* 2013; 70: 1267–1275

LaPorta LA. Relief from migraine headache with aripiprazole treatment. *Headache* 2007; 47: 922–926

Laporte S, Chapelle C, Caillet P, et al. Bleeding risk under selective serotonin reuptake inhibitor (SSRI) antidepressants: a meta-analysis of observational studies. *Pharmacol Res* 2017; 118: 19–32

Larsen JR, Vedtofte L, Jacobsen MSL, et al. Effect of liraglutide treatment on prediabetes and overweight or obesity in clozapine- or olanzapine-treated patients with schizophrenia spectrum disorder: a randomized clinical trial. *JAMA Psychiatry* 2017; 74: 719–728

Larsson H, Rydén E, Boman M, et al. Risk of bipolar disorder and schizophrenia in relatives of people with attention-deficit hyperactivity disorder. *Br J Psychiatry* 2013; 203: 103–106

Lasser RA, Dirks B, Nasrallah H, et al. Adjunctive lisdexamfetamine dimesylate therapy in adult outpatients with predominant negative symptoms of schizophrenia: open-label and randomized-withdrawal phases. *Neuropsychopharmacology* 2013; 38: 2140–2149

Lavretsky H, Park S, Siddarth P, et al. Methylphenidate-enhanced antidepressant response to citalopram in the elderly: a double-blind, placebo-controlled pilot trial. *Am J Geriatr Psychiatry* 2006; 14: 181–185

Lavretsky H, Reinlieb M, St Cyr N, et al. Citalopram, methylphenidate, or their combination in geriatric depression: a randomized, double-blind, placebo-controlled trial. *Am J Psychiatry* 2015; 172: 561–569

Lawn W, Freeman TP, Pope RA, et al. Acute and chronic effects of cannabinoids on effort-related decision-making and reward learning: an evaluation of the cannabis "amotivational'" hypotheses. *Psychopharmacol (Berl)* 2016; 233: 3537–3552

Lazarus LW, Moberg PJ, Langsley PR, et al. Methylphenidate and nortriptyline in the treatment of poststroke depression: a retrospective comparison. *Arch Phys Med Rehabil* 1994; 75: 403–406

Lazarus LW, Winemiller DR, Lingam VR, et al. Efficacy and side effects of methylphenidate for poststroke depression. *J Clin Psychiatry* 1992; 53: 447–449

Leach MJ, Page AT. Herbal medicine for insomnia: a systematic review and meta-analysis. *Sleep Med Rev* 2015; 24: 1–12

Lecrubier Y, Judge R. Long-term evaluation of paroxetine, clomipramine and placebo in panic disorder. Collaborative Paroxetine Panic Study Investigators. *Acta Psychiatr Scand* 1997; 95: 153–160

Lee DJ, Schnitzlein CW, Wolf JP, et al. Psychotherapy versus pharmacotherapy for posttraumatic stress disorder: systematic review and meta-analyses to determine first-line treatments. *Depress Anxiety* 2016; 33: 792–806

Lee EE, Della Selva MP, Liu A, et al. Ketamine as a novel treatment for major depressive disorder and bipolar depression: a systematic review and quantitative meta-analysis. *Gen Hosp Psychiatry* 2015; 37: 178–184

Lee SY, Wang TY, Chen SL, et al. Add-on memantine treatment for bipolar II disorder comorbid with alcohol dependence: a 12-week follow-up study. *Alcohol Clin Exp Res* 2018; 42: 1044–1050

Lehman AF, Lieberman JA, Dixon LB, et al. Practice guideline for the treatment of patients with schizophrenia, second edition. *Am J Psychiatry* 2014; 161 (2 Suppl): 1–56

Leiberich P, Nickel MK, Tritt K, et al. Lamotrigine treatment of aggression in female borderline patients, part II: an 18-month follow-up. *J Psychopharmacol* 2008; 22: 805–808

Leibowitz M, Klein DF. Interrelationship of hysteroid dysphoria and borderline personality disorder. *Psych Clin N Amer* 1981; 4: 67–87

Lejoyeux M, Weinstein A. Compulsive buying. *Am J Drug Alcohol Abuse* 2010; 36: 248–253

Lenhard, W, Lenhard A. Calculation of Effect Sizes. *Psychometrica* 2016; DOI: 10.13140/RG.2.2.17823.92329. www.psychometrica.de/effect_size.html (accessed August 2020)

Lenze EJ, Mulsant BH, Blumberger DM, et al. Efficacy, safety, and tolerability of augmentation pharmacotherapy with aripiprazole for treatment-resistant depression in late life: a randomised, double-blind, placebo-controlled trial. *Lancet* 2015; 386: 2404–2412

Leonard HL, Lenane MC, Swedo SE, et al. A double-blind comparison of clomipramine and desipramine treatment of severe onychophagia (nail biting). *Arch Gen Psychiatry* 1991; 48: 821–827

Lépine J-P, Caillard V, Bisserbe J-C, et al. A randomized, placebo-controlled trial of sertraline for prophylactic treatment of highly recurrent major depression. *Am J Psychiatry* 2004; 161: 836–842

Lepkifiker E, Sverdlik A, Iancu I, et al. Renal insufficiency in long-term lithium treatment. *J Clin Psychiatry* 2004; 65: 850–856

Lepola U, Bergtholdt B, St Lambert J, et al. Controlled-release paroxetine in the treatment of patients with social anxiety disorder. *J Clin Psychiatry* 2004; 65: 222–229

Lepola U, Heftling N, Zhang D, et al. Adjunctive brexpiprazole for elderly patients with major depressive disorder: an open-label, long-term safety and tolerability study. *Int J Geriatr Psychiatry* 2018; 33: 1403–1410

Lerer B, Segman RH, Fangerau H, et al. Pharmacogenetics of tardive dyskinesia: combined analysis of 780 patients supports association with dopamine D3 receptor gene Ser9Gly polymorphism. *Neuropsychopharmacology* 2002; 27: 105–119

Lerner V, Miodownik C, Kaptsan A, et al. Vitamin B6 in the treatment of tardive dyskinesia: a double-blind, placebo-controlled, crossover study. *Am J Psychiatry* 2001; 158: 1511–1514

Lerner V, Miodownik C, Kaptsan A, et al. Vitamin B6 as add-on treatment in chronic schizophrenic and schizoaffective patients: a double-blind, placebo-controlled study. *J Clin Psychiatry* 2002; 63: 54–58

Leucht S, Arbter D, Engel RR, et al. How effective are second generation antipsychotic drugs? A meta-analysis of placebo controlled trials. *Mol Psychiatry* 2009; 4: 429–447

Leucht S, Busch R, Kissling W, et al. Early prediction of antipsychotic nonresponse among patients with schizophrenia. *J Clin Psychiatry* 2007; 68: 352–360

Leucht S, Chaimani A, Leucht C, et al. 60 years of placebo-controlled antipsychotic drug trials in acute schizophrenia: meta-regression of predictors of placebo response. *Schizophr Res* 2018; 201: 315–323

Leucht S, Cipriani A, Spinelli L, et al. Comparative efficacy and tolerability of 15 antipsychotic drugs in schizophrenia: a multiple-treatments meta-analysis. *Lancet* 2013a; 382: 951–962

Leucht S, Crippa A, Siafis S, et al. Dose-response meta-analysis of antipsychotic drugs for acute schizophrenia. *Am J Psychiatry* 2020; 177: 342–353

Leucht S, Helfer B, Dold M, et al. Lithium for schizophrenia. *Cochrane Database Syst Rev* 2015; (10): CD003834

Leucht S, Helfer B, Dold M, Kissling W, McGrath J. Carbamazepine for schizophrenia. *Cochrane Database Syst Rev* 2014; (5): CD001258

Leucht S, Heres S, Davis JM. Increasing placebo response rates in antipsychotic drug trials: let's stop the vicious cycle. *Am J Psychiatry* 2013b; 170: 1232–1234

Leucht S, Leucht C, Huhn M, et al. Sixty years of placebo-controlled antipsychotic drug trials in acute schizophrenia: systematic review, Bayesian meta-analysis, and meta-regression of efficacy predictors. *Am J Psychiatry* 2017; 174: 927–942

Leucht S, Samara M, Heres S, et al. Dose equivalents for second-generation antipsychotics: the minimum effective dose method. *Schizophr Bull* 2014; 40: 314–326

Leucht S, Samara M, Heres S, et al. Dose equivalents for second-generation antipsychotic drugs: the classical mean dose method. *Schizophr Bull* 2015; 41: 1367–1402

Leucht S, Tardy M, Komossa K, et al. Maintenance treatment with antipsychotic drugs for schizophrenia. *Cochrane Database Syst Rev* 2012; (5): CD008016

Leuchter AF, McCracken JT, Hunter AM, et al. Monoamine oxidase A and catechol-o-methyltransferase functional polymorphisms and the placebo response in major depressive disorder. *J Clin Psychopharmacol* 2009; 29: 372–377

Levin FR, Evans SM, Kleber HD. Prevalence of adult attention-deficit hyperactivity disorder among cocaine abusers seeking treatment. *Drug Alcohol Depend* 1998; 52: 15–25

Levin FR, Mariani JJ, Brooks DJ, et al. Dronabinol for the treatment of cannabis dependence: a randomized, double-blind, placebo-controlled trial. *Drug Alcohol Depend* 2011; 116: 142–150

Levin FR, Mariani J, Brooks DJ, et al. A randomized double-blind, placebo-controlled trial of venlafaxine-extended release for co-occurring cannabis dependence and depressive disorders. *Addiction* 2013; 108: 1084–1094

Levine S, Saltzman A. Pyridoxin (vitamin B6) neurotoxicity: enhancement by protein-deficient diet. *J Appl Toxicol* 2004; 24: 497–500

Li N, Wu X, Li L. Chronic administration of clozapine alleviates reversal-learning impairment in isolation-reared rats. *Behav Pharmacol* 2007; 18: 135–145

Li X, Moore S, Olson C. Urine drug tests: how to make the most of them. *Curr Psychiatry* 2019; 18: 11–20

Li R, Wu R, Chen J, et al. A randomized, placebo-controlled pilot study of quetiapine-XR monotherapy or adjunctive therapy to antidepressant in acute major depressive disorder with current generalized anxiety disorder. *Psychopharmacol Bull* 2016; 46: 8–23

Li X, Zhu L, Su Y, et al. Short-term efficacy and tolerability of venlafaxine extended release in adults with generalized anxiety disorder without depression: a meta-analysis. *PLoS One* 2017; 12: e0185865

Li X, Zhu L, Zhou C, et al. Efficacy and tolerability of short-term duloxetine treatment in adults with generalized anxiety disorder: a meta-analysis. *PLoS One* 2018; 13: e0194501

Lieberman JA, Davis RE, Correll CU, et al. ITI-007 for the treatment of schizophrenia: a 4-week randomized, double-blind, controlled trial. *Biol Psychiatry* 2016; 79: 952–961

Lieberman JA, Stroup JS, McEvoy JP, et al. Effectiveness of antipsychotic drugs in patients with chronic schizophrenia. *N Engl J Med* 2005; 353: 1209–1223

Lieberman JA, Tollefson G, Tohen M, et al. Comparative efficacy and safety of atypical and conventional antipsychotic drugs in first-episode psychosis: a randomized, double-blind trial of olanzapine versus haloperidol. *Am J Psychiatry* 2003; 160: 1396–1404

Liebowtizt MR. Social Phobia. *Mod Probl Pharmacopsychiatry* 1987; 22: 141–173

Liebowitz MR, Gelenberg AJ, Munjack D. Venlafaxine extended release vs placebo and paroxetine in social anxiety disorder. *Am J Psychiatry* 2005; 62: 190–198

Liebowitz MR, Careri J, Blatt K, et al. Vortioxetine versus placebo in major depressive disorder comorbid with social anxiety disorder. *Depress Anxiety* 2017; 34: 1164–1172

Liebowitz MR, Schneier FR, Campeas R, et al. Phenelzine vs. atenolol in social phobia: a controlled comparison. *Arch Gen Psychiatry* 1992; 49: 290–300

Lim SW, Ko EM, Shin DW, et al. Clinical symptoms associated with suicidality in patients with panic disorder. *Compr Psychiatry* 2015; 48: 137–144

Lin CH, Lin CH, Chang YC, et al. Sodium benzoate, a D-amino acid oxidase inhibitor, added to clozapine for the treatment of schizophrenia: a randomized, double-blind, placebo-controlled trial. *Biol Psychiatry* 2018; 84: 422–432

Lin CY, Liang SY, Chang YC, et al. Adjunctive sarcosine plus benzoate improved cognitive function in chronic schizophrenia patients with constant clinical symptoms: a randomised, double-blind, placebo-controlled trial. *World J Biol Psychiatry* 2017; 18: 357–386

Linde M, Muelleners WM, Chronicle EP, et al. Antiepileptics other than gabapentin, pregabalin, topiramate, and valproate for the prophylaxis of episodic migraine in adults. *Cochrane Database Syst Rev* 2013; (6): CD010608

Lindenmayer J-P, Nasrallah H, Pucci M, et al. A systematic review of psychostimulant treatment of negative symptoms of schizophrenia: challenges and therapeutic opportunities. *Schizophr Res* 2013; 137: 241–252

Lindley SE, Carlson EB, Hill K. A randomized, double-blind, placebo-controlled trial of augmentation topiramate for chronic combat-related posttraumatic stress disorder. *J Clin Psychopharmacol* 2007; 27: 677–681

Linehan MM, McDavid JD, Brown MZ, et al. Olanzapine plus dialectical behavior therapy for women with high irritability who meet criteria for borderline personality disorder: a double-blind, placebo-controlled pilot study. *J Clin Psychiatry* 2008; 69: 999–1005

Ling J, Kritikos M, Tiplady B. Cognitive effects of creatine ethyl ester supplementation. *Behav Pharmacol* 2009; 20: 673–679

Links P, Steiner M, Boiago I, et al. Lithium therapy for borderline patients: preliminary findings. *J Pers Disord* 1990; 4: 173–181

Lipkovich I, Mallinckrodt CH, Faries DE. The challenges of evaluating dose response in flexible-dose trials using marginal structural models. *Pharm Stat* 2012; 11: 485–493

Lipper S, Davidson JR, Grady TA, et al. Preliminary study of carbamazepine in post-traumatic stress disorder. *Psychosomatics* 1986; 27: 849–854

Litt MD, Babor TK, DelBoca FK, et al. Types of alcoholics, II: application of an empirically derived typology to treatment matching. *Arch Gen Psychiatry* 1992; 49: 609–614

Litten RZ, Castle IJ, Falk D, et al. The placebo effect in clinical trials for alcohol dependence: an exploratory analysis of 51 naltrexone and acamprosate studies. *Alcohol Clin Exp Res* 2013; 37: 2128–2137

Liu J, Wan GB, Huang MS, et al. Probiotic therapy for treating behavioral and gastrointestinal symptoms in autism spectrum disorder: a systematic review of clinical trials. *Curr Med Sci* 2019a; 39: 173–184

Liu RT, Walsh RFL, Sheehan A. Prebiotics and probiotics for depression and anxiety: a systematic review and meta-analysis of controlled clinical trials. *Neurosci Biobehav Rev* 2019b; 102: 13–23

Liu XH, Xiw XH, Wang KY, et al. Efficacy and acceptability of atypical antipsychotics for the treatment of post-traumatic stress disorder: a meta-analysis of randomized, double-blind, placebo-controlled clinical trials. *Psychiatr Res* 2014; 219: 543–549

Liu Y, Zhou X, Zhu D, et al. Is pindolol augmentation effective in depressed patients resistant to selective serotonin reuptake inhibitors? A systematic review and meta-analysis. *Hum Psychopharmacol* 2015; 30: 132–142

Lloret-Linares C, Bellivier F, Heron K, et al. Treating mood disorders in patients with a history of intestinal surgery: a systematic review. *Int Clin Psychopharmacol* 2015; 30: 119–128

Lo M-T, Hinds DA, Tung JY, et al. Genome-wide analyses for personality traits identify six genomic loci and show correlations with psychiatric disorders. *Nat Genet* 2017; 49: 152–156

Locher C, Koechlin H, Zion SR, et al. Efficacy and safety of selective serotonin reuptake inhibitors, serotonin-norepinephrine reuptake inhibitors, and placebo for common psychiatric disorders among children and adolescents: a systematic review and meta-analysis. *JAMA Psychiatry* 2017; 74: 1011–1020

Locher C, Kossowsky J, Gaab J, et al. Moderation of antidepressant and placebo outcomes by baseline severity in late-life depression: a systematic review and meta-analysis. *J Affect Disord* 2015; 181: 50–60

Loebel A, Cucchiaro J, Sarma K, et al. Efficacy and safety of lurasidone 80 mg/day and 160 mg/day in the treatment of schizophrenia: a randomized, double-blind, placebo- and active-controlled trial. *Schizophr Res* 2013; 145: 101–109

Loebel A, Cucchiaro J, Silva R, et al. Lurasidone monotherapy in the treatment of bipolar I depression: a randomized, double-blind, placebo-controlled study. *Am J Psychiatry* 2014a; 171: 160–168

Loebel A, Cucchiaro J, Silva R, et al. Lurasidone as adjunctive therapy with lithium or valproate for the treatment of bipolar I depression: a randomized, double-blind, placebo-controlled study. *Am J Psychiatry* 2014b; 171: 169–177

Loebel A, Cucchiaro I, Silva R, et al. Efficacy of lurasidone across five symptom dimensions of schizophrenia: pooled analysis of short-term, placebo-controlled studies. *Eur Psychiatry* 2015; 30: 26–31

Loebel A, Silva R, Goldman R, et al. Lurasidone dose escalation in early nonresponding patients with schizophrenia: a randomized, placebo-controlled study. *J Clin Psychiatry* 2016; 77: 1672–1680

Loew TH, Nickel MK, Muehlbacher M, et al. Topiramate treatment for women with borderline personality disorder: a double-blind, placebo-controlled study. *J Clin Psychopharmacol* 2006; 26: 61–66

Lohoff FW, Etemad B, Mandos LA, et al. Ziprasidone treatment of refractory generalized anxiety disorder: a placebo-controlled, double-blind study. *J Clin Psychopharmacol* 2010; 30: 185–189

Lombardo I, Sachs G, Kolluri S, et al. Two 6-week, randomized, double-blind, placebo-controlled studies of ziprasidone in outpatients with bipolar I depression: did baseline characteristics impact trial outcome? *J Clin Psychopharmacol* 2012; 32: 470–478

Loonen AJM, Stahl SM. The mechanism of drug-induced akathisia. *CNS Spectrums* 2011; 16: 7–10

Lopez LV, Kane JM. Plasma levels of second-generation antipsychotics and clinical response in acute psychosis: a review of the literature. *Schizophr Res* 2013; 147: 368–374

Lopez LM, Kaptein AA, Helmerhorst FM. Oral contraceptives containing drospirenone for premenstrual syndrome. *Cochrane Database Syst Rev.* 2012; (2): CD006586

Lu ML, Lane HY, Chen KP, et al. Fluvoxamine reduces the clozapine dosage needed in refractory schizophrenic patients. *J Clin Psychiatry* 2000; 61: 594–599

Lu ML, Lane HY, Lin SK, et al. Adjunctive fluvoxamine inhibits clozapine-related weight gain and metabolic disturbance. *J Clin Psychiatry* 2004; 65: 766–771

Lynch JH, Mulvaney SW, Kim EH, et al. Effect of stellate ganglion block on specific symptom clusters for treatment of post-traumatic stress disorder. *Mil Med* 2016; 181: 1135–1141

Lyoo IK, Soon S, Kim TS, et al. A randomized, double-blind placebo controlled trial of oral creatine monohydrate augmentation for enhanced response to a selective serotonin reuptake inhibitor in women with major depressive disorder. *Am J Psychiatry* 2012; 169: 937–945

Macaluso M, Preskorn SH. Knowledge of the pharmacology of antidepressants and antipsychotics yields results comparable with pharmacogenetic testing. *J Psychiatr Pract* 2018; 24: 416–419

Mace S, Taylor D. Aripiprazole: dose-response relationship in schizophrenia and schizoaffective disorder. *CNS Drugs* 2009; 23: 773–780

MacKinnon DF, Zandi PP, Cooper J, et al. Comorbid bipolar disorder and panic disorder in families with a high prevalence of bipolar disorder. *Am J Psychiatry* 2002; 159: 30–35

MacQueen GM, Young LT, Marriott M, et al. Previous mood state predicts response and switch rates in patients with bipolar depression. *Acta Psychiatr Scand* 2002; 105: 414–418

Maddux RE, Riso LP, Klein DN, et al. Select comorbid personality disorders and the treatment of chronic depression with nefazodone, targeted psychotherapy, or their combination. *J Affect Disord* 2009; 117: 174–179

Mahabir M, Ashbaugh AR, Saumier D, et al. Propranolol's impact on cognitive performance in post traumatic stress disorder. *J Affect Disord* 2016; 192: 98–103

Mahmoud RA, Pandina GJ, Turkoz I, et al. Risperidone for treatment-refractory major depressive disorder: a randomized trial. *Ann Intern Med* 2007; 147: 593–602

Maisel NC, Blodgett JC, Wilbourne PL, et al. Meta-analysis of naltrexone and acamprosate for treating alcohol use disorders: when are these medications most helpful? *Addiction* 2013; 108: 275–293

Malhotra AK, Pinals DA, Adler CM, et al. Ketamine-induced exacerbation of psychotic symptoms and cognitive impairment in neuroleptic-free schizophrenics. *Neuropsychopharmacology* 1997; 17: 141–150

Maller JJ, Broadhouse K, Rush AJ, et al. Increased hippocampal tail volume predicts depression status and remission to anti-depressant medications in major depression. *Mol Psychiatry* 2018; 23: 1737–1744

Mallikaarjun S, Kane JM, Brincmont P, et al. Pharmacokinetics, tolerability and safety of aripiprazole once monthly in adult schizophrenia: an open-label, parallel-arm, multiple-dose study. *Schizophr Res* 2013; 150: 281–288

Mallinckrodt CH, Zhang L, Prucka WR, et al. Signal detection and placebo response in schizophrenia: parallels with depression. *Psychopharmacol Bull* 2010; 43: 53–72

Malone RP, Delaney MA, Luebbert F, et al. Double-blind placebo-controlled study of lithium in hospitalized aggressive children and adolescents with conduct disorder. *Arch Gen Psychiatry* 2000; 57: 649–654

Mammen G, Rueda S, Roerecke M, et al. Association of cannabis with long-term clinical symptoms in anxiety and mood disorders: a systematic review of prospective studies. *J Clin Psychiatry* 2018; 79: 17r11839

Mancino MJ, McGaugh J, Chopra MP, et al. Clinical efficacy of sertraline alone and augmented with gabapentin in recently abstinent cocaine-dependent patients with depressive symptoms. *J Clin Psychopharmacol* 2014; 34: 234–239

Maneeton N, Maneeton B, Woottiluk P, et al. Quetiapine monotherapy in acute treatment of generalized anxiety disorder: a systematic review and meta-analysis of randomized controlled trials. *Drug Des Devel Ther* 2016; 10: 259–276

Mann JJ, Aarons SF, Wilner PJ, et al. A controlled study of the antidepressant efficacy and side effects of (-)-deprenyl. A selective monoamine oxidase inhibitor. *Arch Gen Psychiatry* 1989; 46: 45–50

Mannucci C, Calapai F, Cardia L, et al. Clinical pharmacology of *Citrus aurantium* and *Citrus sinensis* for the treatment of anxiety. *Evid Based Complement Alternat Med* 2018; 2018: 3624094

Mannuzza S, Klein RG, Truong NL, et al. Age of methylphenidate treatment initiation in children with ADHD and later substance abuse: prospective follow-up into adulthood. *Am J Psychiatry* 2008; 165: 604–609

Manos GH. Possible serotonin syndrome associated with buspirone added to fluoxetine. *Ann Pharmacother* 2000; 34: 871–874

Manteghi AA, Hebrani P, Mortezania M, et al. Baclofen add-on to citalopram in treatment of posttraumatic stress disorder. *J Clin Psychopharmacol* 2014; 34: 240–243

Manu P, Lapitskaya Y, Shaikh A, et al. Clozapine rechallenge after major adverse effects: clinical guidelines based on 259 cases. *Am J Ther* 2018; 25: e218–e223

Manwani SG, Pardo TB, Albanese MJ, et al. Substance use disorder and other predictors of antidepressant-induced mania: a retrospective chart review. *J Clin Psychiatry* 2006; 67: 1341–1345

Mao JJ, Xie SX, Keefe JR, et al. Long-term chamomile (*Matricaria chamomilla* L.) treatment for generalized anxiety disorder: a randomized clinical trial. *J Clin Phytomedicine* 2016; 23: 1735–1742

Marazziti D, Baroni S, Faravelli L, et al. Plasma clomipramine levels in adult patients with obsessive-compulsive disorder. *Int Clin Psychopharmacol* 2012a; 27: 55–60

Marazziti D, Baroni S, Giannaccini G, et al. Plasma fluvoxamine levels and OCD symptoms/response in adult patients. *Hum Psychopharmacol* 2012b; 27: 397–402

Marcus R, Khan A, Rollin L, et al. Efficacy of aripiprazole adjunctive to lithium or valproate in long-term treatment of patients with bipolar I disorder with an inadequate response to lithium or valproate monotherapy: a multicenter, double-blind, randomized study. *Bipolar Disord* 2011; 13: 133–144

Marcus RN, McQuade RD, Carso WH, et al. The efficacy and safety of aripiprazole as adjunctive therapy in major depressive disorder: a second multicenter, randomized, double-blind, placebo-controlled study. *J Clin Psychopharmacol* 2008; 28: 156–165

Marcus SC, Zummo J, Pettit AR, et al. Antipsychotic adherence and rehospitalization in schizophrenia patients receiving oral versus long-acting injectable antipsychotics following hospital discharge. *J Manag Care Spec Pharm* 2015; 21: 754–768

Marder SR, Davis JM, Chouinard G. The effects of risperidone on the five dimensions of schizophrenia derived by factor analysis: combined results of the North American trials. *J Clin Psychiatry* 1997; 58: 538–546

Marder SR, Kramer M, Ford L, et al. Efficacy and safety of paliperidone extended-release tablets: results of a 6-week, randomized, placebo-controlled study. *Biol Psychiatry* 2007; 62: 1363–1370

Margolin A, Kosten TR, Avants SK, et al. A multicenter trial of bupropion for cocaine dependence in methadone-maintained patients. *Drug Alcohol Depend* 1995; 40: 125–131

Markovitz PJ. Pharmacotherapy of impulsivity, aggression and related disorders. In: Hollander E, Stein D (Eds) *Impulsivity and Aggression*. New York: John Wiley and Sons; 1995, 263–287

Markowitz PJ. Effect of fluoxetine on self-injurious behavior in the developmentally disabled: a preliminary study. *J Clin Psychopharmacol* 1992; 12: 27–31

Markowitz JC, Petkova E, Biyanova T, et al. Exploring personality diagnosis stability following acute psychotherapy for chronic posttraumatic stress disorder. *Depress Anxiety* 2015; 32: 919–926

Markovitz PJ, Calabrese JR, Schulz SC, et al. Fluoxetine in the treatment of borderline and schizotypal personality disorders. *Am J Psychiatry* 1991; 148: 1064–1067

Marks IM, Mathews AM. Brief standard self-rating for phobic patients. *Behav Res Ther* 1979; 17: 263–267

Marriott S, Tyrer P. Benzodiazepine dependence. *Drug Safety* 2012; 9: 93–103

Marshall M, Lewis S, Lockwood A, et al. Association between duration of untreated psychosis and outcome in cohorts of first-episode patients: a systematic review. *Arch Gen Psychiatry* 2005; 62: 975–983

Marshall RD, Lewis-Fernandez R, Blanco C, et al. A controlled trial of paroxetine for chronic PTSD, dissociation, and interpersonal problems in mostly minority adults. *Depress Anxiety* 2007; 24: 77–84

Martinon-Torres G, Fioravanti M, Grimley EJ. Trazodone for agitation in dementia. *Cochrane Database Syst Rev* 2004; (4): CD004990

Marx CE, Bradford DW, Hamer RM, et al. Pregnenolone as a novel therapeutic candidate in schizophrenia: emerging preclinical and clinical evidence. *Neuroscience* 2011; 191: 78–90

Masand P, Murry GB, Pickett P. Psychostimulants in post-stroke depression. *J Neuropsychiatr Clin Neurosci* 1991; 3: 23–27

Masdrakis VG, Papadimitriou GN, Olis P. Lamotrigine administration in panic disorder with agoraphobia. *Clin Neuropharmacol* 2010; 33: 126–128

Masi G, Milone A, Manfredi A, et al. Effectiveness of lithium in children and adolescents with conduct disorder: a retrospective naturalistic study. *CNS Drugs* 2009; 23: 59–69

Maslow AH. A theory of human motivation. *Psychol Rev* 1943; 50: 370–396

Mason M, Cates CJ, Smith I. Effects of opioid, hypnotic and sedating medications on sleep-disordered breathing in adults with obstructive sleep apnoea. *Cochrane Database Syst Rev* 2015; (7): CD011090

Mason BJ, Kocsis JH, Ritvo EC, et al. A double-blind, placebo-controlled trial of desipramine for primary alcohol dependence stratified on the presence or absence of major depression. *J Am Med Assoc* 1996; 275: 761–767

Mason BJ, Quello S, Goodell V, et al. Gabapentin treatment for alcohol dependence: a randomized clinical trial. *JAMA Intern Med* 2014; 174: 70–77

Mathew SJ, Murrough JW, aan het Rot M, et al. Riluzole for relapse prevention following intravenous ketamine in treatment-resistant depression: a pilot randomized, placebo-controlled continuation trial. *Int J Neuropsychopharmacol* 2010; 13: 71–82

Matsuda KT, Cho MC, Lin KM, et al. Clozapine dosage, serum levels, efficacy, and side-effect profiles: a comparison of Korean-American and Caucasian patients. *Psychopharmacol Bull* 1996; 32: 253–257

Matsunaga S, Kishi T, Iwata N. Memantine monotherapy for Alzheimer's disease: a systematic review and meta-analysis. *PLoS One* 2015; 10: e0123289

Mattei C, Rapagnani MP, Stahl SM. Ziprasidone hydrochloride: what role in the management of schizophrenia? J Cent Nerv Syst Dis 2011; 3: 1-16

Matthews JD, Siefert CJ, Blais MA, et al. A double-blind, placebo-controlled study of the impact of galantamine on anterograde memory impairment during electroconvulsive therapy. *J ECT* 2013; 29: 170-178

Maust DT, Lin LA, Blow FC. Benzodiazepine use and misuse among adults in the United States. *Psych Serv* 2019; 70: 98–106

Mavissakalian MR, Perel JM. Imipramine treatment of panic disorder with agoraphobia: dose ranging and plasma level-response relationships. *Am J Psychiatry* 1995; 152: 673–682

Mavissakalian MR, Perel JM. Duration of imipramine therapy and relapse in panic disorder with agoraphobia. *J Clin Psychopharmacol* 2002; 22: 294–299

Mavissakalian M, Perel J, Bowler K, et al. Trazodone in the treatment of panic disorder and agoraphobia with panic attacks. *Am J Psychiatry* 1987; 144: 785–787

Mayberg HS, Silva JA, Brannan SK, et al. The functional neuroanatomy of the placebo effect. *Am J Psychiatry* 2002; 159: 728–737

Mayo-Smith MF. Pharmacological management of alcohol withdrawal: a meta-analysis and evidence-based practice guideline. American Society of Addiction Medicine Working Group on Pharmacological Management of Alcohol Withdrawal. *J Am Med Assoc* 1997; 278: 144–151

Mayoral-van Son J, de la Foz VO, Martinez-Garcia O, et al. Clinical outcome after antipsychotic treatment discontinuation in functionally recovered first-episode nonaffective psychosis individuals: a 3-year naturalistic follow-up study. *J Clin Psychiatry* 2016; 77: 492–500

Mazure CM, Nelson JC, Jatlow PI, et al. The relationship between blood perphenazine levels, early resolution of psychotic symptoms, and side effects. *J Clin Psychiatry* 1990; 51: 330–334

McClure MM, Barch DM, Romero MJ, et al. The effects of guanfacine on context processing abnormalities in schizotypal personality disorder. *Biol Psychiatry* 2007; 61: 1157–1160

McClure MM, Graff F, Triebwasser J, et al. Guanfacine augmentation of a combined intervention of computerized cognitive remediation therapy and social skills training for schizotypal personality disorder. *Am J Psychiatry* 2019; 176: 307-314

McClure MM, Koenigsberg HW, Reynolds D, et al. The effects of risperidone on the cognitive performance of individuals with schizotypal personality disorder. *J Clin Psychopharmacol* 2009; 29: 396–398

McDermott CL, Gray SL. Cholinesterase inhibitor adjunctive therapy for cognitive impairment and depressive symptoms in older adults with depression. *Ann Pharmacother* 2012; 46: 599–605

McDougle CJ, Naylor ST, Cohen DJ, et al. A double-blind, placebo-controlled study of fluvoxamine in adults with autistic disorder. *Arch Gen Psychiatry* 1996; 53: 1001–1008

McDowell D, Nunes EV, Seracini AM, et al. Desipramine treatment of cocaine dependent patients with depression: a placebo-controlled trial. *Drug Alcohol Depend* 2005; 80: 209–221

McElroy SL, Altshuler LL, Suppes T, et al. Axis I psychiatric comorbidity and its relationship to historical illness variables in 288 patients with bipolar disorder. *Am J Psychiatry* 2001; 158: 420–426

McElroy SL, Bowden CL, Collins MA, et al. Relationship of open acute mania treatment to blinded maintenance outcome in bipolar I disorder. *J Affect Disord* 2008; 107: 127–133

McElroy SL, Martens BE, Creech RS, et al. Randomized, double-blind, placebo-controlled study of divalproex extended release loading monotherapy in ambulatory bipolar spectrum disorder patients with moderate-to-severe hypomania or mild mania. *J Clin Psychiatry* 2010a; 71: 557–565

McElroy SL, Martens BE, Mori N, et al. Adjunctive lisdexamfetamine in bipolar depression: a preliminary randomized, placebo-controlled trial. *Int Clin Psychopharmacol* 2015; 30: 6-13

McElroy SL, Weisler RH, Chang W, et al. A double-blind, placebo-controlled study of quetiapine and paroxetine as monotherapy in adults with bipolar depression (EMBOLDEN II). *J Clin Psychiatry* 2010b; 71: 163–174

McGirr A, Vöhringer PA, Ghaemi SN, et al. Safety and efficacy of adjunctive second-generation antidepressant therapy with a mood stabiliser or an atypical antipsychotic in acute bipolar depression: a systematic review and meta-analysis of randomised placebo-controlled trials. *Lancet Psychiatry* 2016; 3: 1138–1146

McGlashan TH, Zipursky RB, Perkins D, et al. Randomized, double-blind trial of olanzapine versus placebo in patients prodromally symptomatic for psychosis. *Am J Psychiatry* 2006; 163: 790–799

McGorry PD, Yung AR, Phillips LJ. Randomized controlled trial of interventions designed to reduce the risk of progression to first-episode psychosis in clinical sample with subthreshold symptoms. *Arch Gen Psychiatry* 2002; 59: 921–928

McGrath PJ, Nunes EV, Stewart JW, et al. Imipramine treatment of alcoholics with primary depression: a placebo-controlled clinical trial. *Arch Gen Psychiatry* 1996; 53: 232–240

McGrath PJ, Stewart JW, Fava M, et al. Tranylcypromine versus venlafaxine plus mirtazapine following three failed antidepressant medication trials for depression: a STAR*D report. *Am J Psychiatry* 2006a; 163: 1531–1541

McGrath PJ, Stewart JW, Quitkin FM, et al. Predictors of relapse in a prospective study of fluoxetine treatment for major depression. *Am J Psychiatry* 2006b; 163: 1542–1548

McGuire P, Robson P, Cubala WJ, et al. Cannabidiol (CBD) as an adjunctive therapy in schizophrenia: a multicenter randomized controlled trial. *Am J Psychiatry* 2018; 175: 225–231

McIntyre A, Gendron A, McIntyre A. Quetiapine adjunct to selective serotonin reuptake inhibitors or venlafaxine in patients with major depression, comorbid anxiety, and residual depressive symptoms: a randomized, placebo-controlled pilot study. *Depress Anxiety* 2007; 24: 487–494

McIntyre RS, Alsuwaidan M, Soczynska JK, et al. The effect of lisdexamfetamine dimesylate on body weight, metabolic parameters, and attention deficit hyperactivity disorder symptomatology in adults with bipolar I/II disorder. *Hum Psychopharmacol* 2013; 28: 421–427

McIntyre RS, Cucchiaro J, Pikalov A, et al. Lurasidone in the treatment of bipolar depression with mixed (subsyndromal hypomanic) features: post hoc analysis of a randomized placebo-controlled trial. *J Clin Psychiatry* 2015; 76: 398–405

McIntyre RS, Harrison J, Loft H, et al. The effects of vortioxetine on cognitive function in patients with major depressive disorder: a meta-analysis of three randomized controlled trials. *Int J Neuropsychopharmacol* 2016; 19: pyw055

McIntyre RS, Subramaniapillai M, Lee Y, et al. Efficacy of adjunctive infliximab vs placebo in the treatment of adults with bipolar I/II depression: a randomized clinical trial. *JAMA Psychiatry* 2019; 76: 783–790

McMahon FJ, Buervenich S, Charney D, et al. Variation in the gene encoding the serotonin 2A receptor is associated with outcome of antidepressant treatment. *Am J Hum Genet* 2006; 78: 804–814

McNeil MJ, Kamal AH, Kutner JS, et al. The burden of polypharmacy in patients near the end of life. *J Pain Symptom Manage* 2016; 51: 178–183

Mech AW, Farah A. Correlation of clinical response with homocysteine reduction during therapy with reduced B vitamins in patients with MDD who are positive for MTHFR C677T or A1298C polymorphism: a randomized, double-blind, placebo-controlled study. *J Clin Psychiatry* 2016; 77: 668–671

Mehyrpooya M, Yasrebifar F, Haghighi M, et al. Evaluating the effect of Coenzyme Q10 augmentation on treatment of bipolar depression: a double-blind controlled clinical trial. *J Clin Psychopharmacol* 2018; 38: 460–466

Meister R, Jansen A, Härter M, et al. Placebo and nocebo reactions in randomized trials of pharmacological treatments for persistent depressive disorder: a meta-regression analysis. *J Affect Disord* 2017; 215: 288–298

Mejer MH, Caspi A, Ambler A, et al. Persistent cannabis users show neuropsychological decline from childhood to midlife. *Proc Natl Acad Sci* 2012; 109: E2657–2664

Mellman TA, Bustamante V, David V, et al. Hypnotic medication in the aftermath of trauma. *J Clin Psychiatry* 2002; 63: 1183–1184

Meltzer HY, Bobo WV, Roy A, et al. A randomized, double-blind comparison of clozapine and high-dose olanzapine in treatment-resistant patients with schizophrenia. *J Clin Psychiatry* 2008; 69: 274–285

Meltzer HY, Cucchiaro J, Silva R, et al. Lurasidone in the treatment of schizophrenia: a randomized, double-blind, placebo- and olanzapine-controlled study. *Am J Psychiatry* 2011; 168: 957–967

Meltzer HY, Matsubara S, Lee JC, et al. Classification of typical and atypical antipsychotic drugs on the basis of dopamine D1, D2 and serotonin 2 pKi values. *J Pharmacol Exper Ther* 1989; 251: 238–246

Mendels J, Krajewski TF, Huffer V, et al. Effective short-term treatment of generalized anxiety disorder with trifluoperazine. *J Clin Psychiatry* 1986; 47: 170–174

Menza MA, Dobkin RD, Marin H. An open-label trial of aripiprazole augmentation for treatment-resistant generalized anxiety disorder. *J Clin Psychopharmacol* 2007; 27: 207–210

Mercer D, Douglass AB, Links PS. Meta-analysis of mood stabilizers, antidepressants and antipsychotics in the treatment of borderline personality disorder: effectiveness for depression and anger symptoms. *J Pers Disord* 2009; 23: 156–174

Merikangas KR, Akiskal HS, Angst J, et al. Lifetime and 12-month prevalence of bipolar spectrum disorder in the National Comorbidity Survey replication. *Arch Gen Psychiatry* 2007; 64: 543–552

Meyer JM. A rational approach to employing high plasma levels of antipsychotics for violence associated with schizophrenia: case vignettes. *CNS Spectr* 2014; 19: 432–438

Meyer JM. Monitoring and improving antipsychotic adherence in outpatient forensic division programs. *CNS Spectr* 2019; 23: 1–9

Meyer JM, Proctor G, Cummings MA, et al. Ciprofloxacin and clozapine: a potentially fatal but underappreciated interaction. *Case Rep Psychiatry* 2016; 2016: 5606098

Meyer TJ, Mill ML, Metzger RL, et al. Development and validation of the Penn State Worry Questionnaire. *Behav Res Ther* 1990; 28: 487–495

Michelson D, Bancroft J, Targum S, et al. Female sexual dysfunction associated with antidepressant administration: a randomized, placebo-controlled study of pharmacologic intervention. *Am J Psychiatry* 2000; 157: 239–243

Michelson D, Kociban K, Tamura R, et al. Mirtazapine, yohimbine or olanzapine augmentation therapy for serotonin reuptake-associated female sexual dysfunction: a randomized, placebo controlled trial. *J Psychiatr Pract* 2002; 36: 147–152

Miller S, McTeague LM, Gyurak A, et al. Cognition-childhood maltreatment interactions in the prediction of antidepressant outcomes in major depressive disorder patients: results from the iSPOT-D trial. *Depress Anxiety* 2015; 32: 594–604

Miller WR, Leckman AL, Delany HD, et al. Long-term follow-up of behavioral self-control training. *J Stud Alcohol* 1992; 53: 249–261

Millon T, Davis RO. *Disorders of Personality: DSM-IV and Beyond, 2nd edn*. Hoboken, New Jersey: John Wiley and Sons; 1996

Mini LJ, Wang-Weigand S, Zhang J. Self-reported efficacy and tolerability of ramelteon 8 mg in older adults experiencing severe sleep-onset difficulty. *Am J Geriatr Pharmacother* 2007; 5: 177–184

Minozzi S, Saulle R, Rösner S. Baclofen for alcohol use disorder. *Cochran Database Syst Rev* 2018; (11): CD012557

Minozzi S, Amato L, Vecchi S, et al. Oral naltrexone maintenance treatment for opioid dependence. *Cochrane Database Syst Rev* 2011; (4): CD001333

Mintz M, Hollenberg E. Revisiting lithium: utility for behavioral stabilization in adolescents and adults with autism spectrum disorder. *Psychopharmacol Bull* 2019; 49: 28–40

Miotto K, McCann M, Basch J, et al. Naltrexone and dysphoria: fact or myth? *Am J Addict* 2002; 11: 151–160

Mitchell AJ, Delaffon V, Vancampfort D, et al. Guideline concordant monitoring of metabolic risk in people treated with antipsychotic medication: systematic review and meta-analysis of screening practices. *Psychol Med* 2012; 42: 125–147

Mithoefer MC, Mithofer AT, Feduccia A, et al. 3,4-methylenedioxymethamphetamine (MDMA)-assisted psychotherapy for post-traumatic stress disorder in military veterans, firefighters, and police officers: a randomised, double-blind, dose-response, phase 2 clinical trial. *Lancet Psychiatry* 2018; 5: 486–497

Mitsikostas DD, Mantonakis L, Chalarakis L. Nocebo in clinical trials for depression: a meta-analysis. *Psychiatry Res* 2014; 215: 82–86

Miura I, Zhang JP, Hagi K, et al. Variants in the DRD2 locus and antipsychotic-related prolactin levels: a meta-analysis. *Psychoneuroendocrinology* 2016; 72: 1–10

Miyaoka T, Furuya M, Yasuda H, et al. Yi-gan san for the treatment of borderline personality disorder: an open-label study. *Prog Neuropsychopharmacol Biol Psychiatry* 2008; 32: 150–154

Modaressi A, Chaibakhsh S, Koulaeinejad N, et al. A systematic review and meta-analysis: memantine augmentation in moderate to severe obsessive-compulsive disorder. *Psychiatry Res* 2019; 282: 112602

Mohamed S, Johnson GR, Chen P, et al. Effect of antidepressant switching vs augmentation on remission among patients with major depressive disorder unresponsive to antidepressant treatment: the VAST-D randomized clinical trial. *JAMA Psychiatry* 2017; 318: 132–145

Mohammadi MR, Kazemi MR, Zia E, et al. Amantadine versus methylphenidate in children and adolescents with attention deficit/hyperactivity disorder: a randomized, double-blind trial. *Hum Psychopharmacol* 2010; 25: 560–565

Mohammadzadeh S, Ahangari TK, Yousefi F, et al. The effect of memantine in adult patients with attention deficit hyperactivity disorder. *Hum Psychopharmacol* 2019; 34: e2687

Mohn C, Rund BR. Neurocognitive profile in major depressive disorders: relationship to symptom level and subjective memory complaints. *BMC Psychiatry* 2016; 16:108

Mojtabai R, Olfson M. National trends in psychotropic medication polypharmacy in office-based psychiatry. *Arch Gen Psychiatry* 2010; 67: 26–36

Molero Y, Larsson H, D'Onofrio BM, et al. Associations between gabapentinoids and suicidal behaviour, unintentional overdoses, injuries, road traffic incidents, and violent crime: population based cohort study in Sweden. *Br Med J* 2019; 365: l2147

Monnelly EP, Ciraulo DA, Knapp C, et al. Low-dose risperidone as adjunctive therapy for irritable aggression in posttraumatic stress disorder. *J Clin Psychopharmacol* 2003; 23: 193–196

Montes JM, Saiz-Ruiz J, Laher G, et al. Lamotriqine for the treatment of bipolar spectrum disorder: chart review. *J Affect Disord* 2005; 86: 69–73

Montgomery SA, Åsberg M. A new depression scale designed to be sensitive to change. *Br J Psychiatry* 1979; 134: 382–389

Montgomery SA, Altamura AC, Katila H, et al. Efficacy of extended release quetiapine fumarate monotherapy in elderly patients with major depressive disorder: secondary analyses in subgroups of patients according to baseline anxiety, sleep disturbance, and pain levels. *Int Clin Psychopharmacol* 2014; 29: 93–105

Montgomery SA, McIntyre A, Osterheider M, et al. A double-blind, placebo-controlled study of fluoxetine in patients with DSM-III-R obsessive-compulsive disorder. *Eur Neuropsychopharmacol* 1993; 3: 143–152

Montgomery SA, Tobias K, Zornberg GL, et al. Efficacy and safety of pregabalin in the treatment of generalized anxiety disorder: a 6-week, multicenter, randomized, double-blind, placebo-controlled comparison of pregabalin and venlafaxine. *J Clin Psychiatry* 2006; 67: 771–782

Morgan CJ, Monaghan L, Curran HV. Beyond the K-hole: a 3-year longitudinal investigation of the cognitive and subjective effects of ketamine in recreational users who have substantially reduced their use of the drug. *Addiction* 2004; 99: 1450–1461

Morrissette DA, Stahl SM. Treating the violent patient with psychosis or impulsivity utilizing antipsychotic polypharmacy and high-dose monotherapy. *CNS Spectr* 2014; 19: 439–448

Mosca D, Zhang M, Prieto R, et al. Efficacy of desvenlafaxine compared with placebo in major depressive disorder patients by age group and severity of depression at baseline. *J Clin Psychopharmacol* 2017; 37: 182–192

Moukhtarian TR, Cooper RE, Vassos E, et al. Effects of stimulants and atomoxetine on emotional lability in adults: a systematic review and meta-analysis. *Eur Psychiatry* 2017; 44: 198–207

Mrkobrada M, Hackam DDG. Selective serotonin reuptake inhibitors and surgery: to hold or not to hold, that is the question: comment on "Perioperative use of selective serotonin reuptake inhibitors and risks for adverse outcomes of surgery." *JAMA Intern Med* 2013; 173: 1082–1083

Muehlbacher M, Nickel MK, Nickel C, et al. Mirtazapine treatment of social phobia in women: a randomized, double-blind, placebo-controlled study. *J Clin Psychopharmacol* 2005; 25: 580–583

Mula M, Pini S, Cassano GB. The role of anticonvulsant drugs in anxiety disorders: a critical review of the evidence. *J Clin Psychopharmacol* 2007; 27: 263–272

Müller U, Rowe JB, Rittman T, et al. Effects of modafinil on non-verbal cognition, task enjoyment and creative thinking in healthy volunteers. *Neuropsychopharmacol* 2013; 64: 490–495

Murphy CC, Fullington HM, Alvarez CA, et al. Polypharmacy and patterns of prescription medication use among cancer survivors. *Cancer* 2018; 124: 2850–2857

Murrough JW, Perez AM, Pillemer S, et al. Rapid and longer-term antidepressant effects of repeated ketamine infusions in treatment-resistant major depression. *Biol Psychiatry* 2013; 74: 250–256

Mushiroda T, Takahashi Y, Onuma T, et al. Association of HLA-A*31:01 screening with the incidence of carbamazepine-induced cutaneous adverse reactions in a Japanese population. *JAMA Neurology* 2018; 75: 842–849

Musil R, Zill P, Seemüller F, et al. Genetics of emergent suicidality during antidepressive treatment: data from a naturalistic study on a large sample of inpatients with a major depressive episode. *Eur Neuropsychopharmacol* 2013; 23: 663–674

Myer BM, Boland JR, Faraone SV. Pharmacogenetics predictors of methylphenidate efficacy in childhood ADHD. *Mol Psychiatry* 2018; 23: 1929–1936

Myrick H, Anton RF, Li X, et al. Effect of naltrexone and ondansetron on alcohol cue-induced activation of the ventral striatum in alcohol-dependent people. *Arch Gen Psychiatry* 2008; 65: 466–475

Myrick H, Anton R, Voronin K, et al. A double-blind evaluation of gabapentin on alcohol effects and drinking in a clinical laboratory paradigm. *Alcohol Clin Exp Res* 2007; 31: 221–227

Myrick H, Malcolm R, Randall PK, et al. A double-blind trial of gabapentin versus lorazepam in the treatment of alcohol withdrawal. *Alcohol Clin Exp Res* 2009; 33: 1582–1588

Naderi S, Faghih H, Aqamolaei A, et al. Amantadine as adjuvant therapy in the treatment of moderate to severe obsessive-compulsive disorder: a double-blind randomized trial with placebo control. *Psychiatry Clin Neurosci* 2019; 83: 169–174

Nair NP. Therapeutic equivalence of risperidone given once daily and twice daily in patients with schizophrenia: the Risperidone Study Group. *J Clin Psychopharmacol* 1998; 18: 103–110

Nair NP, Amin M, Holm P, et al. Moclobemide and nortriptyline in elderly depressed patients: a randomized, multicentre trial against placebo. *J Affect Disord* 1995; 33: 1–9

Nakamura A, Mihara K, Nagai G, et al. Prediction of an optimal dose of lamotrigine for augmentation therapy in treatment-resistant depressive disorder from plasma lamotrigine concentration at week 2. *Ther Drug Monit* 2016; 38: 379–382

Nardi AE, Lopes FL, Valenca AM, et al. Double-blind comparison of 30 and 60 mg tranylcypromine daily in patients with panic disorder comorbid with social anxiety disorder. *Psychiatr Res* 2010; 175: 260–265

Nasrallah HA, Silva R, Phillips D, et al. Lurasidone for the treatment of acutely psychotic patients with schizophrenia: a 6-week, randomized, placebo-controlled study. *J Psychiatry Res* 2013; 47: 670–677

Nasreddine ZS, Phillips NA, Bédirian V, et al. The Montreal Cognitive Assessment (MoCA): a brief screening tool for mild cognitive impairment. *J Am Geriatr Soc* 2005; 53: 695–699

Naugle RI, Kawczak K. Limitations of the mini-mental state examination. *Cleve Clin J Med* 1989; 56: 277–281

Naylor JC, Kilts JD, Bradford JW, et al. A pilot randomized placebo-controlled trial of adjunctive aripiprazole for chronic PTSD in US military veterans resistant to antidepressant treatment. *Int Clin Psychopharmacol* 2015; 30: 167–174

Nelson JC, Byck R. Rapid response to lithium in phenelzine non-responders. *Br J Psychiatry* 1982; 141: 85–86

Nelson JC, Papakostas GI. Atypical antipsychotic augmentation in major depressive disorder: a meta-analysis of placebo-controlled randomized trials. *Am J Psychiatry* 2009; 166: 980–991

Nelson JC, Delucchi K, Schneider LS. Efficacy of second generation antidepressants in late-life depression: a meta-analysis of the evidence. *Am J Geriatr Psychiatry* 2008; 16: 558–567

Nelson JC, Delucchi KL, Schneider LS. Moderators of outcome in late-life depression: a patient-level meta-analysis. *Am J Psychiatry* 2013; 170: 651–659

Nelson CLM, Amsbaugh HM, Reilly JL, et al. Beneficial and adverse effects of antipsychotic medication on cognitive flexibility are related to COMT genotype in first episode psychosis. *Schizophr Res* 2018; 202: 212–216

Nelson JC, Baumann P, Delucchi K, et al. A systematic review and meta-analysis of lithium augmentation of tricyclic and second generation antidepressants in major depression. *J Affect Disord* 2014; 168: 269–275

Nelson JC, Mazure CM, Jatlow PI, et al. Combining norepinephrine and serotonin reuptake inhibition mechanisms for treatment of depression: a double-blind, randomized study. *Biol Psychiatry* 2004; 55: 296–300

Newport DJ, Carpenter LL, McDonald WM, et al. Ketamine and other NMDA receptor antagonists: early clinical trials and possible mechanisms in depression. *Am J Psychiatry* 2015; 172: 950–966

Neylan TC, Lenoci M, Samuelson KW, et al. No improvement of posttraumatic stress disorder symptoms with guanfacine treatment. *Am J Psychiatry* 2006; 163: 2186–2188

Ng CH, Chong S, Lambert T, et al. An inter-ethnic comparison study of clozapine dosage, clinical response and plasma levels. *Int Clin Psychopharmacol* 2005; 20: 163–168

Ng QX, Koh SSH, Chan HW, et al. Clinical use of curcumin in depression: a meta-analysis. *J Am Med Dir Assoc* 2017; 18: 503–508

Ng QX, Soh AY, Venkatanarayanan N, et al. A systematic review of the effect of probiotic supplementation on schizophrenia symptoms. *Neuropsychobiology* 2019; 78: 106

Nickel MK, Muehlbacher M, Nickel C, et al. Aripiprazole in the treatment of patients with borderline personality disorder: a double-blind, placebo-controlled study. *Am J Psychiatry* 2006; 163: 833–838

Nickel MK, Nickel C, Kaplan P, et al. Treatment of aggression with topiramate in male borderline patients: a double-blind, placebo-controlled study. *Biol Psychiatry* 2005; 57: 495–499

Nickel MK, Nickel C, Miterlehner FO, et al. Topiramate treatment of aggression in female borderline personality disorder patients: a double-blind, placebo-controlled study. *J Clin Psychiatry* 2004; 65: 1515–1519

Nielsen J, Jensen SO, Friis RB, et al. Comparative effectiveness of risperidone long-acting injectable vs first-generation antipsychotic long-acting injectables in schizophrenia: results from a nationwide, retrospective inception cohort study. *Schizophr Bull* 2015; 41: 627–636

Nielsen S, Larance B, Degenhardt L, et al. Opioid agonist treatment for pharmaceutical opioid dependent people. *Cochrane Database Syst Rev* 2016; (5): CD01111

Nierenberg AA, Keck PE Jr. Management of monoamine oxidase inhibitor-associated insomnia with trazodone. *J Clin Psychopharmacol* 1989; 9: 42–45

Nierenberg AA, Fava M, Trivedi MH, et al. A comparison of lithium and T(3) augmentation following two failed medication treatments for depression: a STAR*D report. *Am J Psychiatry* 2006; 163: 1519–1530

Nierenberg AA, Friedman ES, Bowden CL, et al. Lithium treatment moderate-dose use study (LiTMUS) for bipolar disorder: a randomized comparative effectiveness trial of optimized personalized treatment with and without lithium. *Am J Psychiatry* 2013; 170: 102–110

Nierenberg AA, Østergaard SD, Iovieno N, et al. Predictors of placebo response in bipolar depression. *Int Clin Psychopharmacol* 2015; 30: 59–66

Niitsu T, Fabbri C, Bentini F, et al. Pharmacogenetics in major depression: a comprehensive meta-analysis. *Prog Neuropsychopharmacol Biol Psychiatry* 2013; 45: 183–194

Nikiforuk A, Popik P. Amisulpride promotes cognitive flexibility in rats: the role of 5-HT7 receptors. *Behav Brain Res* 2013; 248: 136–140

Ninan PT, McElroy SL, Kane CP, et al. Placebo-controlled study of fluvoxamine in the treatment of patients with compulsive buying. *J Clin Psychopharmacol* 2000a; 20: 362–366

Ninan PT, Rothbaum PO, Marsteller FA, et al. A placebo-controlled trial of cognitive-behavioral therapy and clomipramine in trichotillomania. *J Clin Psychiatry* 2000b; 61: 47–50

Nordahl HM, Vogel PA, Morken G, et al. Paroxetine, cognitive therapy or their combination in the treatment of social anxiety disorder with and without avoidant personality disorder: a randomized clinical trial. *Psychother Psychosom* 2016; 85: 346–356

Nordentoft M, Thorup A, Petersen L, et al. Transition rates from schizotypal disorder to psychotic disorder for first-contact patients included in the OPUS Trial: a randomized clinical trial of integrated treatment and standard treatment. *Schizophr Res* 2006; 83: 29–40

Noyes R Jr., Moroz G, Davidson JR, et al. Moclobemide in social phobia: a controlled dose-response trial. *J Clin Psychopharmacol* 1997; 17: 247–254

Nuijten M, Blanken P, van den Brink W, et al. Treatment of crack-cocaine dependence with topiramate: a randomized controlled feasibility trial in the Netherlands. *Drug Alcohol Depend* 2014; 138: 177–184

Nunez NA, Singh B, Romo-Nava F, et al. Efficacy and tolerability of adjunctive modafinil/ armodafinil in bipolar depression: a meta analysis of randomized controlled trials. *Bipolar Disord* 2020; 22: 109–120

O'Connell CP, Goldstein-Piekarski AN, Nemeroff CB, et al. Antidepressant outcomes predicted by genetic variation in corticotropin-releasing hormone binding protein. *Am J Psychiatry* 2018; 175: 251–261

O'Connor CM, Kuchibhatla JW, Silva SG, et al. Safety and efficacy of sertraline for depression in patients with heart failure: results of the SADHART-CHF (Sertraline Against Depression and Heart Disease in Chronic Heart Failure) trial. *J Am Coll Cardiol* 2010; 56: 962–969

O'Donnell CP, Allott KA, Murphy BP, et al. Adjunctive taurine in first-episode psychosis: a phase 2, double-blind, randomized, placebo-controlled study. *J Clin Psychiatry* 2016; 77: e1610–e1617

Office of Management and Budget (OMB) Recommendations from the interagency committee for the review of the race and ethnic standards to the Office of Management and Budget concerning changes to the standards for the classification of federal data on race and ethnicity. *Federal Register* 1997; 62: 36874–36946

Ogasa M, Kimura T, Nakamura M, et al. Lurasidone in the treatment of schizophrenia: a 6-week, placebo-controlled study. *Psychopharmacol (Berl)* 2013; 225: 519–530

Ogawa Y, Takeshima N, Hayasaka Y, et al. Antidepressants plus benzodiazepines for adults with major depression. *Cochrane Database Syst Rev* 2019; 6: CD001026

Olbrich S, Tränkner A, Surova G, et al. CNS- and ANS-arousal predict response to antidepressant medication: findings from the randomized ISPOT-D study. *J Psychiatr Res* 2016; 73: 108–115

Olesen OV, Licht RW, Thomsen E, et al. Serum concentrations and side effects in psychiatric patients during risperidone therapy. *Ther Drug Monit* 1998; 20: 380–384

Oliveira P, Ribeiro J, Donato H, et al. Smoking and antidepressants pharmacokinetics: a systematic review. *Ann Gen Psychiatry* 2017; 16: 17

Oliveto AH, Feingold A, Schottenfeld R, et al. Desipramine in opioid-dependent cocaine abusers maintained on buprenorphine vs methadone. *Arch Gen Psychiatry* 1999; 56: 812–820

Oliveto A, Poling J, Mancino MJ, et al. Sertraline delays relapse in recently abstinent cocaine-dependent patients with depressive symptoms. *Addiction* 2012; 107: 131–141

Olsson EM, von Schéele B, Panossian AG. A randomised, double-blind, placebo-controlled, parallel-group study of the standardised extract SHR-5 of the roots of *Rhodiola rosea* in the treatment of subjects with stress-related fatigue. *Planta Med* 2009; 75: 105–112

Oneta C, Simanowski U, Martinez M, et al. First pass metabolism of ethanol is strikingly influenced by the speed of gastric emptying. *Gut* 1998; 43: 612–619

Orlova Y, Rizzoli P, Loder E. Association of coprescription of triptan antimigraine drugs and selective serotonin reuptake inhibitor or selective serotonin norepinephrine reuptake inhibitor antidepressants with serotonin syndrome. *JAMA Neurol* 2018; 75: 566–572

Ortiz-Orendain J, Castiello-de Obeso S, Colunga-Lozano LE, et al. Antipsychotic combinations for schizophrenia. *Cochrane Database Syst Rev* 2017; (6): CD009005

Oslin DW, Berretini W, Kranzler HR, et al. A functional polymorphism of the mu-opioid receptor gene is associated with naltrexone response in alcohol-dependent patients. *Neuropsychopharmacol* 2003; 28: 1546–1552

Ostacher M, Ng-Mak D, Patel P, et al. Lurasidone compared to other atypical antipsychotic monotherapies for bipolar depression: a systematic review and network meta-analysis. *World J Biol Psychiatry* 2018; 19: 586–601

Ostinelli EG, Jajawi S, Spyridi S, et al. Aripiprazole (intramuscular) for psychosis-induced aggression or agitation (rapid tranquillisation). *Cochrane Database Syst Rev* 2018; (1): CD008074

Ota M, Wakabayashi C, Sato N, et al. Effect of L-theanine on glutamatergic function in patients with schizophrenia. *Acta Neuropsychiatrica* 2015; 27: 291–296

Otasowie J, Castells X, Ehimare UP, et al. Tricyclic antidepressants for attention deficit hyperactivity disorder (ADHD) in children and adolescents. *Cochrane Database Syst Rev* 2014; (9): CD006997

Otto MW, Tuby KS, Gould RA, et al. An effect-size analysis of the relative efficacy and tolerability of selective serotonin reuptake inhibitors for panic disorder. *Am J Psychiatry* 2001; 158: 1989–1992

Ozmenler NK, Karlidere T, Bozkurt A, et al. Mirtazapine augmentation in depressed patients with sexual dysfunction due to selective serotonin reuptake inhibitors. *Hum Psychopharmacol* 2008; 23: 321–326

Pae CU, Kim JJ, Lee CU, et al. Rapid versus conventional initiation of quetiapine in the treatment of schizophrenia: a randomized, parallel-group trial. *J Clin Psychiatry* 2007; 68: 399–405

Pae CU, Lim HK, Peindl K, et al. The atypical antipsychotics olanzapine and risperidone in the treatment of posttraumatic stress disorder: a meta-analysis of randomized, double-blind, placebo-controlled clinical trials. *Int Clin Psychopharmacol* 2008; 23: 1–8

Palac DM, Cornish RD, McDonald WJ, et al. Cognitive function in hypertensives treated with atenolol or propranolol. *J Gen Intern Med* 1990; 5: 310–318

Palhano-Fontes F, Barreto D, Onias H, et al. Rapid antidepressant effects of the psychedelic ayahuasca in treatment-resistant depression: a randomized placebo-controlled trial. *Psychol Med* 2019; 49: 655–663

Pallanti S, Quercioli L, Koran LM. Citalopram intravenous infusion in resistant obsessive-compulsive disorder: an open trial. *J Clin Psychiatry* 2002; 63: 796–801

Pallanti S, Quercioli L, Paiva R, et al. Citalopram for treatment-resistant obsessive-compulsive disorder. *Eur Psychiatry* 1999; 14: 101–106

Palmer SC, Natale P, Ruospo M, et al. Antidepressants for treating depression in adults with end-stage kidney disease treated with dialysis. *Cochrane Database Syst Rev* 2016; (5): CD004541

Palpacuer C, Duprez R, Huneau A, et al. Pharmacologically controlled drinking in the treatment of alcohol dependence or alcohol use disorders: a systematic review with direct and network meta-analyses on nalmefene, naltrexone, acamprosate, baclofen and topiramate. *Addiction* 2018; 113: 220–237

Palpacuer C, Laviolle B, Boussageon R, et al. Risks and benefits of nalmefene in the treatment of adult alcohol dependence: a systematic literature review and meta-analysis of published and unpublished double-blind randomized controlled trials. *PLoS Med* 2015; 12: e1001924

Pande AC, Crockatt JG, Janney CA, et al. Gabapentin in bipolar disorder: a placebo-controlled trial of adjunctive therapy. Gabapentin Bipolar Disorder Study Group. *Bipolar Disord* 2000a; 2: 249–255

Pande AC, Davidson JR, Jefferson JW, et al. Treatment of social phobia with gabapentin: a placebo-controlled study. *J Clin Psychopharmacol* 1999; 19: 341–348

Pande AC, Feltner DE, Jefferson JW, et al. Efficacy of the novel anxiolytic pregabalin in social anxiety disorder: a placebo-controlled, multicenter study. *J Clin Psychopharmacol* 2004; 24: 141–149

Pande AC, Pollack MH, Crockatt J, et al. Placebo-controlled study of gabapentin treatment of panic disorder. *J Clin Psychopharmacol* 2000b; 20: 467–471

Pandina GJ, Canuso CM, Turkoz I, et al. Adjunctive risperidone in the treatment of generalized anxiety disorder: a double-blind, prospective, placebo-controlled, randomized trial. *Psychopharmacol Bull* 2007; 40: 41–57

Pani PP, Trogu E, Pacini M, et al. Anticonvulsants for alcohol dependence. *Cochrane Database Syst Rev* 2014; (2): CD008544

Papakostas GI, Cooper-Kazaz R, Appelhof BC, et al. Simultaneous initiation (coinitiation) of pharmacotherapy with triiodothyronine and a selective serotonin reuptake inhibitor for major depressive disorder: a quantitative synthesis of double-blind studies. *Int Clin Psychopharmacol* 2009; 24: 19–25

Papakostas GI, Fava M. Does the probability of receiving a placebo influence clinical trial outcome? A meta-regression of double-blind, randomized clinical trials in MDD. Eur Neuropsychopharmacol 2009; 19: 34–40

Papakostas GI, Perlis RH, Scalia MJ, et al. A meta-analysis of early sustained response rates between antidepressants and placebo for the treatment of major depressive disorder. *J Clin Psychopharmacol* 2006; 26: 56–60

Papakostas GI, Shelton RC, Zajecka JM, et al. L-methylfolate as adjunctive therapy for SSRI-resistant major depression: results of two randomized, double-blind, parallel-sequential trials. *Am J Psychiatry* 2012a; 169: 1267–1274

Papakostas GI, Shelton RC, Zajecka JM, et al. Effect of adjunctive L-methylfolate 15 mg among inadequate responders to SSRIs in depressed patients who were stratified by biomarker levels and genotype: results from a randomized clinical trial. *J Clin Psychiatry* 2014; 75: 855–863

Papakostas GI, Stahl SM, Kishen A, et al. Efficacy of bupropion and the selective serotonin reuptake inhibitors in the treatment of major depressive disorder with high levels of anxiety (anxious depression): a pooled analysis of 10 studies. *J Clin Psychiatry* 2008; 69: 1287–1292

Papakostas GI, Thase ME, Fava M, et al. Are antidepressant drugs that combine serotonergic and noradrenergic mechanisms of action more effective than the selective serotonin reuptake inhibitors in treating major depressive disorder? A meta-analysis of studies of newer agents. *Biol Psychiatry* 2007; 62: 1217–1227

Papakostas GI, Vitolo OV, Ishak WW, et al. A 12-week, randomized, double-blind, placebo-controlled, sequential parallel comparison trial of ziprasidone as monotherapy for major depressive disorder. *J Clin Psychiatry* 2012b; 73: 1541–1547

Papp LA. Safety and efficacy of levetiracetam for patients with panic disorder: results of an open-label, fixed-flexible dose study. *J Clin Psychiatry* 2006; 67: 1573–1576

Park JY, Kim KH. A randomized, double-blind, placebo-controlled trial of *Schisandra chinensis* for menopausal symptoms. *Climacteric* 2016; 19: 574–580

Park SH, Wackemah RC, Stimmel GL. Serotonin syndrome: is it a reason to avoid the use of tramadol with antidepressants? *J Pharm Pract* 2014; 27: 71–78

Park C, Pan Z, Brietzke E, et al. Predicting antidepressant response using early changes in cognition: a systematic review. *Behav Brain Res* 2018; 353: 154–160

Parker G, Brotchie H, Parker K. Is combination olanzapine and antidepressant medication associated with a more rapid response trajectory than antidepressant alone? *Am J Psychiatry* 2005; 162: 796–798

Parkes L, Tiego J, Aquino K, et al. Transdiagnostic variations in impulsivity and compulsivity in obsessive-compulsive disorder and gambling disorder correlate with effective connectivity in cortical-striatal-thalamic-cortical circuits. *Neuroimage* 2019; 202: 116070

Parsons B, Quitkin FM, McGrath PJ, et al. Phenelzine, imipramine and placebo in borderline patients meeting criteria for atypical depression. *Psychopharmacol Bull* 1989; 25: 524–534

Pasco JA, Jacka FN, Williams LJ, et al. Dietary selenium and major depression: a nested case-control study. *Complement Ther Med* 2012; 20: 119–123

Pascual JC, Soler J, Puigdemont D, et al. Ziprasidone in the treatment of borderline personality disorder: a double-blind, placebo-controlled, randomized study. *J Clin Psychiatry* 2008; 69: 603–608

Patel K, Allen S, Haque MN, et al. Bupropion: a systematic review and meta-analysis of effectiveness as an antidepressant. *Ther Adv Psychopharmacol* 2016; 6: 99–144

Patil ST, Zhang L, Millen BA, et al. Activation of mGlu2/3 receptors as a new approach to treat schizophrenia: a randomized phase 2 clinical trial. *Nat Med* 2007; 13: 1102–1107

Patkar A, Gilmer W, Pae C-U, et al. A 6 week randomized double-blind placebo-controlled trial of ziprasidone for the acute depressive mixed state. *PLoS One* 2012; 7: e34757

Patorno E, Huybrechts KF, Bateman BT, et al. Lithium use in pregnancy and the risk of cardiac malformations. *N Engl J Med* 2017; 376: 2245–2254

Pavlik VM, Doody RS, Rountree SD, et al. Vitamin E use is associated with improved survival in an Alzheimer's disease cohort. *Dement Geriatr Cogn Disord* 2009; 28: 536–540

Pavlova B, Perlis RH, Alda M, et al. Lifetime prevalence of anxiety disorders in people with bipolar disorder: a systematic review and meta-analysis. *Lancet Psychiatry* 2015; 2: 710–717

Pavlovic ZM. Lamotrigine for the treatment of impulsive aggression and affective symptoms in a patient with borderline personality disorder comorbid with body dysmorphic disorder. *J Psychiatry Clin Neurosci* 2008; 20: 121–122

Payne JL, MacKinnon DF, Mondimore FM, et al. Familial aggregation of postpartum mood symptoms in bipolar disorder pedigrees. *Bipolar Disord* 2008; 10: 38–44

Pazzaglia PJ, Post RM, Ketter TA, et al. Preliminary controlled trial of nimodipine in ultra-rapid cycling affective dysregulation. *Psychiatry Res* 1993; 49: 257–272

Peduzzi P, Concato J, Kemper E, et al. A simulation study of the number of events per variable in logistic regression analysis. *J Clin Epidemiol* 1996; 49: 1373–1379

Peet M. The treatment of anxiety with beta-blocking drugs. *Postgrad Med J* 1988; 64(Suppl 2): 45–49

Pelissolo A. Efficacy and tolerability of escitalopram in anxiety disorders: a review. *Encephale* 2008; 34: 400–408

Peng Q, Gizer IR, Libiger O, et al. Association and ancestry analysis of sequence variants in ADH and ALDH using alcohol-related phenotypes in a Native American community sample. *Am J Med Genet B Neuropsychiatr Genet* 2014; 165B: 673–683

Penn DL, Keefe RS, Davis SM, et al. The effects of antipsychotic medications on emotion perception in patients with chronic schizophrenia in the CATIE trial. *Schizophr Res* 2009; 115: 17–23

Pennybaker SJ, Niciu MJ, Luckenbaugh DA, et al. Symptomatology and predictors of antidepressant efficacy in extended responders to a single ketamine infusion. *J Affect Disord* 2017; 208: 560–566

Pérez-Mañá C, Castells X, Torrens M, et al. Efficacy of psychostimulant drugs for amphetamine abuse or dependence. *Cochrane Database Syst Rev* 2013; (9): CD009695

Peritogiannis V. Sensation/novelty-seeking in psychotic disorders: a review of the literature. *World J Psychiatry* 2015; 5: 79–87

Perlis RH, Fraquas R, Fava M, et al. Prevalence and clinical correlates of irritability in major depressive disorder: a preliminary report from the Sequenced Treatment Alternatives to Relieve Depression study. *J Clin Psychiatry* 2005; 66: 159–166

Perlis RH, Laje G, Smoller JW, et al. Genetic and clinical predictors of sexual dysfunction in citalopram-treated depressed patients. *Neuropsychopharmacol* 2009; 34: 1819–1828

Perlis RH, Ostacher M, Miklowitz DJ, et al. Benzodiazepine use and risk of recurrence in bipolar disorder: a STEP-BD report. *J Clin Psychiatry* 2010; 71: 194–200

Perlis RH, Sachs GS, Lafer B, et al. Effect of abrupt change from standard to low serum levels of lithium: a reanalysis of double-blind lithium maintenance data. *Am J Psychiatry* 2002; 159: 1155–1159

Perrella C, Carrus D, Costa E, et al. Quetiapine for the treatment of borderline personality disorder: an open-label study. *Prog Neuropsychopharmacol Biol Psychiatry* 2007; 31: 158–163

Perroud N, Aitchison KJ, Uher R, et al. Genetic predictors of increase in suicidal ideation during antidepressant treatment in the GENDEP project. *Neuropsychopharmacology* 2009; 34: 2517–2528

Perry PJ, Zeilman C, Arndt S. Tricyclic antidepressant concentrations in plasma: an estimate of their sensitivity and specificity as a predictor of response. *J Clin Psychopharmacol* 1994; 14: 230–240

Perry PJ, Alexander B, Prince RA, et al. The utility of a single-point dosing protocol for predicting steady-state lithium levels. *Br J Psychiatry* 1986; 148: 401–405

Perry PJ, Lund BC, Sanger T, et al. Olanzapine plasma concentrations and clinical response: acute phase results of the North American olanzapine trial. *J Clin Psychopharmacol* 2001; 21: 14–20

Perugi G, Toni C, Frare F, et al. Effectiveness of adjunctive gabapentin in resistant bipolar disorder: is it due to anxious-alcohol abuse comorbidity? *J Clin Psychopharmacol* 2002; 22: 584–591

Peselow ED, Dunner DL, Fieve RR, et al. Lithium prophylaxis of depression in unipolar, bipolar II, and cyclothymic patients. *Am J Psychiatry* 1982; 139: 747–752

Peters W, Freeman MP, Kim S, et al. Treatment of premenstrual breakthrough of depression with adjunctive oral contraceptive pills compared with placebo. *J Clin Psychopharmacol* 2017; 37: 609–614

Petersen T, Papakostas GI, Posternak MA, et al. Empirical testing of two models for staging antidepressant treatment resistance. *J Clin Psychopharmacol* 2005; 25: 335–341

Petrakis IL, Ralevski E, Desai N, et al. Noradrenergic vs serotonergic antidepressant with or without naltrexone for veterans with PTSD and comorbid alcohol dependence. *Neuropsychopharmacol* 2012; 37: 996-1004

Petrakis IL, Ralevski E, Nich C, et al. Naltrexone and disulfiram in patients with alcohol dependence and current depression. *J Clin Psychopharmacol* 2007; 27: 160–165

Pettinati HM, Kampman KM, Lynch KG, et al. A double blind, placebo-controlled trial that combines disulfiram and naltrexone for treating co-occurring cocaine and alcohol dependence. *Addict Behav* 2008; 33: 651–657

Pettinati HM, Oslin SW, Kampman KM, et al. A double-blind, placebo-controlled trial combining sertraline and naltrexone for treating co-occurring depression and alcohol dependence. *Am J Psychiatry* 2010; 167: 668–675

Petty F, Davis LL, Nugent AL, et al. Valproate for chronic, combat-induced posttraumatic stress disorder. *J Clin Psychopharmacol* 2002; 22: 100-101

Peuskens J. Risperidone in the treatment of patients with chronic schizophrenia: a multi-national, multi-centre, double-blind, parallel-group study versus haloperidol. Risperidone Study Group. *Br J Psychiatry* 1995; 166: 712–726

Peuskens J, Link CG. A comparison of quetiapine and chlorpromazine in the treatment of schizophrenia. *Acta Psychiatr Scand* 1997; 96: 265-273

Philipsen A, Richter H, Schmahl C, et al. Clonidine in acute aversive inner tension and self-injurious behavior in female patients with borderline personality disorder. *J Clin Psychiatry* 2004a; 65: 1414–1419

Philipsen A, Schmahl C, Lieb K. Naloxone in the treatment of acute dissociative states in female patients with borderline personality disorder. *Pharmacopsychiatry* 2004b; 37: 196–199

Phillips KA. Placebo-controlled study of pimozide augmentation of fluoxetine in body dysmorphic disorder. *Am J Psychiatry* 2005; 162: 377-379

Phillips KA, McElroy SL. Personality disorders and traits in patients with body dysmorphic disorder. *Compr Psychiatry* 2000; 41: 229-236

Pierre JM, Wishing DA, Pierre WC, et al. High dose quetiapine in treatment refractory schizophrenia. *Schizophr Res* 2005; 73: 373–375

Pilkinton P, Berry C, Norrholm S, et al. An open label pilot study of adjunctive asenapine for the treatment of posttraumatic stress disorder. *Psychopharmacol Bull* 2016; 46: 8-17

Pillinger T, McCutcheon RA, Vano L, et al. Comparative effects of 18 antipsychotics on metabolic function in patients with schizophrenia, predictors of metabolic dysregulation, and association with psychopathology: a systematic review and network meta-analysis. *Lancet Psychiatry* 2020; 7: 64–77

Pinquart M, Duberstein PR. Treatment of anxiety disorders in older adults: a meta-analytic comparison of behavioral and pharmacological interventions. *Am J Geriatr Psychiatry* 2007; 15: 639–651

Pitman RK, Sanders KM, Zusman RM, et al. Pilot study of secondary prevention of posttraumatic stress disorder with propranolol. *Biol Psychiatry* 2002; 51: 189–192

Pittler MH, Ernst E. Kava extract for treating anxiety. *Cochrane Database Syst Rev* 2003; (1): CD003383

Pizzagalli DA. Frontocingulate dysfunction in depression: toward biomarkers of treatment response. *Neuropsychopharmacology* 2011; 36: 183-206

Pohl RB, Feltner DE, Fieve RR, et al. Efficacy of pregabalin in the treatment of generalized anxiety disorder: double-blind, placebo controlled comparison of BID versus TID dosing. *J Clin Psychopharmacol* 2005; 25: 151–158

Poling J, Oliveto A, Petry N, et al. Six-month trial of bupropion with contingency management for cocaine dependence in a methadone-maintained population. *Arch Gen Psychiatry* 2006; 63: 219–228

Pollack MH, Allqulander C, Bandelow B, et al. WCA recommendations for the long-term treatment of panic disorder. *CNS Spectr* 2003; 8(8 Suppl 1): 17–30

Pollack MH, Lepola U, Koponen H, et al. A double-blind study of the efficacy of venlafaxine extended-release, paroxetine, and placebo in the treatment of panic disorder. *Depress Anxiety* 2007; 24: 1–14

Pollack MH, Rappaport MH, Fayyad R, et al. Early improvement predicts endpoint remission status in sertraline and placebo treatments of panic disorder. *J Psychiatr Res* 2002; 36: 229–236

Pollack MH, Simon NM, Zalta AK, et al. Olanzapine augmentation of fluoxetine for refractory generalized anxiety disorder: a placebo controlled study. *Biol Psychiatry* 2006; 59: 211–215

Pollack MH, Tiller J, Xie F, et al. Tiagabine in adult patients with generalized anxiety disorder: results from 3 randomized, double-blind, placebo-controlled, parallel-group studies. *J Clin Psychopharmacol* 2008; 28: 308–316

Pollok J, van Agteren JE, Carson-Chahhoud KV. Pharmacological interventions for the treatment of depression in chronic obstructive pulmonary disease. *Cochrane Database Syst Rev* 2018; (12): CD012346

Popiel A, Zawadski B, Praglowska E, et al. Prolonged exposure, paroxetine and the combination in the treatment of PTSD following a motor vehicle accident: a randomized clinical trial – The "TRAKT" study. *J Behav Ther Exp Psychiatry* 2015; 48: 17–26

Popova V, Daly J, Trivedi M, et al. Efficacy and safety of flexibly dosed esketamine nasal spray combined with a newly initiated oral antidepressant in treatment-resistant depression: a randomized double-blind active-controlled study. *Am J Psychiatry* 2019; 176: 428–438

Porcelli S, Drago A, Fabbri C, et al. Pharmacogenetics of antidepressant response. *J Psychiatr Neurosci* 2011; 36: 87–113

Porcelli S, Fabbri C, Serretti A. Meta-analysis of serotonin transporter gene promoter polymorphism (5HTTLPR) association with antidepressant efficacy. *Eur Neuropsychopharmacol* 2012; 22: 239–258

Porsteinsson AP, Drye LT, Pollock BG, et al. Effect of citalopram on agitation in Alzheimer disease: the CitAD randomized clinical trial. *J Am Med Assoc* 2014; 311: 682–691

Portella MJ, de Diego-Adeliño J, Ballesteros J, et al. Can we really accelerate and enhance the selective serotonin reuptake inhibitor antidepressant effect? A randomized clinical trial and a meta-analysis of pindolol in non-resistant depression. *J Clin Psychiatry* 2011; 72: 962–969

Posner J, Kass E, Hulvershorn L. Using stimulants to treat ADHD-related emotional lability. *Curr Psychiatry Rep* 2014; 16: 478

Post RM, Ketter TA, Pazzaglia PJ, et al. Rational polypharmacy in the bipolar affective disorders. *Epilepsy Res Suppl* 1996; 11: 153–180

Potkin SG, Bunny JY, Costa J, et al. Effect of clozapine and adjunctive high-dose glycine in treatment-resistant schizophrenia. *Am J Psychiatry* 1999; 156: 145–147

Potkin SG, Keck PE Jr., Segal S, et al. Ziprasidone in acute bipolar mania: a 21-day randomized, double-blind, placebo-controlled replication trial. *J Clin Psychopharmacol* 2005; 25: 201–310

Potuzak M, Ravichandran C, Lewandowski KE, et al. Categorical versus dimensional classifications of psychotic disorders. *Compr Psychiatry* 2012; 53: 1118–1129

Poulson MB, Damgaard B, Zerahn B, et al. Modafinil may alleviate poststroke fatigue: a randomized, placebo controlled, double-blinded trial. *Stroke* 2015; 46: 3470–3477

Prakash J, Kotwal A, Prabhu H. Therapeutic and prophylactic utility of the memory-enhancing drug donepezil hydrochloride on cognition of patients undergoing electroconvulsive therapy: a randomized trial. *J ECT* 2006; 22: 163–168

Pratte MA, Nanavati KB, Young V, et al. An alternative treatment for anxiety: a systematic review of human trial results reported for the Ayurvedic herb ashwagandha (*Withania somnifera*). *J Altern Complement Med* 2014; 20: 901–908

Preisig M, Fenton BT, Stevens DE, et al. Familial relationship between mood disorders and alcoholism. *Compr Psychiatry* 2001; 42: 87–95

Premachandra BN, Kabir MA, Williams IK. Low T3 syndrome in psychiatric depression. *J Endocrinol Invest* 2006; 29: 568–572

Preskorn SH, Alderman J, Chung M, et al. Pharmacokinetics of desipramine coadministered with sertraline or fluoxetine. *J Clin Psychopharmacol* 1994; 14: 90–98

Primavera D, Bandecchi C, Lepori T, et al. Does duration of untreated psychosis predict very long term outcome of schizophrenic disorders? Results of a retrospective study. *Ann Gen Psychiatry* 2012; 11: 21

Pringsheim T, Marras C. Pimozide for tics in Tourette's syndrome. *Cochrane Database Syst Rev.* 2009; (2): CD006996

Pringsheim T, Holler-Managan Y, Okun MS, et al. Comprehensive systematic review summary: treatment of tics in people with Tourette syndrome and chronic tic disorders. *Neurology* 2019; 92: 907–915

Privitera M, Welty T, Gidal B, et al. How do clinicians adjust lamotrigine doses and use lamotrigine blood levels? A Q-PULSE survey. *Epilepsy Curr* 2014; 14: 218–223

Prosser JM, Yard S, Steele A, et al. A comparison of low-dose risperidone to paroxetine in the treatment of panic attacks: a randomized, single-blind study. *BMC Psychiatry* 2009; 9: 25

Prudic J, Haskett RF, McCall WV, et al. Pharmacological strategies in the prevention of relapse after electroconvulsive therapy. *J ECT* 2013; 29: 3–12.

Pundiak TM, Case BG, Peselow ED, et al. Discontinuation of maintenance selective serotonin reuptake inhibitor monotherapy after 5 years of stable response: a naturalistic study. *J Clin Psychiatry* 2008; 69: 1811–1817

Purdon SE. *The Screen for Cognitive Impairment in Psychiatry (SCIP): Administration Manual and Normative Data*. Edmonton, Alberta: PNL Inc; 2005

Qi W, Gevonden M, Shalev A. Efficacy and tolerability of high-dose escitalopram in posttraumatic stress disorder. *J Clin Psychopharmacol* 2017; 37: 89–93

Quante A, Zeugmann S. Tranylcypromine and bupropion combination therapy in treatment-resistant major depression: a report of 2 cases. *J Clin Psychopharmacol* 2012; 32: 572–574

Quitkin FM, Rabkin JG, Ross D, et al. Identification of true drug response to antidepressants: use of pattern analysis. *Arch Gen Psychiatry* 1984; 41: 782–786

Quitkin FM, Stewart JW, McGrath PJ, et al. Columbia atypical depression: a subgroup of depressives with better response to MAOI than to tricyclic antidepressants or placebo. *Br J Psychiatry* 1993; 21: 30–34

Rabinowitz J, Baruch Y, Barak Y. High-dose escitalopram for the treatment of obsessive-compulsive disorder. *Int Clin Psychopharmacol* 2008; 23: 49–53

Rabkin JG, McElhiney MC, Rabkin R, et al. Modafinil treatment for HIV+ patients: a pilot study. *J Clin Psychiatry* 2004; 65: 1688–1695

Rabkin JG, McElhiney MC, Rabkin R, et al. Placebo-controlled trial of dehydroepiandrosterone (DHEA) for treatment of nonmajor depression in patients with HIV/AIDS. *Am J Psychiatry* 2006; 163: 59–66

Raby WN, Rubin EA, Garawi F, et al. A randomized, double-blind, placebo-controlled trial of venlafaxine for the treatment of depressed cocaine-dependent patients. *Am J Addict* 2014; 23: 68–75

Rae Olmsted KL, Batoszk M, Mulvaney S, et al. Effect of stellate ganglion block treatment in posttraumatic stress disorder symptoms: a randomized clinical trial. *JAMA Psychiatry* 2020; 77: 130–138

Rahman T, Ash DM, Lauriello J, et al. Misleading guidance from pharmacogenomic testing. *Am J Psychiatry* 2017; 174: 922–924

Raison CL, Rutherford RE, Wollwine BJ, et al. A randomized controlled trial of the tumor necrosis factor antagonist infliximab for treatment-resistant depression: the role of baseline inflammatory biomarkers. *JAMA Psychiatry* 2013; 70: 31–41

Rajagopal R, Sundaresan L, Rajkumar AP, et al. Genetic association between the DRD4 promoter polymorphism and clozapine-induced sialorrhea. *Psychiatr Genet* 2014; 24: 273–276

Rajizadeh A, Mozaffari-Khosravi H, Yassini-Ardakani M, et al. Effect of magnesium supplementation on depression status in depressed patients with magnesium deficiency: a randomized, double-blind, placebo-controlled trial. *Nutrition* 2017; 35: 56–60

Rapaport MH, Gharabawi GM, Canuso CM, et al. Effects of risperidone augmentation in patients with treatment-resistant depression: results of open-label treatment followed by double-blind continuation. *Neuropsychopharmacology* 2006; 31: 2505–2513

Rapaport MH, Lydiard RB, Pitts CD, et al. Low doses of controlled-release paroxetine in the treatment of late-life depression: a randomized, placebo-controlled trial. *J Clin Psychiatry* 2009; 70: 46–57

Rapaport MH, Schneider LS, Dunner DL, et al. Efficacy of controlled-release paroxetine in the treatment of late-life depression. *J Clin Psychiatry* 2003; 64: 1065–1074

Raskin J, Wiltse CG, Siegal A, et al. Efficacy of duloxetine on cognition, depression, and pain in elderly patients with major depressive disorder: an 8-week, double-blind, placebo-controlled trial. *Am J Psychiatry* 2007; 164: 900–909

Raskind MA, Peskind ER, Chow B, et al. Trial of prazosin for post-traumatic stress disorder in military veterans. *N Engl J Med* 2018; 378: 507–517

Ratey JJ, Sorgi P, O'Driscoll GA, et al. Nadolol to treat aggression and psychiatric symptomatology in chronic psychiatric inpatients: a double-blind, placebo-controlled study. *J Clin Psychiatry* 1992; 53: 41–46

Rauch SAM, Kim HM, Powell C, et al. Efficacy of prolonged exposure therapy, sertraline hydrochloride, and their combination among veterans with posttraumatic stress disorder: a randomized clinical trial. *JAMA Psychiatry* 2019; 76: 117–126

Ravishankar V, Chowdappa SV, Beneqal V, et al. The efficacy of atomoxetine in treating adult attention deficit hyperactivity disorder (ADHD): a meta-analysis of controlled trials. *Asian J Psychiatry* 2016; 24: 53–58

Ray WA, Chung CP, Murray KT, et al. Atypical antipsychotic drugs and the risk of sudden cardiac death. *N Engl J Med* 2009; 360: 225–235

Reas DL, Grilo CM. Review and meta-analysis of pharmacotherapy for binge-eating disorder. *Obesity* 2008; 16: 2024–2038

Redden L, DelBello M, Wagner KD, et al. Long-term safety of divalproex sodium extended-release in children and adolescents with bipolar I disorder. *J Child Adolesc Psychopharmacol* 2009; 19: 83–89

Reed RC, Dutta S. Does it really matter when a blood sample for valproic acid concentration is taken following once-daily administration of divalproex-ER? *Ther Drug Monit* 2006; 28: 413–418

Reeves H, Batra S, May RS, et al. Efficacy of risperidone augmentation to antidepressants in the management of suicidality in major depressive disorder: a randomized, double-blind, placebo-controlled pilot study. *J Clin Psychiatry* 2008; 69: 1228–1236

Regier DA, Narrow WE, Clarke DE, et al. DSM-5 field trials in the United States and Canada, part II: test-retest reliability of selected categorical diagnoses. *Am J Psychiatry* 2013; 170: 59–70

Reich DB, Zanarini MC, Bieri KA. A preliminary study of lamotrigine in the treatment of affective instability in borderline personality disorder. *Int Clin Psychopharmacol* 2009; 24: 270–275

Reilly TM, Jopling WH, Beard AW. Successful treatment with pimozide of delusional parasitosis. *Br J Dermatol* 1978; 98: 457–459

Reilly-Harrington NA, Sylvia LG, Leon AC, et al. The medication recommendation tracking form: a novel tool for tracking changes in prescribed medication, clinical decision making, and use in comparative effectiveness research. *J Psychiatr Res* 2013; 47: 1686–1693

Reilly-Harrington NA, Sylvia LG, Rabideau DJ, et al. Tracking medication changes to assess outcomes in comparative effectiveness research: a bipolar CHOICE study. *J Affect Disord* 2016; 205: 159–164

Reimherr FW, Williams ED, Strong RE, et al. A double-blind, placebo-controlled, crossover study of osmotic release oral system methylphenidate in adults with ADHD with assessment of oppositional and emotional dimensions of the disorder. *J Clin Psychiatry* 2007; 68: 93–101

Reinares M, Rosa AR, Franco C, et al. A systematic review on the role of anticonvulsants in the treatment of acute bipolar depression. *Int J Neuropsychopharmacol* 2013; 16: 485–496

Reis M, Lundmark J, Bengtsson F. Therapeutic drug monitoring of racemic citalopram: a 5-year experience in Sweden, 1992–1997. *Ther Drug Monit* 2003; 25: 183–191

Reis M, Chermá MD, Carlsson B, et al. Therapeutic drug monitoring of escitalopram in an outpatient setting. *Ther Drug Monit* 2007; 29: 758–766

Reis M, Lundmark J, Björk H, et al. Therapeutic drug monitoring of racemic venlafaxine and its main metabolites in an everyday clinical setting. *Ther Drug Monit* 2002; 24: 545–553

Reist C, Nakamura K, Sagart E, et al. Impulsive aggressive behavior: open-label treatment with citalopram. *J Clin Psychiatry* 2003; 64: 81–85

Remington G, Agid D, Fousslas G, et al. Clozapine and therapeutic drug monitoring: is there sufficient evidence for an upper threshold? *Psychopharmacol (Berl)* 2013; 225: 505–518

Reoux JP, Saxon AJ, Malte CA, et al. Divalproex sodium in alcohol withdrawal: a randomized double-blind placebo-controlled clinical trial. *Alcohol Clin Exp Res* 2001; 25: 1324–1329

Rettenbacher WA, Hofer A, Kemmler G, et al. Neutropenia induced by second generation antipsychotics: a prospective investigation. *Pharmacopsychiatry* 2010; 43: 41–44

Reynolds GP, Hill MJ, Kirk SL. The 5-HT2C receptor and antipsychotic-induced weight gain – mechanisms and genetics. *J Psychopharmacol* 2006; 20(4 Suppl): 15–18

Reynolds GP, Zhang Z, Zhang X. Polymorphism of the promoter region of the serotonin 5-HT(2C) receptor gene and clozapine-induced weight gain. *Am J Psychiatry* 2003; 160: 677–679

Reynolds CF 3rd, Butlers MA, Lopez O, et al. Maintenance treatment of depression in old age: a randomized, double-blind, placebo-controlled evaluation of the efficacy and safety of donepezil combined with antidepressant pharmacotherapy. *Arch Gen Psychiatry* 2011; 68: 51–60

Rickels K, Lipman R, Raab E. Previous medication, duration of illness and placebo response. *J Nerv Ment Dis* 1966; 142: 548–554

Rickels K, DeMartinis N, Gárcia-España F, et al. Imipramine and buspirone in treatment of patients with generalized anxiety disorder who are discontinuing long-term benzodiazepine therapy. *Am J Psychiatry* 2000; 157: 1973–1979

Rickels K, Pollack MH, Feltner DE, et al. Pregabalin for treatment of generalized anxiety disorder: a 4-week, multicenter, double-blind, placebo-controlled trial of pregabalin and alprazolam. *Arch Gen Psychiatry* 2005; 62: 1022–1030

Rief W, Nestoriuc Y, Weiss S, et al. Meta-analysis of the placebo response in antidepressant trials. *J Affect Disord* 2009; 118: 1-8

Rifkin A, Karajgi B, Dicker R, et al. Lithium treatment of conduct disorders in adolescents. *Am J Psychiatry* 1997; 154: 554-555

Rink L, Braun C, Bschor T, et al. Dose increase versus unchanged continuation of antidepressants after initial antidepressant treatment failure in patients with major depressive disorder: a systematic review and meta-analysis of randomized, double-blind trials. *J Clin Psychiatry* 2018; 79: 17r11693

Rinne T, van den Brink W, Wouters L, et al. SSRI treatment of borderline personality disorder: a randomized, placebo-controlled clinical trial for female patients with borderline personality disorder. *Am J Psychiatry* 2002; 159: 2048–2054

Risse S, Whitters A, Burke A, et al. Severe withdrawal symptoms after discontinuation of alprazolam in eight patients with combat-induced posttraumatic stress disorder. *J Clin Psychiatry* 1990; 51: 206–209

Ritsner MS, Bawakny H, Kreinin A. Pregnenolone treatment reduces severity of negative symptoms in recent-onset schizophrenia: an 8-week, double blind, randomized add-on two-center trial. *Psychiatry Clin Neurosci* 2014; 68: 432–440

Ritsner MS, Gibel A, Shleifer T, et al. Pregnenolone and dehydroepiandrosterone as an adjunctive treatment in schizophrenia and schizoaffective disorder: an 8-week, double-blind, randomized, controlled, 2-center, parallel-group trial. *J Clin Psychiatry* 2010; 71: 1351-1362

Ritsner MS, Miodownik C, Ratner Y, et al. L-theanine relieves positive, activation, and anxiety symptoms in patients with schizophrenia and schizoaffective disorder: an 8-week, randomized, double-blind, placebo-controlled, 2-center study. *J Clin Psychiatry* 2011; 72: 34–42

Rivzi SJ, Sproule BA, Gallaugher L, et al. Correlates of benzodiazepine use in major depressive disorder: the effect of anhedonia. *J Affect Disord* 2015; 187: 101–105

Robert S, Hamner MB, Ulmer HG, et al. Open-label trial of escitalopram in the treatment of posttraumatic stress disorder. *J Clin Psychiatry* 2006; 67: 1522–1526

Roberts AC. The importance of serotonin for orbitofrontal function. *Biol Psychiatry* 2011; 69: 1185–1191

Robertson E, Grace S, Wallington T, et al. Antenatal risk factors for postpartum depression: a synthesis of recent literature. *Gen Hosp Psychiatry* 2004; 26: 289–295

Robinson M, Oakes TM, Raskin J, et al. Acute and long-term treatment of late-life major depressive disorder: duloxetine versus placebo. *Am J Geriatr Psychiatry* 2014; 22: 34–45

Robinson RG, Jorge RE, Moser DJ, et al. Escitalopram and problem-solving therapy for prevention of poststroke depression: a randomized controlled trial. *J Am Med Assoc* 2008; 299: 2391–2400

Rocca P, Marchiaro L, Cocuzza E, et al. Treatment of borderline personality disorder with risperidone. *J Clin Psychiatry* 2002; 63: 241–244

Rock EM, Bolognini D, Limebeer CL, et al. Cannabidiol, a non-psychotropic component of cannabis, attenuates vomiting and nausea-like behaviour via indirect agonism of 5-HT(1A) somatodendritic autoreceptors in the dorsal raphe nucleus. *Br J Pharmacol* 2012; 165: 2620–2634

Rodriguez CI, Bender J Jr., Morrison S, et al. Does extended release methylphenidate help adults with hoarding disorder? A case series. *J Clin Psychopharmacol* 2013; 33: 444–447

Roh D, Chang JG, Kim CH, et al. Antipsychotic polypharmacy and high-dose prescription in schizophrenia: a 5-year comparison. *Aust N Z J Psychiatry* 2014; 48: 52–60

Rohde C, Polcwiartek C, Asztalos M, et al. Effectiveness of prescription-based CNS stimulants on hospitalization in patients with schizophrenia: a nation-wide register study. *Schizophr Bull* 2018; 44: 93–100

Rojas-Fernandez CH. Can 5-HT3 antagonists really contribute to serotonin toxicity? A call for clarity and pharmacological law and order. *Drugs Real World Outcomes* 2014; 1: 3–5

Rojtabai R, Olfson M. National trends in psychotropic medication polypharmacy in office-based psychiatry. *Arch Gen Psychiatry* 2010; 67: 26-36

Romanelli RJ, Wu FM, Gamba R, et al. Behavioral therapy and serotonin reuptake inhibitor pharmacotherapy in the treatment of obsessive-compulsive disorder: a systematic review and meta-analysis of head-to-head randomized controlled trials. *Depress Anxiety* 2014; 31: 641–652

Roose SP, Glassman AH, Attia E, et al. Comparative efficacy of selective serotonin reuptake inhibitors and tricyclics in the treatment of melancholia. *Am J Psychiatry* 1994; 151: 1735–1739

Roose SP, Sackeim HA, Krishnan RR, et al. Old-Old Depression Study Group: antidepressant pharmacotherapy in the treatment of depression in the very old. A randomized, placebo-controlled trial. *Am J Psychiatry* 2004; 161: 2050–2059

Rosenbaum JF, Fava M, Hoog SL, et al. Selective serotonin reuptake inhibitor discontinuation syndrome: a randomized clinical trial. *Biol Psychiatry* 1998; 44: 77–87

Rosenberg HC, Chiu TH. Time course for the development of benzodiazepine tolerance and physical dependence. *Neurosci Biobehav Rev* 1985; 9: 123–131

Rosenberg NK, Mellergård M, Rosenberg R, et al. Characteristics of panic disorder patients responding to placebo. *Acta Psychiatr Scand* 1991; 365: 33–38

Rosenblat JD, McIntyre RS. Efficacy and tolerability of minocycline for depression: a systematic review and meta-analysis of clinical trials. *J Affect Disord* 2018; 227: 219–225

Rosenblat JD, Carvalho AF, Li M, et al. Oral ketamine for depression: a systematic review. *J Clin Psychiatry* 2019; 80: 18r12475

Rosenheck R, Dunn L, Peszke M, et al. Impact of clozapine on negative symptoms and on the deficit syndrome in refractory schizophrenia: Department of Veterans Affairs Cooperative Study Group on Clozapine in Refractory Schizophrenia. *Am J Psychiatry* 1999; 156: 88–93

Rosenthal M. Tiagabine for the treatment of generalized anxiety disorder: a randomized, open-label, clinical trial with paroxetine as a positive control. *J Clin Psychiatry* 2003; 64: 1245–1249

Ross DC, Fischhoff J, Davenport B. Treatment of ADHD when tolerance to methylphenidate develops. *Psychiatr Serv* 2002; 53: 102

Roth LS. Posttraumatic stress disorder and benzodiazepines: a myth agreed upon. *Fed Pract* 2010; 27: 12–21

Roth T, Seiden D, Sainati S, et al. Effects of ramelteon on patient-reported sleep latency in older adults with chronic insomnia. *Sleep Med* 2006; 7: 312–318

Rothbaum BO, Killeen TK, Davidson JR, et al. Placebo-controlled trial of risperidone augmentation for selective serotonin reuptake inhibitor-resistant civilian posttraumatic stress disorder. *J Clin Psychiatry* 2008; 69: 520–525

Rothschild AJ, Duval SE. How long should patients with psychotic depression stay on the antipsychotic medication? *J Clin Psychiatry* 2003; 64: 390–396

Rozzini L, Chilovi BV, Conti M, et al. Efficacy of SSRIs on cognition of Alzheimer's disease patients treated with cholinesterase inhibitors. *Int Psychogeriatr* 2010; 22: 114–119

Rucker JH, Jelen LA, Flynn S, et al. Psychedelics in the treatment of unipolar mood disorders: a systematic review. *J Psychopharmacol* 2016; 30: 1220–1229

Ruedrich SL, Swales TP, Rossvanes C, et al. Atypical antipsychotic medication improves aggression, but not self-injurious behaviour, in adults with intellectual disabilities. *J Intellect Disabil Res* 2008; 52: 132–140

Ruhé HG, Huyser J, Swinkels JA, et al. Dose escalation for insufficient response to standard-dose selective serotonin reuptake inhibitors in major depressive disorder: systematic review. *Br J Psychiatry* 2006a; 189: 309–316

Ruhé HG, Huyser J, Swinkels JA, et al. Switching antidepressants after a first selective serotonin reuptake inhibitor in major depressive disorder: a systematic review. *J Clin Psychiatry* 2006b; 67: 1836–1855

Ruiz P, Varner RV, Small DR, et al. Ethnic differences in the neuroleptic treatment of schizophrenia. *Psychiatr Q* 1999; 70: 163–172

Rush AJ, Carmody TJ, Haight BR, et al. Does pretreatment insomnia or anxiety predict acute response to bupropion SR? *Ann Clin Psychiatry* 2005; 17: 1–9

Rush AJ, Kraemer HC, Sackeim HA, et al. Report by the ACNP task force on response and remission in major depressive disorder. *Neuropsychopharmacology* 2006a; 31: 1841–1853

Rush AJ, Trivedi MH, Wisniewski SR, et al. Acute and longer-term outcomes in depressed outpatients requiring one or several treatment steps: a STAR*D report. *Am J Psychiatry* 2006b; 163: 1905–1917

Russo EB, Burnett A, Hall B, et al. Agonistic properties of cannabidiol at 5-HT1a receptors. *Neurochem Res* 2005; 30: 1037–1043

Rutherford BR, Pott E, Tandler JM, et al. Placebo response in antipsychotic clinical trials: a meta-analysis. *JAMA Psychiatry* 2014; 71: 1409–1421

Rutherford BR, Wall MM, Brown PJ, et al. Patient expectancy as a mediator of placebo effects in antidepressant clinical trials. *Am J Psychiatry* 2017; 174: 135–142

Rynn M, Khalid-Kahn S, Garcia-Espana JF, et al. Early response and 8-week treatment outcome in GAD. *Depress Anxiety* 2006; 23: 461–465

Ryszewska-Pokraśniewicz B, Mach A, Skalski M, et al. Effects of magnesium supplementation on unipolar depression: a placebo-controlled study and review of the importance of dosing and magnesium status in the therapeutic response. *Nutrients* 2018; 10(8): E1014

Saad K, Abdel-Rahman AA, Elserogy YM, et al. Vitamin D status in autism spectrum disorders and the efficacy of vitamin D supplementation in autistic children. *Nutr Neurosci* 2016; 19: 346–351

Saavedra-Velez C, Yusim A, Anbarasan D, et al. Modafinil as an adjunctive treatment of sedation, negative symptoms, and cognition in schizophrenia: a critical review. *J Clin Psychiatry* 2009; 70: 104–112

Sachs GS, Chengappa KN, Suppes T, et al. Quetiapine with lithium or divalproex for the treatment of bipolar mania: a randomized, double-blind, placebo-controlled study. *Bipolar Disord* 2004; 6: 213–223

Sachs GS, Greenberg WM, Starace A, et al. Cariprazine in the treatment of acute mania in bipolar I disorder: a double-blind, placebo-controlled, phase III trial. *J Affect Disord* 2015; 174: 296–302

Sachs GS, Grossman F, Ghaemi SN, et al. Combination of a mood stabilizer with risperidone or haloperidol for treatment of acute mania: a double-blind, placebo-controlled comparison of efficacy and safety. *Am J Psychiatry* 2002; 159: 1146-1154

Sachs GS, Ice KS, Chappell PB, et al. Efficacy and safety of adjunctive oral ziprasidone for acute treatment of depression in patients with bipolar I disorder: a randomized, double-blind, placebo-controlled trial. *J Clin Psychiatry* 2011; 72: 1413-1422

Sachs GS, Peters AT, Sylvia L, et al. Polypharmacy and bipolar disorder: what's personality got to do with it? *Int J Neuropsychopharmacol* 2014; 17: 1053-1061

Sachs GS, Vanderburg DG, Karayal ON, et al. Adjunctive oral ziprasidone in patients with acute mania treated with lithium or divalproex, part 1: results of a randomized, double-blind, placebo-controlled trial. *J Clin Psychiatry* 2012; 73: 1412-1419

Sack M, Spieler D, Wizelman L, et al. Intranasal oxytocin reduces provoked symptoms in female patients with posttraumatic stress disorder despite exerting sympathomimetic and positive chronotropic effects in a randomized controlled trial. *BMC Med* 2017; 15: 40

Sackeim HA, Haskett RF, Mulsant BH, et al. Continuation pharmacotherapy in the prevention of relapse following electroconvulsive therapy: a randomized controlled trial. *J Am Med Assoc* 2001; 285: 1299-1307

Sackett DL, Rosenberg WMC, Gray JA, et al. Evidence-based medicine: what it is and what it isn't. *Br Med J* 1996; 312: 71–72

Sackner-Bernstein J, Niebler G, Earl CQ, et al. Cardiovascular profile of modafinil: effects on blood pressure and heart rate. *Chest* 2004; 126: 729S

Saharian A, Ehsaei Z, Mowla A. Aripiprazole as an adjuvant treatment for obsessive and compulsive symptoms in manic phase of bipolar disorder: a randomized, double-blind, placebo-controlled clinical trial. *Prog Neuropsychopharmacol Biol Psychiatry* 2018; 84: 267-271

Sahlholm K, Zeberg H, Nilsson J, et al. The fast-off hypothesis revisited: a functional kinetic study of antipsychotic antagonism of the dopamine D2 receptor. *Eur Neuropsychopharmacol* 2016; 26: 467–476

Sakuma K, Matsunaga S, Nomura I, et al. Folic acid/methylfolate for the treatment of psychopathology in schizophrenia: a systematic review and meta-analysis. *Psychopharmacol (Berl)* 2018; 235: 2303-2314

Salehi B, Imani R, Mohammadi MR, et al. Ginkgo biloba for attention-deficit/hyperactivity disorder in children and adolescents: a double blind, randomized controlled trial. *Prog Neuropsychopharmacol Biol Psychiatry* 2010; 34: 76–80

Salloum IM, Cornelius JR, Daley DC, et al. Efficacy of valproate maintenance in patients with bipolar disorder and alcoholism: a double-blind placebo-controlled study. *Arch Gen Psychiatry* 2005; 62: 37–45

Salzman C, Wolfson AN, Schatzberg A, et al. Effect of fluoxetine on anger in symptomatic volunteers with borderline personality disorder. *J Clin Psychopharmacol* 1994; 15: 23-29

Sämann PG, Höhn D, Chechko N, et al. Prediction of antidepressant treatment response from gray matter volume across diagnostic categories. *Eur Neuropsychopharmacol* 2013; 23: 1503-1515

Samara MT, Goldberg Y, Levine SZ, et al. Initial symptom severity of bipolar I disorder and the efficacy of olanzapine: a meta-analysis of individual participant data from five placebo-controlled studies. *Lancet Psychiatry* 2017; 4: 859-867

Samara MT, Leucht C, Leeflang MM, et al. Early improvement as a predictor of later response to antipsychotics in schizophrenia: a diagnostic test review. *Am J Psychiatry* 2015; 172: 617-629

Samples H, Williams AR, Olfson M, et al. Risk factors for discontinuation of buprenorphine treatment for opioid use disorders in a multi-state sample of Medicaid enrollees. *J Subst Abuse Treat* 2018; 95: 9-16

Sandin S, Lichtstein P, Kuja-Halkola R, et al. The familial risk of autism. *J Am Med Assoc* 2014; 311: 1770-1777

Sandmann J, Lörch B, Bandelow B, et al. Fluvoxamine or placebo in the treatment of panic disorder and relationship to blood concentrations of fluvoxamine. *Pharmacopsychiatry* 1998; 31: 117-121

Sanfilipo M, Wolkin A, Angrist B, et al. Amphetamine and negative symptoms of schizophrenia. *Psychopharmacol (Berl)* 1996; 123: 211-214

Sani G, Gualtieri I, Paolino M, et al. Drug treatment of trichotillomania (hair-pulling disorder), excoriation (skin-picking) disorder, and nail-biting (onychophagia). *Curr Neuropharmacol* 2019; 17: 775-786

Sansone RA, Wiederman MW, Sansone LA. The Self-Harm Inventory (SHI): development of a scale for identifying self destructive behaviors and borderline personality disorder. *J Clin Psychol* 1998; 54: 973-83

Santos B, González-Fraile E, Zabala A, et al. Cognitive improvement of acetylcholinesterase inhibitors in schizophrenia. *J Psychopharmacol* 2018; 32: 1155-1166

Sarpal DK, Argyelan M, Robinson DG, et al. Baseline striatal functional connectivity as a predictor of response to antipsychotic drug treatment. *Am J Psychiatry* 2016; 173: 69-77

Sarris J. Herbal medicines in the treatment of psychiatric disorders: 10-year updated review. *Phytother Res* 2018; 32: 1147-1162

Sarris J, Murphy J, Mischoulon D, et al. Adjunctive nutraceutical for depression: a systematic review and meta-analyses. *Am J Psychiatry* 2016; 173: 575-587

Sarris J, Price LH, Carpenter LL, et al. Is S-adenosyl methionine (SAMe) for depression only effective in males? A re-analysis of data from a randomized clinical trial. *Pharmacopsychiatry* 2015; 48: 141–144

Sartori HE. Lithium orotate in the treatment of alcoholism and related conditions. *Alcohol* 1986; 3: 97–100

Sasson Y, Iancu I, Fux M, et al. A double-blind crossover comparison of clomipramine and desipramine in the treatment of panic disorder. *Eur Neuropsychopharmacol* 1999; 9: 191–196

Saxena S, Sumner J. Venlafaxine extended-release treatment of hoarding disorder. *Int Clin Psychopharmacol* 2014; 29: 266-273

Saxena S, Brody AL, Maidment KM, et al. Paroxetine treatment of compulsive hoarding. *J Psychiatr Res* 2007; 41: 481–487

Scarvalone PA, Cloitre M, Spielman LA, et al. Distress reduction during the structured clinical interview for DSM-III-R. *Psychiatr Res* 1996; 59: 245–249

Schaefer M, Sarkar S, Theophil I, et al. Acute and long-term memantine add-on treatment to risperidone improves cognitive dysfunction in patients with acute and chronic schizophrenia. *Pharmacopsychiatry* 2020; 53: 21–29

Schaffler K, Wolf OT, Burkart M. No benefit adding *Eleutherococcus senticosus* to stress management training in stress-related fatigue/weakness, impaired work or concentration, a randomized controlled study. *Pharmacopsychiatry* 2013; 46: 181–190

Schatzberg A, Roose S. A double-blind, placebo-controlled study of venlafaxine and fluoxetine in geriatric outpatients with major depression. *Am J Geriatr Psychiatry* 2006; 14: 361–370

Schatzberg AF, DeBattista C, Lazzeroni LC, et al. ABCB1 genetic effects on antidepressant outcomes: a report from the iSPOT-D trial. *Am J Psychiatry* 2015; 172: 751–759

Schatzberg AF, Haddad P, Kaplan EM, et al. Possible biological mechanisms of the serotonin reuptake inhibitor discontinuation syndrome. Discontinuation Consensus Panel. *J Clin Psychiatry* 1997; 58 (Suppl 7): 23–27

Schmahl C, Kleindienst N, Limberger M, et al. Evaluation of naltrexone for dissociative symptoms in borderline personality disorder. *Int Clin Psychopharmacol* 2012; 27: 61–68

Schmidt PJ, Daly RC, Bloch M. Dehydroepiandrosterone monotherapy in midlife-onset major and minor depression. *Arch Gen Psychiatry* 2005; 62: 154–162

Schmitt R, Gazelle FK, Lima MS, et al. The efficacy of antidepressants for generalized anxiety disorder: a systematic review and meta-analysis. *Braz J Psychiatry* 2005; 27: 18–24

Schneider LS, Dagerman K, Insel SP. Efficacy and adverse effects of atypical antipsychotics for dementia: meta-analysis of randomized, placebo-controlled trials. *Am J Geriatr Psychiatry* 2006; 14: 191–210

Schneider LS, Nelson JC, Clary CM, et al. An 8-week multicenter, parallel-group, double-blind, placebo controlled study of sertraline in elderly outpatients with major depression. *Am J Psychiatry* 2003; 160: 1277–1285

Schneier FR, Campeas R, Carcamo J, et al. Combined mirtazapine and SSRI treatment of PTSD: a placebo-controlled trial. *Depress Anxiety* 2015; 32: 570–579

Scholey A, Ossoukhova A, Owen L, et al. Effects of American ginseng (Panax quinquefolius) on neurocognitive function: an acute, randomised, double-blind, placebo-controlled, crossover study. *Psychopharmacol (Berl)* 2010; 212: 345–356

Schottenfeld RS, Chawarski MC, Pakes JR, et al. Methadone versus buprenorphine with contingency management or performance feedback for cocaine and opioid dependence. *Am J Psychiatry* 2005; 162: 340–349

Schulz SC, Zanarini MC, Bateman A, et al. Olanzapine for the treatment of borderline personality disorder: variable dose 12-week randomised double-blind placebo-controlled study. *Br J Psychiatry* 2008; 193: 485–492

Schutters SIJ, Van Megan HJGM, Van Veen JF, et al. Mirtazapine in generalized social anxiety disorder: a randomized, double-blind, placebo-controlled study. *Int Clin Psychopharmacol* 2010; 25: 302–304

Schweizer E, Rickels K, Hassman H, et al. Buspirone and imipramine for the treatment of major depression in the elderly. *J Clin Psychiatry* 1998; 59: 175–183

Schwenk ES, Viscusi ER, Buvanendram A, et al. Consensus guidelines on the use of intravenous ketamine infusions for acute pain management from the American Society of Regional Anesthesia and Pain Medicine, the American Academy of Pain Medicine, and the American Society of Anesthesiologists. *Reg Anesth Pain Med* 2018; 43: 456–466

Scoriels L, Jones PB, Sahakian PJ. Modafinil effects on cognition and emotion in schizophrenia and its neurochemical modulation in the brain. *Neuropsychopharmacol* 2013; 64: 168–184

Scuderi C, De Filippis D, Iuvone T, et al. Cannabidiol in medicine: a review of its therapeutic potential in CNS disorders. *Phytother Res* 2009; 23: 597–602

Seedat S, Stein MB. Double-blind, placebo-controlled assessment of combined clonazepam with paroxetine compared with paroxetine monotherapy for generalized social anxiety disorder. *J Clin Psychiatry* 2004; 65: 244–248

Seeman P. All roads to schizophrenia lead to dopamine supersensitivity and elevated dopamine D2(high) receptors. *CNS Neurosci Ther* 2011; 17: 118–132

Seitz DP, Adunuri N, Gill SS, et al. Antidepressants for agitation and psychosis in dementia. *Cochrane Database Syst Rev* 2011; (2): CD008191

Selle V, Schalkwijk S, Vásquez GH, et al. Treatments for acute bipolar depression: meta-analyses of placebo-controlled, monotherapy trials of anticonvulsants, lithium and antipsychotics. *Pharmacopsychiatry* 2014; 47: 43–52

Selles RR, McGuire JF, Small BJ, et al. A systematic review and meta-analysis of psychiatric treatments for excoriation (skin-picking) disorder. *Gen Hosp Psychiatry* 2016; 41: 29–37

Senderovich A, Jeyapragasan G. Is there a role for combined use of gabapentin and pregabalin in pain control? Too good to be true? *Curr Med Res Opin* 2018; 34: 677–682

Sephery AA, Potvin S, Elie R, et al. Selective serotonin reuptake inhibitor (SSRI) add-on therapy for the negative symptoms of schizophrenia: a meta-analysis. *J Clin Psychiatry* 2007; 68: 604–610

Serafini G, Adavastro G, Canepa G, et al. The efficacy of buprenorphine in major depression, treatment-resistant depression and suicidal behavior: a systematic review. *Int J Mol Sci* 2018; 19: E2410

Serban G, Siegel S. Response of borderline and schizotypal patients to small doses of thiothixene and haloperidol. *Am J Psychiatry* 1984; 141: 1455–1458

Servan A, Brunelin J, Poulet E. The effects of oxytocin on social cognition in borderline personality disorder. *Encephale* 2018; 44: 46–51

Shahani L. Venlafaxine augmentation with lithium leading to serotonin syndrome. *J Neuropsychiatry Clin Neurosci* 2012; 24: E47

Shakibaei F, Radmanesh M, Salari E, et al. Ginkgo biloba in the treatment of attention-deficit/hyperactivity disorder in children and adolescents: a randomized, placebo-controlled, trial. *Compl Ther Clin Pract* 2015; 21: 61–67

Shalev AY, Ankri Y, Israeli-Shalev Y, et al. Prevention of posttraumatic stress disorder by early treatment: results from the Jerusalem Trauma Outreach and Prevention Study. *Arch Gen Psychiatry* 2012; 69: 166–176

Shams M, Hiemke C, Härtter S. Therapeutic drug monitoring of the antidepressant mirtazapine and its N-demethylated metabolite in human serum. *Ther Drug Monit* 2004; 26: 78–84

Shapiro HI, Davis KA. Hypercalcemia and "primary" hyperparathyroidism during lithium therapy. *Am J Psychiatry* 2015; 172: 12–15

Shaw P, Stringaris A, Nigg J, et al. Emotion dysregulation in attention deficit hyperactivity disorder. *Am J Psychiatry* 2014; 171: 276–293

Shear MK, Reynolds CF 3rd, Simon NM, et al. Optimizing treatment of complicated grief: a randomized clinical trial. *JAMA Psychiatry* 2016; 73: 685–694

Sheard MH, Marini JL, Bridges CI, et al. The effect of lithium on impulsive aggressive behavior in man. *Am J Psychiatry* 1976; 133: 1409–1413

Sheehan DV, Sheehan KH, Raj BA. The speed of onset of alprazolam-XR compared to alprazolam-CT in panic disorder. *Psychopharmacol Bull* 2007; 40: 63–81

Sheehan DV, Burnham DB, Iyengar MK, et al. Efficacy and tolerability of controlled-release paroxetine in the treatment of panic disorder. *J Clin Psychiatry* 2005; 66: 34–40

Sheehan DV, Harnett-Sheehan K, Hidalgo RB, et al. Randomized, placebo-controlled trial of quetiapine XR and divalproex ER monotherapies in the treatment of the anxious bipolar patient. *J Affect Disord* 2013; 145: 83–94

Sheehan DV, McElroy SL, Harnett-Sheehan K, et al. Randomized, placebo-controlled trial of risperidone for acute treatment of bipolar anxiety. *J Affect Disord* 2009; 115: 376–385

Sheehan DV, Raj AB, Harnett-Sheehan K, et al. The relative efficacy of high-dose buspirone and alprazolam in the treatment of panic disorder: a double-blind placebo-controlled study. *Acta Psychiatr Scand* 1993; 88: 1–11

Sheehan DV, Raj AB, Sheehan KH, et al. The relative efficacy of buspirone, imipramine and placebo in panic disorder: a preliminary report. *Pharmacol Biochem Behav* 1988; 29: 815–817

Sheehan DV, Raj AB, Sheehan KH, et al. Is buspirone effective for panic disorder? *J Clin Psychopharmacol* 1990; 10: 3–11

Shelton RC, Tollefson GD, Tohen M, et al. A novel augmentation strategy for treating resistant major depression. *Am J Psychiatry* 2001; 158: 131–134

Shelton RC, Williamson DJ, Corya SA, et al. Olanzapine/fluoxetine combination for treatment-resistant depression: a controlled study of SSRI and nortriptyline resistance. *J Clin Psychiatry* 2005; 66: 1289–1297

Shergis JL, Zhang AL, Zhou W, et al. Panax ginseng in randomised controlled trials: a systematic review. *Phytother Res* 2013; 27: 949–965

Shi Q, Pavey ES, Carter RE. Bonferroni-based correction factor for multiple, correlated endpoints. *Pharm Stat* 2012; 11: 300–309

Shim J-C, Shin JG, Kelly DL, et al. Adjunctive treatment with a dopamine partial agonist, aripiprazole, for antipsychotic-induced hyperprolactinemia: a placebo-controlled trial. *Am J Psychiatry* 2007; 164: 1404–1410

Shin B-C, Lee MS, Yang EJ, et al. Maca (*L. myenii*) for improving sexual function: a systematic review. *BMC Complement Altern Med* 2010; 10: 44

Shiner B, Westgate CL, Gui J, et al. A retrospective comparative effectiveness study of medications for posttraumatic stress disorder in routine practice. *J Clin Psychiatry* 2018; 79: 18m12145

Shioda K, Nisijima K, Yoshino T, et al. Mirtazapine abolishes hyperthermia in an animal model of serotonin syndrome. *Neurosci Lett* 2010; 482: 216–219

Shiroma PR, Drews MS, Geske JR, et al. SLC6A4 polymorphisms and age of onset in late-life depression on treatment outcomes with citalopram: a Sequenced Treatment Alternatives to Relieve Depression (STAR*D) report. *Am J Geriatr Psychiatry* 2014; 22: 1140–1148

Shlipak MG, Matsushita K, Ärnlöv J, et al. Cystatin C versus creatinine in determining risk based on kidney function. *N Engl J Med* 2013; 369: 932–943

Shulman KI, Walker SE. Refining the MAOI diet: tyramine content of pizzas and soy products. *J Clin Psychiatry* 1999; 60: 191–193

Shulman KI, Walker SE, MacKenzie S, et al. Dietary restriction, tyramine, and the use of monoamine oxidase inhibitors. *J Clin Psychopharmacol* 1989; 9: 397–402

Shuman M, Chukwu A, Van Veldhuizen N, et al. Relationship between mirtazapine dose and incidence of adrenergic side effects: an exploratory analysis. *Mental Health Clin* 2019; 9: 41–47

Schumer MC, Bartley CA, Bloch MH. Systematic review of pharmacological and behavioral treatments for skin picking disorder. *J Clin Psychopharmacol* 2016; 36(2): 147–152

Siassi I. Lithium treatment of impulsive behavior in children. *J Clin Psychiatry* 1982; 43: 482–484

Sidor MM, McQueen GM. Antidepressants for the acute treatment of bipolar depression: a systematic review and meta-analysis, *J Clin Psychiatry* 2011; 72: 156–167

Sievewright H, Tyrer P, Johnson T. Change in personality status in neurotic disorders. *Lancet* 2002; 359: 2253–2254

Silberstein SD, Peres MF, Hopkins MM, et al. Olanzapine in the treatment of refractory migraine and chronic daily headache. *Headache* 2002; 42: 515–518

Silverman BL, Martin W, Memisoglu A, et al. A randomized, double-blind, placebo-controlled proof of concept study to evaluate samidorphan in the prevention of olanzapine-induced weight gain in healthy volunteers. *Schizophr Res* 2018; 195: 245–251

Simeon D, Stein DJ, Gross S, et al. A double-blind trial of fluoxetine in pathologic skin picking. *J Clin Psychiatry* 1997; 58: 341–347

Simeon JF, Ferguson HB, Knott V, et al. Clinical, cognitive, and neurophysiological effects of alprazolam in children and adolescents with overanxious and avoidant disorders. *J Am Acad Child Adolesc Psychiatry* 1992; 31: 29–33

Simhandl C, Denk E, Thau K. The comparative efficacy of carbamazepine low and high serum level and lithium carbonate in the prophylaxis of affective disorders. *J Affect Disord* 1993; 28: 221–231

Simon NM, Connor KM, Lang AJ, et al. Paroxetine CR augmentation for posttraumatic stress disorder refractory to prolonged exposure therapy. *J Clin Psychiatry* 2008; 69: 400–405

Simon NM, Hoge EA, Fischmann D, et al. An open-label trial of risperidone augmentation for refractory anxiety disorders. *J Clin Psychiatry* 2006a; 67: 381–385

Simon NM, Worthington JJ, Doyle AC, et al. An open-label study of levetiracetam for the treatment of social anxiety disorder. *J Clin Psychiatry* 2004; 65: 1219–1222

Simon NM, Zalta AK, Worthington JJ 3rd, et al. Preliminary support for gender differences in response to fluoxetine for generalized anxiety disorder. *Depress Anxiety* 2006b; 23: 373–376

Simpson EB, Yen S, Costello E, et al. Combined dialectical behavior therapy and fluoxetine in the treatment of borderline personality disorder. *J Clin Psychiatry* 2005; 65: 379–385

Sinclair DJ, Zhao S, Qi F, et al. Electroconvulsive therapy for treatment-resistant schizophrenia. *Cochrane Database Syst Rev* 2019; (3): CD011847

Singer S, Tkachenko E, Sharon P, et al. Psychiatric adverse events in patients taking isotretinoin as reported in a Food and Drug Administration database from 1997–2017. *JAMA Dermatol* 2019; 155: 1162–1166

Singh SP, Singh V. Meta-analysis of the efficacy of adjunctive NMDA receptor modulators in chronic schizophrenia. *CNS Drugs* 2011; 25: 859–885

Singh M, Keer D, Klimas J, et al. Topiramate for cocaine dependence: a systematic review and meta-analysis of randomized controlled trials. *Addiction* 2016; 111: 1337–1346

Singh NP, Despars JA, Stansbury DW, et al. Effects of buspirone on anxiety levels and exercise tolerance in patients with chronic airflow obstruction and mild anxiety. *Chest* 1993; 103: 800–804

Singh SP, Singh V, Kar N, et al. Efficacy of antidepressants in treating the negative symptoms of chronic schizophrenia: meta-analysis. *Br J Psychiatry* 2010; 197: 174–179

Siris SG, Adan F, Cohen M, et al. Postpsychotic depression and negative symptoms: an investigation of syndromal overlap. *Am J Psychiatry* 1988; 145: 1532–1537

Siskind D, McCartney L, Goldschlager R, et al. Clozapine v. first- and second-generation antipsychotics in treatment-refractory schizophrenia: systematic review and meta-analysis. *Br J Psychiatry* 2016; 209: 385–392

Siskind DJ, Lee M, Ravindran A, et al. Augmentation strategies for clozapine refractory schizophrenia: a systematic review and meta-analysis. *Aust N Z J Psychiatry* 2018; 52: 751–767

Skapinakis P, Caldwell DM, Hollingworth W, et al. Pharmacological and psychotherapeutic interventions for management of obsessive-compulsive disorder in adults: a systematic review and network meta-analysis. *Lancet Psychiatry* 2016; 3: 730–739

Skelley JW, Deas CM, Curren Z, Ennis J. Use of cannabidiol in anxiety and anxiety-related disorders. *J Am Pharm Assoc (2003)* 2020; 60: 253–261

Skinner MD, Lahmek P, Pham H, et al. Disulfiram efficacy in the treatment of alcohol dependence: a meta-analysis. *PLoS One* 2014; 9: e87366

Skoglund C, Chen Q, Franck J, et al. Attention-deficit/hyperactivity disorder and risk for substance use disorders in relatives. *Biol Psychiatry* 2015; 77: 880–886

Slee A, Nazareth I, Bondaronek P, et al. Pharmacological treatments for generalised anxiety disorder: a systematic review and network meta-analysis. *Lancet* 2019; 393: 768–777

Small JG, Hirsch SR, Arvinitis LA, et al. Quetiapine in patients with schizophrenia: a high- and low-dose double-blind comparison with placebo. Seroquel Study Group. *Arch Gen Psychiatry* 1997; 54: 549–557

Smith GC, Pell JP. Parachute use to prevent death and major trauma related to gravitational challenge: systematic review of randomised controlled trials. *Br Med J* 2003; 237: 1459–1461

Smith DF, Schou M. Kidney function and lithium concentrations in rats given an injection of lithium orotate or lithium carbonate. *J Pharm Pharmacol* 1979; 31: 161–163

Snyderman SH, Rynn MA, Rickels K. Open-label pilot study of ziprasidone for refractory generalized anxiety disorder. *J Clin Psychopharmacol* 2005; 25: 497–499

Soares-Weiser K, Rathbone J. Neuroleptic reduction and/or cessation and neuroleptics as specific treatments for tardive dyskinesia. *Cochrane Database Syst Rev.* 2006; (1): CD000459

Soares-Weiser K, Maayan N, Bergman H. Vitamin E for antipsychotic-induced tardive dyskinesia. *Cochrane Database Syst Rev* 2018; (1): CD000209

Sobanski T, Bagli M, Laux G, et al. Serotonin syndrome after lithium add-on medication to paroxetine. *Pharmacopsychiatry* 1997; 30: 106–107

Sobotka JL, Alexander B, Cook BL. A review of carbamazepine's hematologic reactions and monitoring recommendations. *DICP* 1990; 24: 1214–1219

Soler J, Pascual JC, Campins J, et al. Double-blind, placebo-controlled study of dialectical behavior therapy plus olanzapine for borderline personality disorder. *Am J Psychiatry* 2005; 162: 1221–1224

Solmi M, Fornaro M, Toyoshima K, et al. Systematic review and exploratory meta-analysis of the efficacy, safety, and biological effects of psychostimulants and atomoxetine in patients with schizophrenia or schizoaffective disorder. *CNS Spectrums* 2019; 24: 479–495

Solmi M, Pigato G, Kane JM, et al. Treatment of tardive dyskinesia with VMAT-2 inhibitors: a systematic review and meta-analysis of randomized controlled trials. *Drug Des Devel Ther* 2018; 12: 1215–1238

Solmi M, Veronese N, Thapa N, et al. Systematic review and meta-analysis of the efficacy and safety of minocycline in schizophrenia. *CNS Spectr* 2017; 22: 415–426

Soloff PH, Cornelius J, George A, et al. Efficacy of phenelzine and haloperidol in borderline personality disorder. *Arch Gen Psychiatry* 1993; 50: 377–385

Soloff PH, George A, Nathan RS, et al. Progress in pharmacotherapy of borderline disorders: a double-blind study of amitriptyline, haloperidol, and placebo. *Arch Gen Psychiatry* 1986; 43: 691–697

Soloff PH, George A, Nathan S, et al. Amitriptyline versus haloperidol in borderlines: final outcomes and predictors of response. *J Clin Psychopharmcol* 1989; 9: 238–246

Solomon DA, Leon AC, Coryell WH, et al. Longitudinal course of bipolar I disorder: duration of mood episodes. *Arch Gen Psychiatry* 2010; 67: 339–347

Solomon M, Ozonoff S, Carter C, et al. Formal thought disorder and the autism spectrum: relationship with symptoms, executive control, and anxiety. *J Autism Dev Disord* 2008; 38: 1474–1484

Sommer IE, de Witte L, Begemann M, et al. Nonsteroidal anti-inflammatory drugs in schizophrenia: ready for practice or a good start? A meta-analysis. *J Clin Psychiatry* 2012; 73: 414–419

Sonne S, Rubey R, Brady K, et al. Naltrexone treatment of self-injurious thoughts and behaviors. *J Nerv Ment Dis.* 1996;184:192–195

Sood S. Neutropenia with multiple antipsychotics including dose dependent neutropenia with lurasidone. *Clin Psychopharmacol Neurosci* 2017; 15: 413–415

Soomro GM, Altman D, Rajagopal S, et al. Selective serotonin re-uptake inhibitors (SSRIs) versus placebo for obsessive compulsive disorder (OCD). *Cochrane Database Syst Rev* 2008; (1): CD001765

Southwick SM, Pietrzak RH, Charney DS, et al. Resilience: the role of accurate appraisal, thresholds, and socioenvironmental factors. *Behav Brain Sci* 2015; 38: e122

Soutif-Veillon A, Ferland G, Rolland Y, et al. Increased dietary vitamin K intake is associated with less severe subjective memory complaint among older adults. *Maturitas* 2016; 93: 131–136

Soyka M. Othello syndrome: jealousy and jealous delusions as symptoms of psychiatric disorders. *Fortschr Neurol Psychiatr* 1995; 63: 487–494

Soyka M. Neurobiology of aggression and violence. *Schizophr Bull* 2011; 37: 913–920

Sparshatt A, Taylor D, Patel MX, Kapur S. A systematic review of aripiprazole: dose, plasma concentration, receptor occupancy, and response: implications for therapeutic drug monitoring. *J Clin Psychiatry* 2010; 71: 1447–1456

Sparshatt A, Taylor D, Patel MX, Kapur S. Relationship between daily dose, plasma concentrations, dopamine receptor occupancy, and clinical response to quetiapine: a review. *J Clin Psychiatry* 2011; 72: 1108–1123

Sperling H, Eisenhardt A, Virchow S, et al. Sildenafil response is influenced by the G protein beta 3 subunit GNB3 C825T polymorphism: a pilot study. *J Urol* 2003; 169: 1048–1051

Spielberger CD, Gorsuch RL, Lushene PR, et al. *Manual for the State-Trait Anxiety Inventory*. Palo Alto, California: Consulting Psychologists Press; 1983

Spina E, De Domenico P, Ruello C, et al. Adjunctive fluoxetine in the treatment of negative symptoms in chronic schizophrenic patients. *Int Clin Psychopharmacol* 1994; 9: 281–285

Sprouse AA, van Breemen RB. Pharmacokinetic interactions between drugs and botanical dietary supplements. *Drug Metab Dispos* 2016; 44: 162–171

Sramek JJ, Pi EH. Ethnicity and antidepressant response. *Mt Sinai J Med* 1996; 63: 320–325

Sramek JJ, Murphy MF, Cutler NR. Sex differences in the psychopharmacological treatment of depression. *Dialogues Clin Neurosci* 2016; 18: 447–457

Stahl SM. Drugs for psychosis and mood: unique actions at D3, D2 and D1 dopamine receptor subtypes. *CNS Spectr* 2017; 22: 375–384

Stahl SM. Comparing pharmacologic mechanism of action for the vesicular monoamine transporter 2 (VMAT2) inhibitors valbenazine and deutetrabenazine in treating tardive dyskinesia: does one have advantages over the other? *CNS Spectr* 2018; 23: 239–243

Stahl SM, Morrissette DA, Faedda G, et al. Guidelines for the recognition and management of mixed depression. *CNS Spectr* 2017; 22: 203–219

Stamm TJ, Becker D, Sondergeld LM, et al. Prediction of antidepressant response to venlafaxine by a combination of early response to assessment and therapeutic drug monitoring. *Pharmacopsychiatry* 2014a; 47: 174–179

Stamm TJ, Lewitzka U, Sauer C, et al. Supraphysiologic doses of levothyroxine as adjunctive therapy in bipolar depression: a randomized, double-blind, placebo-controlled study. *J Clin Psychiatry* 2014b; 75: 162–168

Stanley B, Sher L, Wilson S, et al. Non-suicidal self-injurious behavior, endogenous opioids and monoamine neurotransmitters. *J Affect Disord* 2010; 124: 134–140

Starzer MSK, Nordentoft M, Hjorthøj C. Rates and predictors of conversion to schizophrenia or bipolar disorder following substance-induced psychosis. *Am J Psychiatry* 2018; 175: 343–350

Steen NE, Aas M, Simonsen C, et al. Serum level of venlafaxine is associated with better memory in psychotic disorders. *Schizophr Res* 2015; 160: 386–392

Steen NE, Aas M, Simonsen C, et al. Serum levels of second-generation antipsychotics are associated with cognitive function in psychotic disorders. *World J Biol Psychiatry* 2017; 18: 471–482

Stein DJ. Pharmacotherapy of adjustment disorder: a review. *World J Biol Psychiatry* 2018; 19(Suppl 1): S46–S52

Stein DJ, Spadaccini E, Hollander E. Meta-analysis of pharmacotherapy trials for obsessive-compulsive disorder. *Int Clin Psychopharmacol* 1995; 10: 11–18

Stein MB, Kline NA, Matloff JL. Adjunctive olanzapine for SSRI-resistant combat-related PTSD: a double-blind, placebo-controlled study. *Am J Psychiatry* 2002b; 159: 1777–1779

Stein DJ, Baldwin DS, Dolberg OT, et al. Which factors predict placebo response in anxiety disorders and major depression? An analysis of placebo-controlled studies of escitalopram. *J Clin Psychiatry* 2006; 67: 1741–1746

Stein DJ, Hollander E, Anthony DT, et al. Serotonergic medications for sexual obsessions, sexual addictions, and paraphilias. *J Clin Psychiatry* 1992; 53: 267–271

Stein DJ, Simeon D, Frenkel M, et al. An open trial of valproate in borderline personality disorder. *J Clin Psychiatry* 1995a; 56: 506–510

Stein DJ, Versiani M, Hair T, et al. Efficacy of paroxetine for relapse prevention in social anxiety disorder: a 24-week study. *Arch Gen Psychiatry* 2002a; 59: 1111–1118

Stein MB, Chartier MJ, Hazen AL, et al. Paroxetine in the treatment of generalized social phobia: open-label treatment and double-blind placebo-controlled discontinuation. *J Clin Psychopharmacol* 1996; 16: 218–222

Stein MB, Liebowitz MR, Lydiard RB, et al. Paroxetine treatment of generalized social phobia (social anxiety disorder): a randomized controlled trial. *J Am Med Assoc* 1998; 280: 708–713

Stein MB, Ravindran LN, Simon NM, et al. Levetiracetam in generalized social anxiety disorder: a double-blind, randomized controlled trial. *J Clin Psychiatry* 2010; 71: 627–631

Stein MB, Sareen J, Hami S, et al. Pindolol potentiation of paroxetine for generalized social phobia: a double-blind, placebo-controlled, crossover study. *Am J Psychiatry* 2001; 158: 1725–1727

Sterne JA, Gavaghan D, Egger M. Publication and related bias in meta-analysis: power of statistical tests and prevalence in the literature. *J Clin Epidemiol* 2000; 53: 1119–1129

Stevinson C, Ernst E. Valerian for insomnia: a systematic review of randomized clinical trials. *Sleep Med* 2000; 1: 91–99

Stewart JW, Deliyannides DA, McGrath PJ. How treatable is refractory depression? *J Affect Disord* 2014; 167: 148–152

Stewart JW, Quitkin FM, McGrath PJ, et al. Use of pattern analysis to predict differential relapse of remitted patients with major depression during 1 year of treatment with fluoxetine or placebo. *Arch Gen Psychiatry* 1998; 55: 334–343

Stock CJ, Carpenter L, Ying J, et al. Gabapentin versus chlordiazepoxide for outpatient alcohol detoxification treatment. *Ann Pharmacother* 2013; 47: 961–969

Stoffers J, Völlm BA, Rücker G, et al. Pharmacological interventions for borderline personality disorder. *Cochrane Database Syst Rev* 2010; (6): CD005653

Stoll AL, Sachs GS, Cohen BM, et al. Choline in the treatment of rapid-cycling bipolar disorder: clinical and neurochemical findings in lithium-treated patients. *Biol Psychiatry* 1996; 40: 382–388

Stone JM, Roux S, Taylor D, et al. First-generation *versus* second-generation long-acting injectable antipsychotic drugs and time to relapse. *Ther Adv Psychopharmacol* 2018; 8: 333–336

Storch EA, Larson MJ, Shapira NA, et al. Clinical predictors of early fluoxetine treatment response in obsessive-compulsive disorder. *Depress Anxiety* 2006; 23: 429–433

Storebø OJ, Ramstad E, Krogh HB, et al. Methylphenidate for children and adolescents with attention deficit hyperactivity disorder (ADHD). *Cochrane Database Syst Rev* 2015; (11): CD009885

Stough C, Lloyd J, Clarke J, et al. The chronic effects of an extract of *Bacopa monniera* (Brahmi) on cognitive function in healthy human subjects. *Psychopharmacol (Berl)* 2001; 156: 481–484

Strain EC, Stitzer ML, Liebson IA, et al. Comparison of buprenorphine and methadone in the treatment of opioid dependence. *Am J Psychiatry* 1994; 151: 1025–1030

Streichenwein SM, Thornby JA. A long-term, double-blind, placebo-controlled, crossover trial of the efficacy of fluoxetine for trichotillomania. *Am J Psychiatry* 1995; 152: 1192–1196

Stübner S, Grohman R, Engel R, et al. Blood dyscrasias induced by psychotropic drugs. *Pharmacopsychiatry* 2004; 37 (Suppl 1): S70–S78

Sugarman MA, Kirsch I, Huppert JD. Obsessive-compulsive disorder has a reduced placebo (and antidepressant) response compared to other anxiety disorders: a meta-analysis. *J Affect Disord* 2017; 218: 217–226

Suliman S, Seedat S, Pingo J, et al. Escitalopram in the prevention of posttraumatic stress disorder: a pilot randomized controlled trial. *BMC Psychiatry* 2015; 15: 24

Sullivan PF, Daly MJ, O'Donovan M. Genetic architectures of psychiatric disorders: the emerging picture and its implications. *Nat Rev Genet* 2012; 13: 537–551

Sullivan JT, Sykora K, Schneiderman J, et al. Assessment of alcohol withdrawal: the revised Clinical Institute Withdrawal Assessment for Alcohol scale (CIWA-Ar). *Br J Addict* 1989; 84: 1353–1357

Sultana A, McMonagle T. Pimozide for schizophrenia or related psychoses. *Cochrane Database Syst Rev* 2000; (2): CD001949

Sun Y, Liang Y, Jiao Y, et al. Comparative efficacy and acceptability of antidepressant treatment in poststroke depression: a multiple-treatments meta-analysis. *BMJ Open* 2017; 7: e016499

Sundquist J, Sundquist K, Ji J. Autism and attention deficit/hyperactivity disorder among individuals with a family history of alcohol use disorders. *Elife* 2014; 3: e02917

Suppes T, Hirschfeld RM, Vieta E, et al. Quetiapine for the treatment of bipolar II depression: analysis of data from two randomized, double-blind, placebo-controlled studies. *World J Biol Psychiatry* 2008; 9: 198–211

Suppes T, McElroy SL, Sheehan DV, et al. A randomized, double-blind, placebo-controlled study of ziprasidone monotherapy in bipolar disorder with co-occurring lifetime panic or generalized anxiety disorder. *J Clin Psychiatry* 2014; 75: 77–84

Suppes T, Silva R, Cucchiaro J, et al. Lurasidone for the treatment of major depressive disorder with mixed features: a randomized, double-blind, placebo-controlled study. *Am J Psychiatry* 2016; 173: 400–407

Sutherland SM, Davidson JR. Pharmacotherapy for posttraumatic stress disorder. *Psychiatr Clin N Amer* 1994; 17: 409–423

Swann AC, Anderson JC, Dougherty DM, et al. Measurement of inter-episode impulsivity in bipolar disorder. *Psychiatry Res* 2001; 101: 195–197

Swann AC, Bowden CL, Calabrese JR, et al. Differential effect of number of previous episodes of affective disorder on response to lithium or divalproex in acute mania. *Am J Psychiatry* 1999; 156: 1264–1266

Swedo SE, Leonard HL, Rapoport JL, et al. A double-blind comparison of clomipramine and desipramine in the treatment of trichotillomania (hair pulling). *N Engl J Med* 1989; 321: 497–501

Sweet RA, Pollock BG, Mulsant BH, et al. Pharmacological profile of perphenazine's metabolites. *J Clin Psychopharmacol* 2000; 20: 181–187

Szegedi A, Durgam S, Mackle M, et al. Randomized, double-blind, placebo-controlled trial of asenapine maintenance therapy in adults with an acute manic or mixed episode associated with bipolar I disorder. *Am J Psychiatry* 2018; 175: 71–79

Szegedi A, Jansen WT, van Willigenburg AP, et al. Early improvement in the first 2 weeks as a predictor of treatment outcome in patients with major depressive disorder: a meta-analysis including 6562 patients. *J Clin Psychiatry* 2009; 70: 344–353

Szegedi A, Wetzel H, Leal M, et al. Combination treatment with clomipramine and fluvoxamine: drug monitoring, safety and tolerability data. *J Clin Psychiatry* 1996; 57: 257–264

Szegedi A, Zhao J, van Willigenburg A, et al. Effects of asenapine on depressive symptoms in patients with bipolar I disorder experiencing acute manic or mixed episodes: a post hoc analysis of two 3-week clinical trials. *BMC Psychiatry* 2011; 11: 101

Szeszko PR, Bilder RM, Dunlop JA, et al. Longitudinal assessment of methylphenidate effects on oral word production and symptoms in first-episode schizophrenia at acute and stabilized phases. *Biol Psychiatry* 1999; 45: 680–686

Szuba MP, Hornig-Rohan M, Amsterdam JD. Rapid conversion from one monoamine oxidase inhibitor to another. *J Clin Psychiatry* 1997; 58: 307–310

Tait DS, Marston HM, Shahid M, et al. Asenapine restores cognitive flexibility in rats with medial prefrontal cortex lesions. *Psychopharmacol (Berl)* 2009; 202: 295–306

Takano A, Ono S, Yamana H, et al. Factors associated with long-term prescription of benzodiazepine: a retrospective cohort study using a health insurance database in Japan. *BMJ Open* 2019; 9: e029641

Takeshima N, Ogawa Y, Hayasaka Y, et al. Continuation and discontinuation of benzodiazepine prescriptions: a cohort study based on a large claims database in Japan. *Psychiatr Res* 2016; 237: 201–207

Tang TZ, DeRubeis RJ, Hollon SD, et al. Personality change during depression treatment: a placebo-controlled trial. *Arch Gen Psychiatry* 2009; 66: 1322–1330

Tanzer T, Shah S, Benson C, et al. Varenicline for cognitive impairment in people with schizophrenia: systematic review and meta-analysis. *Psychopharmacol Berl* 2020; 237: 11–19

Tardy M, Dold M, Engel RR, et al. Trifluoperazine versus low-potency first-generation antipsychotic drugs for schizophrenia. *Cochrane Database Syst Rev* 2014c; (7): CD009396

Tardy M, Huhn M, Engel RR, et al. Perphenazine versus low-potency first-generation antipsychotic drugs for schizophrenia. *Cochrane database Syst Rev* 2014a; 7: CD009369

Tardy M, Huhn M, Engel RR, et al. Fluphenazine versus low-potency first-generation antipsychotic drugs for schizophrenia. *Cochrane Database Syst Rev* 2014b; 3: CD009230

Targownik LE, Bolton JM, Metge CJ, et al. Selective serotonin reuptake inhibitors are associated with a modest increase in the risk of upper gastrointestinal bleeding. *Am J Gastroenterol* 2009; 104: 1475–1482

Tarleton EK, Littenberg B, MacLean CD, et al. Role of magnesium supplementation in the treatment of depression: a randomized clinical trial. *PLoS One* 2017; 12: e0180067

Taylor D. Selective serotonin reuptake inhibitors and tricyclic antidepressants in combination: interactions and therapeutic uses. *Br J Psychiatry* 1995; 167: 575–580

Taylor D, Paton C, Kapur S (Eds). *The Maudsley Prescribing Guidelines in Psychiatry, 11th Edn*. London: Wiley Blackwell; 2015

Taylor CB, Youngblood ME, Catellier D, et al. Effects of antidepressant medication on morbidity and mortality in depressed patients after myocardial infarction. *Arch Gen Psychiatry* 2005; 62: 792–798

Taylor CP, Traynelis SF, Siffert J, et al. Pharmacology of dextromethorphan: relevance to dextromethorphan/quinidine (Nuedexta®) clinical use. *Pharmacol Ther* 2016; 164: 170–182

Tedeschini E, Levkovitz Y, Iovieno N, et al. Efficacy of antidepressants for late-life depression: a meta-analysis and meta-regression of placebo-controlled randomized trials. *J Clin Psychiatry* 2011; 72: 1660–1668

Teicher MH, Glod CA, Aaronson ST, et al. Open assessment of the safety and efficacy of thioridazine in the treatment of patients with borderline personality disorder. *Psychopharmacol Bull* 1989; 25: 535–549

Terao T, Ishida A, Kimura T, et al. Preventive effects of lamotrigine in bipolar II versus bipolar I disorder. *J Clin Psychiatry* 2017; 78: e1000–e1005

Thase ME, Chen D, Edwards J, et al. Effect of vilazodone on anxiety symptoms in patients with major depressive disorder. *Int Clin Psychopharmacol* 2014; 29: 351–356

Thase ME, Corya SA, Ountokun O, et al. A randomized, double-blind comparison of olanzapine/fluoxetine combination, olanzapine, and fluoxetine in treatment-resistant major depressive disorder. *J Clin Psychiatry* 2007; 68: 224–236

Thase ME, Jonas A, Khan A, et al. Aripiprazole monotherapy in nonpsychotic bipolar I depression: results of 2 randomized, placebo-controlled studies. *J Clin Psychopharmacol* 2008; 28: 13–20

Thase ME, Parikh SV, Rothschild AJ, et al. Impact of pharmacogenomics on clinical outcomes for patients taking medications with gene-drug interactions in a randomized controlled trial. *J Clin Psychiatry* 2019a; 80: 19m12910

Thase ME, Youakim JM, Skuban A, et al. Efficacy and safety of adjunctive brexpiprazole 2 mg in major depressive disorder: a phase 3, randomized, placebo-controlled study in patients with inadequate response to antidepressants. *J Clin Psychiatry* 2015a; 76: 1224–1231

Thase ME, Youakim JM, Skuban A, et al. Adjunctive brexpiprazole 1 and 3 mg for patients with major depressive disorder following inadequate response to antidepressants: a phase 3, randomized, double-blind study. *J Clin Psychiatry* 2015b; 76: 1232–1240

Thase ME, Zhang P, Weiss C, et al. Efficacy and safety of brexpiprazole as adjunctive treatment in major depressive disorder: overview of four short-term studies. *Expert Opin Pharmacother* 2019b; 20: 1907–1916

Thomas A, Baillie GL, Phillips AM, et al. Cannabidiol displays unexpectedly high potency as an antagonist of CB1 and CB2 receptor agonists in vitro. *Br J Pharmacol* 2007; 150: 613–623

Thomas SE, Randall PK, Book SW, et al. A complex relationship between co-occurring social anxiety and alcohol use disorders: what effect does treating social anxiety have on drinking? *Alcohol Clin Exp Res* 2008; 32: 77–84

Thone J. Worsened agitation and confusion in schizophrenia subsequent to high-dose aripiprazole. *J Neuropsychiatry Clin Neurosci* 2007; 19: 481–482

Thorlund K, Druyts E, Wu P, et al. Comparative efficacy and safety of selective serotonin reuptake inhibitors and serotonin-norepinephrine reuptake inhibitors in older adults: a network meta-analysis. *J Am Geriatr Soc* 2015; 63: 1002–1009

Thys-Jacobs S, Starkey P, Bernstein D, et al. Calcium carbonate and the premenstrual syndrome: effects on premenstrual and menstrual symptoms. Premenstrual Syndrome Study Group. *Am J Obstet Gynecol* 1998; 179: 444–452

Tiihonen J, Wahlbeck K, Kiviniemi V. The efficacy of lamotrigine in clozapine-resistant schizophrenia: a systematic review and meta-analysis. *Schizophr Res* 2009; 109: 10–14

Tiihonen J, Ryynänen OP, Kauhanen J, et al. Citalopram in the treatment of alcoholism: a double-blind placebo-controlled study. *Pharmacopsychiatry* 1996; 29: 27–29

Timmer CJ, Sitsen JM, Delbressine LP. Clinical pharmacokinetics of mirtazapine. *Clin Pharmacokinet* 2000; 38: 461–474

Tohen M, Calabrese JR, Sachs GS, et al. Randomized, placebo-controlled trial of olanzapine as maintenance therapy in patients with bipolar I disorder responding to acute treatment with olanzapine. *Am J Psychiatry* 2006; 163: 247–256

Tohen M, Chengappa KNR, Suppes T, et al. Efficacy of olanzapine in combination with valproate or lithium in the treatment of mania in patients partially nonresponsive to valproate or lithium monotherapy. *Arch Gen Psychiatry* 2002; 59: 62–69

Tohen M, Chengappa KNR, Suppes T, et al. Relapse prevention in bipolar I disorder: 18-month comparison of olanzapine plus mood stabiliser v. mood stabiliser alone. *Br J Psychiatry* 2004; 184: 337–345

Tohen M, Frank E, Bowden CL, et al. The International Society for Bipolar Disorders (ISBD) task force report on the nomenclature of course and outcome in bipolar disorders. *Bipolar Disord* 2009; 11: 453–473

Tohen M, Goldberg JF, Gonzalez-Pinto Arrillaga AM, et al. A 12-week, double-blind comparison of olanzapine vs haloperidol in the treatment of acute mania. *Arch Gen Psychiatry* 2003a; 60: 1218–1226

Tohen M, Katagiri H, Fujikoshi S, et al. Efficacy of olanzapine monotherapy in acute bipolar depression: a pooled analysis of controlled studies. *J Affect Disord* 2013; 149: 196–201

Tohen M, Vieta E, Calabrese J, et al. Efficacy of olanzapine and olanzapine-fluoxetine combination in the treatment of bipolar I depression. *Arch Gen Psychiatry* 2003b; 60: 1079–1088

Tollefson GD, Beasley CM Jr., Tran PV, et al. Olanzapine versus haloperidol in the treatment of schizophrenia and schizoaffective and schizophreniform disorders: results from an international collaborative trial. *Am J Psychiatry* 1997; 154: 457–467

Tollefson GD, Bosomworth JC, Heiligenstein JH, et al. A double-blind, placebo-controlled clinical trial of fluoxetine in geriatric patients with major depression: the Fluoxetine Collaborative Study Group. *Int Geropsychiatr* 1995; 7: 89–104

Tollefson GD, Greist JH, Jefferson JW, et al. Is baseline agitation a relative contraindication for a selective serotonin reuptake inhibitor? A comparative trial of fluoxetine versus imipramine. *J Clin Psychopharmacol* 1994a; 14: 385–391

Tollefson GD, Rampey AH, Potvin JH, et al. A multicenter investigation of fixed-dose fluoxetine in the treatment of obsessive-compulsive disorder. *Arch Gen Psychiatry* 1994b; 51: 559–567

Tomita T, Yasui-Furukori N, Nakagami T, et al. Therapeutic reference range for plasma concentrations of paroxetine in patients with major depressive disorder. *Ther Drug Monit* 2014; 36: 480–485

Tondo L, Vázquez G, Baldessarini RJ. Mania associated with antidepressant treatment: comprehensive meta-analytic review. *Acta Psychiatr Scand* 2010; 121: 404–414

Tondo L, Burrai C, Scamonatti L, et al. Carbamazepine in panic disorder. *Am J Psychiatry* 1989; 146: 558–559

Toniolo RA, Fernandes FBF, Silva M, et al. Cognitive effects of creatine monohydrate adjunctive therapy in patients with bipolar depression: results from a randomized, double-blind, placebo-controlled trial. *J Affect Disord* 2017; 224: 69–75

Toth C. Substitution of gabapentin therapy with pregabalin therapy in neuropathic pain due to peripheral neuropathy. *Pain Med* 2010; 11: 456–465

Touma KTB, Zoucha AM, Scarff JR. Liothyroine for depression: a review and guidance for safety monitoring. *Innov Clin Neurosci* 2017; 14: 24–29

Trichard C, Paillère-Martinot M-L, Attar-Levy D, et al. Binding of antipsychotic drugs to cortical $5HT_{2A}$ receptors: a PET study of chlorpromazine, clozapine, and amisulpride in schizophrenic patients. *Am J Psychiatry* 1998; 155: 505–508

Tritt K, Nickel C, Lahman C, et al. Lamotrigine treatment of aggression in female borderline-patients: a randomized, double-blind, placebo-controlled study. *J Psychopharmacol* 2005; 19: 287–291

Trivedi MH, Rush AJ, Carmody TJ, et al. Do bupropion SR and sertraline differ in their effects on anxiety in depressed patients? *J Clin Psychiatry* 2001; 62: 776–781

Trivedi MH, Thase ME, Osuntokun O, et al. An integrated analysis of olanzapine/fluoxetine combination in clinical trials of treatment-resistant depression. *J Clin Psychiatry* 2009; 70: 387–396

Truman CJ, Goldberg JF, Ghaemi SN, et al. Self-reported history of manic/hypomanic switch associated with antidepressant use: data from the Systematic Treatment Enhancement Program for Bipolar Disorder (STEP-BD). *J Clin Psychiatry* 2007; 68: 1472–1479

Tucker P, Trautman RP, Wyatt DB, et al. Efficacy and safety of topiramate monotherapy in civilian posttraumatic stress disorder: a randomized, double-blind, placebo-controlled study. *J Clin Psychiatry* 2007; 68: 201–206

Tueth MJ, Cheong JA. Successful treatment with pimozide of Capgras syndrome in an elderly male. *J Geriatr Psychiatry Neurol* 1992; 5: 217–219

Turkmen S, Backstrom T, Wahlstrom G, et al. Tolerance to allopregnanolone with focus on the GABA-A receptor. *Br J Pharmacol* 2011; 162: 311–327

Turkoz I, Daly E, Sigh J, et al. Treatment response with esketamine nasal spray plus an oral antidepressant in patients with treatment-resistant depression without evidence of early response: a pooled post hoc analysis of the TRANSFORM Studies. *J Clin Psychiatry*, 2021; 82(4):20m13800

Turner DC, Clark L, Dowson J, et al. Modafinil improves cognition and response inhibition in adult attention-deficit/hyperactivity disorder. *Biol Psychiatry* 2004a; 55: 1031–1040

Turner DC, Clark L, Pomarol-Clotet E, et al. Modafinil improves cognition and attentional set shifting in patients with chronic schizophrenia. *Neuropsychopharmacology* 2004b; 29: 1363–1373

Turner DC, Robbins TW, Clark L, et al. Cognitive enhancing effects of modafinil in healthy volunteers. *Psychopharmacology (Berl)* 2003, 165. 260–269

Turner H, Matthews AM, Linardatos E, et al. Selective publication of antidepressant trials and its influence on apparent efficacy. *N Engl J Med* 2008; 358: 252–260

Turner SM, Beidel DC, Dancu C, et al. An empirically derived inventory to measure social fears and anxiety: the Social Phobia and Anxiety Inventory. *Psychol Assess* 1989; 1: 35–40

Uguz F. Second-generation antipsychotics during the lactation period: a comparative systematic review on infant safety. *J Clin Psychopharmacol* 2016; 36: 244–252

Uhde T, Stein MB, Post RM. Lack of efficacy of carbamazepine in the treatment of panic disorder. *Am J Psychiatry* 1988; 145: 1104–1109

Uher R, Perlis RH, Henigsberg N, et al. Depression symptom dimensions as predictors of antidepressant treatment outcome: replicable evidence for interest-activity symptoms. *Psychol Med* 2012; 42: 967–980

Uher R, Perroud N, Ng MYM, et al. Genome-wide pharmacogenetics of antidepressant response in the GENDEP project. *Am J Psychiatry* 2010; 167: 555–564

Uher R, Tansey KE, Dew T, et al. An inflammatory biomarker as a differential predictor of outcome of depression treatment with escitalopram or nortriptyline. *Am J Psychiatry* 2014; 171: 1278–1286

Ujike H, Nomura A, Morita Y, et al. Multiple genetic factors in olanzapine-induced weight gain in schizophrenia patients: a cohort study. *J Clin Psychiatry* 2008; 69: 1416–1422

Ulrich S, Wurthmann C, Brosz M, et al: The relationship between serum concentration and therapeutic effect of haloperidol in patients with acute schizophrenia. *Clin Pharmacokinet* 1998; 34: 227–263

Umbricht D, Alberati D, Martin-Facklam M, et al. Effect of bitopertin, a glycine reuptake inhibitor, on negative symptoms of schizophrenia: a randomized, double-blind, proof-of-concept study. *JAMA Psychiatry* 2014a; 71: 637–646

Umbricht A, DeFulio A, Winstanley EL, et al. Topiramate for cocaine dependence during methadone maintenance treatment: a randomized controlled trial. *Drug Alcohol Depend* 2014b; 140: 92–100

Ungvari GS, Hollokoi RI. Successful treatment of litigious paranoia with pimozide. *Can J Psychiatry* 1993; 38: 4–8

Unterecker S, Deckert J, Pfuhlman B. No influence of body weight on serum levels of antidepressants. *Ther Drug Monit* 2011; 33: 730–744

Unterecker S, Riederer P, Proft F, et al. Effects of gender and age on serum concentrations of antidepressants under naturalistic conditions. *J Neural Transm (Vienna)* 2013; 120: 1237–1246

Usmani ZA, Carson-Chahhoud KV, Esterman AJ, et al. A randomized placebo-controlled trial of paroxetine for the management of anxiety in chronic obstructive pulmonary disease (PAC Study). *J Multidiscip Health* 2018; 11: 287–293

Vahedi H, Merat S, Rashidioon A, et al. The effect of fluoxetine in patients with pain and constipation-predominant irritable bowel syndrome: a double-blind randomized-controlled study. *Alim Pharmacol Ther* 2005; 22: 381–385

Vaishnavi S, Alamy S, Zhang W, et al. Quetiapine as monotherapy for social anxiety disorder: a placebo-controlled study. *Prog Neuropharmacol Biol Psychiatry* 2007; 31: 1464–1469

Vaiva G, Ducrocq F, Jezquel K, et al. Immediate treatment with propranolol decreases posttraumatic stress disorder two months after trauma. *Biol Psychiatry* 2003; 54: 947–949

Vallée M, Vitiello S, Bellocchio L, et al. Pregnenolone can protect the brain from cannabis intoxication. *Science* 2014; 343: 94–98

Valles-Colomer M, Falony G, Darzi Y, et al. The neuroactive potential of the human gut microbiota in quality of life and depression. *Nat Microbiol* 2019; 4: 623–632

Van Ameringen M, Lane RM, Walker JR, et al. Sertraline treatment of generalized social phobia: a 20-week, double-blind, placebo-controlled study. *Am J Psychiatry* 2001; 158: 275–281

Van Ameringen M, Mancini C, Pipe B, et al. An open trial of topiramate in the treatment of generalized social phobia. *J Clin Psychiatry* 2004; 64: 1674–1678

van Broekhoven KEM, Karreman A, Hartman EE, et al. Obsessive-compulsive personality disorder symptoms as a risk factor for postpartum depressive symptoms. *Arch Womens Ment Health* 2019; 22: 475–483

VanderZwaag C, McGee M, McEvoy JP, et al. Response of patients with treatment-refractory schizophrenia to clozapine within three serum level ranges. *Am J Psychiatry* 1996; 153: 1579–1584

Van den Eynde F, Senturk V, Naudts K, et al. Efficacy of quetiapine for impulsivity and affective symptoms in borderline personality disorder. *J Clin Psychopharmacol* 2008; 28: 147–155

Van der Loos ML, Mulder PG, Hartong EG, et al. Efficacy and safety of lamotrigine as add-on treatment to lithium in bipolar depression: a multi-center, double-blind, placebo-controlled trial. *J Clin Psychiatry* 2009; 70: 223–231

van Dinteren R, Arns M, Kenemans L, et al. Utility of event-related potentials in predicting antidepressant treatment response: an iSPOT-D report. *Eur Neuropsychopharmacol* 2015; 25: 1981–1990

Van Haelst IM, van Klei WA, Doodeman HJ, et al. Antidepressant treatment with monoamine oxidase inhibitors and the occurrence of intraoperative hemodynamic events: a retrospective observational cohort study. *J Clin Psychiatry* 2012; 73: 1103–1109

van Kammen DP, Boronow JJ. Dextro-amphetamine diminishes negative symptoms in schizophrenia. *Int Clin Psychopharmacol* 1988; 3: 111–121

Van Os J. Is there a continuum of psychotic experiences in the general population? *Epidemiol Psichiatr Soc* 2003; 12: 242–252

van Vliet IM, den Boer JA, Westenberg HG. Psychopharmacological treatment of social phobia: a double-blind placebo controlled study with fluvoxamine. *Psychopharmacology (Berl)* 1994; 115: 128–134

van Vliet IM, den Boer JA, Westenberg HG, et al. Clinical effects of buspirone in social phobia: a double-blind, placebo-controlled study. *J Clin Psychiatry* 1997; 58: 164–168

van Zuiden M, Frijling JL, Nawijn L, et al. Intranasal oxytocin to prevent posttraumatic stress disorder symptoms: a randomized controlled trial in emergency department patients. *Biol Psychiatry* 2017; 81: 1030–1040

Varma A, Moore MB, Miller CWT, et al. Topiramate as monotherapy or adjunctive treatment for posttraumatic stress disorder: a meta-analysis. *J Trauma Stress* 2018; 31: 125–133

Vasudev K, Goswami U, Kohli K. Carbamazepine and valproate monotherapy: feasibility, relative safety and efficacy, and therapeutic drug monitoring in manic disorder. *Psychopharmacol (Berl)* 2000; 150: 15–23

Veale D, Miles S, Smallcombe N, Atypical antipsychotic augmentation in SSRI treatment-refractory obsessive-compulsive disorder: a systematic review and meta-analysis. *BMC Psychiatry* 2014; 14: 317

Veefkind AH, Haffmans PMJ, Hoencamp E. Venlafaxine serum levels and CYP2D6 genotype. *Ther Drug Monit* 2000; 22: 202–208

Veerman SR, Schulte PF, Deijen JB, et al. Adjunctive memantine in clozapine-treated refractory schizophrenia: an open-label 1-year extension study. *Psychol Med* 2017; 47: 363–375

Veerman SR, Schulte PF, Smith JD, et al. Memantine augmentation in clozapine-refractory schizophrenia: a randomized, double-blind, placebo-controlled crossover study. *Psychol Med* 2016; 46: 1909–1921

Vellekkatt F, Menon V. Efficacy of vitamin D supplementation in major depression: a meta-analysis of randomized controlled trials. *J Postgrad Med* 2019; 65: 74–80

Verbeeck W, Bekkering GE, Van den Noortgate W, et al. Bupropion for attention deficit hyperactivity disorder (ADHD) in adults. *Cochrane Database Syst Rev* 2017; (10): CD009504

Verheul R, Lehert P, Geerlings PJ, et al. Predictors of acamprosate efficacy: results from a pooled analysis of seven European trials including 1485 alcohol-dependent patients. *Psychopharmacol (Berl)* 2005; 178: 167–173

Verhulst FC, Van der Ende J. The eight-year stability of problem behavior in an epidemiologic sample. *Ped Res* 1995; 38: 612–617

Vernon JA, Grudnikoff E, Seidman AJ, et al. Antidepressants for cognitive impairment in schizophrenia: a systematic review and meta-analysis. *Schizophr Res* 2014; 159: 385–394

Veroniki AA, Cogo E, Rios P, et al. Comparative safety of anti-epileptic drugs during pregnancy: a systematic review and network meta-analysis of congenital malformations and prenatal outcomes. *BMC Med* 2017; 15: 95

Versiani M, Nardi AE, Mundim FD, et al. Pharmacotherapy of social phobia: a controlled study with moclobemide and phenelzine. *Br J Psychiatry* 1992; 161: 353–360

Victoroff J, Coburn K, Reeve A, et al. Pharmacological management of persistent hostility and aggression in persons with schizophrenia spectrum disorders: a systematic review. *J Neuropsychiatry Clin Neurosci* 2014; 26: 283–312

Vieta E, Calabrese JR, Goikolea JM, et al. Quetiapine monotherapy in the treatment of patients with bipolar I or II depression and a rapid cycling disease course: a randomized, double-blind, placebo-controlled study. *Bipolar Disord* 2007; 9: 413–425

Vieta E, Cruz N, García-Campayo J, et al. A double-blind, randomized, placebo-controlled prophylaxis study of oxcarbazepine as adjunct treatment to lithium in the long-term treatment of bipolar I and II disorder. *Int J Neuropsychopharmacol* 2008a; 11: 445–452

Vieta E, Nuamah IF, Lim P, et al. A randomized, placebo- and active-controlled study of paliperidone extended release for the treatment of acute manic and mixed episodes of bipolar I disorder. *Bipolar Disord* 2010; 12: 230–243

Vieta E, T'Joen C, McQuade RD, et al. Efficacy of adjunctive aripiprazole to either valproate or lithium in bipolar mania patients partially nonresponsive to valproate/lithium monotherapy: a placebo-controlled study. *Am J Psychiatry* 2008b; 165: 1316–1325

Vigen CL, Mack WJ, Keefe RS, et al. Cognitive effects of atypical antipsychotic medications in patients with Alzheimer's disease: outcomes from CATIE-AD. *Am J Psychiatry* 2011; 168: 831–839

Viguera AC, Nunacs R, Cohen LS, et al. Risk of recurrence of bipolar disorder in pregnant and nonpregnant women after discontinuing lithium maintenance. *Am J Psychiatry* 2000; 157: 179–184

Viguera AC, Tondo L, Koukopoulos AE, et al. Episodes of mood disorders in 2,252 pregnancies and postpartum periods. *Am J Psychiatry* 2011; 168: 1179–1185

Viktorin A, Rydén E, Thase ME, et al. The risk of treatment-emergent mania with methylphenidate in bipolar disorder. *Am J Psychiatry* 2017; 174: 341–348

Villarreal G, Hamer MB, Cañive JM, et al. Efficacy of quetiapine monotherapy in posttraumatic stress disorder: a randomized, placebo-controlled trial. *Am J Psychiatry* 2016; 173: 1205–1212

Villeneuve E, Lemelin S. Open-label study of atypical neuroleptic quetiapine for treatment of borderline personality disorder: impulsivity as main target. *J Clin Psychiatry* 2005; 66: 1298–1303

Vita D, De Peri L, Siracusano A, et al. Efficacy and tolerability of asenapine for acute mania in bipolar I disorder: meta-analyses of randomized-controlled trials. *Int Clin Psychopharmacol* 2013; 28: 219–227

Voican CS, Corruble E, Naveau S, et al. Antidepressant-induced liver injury: a review for clinicians. *Am J Psychiatry* 2014; 171: 404–415

Volavka J, Citrome L. Pathways to aggression in schizophrenia affect results of treatment. *Schizophr Bull* 2011; 37: 921–929

Volavka J, Czobor P, Citrome L, et al. Effectiveness of antipsychotic drugs against hostility in patients with schizophrenia in the Clinical Antipsychotic Trials of Intervention Effectiveness (CATIE) study. *CNS Spectr* 2014; 19: 374–381

von Wolff A, Hölzel P, Westphal A, et al. Selective serotonin reuptake inhibitors and tricyclic antidepressants in the acute treatment of chronic depression and dysthymia: a systematic review and meta-analysis. *J Affect Disord* 2013; 144: 7–15

Wagner GJ, Rabkin R. Effects of dextroamphetamine on depression and fatigue in men with HIV: a double-blind, placebo-controlled trial. *J Clin Psychiatry* 2000; 61: 436–440

Wagner J, Wagner ML. Non-benzodiazepines for the treatment of insomnia. *Sleep Med Rev* 2000; 4: 551–581

Wagner KD, Kowatch R, Emslie GJ, et al. A double-blind, randomized, placebo-controlled trial of oxcarbazepine in the treatment of bipolar disorder in children and adolescents. *Am J Psychiatry* 2006; 163: 1179–1186

Waldschmitt C, Vogel F, Pfuhlmann B, et al. Duloxetine serum concentrations and clinical effects. Data from a therapeutic drug monitoring (TDM) survey. *Pharmacopsychiatry* 2009; 42: 189–193

Walker SE, Shulman KI, Tailor SA, et al. Tyramine content of previously restricted foods in monoamine oxidase inhibitor diets. *J Clin Psychopharmacol* 1996; 16: 383–388

Walshaw PD, Gyulai L, Bauer M, et al. Adjunctive thyroid hormone treatment in rapid cycling bipolar disorder: a double-blind placebo-controlled trial of levothyroxine (L-T_4) and triiodothyronine (T_3). *Bipolar Disord* 2018; 20: 594–603

Walther A, Breidenstein J, Miller R. Association of testosterone treatment with alleviation of depression symptoms in men: a systematic review and meta-analysis. *JAMA Psychiatry* 2019; 76: 31–40

Wang G-J, Volkow N, Wigal T, et al. Chronic treatment with methylphenidate increases dopamine transporter density in patients with attention deficit hyperactivity disorder. *J Nucl Med* 2009; 50(Suppl 2): 1283

Wang MT, Tsai CL, Lin CW, et al. Association between antipsychotic agent and risk of acute respiratory failure in patients with chronic obstructive pulmonary disease. *JAMA Psychiatry* 2017b; 74: 252–260

Wang PW, Hill SJ, Childers ME, et al. Open adjunctive ziprasidone associated with weight loss in obese and overweight bipolar disorder patients. *J Psychiatr Res* 2011; 45: 1128–1132

Wang SM, Han C, Lee SJ, et al. Modafinil for the treatment of attention-deficit/hyperactivity disorder: a meta-analysis. *J Psychiatr Res* 2017a; 84: 292–300

Warner MD, Dorn MR, Peabody CA. Survey on the usefulness of trazodone in patients with PTSD with insomnia or nightmares. *Pharmacopsychiatry* 2001; 34: 128–131

Watanabe T, Ueda M, Saeki Y, et al. High plasma concentrations of paroxetine impede clinical response in patients with panic disorder. *Ther Drug Monit* 2007; 29: 40–44

Watts BV, Schnurr PR, Mayo L, et al. Meta-analysis of the efficacy of treatments for posttraumatic stress disorder. *J Clin Psychiatry* 2013; 74: e541–e550

Waxmonsky JG, Waschbusch DA, Glatt SJ, et al. Prediction of placebo response in 2 clinical trials of lisdexamfetamine dimesylate for the treatment of ADHD. *J Clin Psychiatry* 2011; 72: 1366–1375

Weathers FW, Keane TM, Davidson JR. Clinician-administered PTSD scale: a review of the first ten years of research. *Depress Anxiety* 2001; 13: 132–156

Weimer K, Colloca L, Enck P, et al. Placebo effects in psychiatry: mediators and moderators. *Lancet Psychiatry* 2015; 2: 246–257

Weinstock LM, Gaudino BA, Epstein-Lubow G, et al. Medication burden in bipolar disorder: a chart review of patients at psychiatric hospital admission. *Psychiatry Res* 2014; 216: 24–30

Weiser M, Heresco-Levy U, Davidson M, et al. A multicenter, add-on randomized controlled trial of low-dose d-serine for negative and cognitive symptoms of schizophrenia. *J Clin Psychiatry* 2012; 73: e728–e734

Weisler R, Ginsberg L, Dirks B, et al. Treatment with lisdexamfetamine dimesylate improves self- and informant-rated executive function behaviors and clinician- and informant-rated ADHD symptoms in adults: data from a randomized, double-blind, placebo-controlled study. *J Atten Disord* 2017; 21: 1198–1207

Weisler R, Joyce M, McGill L, et al. Extended release quetiapine fumarate monotherapy for major depressive disorder: results of a double-blind, randomized, placebo-controlled study. *CNS Spectr* 2009; 14: 299–313

Weisler RH, Keck P Jr., Swann AC, et al. Extended-release carbamazepine capsules as monotherapy for acute mania in bipolar disorder: a multicenter, randomized, double-blind, placebo-controlled trial. *J Clin Psychiatry* 2005; 66: 323–330

Weiss RD, O'Malley SS, Hosking JD, et al. Do patients with alcohol dependence respond to placebo? Results from the COMBINE Study. *J Stud Alcohol Drugs* 2008; 69: 878–884

Weissman H, Qureshi IA. Systematic review: pharmacological treatment of tic disorders: efficacy of antipsychotic and alpha-2 adrenergic agonist agents. *Neurosci Biobehav Rev* 2013; 37: 1162–1171

Weissman AM, Levy BT, Hartz AJ, et al. Pooled analysis of antidepressant levels in lactating mothers, breast milk, and nursing infants. *Am J Psychiatry* 2004; 161: 1066–1078

Welge J, Keck PE Jr. Moderators of placebo response to antipsychotic treatment in patients with schizophrenia: a meta-regression. *Psychopharmacol (Berl)* 2003; 166: 1–10

Welten CCM, Koeter MJW, Wohlfarth T, et al. Placebo response in antipsychotic trials of patients with acute mania. Results of an individual patient data meta-analysis. *Eur Neuropsychopharmacol* 2015; 25: 1018–1026

Wesson DR, Ling W. The Clinical Opiate Withdrawal Scale (COWS). *J Psychoactive Drugs* 2003; 35: 253–259

Wheeler SD. Donepezil treatment of topiramate-related cognitive dysfunction. *Headache* 2006; 46: 332–335

Whitaker LR, Degulet M, Morikawa H. Social deprivation enhances VTA synaptic plasticity and drug-induced contextual learning. *Neuron* 2013; 77: 335–345

White K, Simpson G. Combined MAOI-tricyclic antidepressant treatment: a reevaluation. *J Clin Psychopharmacol* 1981; 1: 264–282

White K, Razani J, Simpson G. Combined MAOI-tricyclic antidepressant treatment: a controlled trial. *Psychopharmacol Bull* 1982; 18: 180–181

Wigal SB, Biederman J, Swanson JM, et al. Efficacy and safety of modafinil film-coated tablets in children and adolescents with or without prior stimulant treatment for attention-deficit/hyperactivity disorder: pooled analysis of 3 randomized, double-blind, placebo-controlled studies. *Prim Care Companion J Clin Psychiatry* 2006; 8: 352–360

Wijkstra J, Lijmer J, Burger H, et al. Pharmacological treatment for psychotic depression. *Cochrane Database Syst Rev* 2015; (7): CD004044

Wilens T, McBurnett K, Stein M, et al. ADHD treatment with once-daily OROS methylphenidate: final results from a long-term open-label study. *J Am Acad Child Adolesc Psychiatry* 2005b; 44: 1015–1023

Wilens TE, Faraone SV, Biederman J, et al. Does stimulant therapy of attention-deficit/hyperactivity disorder beget later substance abuse? A meta-analytic review of the literature. *Pediatrics* 2003a; 111: 179–185

Wilens TE, Haight BR, Horrigan JP, et al. Bupropion XL in adults with attention-deficit/hyperactivity disorder: a randomized, placebo-controlled study. *Biol Psychiatry* 2005a; 57: 793–801

Wilens TE, Prince JB, Spencer T, et al. An open trial of bupropion for the treatment of adults with attention-deficit/hyperactivity disorder and bipolar disorder. *Biol Psychiatry* 2003b; 54: 9–16

Wilens TE, Spencer TJ, Biederman J, et al. A controlled clinical trial of bupropion for attention deficit hyperactivity disorder in adults. *Am J Psychiatry* 2001; 158: 282–288

Williams AM. Coadministration of intramuscular olanzapine and benzodiazepines in agitated patients with mental illness. *Ment Health Clin* 2018; 8: 208–213

Williams J, Ziedonis DM. Naltrexone-bupropion combination therapy for protracted abstinence dysphoria. *Am J Addict* 2003; 12: 270–272

Williams LM, Debattista C, Duchemin AM, et al. Childhood trauma predicts antidepressant response in adults with major depression: data from the Randomized International Study to Predict Optimized Treatment for Depression. *Mol Psychiatry* 2016; 6: e799

Williams NR, Heifets BD, Blasey C, et al. Attenuation of antidepressant effects of ketamine by opioid receptor antagonism. *Am J Psychiatry* 2018; 175: 1205–1215

Wils RS, Gotfredsen DR, Hjorthøj C, et al. Antipsychotic medication and remission of psychotic symptoms 10 years after a first-episode psychosis. *Schizophr Res* 2017; 182: 42–48

Wilson W. The brief social phobia scale. *J Clin Psychiatry* 1993; (52 Suppl): 48–51

Wingård L, Taipale H, Reutfors J, et al. Initiation and long-term use of benzodiazepines and Z-drugs in bipolar disorder. *Bipol Disord* 2018; 20: 634–646

Winhusen T, Somoza E, Ciraulo DA, et al. A double-blind, placebo-controlled trial of tiagabine for the treatment of cocaine dependence. *Drug Alcohol Depend* 2007; 91: 141–148

Wink LK, Pedapati EV, Horn PS, et al. Multiple antipsychotic medication use in autism spectrum disorder. *J Child Adolsc Psychopharmacol* 2017; 27: 91–94

Winkler A, Auer C, Doering BK, et al. Drug treatment of primary insomnia: a meta-analysis of polysomnographic randomized controlled trials. *CNS Drugs* 2014; 28: 799–816

Winstanley EL, Bigelow GE, Silverman K, et al. A randomized controlled trial of fluoxetine in the treatment of cocaine dependence among methadone-maintained patients. *J Subst Abuse Treat* 2011; 40: 255–264

Winter H, Irle E. Hippocampal volume in adult burn patients with and without posttraumatic stress disorder. *Am J Psychiatry* 2004; 161: 2194–2200

Witcomb GL, Bouman WP, Claes L, et al. Levels of depression in transgender people and its predictors: results of a large matched control study with transgender people accessing clinical services. *J Affect Disord* 2018; 235: 308–315

Wittenborn JR, Weber ESP, Brown M. Niacin in the long-term treatment of schizophrenia. *Arch Gen Psychiatry* 1973; 28: 308–315

Woelk H, Arnoldt KH, Keiser M, et al. Ginkgo biloba special extract EGb 761 in generalized anxiety disorder and adjustment disorder with anxious mood: a randomized, double-blind, placebo-controlled trial. *J Psychiatry Res* 2007; 41: 472–480

Wolf EJ, Lunney CA, Schnurr PP. The influence of the dissociative subtype of posttraumatic stress disorder on treatment efficacy in female veterans and active duty service members. *J Consult Clin Psychol* 2016; 84: 95–100

Wolkowitz OM, Reus VI, Keebler A, et al. Double-blind treatment of major depression with dehydroepiandrosterone. *Am J Psychiatry* 1999; 156: 646–649

Wollweber B, Keck ME, Schmidt U. Improvement of nonsuicidal self-injury following treatment with antipsychotics possessing strong D1 antagonistic activity: evidence from a report of three cases. *Ther Adv Pharmacol* 2015; 5: 208–213

Woodman CL, Noyes R Jr. Panic disorder: treatment with valproate. *J Clin Psychiatry* 1994; 55: 134–136

Woodruff-Pak DS, Lander C, Geerts H. Nicotinic cholinergic modulation: galantamine as a prototype. *CNS Drug Rev Winter* 2002; 8: 405Y426

Woon FL, Sood S, Hedges DW. Hippocampal volume deficits associated with exposure to psychological trauma and posttraumatic stress disorder in adults: a meta-analysis. *Prog Neuropsychopharmacol Biol Psychiatry* 2010; 24: 1181–1188

Wu YL, Ding XX, Sun YH, et al. Association between MTHFR C677T polymorphism and depression: an updated meta-analysis of 26 studies. *Prog Neuropsychopharmacol Biol Psychiatry* 2013; 46: 78–85

Wunderink L, Nieboer RM, Wiersma D, et al. Recovery in remitted first-episode psychosis at 7 years of follow-up of an early dose reduction/discontinuation or maintenance treatment strategy: long-term follow-up of a 2-year randomized clinical trial. *JAMA Psychiatry* 2013; 70: 913–920

Xie C, Tang Y, Wang Y, et al. Efficacy and safety of antidepressants for the treatment of irritable bowel syndrome: a meta-analysis. *PLoS One* 2015; 10: e0127815

Yamatsu A, Yamashita Y, Manu I, et al. The improvement of sleep by oral intake of GABA and Apocynum venetum leaf extract. *J Nutr Sci Vitaminol (Tokyo)* 2015; 61: 182–187

Yang C, Hao Z, Tian J, et al. Does antipsychotic drug use increase the risk of long term mortality? A systematic review and meta-analysis of observational studies. *Oncotarget* 2018; 9: 15101–15110

Yang CS, Zhang LL, Zeng LN, et al. Topiramate for Tourette's syndrome in children: a meta-analysis. *Pediatr Neurol* 2013; 49: 344–350

Yargic LI, Corapcioglu A, Kocabesoglu N, et al. A prospective randomized single-blind, multicenter trial comparing the efficacy and safety of paroxetine with and without quetiapine therapy in depression associated with anxiety. *Int J Clin Pract* 2004; 8: 205–211

Yasui-Furukori N, Saito M, Nakagami T, et al. Clinical response to risperidone in relation to plasma drug concentrations in acutely exacerbated schizophrenic patients. *J Psychopharmacol* 2010; 24: 987–994

Yasui-Furukori N, Tsuchimine S, Nakagami T, et al. Association between plasma paroxetine concentration and changes in plasma brain-derived neurotrophic factor levels in patients with major depressive disorder. *Psychopharmacology* 2011; 26: 194–200

Yatham LN, Beaulieu S, Schaffer A, et al. Optimal duration of risperidone or olanzapine adjunctive therapy to mood stabilizer following remission of a manic episode: a CANMAT randomized double-blind trial. *Mol Psychiatry* 2016; 21: 1050–1056

Yatham LN, Grossman F, Augustyns I, et al. Mood stabilisers plus risperidone or placebo in the treatment of acute mania: international, double-blind, randomised controlled trial. *Br J Psychiatry* 2003; 182: 141–147

Yatham LN, Mackala S, Basivireddy J, et al. Lurasidone versus treatment as usual for cognitive impairment in euthymic patients with bipolar I disorder: a randomised, open-label, pilot study. *Lancet Psychiatry* 2017; 4: 208–217

Yazici O, Kora K, Polat A, et al. Controlled lithium discontinuation in bipolar patients with good response to long-term lithium prophylaxis. *J Affect Disord* 2004; 80: 269–271

Yeh MS, Mari JJ, Costa MC, et al. A double-blind randomized controlled trial to study the efficacy of topiramate in a civilian sample of PTSD. *CNS Neurosci Ther* 2011; 17: 305–310

Yeh RW, Valsdottir LR, Yeh M, et al. Parachute use to prevent death and major trauma when jumping from aircraft: randomized controlled trial. *Br Med J* 2018; 363: k5094

Yehuda R, Bierer LM, Pratchett LC, et al. Cortisol augmentation of a psychological treatment for warfighters with posttraumatic stress disorder: randomized trial showing improved treatment retention and outcome. *Psychoneuroendocrinology* 2015; 51: 589–597

Yeung CK, Chan HH. Cutaneous adverse effects of lithium: epidemiology and management. *Am J Clin Dermatol* 2004; 5: 3–8

Yildiz A, Nikodem M, Vieta, et al. A network meta-analysis on comparative efficacy and all-cause discontinuation of antimanic treatments in acute bipolar mania. *Psychol Med* 2015; 45: 299–317

Yildiz A, Vieta E, Leucht S, et al. Efficacy of antimanic treatments: meta-analysis of randomized, controlled trials. *Neuropsychopharmacology* 2011a; 36: 375–389

Yildiz A, Vieta E, Tohen M, et al. Factors modifying drug and placebo responses in randomized trials for bipolar mania. *Neuropsychopharmacology* 2011b; 14: 863–875

Yokoi F, Gründner G, Biziere K, et al. Dopamine D_2 and D_3 receptor occupancy in normal humans treated with the antipsychotic drug aripiprazole (OPC 14597): a study using positron emission tomography and [^{11}C] raclopide. *Neuropsychopharmacology* 2002; 27: 248–259

Yolland CO, Hanratty Y, Neill E, et al. Meta-analysis of randomised controlled trials with *N*-acetylcysteine in the treatment of schizophrenia. *Aust N Z J Psychiatry* 2020; 54: 453–466

Yonkers KA, Pearlstein TB, Gotman N. A pilot study to compare fluoxetine, calcium, and placebo in the treatment of premenstrual syndrome. *J Clin Psychopharmacol* 2013; 33: 614–620

Yonkers KA, Gotman N, Smith MV, et al. Does antidepressant use attenuate the risk of a major depressive episode in pregnancy? *Epidemiology* 2011; 22: 848–854

Yonkers KA, Kornstein SG, Gueorquieva R, et al. Symptom-onset dosing of sertraline for the treatment of premenstrual dysphoric disorder: a randomized clinical trial. *JAMA Psychiatry* 2015; 72: 1037–1044

Yu H, Yan H, Wang L, et al. Five novel loci associated with antipsychotic treatment response in patients with schizophrenia: a genome-wide association study. *Lancet Psychiatry* 2018; 5: 327–338

Yudofsky S, Williams D, Gorman J. Propranolol in the treatment of rage and violent behavior in patients with chronic brain syndromes. *Am J Psychiatry* 1981; 138: 218–220

Yun LWH, Maravi M, Koayashi JS, et al. Antidepressant treatment improves adherence to antiretroviral therapy among depressed HIV-infected patients. *J Acquired Immune Defic Syndr* 2005; 38: 432–438

Yung AR, Phillips LJ, Nelson B, et al. Randomized controlled trial of interventions for young people at ultra high risk for psychosis: a 6-month analysis. *J Clin Psychiatry* 2011; 72: 430–440

Yury CA, Fisher JE. Meta-analysis of the effectiveness of atypical antipsychotics for the treatment of behavioural problems in persons with dementia. *Psychother Psychosom* 2007; 76: 213–218

Zajecka JM. The effect of nefazodone on comorbid anxiety symptoms associated with depression: experience in family practice and psychiatric outpatient settings. *J Clin Psychiatry* 1996; 57(Suppl 2): 10–14

Zajecka J, Tracy KA, Mitchell S. Discontinuation symptoms after treatment with serotonin reuptake inhibitors: a literature review. *J Clin Psychiatry* 1997; 58: 291–297

Zanarini MC, Frankenburg FR. Olanzapine treatment of female borderline personality disorder patients: a double-blind, placebo-controlled pilot study. *J Clin Psychiatry* 2001; 62: 849–854

Zanarini MC, Frankenburg FR, Parchini A. A preliminary, randomized trial of fluoxetine, olanzapine, and the olanzapine-fluoxetine combination in women with borderline personality disorder. *J Clin Psychiatry* 2004; 65: 903–907

Zanarini MC, Schulz SC, Detke HC, et al. A dose comparison of olanzapine for the treatment of borderline personality disorder: a 12-week randomized, double-blind, placebo-controlled study. *J Clin Psychiatry* 2011; 72: 1353–1362

Zanarini MC, Schulz SC, Detke HC, et al. Open-label treatment with olanzapine for patients with borderline personality disorder. *J Clin Psychopharmacol* 2012; 32: 398–402

Zanarini MC, Vujanovic AA, Parachini EA, et al. Zanarini Rating Scale for Borderline Personality Disorder (ZAN-BPD): a continuous measure of DSM-IV borderline psychopathology. *J Pers Disord* 2003; 17: 233–242

Zanos P, Moaddel R, Morris PJ, et al. NMDAR inhibition-independent antidepressant actions of ketamine metabolites. *Nature* 2016; 533: 481–486

Zarate CA Jr., Tohen M. Double-blind comparison of the continued use of antipsychotic treatment versus its discontinuation in remitted manic patients. *Am J Psychiatry* 2004; 161: 169–171

Zareifopoulos N, Dylja I. Efficacy and tolerability of vilazodone for the acute treatment of generalized anxiety disorder: a meta-analysis. *Asia J Psychiatry* 2017; 26: 115–122

Zaremba D, Schulze Kalthoff I, Förster K, et al. The effects of processing speed on memory impairment in patients with major depressive disorder. *Prog Neuropsychopharmacol Biol Psychiatry* 2019; 92: 494–500

Zedler BK, Mann HL, Kim MM, et al. Buprenorphine compared with methadone to treat pregnant women with opioid use disorder: a systematic review and meta-analysis of safety in the mother, fetus and child. *Addiction* 2016; 111: 2115–2128

Zeier Z, Carpenter LL, Kalin NH, et al. Clinical implementation of pharmacogenetic decision support tools for antidepressant drug prescribing. *Am J Psychiatry* 2018; 175: 873–886

Zeng T, Long Y-S, Min F-L, et al. Association of HLA-B*1502 alleles with lamotrigine-induced Stevens-Johnson syndrome and toxic epidermal necrolysis in Han Chinese subjects: a meta-analysis. *Int J Dermatol* 2015; 54: 488–493

Zetin M, Garber D, De Antonio M, et al. Prediction of lithium dose: a mathematical alternative to the test-dose method. *J Clin Psychiatry* 1986; 47: 175–178

Zhang J-P, Lencz T, Malhotra AK. D_2 receptor genetic variation and clinical response to antipsychotic drug treatment: a meta-analysis. *Am J Psychiatry* 2010; 167: 763–772

Zhang W, Connor KM, Davidson JR. Levetiracetam in social phobia: a placebo controlled pilot study. *J Psychopharmacol* 2005; 19: 551–553

Zhang JP, Lencz T, Zhang RX, et al. Pharmacogenetic associations of antipsychotic drug-related weight gain: a systematic review and meta-analysis. *Schizophr Bull* 2016; 42: 1418–1437

Zhang XY, Tan YL, Zhou DF, et al. Association of clozapine-induced weight gain with polymorphism in the leptin promoter region in patients with chronic schizophrenia in a Chinese population. *J Clin Psychopharmacol* 2007a; 27: 246–251

Zhang ZJ, Kang WH, Li Q, et al. Beneficial effects of ondansetron as an adjunct to haloperidol for chronic, treatment-resistant schizophrenia: a double-blind, randomized, placebo-controlled study. *Schizophr Res* 2006; 88: 102–110

Zhang ZJ, Kang WH, Li Q, et al. The beneficial effects of the herbal medicine Free and Easy Wanderer Plus (FEWP) for mood disorders: double-blind, placebo-controlled studies. *J Psychiatry Res* 2007b; 41: 828–836

Zhang ZJ, Kang WT, Tan QR, et al. Adjunctive herbal medicine with carbamazepine for bipolar disorders: a double-blind, randomized, placebo-controlled study. *J Psychiatr Res* 2007c; 41: 360–369

Zheng W, Cai DB, Zhang Q-E, et al. Adjunctive ondansetron for schizophrenia: a systematic review and meta-analysis of randomized controlled trials. *J Psychiatry Res* 2019; 113: 27–33

Zheng W, Cao XL, Ungvari GS, et al. Electroconvulsive therapy added to non-clozapine antipsychotic medication for treatment resistant schizophrenia: meta-analysis of randomized controlled trials. *PLoS One* 2016a; 11: e0156510

Zheng W, Wang S, Ungvari GS, et al. Amantadine for antipsychotic-related weight gain: meta-analysis of randomized placebo-controlled trials. *J Clin Psychopharmacol* 2017a; 37: 341–346

Zheng W, Xiang Y-T, Xiang Y-Q, et al. Efficacy and safety of adjunctive topiramate for schizophrenia: a meta-analysis of randomized controlled trials. *Acta Psychiatr Scand* 2016b; 134: 385–398

Zheng W, Xiang YT, Yang XH, et al. Clozapine augmentation with antiepileptic drugs for treatment-resistant schizophrenia: a met-analysis of randomized controlled trials. *J Clin Psychiatry* 2017b; 78: e498–e505

Zhong G, Wang Y, Zhang Y, et al. Association between benzodiazepine use and dementia: a meta-analysis. *PLoS One* 2015; 10: e0127836

Zhou X, Ravindran AV, Qin B, et al. Comparative efficacy, acceptability, and tolerability of augmentation agents in treatment-resistant depression: systematic review and network meta-analysis. *J Clin Psychiatry* 2015; 76: e487–e498

Zhu J, Cai H, Yuan Y, et al. Variance of the global signal as a pretreatment predictor of antidepressant treatment response in drug-naïve major depressive disorder. *Brain Imaging Behav* 2018; 12: 1768–1774

Zhu ZG, Sun MX, Zhang WL, et al. The efficacy and safety of coenzyme Q10 in Parkinson's disease: a meta-analysis of randomized controlled trials. *Neurol Sci* 2017; 38: 215–224

Zilcha-Mano S, Roose SP, Barber JP, et al. Therapeutic alliance in antidepressant treatment: cause or effect of symptomatic levels? *Psychother Psychosom* 2015; 84: 177–182

Zipursky RB, Menezes NM, Streiner DL, et al. Risk of symptom recurrence with medication discontinuation in first-episode psychosis: a systematic review. *Schizophr Res* 2014; 152: 408–414

Zisook S, Johnson GR, Tal I, et al. General predictors and moderators of depression remission: a VAST-D report. *Am J Psychiatry* 2019; 176: 348–357

Zisook S, Lesser IM, Lebowitz B, et al. Effects of antidepressant medication treatment on suicidal ideation and behavior in a randomized trial: an exploratory report from the combining medications to enhance depression outcomes study. *J Clin Psychiatry* 2011; 72: 1322–1332

Zisook S, Rush AJ, Haight BR, et al. Use of bupropion in combination with serotonin reuptake inhibitors. *Biol Psychiatry* 2006; 59: 203–210

Zisook S, Shuchter SR, Pedrelli P, et al. Bupropion sustained release for bereavement: results of an open trial. *J Clin Psychiatry* 2001; 62: 227–230

Zohar J, Amital D, Miodownik C, et al. Double-blind placebo-controlled pilot study of sertraline in military veterans with posttraumatic stress disorder. *J Clin Psychopharmacol* 2002; 22: 190–195

Zohar J, Fostick L, Juven-Wetzler A, et al. Secondary prevention of chronic PTSD by early- and short-term administration of escitalopram: a prospective randomized, placebo-controlled, double-blind trial. *J Clin Psychiatry* 2018; 79: 16m10730

Zung WWK. A rating instrument for anxiety disorders. *Psychosomatics* 1971; 12: 371–379

Zweifel JE, O'Brien WH. A meta-analysis of the effect of hormone replacement therapy upon depressed mood. *Psychoneuroendocrinology* 1997; 22: 189–212

Index

Locators in **bold** refer to tables; those in *italic* to figures